DIAGNOSTIC PATHOLOGY
KIDNEY DISEASES

AMIRSYS®

i

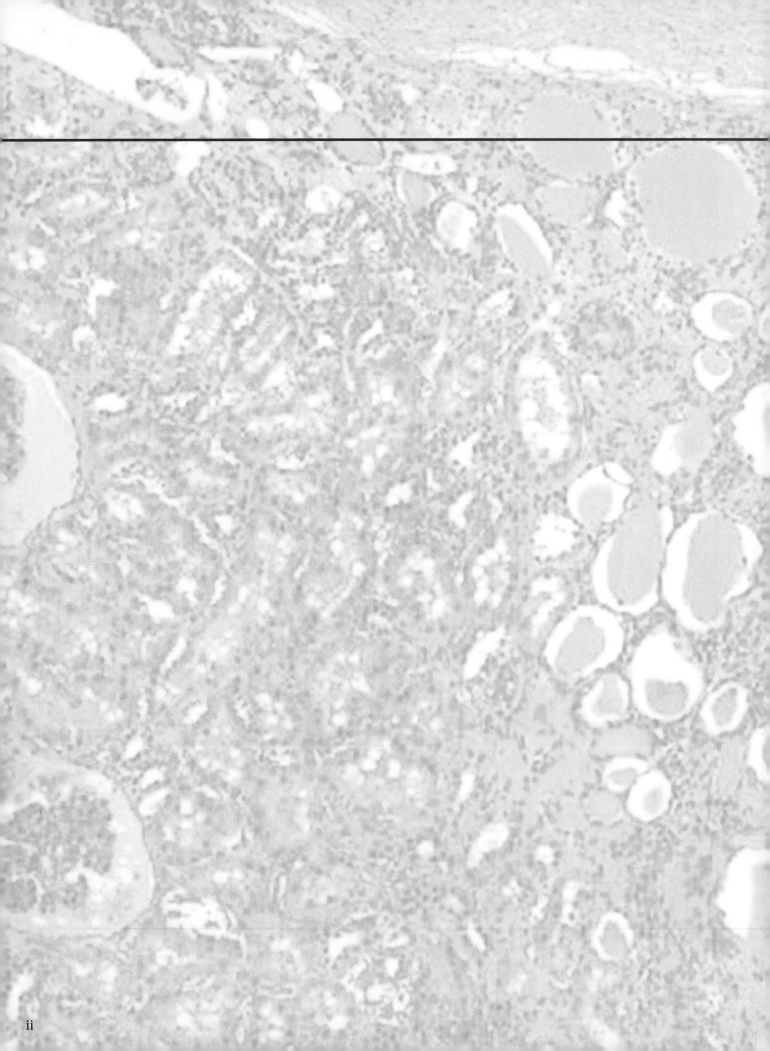

DIAGNOSTIC PATHOLOGY
KIDNEY DISEASES

AMIRSYS®

Robert B. Colvin, MD
Benjamin Castleman Distinguished Professor of Pathology
Department of Pathology
Harvard Medical School
Massachusetts General Hospital
Boston, MA

Anthony Chang, MD
Associate Professor of Pathology
University of Chicago Medical Center
Chicago, IL

Neeraja Kambham, MD
Associate Professor of Pathology
Stanford University School of Medicine
Stanford, CA

Shane M. Meehan, MBBCh
Professor of Pathology
University of Chicago Medical Center
Chicago, IL

Joseph Gaut, MD, PhD
Instructor of Pathology and Immunopathology
Washington University School of Medicine
Saint Louis, MO

Surya V. Seshan, MD
Professor of Clinical Pathology
Weill Cornell Medical College
Cornell University
New York, NY

Sanjay Jain, MD, PhD
Assistant Professor of Medicine (Renal Division),
Pathology, and Immunopathology
Co-director, Kidney Translational Research Core
Washington University School of Medicine
Saint Louis, MO

Alton B. "Brad" Farris III, MD
Assistant Professor of Pathology
Department of Pathology
Emory University School of Medicine
Atlanta, GA

Lynn D. Cornell, MD
Assistant Professor of Laboratory Medicine and Pathology
Consultant, Division of Anatomic Pathology
Mayo Clinic College of Medicine
Rochester, MN

Helen Liapis, MD
Professor of Medicine (Renal Division), Pathology,
and Immunology
Washington University School of Medicine
Saint Louis, MO

Stephen M. Bonsib, MD
Albert G. and Harriet G. Smith Endowed Professor
Chair, Department of Pathology
Louisiana State University Health Sciences Center
Shreveport, LA

Aleksandr Vasilyev, MD, PhD
Instructor of Pathology
Harvard Medical School
Assistant in Molecular Pathology
Massachusetts General Hospital
Boston, MA

AMIRSYS®
Names you know. Content you trust.®

First Edition

© 2011 Amirsys, Inc.

Compilation © 2011 Amirsys Publishing, Inc.

All rights reserved. No part of this publication may be reproduced, stored in a retrieval system, or transmitted, in any form or media or by any means, electronic, mechanical, photocopying, recording, or otherwise, without prior written permission from Amirsys, Inc.

Printed in Canada by Friesens, Altona, Manitoba, Canada

ISBN: 978-1-931884-53-2

Notice and Disclaimer

Library of Congress Cataloging-in-Publication Data

Diagnostic pathology. Kidney diseases / [edited by] Robert B. Colvin. -- 1st ed.
    p. ; cm.
Kidney diseases
Includes bibliographical references and index.
ISBN 978-1-931884-53-2
1. Kidneys--Diseases--Diagnosis--Atlases. I. Colvin, Robert B. II. Title: Kidney diseases.
[DNLM: 1. Kidney Diseases--diagnosis--Atlases. 2. Kidney Diseases--pathology--Atlases.
WJ 17]
RC904.D519 2011
616.6'1075--dc22

                  2011007177

The authors thank our teachers, students, and families, who gave us guidance, inspiration, and love. We owe you everything. You know who you are!

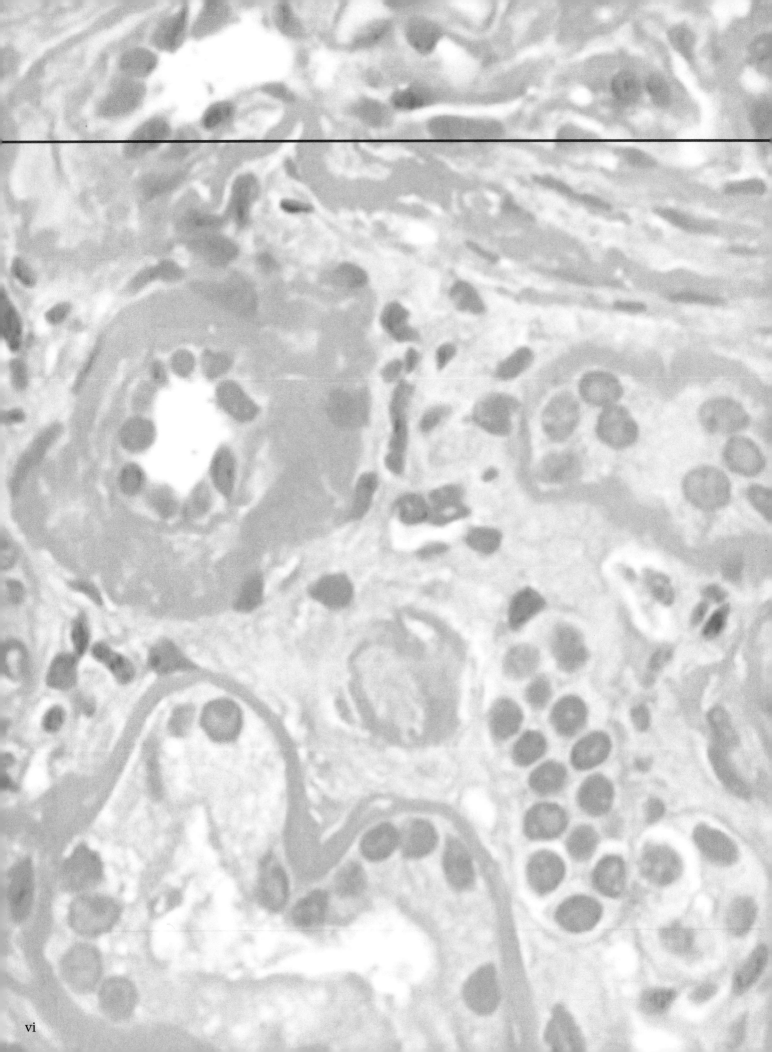

CONTRIBUTORS

We are grateful to the collaborators listed below who kindly and without hesitation shared their digital images of unusual or unique cases, published and unpublished. They are cited individually in the figure legends, but we also wish to acknowledge them as a group. Their help was essential in our endeavor to create a comprehensive text. We are also indebted to our patients who contributed their specimens for research to find better treatment, diagnosis, and understanding of renal diseases.

Anil Abraham, MD
Cyril Abrahams, MD
Shreeram Akilesh, MD
Niaz Banaei, MD
Laura Barisoni-Thomas, MD
Jay Bernstein, MD
Gerald Berry, MD
Athanase Billis, MD
Erika Bracamonte, MD
Helen Catthro, MD
Jacob Churg, MD
Arthur Cohen, MD
A. Bernard Collins, BS
Terence Cook, MD
Vivette D'Agati, MD
Cinthia Drachenberg, MD
Andrew Evan, MD
Luis Fajardo, MD
Dusan Ferluga, MD
Judith A. Ferry, MD
Mary Fidler, MD
Andreas Friedl, MD
Billie Fyfe, MD
Nancy L. Harris, MD
Joel Henderson, MD
Randolph A. Hennigar, MD, PhD
Leal Herlitz, MD
Guillermo Herrara, MD
Bela Ivanyi, MD
George Jarad, MD
J. Charles Jennette, MD
Jason Karamchadani, MD
Jolanta Kowalewska, MD
Yaël B. Kushner, MD
Reinhold Linke, MD
Alexander Magil, MD
Cynthia Magro, MD

Christine Menias, MD
Michael Mihatsch, MD
Jeffery Miner, PhD
Guido Monga, MD
Jose Montoya, MD
Jocelyn Moore, MD
Tibor Nadasdy, MD
Samih Nasr, MD
Cynthia Nast, MD
Volker Nickeleit, MD
Louis Novea-Takara, MD
Ryuji Ohashi, MD
Juan Olano, MD
Victor Pardo, MD
Kwan-Kyu Park, MD
Vesna Petronic-Rosic, MD
Maria M. Picken, MD, PhD
Lorraine Racusen, MD
Emilio Ramos, MD
Parmjeet Randhawa, MD
Ian Roberts, MD
Seymour Rosen, MD
Virginie Royal, MD
Luis Salinas-Madrigal, MD
Josef Schroeder, MD, PhD
Eveline Schneeberger, MD
Akira Shimizu, MD, PhD
R. Neal Smith, MD, PhD
Keyoumars Soltani, MD
Jie Song, MD
Gerald Spear, MD
Jerome Taxy, MD
Diana Taheri, MD
Nguyen Trang, MD
Megan Troxell, MD
Rosemary Wieczorek, MD

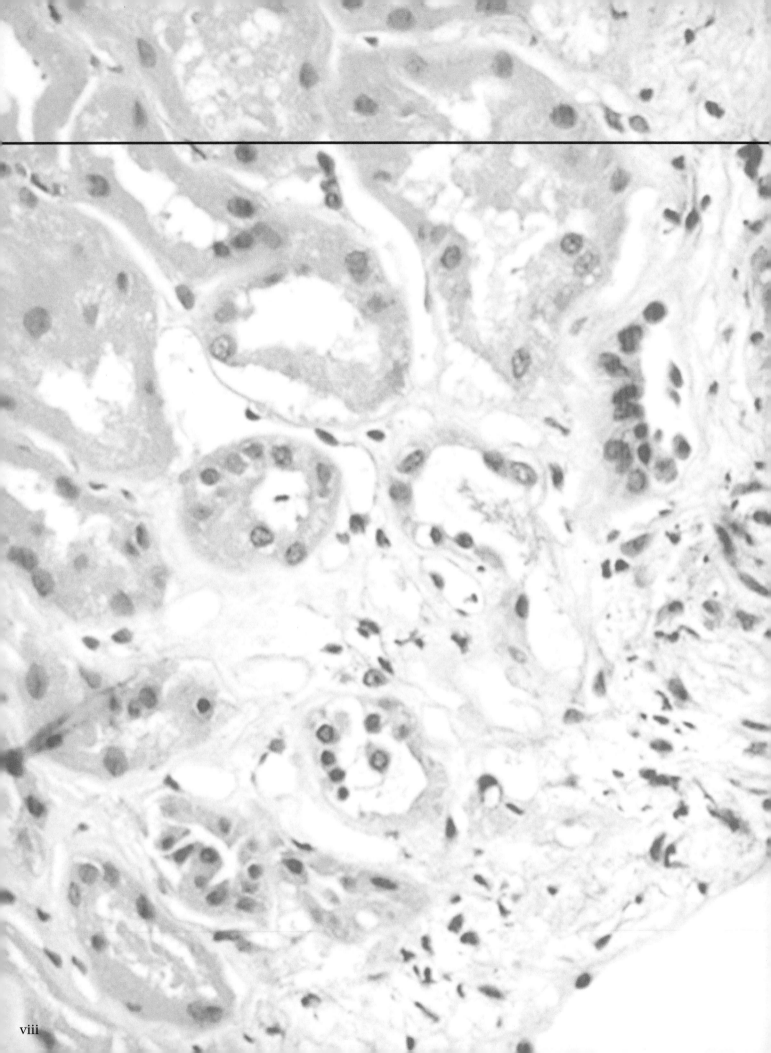

DIAGNOSTIC PATHOLOGY
KIDNEY DISEASES

AMIRSYS®

Amirsys, creators of the highly acclaimed radiology series Diagnostic Imaging, proudly introduces its new Diagnostic Pathology series, designed as easy-to-use reference texts for the busy practicing surgical pathologist. Written by world-renowned experts, the series will consist of 15 titles in all the crucial diagnostic areas of surgical pathology.

The newest book in this series, *Diagnostic Pathology: Kidney Diseases*, contains approximately 950 pages of comprehensive, yet concise, descriptions of more than 210 specific diagnoses. Amirsys's pioneering bulleted format distills pertinent information to the essentials. Each chapter has the same organization providing an easy-to-read reference for making rapid, efficient, and accurate diagnoses in a busy surgical pathology practice. A highlighted Key Facts box provides the essential features of each diagnosis. Detailed sections on Terminology, Etiology/Pathogenesis, Clinical Issues, Macroscopic and Microscopic Findings, and the all important Differential Diagnoses follow so you can find the information you need in the exact same place every time.

Most importantly, every diagnosis features numerous high-quality images, including gross pathology, H&E and immunohistochemical stains, correlative radiographic images, and richly colored graphics, all of which are fully annotated to maximize their illustrative potential.

We believe that this lavishly illustrated series, with its up-to-date information and practical focus, will become the core of your reference collection. Enjoy!

Elizabeth H. Hammond, MD
Executive Editor, Pathology
Amirsys, Inc.

Paula J. Woodward, MD
President
Amirsys Publishing, Inc.

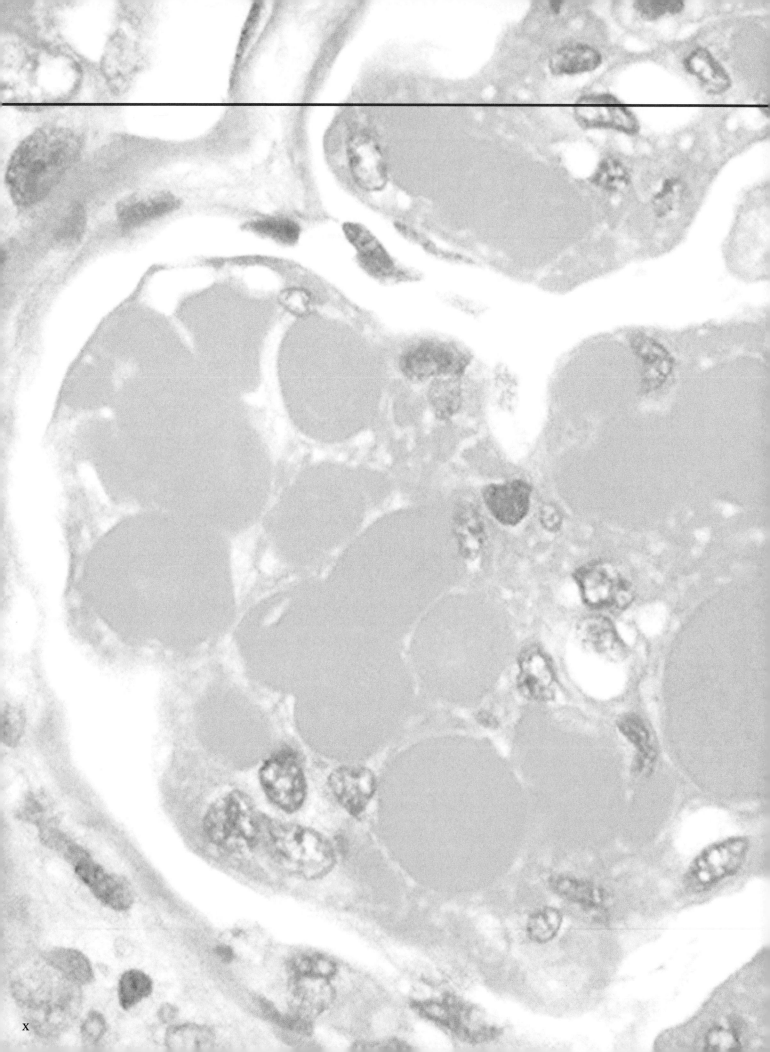

x

PREFACE

Welcome to the world of renal pathology! The team of renal pathologists who developed *Diagnostic Pathology: Kidney Diseases* has 200 years combined experience. We were motivated by the desire to create a comprehensive, accessible, succinct, and diagnostically useful resource for practicing pathologists, nephrologists, and all students of kidney diseases. In these pages you will find the most complete survey available of nonneoplastic diseases of native and transplant kidneys, amply illustrated by over 3,200 pathology images of classic and variant features.

This is a highly *structured* book with consistent categories of information in succinct outline form. Each disease is given a separate chapter. In each chapter you will find relevant light, immunofluorescent, and electron microscopic findings, as well as clinical presentation, pathogenesis, molecular genetics, gross features, and differential diagnosis. Key facts are highlighted for easy review, and many tables and custom diagrams are provided to synthesize the information.

Of considerable importance, this is a *living* book. With Amirsys eBook Advantage™, the web-accessible version is available to all owners of the book and will be kept current. New diseases and newly appreciated features of old diseases will be added by the authors and collaborators.

Renal pathology has certain features that differentiate it from much of diagnostic pathology, in that the routine analysis of the biopsy typically includes a consideration of pathogenesis and etiology. Renal pathologists are concerned with mechanisms, as well as the "diagnosis," and require the knowledge of the clinical presentation and relevant laboratory tests in their diagnostic assessment. All of these elements critical for diagnosis are provided for each disease entity discussed in *Diagnostic Pathology: Kidney Diseases*.

We hope you will find this text and internet resource useful. We welcome your feedback (feedback@amirsys.com) so that we can continue to enhance its value.

Robert B. Colvin, MD
Benjamin Castleman Distinguished Professor of Pathology
Department of Pathology
Harvard Medical School
Massachusetts General Hospital
Boston, MA

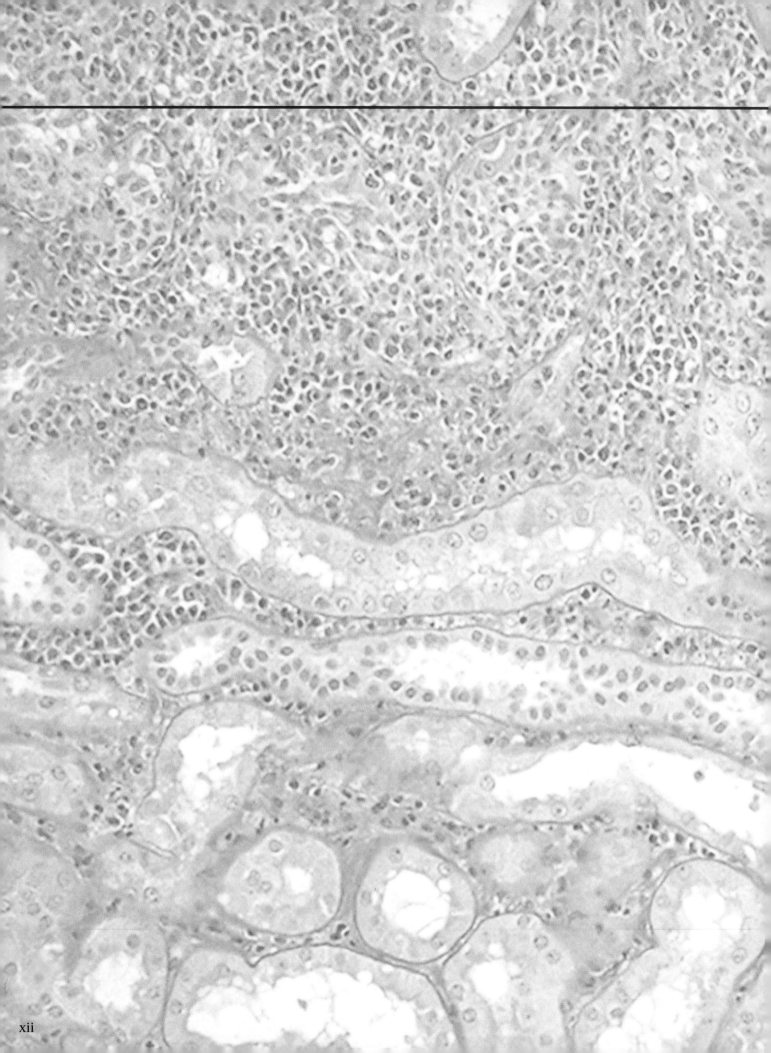

ACKNOWLEDGMENTS

Contributing Authors

Xin Gu, MD

Ami Bhalodia, MD

Text Editing

Ashley R. Renlund, MA

Arthur G. Gelsinger, MA

Matthew R. Connelly, MA

Lorna Morring, MS

Alicia M. Moulton, BA

Image Editing

Jeffrey J. Marmorstone, BS

Lisa A. Magar, BS

Medical Text Editing

Yaël B. Kushner, MD

Sara Cuadra Acree, MD

Illustrations

Laura C. Sesto, MA

Richard Coombs, MS

Lane R. Bennion, MS

Art Direction and Design

Laura C. Sesto, MA

Assistant Editor

Dave L. Chance, MA

Publishing Lead

Kellie J. Heap, BA

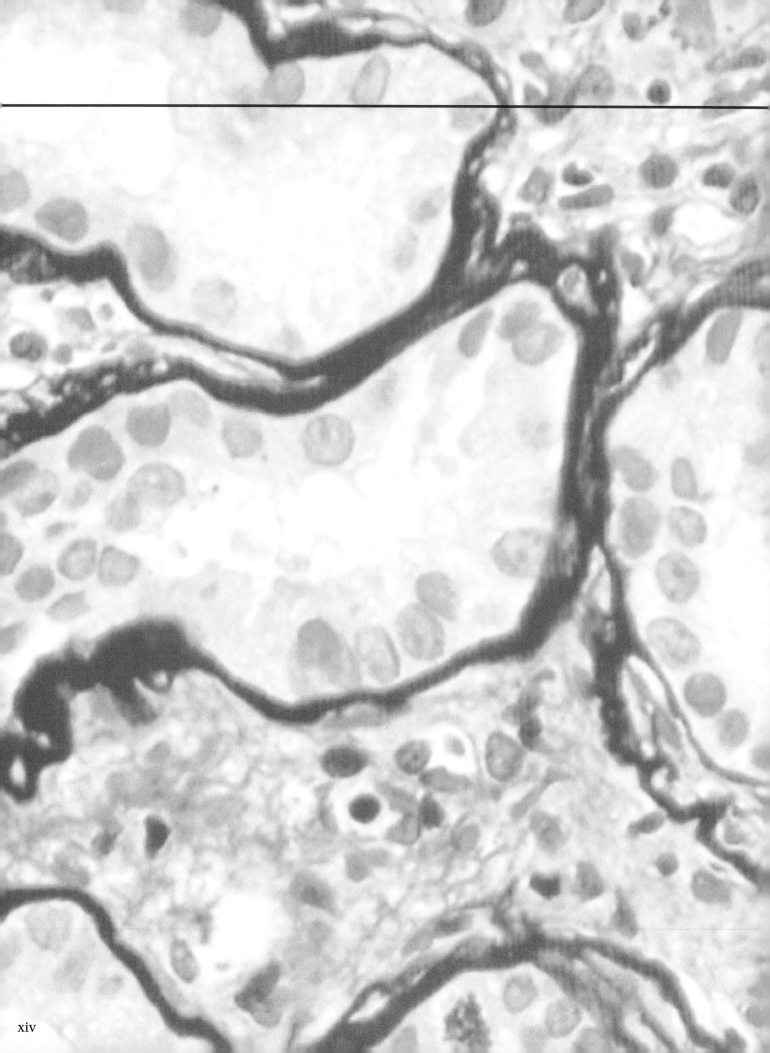

SECTIONS

Introduction

Glomerular Diseases

Vascular Diseases

Tubulointerstitial Diseases

Infections of the Kidney

Developmental and Cystic Diseases

Diseases of the Collecting System

Diseases of the Renal Allograft

Antibody Index

TABLE OF CONTENTS

C20449420

SECTION 5
Infections of the Kidney

Bacterial Infections of the Kidney

Fungal, Rickettsial, and Parasitic Infections of the Kidney

SECTION 6
Developmental and Cystic Diseases

SECTION 7
Diseases of the Collecting System

SECTION 8
Diseases of the Renal Allograft

Rejection

Recurrent and de Novo Diseases

Nonimmunologic Injury

Stable and Accepted Grafts

SECTION 9
Antibody Index

DIAGNOSTIC PATHOLOGY
KIDNEY DISEASES

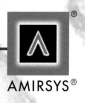

AMIRSYS®

Introduction

INTRODUCTION TO RENAL PATHOLOGY

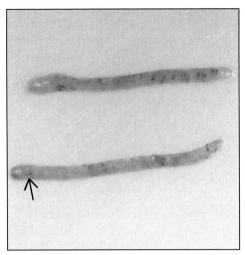

Renal biopsy cores from 16-g needle are typically 1 mm in diameter, 10-20 mm long (these are ~ 13 mm). Glomeruli appear as pale or congested bulges; red cell casts as brown streaks ➡ or dots. (Courtesy C. Swetts, MD.)

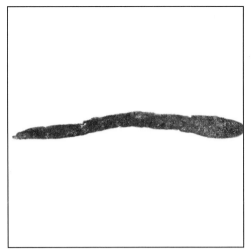

Renal biopsy core is divided into portions for LM, IF, and EM. The biopsy is 1st examined under low power to determine the nature of the sample and search for focal lesions.

VALUE OF RENAL BIOPSY

Provides Diagnosis
- Alters clinical diagnosis in 25-50%

Guides Treatment
- Changes therapy in 30-40%
- Determines reversibility and activity

Predicts Prognosis
- Specific pathologic features and extent of changes

Reveals Pathogenesis
- Molecular and cellular mechanisms

Validates Outcome
- Used as endpoint in clinical trials

INDICATIONS FOR RENAL BIOPSY

Elevated Cr or BUN
- Elevated with decreased renal filtration
- Measure creatinine clearance or estimate glomerular filtration rate (GFR) based on gender, body weight, race, age

Proteinuria
- May be asymptomatic or symptomatic
- Usually a sign of increased permeability of glomerulus
  - Failure of reabsorption by tubules can lead to low-level proteinuria
- 1-3 g/d usually asymptomatic
- Higher levels lead to edema and nephrotic syndrome

Nephrotic Syndrome
- Proteinuria > 3.5 g/d, hypoalbuminemia, edema, hyperlipidemia, lipiduria
- Increased glomerular permeability to albumin and other plasma proteins

Hematuria
- May be asymptomatic or symptomatic (gross hematuria)
- Usually a sign of glomerular inflammation and ruptured GBM, especially with RBC casts
- When combined with acute renal failure and red cell casts, termed nephritic syndrome

Nephritic Syndrome
- Hematuria, proteinuria, elevated Cr, hypertension, edema
- Loss of function due to decreased glomerular blood flow, salt retention

BIOPSY TECHNIQUE AND SAFETY

Percutaneous (Needle) Biopsy
- Ultrasound guided, automated gun
- 16-18-gauge needle is usual
- Generally regarded as safe outpatient procedure
  - Microhematuria usual, macrohematuria ~ 5%
    - Major complications in 1-3% (varies with technique)
  - No loss of kidney or death in recent series
- Diagnostic yield in 90-100% (~ 10-16 glomeruli/16g core, about 50% less with 18g)

Open (Wedge) Biopsy
- Primarily samples outer cortex

Transjugular Vein Biopsy
- High-risk patients

PROCESSING OF TISSUE

Gross Examination
- Determine whether glomeruli in sample
- Dissecting microscope, loupe

INTRODUCTION TO RENAL PATHOLOGY

Division of Sample
- Divide into 3 parts for light (LM), immunofluorescence (IF), and electron microscopy (EM)
  - If 2 cores, 1/2 of each for LM, 1/2 of 1 for IF, 1/2 of other for EM
  - If 1 core, ends for EM, split rest for LM and EM with larger gauge needles (15-16-gauge)

Light Microscopy
- Formalin-fixed, paraffin-embedded, 2-3 μm sections
  - Multiple levels
- H&E, PAS, and silver and trichrome stains usual
  - Other stains as indicated

Immunofluorescence
- Quick freeze on cryostat chuck or liquid N_2
- Frozen sections cut at 3-4 μm
- Stain for IgG, IgA, IgM, kappa, lambda, C1q, C3, fibrinogen, albumin
  - C4d on transplant biopsies

Electron Microscopy
- 2% paraformaldehyde/2.5% glutaraldehyde in cacodylate or phosphate buffered fixative (Karnovsky half strength, "K2")
  - Osmium post-fix
- 1 μm toluidine blue stained sections to screen for glomeruli
- Choose 1-2 blocks with glomeruli and trim for EM sectioning and staining (Pb/Ur)

Recording Results
- Digital cameras commonly used for both IF and EM
- Whole slide scans for LM (research)
- EM morphometry to measure GBM thickness

SYSTEMATIC APPROACH

Light Microscopy
- Examine each of 4 components
  - Glomeruli, tubules, interstitium, and vessels
  - Try to decide which component is primarily affected
- Describe and quantitate changes in each compartment
  - Distinguish acute and chronic changes
  - Examine each section

Immunofluorescence
- Assess pattern, extent, and intensity of glomerular staining
- Assess presence and pattern of deposits in other sites (TBM, vessels, interstitium)

Electron Microscopy
- GBM thickness and appearance
- Presence and location of electron dense deposits
  - Substructure and periodicity, if any
- Podocyte changes (effacement)
- Endothelial changes
- Mesangial features
- TBM, interstitium, peritubular capillaries

ISSUES IN INTERPRETATION

Sampling
- Adequacy of sample is dependent on nature of disease
  - Small samples are adequate for diffuse diseases
  - Large samples are needed for focal diseases
- The rarer the lesion, the greater the sample needed
  - $S = 1 - (1 - p) \char94 n$, where S = probability of obtaining at least 1 affected glomerulus, p = fraction of affected glomeruli in kidney, and n = number of glomeruli in sample (binomial distribution)
  - For example, if 10% of glomeruli are affected, need 30 glomeruli to have > 95% chance of sampling at least 1 affected glomerulus
- Estimation of % affected glomeruli in kidney is similarly subject to sampling error (e.g., distinction between > 50% and < 50%)
- Distribution of lesions is not random in some diseases (e.g., FSGS)
- Options when inadequate
  - Reprocess paraffin or frozen block for EM or frozen for paraffin
  - Immunohistochemistry for Ig in paraffin block

Scoring Systems and Definitions
- Described by several classification systems
  - Lupus (ISN/RPS), IgA (Oxford), transplants (Banff)
- Do not always agree on definitions or method of scoring for same features

Complex Biopsies
- > 1 disease may be present
  - Common in allografts
  - Residue from past disease persists

Functional Interrelationships
- Disease of 1 component affects others
  - Loss of glomeruli affects blood supply of tubules
  - Vascular disease affects tubules and glomeruli

REPORTING RECOMMENDATIONS

Diagnosis
- Include severity and activity whenever possible
- Use current classification system for particular disease (e.g., lupus, IgA, diabetes, transplant)

Description
- Indicate sample (number of cores, cortex, medulla, corticomedullary junction)
- Glomeruli
  - Count number in sample (can count section with greatest number)
  - Give % of globally and segmentally sclerotic glomeruli
  - Mesangial cellularity
  - Thickening of capillary wall/GBM
  - Presence or absence of inflammation, necrosis, crescents, thrombi, adhesions, hyaline, periglomerular fibrosis
    - Indicate fraction of glomeruli involved
  - Useful to give the % of normal glomeruli

- Tubules
  - Acute injury, necrosis
  - Atrophy (give %)
  - Casts (RBC, protein, pigment, neutrophils)
  - Tubular reabsorption droplets
  - Vacuolization, nuclear inclusions, giant mitochondria
- Interstitium
  - Inflammation, type of cells, granuloma
  - Fibrosis, pattern, extent (%)
- Vessels
  - Count arteries
  - Intimal fibrosis, arteries (% luminal occlusion)
  - Arteriolar hyalinization (extent)
  - Vasculitis
  - Peritubular capillaritis
- Immunofluorescence
  - Indicate number of glomeruli in sample
  - Give pattern and intensity of glomerular staining for each positive reactant and score 0-4(+)
  - Note other relevant staining: TBM, interstitium, vessels, reabsorption droplets
  - List all stains used, including negative
- Electron microscopy
  - Indicate number of glomeruli
  - Status of podocytes (effacement, hypertrophy)
  - GBM (thickness, lamination, deposits)
  - Extent and position of deposits
    - Give substructure, if any, and dimensions
  - Mesangial features (fibrils, cells, deposits)

Summary

- Compare with previous biopsy, if any
- Link to clinical information
- Discuss differential and basis of conclusion

DEFINITIONS FOR GLOMERULI

Adhesion

- Abnormal attachment of glomerular tuft to Bowman capsule; area of continuity between glomerular tuft and Bowman capsule separate from extracapillary lesion or from area of segmental sclerosis

Bowman Capsule

- Layer of basement membrane surrounding Bowman space on which parietal epithelial cells rest; continuous with GBM at base of glomerulus

Bowman Space

- Space between glomerular tuft and surrounding Bowman capsule, in continuity with lumen of proximal tubule

Capillary Wall Thickening

- Used for H&E sections in which GBM, deposits, and cellular elements all contribute to thickness

Collapsing Lesion

- Collapse of glomerular capillaries with overlying podocyte hypercellularity

Crescent

- Extracapillary proliferation of > 2 cell layers occupying 25% or more of glomerular capsular circumference or > 10%
  - Sometimes graded: < 10% (tiny focus), 10-25%, 25-50%, > 50% of glomerular capsular circumference

Crescent, Cellular

- Crescent with cells and no fibrosis; usually have fibrin and inflammatory cells

Crescent, Fibrocellular

- Crescent with mixture of cellular and fibrous components

Crescent, Fibrous

- Predominantly fibrous tissue in Bowman space; no fibrin or inflammatory cells

Diffuse

- Majority of glomeruli (≥ 50%)

Duplication of GBM

- Double layer of GBM separated by clear zone on silver or PAS stains; sometimes likened to "tram tracks"; sometimes redundantly called "reduplication"

Endocapillary Hypercellularity (Proliferation)

- Increased numbers of intracapillary cells causing narrowing of glomerular capillary lumina

Extracapillary Hypercellularity (Proliferation)

- Synonym for crescent

Fenestrations (Fenestrae)

- Openings through endothelial cells, ~ 50 nm in diameter, that allow fluid passage but retain formed elements

Fibrinoid Necrosis

- Area of necrosis that stains brick red with eosin due to denatured proteins and fibrin

Filtration Slit Diaphragm

- Connection between podocyte foot processes consisting of nephrin and other components; thought to be responsible for macromolecular filtration; a.k.a. "zipper" for its en face appearance

Focal

- Minority of glomeruli (< 50%)

Glomerular Basement Membrane

- Continuous layer of collagen type IV and matrix components on which podocytes and endothelial cells rest; does not include Bowman capsule

GBM Thickening

- Used for PAS and silver stains that distinguish GBM elements

Hyaline Deposits

- Homogeneous, dense eosinophilic deposits, often with clear fine lipid droplets; composition not well defined

INTRODUCTION TO RENAL PATHOLOGY

Hyaline Thrombi
- Synonym for pseudothrombi

Hypertrophy
- Increase in size (diameter) of glomerulus (normally < 1/2 diameter of a 40x field); typically accompanied by increased mesangium and thickened GBM

Inflammation
- Increased numbers of leukocytes (granulocytes, monocytes, lymphocytes) in capillaries (normally < 2/ glomerulus)

Global
- Entire glomerulus involved (> 50% in lupus)

Ischemic Collapse (Sclerosis)
- Glomerulus showing collapse of capillary tuft ± thickening of Bowman capsule and fibrosis in Bowman space

Karyorrhexis
- Pyknotic and fragmented nuclei

Mesangial Cell
- Normal resident of mesangium in glomerulus; has contractile and phagocytic properties

Mesangial Hypercellularity
- 3 or 4 mesangial nuclei or more in 1 mesangial area in a 3 micron section; lupus classification uses 3; IgA classification uses 4
  - Subdivided into mild (4-5), moderate (6-7), and severe (8 or more)

Mesangial Matrix
- Extracellular component of normal mesangium, includes collagen III, fibronectin, and variety of glycosaminoglycans

Mesangial Matrix Expansion
- Width of mesangial interspace exceeds 2 mesangial cell nuclei in at least 2 glomerular lobules (IgA)

Mesangiolysis
- Loss of integrity of mesangium so that glomerular capillary forms aneurysmal dilation

Necrosis
- Loss of integrity of glomerulus; typically manifested by fragmented nuclei (karyorrhexis), disruption of GBM, and deposition of fibrin; minimum requirement is extravascular fibrin (IgA)

Nodules
- Rounded expansion of mesangial matrix &/or cells with peripheral necklace of capillaries

Nuclear Dust
- Fragments of neutrophil nuclei (karyorrhexis) in site of inflammation

Parietal Epithelium
- Cells that line Bowman capsule

Pseudothrombi
- Eosinophilic, rounded aggregates in glomerular capillaries due to immune complex precipitates rather than fibrin (typically due to cryoglobulins with IgG, IgM, and C3); a.k.a. hyaline thrombi

Podocyte
- Cell on outside of GBM with extensive foot processes connected with filtration slit diaphragms; terminally differentiated

Sclerosis
- Obliteration of capillary lumen by increased extracellular matrix, ± hyalinosis or foam cells

Segmental
- Part of a glomerulus involved; definitions varies from any amount to < 50%

Spikes
- "Hair on end" pattern of subepithelial GBM on silver or PAS stain; need 40-100x to appreciate

DEFINITIONS FOR TUBULES

Acute Tubular Injury
- Loss of brush border on PAS stain, thin cytoplasm, loss of nuclei; simplification of epithelium without tubular basement membrane thickening (IgA)

Acute Tubular Necrosis
- Epithelial cell death, as manifested by loss of or pale-staining nuclei and eosinophilic cytoplasm; usually not conspicuous unless toxin or vessel occlusion; sometimes used as a synonym for acute tubular injury

Apoptosis
- Epithelial cell death, as manifested by hyperchromatism and dissolution of nuclei

Casts
- Presence of protein or cells in tubular lumen, taking shape of tubule

Casts, Red Cell
- Presence of compacted red cells in tubular lumen; may be hemolyzed or fragmented; need to distinguish from biopsy artifact

Casts, Tamm-Horsfall
- Cast of protein normally produced in distal tubule; pale on H&E, strongly PAS positive

Dystrophic Calcification
- Calcification of necrotic cells or debris; typically in casts as variably sized basophilic granules

Fatty Change
- Tubules with clear cytoplasm containing lipid (demonstrable in Oil red O stained frozen sections); a feature of nephrotic syndrome

Granuloma
- Nodular collection of epithelioid macrophages, sometimes with multinucleated macrophages (a.k.a "histocytes"), usually with lymphocytes

Intranuclear Inclusions
- Homogeneous dense or pale transformation of nucleus, indicative of active viral replication

Isometric Vacuolization
- Abundant clear vacuoles of same size in cytoplasm

Nephrocalcinosis
- Accumulation of calcium salts, typically in TBM as basophilic, linear deposit; also present in casts

Osmotic Nephrosis
- Fine clear vacuolization in tubules

Thyroidization
- Dilated tubular segments with eosinophilic proteinaceous casts and thin epithelial lining

Tubular Atrophy
- Loss of cytoplasmic organelles (pale cytoplasm) accompanied by shrinkage of tubular diameter and often thickened TBM

Tubular Hypertrophy
- Increased diameter of tubules with increased size of epithelial cells

Tubular Reabsorption Droplets
- PAS(+) small round granules in tubular cells; contain albumin and often other plasma proteins and indicate glomerular proteinuria

Tubular Rupture
- Disruption of TBM with localized inflammatory response; may have granulomatous reaction and spilling of Tamm-Horsfall protein into interstitium ("piss granuloma")

Tubulitis
- Mononuclear leukocytes within epithelial layer of tubules

DEFINITIONS FOR INTERSTITIUM

Abscess
- Localized collection of neutrophils in area of destruction of normal tissue components

Interstitial Fibrosis
- Expansion of normal interstitial connective tissue by increased collagen (I and III, typically); may or may not be accompanied by tubular atrophy; may be diffuse or focal
  - Scored by % of cortex involved or area of fibrosis

Interstitial Inflammation
- Increased numbers of leukocytes between tubules; may be focal or diffuse, nodular, perivascular, subcapsular

- Should be noted whether or not inflammation is confined to areas of interstitial fibrosis

DEFINITIONS FOR VESSELS

Arteriolar Hyalinosis
- Accumulation of eosinophilic, amorphous material (usually containing plasma proteins) in arteriolar wall; may be subendothelial, peripheral nodular, or transmural; focal or circumferential

Capillaritis
- Accumulation of leukocytes in peritubular capillaries

Endarteritis
- Mononuclear inflammatory cells under endothelium of arteries and arterioles

Fibrinoid Necrosis
- Brick red staining of vessel wall on H&E with loss of smooth muscle nuclei; may have inflammatory component

Intimal Fibroelastosis
- Thickening of arterial intima with multiple layers of elastic fibers and collagen; usually not very cellular

Intimal Fibrosis
- Accumulation of fibrous tissue in intima, usually concentric, causing stenosis of lumen

Mucoid Intimal Thickening
- Accumulation of edematous extracellular matrix in intima resembling mucus; pale blue on H&E, Alcian blue positive

"Onion Skinning"
- Multilayered cells and matrix in intima of small arteries and arterioles

Vasculitis
- Inflammation in wall of vessel, as manifested by neutrophil karyorrhexis, fibrinoid necrosis of media; may occur in any sized vessel, artery, capillary, or vein

SELECTED REFERENCES

1. Sis B et al: Banff '09 meeting report: antibody mediated graft deterioration and implementation of Banff working groups. Am J Transplant. 10(3):464-71, 2010
2. Working Group of the International IgA Nephropathy Network and the Renal Pathology Society et al: The Oxford classification of IgA nephropathy: pathology definitions, correlations, and reproducibility. Kidney Int. 76(5):546-56, 2009
3. Weening JJ et al: The classification of glomerulonephritis in systemic lupus erythematosus revisited. J Am Soc Nephrol. 15(2):241-50, 2004
4. Corwin HL et al: The importance of sample size in the interpretation of the renal biopsy. Am J Nephrol. 8(2):85-9, 1988

Normal Glomerulus and Mesangial Hypercellularity

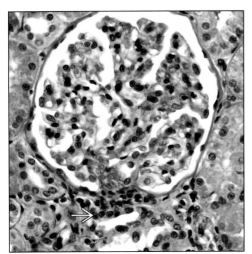

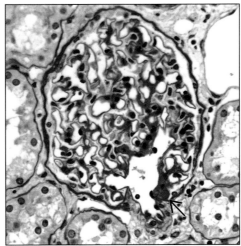

(Left) H&E shows a normal glomerulus from a biopsy for asymptomatic microhematuria. The juxtaglomerular apparatus is at the base ➡. The capillaries are open, and the cellularity is normal although it is difficult to define the mesangium. *(Right)* Glomerulus in a donor biopsy stained with PAS reveals a thin GBM, open capillaries, an inconspicuous mesangium, and normal podocytes. A small hyaline deposit is present at the hilum ➡, but it is otherwise normal.

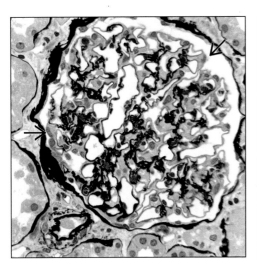

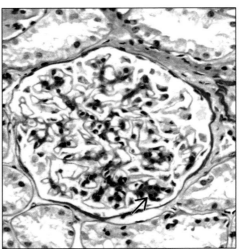

(Left) Donor biopsy stained with Jones silver stain highlights the normal GBM. The podocytes ➡ are well seen, but the mesangial cells are lost in the densely stained mesangial matrix. This and the PAS stain are most valuable for appreciating the LM glomerular anatomy. *(Right)* Minimal mesangial hypercellularity ➡ from a patient with lupus nephritis is shown. The threshold for mesangial hypercellularity is 3-4 mesangial cells per mesangial area in a 2-3 μm section.

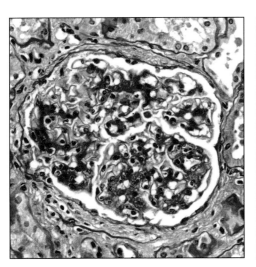

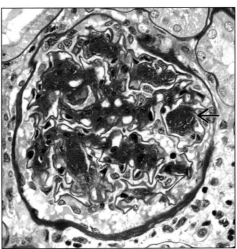

(Left) Moderate global mesangial hypercellularity in a patient with IgA nephropathy is shown. All segments of the glomerulus have increased mesangial cells and matrix. *(Right)* Marked global expansion of the mesangial matrix and cellularity with a segmental nodular pattern ➡ is evident in this glomerulus with diabetic glomerulosclerosis.

Glomerular Inflammation

(Left) Neutrophils can be seen in glomerular capillaries ➡ with swollen endothelial cells that occlude the capillary lumina in a lupus nephritis case. Fragments of nuclei (nuclear dust) or karyorrhexis are present ➡. *(Right)* Necrosis of a glomerulus is shown, with loss of nuclei and obliteration of the normal architecture of the glomerulus ➡. Thrombi are evident in arterioles ➡ in this case of thrombotic microangiopathy.

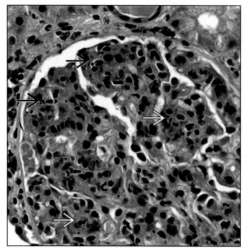 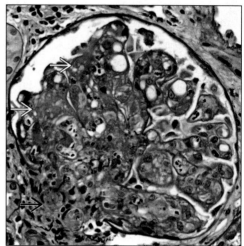

(Left) Fibrinoid necrosis is best seen on H&E stained sections in which the fibrin and denatured protein stain brick red ➡ with nearby nuclear dust. An area of old necrosis with loss of the normal architecture but without fibrin is also present ➡. Patient has ANCA-related glomerulonephritis. *(Right)* This glomerulus has an infiltrate of monocytes in the capillaries, occluding the lumina. Patient has mixed cryoglobulinemia.

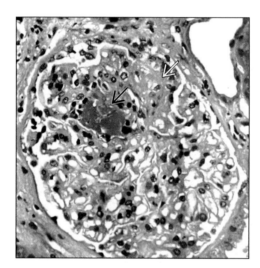 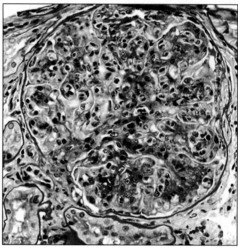

(Left) Thrombi in capillaries ➡ and fibrinoid necrosis ➡ are shown in a glomerular tuft from a patient with endocarditis. *(Right)* Endocapillary hypercellularity ➡ illustrated in this glomerulus from a patient with lupus nephritis is defined as leukocytes or other cells filling the capillary loops. Here there are both mononuclear and polymorphonuclear cells. The capillary walls are also thickened, but this is better appreciated in PAS or silver stains.

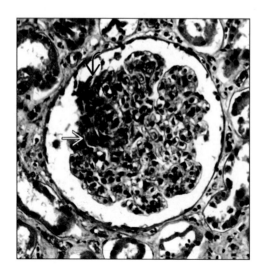 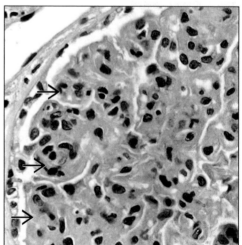

Crescents

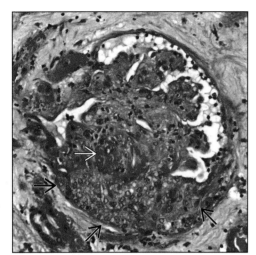 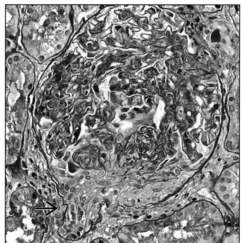

(Left) H&E shows a cellular crescent ⊟ occupying 1/3 of the circumference of Bowman capsule with associated fibrinoid necrosis ⊟. A crescent is defined as a layer of more than 2 cells in Bowman space occupying ≥ 25% of the circumference of Bowman capsule. Crescents are also known as extracapillary proliferation. *(Right)* Crescents interfere with glomerular function by compressing the tuft and blocking the outlet of Bowman space into the proximal tubule ⊟.

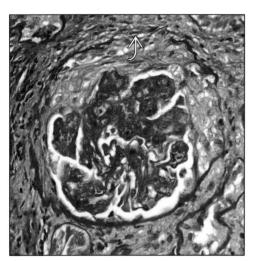 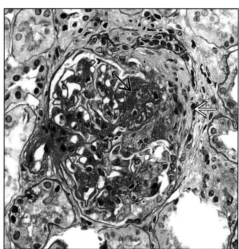

(Left) Crescents start as a cellular proliferation of parietal epithelial cells and evolve into fibrocellular crescents (shown here), which have less cellularity and more collagen deposition. Disruption ⊟ of Bowman capsule is present, a typical feature of crescents. *(Right)* A fibrous crescent remains in this glomerulus with associated adherent segmental sclerosis ⊟ of the tuft due to prior necrosis. Bowman capsule is disrupted ⊟.

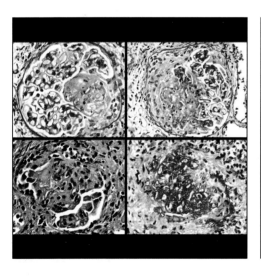 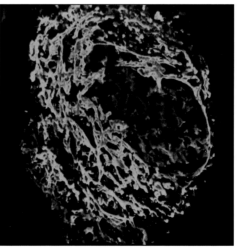

(Left) Evolution of crescents is shown, from cellular (upper L), to destruction of the tuft (upper R), to scarring of the tuft (lower L), to end-stage destroyed glomerulus with remnants of GBM and disrupted Bowman capsule (lower R). *(Right)* Crescents typically have deposition of fibrin among the proliferating parietal epithelial cells. Activation of the clotting system in Bowman space is a general mechanism of formation of crescents, whatever the underlying glomerular disease.

GBM Abnormalities and Adhesions

(Left) The silver stain is useful to demonstrate abnormalities of the GBM, as shown here in a glomerulus with prominent duplication of the GBM ("tram tracks") ➡. Image is from an allograft with transplant glomerulopathy. *(Right)* GBM "spikes" can be appreciated in membranous glomerulonephritis on a thin (2 μm) silver stained section ➡. These protrusions of the GBM surround the silver negative immune complex deposits.

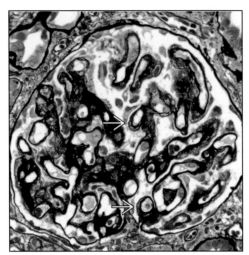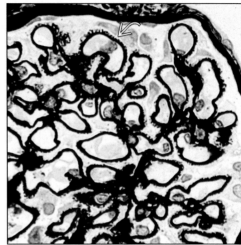

(Left) Wire loops ➡ are eosinophilic thickening of the glomerular capillary wall due to subendothelial deposits, shown here in a case of active lupus nephritis, class IV. *(Right)* Adhesion of a sclerotic glomerular segment to Bowman capsule (BC) is shown in a patient with idiopathic focal segmental glomerulosclerosis (FSGS). A useful feature to distinguish an adhesion from artifactual compression of the tuft against the BC is the tenting of BC ➡ toward the glomerulus.

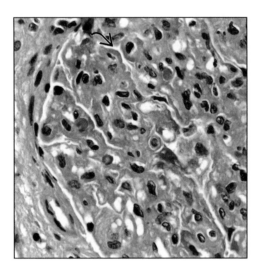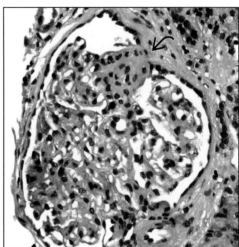

(Left) Abundant hyaline deposition ➡ in an adhesion with scarred segment of the glomerulus is shown. Lipid droplets ➡ (unstained) help distinguish this from fibrin. *(Right)* Periodic acid-Schiff shows a pseudocrescent ➡ caused by bridging of parietal (or visceral) epithelial cells from Bowman capsule to the GBM in a patient with collapsing glomerulopathy.

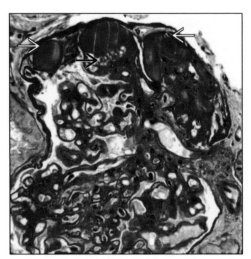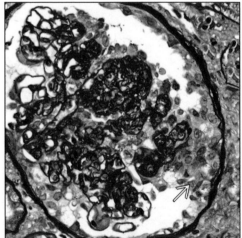

Light Microscopy Tubules

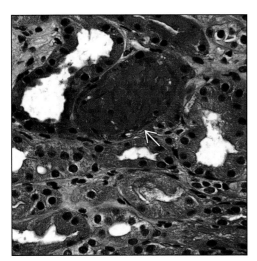 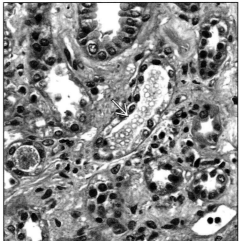

(Left) Red cell cast in a tubule ➡ is shown. The compaction of the erythrocytes and complete filling of the tubule indicate that this is not an artifact of the biopsy procedure. (Right) Hemolyzed red cell cast in a tubule is shown ➡. The ghost cells can still be recognized on H&E. Hemolysis indicates that these are not artifacts of the biopsy. Patient has Henoch-Schönlein purpura.

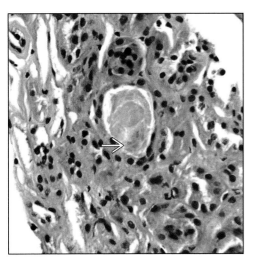 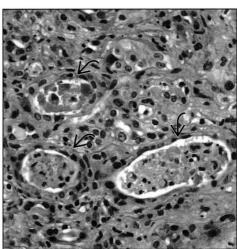

(Left) A pigmented cast ➡ was all that remained as evidence of prior glomerular bleeding in a patient with IgA nephropathy. (Right) Casts ➡ in acute tubular necrosis typically contain nuclear fragments and eosinophilic cytoplasmic debris derived from necrotic tubular epithelial cells.

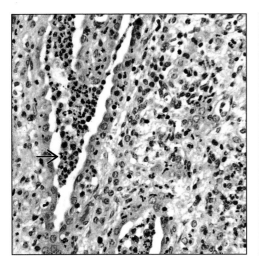 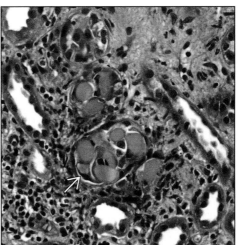

(Left) In acute pyelonephritis (not often diagnosed in biopsy), prominent neutrophil casts ➡ can be seen (as in this case) where they are in a collecting duct identifiable by its branching. (Right) Eosinophilic casts with attached mononuclear cells ➡ should raise suspicion of myeloma cast nephropathy, as illustrated in this case.

Light Microscopy Tubules

(Left) Normal tubules and interstitium in a donor biopsy stained with PAS are shown. Tubules are separated by peritubular capillaries, and there is minimal fibrous tissue. **(Right)** Tubular reabsorption droplets in the cytoplasm of proximal tubular cells are round granules that are positive with PAS stain ➡. The distal tubules are negative ➡. Patient had minimal change disease.

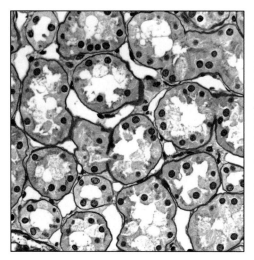
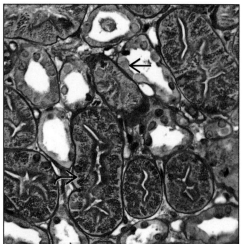

(Left) Periodic acid-Schiff shows acute tubular injury with thinned cytoplasm ➡ with loss of brush border, decreased numbers of nuclei ➡, and granular casts ➡. **(Right)** Myoglobin casts are typically strongly eosinophilic and granular. They can be identified with antimyoglobin immunohistochemistry.

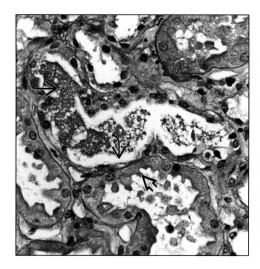
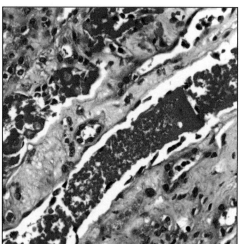

(Left) Thyroidization is a term applied to the eosinophilic casts in atrophic, microcystic tubules. These are generally associated with chronic pyelonephritis but are not specific. They are caused by disruption of the tubules by scar and retention of Tamm-Horsfall protein. **(Right)** Nephrocalcinosis is manifested by TBM deposits of basophilic calcium salts ➡. Nephrocalcinosis can be seen in a variety of conditions with hypercalcemia and in nephrogenic systemic sclerosis related to gadolinium scans.

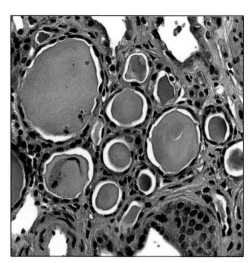
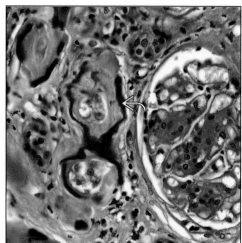

Light Microscopy Tubules and Interstitium

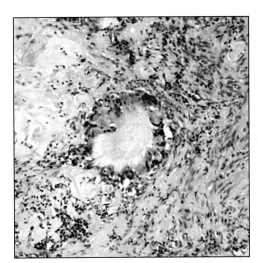

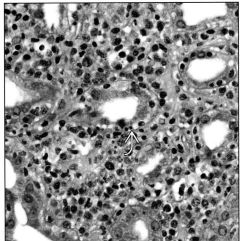

(Left) H&E shows a urate deposit with a giant cell reaction in the medulla of kidney from a patient with gout. The crystals dissolve, in contrast to oxalates, but can be seen in frozen tissue. (Right) Acute interstitial inflammation with mononuclear cells separates and invades the tubules (tubulitis) ➤. This pattern can be seen in acute rejection (as in this case) or in drug allergy and other conditions.

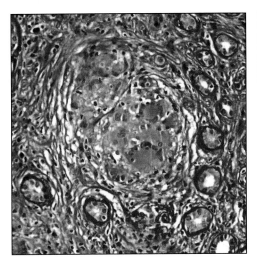

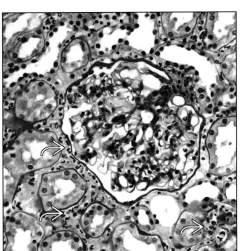

(Left) Interstitial granuloma with multinucleated giant cells is shown. Granulomatous interstitial nephritis has a broad differential, including infection (mycobacteria, adenovirus), sarcoidosis, Crohn disease, and drug allergy. (Right) Neutrophils in peritubular capillaries (capillaritis) ➤ are a sign of acute antibody-mediated rejection. Neutrophils can be relatively inconspicuous.

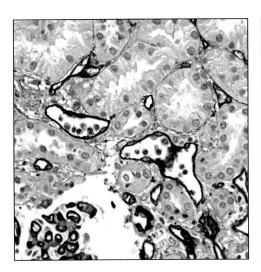

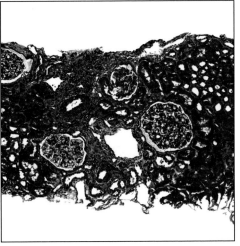

(Left) Intracapillary mononuclear cells and positive staining for C4d in peritubular capillaries are defining characteristics of chronic humoral rejection. (Right) Trichrome stain allows more accurate assessment of interstitial fibrosis; illustrated here is focal fibrosis that is typical of vascular disease, with loss of tubules and relative preservation of glomeruli.

Light Microscopy Arteries

(Left) Arteriolar hyalinosis is PAS positive and may be focal, circumferential, or nodular ➔. This case is a donor biopsy. Arteriolar hyalinosis is caused by hypertension, diabetes, aging, and calcineurin inhibitors. *(Right)* Leukocytoclastic vasculitis with nuclear dust and fibrinoid necrosis is evident in a small artery ➔. Microscopic polyangiitis in a renal biopsy is associated with ANCA(+), cryoglobulinemia, and Henoch-Schönlein purpura.

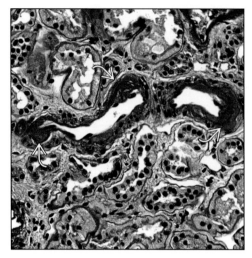
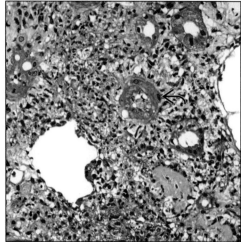

(Left) Mucoid intimal thickening appears as a loose, slightly basophilic accumulation of matrix in the intima, a sign of thrombotic microangiopathy. In this case, it was related to a factor H mutation. *(Right)* Organized thrombus in an arcuate-sized artery in a patient with thrombotic microangiopathy is shown.

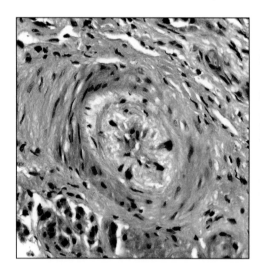
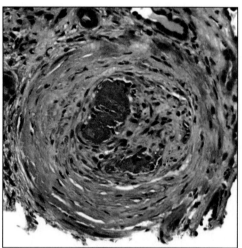

(Left) "Onion skin" pattern of intimal thickening in a small artery in a patient with severe hypertension is shown. *(Right)* Elastic fiber stain highlights the fibroelastosis of the intima that occurs in longstanding hypertension.

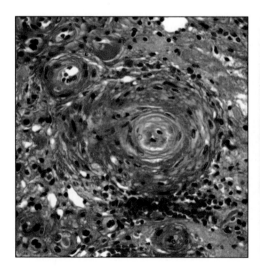
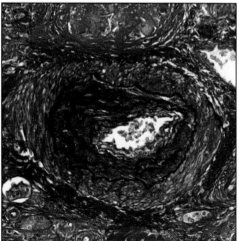

Immunofluorescence Glomeruli

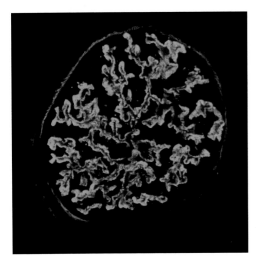
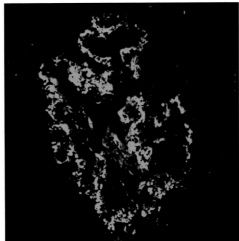

(Left) Fine, uniform, granular deposits all along the GBM are typical of subepithelial deposits in membranous glomerulonephritis, here stained for IgG. Some appear to be in the mesangium, but these may be tangential cuts of the GBM. *(Right)* Rounded granular deposits of IgG along the GBM are typical of the "humps" of post-infectious glomerulonephritis (GN), as in this case of post-streptococcal GN.

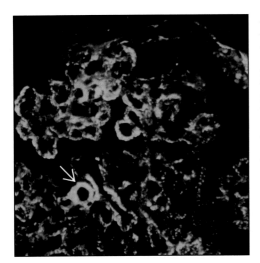
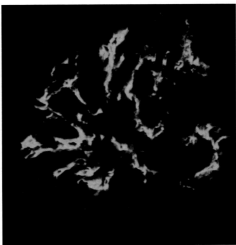

(Left) Coarse, granular, and elongated deposits ➡ along the GBM (sometimes referred to as "wire loop" lesions) are typical of subendothelial deposits, as in this case of lupus nephritis. *(Right)* Classical mesangial deposition pattern in glomerulus resembles the branches of a tree, as in this IgA stain in IgA nephropathy.

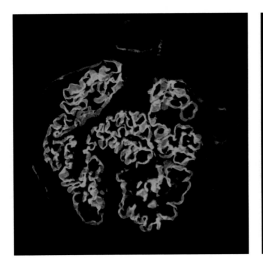
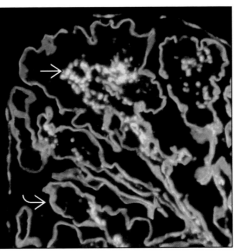

(Left) Linear IgG in the GBM is characteristic of anti-GBM disease, as shown in this case. Diabetes can also have prominent linear IgG, but in that case, albumin is similarly present. *(Right)* Dense deposit disease has a unique IF pattern. C3 is deposited in coarse, brightly staining granules ➡ in the mesangium, sometimes with a dark center. Linear GBM staining ➡ is also present.

Immunofluorescence Glomeruli

(Left) Glomerular pseudothrombi (hyaline thrombi) ➡ of mixed cryoglobulinemia appear as rounded, brightly stained deposits in glomerular capillaries when stained for IgM. These are not fibrin thrombi but rather are precipitates of immune complexes. *(Right)* IgM and C3 commonly are present in segments of glomeruli that are sclerotic, as shown here in a case of FSGS stained for IgM.

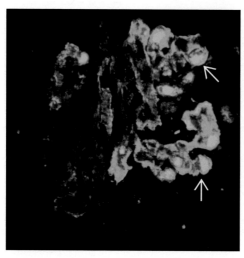
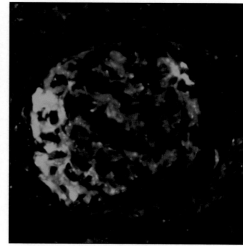

(Left) C3 is deposited in the mesangium and along the GBM in a coarse, granular pattern in membranoproliferative glomerulonephritis, type I (shown here) accompanied by immunoglobulin. *(Right)* A mesangial pattern of IgG is evident in this patient with lupus nephritis (class II). The GBM has rare speckles.

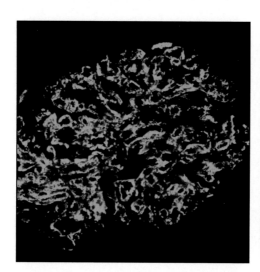
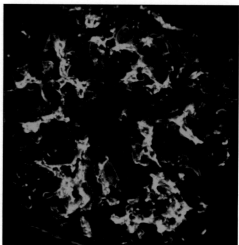

(Left) Fibrillary GN has a distinctive pattern with deposits of IgG in the mesangium and segmentally along the GBM in a broad linear distribution. *(Right)* Amyloid deposits in the glomeruli have broad, fairly homogeneous staining in the mesangium and GBM for the components of the amyloid (light chains, amyloid A protein, fibrinogen, etc.). This case is stained for amyloid A protein.

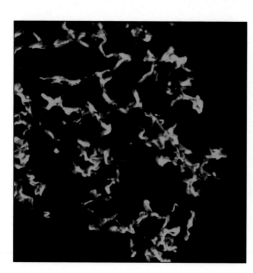
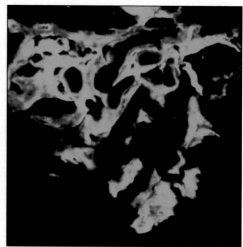

1

Immunofluorescence Tubules and Vessels

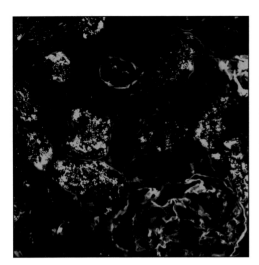
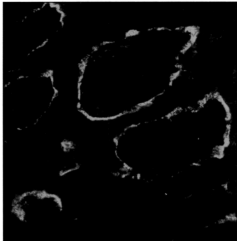

(Left) Tubular reabsorption droplets stain for albumin (as in this image) and other plasma proteins (IgG, C3, fibrinogen, etc.). This is an indication of glomerular proteinuria. Minimal change disease. *(Right)* Granular deposits of IgG along the TBM can be seen in lupus nephritis and occasionally in other diseases, such as polyoma infections. In contrast, C3 deposits segmentally in the TBM are common and should not be taken as evidence of immune complex deposition.

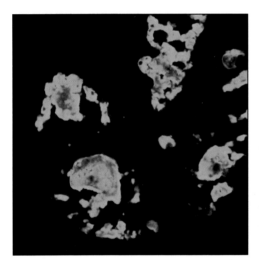
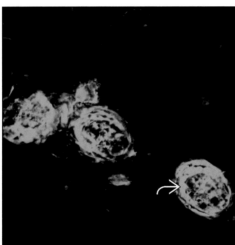

(Left) Light chain staining is essential for the diagnosis of monoclonal gammopathies. In this patient with myeloma cast nephropathy, kappa, but not lambda, was detected in the casts in the tubules. *(Right)* Fibrin ➡ is detected in the arterioles in this case of thrombotic microangiopathy due to Avastin therapy. Fibrin also permeates the wall, a reflection of fibrinoid necrosis of the vessels.

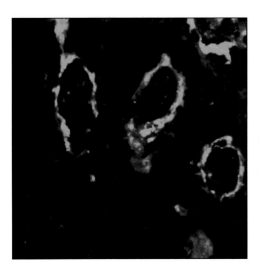
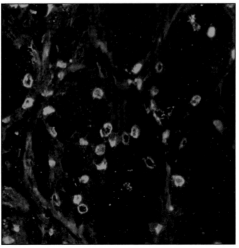

(Left) C3 is not uncommonly detected in the tubular basement membrane, as in this case of calcineurin inhibitor toxicity in an allograft. Tubular cells activate the alternative complement pathway, and this is probably a manifestation of tubular injury. *(Right)* Lupus biopsies sometimes show antinuclear antibody (ANA) in tubular cells, here stained with anti-IgM. These are probably due to plasma ANA artifactually depositing during the IF staining procedure in permeabilized cells.

INTRODUCTION TO RENAL PATHOLOGY

Electron Microscopy GBM

(Left) EM shows normal glomerulus with podocyte foot processes ➘ and a normal GBM ➘. The normal GBM is thicker than a typical foot process. *(Right)* Widespread effacement of foot processes ➘ is a feature of minimal change disease and, to some degree, of other diseases with glomerular proteinuria.

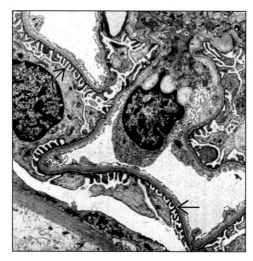
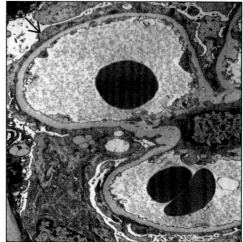

(Left) Thin basement membrane disease has thin but otherwise normal GBM. The measurements are taken using a grid overlay. The distance is measured where the grid crosses the GBM, and the harmonic mean is calculated (normal mean ± 2 s.d. is 373 ± 84 nm for males, 326 ± 90 nm for females). *(Right)* Diabetes has a uniformly thickened but otherwise normal GBM. The thickness has been measured using a grid overlay (normal mean ± 2 s.d. is 373 ± 84 nm for males, 326 ± 90 nm for females).

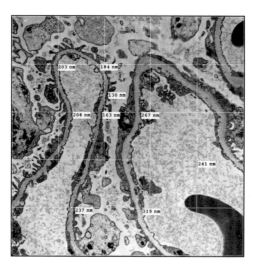
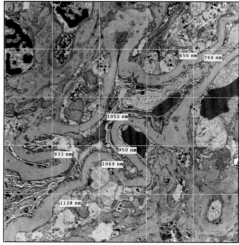

(Left) Podocyte injury is sometimes reflected by new subepithelial layers of basement membrane matrix ➘ between the podocyte ➘ and original GBM ➘. This is a characteristic feature of collapsing glomerulopathy. Intracapillary endothelial cells or macrophages contain lipid (foam cells) ➘. *(Right)* Fine reticulated lamination of a thickened GBM ➘ with scalloping of the subepithelial surface is a characteristic feature of Alport syndrome.

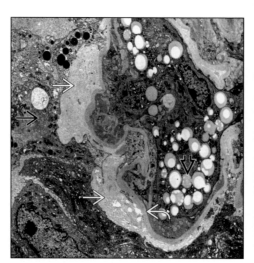
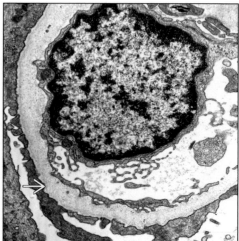

Electron Microscopy Organized Deposits

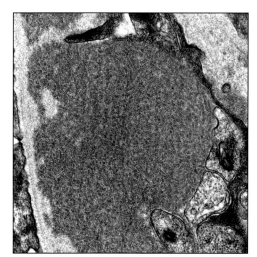
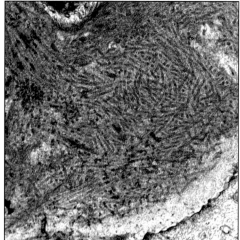

(Left) EM shows an organized mesangial deposit in a patient with mixed cryoglobulinemia (34,000x). (Right) Immunotactoid glomerulopathy has tubular deposits typically > 25 nm in diameter; in this case they measured ~ 35 nm (34,000x).

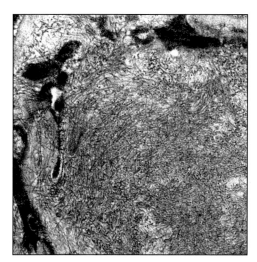
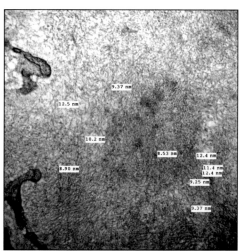

(Left) Fibrillary glomerulonephritis has nonperiodic fibrils that are typically 10-20 nm in diameter; in this case they were ~ 13 nm in diameter (34,000x). (Right) Amyloid fibrils are typically 8-12 nm in diameter without periodicity. These averaged ~ 10 nm. The appearance is similar to fibrillary GN, and a Congo red stain is necessary to confirm their identity (34,000x).

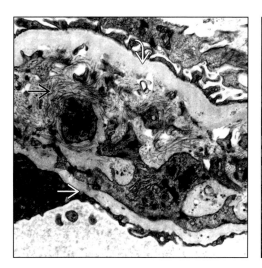
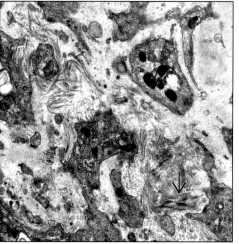

(Left) Type III collagen glomerulopathy (collagenofibrotic glomerulopathy) has deposits of fibrillar collagen with a periodicity of 62 nm ⮕. The GBM is duplicated; original ⮕ and new ➡ subendothelial layers are indicated. (Right) Fibrillar collagen ➡ is sometimes detected in the mesangium as part of a pathologic process of sclerosis. Here the fibrils are seen in a case of IgA nephropathy. This should not be confused with type III collagen glomerulopathy.

Introduction

Electron Microscopy Immune Complex Deposits

(Left) EM of a glomerulus from a patient with post-streptococcal GN shows the characteristic "humps" located along the GBM in the subepithelial space ➡. These do not elicit a GBM response of "spikes" in contrast to membranous GN. (Right) A glomerular capillary has subepithelial deposits with spikes of GBM between them ➡. This is a typical feature of membranous GN in contrast to postinfectious GN. The neutrophil ➡ in the capillary may be a sign of renal vein thrombosis.

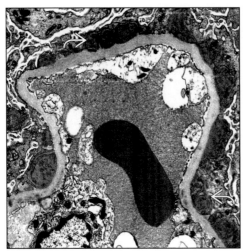 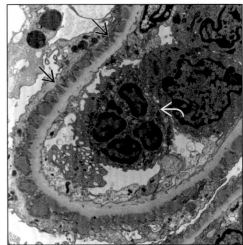

(Left) Mesangial deposits ➡ in IgA nephropathy typically hug the mesangial cells ➡ and are amorphous. (Right) Subendothelial deposits ➡ are present in many glomerular diseases and usually elicit a new layer of GBM over their surface, as in this case from a patient with lupus nephritis. Subepithelial deposits are also present and penetrate the GBM ➡.

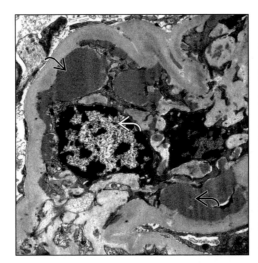 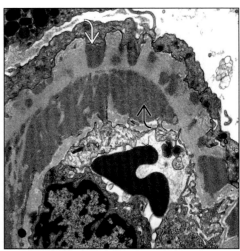

(Left) Immune complex deposits can be reabsorbed or dissolved with time, in which case they begin to lose their electron density ➡, as in this case of membranous GN. (Right) The reabsorption of deposits occurs with time in most diseases; here, a subepithelial deposit in membranous GN is almost completely removed ➡ and resurfaced with a new layer of subepithelial GBM ➡.

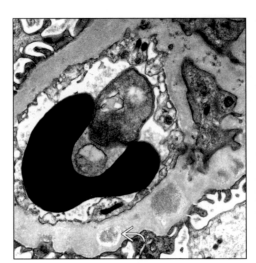 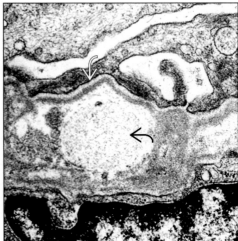

1

Electron Microscopy Distinctive Deposits

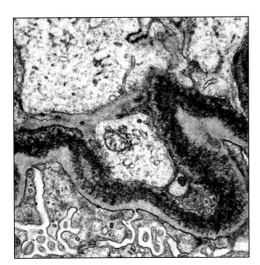
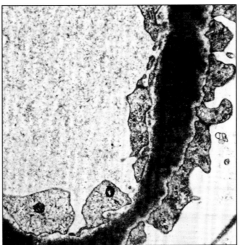

(Left) Granular dense deposits in the GBM, mesangium, TBM, and vascular BM characterize systemic light chain deposition, here shown in a glomerular capillary in a patient with kappa light chain deposition by IF. (Right) The densest deposit in renal pathology by EM is that in dense deposit disease (DDD), here shown replacing the GBM in a glomerular capillary in a child with DDD. The deposits contain C3 and factor H.

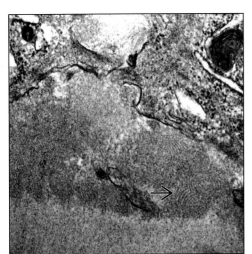
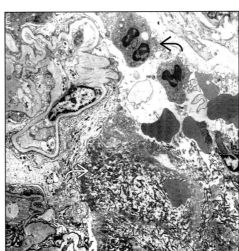

(Left) Deposits with periodicity are sometimes evident in lupus nephritis, where they have been called "Churg's thumbprints" ➡ for the renal pathologist who 1st described them. (Right) Fibrin by EM appears denser than the usual immune complex deposit and has a fibrillar "tactoid" pattern; sometimes the 22 nm periodicity is evident. Shown here are fibrin ➡ and neutrophils ➡ in Bowman space in a patient with ANCA-related GN and crescents.

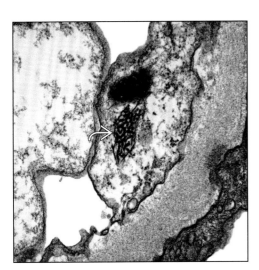
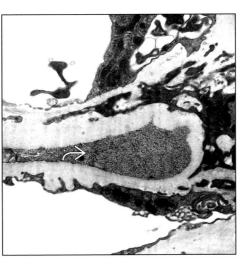

(Left) Once thought to be a virus, this intracellular tubular aggregate in a glomerular endothelial cell is known as a "tubuloreticular structure" ➡. This is a cellular response to interferons and is most often found in lupus and in patients treated with interferons. (Right) A particulate subepithelial deposit ➡ of unknown nature is sometimes found without clear explanation. This is almost certainly not a virus; theories include lipoproteins or components of the podocyte.

NORMAL KIDNEY DEVELOPMENT

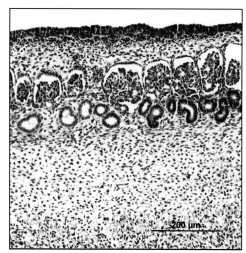

Hematoxylin & eosin stained section shows linear organization of mesonephros in a human fetus. Note the recognizable glomeruli and tubules.

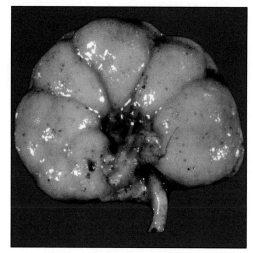

Gross photograph of a normal human fetal kidney shows prominent lobulations. These lobulations disappear with continued growth postnatally to give rise to a smooth-surfaced kidney.

TERMINOLOGY

Abbreviations
- Wolffian duct (WD) (a.k.a. nephric duct)
- Ureteric bud (UB)
- Collecting duct (CD)
- Metanephric mesenchyme (MM)
- Intermediate mesoderm (IM)
- Mesenchymal to epithelial transition (MET)

STAGES OF KIDNEY DEVELOPMENT

Overview
- Embryonic kidney development begins from collection of cells in IM, a layer of tissue between paraxial mesoderm and lateral plate mesoderm
- 3 sets of embryonic kidneys (pronephros, mesonephros, and metanephros) develop in anterior (rostral) to posterior (caudal) direction
- Pronephros and mesonephros precede definitive kidney (metanephros)

Pronephros
- Transient collection of cells in IM at about 3 weeks of gestation undergo MET to initiate induction of each nephric duct
- Nephric duct grows in rostrocaudal direction toward cloaca
- As nephric duct extends caudally, it induces formation of tubules in IM that degenerate by 4 weeks gestation
- Involution of pronephros coincides with beginning of mesonephros
- Without the WD, kidneys, ureters, and male genital tract do not develop

Mesonephros
- Continued WD growth progressively induces adjacent mesenchyme to form mesonephros, starting at about 3.5 weeks

- Transient **linear organization** of functional nephrons connected to nephric duct (about 34)
- Regresses at about 16 weeks gestation in humans except most of the anterior/cranial mesonephric tubules, which in males, become part of epididymis
- WD becomes vas deferens in males
- Many genes/processes that regulate mesonephros and metanephros development are thought to be similar

Metanephros
- Definitive kidney
- Begins at about 4th-5th week of gestation, giving rise to about 1 million nephrons/kidney
- Starts from distal end of WD as diverticulum
- **Branched organization** of urinary collecting system and proximal nephrons (tubules and glomeruli)
- Fetal and embryonic kidneys have **lobulated** appearance
- As nephrons are added, grooves distend, and kidney surface becomes smooth
- Lateral fusion of cortex of lobules produces columns of Bertin

Comparative Development
- Mouse
  - Nephric ducts extend caudally beginning at embryonic (E) 8.5d to induce formation of tubules in IM, which regresses by E9.5d
  - WD growth induces adjacent mesenchyme to form mesonephros starting at E9d
  - Mesonephros regresses about E15.5d
    - Only rostral mesonephric tubules connect to WD
  - Metanephros formation begins at about E10.5d

MAJOR COMPONENTS OF DEVELOPING METANEPHROS, ORIGIN, AND DERIVATIVES

Overview
- About 30 different cell types in mammalian kidney
- Origin of some is known
- Fate mapping and lineage tracing studies help determine origin and destiny of various cell types

Ureteric Bud
- Derived from WD
- Produces cortical and medullary CDs (principal and intercalated cells), calices, pelvis, and ureter

Metanephric Mesenchyme
- Derived from IM; produces glomeruli (podocytes, parietal and visceral epithelium of Bowman capsule), proximal tubules, loop of Henle, distal tubules, connecting tubules

Stroma
- Likely originates from paraxial mesoderm
- Source for interstitial cells, pericytes, smooth muscle cells, mesangium, capsule, likely angioblasts, and nerves

Vasculature
- Blood vessels derived from sacral branches of descending aorta
- Lymphatics follow vessels and drain into lumbar lymph nodes

Innervation
- Sympathetic innervation from renal ganglia regulates blood flow (activation reduces flow)
- Afferent or sensory nerve fibers follow along sympathetic tracts to lower thoracic levels
- Parasympathetic innervation to ureter and lower urinary tract by pelvic ganglia located adjacent to bladder neck

STEPS IN METANEPHRIC KIDNEY DEVELOPMENT

UB Induction
- Signals from MM induce UB outgrowth from caudal end of each WD

UB Invasion into MM
- Inductive signals induce initial branching as T-shaped structure
  - Trunk of this structure is UB stalk, which will become ureter
  - Tips are called UB tips or ampulla
  - Rapid proliferation and subsequent branching occur in UB tips
  - UB tips regulate subsequent nephrogenesis

Mesenchymal Condensation
- Process necessary for nephrogenesis, occurs by virtue of aggregation of mesenchymal cells around UB tips
- MM signals UB to branch; signals from UB instruct MM to undergo mesenchymal condensation (reciprocal interactions)

Branching Morphogenesis
- Factors from stroma and condensed mesenchyme stimulate repetitive branching of UB tip, giving rise to new stalks and UB tips in each cycle (branching morphogenesis), resulting in centripetal growth of developing kidney
  - 1st few generations of branching produce pelvis and major and minor calices; later generations of branching produce collecting duct system in kidney
  - Lateral branching may also occur from stalks
- Can be divided into 3 main stages
  - Initial rapid branching
  - Period of slower rate of branching to promote lengthening of stalks
  - Rapid branching toward end where many nephrons are stimulated from each UB tip, forming arcades

Pretubular Aggregates
- Form next to junction of UB stalk and node from a subset of cap mesenchyme cells that have undergone mesenchymal to epithelial transition

Comma-shaped Body
- Formed from pretubular aggregates
- Cleft in comma-shaped body is infiltrated by capillaries, mainly from extrarenal sites, although stromal endothelial progenitors may participate

S-shaped Body (Tubulogenesis and Glomerulogenesis)
- Formed from proliferation of comma-shaped body; indicates that patterning of nephron has occurred
  - Outer portion of proximal end of this structure (farther from UB stalk) becomes parietal layer of Bowman capsule and inner layer (visceral layer); cleft is invaded by capillaries (glomerular tuft)
  - Proximal end gives rise to podocytes
  - Distal ends produce proximal and distal tubules (closer to UB stalk); distal end fuses with collecting ducts
- Glomerulogenesis begins at about 8 weeks of gestation
  - Developing glomeruli grow in rows (generations) from tips of UB
  - Due to centripetal branching and subsequent nephrogenesis, more mature or older glomeruli are located toward corticomedullary area and newer ones toward periphery
  - Between 23-33 weeks of gestation, gestational age can be determined by counting number of glomerular rows in cortex
  - Glomerular generation is precise and can be used to identify gestational age in autopsy or products of conception
    - Gestational age (weeks) = 4.7 x number of glomerular layers + 0.1
  - Total of 9-14 glomerular generations by end of gestation (variation due to methodology)
- Glomerulogenesis is complete about 2 weeks before birth in humans

- Fetal glomeruli appear compact with closely aligned podocytes, known as immature glomeruli
- Tubulogenesis continues for a few weeks after birth
- After birth, kidney growth occurs by adding length and diameter to tubules and diameter to glomeruli
  - No more glomeruli are added after birth, with total numbers of 227,000-1,825,000/kidney
  - Varies by birth weight

Collecting Ducts
- UB stalk and tip differentiate into CDs
  - Principal cells (ion pumps, Na, K)
  - Intercalated cells (acid-base balance)

FINAL POSITION OF KIDNEYS

Kidney Ascent: Pelvis to Abdomen
- Not true migration
  - Apparent ascent due to disparate caudal growth of fetus relative to trunk leaving kidneys behind
- Begins at about 6 weeks of gestation
  - Initially, kidneys posteriorly located and hila pointing anteriorly
- By 7-8 weeks, kidneys start medial rotation and apparent ascent
- By 9 weeks, hila anteromedially positioned and kidneys in retroperitoneal cavity in abdomen
  - Approximately located at T12-L1
  - Positioned underneath adrenal glands, result in flattening of adrenal inferior surface

Blood Supply of Ascending Kidneys
- Derives from closest vessel, aorta
- Blood vessels change with ascent, thus are transient until final location in abdomen
  - While located in pelvis, kidneys derive blood supply from lower segments of aorta
  - Abdominally positioned kidneys derive from higher segments of aorta and caudal branches degenerate
- Accessory blood supply and variations may be partly due to persistence of early vessels
- Failure of lower vessels to degenerate can lead to ureteral obstruction as they may cross over ureter

GENES IMPORTANT IN KIDNEY DEVELOPMENT

Major Genes by Stage Identified from Model Organisms
- WD growth or development
  - *LIM1, PAX2, GATA3, Emx2, EYA1, FOXC1, Odd1*
- Ensuring single UB outgrowth
  - *RET, Gdnf, Spry1, ROBO2, Slit2, LIM1, Bmp4, GATA3*
- UB induction
  - *RET, Gfrα1, GDNF*
- UB branching
  - *RET, Ralph2, FoxB2, WT1, PAX2, Gdnf, Wnt11, BMP7, Wnt4, Foxd1, SAL1, Bcl2, Fgf7, Fgf10, Fgfrl1, Fgfr2IIIb, Fgfr1, Fgfr2, FRAS1*
- MM condensation, nephrogenesis (tubulogenesis, glomerulogenesis)
  - *AGT, AGTR1, Notch1, Notch2, Fgf2, Fgf8, Fgfr1, Six2, BMP7, PdgfB, CD2AP, Vegf, Wnt4, A3b1, At2, LAMB2, WT1, PAX2, Wnt9*

CELLULAR PROCESSES IN KIDNEY DEVELOPMENT

Stages and Different Compartments
- WD growth: Proliferation, migration, and cell structure changes, particularly at distal tip
- UB outgrowth and branching
  - Proliferation occurs mainly in UB tip and differentiation at end
  - Cell death is low
- MM and nephrogenesis
  - In absence of mesenchymal induction or proper branching, **apoptosis is default**
  - Initially proliferates to synchronize with UB branching
  - Cell death occurs in both MM and stroma
  - Balance maintained between cell death and proliferation as growth continues
  - Migration involved in generation of pretubular aggregates and various cell types of tubules and glomerulus

SELECTED REFERENCES

1. Chi X et al: Ret-dependent cell rearrangements in the Wolffian duct epithelium initiate ureteric bud morphogenesis. Dev Cell. 17(2):199-209, 2009
2. Dressler GR: Advances in early kidney specification, development and patterning. Development. 136(23):3863-74, 2009
3. Guillaume R et al: Paraxial mesoderm contributes stromal cells to the developing kidney. Dev Biol. 329(2):169-75, 2009
4. Grote D et al: Gata3 acts downstream of beta-catenin signaling to prevent ectopic metanephric kidney induction. PLoS Genet. 4(12):e1000316, 2008
5. Jennette JC et al: Heptinstall's Pathology of the Kidney. 6th ed. Philadelphia: Lippincott Williams & Wilkins. 2007
6. Kopan R et al: Molecular insights into segmentation along the proximal-distal axis of the nephron. J Am Soc Nephrol. 18(7):2014-20, 2007
7. Basson MA et al: Branching morphogenesis of the ureteric epithelium during kidney development is coordinated by the opposing functions of GDNF and Sprouty1. Dev Biol. 299(2):466-77, 2006
8. Costantini F: Renal branching morphogenesis: concepts, questions, and recent advances. Differentiation. 74(7):402-21, 2006
9. dos Santos AM et al: Assessment of renal maturity by assisted morphometry in autopsied fetuses. Early Hum Dev. 82(11):709-13, 2006
10. Dressler GR: The cellular basis of kidney development. Annu Rev Cell Dev Biol. 22:509-29, 2006
11. Jain S et al: Critical and distinct roles for key RET tyrosine docking sites in renal development. Genes Dev. 20(3):321-33, 2006
12. Basson MA et al: Sprouty1 is a critical regulator of GDNF/RET-mediated kidney induction. Dev Cell. 8(2):229-39, 2005
13. Grieshammer U et al: SLIT2-mediated ROBO2 signaling restricts kidney induction to a single site. Dev Cell. 6(5):709-17, 2004

NORMAL KIDNEY DEVELOPMENT

Expression of Selected Genes in Developing Murine Kidney

Mesonephros and WD	UB Stalk	UB Tip	Metanephric Mesenchyme	Stroma	C-, S-shaped Bodies, Tubules	Glomerulus
Pax2	Met	Ret	Gfrα1	Foxd1	Pax2	Wt1
Lim1	Wnt9b	Gfrα1	Gdnf	Pod1	Wnt4	Pax2
Odd1	Wnt7	Wnt11	Robo2	Bmp5	Lhx1	Pod1
Ret		Spry1	Wt1	Fgf7	Brn1	Glepp1
Gfrα1		Slit2	Pax2	Fgf10	Dll1	Neph
Spry1		Pax2	Foxc1	Rarα1	Notch1	Vegf
Bmp4		Lim1	Eya1	Rarβ2	Notch2	Pdgf
Pax8		Hspg	Sal1	Raraldh2	Jag1	Lmx1b
Robo2		Emx2	Six2		Hes	Cd2AP
Slit2		Agt	Pax3		Hey	Nck
FoxC1		Fgfr2(IIIb)	Bmp7		Cdh6, 11	ColIV
Gata3		Gpc3	Hox11		Jnk	
α3β1		Erm	Pleiotrophin			
		Pea3	Bmp4			
		Wnt9b	Agtr2			
		Spry2	Midkine			
		Grip1	Pbx1			

For a more detailed list, see www.gudmap.org.

Human Fetal Gestational Age and Glomerular Development

Gestational Age (in Weeks)	Rows of Glomeruli in Cortex from Medulla to Capsule*	Number of Mature Glomerular Layers (NGL)**
16-23	3	
24	3-5	4.3 ± 0.8
25	4-6	4.6 ± 0.7
26	5-7	
27	6-8	6.1 ± 1.1
28	7-9	6.0 ± 1.2
29	8-10	6.3 ± 1.3
30	9-11	
31	10-12	7.1 ± 0.9
32	11-13	
33	12-13	7.7 ± 0.8
34	12-14	
35-42	12-14	7.6 ± 0.4 - 8.6 ± 1.3
Newborn-adult	12-14	
	Cortex between columns of Bertin	Radial counts; excludes columns of Bertin

*Adapted from Dorovini-Zis K et al: Gestational development of brain. Arch Pathol Lab Med. 101(4):192-5, 1977. **Adapted from dos Santos AM et al: Assessment of renal maturity by assisted morphometry in autopsied fetuses. Early Hum Dev. 82(11):709-13, 2006.

14. Hughson M et al: Glomerular number and size in autopsy kidneys: the relationship to birth weight. Kidney Int. 63(6):2113-22, 2003

15. Vize PD et al: The Kidney: From Normal Development to Congenital Disease. London: Academic Press. 2003

16. Lechner MS et al: The molecular basis of embryonic kidney development. Mech Dev. 62(2):105-20, 1997

17. Kriz W et al: Structural organization of the mammalian kidney. In Seldin DW et al: The Kidney: Physiology and Pathophysiology. New York: Raven Press. 2nd ed. 661-698,1992

18. Saxen L: Organogenesis of the Kidney. Cambridge: Cambridge University Press. 1987

19. Dorovini-Zis K et al: Gestational development of brain. Arch Pathol Lab Med. 101(4):192-5, 1977

Embryonic Kidney Development

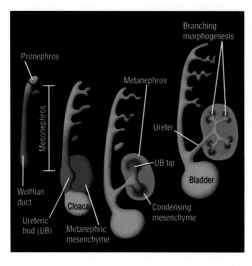

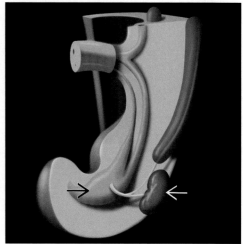

(Left) Graphic depicts early events in kidney development. Pronephros: Transient, nonfunctional kidneys begin at ~ 3rd gestational week from intermediate mesoderm. Mesonephros: Second set of transient kidneys begin at 3.5 weeks, consisting of Wolffian (mesonephric) duct with a linear arrangement of nephrons. Metanephros: Definitive kidney begins at 4 weeks with UB outgrowth that invades into metanephric mesenchyme and undergoes branching morphogenesis. (Right) Graphic shows cloaca ⊡ & kidney ➡.

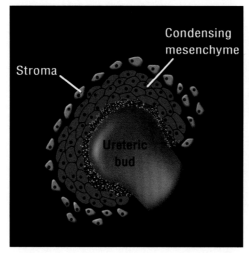

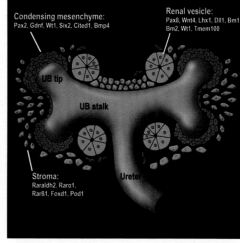

(Left) Initial UB invasion into mesenchyme results in mesenchymal condensation around the UB tip. (Right) Reciprocal interactions between the condensing mesenchyme, stroma, and UB lead to UB branching and initiation of renal vesicle formation (through epithelial to mesenchymal transformation). The initial UB stalk that grows from the Wolffian duct becomes the ureter. Some of the important genes in the development of each structure are indicated.

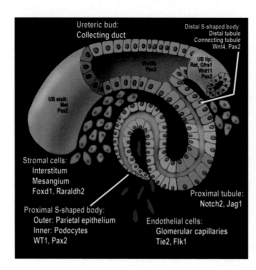

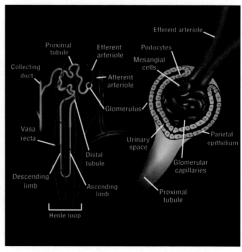

(Left) A renal vesicle undergoes further patterning and differentiation to form a comma-shaped body and then an S-shaped structure. Endothelial cells invade the proximal cleft of the S-shaped body, the proximal end becomes the glomerulus, and the distal end becomes the connecting tubule, which joins to the collecting ducts. (Right) Illustration depicts the relationship between blood vessels and the nephron. The major cell types in the glomerulus are shown. Modified from Dressler 2009.

NORMAL KIDNEY DEVELOPMENT

Ascent of the Kidneys

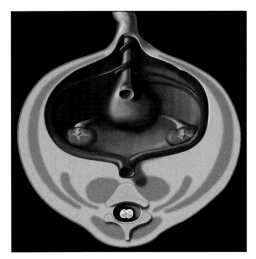 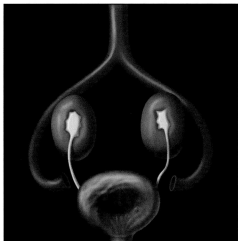

(Left) Axial view shows posteriorly facing kidneys in the pelvic cavity during early development (about 6 weeks). *(Right)* Coronal view at 6 weeks shows posteriorly facing kidneys in the pelvis with the hila point anteriorly. The blood supply is from the lower transient branches of the aorta.

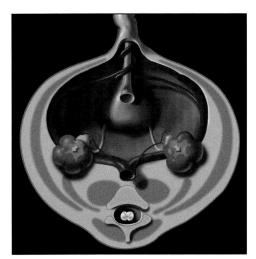 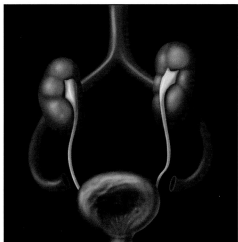

(Left) Axial view during the middle stages of kidney development (7 weeks) shows kidneys beginning ascent and medial rotation. *(Right)* Illustration depicts middle stages of kidney ascent as they begin medial rotation (7 weeks), with the blood supply from more superiorly located transient vessels from the aorta than in previous stages. There is actually no true migration but apparent ascent due to disparate caudal growth of the fetus leaving the kidney behind.

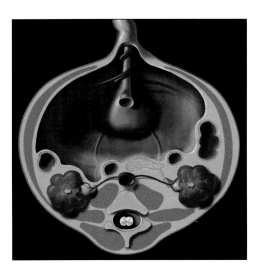 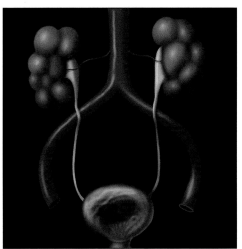

(Left) Axial view shows that the kidneys have completed the ascent and are located retroperitoneally. *(Right)* The final retroperitoneal location of the kidneys in the abdomen is shown. The hila face anteromedially. The blood supply is from renal arteries emanating from the aorta before aortic bifurcation.

Stages of Early Kidney Development

(Left) Low-power image from a sagittal section of 1st trimester human products of conception shows the location of the developing mesonephros and its organization in a linear fashion ➡️. The rostral side is on the left and the caudal end is on the right. Note the relationship of the mesonephros with respect to other organs such as the liver ⮊, heart ⮊, and somites ⮕. *(Right)* High-power view of human fetal mesonephros shows a primitive glomerulus ➡️ and tubules ⮊.

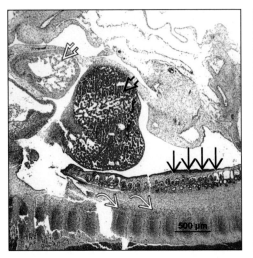
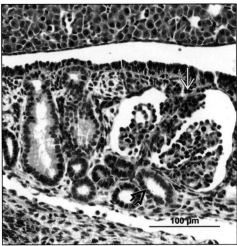

(Left) Live detection of 1st UB branching to produce T-shaped structure, visualized by green fluorescent protein (GFP) from the Ret locus in mice. The image is from E11.5d mouse urinary tract. The intense green signal in the UB tip ➡️ represents sites of Ret expression that regulate UB branching. The initial UB stalk ⮊ will become the ureter. *(Right)* Shown here is branching morphogenesis depicted by GFP expression in UB tips in a mouse metanephric kidney organ culture.

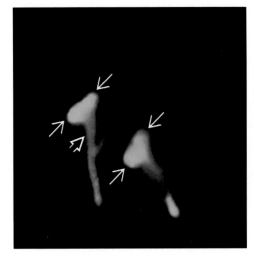
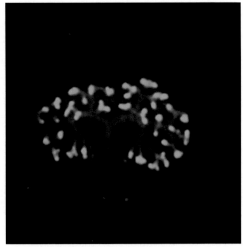

(Left) Early stage of metanephric development shows UB invasion into the MM from human products of conception. Note that the collection of cells surrounding a cross section of UB tips ➡️ is the condensing mesenchyme ⮊ that undergoes mesenchymal to epithelial transformation to produce tubules and glomeruli. *(Right)* Branching UB shows tips ➡️, mesenchymal condensation ⮊, pretubular aggregates ➡️, and renal vesicles ⮕ in later stages of human metanephros development.

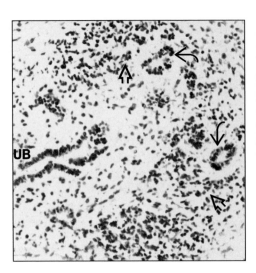
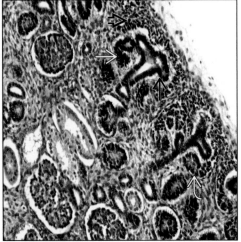

Stages of Later Kidney Development

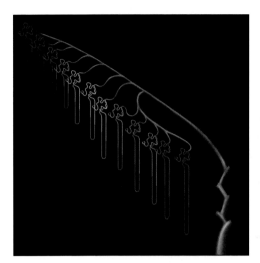

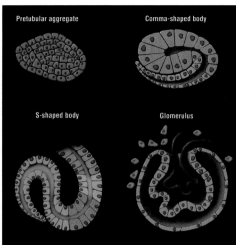

(Left) Diagram depicts glomerulogenesis. A total of 12-14 glomerular generations develop centripetally, with older glomeruli toward the corticomedullary junction. Glomerulogenesis is complete by birth with no new glomeruli forming postnatally in humans. (Right) In stages of proximal nephron development, pretubular aggregates lead to comma-shaped bodies that give rise to S-shaped bodies. The proximal part of these become tubules and the distal part glomerular epithelial cells.

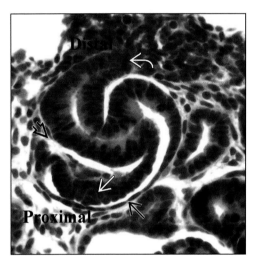

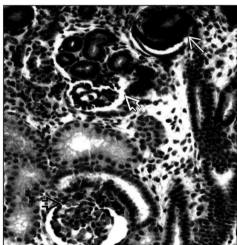

(Left) Image of a human S-shaped body shows the proximal end, glomerulus, distal end, and connecting tubule ➡. The cleft ➡ is where the endothelial cells migrate to form the glomerular tuft. The outer layer becomes the parietal epithelium ➡ of Bowman capsule, and the inner cells become podocytes ➡. (Right) Image of human metanephros shows different stages of nephrogenesis: Early comma-shaped body ➡, intermediate ➡, and more advanced stage ➡.

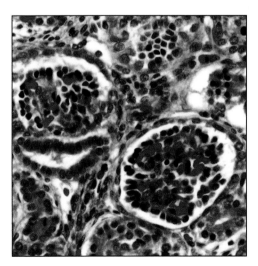

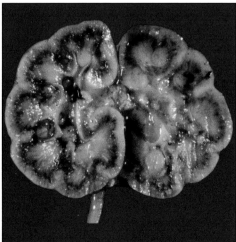

(Left) Image shows features of human fetal glomeruli. Note that they are not fully vascularized; eventually, 10-12 capillary loops will fill each glomerulus. Podocytes are densely arranged, forming a corona at the periphery of the capillary loops. As the loops develop, the podocytes flatten. (Right) Coronal section of a fetal kidney is shown. Note that the cut surface shows lobulations and a well-organized cortex and medulla.

NORMAL KIDNEY STRUCTURE

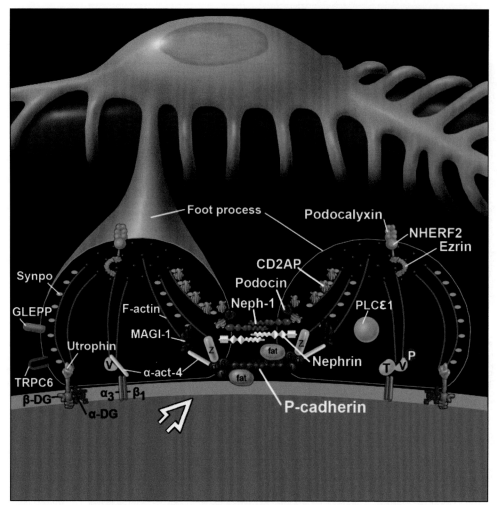

A schematic representation of podocyte and slit diaphragm proteins in relation to each other and to the GBM ➡. α3β1-integrins and dystroglycans (α-DG and β-DG) anchor foot processes to GBM. Podocalyxin and synaptopodin (synpo) regulate the plasticity of actin-based cytoskeleton (F-actin, α-actinin-4). The podocyte-slit diaphragm complex molecules nephrin, podocin, ZO-1 (Z), mFAT1 (fat), Neph-1, CD2AP, P-cadherin, and others regulate the glomerular filtration barrier. Other molecules include PLCε1(phospholipase C epsilon 1), TRPC6 (transient receptor potential 6 ion channel), GLEPP (glomerular epithelial protein 1), talin (T), vinculin (V), and NHERF2 (Na⁺/H⁺ exchanger regulatory factor).

TERMINOLOGY

Abbreviations
- Glomerular basement membrane (GBM)
- Peritubular capillaries (PTC)

MACROSCOPIC FINDINGS

Anatomic Features
- Kidneys are paired, bean-shaped organs
  - Each kidney weighs 150 g each, measures 11 cm in length, is 5-7 cm wide, and 3 cm thick
    - Kidneys in women are smaller, but size best correlates with body surface area and weight
    - After 3rd decade, there is progressive decline in renal mass due to glomerulosclerosis
  - Located in retroperitoneal space, extending from 12th thoracic to 3rd lumbar vertebrae, with hilum oriented slightly anteriorly

- Renal sinus refers to concave space at hilum composed of adipose tissue, renal pelvis, and neurovascular structures
- Pelvic calyces converge into renal pelvis, which narrows inferiorly as ureter
  - Outer surface is smooth and covered by translucent, fibrous capsule surrounded by perinephric fat
  - Fetal lobulations demarcated by surface grooves may be seen mostly in infants

Longitudinal Cross Section of Kidney
- Kidney has dark brown outer cortex and paler inner medullary "pyramids"
- Cortex is approximately 1 cm in thickness
  - Cortex that extends in between medullary pyramids is referred to as "columns of Bertini"
- Pyramid and surrounding cortex constitute renal lobe; normal kidney has 11-14 lobes
- Each kidney has 7-10 medullary pyramids
  - Papillae are tips of medullary pyramids

1

NORMAL KIDNEY STRUCTURE

○ Most papillae in central portion drain single lobe and are termed "simple papillae"
  ■ They have slit-like openings of ducts of Bellini
  ■ Convex tips aid in prevention of urinary reflux from pelvis into kidney
○ Papillae in superior and inferior poles drain 2-3 lobes and are termed "compound papillae"
  ■ Orifices of ducts of Bellini are rounded and gaping open, thus susceptible to intrarenal reflux

Vascular Supply and Nerve Innervation

- Arterial supply
  ○ Kidney receives up to 1/4 of cardiac output
  ○ Renal end arteries have no collateral blood flow
  ○ Renal artery from aorta enters hilum and divides into anterior and posterior segmental branches
  ○ Segmental arteries divide into 6-8 interlobar arteries, which traverse between renal lobes and penetrate renal parenchyma at corticomedullary junction
  ○ Interlobar arteries continue as arcuate arteries at right angles along corticomedullary junction
  ○ Arcuate arteries give rise to interlobular arteries that extend into outer cortex at right angles
  ○ Interlobular arteries further branch out as afferent arterioles that terminate as glomerular capillary tufts
- Venous drainage
  ○ Blood from PTCs and vasa recta drains sequentially into interlobular, arcuate, and interlobar veins
  ○ Larger veins traverse parallel to arteries, merge into renal veins, and drain into inferior vena cava
  ○ Due to high perfusion rates, renal arteriovenous oxygen gradient is much lower than in other organs
- Lymphatic supply
  ○ Lymphatic drainage follows vasculature
    ■ Lymphatics begin in adventitia of interlobular arteries, merge with other lymphatics, and exit from renal hilus
    ■ Lymphatics eventually drain into hilar and para-aortic lymph nodes
    ■ There are no periglomerular or peritubular lymphatic vessels
  ○ Superficial outer cortex is drained by transcapsular lymphatics that join hilar lymphatics
- Nerve supply
  ○ Sympathetic fibers from celiac plexus traverse via splanchnic nerves to ganglia in renal plexus
  ○ Nerve fibers traverse along arterial system and innervate blood vessels, cortical tubules, and juxtaglomerular apparatus
  ○ Sensory fibers from kidney also travel along sympathetic pathways to T10-T11 nerves

MICROSCOPIC FINDINGS

Architectural Organization

- Cortex is organized into 2 architectural components
  ○ Cortical labyrinth
    ■ Composed of glomeruli, proximal tubules and distal convoluted tubules, and initial portions of collecting ducts
    ■ Vasculature includes interlobular arteries and veins, arterioles, venules, and capillaries

    ■ Interstitium is scant and has PTCs and interstitial cells
  ○ Medullary rays
    ■ Elongated projections of medullary tissue extending into cortex
    ■ Composed of tubular segments arranged at right angles to corticomedullary junction
    ■ Tubular segments include collecting ducts and straight segments of proximal and distal tubules
- Medulla is composed of inner and outer segments
  ○ Outer medulla has outer and inner stripes
    ■ Outer stripe is composed of straight portions of proximal tubule, collecting ducts, and thick ascending loops of Henle
    ■ Inner stripe has thin descending and thick ascending loops of Henle and collecting ducts
  ○ Inner medulla has thin descending and ascending loops of Henle and collecting ducts of Bellini

Nephron

- Nephron is functional unit of kidney derived from metanephric blastema
- Each kidney has approximately 1,000,000 nephrons
- Each nephron contains glomerulus and tubule
  ○ Glomeruli are confined to cortex
  ○ Tubule is comprised of proximal tubule, loop of Henle, and distal tubule
  ○ Outer and midcortical glomeruli extend short loops of Henle into inner stripe of outer medulla
  ○ Glomeruli at corticomedullary junction (juxtamedullary glomeruli) have long loops of Henle that dip deep into inner medulla
- Distal nephron tubule drains into collecting ducts and eventually into renal pelvis; both are embryologically derived from ureteric bud

Glomerulus

- Glomerulus is composed of capillary tuft that floats within Bowman space, is anchored at vascular pole, and is surrounded by Bowman capsule
- Mean adult diameter of glomerulus is 200 μm; juxtamedullary glomeruli are slightly larger
- Cellular components include endothelial cell, mesangial cell, podocyte, and parietal epithelial cell
  ○ There is evidence for cross talk via signaling pathways between various glomerular cells
  ○ Cytokines synthesized by one cell type may influence receptors on other cells
  ○ For example, vascular endothelial growth factor (VEGF) produced by podocytes has significant effects on endothelial cells
- Extracellular matrix includes mesangial matrix, GBM, and Bowman capsule
- Glomerular filtration barrier is composed of endothelial cell surface layer, endothelial cells, GBM, slit diaphragm, and subpodocyte space
  ○ These compartments restrict flow of molecules in filtrate on basis of charge, shape, and size
- Endothelial cells
  ○ Endothelial cytoplasm completely surrounds inner aspect of capillary loop and has microtubules and filaments that provide cytoskeletal support

1

NORMAL KIDNEY STRUCTURE

- Nucleus and nonfenestrated cytoplasm usually reside over mesangial interface
- Thin, attenuated layer of fenestrated cytoplasm extends along GBM
  - Fenestrations are 70-100 nm in diameter
- Surface polyanionic glycoproteins, such as podocalyxin, impart negative charge and thus restrict filtration of plasma molecules
- "Endothelial surface layer" is carbohydrate-rich meshwork coating luminal aspect of endothelial cells and is being recognized as important component of glomerular filtration barrier
- Endothelial cells secrete several molecules involved in immune response and coagulation system and express MHC class II molecules
- Mesangial cells
  - Restricted to 1-2 per matrix area
  - Numerous cytoplasmic processes extend to endothelial cells, mesangial GBM, and other mesangial cells
    - Make direct contact and form gap junctions with endothelial cells through fenestrations at interface
  - Smooth muscle properties of mesangial cells are mediated by vimentin intermediate filaments, actin-based cytoskeleton, and contractile proteins
  - The phagocytic properties enable them to participate in degradation of immune complexes
  - Secrete molecules that participate in matrix production and degradation in response to injury
- Podocytes or visceral epithelial cells
  - Podocyte is specialized cell with large cell body and multiple elongated arborizing cell processes that end in terminal structures called foot processes
  - These terminally differentiated cells have tightly controlled cell cycles but are capable of proliferation (dysregulation) on exposure to injury
  - Podocytes participate in GBM synthesis, contribute to glomerular filtration barrier, and help maintain hydraulic regulation of capillary loop diameter
  - They express unique set of molecules including WT1, C3b receptors, and vimentin, but not cytokeratin intermediate filaments
  - Podocytes reside in urinary space and and are attached to GBMs via foot processes
  - Cell body resides near GBM reflection of adjacent capillary loops and consists of major organelles
    - Cell body is separated from GBM by subpodocyte space and layer of foot processes
    - Subpodocyte space is dynamic and restrictive compartment that covers 60% of glomerular filtration barrier and thus helps podocytes modulate glomerular permeability
  - Cell processes are rich in microtubules and intermediate filaments
  - Foot processes are cytoplasmic extensions arranged at right angles to long axis of GBM
    - They extensively interdigitate with foot processes of adjacent podocytes
    - Foot processes anchored to GBM by α3β1-integrins and dystroglycans
    - Between foot processes are slits bridged by zipper-like slit diaphragms

- Foot process structure is maintained by its actin-based cytoskeleton
- Several molecules have been described in podocyte foot processes and slit diaphragms that contribute to structural integrity and permselectivity of filtration barrier
- Parietal epithelial cells
  - Flattened cells that line inner surface of Bowman capsule
  - In continuity with podocytes at vascular pole and with tubular epithelial cells at urinary pole
  - Contain cytokeratin intermediate filaments and are capable of proliferation in response to injury
- Mesangial matrix
  - Mesangial matrix and cells form supporting infrastructure of glomerulus
  - Composed of microfibrils, type IV (α1 and α2) and V collagen, laminin, and fibronectin
  - Is more porous to macromolecules than GBM
- Glomerular basement membrane
  - GBM is composed of fused basal lamina of endothelial cells and podocytes
  - Has 3 layers (i.e., inner lamina rara interna, central lamina densa, and outer lamina rara externa)
  - Measures approximately 300-350 nm in thickness with slightly thicker GBM in males
  - Children have thinner basement membranes but achieve adult thickness by age 10-12 years
  - GBM is composed predominantly of type IV collagen, noncollagenous glycoproteins (laminin, entactin), and sulfated proteoglycans
    - Collagen type IV is triple helix substructure composed of heterodimers of 3 α chain combinations (from α1-α6)
    - GBM is composed of collagen type IV with α3.α4.α5 chain network
    - Collagen type IV structure has attachment sites for other basement membrane molecules
    - Noncollagenous glycoproteins and collagen type IV are crosslinked for structural integrity
    - Sulfated proteoglycans impart anionic charge
  - GBM restricts flow of molecules in filtrate, provides structural support, and has attachment sites for various molecules that affect cell signaling and polarity
- Bowman capsule
  - Bowman capsule is connective tissue barrier between interstitium and urinary space
  - It is continuous with proximal tubular basement membrane at urinary pole and with GBM at vascular pole
  - Components include collagen type IV (α1, α2, α5, α6), laminin, and entactin

Juxtaglomerular Apparatus

- Located at glomerular vascular pole that comes in contact with distal tubule as it ascends toward its glomerulus
- Glomerular component includes terminal afferent arteriole and initial portion of efferent arteriole
- Tubular component includes "macula densa," which refers to specialized distal tubular epithelial cells

- ○ Macula densa cells are elongated with reverse polarity of apical nuclei
- ○ It is responsible for "tubuloglomerular feedback," which regulates glomerular blood flow based on NaCl concentration in distal tubular lumen
- Extraglomerular mesangial cells are in continuity with arteriolar smooth muscle cells
- Renin-secreting juxtaglomerular granular cells are mostly within muscularis of afferent arterioles
  - ○ They receive rich sympathetic innervation, which regulates renin secretion
  - ○ Renin secretion is also regulated by NaCl within tubular lumens near macula densa

Tubules

- Tubular segments of nephron include proximal tubule, loop of Henle, and distal convoluted tubule
- Collecting duct is derived from ureteric bud and is not embryologically part of nephron
- Connecting duct segment between distal tubule and collecting duct is not well delineated in humans
- Proximal tubule
  - ○ Begins at tubular pole of glomerulus and is composed of proximal convoluted segment in cortex and straight segment residing in medulla
  - ○ Lining cells are eosinophilic with abundant mitochondria and have prominent brush border
- Loop of Henle
  - ○ Proximal tubule descends as thin descending limb, thin ascending limb, and thick ascending limb
  - ○ Thick ascending limb merges with distal tubule at junction of macula densa
  - ○ Glomeruli from outer and middle cortex have short descending thin loops extending only to outer medulla
  - ○ Juxtamedullary glomeruli have long descending thin loops that extend deep into papillary tips
  - ○ Epithelium of thin limbs is flattened and may mimic capillaries
- Distal tubule
  - ○ Distal tubules drain into collecting ducts
  - ○ Epithelium is composed of small paler cells without brush borders
- Collecting duct
  - ○ Epithelium is cuboidal; cells increase in height as ducts descend into medulla
  - ○ Lining cells include principal and intercalated cells
  - ○ Intercalated cells are mainly in cortex and outer medulla and are progressively fewer in deep medulla
  - ○ Collecting dusts coalesce into larger ducts of Bellini

Interstitium

- Renal cortex has minimal amounts of interstitium
- Medullary interstitium is quite prominent in inner medulla and papillary tips

Capillary Network

- Renal circulation has dual capillary beds in series: Glomerular network and PTC network
- Glomerular capillary network
  - ○ Afferent arteriole breaks into glomerular capillaries
  - ○ Glomerular capillaries coalesce into efferent arteriole, which immediately bifurcates to form PTC network
  - ○ Maintains higher pressures (40-50 mmHg) compared with other capillary beds, including PTCs (5-10 mmHg)
  - ○ Usually, efferent arterioles are slightly smaller than afferent arterioles, but converse is true for juxtamedullary arterioles
- Peritubular capillaries
  - ○ Form extensive vascular network in cortex
  - ○ Return reabsorbed fluid from tubules into circulation
  - ○ Receive postglomerular blood with high oncotic pressure due to increased concentration of proteins and red blood cells
  - ○ Specialized PTC in medulla are called vasa recta
    - ■ Arise from postglomerular efferent arterioles of juxtamedullary glomeruli
    - ■ Form hairpin loops that descend into outer renal medulla forming rich vascular bundles
    - ■ Countercurrent mechanism in vasa recta is responsible for high osmotic concentration of medullary interstitium relative to collecting duct lumens and plasma
    - ■ Are seen throughout medulla except in papillae
  - ○ PTC coalesce to form venules and, eventually, renal vein

SELECTED REFERENCES

1. Mathieson PW: Update on the podocyte. Curr Opin Nephrol Hypertens. 18(3):206-11, 2009
2. Salmon AH et al: New aspects of glomerular filtration barrier structure and function: five layers (at least) not three. Curr Opin Nephrol Hypertens. 18(3):197-205, 2009
3. Satchell SC et al: Glomerular endothelial cell fenestrations: an integral component of the glomerular filtration barrier. Am J Physiol Renal Physiol. 296(5):F947-56, 2009
4. Schlöndorff D et al: The mesangial cell revisited: no cell is an island. J Am Soc Nephrol. 20(6):1179-87, 2009
5. Bonsib SM: Renal anatomy and histology. In Jennette JC et al: Heptinstall's pathology of the kidney. 6th edition. Philadelphia: Lippincott Williams & Wilkins. 1-70, 2007
6. Barisoni L et al: Update in podocyte biology: putting one's best foot forward. Curr Opin Nephrol Hypertens. 12(3):251-8, 2003
7. Kurokawa K: Tubuloglomerular feedback: its physiological and pathophysiological significance. Kidney Int Suppl. 67:S71-4, 1998
8. Pesce C: Glomerular number and size: facts and artefacts. Anat Rec. 251(1):66-71, 1998
9. Epstein M: Aging and the kidney. J Am Soc Nephrol. 7(8):1106-22, 1996
10. Hudson BG et al: Structure and organization of type IV collagen of renal glomerular basement membrane. Contrib Nephrol. 107:163-7, 1994
11. Lingrel JB et al: Structure-function studies of the Na,K-ATPase. Kidney Int Suppl. 44:S32-9, 1994
12. Latta H: An approach to the structure and function of the glomerular mesangium. J Am Soc Nephrol. 2(10 Suppl):S65-73, 1992

NORMAL KIDNEY STRUCTURE

Podocyte and Slit Diaphragm Molecules

Molecule	Gene	Functional Properties
Podocyte-Slit Diaphragm Complex		
Nephrin	NPHS1	Major transmembrane structural protein of slit diaphragm and member of immunoglobulin superfamily; nephrin molecules associate with signaling microdomains of foot process cell membranes (lipid rafts) and can also interact with other molecules such as CD2AP and podocin to enhance signaling process
Podocin	NPHS2	Podocyte transmembrane molecule of stomatin family that maintains structural integrity of slit diaphragm; interacts with nephrin, CD2AP, and neph1, and is thus involved in signaling
CD2AP	CD2AP	Intracellular adapter podocyte protein binds to cytoplasmic domain of nephrin and links it to actin-based cytoskeleton
NEPH-1	KIRREL	Transmembrane podocyte protein of immunoglobulin superfamily; neph-1 interacts with podocin, ZO-1, and nephrin
ZO-1	TJP1	Podocyte membrane protein located at point of attachment between slit diaphragm and foot process; interacts with neph-1 and actin-based cytoskeleton; may participate in signaling events through tyrosine phosphorylation
mFAT1	FAT	Protocadherin within slit diaphragm that may be involved in its development; functions may include cell adhesion and role as spacer molecule to maintain extracellular space
P-cadherin	CDH3	Slit diaphragm molecule involved in cell adhesion
Podocyte-Glomerular Basement Membrane (GBM) Complex		
α3β1-integrin		Helps anchor podocyte foot processes to GBM; integrins bridge structural proteins of GBM such as collagen IV, laminin, entactin, and fibronectin to podocyte actin-based cytoskeleton
Dystroglycan		Podocyte transmembrane molecule with α and β subunits; α subunit binds to cationic components of GBM, and intracellular β subunit binds to actin cytoskeleton
Podocyte		
Podocalyxin	PODXL	Major determinant of podocyte anionic glycocalyx located along luminal (facing urinary space) aspect of podocyte; maintains glomerular architecture and foot process integrity via its connections to actin-based cytoskeleton
GLEPP-1		Transmembrane protein along luminal aspect and a receptor tyrosine phosphatase; may help regulate glomerular filtration rate through effects on podocyte structure and function
WT-1	WT-1	Transcription factor restricted to podocytes in adult kidney
Actin-based cytoskeleton		Includes actin, myosin, α-actinin, and synaptopodin, which maintain structural integrity of foot processes
Other		C3b receptor, vimentin, TRPC6 ion channel, cell cycling molecules such as p27, p57, cyclin D3; transcription factors such as PAX2, Pod1, LMX1B are involved in podocyte development and differentiation but are downregulated in adult kidney

Characteristics of Tubular Segments of Nephron

Structural Characteristics	Functional Considerations	Other Comments
Proximal Tubule		
Eosinophilic cytoplasm and prominent apical brush border best seen on PAS stain; abundant mitochondria and basolateral infoldings that interdigitate with adjacent cells	Absorb bulk of solutes in glomerular filtrate including 60% of Na+, Cl-, K+, Ca2+, and water, and 90% of HCO3-, glucose, and amino acids	Site of Na+/K+ ATPase pump in basolateral membrane that derives energy from abundant mitochondria; water channel aquaporin I in microvilli
Have tight intercellular junctions with zona occludens	Secretion of solutes, such as organic anions and cations, into lumens	Also has Na+/H+ exchanger (sensitive to angiotensin II), Cl- anion exchanger
Loop of Henle		
Includes thin descending, thin ascending limb; thick ascending limb terminates with macula densa; epithelium of thin limbs is flattened	Maintains high concentrations of medullary interstitium and countercurrent mechanisms	Thick ascending limb has Na+K+2Cl- (NKCC2) membrane cotransporter, target of furosemide
Basolateral infolding and mitochondria are fewer, more so in thin descending and ascending loops	Thick ascending limb is water impermeable (diluting segment), site of Mg+2 reabsorption, & secretes T-H protein	Thin descending limb has Na+/K+ ATPase, carbonic anhydrase, and aquaporin I
Distal Convoluted Tubule		
Lining cells are smaller, less eosinophilic than proximal tubular cells, and lack brush border	Determines final urine tonicity, volume, and concentrations of Na+, K+, and Cl-	Site of Na+/Cl- cotransporter (NCCT), a thiazide diuretic-sensitive carrier protein
Basolateral infoldings are well developed, and mitochondria are quite abundant	Site of action of regulatory hormones such as aldosterone and vasopressin	
Collecting Duct		
Have principal (paler cytoplasm) and intercalated cells (darker cells with more organelles)	Principal cells are mainly involved in Na+ and water transport	Principal cells have vasopressin receptors and water channel aquaporins 2, 3, and 4
Epithelial cells are cuboidal with mild basal infolding	Intercalated cells are site of acid base regulation	Intercalated cells have H+ ATPase, HCO3-/Cl- exchanger and carbonic anhydrase
Lining epithelium of papillary tips resembles urothelium		Distal tubule has epithelial Na+ channel (ENaC), amiloride diuretic-sensitive channel

1

NORMAL KIDNEY STRUCTURE

Architectural Organization of Kidney

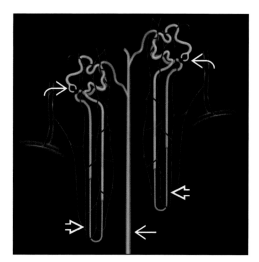

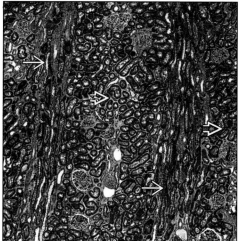

(Left) Glomeruli ⇗ are located in the cortex while loops of Henle dip into the medulla ⇥. The collecting duct ⇥ extends from the cortex to the inner medulla. The vasculature (red) forms glomerular and peritubular plexus. (Right) A longitudinal section of the cortex shows a cortical labyrinth ⇥ composed predominantly of glomeruli and proximal and distal convoluted tubules. The labyrinth is flanked by medullary rays ⇥ composed of collecting ducts and straight segments of tubules.

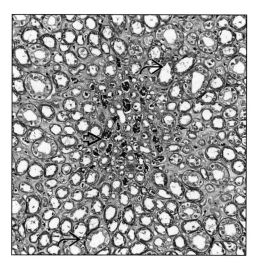

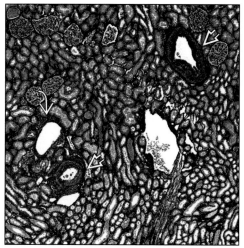

(Left) The vascular bundles in the outer medulla are composed of descending and ascending vasa recta ⇥ and are surrounded by loops of Henle ⇗. (Right) The arcuate arteries ⇥ curve along the corticomedullary junction and give rise to interlobular arteries. The arcuate veins ⇗ run parallel to the corresponding arteries. Note the cortex on the top with the glomeruli and medulla on the bottom with only tubular segments.

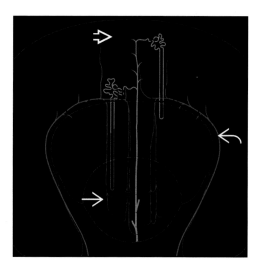

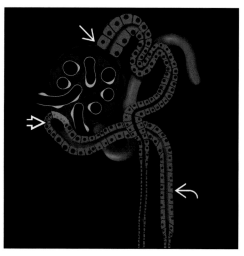

(Left) The arcuate arteries ⇗ (red) arch along the corticomedullary junction and eventually give rise to glomerular afferent arterioles ⇥. The efferent arterioles from glomeruli form peritubular plexus extending into medulla ⇥. These vasa recta converge into arcuate veins ⇗ (blue). (Right) The proximal tubule originates at the glomerular tubular pole ⇥ and merges with the loop of Henle. The thick ascending limb of the loop ⇗ ends with the macula densa ⇥ and extends as the distal tubule.

Introduction

Glomerular Structure

(Left) The Jones methenamine silver stain highlights the mesangium ➡, glomerular basement membranes ➡, and Bowman capsule ➡. Note the scant mesangial matrix in a normal glomerulus. An arteriole is seen near the vascular pole of the glomerulus ➡. (Right) Antisera to WT1 protein highlights only glomerular podocytes ➡. WT1 is required for normal kidney development, but expression is restricted to podocytes in adults.

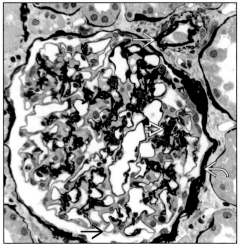
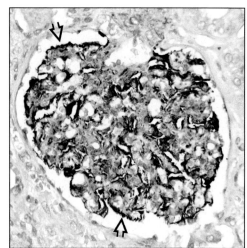

(Left) The glomerular vascular pole has a juxtaglomerular apparatus at the confluence of an afferent arteriole ➡, efferent arteriole ➡, and distal tubule ➡. Specialized elongated cells within the distal tubule are referred to as the macula densa. The proximal tubule arises opposite to the vascular pole. (Right) The capillary loop is covered by interdigitating foot processes of the podocyte ➡, and the fenestrated endothelial cell ➡ extends along the GBM. The mesangial cells ➡ and adjacent matrix support the glomerular capillary tuft.

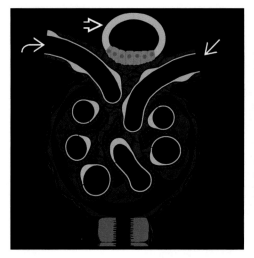
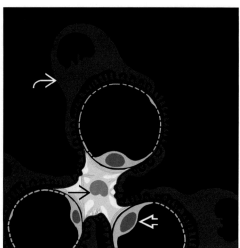

(Left) Electron micrograph shows thin fenestrated cytoplasm of the endothelial cell ➡ lining the capillary loop and podocyte foot processes ➡ within the urinary space. Endothelial nucleus ➡ and podocyte nucleus ➡ are also seen. (Right) Electron micrograph of the glomerular filtration barrier shows podocyte foot processes ➡ with intervening slit diaphragms ➡. The lamina densa ➡ of the glomerular basement membrane and the fenestrated cytoplasm of the endothelial cell ➡ are also seen.

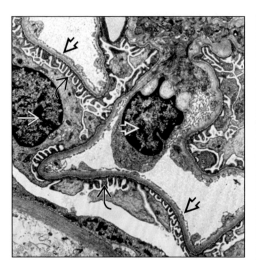
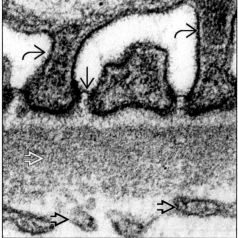

1

NORMAL KIDNEY STRUCTURE

Tubular Structure

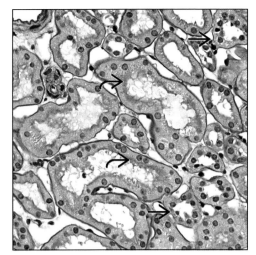
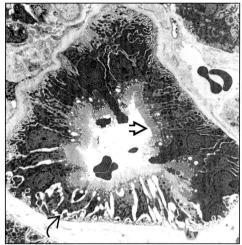

(Left) The normal proximal tubules have abundant cytoplasm of the epithelial cells and an apical brush border ➡ highlighted by PAS stain. In contrast, the distal tubules are smaller in diameter and lack the brush border ➡. Note the back-to-back arrangement of the tubules with scant interstitial matrix. *(Right)* Electron micrograph of the proximal tubule shows numerous basolateral interdigitations of the cytoplasm ➡, abundant mitochondria, and tall luminal brush border ➡.

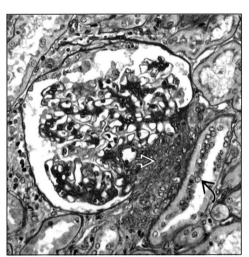
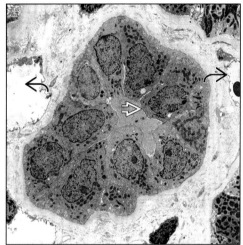

(Left) Juxtaglomerular apparatus is responsible for "tubuloglomerular" feedback and is composed of the macula densa ➡, a specialized portion of the distal convoluted tubule, periglomerular portions of the afferent and efferent arterioles, and juxtaglomerular cells ➡. *(Right)* Distal convoluted tubules have basolateral interdigitations of the cytoplasm but sparse apical microvilli ➡. Note the peritubular capillaries ➡ next to the tubules.

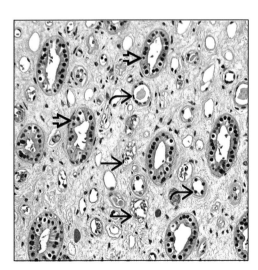
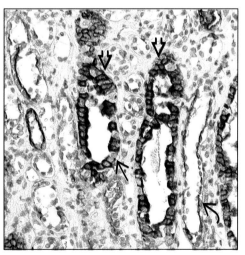

(Left) A cross section of the inner medulla shows prominent collecting ducts ➡ and thin loops of Henle ➡ embedded in abundant interstitial stroma. The peritubular capillaries ➡ in the medulla form a network of vasa recta. *(Right)* An immunostain for cytokeratin 7 highlights the collecting ducts ➡ where the probable principal cells show diffuse cytoplasmic staining and the intercalated cells fail to do so ➡. CK7 expression is also seen in the loops of Henle ➡.

Glomerular Diseases

MINIMAL CHANGE DISEASE

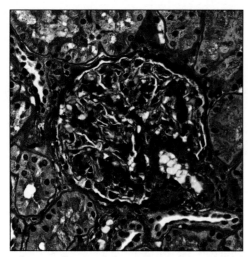

A biopsy with minimal change disease shows a normal glomerulus on PAS stain without GBM thickening or inflammatory cells and with minimal mesangial hypercellularity.

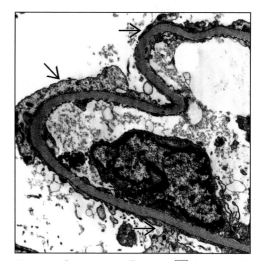

Prominent foot process effacement ⊇ is present in this case of minimal change disease. The glomerular basement membrane has a normal thickness, and no electron-dense deposits are present.

TERMINOLOGY

Abbreviations
- Minimal change disease (MCD)

Synonyms
- Lipoid nephrosis
- Nil disease
- Minimal change nephrotic syndrome
- Minimal change glomerulopathy

Definitions
- Idiopathic glomerular disease that causes nephrotic syndrome, with little or no light or immunofluorescent microscopic abnormalities and podocyte foot process effacement on electron microscopy
- Occurs as primary (idiopathic) disease, especially in children, and secondary to drugs, allergic reactions, and neoplasia at all ages

ETIOLOGY/PATHOGENESIS

Idiopathic (Primary)
- Classified as disease of podocytes, a "podocytopathy"
- Loss of podocyte negatively charged glycocalyx a central feature
  - Cause unknown; possibilities include
    - Enzymatic cleavage (e.g., neuraminidase)
    - Neutralizing positively charged molecule
    - Decreased synthesis
  - Loss of negative (anionic) charge leads to
    - Selective leakage of albumin
    - Albumin is most negatively charged of major plasma proteins
    - Foot process effacement
- Circulating permeability factor or cytokine abnormality postulated

- Various substances have been suggested, ranging in molecular weight from 12-160 kDa
- IL-13, an anti-inflammatory Th2 cytokine for B cells and monocytes, is implicated
- T-cell IL-13 content increases during relapse
- Increased serum IgE, IgG4 in some patients

Secondary Forms of MCD
- Infection
  - Human immunodeficiency virus (HIV)
  - Upper respiratory tract infection
- Hodgkin disease and other lymphoproliferative disorders (lymphoma)
  - Possibly related to abnormal T-cell function
- Allergy
  - Drugs, especially nonsteroidal anti-inflammatory drugs
  - Bee venom
  - Immunization
  - Mononucleosis
- Systemic lupus erythematosus
- Graft vs. host disease
- Acute renal allograft rejection (rare manifestation)

Experimental Studies
- Key features of MCD (e.g., foot process effacement [FPE], proteinuria) reproduced in rats or mice by
  - Overexpression of IL-13
  - Administration of puromycin aminonucleoside or Adriamycin
  - Supernatants from hybridomas made from T cells from patients with MCD
  - Administration of neuraminidase or protamine sulfate (removes sialic acid or neutralizes anionic charge, respectively)

CLINICAL ISSUES

Epidemiology
- Age

MINIMAL CHANGE DISEASE

Key Facts

Terminology
- Synonyms: Lipoid nephrosis, nil disease

Etiology/Pathogenesis
- Usually idiopathic
- Involves loss of glomerular negative charge
- Circulating permeability factor
- Secondary forms due to virus, drugs, lymphoma

Clinical Issues
- Nephrotic syndrome
- Most common in young children, boys > girls
- 90-95% respond to corticosteroids
- Can present as acute renal insufficiency in adults

Microscopic Pathology
- Glomerulus normal by light microscopy except for variable podocyte hypertrophy

- Resorption droplets in tubules

Ancillary Tests
- IF negative except for variable focal IgM ± C3
- EM shows podocyte foot process effacement, normal GBM, and no deposits

Top Differential Diagnoses
- Focal segmental glomerulosclerosis (FSGS)
- Diffuse mesangial hypercellularity (DMH)
- IgA, IgM, or C1q nephropathy

Diagnostic Checklist
- Examination of biopsy at multiple levels may prevent missed diagnosis of FSGS
- Note whether biopsy includes corticomedullary junction, the site initially affected by FSGS

- Most common in children (65-75% of cases)
  - Median age of onset is 2.5 years
  - Peak incidence is at 2-3 years
  - Causes ~ 90% of nephrotic syndrome in preadolescents and ~ 50% in adolescents
- Adults have late peak incidence, > 80 years old
  - 26% of adults with nephrotic syndrome are < 65 years
  - 20% are 65-79 years
  - 46% are 80-91 years
- Gender
  - In children, 2:1 ratio of males to females
  - In adults: Equal gender distribution
- Ethnicity
  - More common in whites and Asians than in blacks

Presentation
- Sudden (days) onset of nephrotic syndrome
- Nephrotic syndrome
  - Proteinuria defined as ≥ 3.5 g/d in adults and ≥ 40 mg/m² body surface area (BSA)/hr in timed overnight collection in children
    - Selective proteinuria (chiefly albumin)
  - Edema
  - Hypoalbuminemia defined as serum albumin < 3.5 g/dL in adults and < 2.5 g/dL in children
  - Hypercholesterolemia
  - Lipiduria
    - Lipid-laden enucleated tubular cells may be seen as "oval fat bodies" in urinary sediment, with polarizable lipid
    - Gave rise to the term "lipoid nephrosis," original term for MCD
- Hematuria
  - Microscopic hematuria (10-30% of cases)
- Renal dysfunction
  - Acute renal insufficiency may occur in adults with MCD from acute ischemic tubular injury due to poor perfusion
    - Associated with extreme hypoalbuminemia
    - May be accompanied by anasarca
    - Most recover with steroids and diuretics

- Renal insufficiency (plasma creatinine > 98th percentile) in < 1/3 of children with MCD, typically mild
  - Due to reduced glomerular hydraulic conductivity secondary to loss of filtration slit pores, which are responsible for allowing flux of small molecules

Treatment
- Drugs
  - Corticosteroids
    - 90-95% respond over 4-6 weeks
    - 8-week course of steroids often used as 1st treatment of nephrotic syndrome in children
    - If no response to steroids, renal biopsy typically performed to rule out other diseases
    - Up to 50% of children and 30% of adults relapse after steroid treatment within 1st year; usually treated with another course of steroids
  - 2nd line of treatment for steroid failures
    - Alkylating agents (e.g., chlorambucil or cyclophosphamide)
    - Levamisole
    - Cyclosporine

Prognosis
- Primary (idiopathic)
  - Rarely, if ever, leads to renal failure
  - Before steroids and antibiotics, fatalities from infection
  - Adults with MCD and acute renal failure also usually fully recover
- Secondary
  - Remits if underlying condition can be cured
- MCD may be initial manifestation of focal segmental glomerulosclerosis (FSGS) (~ 5%), in which case prognosis is that of FSGS

MACROSCOPIC FEATURES

General Features
- Enlarged, waxy, yellow cortex because of lipid accumulation in proximal tubules

2

3

- Gross examination is rare since advent of treatment with corticosteroids and comorbid conditions with antibiotics

MICROSCOPIC PATHOLOGY

Histologic Features
- Glomeruli
  - Normal appearance by light microscopy
    - Slight increases in mesangial cellularity and matrix in minority
    - Glomerular basement membranes are normal
  - Podocytes may be swollen and prominent with basophilic cytoplasm, resembling plasma cells
    - Resorption droplets in visceral epithelial cells
  - Loss of normal negative charge revealed by decreased colloidal iron stain of podocytes
  - Globally sclerotic glomeruli may be seen in MCD in adults
    - 10% of glomeruli may be sclerotic by age 40 and 30% by age 80
  - In children, involuted glomeruli are sometimes present
    - Lack of atrophic tubules indicates developmental rather than acquired glomerular sclerosis
- Tubules
  - Protein resorption droplets ("hyaline droplets")
    - PAS(+) and red on trichrome stain
  - Lipid droplets
    - Origin of term "lipoid nephrosis"
    - Clear vacuoles on H&E, PAS, and trichrome
    - Red droplets on oil red O stained frozen sections
  - Usually little to no tubular atrophy
    - Older patients with concurrent arteriosclerosis may have underlying glomerular obsolescence and tubular atrophy
  - Tubular regenerative changes and injury in adults with acute renal failure
- Interstitial inflammation and fibrosis are usually absent
  - Interstitial foam cells may be seen but are rare

ANCILLARY TESTS

Immunofluorescence
- Typically no deposits of immunoglobulin or complement
- Minority have faint (≤ 1+) staining in glomeruli for IgM ± C3
  - < 5% of MCD cases have mesangial staining for IgG, IgM, IgA, C1q, &/or C3, particularly in children
    - Prognosis may be worse in these cases, with higher rate of steroid resistance
    - Paramesangial pattern suggests nonspecific entrapment
- Renal tubular resorption droplets stain for albumin
  - Usually, there is little immunoglobulin or C3 droplets in tubules (variable)

Electron Microscopy
- Transmission

- Podocyte foot process effacement (FPE) is widespread and the only major change by EM
  - Usually, FPE is diffuse and severe, involving > 75% of capillary surface
  - "Effacement" preferred to "fusion" since foot processes retract rather than fuse and cell body spreads on GBM
  - Extent of FPE (% of surface) correlates with severity of proteinuria
  - Filtration slit diaphragms are lost
  - After remission, foot processes return to normal
  - Although FPE is primary feature of MCD, it occurs in any renal disease with severe glomerular proteinuria
- Podocytes may be "swollen"
  - Vacuolization and microvillous transformation
  - Contain resorption droplets and increased cellular organelles
- Mild mesangial expansion in minority of cases
  - Vague mesangial and paramesangial electron densities may be seen, representing nonspecific protein insudation rather than true immune complex deposition
- Tubules
  - Proximal tubules contain electron-dense resorption droplets (secondary lysosomes) and electron-lucent lipid droplets

Immunohistochemistry
- Decreased nephrin along GBM, corresponding with loss of slit diaphragms
  - Nephrin loss is seen in other diseases with FPE, and this stain is not routinely performed

DIFFERENTIAL DIAGNOSIS

Focal Segmental Glomerulosclerosis (FSGS)
- Serial sectioning required to detect sclerotic glomeruli to diagnose or exclude FSGS
  - Segmental hyalinosis or synechiae to Bowman capsule indicative of FSGS
  - Endocapillary foam cells are rare in MCD and should raise possibility of FSGS
  - Sclerotic glomeruli in FSGS are most common at corticomedullary junction
  - Sections of segmentally sclerotic glomeruli may appear normal if plane of section does not include segmental sclerosis
  - FSGS cases with unsampled sclerotic glomeruli may be misdiagnosed as MCD
- Glomerular hypertrophy or tubular atrophy may be an indicator of underlying FSGS
- Idiopathic FSGS considered to be in spectrum with MCD by many investigators
  - Many cases that show MCD on initial biopsy show FSGS later
    - This sequence has been documented in recurrent FSGS in transplants in which MCD present on initial biopsies after transplant is followed by FSGS in later biopsies
    - Animal models also suggest similar circulating factor in both MCD and FSGS

MINIMAL CHANGE DISEASE

Diffuse Mesangial Hypercellularity (DMH)
- Variant of MCD
- Affects primarily children, accounting for ~ 3% of pediatric cases of idiopathic nephrotic syndrome
  - Are more likely to have hematuria and hypertension
- > 4 mesangial cells per mesangial region in ≥ 80% of glomeruli in 2-3 μm tissue sections
  - Capillary lumens are not occluded
  - GBM is not duplicated
  - No mesangial interposition
- IF may show IgM or C3
- EM shows podocyte FPE and electron-dense deposits in 50% of cases
- Higher rate of steroid resistance

IgM Nephropathy
- Considered to be variant of MCD by some renal pathologists; however, occurrence as familial disease suggests it is distinct entity
- Diffuse, global mesangial IgM staining is present on IF at moderate intensity or greater (≥ 2+)
- C3 deposits may also be seen (30-100% of cases), sometimes accompanied by other immunoglobulins
- EM shows FPE and occasional scanty paramesangial deposits
- Hematuria and hypertension more common than in MCD
- 6x increased rate of progression to FSGS in children compared with MCD

IgA Nephropathy
- Usually not difficult because of prominent mesangial IgA deposits and electron-dense deposits in mesangium
- MCD superimposed on IgA nephropathy diagnosis should be entertained if nephrotic syndrome is of rapid onset and complete FPE is present

C1q Nephropathy
- May display MCD-like lesion with podocytopathy, typically accompanied by nephrotic syndrome (generally unresponsive to steroids) and hematuria in ~ 40%
- Dominant C1q in mesangium (≥ 2+) ± immunoglobulins on IF distinguishes from MCD (sometimes can be "full house")
- Occasional electron-dense deposits can be found on EM, further differentiating C1q nephropathy from MCD
- No diagnostic evidence of lupus nephritis (e.g., autoantibodies, extrarenal manifestations, tubuloreticular structures, etc.)

DIAGNOSTIC CHECKLIST

Pathologic Interpretation Pearls
- Examination of biopsy at multiple levels may prevent missed diagnosis of FSGS
- Note whether biopsy includes corticomedullary junction, the site initially affected by FSGS

- Acute tubular necrosis may be present and account for acute renal failure
- Podocyte hypertrophy (basophilia and smudged chromatin) and tubular reabsorption droplets in otherwise normal biopsy are clues to diagnosis

SELECTED REFERENCES

1. IJpelaar DH et al: Fidelity and evolution of recurrent FSGS in renal allografts. J Am Soc Nephrol. 19(11):2219-24, 2008
2. Vizjak A et al: Pathology, clinical presentations, and outcomes of C1q nephropathy. J Am Soc Nephrol. 19(11):2237-44, 2008
3. Lai KW et al: Overexpression of interleukin-13 induces minimal-change-like nephropathy in rats. J Am Soc Nephrol. 18(5):1476-85, 2007
4. Mathieson PW: Minimal change nephropathy and focal segmental glomerulosclerosis. Semin Immunopathol. 29(4):415-26, 2007
5. Olson JL: The nephrotic syndrome and minimal change disease. In Jennette JC et al: Heptinstall's Pathology of the Kidney. 6th ed. Philadelphia: Lippincott Williams & Wilkins. 125-154, 2007
6. D'Agati VD et al: Non-Neoplastic Kidney Diseases. Washington, DC: American Registry of Pathology, 2005
7. Nair R et al: Renal biopsy in patients aged 80 years and older. Am J Kidney Dis. 44(4):618-26, 2004
8. Stokes MB et al: Glomerular tip lesion: a distinct entity within the minimal change disease/focal segmental glomerulosclerosis spectrum. Kidney Int. 65(5):1690-702, 2004
9. van den Berg JG et al: Role of the immune system in the pathogenesis of idiopathic nephrotic syndrome. Clin Sci (Lond). 107(2):125-36, 2004
10. Filler G et al: Is there really an increase in non-minimal change nephrotic syndrome in children? Am J Kidney Dis. 42(6):1107-13, 2003
11. Howie AJ: Pathology of minimal change nephropathy and segmental sclerosing glomerular disorders. Nephrol Dial Transplant. 18 Suppl 6:vi33-8, 2003
12. Fogo AB: Minimal change disease and focal segmental glomerulosclerosis. Nephrol Dial Transplant. 16 Suppl 6:74-6, 2001
13. Koyama A et al: A glomerular permeability factor produced by human T cell hybridomas. Kidney Int. 40(3):453-60, 1991
14. Fogo A et al: Glomerular hypertrophy in minimal change disease predicts subsequent progression to focal glomerular sclerosis. Kidney Int. 38(1):115-23, 1990
15. Jennette JC et al: Adult minimal change glomerulopathy with acute renal failure. Am J Kidney Dis. 16(5):432-7, 1990
16. Bertani T et al: Adriamycin-induced nephrotic syndrome in rats: sequence of pathologic events. Lab Invest. 46(1):16-23, 1982

MINIMAL CHANGE DISEASE

Light Microscopy

(Left) This low-power view of a trichrome shows no appreciable glomerular abnormality, and the tubulointerstitium is unremarkable with only fine strands of connective tissue between tubules, compatible with absent interstitial fibrosis and tubular atrophy. *(Right)* A glomerulus ⇨ is relatively normal in this case of minimal change disease. Vacuoles ⇨ due to lipid accumulation are seen in the renal proximal tubules, which would be shown by oil red O staining of frozen sections.

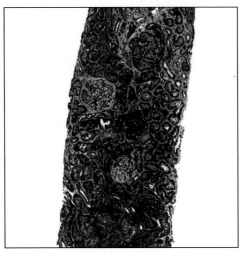 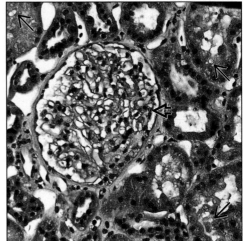

(Left) This Jones methenamine silver stain shows that the glomerular basement membranes have a normal thickness in minimal change disease ⇨ with no duplication or glomerular hypercellularity. *(Right)* Glomerulus from a patient with minimal change disease appears normal by light microscopy. The only clue that there is proteinuria is the presence of hypertrophied podocytes ⇨, which have increased, basophilic cytoplasm.

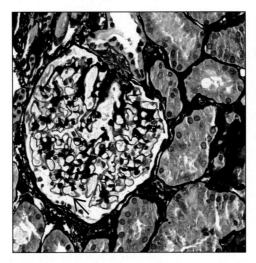 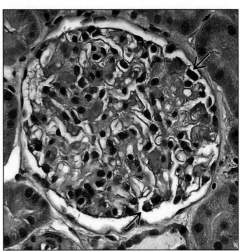

(Left) PAS positive tubular resorption droplets ⇨ in minimal change disease are predominantly in the proximal renal tubules. These are found in any disease with glomerular proteinuria. *(Right)* Oil red O stain of a frozen section from a patient with MCD shows the characteristic lipid ⇨ in proximal tubules. These accumulate in tubules in all diseases with nephrotic range proteinuria, but since the lipid was the only feature noted originally in MCD it lead to the term "lipoid nephrosis."

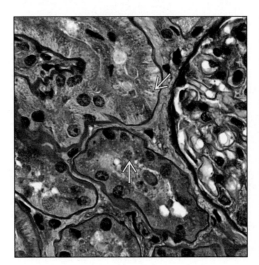 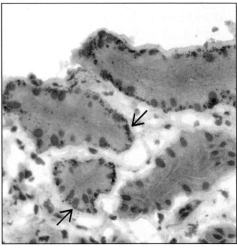

MINIMAL CHANGE DISEASE

Immunofluorescence

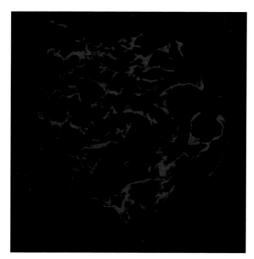
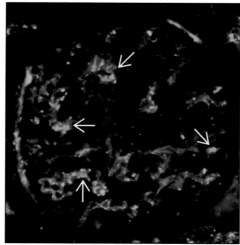

(Left) A case of minimal change disease is stained for IgG. Little or no IgG is present in MCD in the form of immune complexes. However, IgG and other plasma proteins may be found in podocytes as reabsorption droplets, which may be confused with deposits. *(Right)* In minimal change disease, there can be minimal mesangial staining for IgM in a minority of cases, as seen in this case ➡.

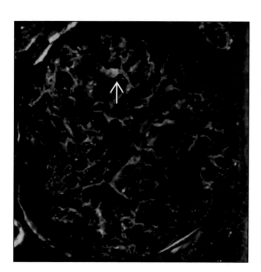
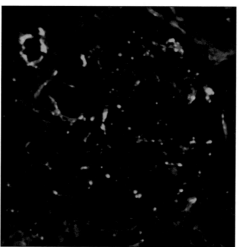

(Left) In minimal change disease, there is usually little or no deposition of immunoglobulin or complement components. However, minor degrees of staining in the mesangium and Bowman capsule ➡ for C3 can be seen, as in this case. *(Right)* This patient with minimal change disease has more prominent C3 in the glomerulus. Most is probably in podocyte reabsorption droplets, and some is in the mesangium. The arterial wall also has C3, a common, nonspecific finding.

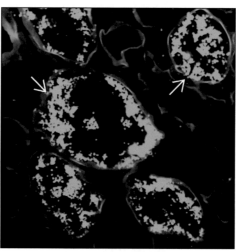

(Left) In minimal change disease (MCD), little or no immunoglobulin is typically present. In this MCD case, no IgA is detected in the glomerulus aside from a few faint granules that are probably protein reabsorption droplets in the podocyte ➡. *(Right)* Immunofluorescence for albumin demonstrates abundant resorption droplets ➡ in proximal tubules in minimal change disease. Other plasma proteins may also be present, presumably a function of the selectivity of the proteinuria.

MINIMAL CHANGE DISEASE

Electron Microscopy

(Left) Electron microscopy shows markedly swollen podocytes ➡ with diffuse foot process effacement ➡ in this patient with minimal change disease. No deposits are present, and the GBM and endothelial cells appear normal. *(Right)* This patient with minimal change disease shows expansion of the cell body surface area, a classic feature of the podocyte reaction to heavy proteinuria that produces villous hypertrophy ➡. Foot processes are effaced, and the GBM is normal.

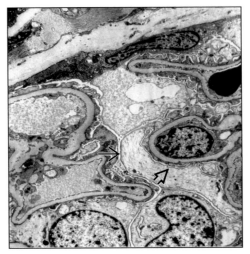
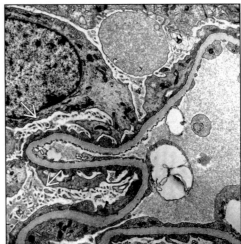

(Left) In minimal change disease, podocytes can have prominent microvillous hypertrophy ➡, as seen here. *(Right)* In minimal change disease, the mesangium can be mildly expanded with cellular debris ➡. Vague densities ➡ may be present although these are not considered evidence of an immune complex-mediated disorder but rather of nonspecific entrapment.

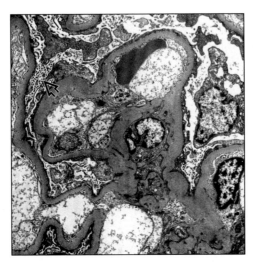
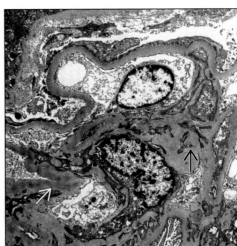

(Left) Patient with minimal change disease has swollen podocytes ➡ but only patchy foot process effacement in this capillary. *(Right)* The tubules in minimal change disease may have frequent resorption droplets, some of which are clear ➡ on EM, representing lipid vacuoles, and some of which are electron dense ➡, representing proteinaceous droplets.

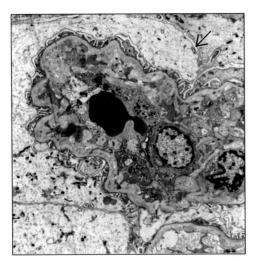
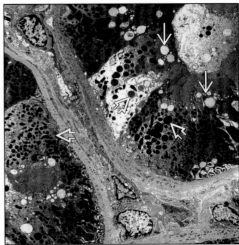

MINIMAL CHANGE DISEASE

Variant Microscopic Features

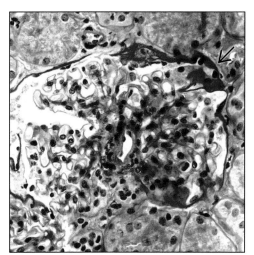

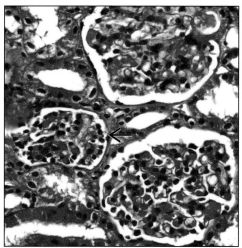

(Left) This "pseudo-adhesion" ⮕ is due to a tangential section through the GBM in a patient with minimal change disease. In presumed MCD, it is essential to search for evidence of FSGS in multiple levels, as adhesions and artifacts such as this can confound interpretation. **(Right)** This specimen is from a 5-year-old boy who presented with MCD. Glomeruli with an immature appearance are present, with crowded podocytes ⮕. This should not be confused with collapsing glomerulopathy.

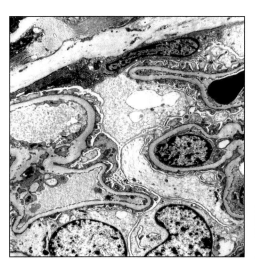

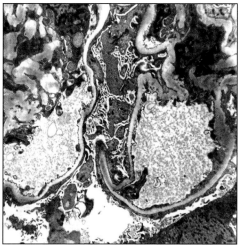

(Left) This specimen is from an 18-year-old boy who presented with nephrotic syndrome due to MCD associated with retroperitoneal masses, later shown to be Hodgkin disease. Lymphoma is a cause of MCD but usually remits with remission of the lymphoma. **(Right)** A 68-year-old woman presented with 3.4 g protein/day and edema associated with NSAIDs. Acute interstitial nephritis was also present. Drugs, especially NSAIDs, are associated with MCD.

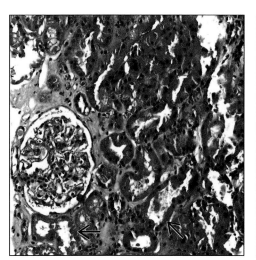

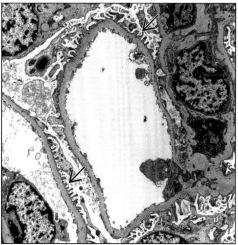

(Left) Acute tubular injury can complicate MCD in the elderly. This biopsy shows mild tubular injury with dilated proximal tubules and loss of brush borders ⮕. This 77-year-old man had 5.7 g/d proteinuria, a serum albumin of 2.2 g/dL, and an acute rise of Cr from 1.4 to 2.9 mg/dL. **(Right)** A 9-year-old girl with nephrotic syndrome was treated successfully with corticosteroids and biopsied when the proteinuria was in remission. The EM shows complete recovery of foot processes ⮕.

MINIMAL CHANGE DISEASE

MCD Superimposed on IgA Nephropathy

(Left) Periodic acid-Schiff shows a biopsy from a 48-year-old man with acute onset of nephrotic syndrome with anasarca, hypoalbuminemia (1 g/dL), hyperlipidemia, and 15 g/d proteinuria. He had acutely elevated creatinine at 1.5 mg/dL. The glomeruli show mild mesangial hypercellularity. Acute tubular injury is present, with dilated tubules showing flattened epithelium ➡. *(Right)* A glomerulus shows mild mesangial hypercellularity ➡. No segmental scars were identified in the sample.

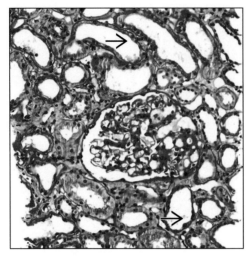
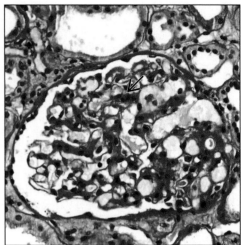

(Left) Protein reabsorption droplets are seen within tubular epithelial cells, indicative of proteinuria ➡. *(Right)* Immunofluorescence staining for IgA reveals bright granular mesangial staining ➡. The glomeruli showed similar staining for C3 and kappa and lambda light chains. The presence of IgA-dominant immune complex deposits is unexpected in the setting of acute nephrotic syndrome clinically suspicious for minimal change disease.

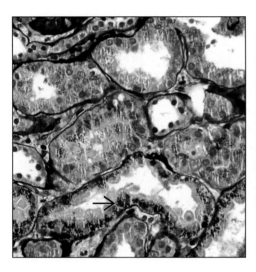
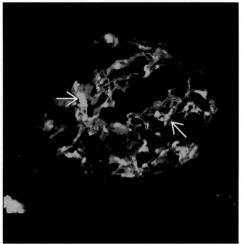

(Left) Ultrastructural studies reveal diffuse podocyte foot process effacement, typical of minimal change disease ➡. Mesangial and paramesangial electron-dense deposits are present as well, part of IgA nephropathy ➡. *(Right)* Mesangial immune complex-type electron-dense deposits ➡ are more visible at higher magnification, along with diffuse podocyte foot process effacement ➡.

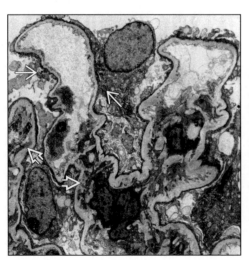
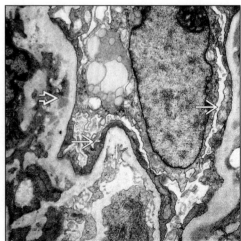

MINIMAL CHANGE DISEASE

C1q Nephropathy with a Minimal Change Disease Pattern

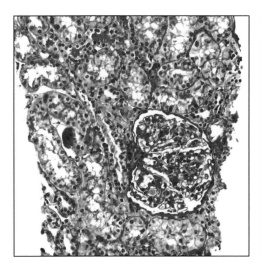

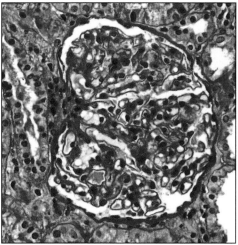

(Left) This biopsy was taken from a 20-year-old man with sudden onset of nephrotic syndrome, including anasarca and 10 g/d proteinuria. All sampled glomeruli appeared normal, and no segmental scars or proliferative features were identified. *(Right)* On higher magnification of a glomerulus, mesangial hypercellularity is not present in this case of C1q nephropathy with a minimal change disease pattern.

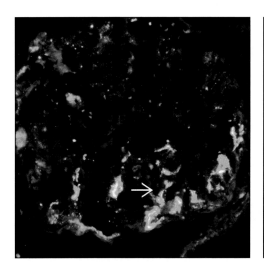

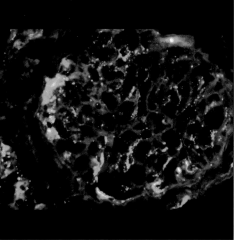

(Left) Immunofluorescence staining for C1q reveals 2+ granular mesangial staining ➡. C1q was the dominant immunoreactant in this case; there was lesser staining of glomeruli for IgG, kappa, and lambda, and stains for IgA were negative. The patient did not have clinical or laboratory evidence of systemic lupus erythematosus and otherwise had MCD. *(Right)* Immunofluorescence staining for C3 reveals dimmer granular mesangial staining.

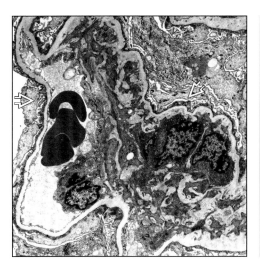

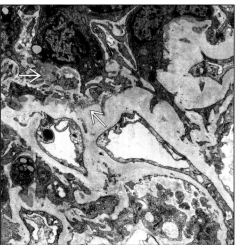

(Left) By electron microscopy, there is diffuse podocyte foot process effacement with villous hypertrophy of the podocytes, typical of minimal change disease ➡. *(Right)* There are scattered small amorphous mesangial electron-dense deposits segmentally within glomeruli in this patient with minimal change disease and C1q deposits ➡.

DRUG-INDUCED MINIMAL CHANGE DISEASE

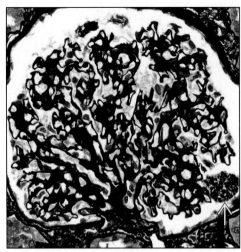

Jones methenamine silver reveals a normal glomerulus with delicate basement membranes and normal cellularity. Prominent podocyte protein droplets ➡ correlate with severe proteinuria (13 g/d).

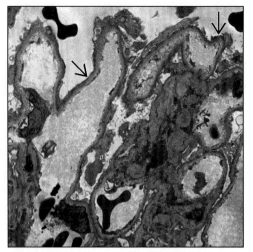

Electron micrograph reveals extensive effacement of the podocyte foot processes ➡ in this glomerulus in a patient with severe proteinuria (17 g/d) after administration of nonsteroidal anti-inflammatory drugs.

TERMINOLOGY

Abbreviations
- Minimal change disease (MCD)

ETIOLOGY/PATHOGENESIS

Implicated Drugs
- Nonsteroidal anti-inflammatory drugs (NSAIDs)
  - Diclofenac
  - 5-aminosalicylic acid (ASA)
- Cyclooxygenase 2 inhibitor
  - Celecoxib
- Pamidronate
  - Can also result in focal segmental glomerulosclerosis or collapsing glomerulopathy
- Interferon-α
- Interferon-β
- Lithium
- Gold
- Penicillamine
- Rifampin
- Amoxicillin

Mechanism Unknown
- T lymphocytes and chemokines have been implicated in pathogenesis of MCD
  - Not clear if these play a role in drug-induced MCD

CLINICAL ISSUES

Epidemiology
- Ethnicity
  - No ethnic predilection

Presentation
- Nephrotic syndrome
- Acute renal failure
  - Occasionally present

Laboratory Tests
- Urine dipstick
- 24-hour urine collection

Treatment
- Drugs
  - Steroids
    - Rarely needed
- Discontinuation of offending pharmacologic agent

Prognosis
- Good
  - Rapid remission after drug withdrawal

MICROSCOPIC PATHOLOGY

Histologic Features
- Normal glomeruli by light microscopy
- Interstitial inflammation
  - Often present
  - Acute tubular injury may be present

ANCILLARY TESTS

Immunofluorescence
- No immune deposits

Electron Microscopy
- Transmission
  - Extensive effacement of podocyte foot processes
  - No electron-dense deposits present

DIFFERENTIAL DIAGNOSIS

Minimal Change Disease
- Absence of administration of new pharmacologic agent would distinguish idiopathic form from drug-induced MCD

DRUG-INDUCED MINIMAL CHANGE DISEASE

Key Facts

Etiology/Pathogenesis
- Common offending agents
  - Nonsteroidal anti-inflammatory drugs (NSAIDs)
  - Cyclooxygenase 2 inhibitors
  - Pamidronate
  - Interferon-α and interferon-β
  - Rifampin

Clinical Issues
- Nephrotic syndrome

- Treatment
  - Discontinue offending pharmacologic agent

Microscopic Pathology
- Normal glomeruli by light microscopy
- Diffuse podocyte foot process effacement

Top Differential Diagnoses
- Minimal change disease
- Focal segmental glomerulosclerosis

Focal Segmental Glomerulosclerosis
- Diffuse effacement of podocyte foot processes should always raise this diagnostic consideration
- Sampling issue if < 20 glomeruli are present for evaluation or if corticomedullary junction is absent
- Interstitial fibrosis and tubular atrophy may be related to aging but also raise this consideration

Acute Interstitial Nephritis
- Prominent interstitial inflammation with tubulitis
- May occur concurrently with drug-induced MCD

IgM Nephropathy
- Normal glomeruli by light microscopy
- Mesangial IgM immune complexes detected by immunofluorescence and electron microscopy

Lithium Nephrotoxicity
- Severe proteinuria may be present
- Cystic dilatation of distal nephron segments
- Clinical history of bipolar or other psychiatric disorder

DIAGNOSTIC CHECKLIST

Pathologic Interpretation Pearls
- Knowledge of clinical history of medications is critical
- Electron microscopy is essential to establish diagnosis

SELECTED REFERENCES

1. Galesic K et al: Minimal change disease and acute tubular necrosis caused by diclofenac. Nephrology (Carlton). 13(1):87-8, 2008
2. Almansori M et al: Cyclooxygenase-2 inhibitor-associated minimal-change disease. Clin Nephrol. 63(5):381-4, 2005
3. Kohno K et al: Minimal change nephrotic syndrome associated with rifampicin treatment. Nephrol Dial Transplant. 15(7):1056-9, 2000
4. Tam VK et al: Nephrotic syndrome and renal insufficiency associated with lithium therapy. Am J Kidney Dis. 27(5):715-20, 1996
5. Warren GV et al: Minimal change glomerulopathy associated with nonsteroidal antiinflammatory drugs. Am J Kidney Dis. 13(2):127-30, 1989
6. Savill JS et al: Minimal change nephropathy and pemphigus vulgaris associated with penicillamine treatment of rheumatoid arthritis. Clin Nephrol. 29(5):267-70, 1988
7. Wolters J et al: Minimal change nephropathy during gold treatment. A case with unusual histopathological and immunopathological features. Neth J Med. 31(5-6):234-40, 1987
8. Hannedouche T et al: Nephrotic syndrome due to isolated minimal change glomerular disease in a patient taking pirprofen. Clin Nephrol. 25(6):314, 1986
9. Bander SJ: Reversible renal failure and nephrotic syndrome without interstitial nephritis from zomepirac. Am J Kidney Dis. 6(4):233-6, 1985

IMAGE GALLERY

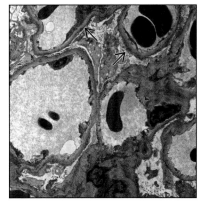 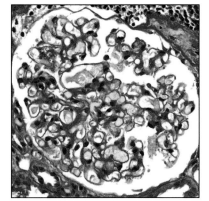 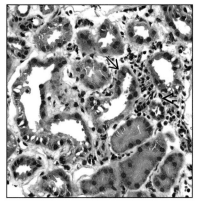

(Left) Electron micrograph shows diffuse effacement of the visceral epithelial cell foot processes ➡ in this glomerulus. *(Center)* Periodic acid-Schiff shows a normal glomerulus by light microscopy. Diagnostic findings can only be observed by electron microscopy. *(Right)* Hematoxylin & eosin shows diffuse interstitial inflammation ➡ and edema, which is often present in cases of drug-induced MCD. A mitotic figure ➡ indicates acute tubular injury and correlates with the presence of acute renal failure. Rare eosinophils (not shown) were also noted.

FOCAL SEGMENTAL GLOMERULOSCLEROSIS CLASSIFICATION

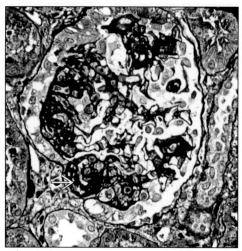

Light microscopy of a case of collapsing FSGS shows a glomerulus with areas of sclerosis ➡ (silver stain).

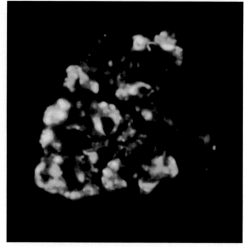

Immunofluorescence for C3 shows a predominantly segmental pattern of staining in the mesangium and in areas of glomerular capillary loop collapse in a case of FSGS.

TERMINOLOGY

Abbreviations
- Focal segmental glomerulosclerosis (FSGS)

Definitions
- Group of podocytopathies (of varied etiology) that share the feature of focal segmental glomerulosclerosis, typically with moderate to heavy proteinuria

CLASSIFICATION SYSTEMS

Morphologic Classification
- Based on glomerular morphology categories defined by the Columbia classification
  - Collapsing variant
  - Glomerular tip lesion
  - Cellular variant
  - Perihilar variant
  - FSGS not otherwise specified (NOS)

Etiologic Classification
- Based on identified causes of FSGS: Some correspondence with morphologic variants
- Familial/genetic
  - Increasing number of genes identified
    - β-integrin mutations
    - α-actinin-4 mutations
    - *WT-1* mutations
    - Podocin mutations
- Drug-induced
  - Pamidronate
  - Heroin (heroin nephropathy)
  - Lithium
  - Interferon-α and -β
- Virus
  - HIV (HIV-associated nephropathy [HIVAN])
  - Parvovirus B19

- Adaptive, structural-functional responses
  - Secondary to congenital or acquired reduction in nephrons relative to body mass
    - Oligomeganephronia, unilateral renal agenesis, renal dysplasia, reflux nephropathy, hypertension, anabolic steroids
- Vascular
  - Hypertension
  - Thrombotic microangiopathy
  - Atheromatous emboli
  - Calcineurin inhibitor toxicity
- Idiopathic
  - Usual primary form, either NOS or collapsing variant
  - Plasma factor responsible, identity sought

EPIDEMIOLOGY

Incidence
- Most common cause of nephrotic syndrome in adults
- Apparent increased incidence over past 2 decades
  - ~ 25% of adult nephropathies, compared with < 10% 20 years ago

History
- Focal and segmental glomerular hyalinization and capillary loop degradation described by Fahr in 1925
- Arnold Rich described juxtamedullary glomerulosclerosis in children dying with nephrotic syndrome in 1957
- FSGS was recognized as a distinct entity by International Study of Kidney Diseases in Children in the 1970s
- Collapsing variant was recognized by Mark Weiss in the 1980s and later as usual pattern of HIVAN

FOCAL SEGMENTAL GLOMERULOSCLEROSIS CLASSIFICATION

ETIOLOGY/PATHOGENESIS

Pathogenesis
- Now classified as podocytopathies
  - Familial podocyte protein defects
    - Mutations in *TRPC6*, a calcium-permeable cation channel, lead to abnormal podocyte function and hereditary FSGS
    - FSGS with defects in α-actinin-4 (*ACTN4*), podocin (*NPHS2*, defective in corticosteroid-resistant nephrotic syndrome), and nephrin (*NPHS1*, defective in congenital nephrotic syndrome of the Finnish type) are relatively rare familial forms of FSGS
    - Nephrin interacts with CD2-associated protein (CD2AP), and podocin interacts with the nephrin-CD2AP complex
    - Mutations in WT1 transcription factor, which regulates several podocyte genes, lead to FSGS syndromes (Denys-Drash and Frasier syndromes)
  - Abnormal cytokines are now thought to play major role in idiopathic FSGS development
    - Circulating factor identified in patients who have recurrent FSGS after transplant, typically occurring within months after transplantation
  - Podocyte dysregulation/dysfunction
    - Differentiation markers of podocytes (e.g., Wilms tumor WT-1 protein, podocalyxin, and synaptopodin) disappear in collapsing FSGS and HIVAN
  - Loss of podocytes leads to adhesions
  - Risk factor in African descent is *APOL1* gene
- Relationship with minimal change disease (MCD) unclear
  - Dystroglycan, an integral component of the GBM, is decreased in MCD but maintained in nonsclerotic segments in FSGS

CLINICAL IMPLICATIONS

Prognosis
- Generally poor with substantial fraction progressing to end-stage renal disease

Clinical Presentation
- Proteinuria
- Nephrotic syndrome
- Azotemia

Treatment
- Plasmapheresis has been used to induce remission in some patients with recurrent FSGS

MACROSCOPIC FINDINGS

General Features
- Pale yellow kidneys due to lipid in tubules

MICROSCOPIC FINDINGS

General Features
- Glomeruli
  - Sclerosis involves some glomeruli (focal) and only a portion of glomerular tuft (segmental)
    - Diagnosed even when only 1 glomerulus involved
    - Global sclerosis may be an incidental finding and is not particularly useful in making diagnosis of FSGS
  - Adhesions (synechiae) of glomerular tuft to Bowman space often accompany segmental sclerosis and are often seen early in sclerosis process
  - Hyalinosis
    - Portion of glomerular involvement has a smooth, glassy (hyaline) appearance
    - Typically thought to occur from insudation of plasma proteins
  - Increased matrix with obliteration of glomerular capillary lumen
  - FSGS has zonal distribution, beginning in corticomedullary (juxtamedullary) junction (CMJ)
    - Important to note whether sampling of CMJ is included
  - Glomerular hypertrophy often accompanies FSGS
    - Potential surrogate marker in cases without sampled segmental sclerosis
- Tubules
  - Tubular epithelial cells contain PAS(+) reabsorption droplets due to glomerular proteinuria
  - Tubular atrophy is typically only focal early in course of FSGS
    - TBM thickened in areas of atrophy
    - Tubular atrophy may be more prominent late in course of the disease
  - Tubulointerstitial changes pronounced in collapsing variants of FSGS and in HIVAN
    - Cystic dilatation and more prominent lymphoid infiltrate
- Interstitium
  - Interstitial fibrosis (IF) may be present and is typically focal
    - Some cases have extensive IF ± tubular atrophy (TA), and IF/TA in young patients may indicate unsampled FSGS in patients without identified glomerulosclerosis
  - Interstitial inflammation is absent or minimal
- Vessels
  - Arteriolar hyalinosis and arterial intimal fibrosis may be prominent late in course of FSGS

ANCILLARY TESTS

Immunofluorescence
- IgM and C3 often positive in sclerotic areas or areas of mesangial matrix increase
  - Thought to be nonspecific entrapment
  - IgM staining without EM deposits does not appear to have etiologic, prognostic, or diagnostic significance

FOCAL SEGMENTAL GLOMERULOSCLEROSIS CLASSIFICATION

FSGS Morphologic Classification Algorithm

Variant	Diagnostic Criteria	Exclude	Prognosis
Collapsing	≥ 1 glomerulus with collapse with segmental or global collapse and podocyte hyperplasia and hypertrophy	None	Poor
Tip	≥ 1 segmental lesion in tip domain (outer 25% of the tuft next to proximal tubule origin), adhesion is required at tubular lumen or neck	Collapsing variant, perihilar sclerosis	Possibly better prognosis
Cellular	≥ 1 glomerulus with segmental or global endocapillary hypercellularity occluding lumina, ± karyorrhexis and foam cells	Collapsing and tip variants	Possibly early-stage lesion
Perihilar	≥ 1 glomerulus with perihilar hyalinosis, ± sclerosis	Collapsing, tip, and cellular variants	Might often be a secondary type of FSGS
FSGS (NOS)	≥ 1 glomerulus with segmental increase in matrix obliterating capillary lumina	Collapsing, tip, cellular, and perihilar variants	Usual course

FSGS Morphologic Features

Variant	Location	Distribution	Hyaline	Adhesion	PCH	MHC	GM	AH
Collapsing	Anywhere	Segmental or global	-/+	-/+	+++	-/+	-/+	-/+
Tip	Tip domain	Segmental	+/-	+++/-	-	-/+	-/+	-/+
Cellular	Anywhere	Segmental	-/+	-/+	-	-/+	-/+	-/+
Perihilar	Perihilar	Segmental	++/-	+++/-	-	-/+	+++/-	++/-
FSGS (NOS)	Anywhere	Segmental	+/-	++/-	-/+	-/+	+/-	+/-

AH = arteriolar hyalinosis, GM = glomerulomegaly, MHC = mesangial hypercellularity, PCH = podocyte hyperplasia. Features are expressed as "most common/least common presentation." Each (+) denotes the approximate frequency at which the features occur; (-) denotes that this feature may be absent. Adapted from D'Agati et al: Pathologic classification of focal segmental glomerulosclerosis: a working proposal. Am J Kidney Dis. 43(2):368-82, 2004.

Electron Microscopy

- Foot process effacement (FPE) typically not complete
- Secondary FSGS usually shows less FPE than idiopathic forms of FSGS
- In HIVAN, tubuloreticular inclusions can sometimes be identified
- Subepithelial multilamination of GBM in collapsing variant

DIFFERENTIAL DIAGNOSIS

Focal Glomerulonephritis (GN)

- IgA nephropathy, lupus, and other inflammatory GNs can result in segmental scars in glomeruli

Minimal Change Disease (MCD)

- No segmental sclerosis
- FPE is usually complete in MCD but is typically less in most cases of FSGS
- Numerous globally sclerotic glomeruli, interstitial fibrosis, and vascular changes in a patient with nephrotic syndrome are suggestive of FSGS even if no segmental lesions are seen

DIAGNOSTIC CHECKLIST

Pathologic Interpretation Pearls

- Difference in outcome between MCD and FSGS equivalent to difference between benign & malignant
- Multiple levels (step sections) may be needed to identify focal segmental lesions

- Adequate sample of glomeruli is crucial to make diagnosis of FSGS since focal lesions may be missed with small samples
  - For example, biopsy with only 10 glomeruli has 35% probability of missing the focal lesion present in only 10% of glomeruli; whereas, probability decreases to 12% if 20 glomeruli are sampled
- Note whether CMJ is included in sample

SELECTED REFERENCES

1. Freedman BI et al: The apolipoprotein L1 (APOL1) gene and nondiabetic nephropathy in African Americans. J Am Soc Nephrol. 21(9):1422-6, 2010
2. Tryggvason K et al: Hereditary proteinuria syndromes and mechanisms of proteinuria. N Engl J Med. 354(13):1387-401, 2006
3. D'Agati VD et al: Pathologic classification of focal segmental glomerulosclerosis: a working proposal. Am J Kidney Dis. 43(2):368-82, 2004
4. Ichikawa I et al: Focal segmental glomerulosclerosis. Pediatr Nephrol. 10(3):374-91, 1996
5. Corwin HL et al: The importance of sample size in the interpretation of the renal biopsy. Am J Nephrol. 8(2):85-9, 1988
6. Churg J et al: Pathology of the nephrotic syndrome in children: a report for the International Study of Kidney Disease in Children. Lancet. 760(1):1299-302, 1970
7. Rich AR: A hitherto undescribed vulnerability of the juxtamedullary glomeruli in lipoid nephrosis. Bull Johns Hopkins Hosp. 100(4):173-86, 1957
8. Fahr T: Pathologische Anatomie des morbus brightii. In Henke F et al: Handbuch der speziellen pathologischen Anatomie and Histologie. Berlin: Springer. 156, 1925

Diagrammatic Features

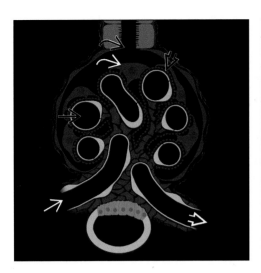 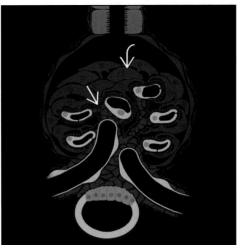

(Left) In a schematic of a glomerulus, features that are important to consider in FSGS include the podocytes ➡, the hilar region with the afferent ➡ and efferent ➡ arterioles, the endocapillary cells ➡, sclerosis along glomerular basement membranes ➡, & the "tip" of the glomerulus at the tubular pole ➡. *(Right)* In FSGS collapsing variant, at least 1 glomerulus has collapse & an overlying podocyte hypertrophy/hyperplasia ➡, together with glomerulosclerosis ➡.

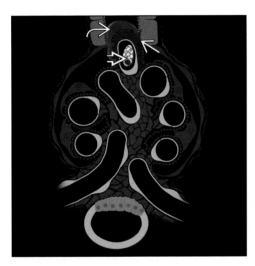 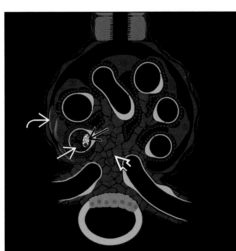

(Left) In FSGS "tip" variant, there is at least 1 segmental lesion involving the tip domain, often coupled with an adhesion ➡, podocyte hypertrophy ➡, and intraluminal foam cells ➡. *(Right)* In FSGS cellular variant, there is at least 1 glomerulus with segmental endocapillary hypercellularity occluding lumina, often with inflammatory cells, foam cells ➡, karyorrhexis ➡, overlying podocyte hyperplasia ➡, and mesangial hypercellularity ➡.

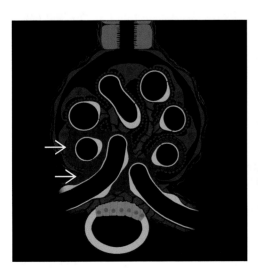 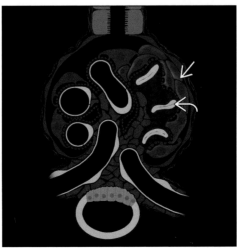

(Left) In FSGS perihilar variant, at least 1 glomerulus has perihilar hyalinosis/sclerosis ➡, which must be present in > 50% of glomeruli with segmental lesions. *(Right)* In FSGS (NOS), at least 1 glomerulus must have segmental increase in the matrix that obliterates the capillary lumina. This is often in a peripheral, nonspecific pattern of sclerosis ➡ ± overlying podocyte hypertrophy ➡.

FOCAL SEGMENTAL GLOMERULOSCLEROSIS, PRIMARY

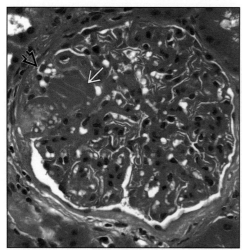

Focal segmental glomerulosclerosis (FSGS) has segmental scars in some glomeruli, typically with hyaline ➡ and adhesion ⧉ to Bowman capsule. Most of the glomerulus appears normal.

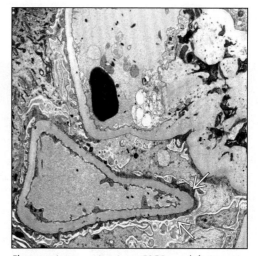

Electron microscopy in primary FSGS reveals foot process effacement ➡, which can be patchy or global. The GBM is normal unless there is glomerular hypertrophy. Deposits are not prominent.

TERMINOLOGY

Abbreviations
- Focal segmental glomerulosclerosis (FSGS)

Definitions
- Idiopathic glomerular disease manifested by marked proteinuria, often nephrotic syndrome, with focal segmental glomerulosclerosis, adhesion to Bowman capsule (BC), and foot process effacement (FPE), without evidence of other underlying glomerular or renal disease
  - Classified separately from FSGS due to known genetic disorders, infection, drugs, hyperperfusion, and other renal diseases
  - As more specific genetic, metabolic, and microbial causes are identified, this category will diminish and be replaced by FSGS of known etiologies

ETIOLOGY/PATHOGENESIS

Idiopathic Disease
- Putative plasma factor plus genetic predisposition
- May have multiple etiologies leading to common end pathology
  - Podocyte foot process effacement and segmental glomerular scarring

Podocyte Disease
- Podocyte depletion is believed to be a central mechanism (podocytopenia)
  - Podocytes have limited replicative ability
  - Loss of podocytes leads to bare GBM, which promotes adhesion and repopulation by progenitor cells from BC
  - Cause of podocytopenia not established
    - TGF-β is mediator in animal models

Plasma Factor
- Proteinuria often recurs after renal transplant

- Sometimes within minutes of reperfusion
- Identification of plasma factor remains elusive
  - Adaptive transfer of proteinuria in rats by protein fractions of patient serum
  - Recent evidence that urokinase receptor may be mediator

Genetic Factors
- Several forms of FSGS with similar morphology have genetic defect (podocin, α-actinin-4)
- Increased risk of FSGS in African-Americans, with variant of *APOL-1* gene
  - Provides selective advantage in regions with trypanosomiasis
    - ApoL-1 protein variant is trypanocidal

Tubulointerstitial Injury
- Proteinuria thought to cause tubulointerstitial damage by ↑ tubular chemokine expression and endoplasmic stress response
  - Monocyte chemoattractant protein-1, osteopontin, and tubular endothelin-1

CLINICAL ISSUES

Epidemiology
- Incidence
  - Most common cause of nephrotic syndrome (NS) in adults
    - ~ 20% of renal biopsies
  - 1.8/100,000 per year among a largely white Minnesota population
    - Incidence increased 13x from 1973 to 2003
  - FSGS-related end-stage renal disease (ESRD)
    - Increased 49x from 1980 to 2000
    - Blacks: 23.6/million per year in 2000; lifetime risk is 1:556
    - Whites: 5.4/million per year in 2000; lifetime risk is 1:2,500
  - NOS and tip variants have about equal frequency

FOCAL SEGMENTAL GLOMERULOSCLEROSIS, PRIMARY

Key Facts

Etiology/Pathogenesis
- Idiopathic podocyte disease
- Plasma factor and genetic predisposition

Clinical Issues
- Nephrotic-range proteinuria or nephrotic syndrome
- More common in blacks
- Minority (~ 33%) respond to steroids
  - Tip variant often behaves like MCD
  - Cellular variant has ↑ ESRD incidence

Microscopic Pathology
- Focal segmental glomerulosclerosis
  - Adhesion to BC, randomly distributed in glomerulus
  - Juxtamedullary glomeruli affected early
  - IgM and C3 in segmental scars by IF

- Foot process effacement by EM
- Tip variant has adhesion at inlet of proximal tubule
- Cellular variant had endocapillary hypercellularity occluding lumina

Top Differential Diagnoses
- Scar from focal glomerulonephritis
- Focal proliferative GN (cellular variant)
- Minimal change disease if no segmental scar

Diagnostic Checklist
- Multiple levels may be necessary to demonstrate segmental lesion
- FSGS, NOS is diagnosis of exclusion since other diseases can cause segmental glomerular scars

---

- Cellular variant much rarer
- Age
  - FSGS NOS mean age of onset: ~ 50 years
  - Tip variant younger; age of onset: mean 44-47 years (range: 12-79 years)
- Gender
  - Male preponderance (1.5- to 3.0-fold)
- Ethnicity
  - All ethnic groups
  - FSGS more common in blacks (e.g., African-Americans)
    - 4x higher frequency of FSGS-related ESRD in blacks than in whites or Asians
    - Cellular and collapsing variants also show a black predominance

Presentation
- Proteinuria
  - Usually nephrotic range (> 3.5 g/d) in ~ 60% of NOS variant
  - Tip lesion: Almost all have NS (97%)
    - NS often presents suddenly, as in minimal change disease (MCD)
  - More severe proteinuria in cellular variant than in conventional FSGS NOS
- Hypertension (~ 65%)

Treatment
- Drugs
  - NOS variant
    - ~ 33% respond to steroids
  - Tip variant sometimes shows excellent steroid response, similar to MCD
  - Cellular variant sometimes responds to immunosuppressive therapy (e.g., cyclophosphamide or cyclosporine)
  - Angiotensin-converting enzyme (ACE) inhibitors to ↓ proteinuria and tubular injury

Prognosis
- NOS variant: ~ 50% renal survival at ~ 7 years
- Tip variant: ~ 80% renal survival at 10 years

- Often behaves like MCD; however, some studies show eventual FSGS and ESRD
- Cellular variant has ↑ ESRD prevalence but may remit with therapy

MACROSCOPIC FEATURES

General Features
- Yellow cortex due to increased lipid in proximal tubular epithelium
- Late stage
  - Thin cortex
  - Finely granular surface

MICROSCOPIC PATHOLOGY

Histologic Features
- Glomeruli (NOS variant)
  - Adhesion of glomerular capillaries to BC
    - Randomly distributed (by definition, not at tip or perihilar)
    - Sometimes observe cells from BC bridging between BC and GBM
  - Accumulation of hyaline at site of adhesion
  - Segmental sclerosis of glomerular capillaries
  - Zonal distribution in cortex
    - Most severe at corticomedullary junction
  - Mild, variable mesangial hypercellularity
  - Normal GBM by light microscopy
  - By definition, no glomerular collapse with podocyte proliferation (a feature of collapsing variant)
- Tubules
  - Tubular resorption droplets
  - Focal atrophy, associated with areas of glomerulosclerosis
- Interstitium
  - Fibrosis, correlated with FSGS lesions
- Vessels
  - Arteriolar hyalinosis
  - Intimal fibrosis

FOCAL SEGMENTAL GLOMERULOSCLEROSIS, PRIMARY

Variants

- Tip variant (Howie and Brewer)
  - Tip region: Outer 25% of glomerulus next to proximal tubule origin
    - Podocyte adhesion or confluence with parietal or tubular cells and tubular neck or lumen
    - Affected segment may "herniate" into tubular lumen
  - Segmental lesions contain endocapillary hypercellularity or sclerosis
    - Usually intracapillary foam cells
  - ~ 80% of tip lesion cases also had cellular variant features in 1 study
  - Tip lesion can be seen in glomerular diseases other than primary FSGS (e.g., TMA, GN)
- Cellular variant
  - Endocapillary hypercellularity occluding lumina
    - Intracapillary endothelial cells and macrophage-type foam cells ± neutrophils and lymphocytes
    - ± apoptosis with pyknotic or karyorrhectic debris
    - ± fibrin within glomerular capillaries
  - Some consider FSGS cellular lesion and collapsing glomerulopathy to be same entity

ANCILLARY TESTS

Immunofluorescence

- IgM and C3 in segments with focal glomerulosclerosis
- Other stains typically negative or minimal scattered deposits (IgG, IgA, C1q, fibrin)
- Kappa and lambda stain equivalent and similar to IgM
- Tubular resorption droplets stain for most plasma proteins

Electron Microscopy

- Podocyte foot process effacement (FPE), variable in extent
  - Foot process width > 1,500 μm distinguishes primary FSGS from secondary FSGS due to nephron overload
- Normal GBM, no rupture
- No or minor deposits
- In adhesion
  - Loss of podocytes with bridging of parietal epithelium to GBM
- Cellular variant
  - Endocapillary hypercellularity leads to segmental glomerular capillary occlusion

DIFFERENTIAL DIAGNOSIS

Segmental Scar from Focal Glomerulonephritis

- PAS stain may show disrupted GBM in GN (e.g., IgA nephropathy)
- Usually more of a stronger reaction of BC than seen in primary FSGS
- Prominent immune complexes by IF, deposits on EM
- Clinical history (infection, serology)

Secondary FSGS

- Glomerular hypertrophy
- Less extensive FPE (through measure of foot process width)
- Perihilar distribution of adhesions and hyaline

Other Glomerular Diseases

- Tip lesion occurs other glomerular diseases (e.g., membranous GN, IgA nephropathy, diabetes)

Minimal Change Disease

- Cannot distinguish without presence of segmental glomerulosclerosis
- Sampling is an issue, particularly without corticomedullary junction

DIAGNOSTIC CHECKLIST

Pathologic Interpretation Pearls

- In setting of nephrotic syndrome and lesions of minimal change disease, FSGS cannot be ruled out
  - Presence of tubular atrophy even without glomerular scar is suspicious
  - Multiple levels may be necessary to demonstrate segmental lesion
- FSGS NOS is diagnosis of exclusion since other diseases can cause segmental glomerular scars

SELECTED REFERENCES

1. Cybulsky AV: Endoplasmic reticulum stress in proteinuric kidney disease. Kidney Int. 77(3):187-93, 2010
2. Freedman BI et al: The apolipoprotein L1 (APOL1) gene and nondiabetic nephropathy in African Americans. J Am Soc Nephrol. 21(9):1422-6, 2010
3. Gbadegesin R et al: Pathogenesis and therapy of focal segmental glomerulosclerosis: an update. Pediatr Nephrol. Epub ahead of print, 2010
4. D'Agati VD: Podocyte injury in focal segmental glomerulosclerosis: Lessons from animal models (a play in five acts). Kidney Int. 73(4):399-406, 2008
5. Deegens JK et al: Pathological variants of focal segmental glomerulosclerosis in an adult Dutch population--epidemiology and outcome. Nephrol Dial Transplant. 23(1):186-92, 2008
6. Deegens JK et al: Podocyte foot process effacement as a diagnostic tool in focal segmental glomerulosclerosis. Kidney Int. 74(12):1568-76, 2008
7. Wei C et al: Modification of kidney barrier function by the urokinase receptor. Nat Med. 14(1):55-63, 2008
8. D'Agati VD et al: Pathologic classification of focal segmental glomerulosclerosis: a working proposal. Am J Kidney Dis. 43(2):368-82, 2004
9. Stokes MB et al: Glomerular tip lesion: a distinct entity within the minimal change disease/focal segmental glomerulosclerosis spectrum. Kidney Int. 65(5):1690-702, 2004

Microscopic Features

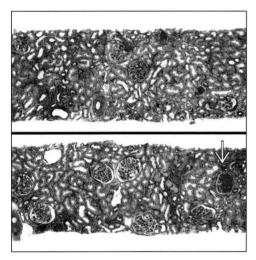

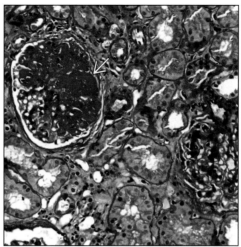

(Left) Low-power view of a biopsy from an African-American male with FSGS reveals 1 glomerulus ➡️ with focal segmental glomerulosclerosis. These glomeruli are preferentially located at the corticomedullary junction, which should be included to consider the sample adequate. (Right) Defining features of FSGS are sparing of some glomeruli ("focal") & partial involvement of affected tufts ("segmental"). Affected glomerulus has broad adhesion & hyalinosis ➡️.

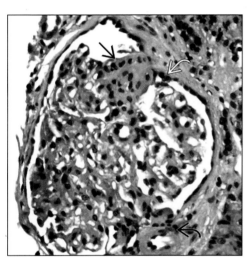

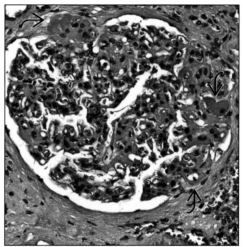

(Left) Adhesion of a glomerular tuft segment ➡️ to Bowman capsule (BC) is shown. Note the tenting of BC ➡️, a useful feature to indicate that the adhesion is not an artifact. Identification of the glomerular base ➡️ helps exclude that structure, which can sometimes resemble an adhesion. (Right) This glomerulus has 3 sites of adhesion to BC with accompanying deposition of hyaline ➡️. The rest of the glomerulus has mild mesangial hypercellularity but is otherwise unremarkable.

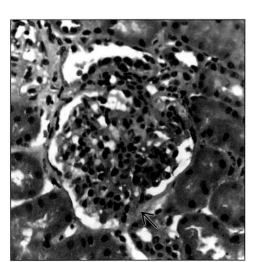

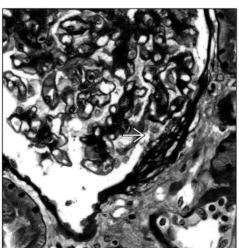

(Left) Subtle adhesion ➡️ in a 6 year old with nephrotic syndrome is shown. The tenting of Bowman capsule is useful to distinguish real from artifactual adhesions. (Right) An adhesion appears to have a cell ➡️ bridging between the laminated Bowman capsule and the GBM. The presence of a Bowman capsule reaction helps distinguish a real adhesion from one created as a biopsy artifact, with compression of the tuft against the capsule.

FOCAL SEGMENTAL GLOMERULOSCLEROSIS, PRIMARY

Immunofluorescence

(Left) Segmental IgM deposits ➡ in the sclerotic segments of the involved glomeruli in FSGS are shown. Mesangial IgM is also not uncommon. *(Right)* C3 deposits in sclerotic segments of glomeruli ➡ in FSGS are seen here. C3 is also present in the rest of the glomerulus in the mesangium ➡. Mesangial IgM and C3 are variably present in FSGS but typically not prominent. Glomeruli with sclerosis, whatever the cause, may have IgM and C3 deposits, presumed due to nonspecific trapping.

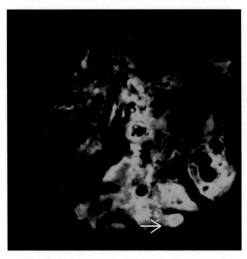 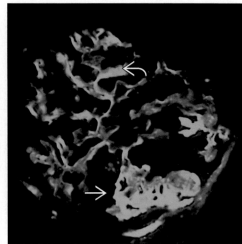

(Left) Segmental IgM ➡ in a case of FSGS is shown. Typical of FSGS, this case also had C3 but no IgG or IgA staining. *(Right)* C3 is present in a capsular adhesion. Whether this has a role in the pathogenesis is unknown, but it is almost invariably present, along with IgM.

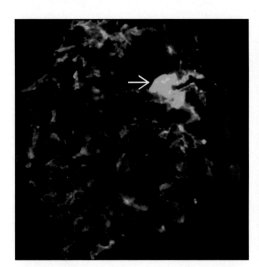 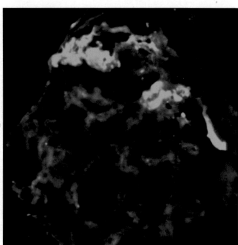

(Left) FSGS typically has little or no IgG, as illustrated here. The faint linear IgG in this case is probably related to the patient's diabetes. *(Right)* A negative stain for IgA, as illustrated, is reassuring that the underlying cause of the segmental glomerulosclerosis is not IgA nephropathy but rather FSGS.

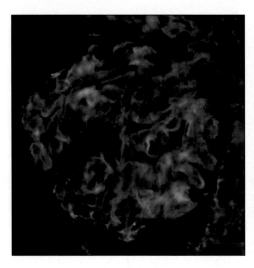 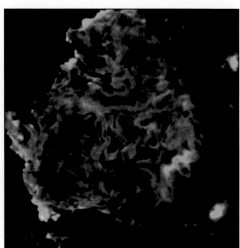

FOCAL SEGMENTAL GLOMERULOSCLEROSIS, PRIMARY

Electron Microscopy

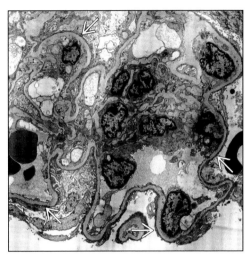
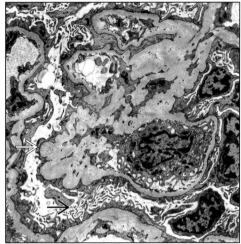

(Left) Electron microscopy at low power in FSGS reveals extensive foot process effacement ➡ and a normal GBM in a 25 year old with nephrotic-range proteinuria and FSGS seen in the light microscopic portion of the biopsy. (Right) Villous hypertrophy of podocyte surfaces ➡ is prominent in this case of FSGS that followed a previous biopsy showing minimal change-like lesions without sclerosis. The GBM is segmentally wrinkled ➡.

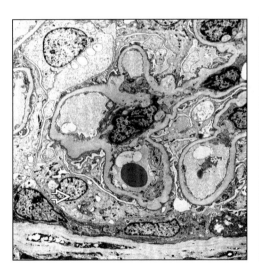
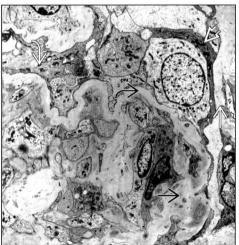

(Left) In this 22-year-old African-American with 1.8 g/d proteinuria and FSGS, patchy foot process effacement affects ~ 20% of glomerular capillaries. A podocyte ➡ is stretched & is in close contact with parietal epithelium but not the Bowman capsule (BC). (Right) Segmental glomerulosclerosis ➡ with adhesion to BC ➡ in a 25-year-old African-American with nephrotic syndrome is shown. A cell ➡ bridges the GBM ➡ & BC. Podocyte foot process effacement is widespread ➡.

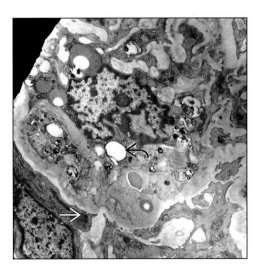
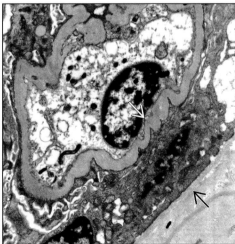

(Left) Segmental scar shows lipid in mesangial cells ➡ and loss of the podocytes ➡. (Right) An apparent single cell bridges the Bowman capsule ➡ and the GBM ➡, probably the earliest phase of an adhesion in FSGS. The nature of the cell is not certain, but based on experimental evidence, it is probably a parietal epithelial cell that attached to a bare GBM.

FOCAL SEGMENTAL GLOMERULOSCLEROSIS, PRIMARY

FSGS, Tip Variant

(Left) In this case of FSGS, tip variant, there is herniation of the glomerular tuft ➡ into the proximal tubule where it exits the Bowman space. *(Right)* In this case of FSGS, tip variant, a glomerular capillary contains foam cells and is adherent to Bowman capsule ➡ at the inlet of the proximal tubule ➡. Enlarged, reactive podocytes are also at the site ➡.

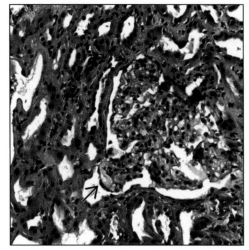
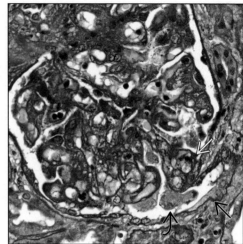

(Left) In this case of FSGS, tip variant, the glomerular tuft is "herniating" through the site at which the tubular pole exits ➡, and adjacent glomerular capillary loops are thickened ➡. Hypertrophic podocytes ➡ are also present. *(Right)* Immunofluorescence of a case of FSGS, tip variant shows nonspecific entrapment of kappa at the tubular pole.

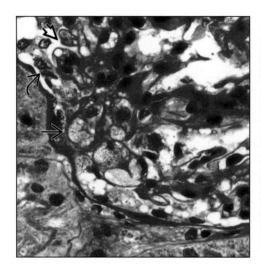
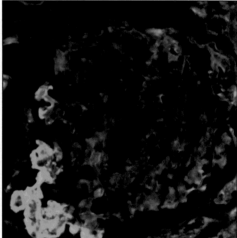

(Left) In this case of FSGS, tip variant, EM shows wrinkled glomerular basement membranes ➡ and endocapillary hypercellularity ➡ at the portion adjacent to the tubular pole. *(Right)* In this case of FSGS, tip variant, there is widespread podocyte foot process effacement ➡ by electron microscopy.

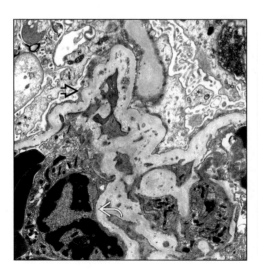
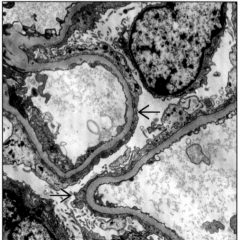

FSGS, Cellular Variant

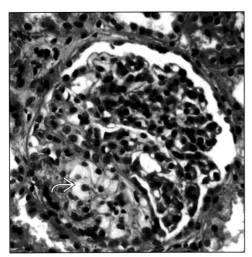
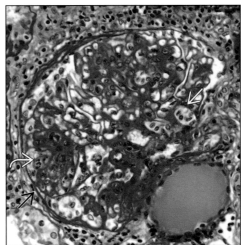

(Left) The cellular variant is defined as having at least 1 glomerulus with segmental endocapillary hypercellularity occluding lumina, ± foam cells, and ± karyorrhexis. Foam cells ⇶ are prominent in the area of adhesion. This is probably related to severe hyperlipidemia. (Right) In this case of FSGS, cellular variant, the glomerulus shows intracapillary cells ➡ and adhesions to Bowman capsule ➡. Karyorrhexis is also present ⇶.

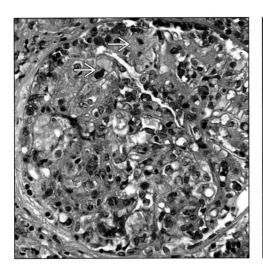
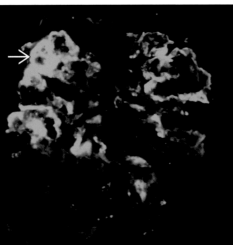

(Left) Trichrome stain of a biopsy with the cellular variant of FSGS shows most glomerular capillaries filled with mononuclear cells with abundant, sometimes foamy cytoplasm ⇶. (Right) In this case of FSGS, cellular variant, there is segmental deposition of C3 ➡ by immunofluorescence.

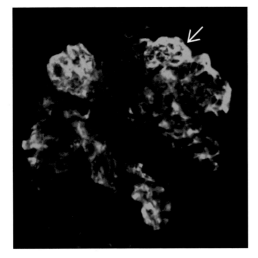
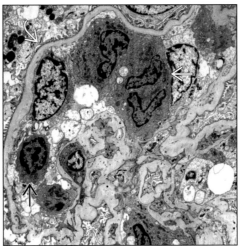

(Left) IgM by immunofluorescence shows segmental positivity ➡ in the cellular variant of FSGS. (Right) The cellular variant of FSGS is defined by intracapillary cells, here shown to be monocytes ➡ and lymphocytes ➡. Foam cells, either macrophages or endothelial cells, can also be conspicuous. Foot process effacement is present but patchy ⇶.

FOCAL SEGMENTAL GLOMERULOSCLEROSIS, SECONDARY

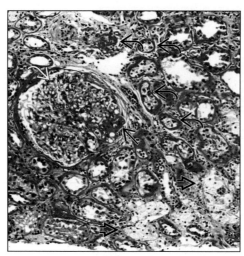

Secondary FSGS is often manifested by glomerulomegaly ⇉ and a perihilar distribution of the glomerular adhesions ➡. This case also shows interstitial foam cells ⊳ and tubular atrophy ➡.

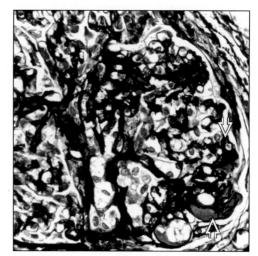

High-power view of a silver stain in a 21-year-old man with nephrotic syndrome and perihilar segmental GS shows that intracapillary hyaline ⇉ is present in the segmental sclerosis lesion.

TERMINOLOGY

Abbreviations
- Secondary focal segmental glomerulosclerosis (2° FSGS)

Definitions
- "Primary" and "secondary" FSGS terminology confusing since specific causal mechanisms are being identified in both
- Here, 2° FSGS is defined as FSGS that arises as maladaptive response to loss of nephrons or increased demand, probably due to increased filtration/perfusion of glomeruli and podocyte stress

ETIOLOGY/PATHOGENESIS

Adaptive Structural-Functional Response
- Imbalance between glomerular capacity and metabolic demands
  - Thought to act through glomerular hypertension (HTN), increased filtration, and podocyte stress
  - ↑ glomerular capillary pressures and flow rates
- Arises from several pathways
  - Failure to develop normal number of glomeruli
    - Unilateral renal agenesis, dysplasia, oligomeganephronia, and other congenital renal developmental diseases
  - Acquired disease that causes ↓ of functional nephrons
    - Sequelae of chronic renal disease of any etiology that destroys nephrons: Final common pathway
    - Reflux nephropathy, Alport syndrome, HTN, cortical necrosis, and virtually any other chronic renal disease
  - Normal number of glomeruli but increased "demand"
    - Obesity, body builders, anabolic steroids, possibly HTN

Specific Mechanisms
- Obesity-related glomerulopathy (ORG)
  - Receptor for advanced glycation end products (RAGE) may mediate obesity-associated renal injury
  - RAGE may also be important to diabetes, doxorubicin-induced nephropathy, HTN, lupus nephritis, ischemic renal injury, and renal amyloidosis
  - RAGE antagonism may be useful in treating chronic kidney disease
- Calcineurin inhibitors (CNIs)
  - Arteriolar constriction leads to variable glomerular perfusion
  - Particularly important in renal transplant recipients since FSGS can sometimes be ascribed to CNIs
- Anabolic steroids used in bodybuilding
  - Possibly due to direct nephrotoxic effect of anabolic steroids and ↑ lean body mass
- Sleep apnea
  - Hypoxia leads to sympathetic nervous system activation and stimulates renin-angiotensin system
- Unilateral renal agenesis
  - Higher risk of FSGS than general population
    - Loss of 1 kidney later in life does not appear to cause same risk for FSGS in remaining kidney
    - When 1 kidney and portion of other are lost in adults, ↑ risk of FSGS development

Pathologic Consequences
- Glomerular hypertrophy
  - ↑ diameter and number of mesangial cells
  - Thickened GBM
  - Relative deficiency of podocytes, which have limited replicative ability
- Segmental glomerular capillary scars and adhesions to Bowman capsule
  - Classically, adhesion and hyaline in perihilar region
  - Known as the "hilar" variant of FSGS

FOCAL SEGMENTAL GLOMERULOSCLEROSIS, SECONDARY

Key Facts

Terminology
- FSGS secondary to imbalance of glomerular functional capacity and demand

Etiology/Pathogenesis
- Adaptive structural-functional response
  - Reduced nephron mass: Oligomeganephronia, reflux nephropathy, renal agenesis/dysplasia/ablation/necrosis, advanced renal disease
  - Normal nephron mass: HTN, obesity, atheroemboli/vaso-occlusion, sickle cell anemia, congenital heart disease, drugs (anabolic steroids, calcineurin inhibitors)
- Glomerular HTN

Clinical Issues
- Proteinuria and systemic HTN

Microscopic Pathology
- Glomerulomegaly
- FSGS in perihilar distribution
- Compensatory tubular hypertrophy
- Often arteriolar hyalinosis, arteriosclerosis
- IF: Most notable for segmental IgM and C3
- EM: Segmental podocyte foot process effacement (FPE)
  - Increased thickness of otherwise normal GBM

Top Differential Diagnoses
- Primary FSGS
- Segmental scars from GN

Diagnostic Checklist
- Routinely assess glomerular size in biopsies
- Normal is < 50% of diameter of 40x field

Animal Models
- 5/6 nephrectomy in rats
  - Widely used model
  - Removal/infarction of upper and lower pole of kidney followed by contralateral nephrectomy
  - Results in HTN, glomerulomegaly, and, later, FSGS over 8-12 weeks with proteinuria and loss of renal function
  - Ameliorated by inhibitors of renin-angiotensin system (angiotensin II receptor inhibitors)
  - Strain differences in rats and mice

CLINICAL ISSUES

Epidemiology
- Incidence
  - Coincident with ↑ in obesity incidence: Apparent ↑ incidence of ORG

Presentation
- Proteinuria
  - Proteinuria is often > 3.5 g/d but usually without hypoalbuminemia, hypercholesterolemia, and edema
  - Specifically, ORG shows lower incidence of nephrotic syndrome than idiopathic FSGS
- Renal dysfunction
  - Most have ↑ serum creatinine and ↓ GFR preceding development of nephrotic proteinuria
    - ORG is notable exception since it may have ↑ GFR (supernormal, > 120 mL/min) 2° to hyperfiltration/overwork state caused by ↑ ratio of body mass to renal mass
- Hypertension
- ORG patients typically have a BMI > 30
  - BMI 30-34.9, grade 1 obesity; BMI 35.0-39.9, grade 2 obesity; and BMI ≥ 40, grade 3 obesity (morbid obesity)

Treatment
- Drugs

  - Angiotensin II receptor antagonists
  - Steroids are not typically effective
    - Often contraindicated in many patients (e.g., in obesity) due to stimulation of weight gain and diabetes
  - ACE inhibitors
  - Low-protein diet
- Other treatment
  - Bariatric surgery may normalize proteinuria associated with ORG
  - Stop anabolic steroid use

Prognosis
- 2° FSGS is typically thought to be more indolent than 1° FSGS
- Studies regarding prognosis of perihilar variant of FSGS are mixed
  - Probably relates to underlying causes

MICROSCOPIC PATHOLOGY

Histologic Features
- Glomeruli
  - Glomerulomegaly
    - Glomeruli enlarged with expanded hypercellular mesangium
    - Universal definition of glomerulomegaly not established, even by "gold standard" morphometric methods, since there is significant population variability
    - Rule of thumb: Glomerular diameter > 220 μm (~ 1/2 diameter of typical 40x objective field)
    - Variable degrees, heterogeneity
  - Segmental glomerulosclerosis (GS)
    - Loss of intrinsic cells and structure
  - Adhesion to Bowman capsule
    - Typically in perihilar region
    - Contains hyaline deposits in capillary loops
    - Hyalinosis composed of protein insudation between GBM and endothelial cells

FOCAL SEGMENTAL GLOMERULOSCLEROSIS, SECONDARY

- To qualify for hilar variant, > 50% of glomeruli with segmental lesions must have perihilar GS &/ or hyalinosis
  - Foam cells may be entrapped in sclerotic lesions
  - Global GS may be present
  - Podocyte hypertrophy and hyperplasia may be present
- Vessels
  - Arteriolar hyalinosis may be in continuity with perihilar segment of arteriole
- Tubules and interstitium
  - Tubular hypertrophy (increased diameter of tubule and size of tubular cells)
  - Atrophy and interstitial fibrosis (IF) related to loss of nephrons

Specific Features by Cause

- Obesity
  - Mesangial expansion, GBM thickening, and glomerulomegaly
  - Segmental lesions often perihilar with associated hyalinosis
  - Tubulointerstitial disease often mild in comparison with glomerular changes
- Hypertension
  - GS typically occurs in outer cortex, forming subcapsular scars
  - Glomerular hypertrophy
  - Segmental sclerosis often perihilar
  - Atubular glomeruli often form, leading to cystic dilatation of Bowman space
  - Interstitial fibrosis and tubular atrophy prominent
  - Arteriosclerosis and arteriolar hyalinosis (arteriolosclerosis) present
- Reflux nephropathy
  - Reflux nephropathy shows prominent periglomerular fibrosis and thickening of Bowman capsule
  - Interstitial fibrosis in "geographic" pattern
- Heroin use
  - Global GS, epithelial cell changes, IF, and tubular injury are more prominent than in idiopathic FSGS
- Sickle cell disease
  - Glomerular hypertrophy and capillary loop congestion by sickled erythrocytes
  - Glomerular capillaries may have double contours due to chronic thrombotic microangiopathy-type picture
- Oligomeganephronia
  - Oligomeganephronia results from ↓ glomerular number and resultant enlargement of remaining glomeruli

ANCILLARY TESTS

Immunofluorescence

- Segmental IgM and C3 in glomerulosclerotic lesions
- Little or no immunoglobulin otherwise

Electron Microscopy

- Podocyte foot process effacement (FPE) is cardinal feature
  - Typically segmental FPE (often < 50%) in 2° forms of FSGS
  - Podocyte hypertrophy and hyperplasia typically less than in 1° FSGS
  - Podocytes may detach from GBM and may contain protein resorption droplets
  - Podocytes may eventually detach, leaving bare GBM segments
- Features of particular etiologies
  - Obesity-associated FSGS: Subtotal FPE and marked glomerulomegaly
  - HTN: Ischemic wrinkling and thickening of GBM

DIFFERENTIAL DIAGNOSIS

Primary FSGS

- Typically greater proteinuria (nephrotic syndrome)
- More diffuse FPE

Identification of Underlying Renal Disease

- 2° FSGS is chronic stage of many immune complex, proliferative, or nonimmune diseases
- Immune complexes may be difficult to find in end-stage kidneys, making diligent search necessary

Focal Glomerulonephritis

- Segmental scars may be residue of past inflammatory GN

DIAGNOSTIC CHECKLIST

Clinically Relevant Pathologic Features

- Assessment of clinical history is important in finding 2° cause

Pathologic Interpretation Pearls

- Perihilar GS is clue for 2° FSGS
- Routinely assess glomerular size in biopsies
  - Normal is < 50% of diameter of 40x field

SELECTED REFERENCES

1. Puelles VG et al: Glomerular number and size variability and risk for kidney disease. Curr Opin Nephrol Hypertens. 20(1):7-15, 2011
2. Fogo AB: The spectrum of FSGS: does pathology matter? Nephrol Dial Transplant. 25(4):1034-6, 2010
3. Herlitz LC et al: Development of focal segmental glomerulosclerosis after anabolic steroid abuse. J Am Soc Nephrol. 21(1):163-72, 2010
4. D'Agati VD et al: Pathologic classification of focal segmental glomerulosclerosis: a working proposal. Am J Kidney Dis. 43(2):368-82, 2004
5. Fogo AB: Animal models of FSGS: lessons for pathogenesis and treatment. Semin Nephrol. 23(2):161-71, 2003
6. Kambham N et al: Obesity-related glomerulopathy: an emerging epidemic. Kidney Int. 59(4):1498-509, 2001

FOCAL SEGMENTAL GLOMERULOSCLEROSIS, SECONDARY

Microscopic Features

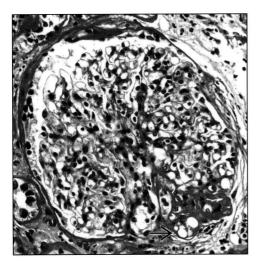
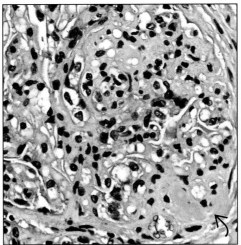

(Left) Striking glomerulomegaly is evident in this 21-year-old man with nephrotic syndrome who has secondary FSGS with a perihilar adhesion ➡. The hyaline in the adhesion stains strongly for PAS and contains lipid droplets. (Right) The adhesions in secondary FSGS typically contain hyaline ➡, which is usually homogeneous. The adhesions and hyaline material sometimes also contain clear fine lipid droplets.

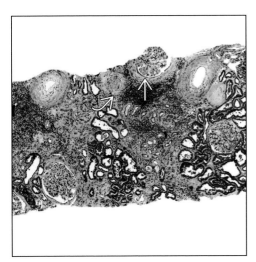
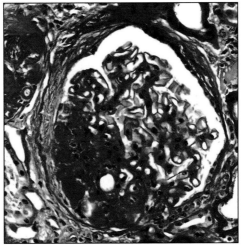

(Left) One of the more common causes of 2° FSGS in current renal biopsies is HTN, which causes progressive loss of functional nephrons and produces global ➡ & segmental ➡ glomerulosclerosis, shown in a 63-year-old woman with poorly controlled HTN for 30 years. (Right) Secondary FSGS can arise from many causes; in this case, hilar sclerosis & adhesions were due to chronic renal disease presumed to be hypertensive nephropathy. Cr was 2.2, and the urine protein/Cr ratio was 2.8.

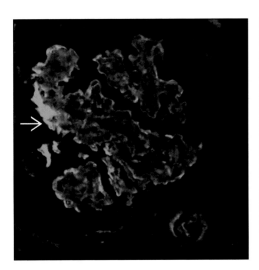
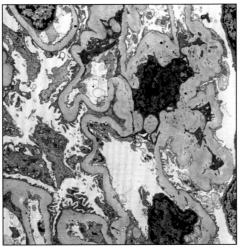

(Left) The main value of IF in cases with FSGS is to rule out underlying glomerular disease. In FSGS of all types, segmental deposits of IgM ➡ & C3 are in the segmental lesions, sometimes with segmental granular deposits along the GBM. (Right) The manifestation of glomerular hypertrophy by EM is a diffusely thickened GBM. Secondary FSGS often has relatively little foot process effacement despite moderately heavy proteinuria (in this case due to hypertension, ~ 3 g/d).

Obesity-related Glomerulopathy

(Left) H&E from a 37-year-old African-American woman with morbid obesity (> 350 lb), HTN, and proteinuria shows a hypertrophic glomerulus ➡ and a relatively normal-sized glomerulus with periglomerular fibrosis ➡. Overall, this is clinicopathologically compatible with obesity-related glomerulopathy (ORG). *(Right)* In an ORG case, there is peripheral condensation of the glomerular capillary loops ➡, suggestive of evolving focal segmental GS.

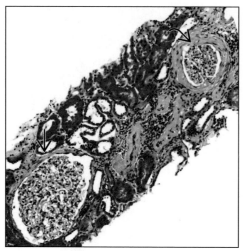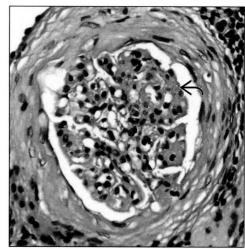

(Left) A PAS stain shows the peripheral irregularities in glomerular capillary loops ➡ in a case most compatible with obesity-related glomerulopathy in a 37 year old with morbid obesity. *(Right)* A periodic acid-methenamine-silver (PAMS) stain shows peripheral irregularities ➡ in the glomerular capillary loops in a case of obesity-related glomerulopathy.

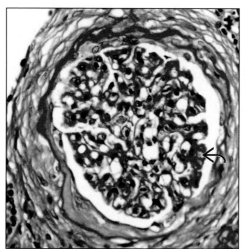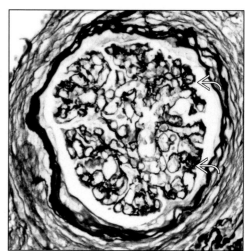

(Left) In a case of obesity-related glomerulopathy, a glomerulus shows marked hypertrophy in a 37 year old with morbid obesity. *(Right)* A glomerulus shows marked hypertrophy in a case of obesity-related glomerulopathy. Normally, a glomerulus should fit into a 40x field, but in this case, less than 2/3 of the glomerulus fits.

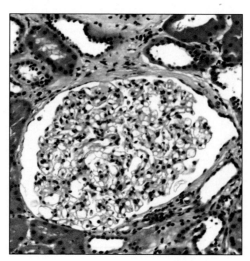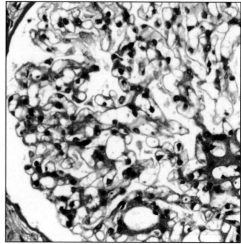

Obesity- and Anabolic Steroid-related Glomerulopathy

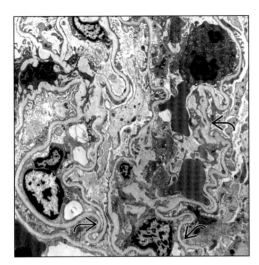
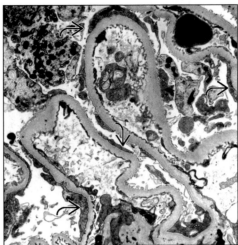

(Left) In a 53-year-old man with morbid obesity (BMI 41.9), creatinine 10 mg/dL, and a urine protein/creatinine ratio of 12.96, GBMs show marked wrinkling with segmental near-occlusion of glomerular capillary loops ➔. *(Right)* In a 53-year-old man with obesity-related glomerulopathy (ORG) (BMI 41.9), there was segmental effacement of foot processes ➔, compatible with a 2° case of focal segmental GS (FSGS).

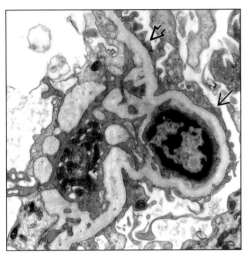
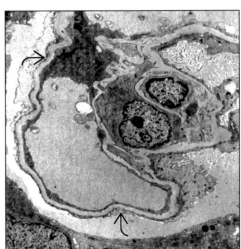

(Left) In a 53-year-old man with a BMI of 41.9, there was prominent segmental podocyte foot process effacement (FPE) ➔, together with more preserved foot processes ➔, compatible with obesity-related 2° FSGS, attributed in this case to ORG. *(Right)* In a 40-year-old male bodybuilder with years of anabolic steroid use, there is prominent segmental podocyte FPE ➔. This feature leads to a diagnosis of 2° focal segmental GS attributed to anabolic steroid use.

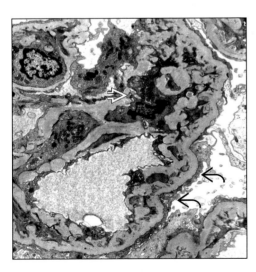
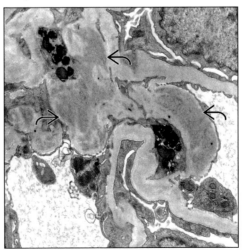

(Left) In a 40 year old with a history of years of anabolic steroid use for bodybuilding, there is segmental podocyte FPE ➔, compatible with a 2° FSGS attributed, in this case, to the anabolic steroids. In addition, there is mesangial expansion ➔. *(Right)* In FSGS attributed to anabolic steroids, there were occasional vague densities ➔, some having a hyaline quality. IF did not impart specificity to the densities, suggesting that their presence is 2° to entrapment.

COLLAPSING GLOMERULOPATHY

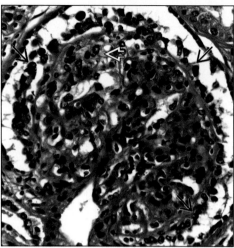

In collapsing glomerulopathy, glomerular capillary loops are not well defined ⬆, and a rim of crowded, reactive podocytes is present ➡.

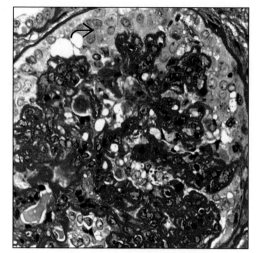

Podocyte proliferation in collapsing glomerulopathy can resemble a cellular crescent ➡. However, the cells are more rounded than the more spindle-shaped parietal epithelial cells typically seen in a crescent.

TERMINOLOGY

Abbreviations
- Collapsing glomerulopathy (CG)
- Focal segmental glomerulosclerosis (FSGS)

Synonyms
- Primary FSGS, collapsing variant
- Idiopathic collapsing FSGS

Definitions
- "Podocytopathy" defined pathologically by prominent capillary loop collapse, podocyte hypercellularity, and proliferation
  - Many different causes of collapsing podocyte phenotype
  - Target not limited to podocytes: Proximal tubular cells proliferate, and tubules are dilated

ETIOLOGY/PATHOGENESIS

Many Causes
- Idiopathic (usual)
- Infection
- Drugs
- Vascular disease
- Autoimmune disease
- Malignancy
- Genetic disorders

Idiopathic (Primary)
- Cause unknown
  - Circulating permeability factor suspected but has limited experimental evidence
- Genetic factors may contribute
  - Prevalent *APOL1* in blacks has strong association with HIV-associated nephropathy and FSGS (and possibly with idiopathic CG)
    - Closely linked to *MYH9* E1 haplotype (nonmuscle myosin heavy chain IIA)

Podocyte Proliferation
- CG is thought to be disorder resulting from podocyte proliferation and dedifferentiation
  - Normally, podocytes have low rate of turnover
    - WT-1 transcription factor inhibits proliferation
    - Podocytes in CG characteristically lose expression of WT-1 and increase expression of proteins involved in cell division (e.g., Ki-67)
- Because of this, authors argue that CG may not be a form of FSGS since other forms of FSGS are considered to be due to loss of podocytes (podocytopenia)
  - FSGS consists of sclerosis (segmental solidification) of glomerulus and adhesions to Bowman capsule
  - In contrast, CG consists of pseudocrescent collapse of tuft with increased numbers of podocytes with few adhesions
  - CG also does not respond to typical therapies used for FSGS, suggesting different pathogenesis

Mitochondrial Dysfunction
- Mitochondrial phenyltransferase-like protein mutations have been identified in *kd/kd* mice and associated with CG
- May be involved in damage induced by some bisphosphonates

CLINICAL ISSUES

Epidemiology
- Ethnicity
  - Blacks are disproportionately affected (20-50x)

Presentation
- Proteinuria, nephrotic range
- Nephrotic syndrome
  - Hypoalbuminemia
  - Hypercholesterolemia
- Renal dysfunction

COLLAPSING GLOMERULOPATHY

Key Facts

Etiology/Pathogenesis
- Podocyte proliferation and dedifferentiation are thought to play a role
- Idiopathic most common form
- Heterogeneous secondary forms
  - Infection: HIV, parvovirus B19, and many others
  - Medications: Interferon, bisphosphonates (pamidronate), calcineurin inhibitors, and others
  - Miscellaneous: Autoimmune disease, thrombotic microangiopathy, genetic diseases

Clinical Issues
- Blacks disproportionately affected in idiopathic and HIV-associated forms
- Nephrotic syndrome and nephrotic-range proteinuria
- Renal dysfunction
- Often refractory to steroid therapy

- Rapid progression to renal failure

Microscopic Pathology
- At least 1 glomerulus with
  - Global or segmental collapse
  - Overlying podocyte hyperplasia and hypertrophy
- Tubulointerstitial fibrosis, cysts, and inflammation
- Immunofluorescence: Segmental IgM and C3
- Electron microscopy
  - Wrinkled glomerular basement membranes with capillary loop collapse
  - Segmental foot process effacement

Top Differential Diagnoses
- FSGS, cellular variant
- Crescentic glomerulonephritis
- FSGS, not otherwise specified (NOS)

  - Elevated serum creatinine at presentation, higher than FSGS controls

Treatment
- Drugs
  - None effective
  - Steroid therapy may be used, but disease may be refractory
  - Retinoic acid derivatives and inhibitors of cyclin-dependent kinesis may inhibit or reverse CG
    - Inhibits proliferation and promotes differentiation

Prognosis
- Rapid progression to renal failure (6 months) is usual course of idiopathic CG, more rapid than other types of FSGS
  - Described as "malignant" FSGS variant when initially recognized in 1978 by Brown and colleagues
- Other causes of CG also typically have rapid loss of renal function although improvement can occur with recovery from or removal of etiologic agent

MICROSCOPIC PATHOLOGY

Histologic Features
- Glomeruli
  - At least 1 glomerulus with global or segmental collapse and overlying podocyte hyperplasia and hypertrophy, according to Columbia Working Proposal
    - This is lowest possible threshold and has led to marked increase in diagnosis of CG
  - Podocytes with hypertrophy and hyperplasia
    - Urinary space may be filled with podocytes, forming pseudocrescents
    - Enlarged nuclei with open, vesicular chromatin and frequent nucleoli
    - Binucleate forms may be seen
    - Mitotic figures may rarely be seen
    - Protein resorption droplets may be seen in pseudocrescent podocytes

  - Glomerular basement membranes are wrinkled in areas of collapse
    - PAS and Jones methenamine silver stains are useful in highlighting basement membrane collapse
  - Mesangial and intracapillary matrix are not appreciably increased
- Tubules
  - Tubular microcysts (in 40% of cases)
    - Proximal tubules dilated with proteinaceous casts, sometimes with "peripheral scalloping"
    - Proliferation of tubular cells
    - Enlarged hyperchromatic nuclei, mitotic figures, nucleoli, and focal apoptosis
  - Tubular atrophy/injury
    - Tubular epithelial simplification and flattening
  - Tubulitis can be present, often composed of neutrophilic tubulitis
- Interstitium
  - Inflammation
    - Interstitial mononuclear inflammation can be prominent
  - Edema
- Arteries/arterioles
  - Renal vessels may have changes of thrombotic microangiopathy if etiology involves TMA

ANCILLARY TESTS

Immunofluorescence
- IgM and C3 with segmental or global deposits in collapsed segments with less common deposits of C1q
- IgG, IgA, and albumin in visceral epithelial protein resorption droplets
- Tubules have epithelial protein resorption droplets containing plasma proteins (IgG, IgA, C3, albumin, and others)

Electron Microscopy
- Podocyte hypertrophy overlying areas of collapse
  - Foot processes are extensively effaced

- Contain electron-dense protein resorption droplets, electron-lucent transport vesicles, and increased numbers of organelles, including prominent rough endoplasmic reticulum
- Podocytes detached from glomerular basement membrane with interposition of newly formed extracellular matrix
- Multiple layers of newly formed GBM between podocyte and original GBM
- Actin cytoskeleton is disrupted, making cytoplasm appear open and pale
- Podocytes become cuboidal
- Glomerular basement membrane
  - Wrinkled GBM in areas of collapse
  - GBM not appreciably thickened
  - Absent electron-dense deposits except for small, rare paramesangial deposits
- Glomerular endothelium
  - Absent tubuloreticular inclusions in all forms except for HIV-associated CG, interferon-mediated forms, and lupus-associated forms

Immunohistochemistry

- Ki-67 (MIB-1), a proliferation marker, is positive in podocytes, indicating that they are engaged in proliferation
  - Normal podocytes have no or rare Ki-67(+) podocytes (< 1/glomerulus)
- Podocyte differentiation markers are lost (e.g., WT-1, synaptopodin, podocin, podocalyxin, glomerular epithelial protein 1 [GLEPP1], C3b receptor, and CALLA [CD10]), suggesting that dedifferentiation plays a role in CG

DIFFERENTIAL DIAGNOSIS

FSGS, Cellular Variant

- CG lacks endocapillary hypercellularity seen in FSGS, cellular variant
- Some authors consider cellular variant or "cellular lesion" to be same entity as CG
  - However, Columbia working proposal for FSGS classification (D'Agati et al) specifies that endocapillary hypercellularity is more evident in "cellular variant"
  - Endocapillary cells may even appear decreased in CG

FSGS, Not Otherwise Specified (NOS)

- Podocyte proliferation and hypercellularity absent
- CG typically has less hyalinosis and adhesions to BC
- Segmental and global sclerosis of usual type can be seen together with collapsing lesions, but collapsing features are considered to trump others and force classification to CG

Crescentic Glomerulonephritis

- Crescent cells generally do not have prominent reabsorption droplets
- Hypertrophic podocytes of CG do not have spindled morphology of true crescents
- True crescents also contain fibrin and matrix material not seen in pseudocrescents of CG

- Necrotizing lesions in capillary tuft and glomerular basement membrane breaks

HIV-associated Nephropathy

- Prominent tubuloreticular structures in endothelial cells
- May have mitochondrial abnormalities in tubules due to HAART

CG Related to Other Diseases

- Evidence of thrombotic microangiopathy
- Cholesterol emboli
- Underlying glomerular disease
  - Lupus nephritis

SELECTED REFERENCES

1. Lasagni L et al: Glomerular epithelial stem cells: the good, the bad, and the ugly. J Am Soc Nephrol. 21(10):1612-9, 2010
2. Winkler CA et al: Genetics of focal segmental glomerulosclerosis and human immunodeficiency virus-associated collapsing glomerulopathy: the role of MYH9 genetic variation. Semin Nephrol. 30(2):111-25, 2010
3. Albaqumi M et al: Current views on collapsing glomerulopathy. J Am Soc Nephrol. 19(7):1276-81, 2008
4. Kopp JB et al: MYH9 is a major-effect risk gene for focal segmental glomerulosclerosis. Nat Genet. 40(10):1175-84, 2008
5. Albaqumi M et al: Collapsing glomerulopathy. J Am Soc Nephrol. 17(10):2854-63, 2006
6. D'Agati VD et al: Atlas of Nontumor Pathology: Non-neoplastic Kidney Diseases. Washington, DC: American Registry of Pathology, 2005
7. D'Agati VD et al: Pathologic classification of focal segmental glomerulosclerosis: a working proposal. Am J Kidney Dis. 43(2):368-82, 2004
8. Moudgil A et al: Association of parvovirus B19 infection with idiopathic collapsing glomerulopathy. Kidney Int. 59(6):2126-33, 2001
9. Valeri A et al: Idiopathic collapsing focal segmental glomerulosclerosis: a clinicopathologic study. Kidney Int. 50(5):1734-46, 1996
10. Carbone L et al: Course and prognosis of human immunodeficiency virus-associated nephropathy. Am J Med. 87(4):389-95, 1989
11. Weiss MA et al: Nephrotic syndrome, progressive irreversible renal failure, and glomerular "collapse": a new clinicopathologic entity? Am J Kidney Dis. 7(1):20-8, 1986
12. Brown CB et al: Focal segmental glomerulosclerosis with rapid decline in renal function ("malignant FSGS"). Clin Nephrol. 10(2):51-61, 1978
13. Cameron JS et al: The long-term prognosis of patients with focal segmental glomerulosclerosis. Clin Nephrol. 10(6):213-8, 1978

Pathogenetic Classification of Collapsing Glomerulopathy

Category	Cause	Comments
Idiopathic	Possible circulating factor	Most common form, higher frequency in blacks; possibly associated with *APOL1* variant
Infection		
	HIV	Widespread recognition in 1980s in HIV-associated nephropathy; higher frequency in blacks; associated with *APOL1* variant
	Parvovirus B19	Viral antigen in podocytes
	Leishmaniasis	
	Loa loa	
	Filariasis	
	Tuberculosis	
	Cytomegalovirus	
	Campylobacter enteritis	
Drugs		
	IV drug abuse (e.g., heroin)	Often associated with HIV
	Bisphosphonates (e.g., pamidronate)	
	Interferons-α and -β	
	Valproic acid	
	Calcineurin inhibitors	May originate through thrombotic microangiopathy-like state
Vascular		
	Thrombotic microangiopathy	
	Atheroemboli	
Autoimmune disease		
	Guillain-Barré syndrome	
	Systemic lupus erythematosus and lupus-like syndromes	
	Mixed connective tissue disease	
	Still disease	
Malignancy		
	Leukemia/lymphoma	
Genetic		
	CoQ2 nephropathy (co-enzyme Q2)	Described in Europeans
	Mandibuloacral dysplasia (zinc metalloproteinase, *ZMPSTE24*)	Metalloproteinase is involved in post-translational cleavage of carboxy-terminal residues of farnesylated prelamin A
	Action-myoclonus renal failure (*SCARB2*)	Myoclonic epilepsy associated with renal failure and preserved cognitive function
	HIV-associated nephropathy, FSGS, and focal global glomerulosclerosis (hypertensive glomerular disease)	Associated with APOL1 variant that promotes resistance to trypanosomiasis
	Familial CG	Unknown genes

COLLAPSING GLOMERULOPATHY

Gross and Microscopic Features

(Left) This nephrectomy specimen from a 7-year-old boy with idiopathic collapsing glomerulopathy was done in preparation for renal transplantation. Yellow areas at the corticomedullary junction ➡ are due to lipid in tubules. *(Right)* This collapsing glomerulopathy was in a 7-year-old boy having a nephrectomy prior to transplantation. Collapse and consolidation of the glomerular tuft is evident ➡. The interstitium is mildly inflamed, and tubules are reactive with occasional mitotic figures ➡.

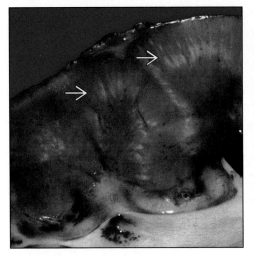 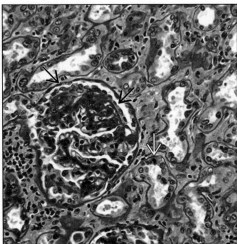

(Left) Low power shows hypercellular glomeruli ➡, prominent interstitial fibrosis and tubular atrophy, tubular microcyst formation ➡, and interstitial inflammation ➡. *(Right)* Glomerular capillary loops are not well defined in this glomerulus with collapsing glomerulopathy. A rim of reactive podocytes ➡ nearly surrounds the glomerulus. Tubules contain debris ➡.

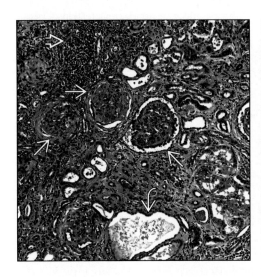 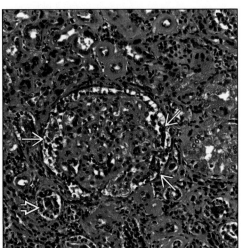

(Left) This glomerulus with glomerular capillary loop collapse has prominent adhesions to Bowman capsule ➡. *(Right)* A higher power image of a glomerulus shows glomerular capillary loop collapse ➡ and many reactive podocytes ➡.

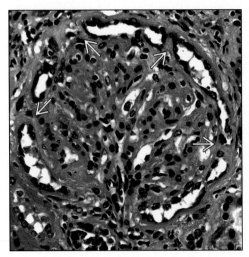 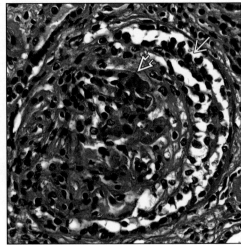

COLLAPSING GLOMERULOPATHY

Microscopic Features

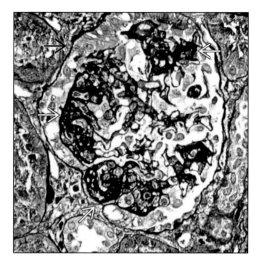 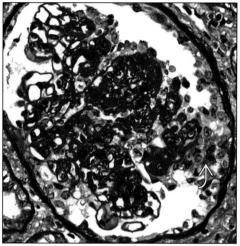

(Left) This Jones methenamine silver (JMS) stain illustrates areas of glomerular capillary loop collapse ➡. The podocytes in the Bowman space resemble a crescent ➡. (Right) Collapsing glomerulopathy with a pseudocrescent is shown. This glomerulus has podocytes that bridge ➡ between the glomerular tuft and BC. These cells may actually arise from the podocyte progenitor cells that normally reside in BC, which are repopulating the glomerular tuft.

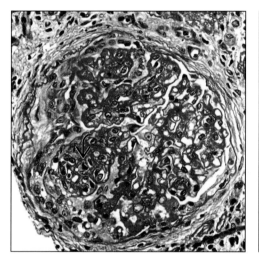 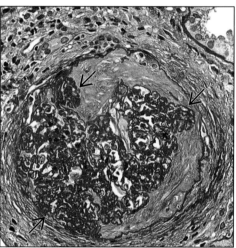

(Left) CG from a 74-year-old Caucasian man with nephrotic syndrome. Severe vascular disease was present in the biopsy as well and may have contributed. An unidentified cell (perhaps a podocyte) is in mitosis ➡. (Right) A globally sclerotic glomerulus in a case of CG shows collapse and occlusion of glomerular capillary loops ➡, illustrating the collapsing process that leads to global sclerosis. The lesion can be confused with a fibrous crescent.

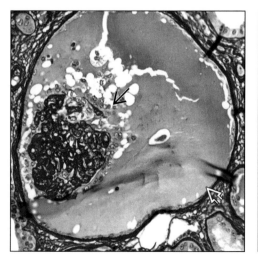 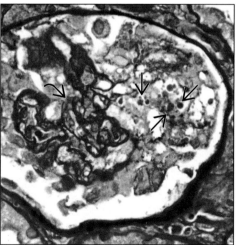

(Left) A glomerulus has undergone prominent collapse with overlying podocyte hypertrophy ➡ and marked dilatation of Bowman space ➡. (Right) This collapsed glomerulus ➡ has prominent podocyte proliferation with tubular reabsorption droplets evident in the podocytes ➡.

COLLAPSING GLOMERULOPATHY

Electron Microscopy and Differential Diagnosis

(Left) Capillary loops are occluded ⇨ in this collapsing glomerulopathy, and podocytes are diffusely effaced ⇨. Endocapillary cells are swollen and reactive; however, this case did not have enough endocapillary cellularity to suggest the "cellular lesion." (Right) EM shows prominent glomerular basement membrane wrinkling with collapse of glomerular capillary loops ⇨.

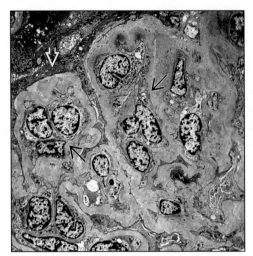 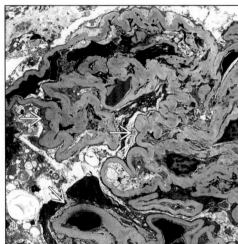

(Left) The GBM is wrinkled ⇨ with collapse of glomerular capillary loops ⇨, diagnostic of collapsing glomerulopathy. Podocytes are segmentally separated ⇨ from the original GBM. Swollen reactive endothelial cells are also present ⇨. (Right) Podocytes ⇨ are separated from the original GBM ⇨ by multiple layers of newly formed matrix ⇨, indicating past podocyte injury and repair. The segmental process was first described in FSGS associated with heroin addiction.

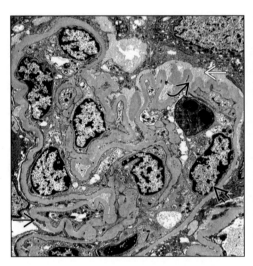 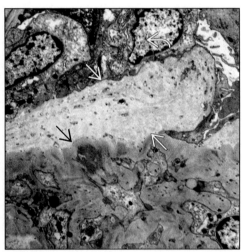

(Left) Prominent laminations ⇨ on the outer aspect of the collapsed GBM are evident in this case of collapsing glomerulopathy. Intracapillary foam cells were present ⇨, a feature more commonly associated with the cellular variant of FSGS. (Right) The main feature that distinguishes HIV-related collapsing glomerulopathy from idiopathic is the presence of endothelial tubuloreticular structures in the former, as illustrated in this case of HIV-associated nephropathy ⇨.

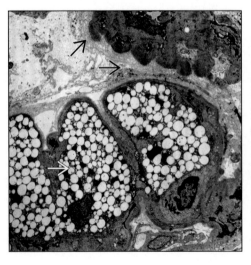 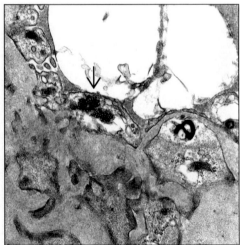

COLLAPSING GLOMERULOPATHY

Immunohistochemistry and Immunofluorescence

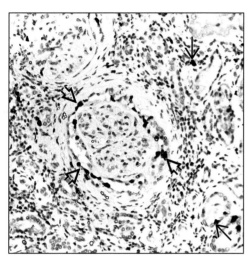 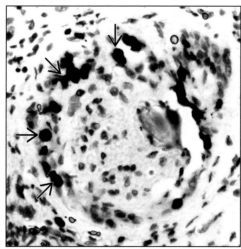

(Left) Ki-67 immunohistochemistry highlights proliferating podocytes ⮑. Occasional Ki-67(+) proliferating tubular epithelial cells → are also present, compatible with the tubular injury that can be seen in collapsing glomerulopathy. (Right) Proliferating podocytes → are highlighted by Ki-67 immunohistochemistry in this case of collapsing glomerulopathy.

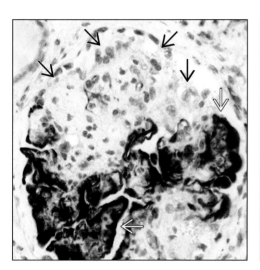 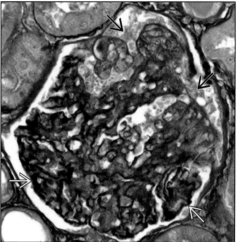

(Left) WT1 stain of glomerulus in collapsing glomerulopathy shows segmental loss of expression in podocytes, a sign of dedifferentiation ⮑. The other 1/2 of the glomerulus stains normally for WT1 ⮑. WT1 inhibits cell proliferation and is characteristically lost in CG. (Right) Loss of the negative charge of the podocytes can be detected by loss of colloidal iron staining as shown segmentally in this glomerulus ⮑. Normal staining is seen in 1/2 of the glomerulus ⮑.

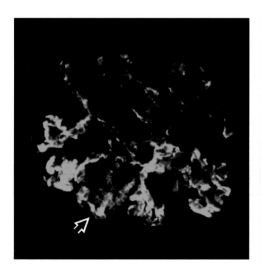 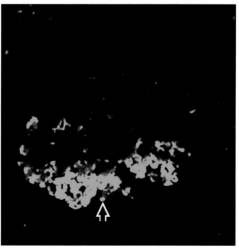

(Left) Immunofluorescence shows segmental IgM deposition in areas of glomerular capillary loop collapse ⮑. (Right) Immunofluorescence shows segmental C3 deposition ⮑ in areas of glomerular capillary loop collapse.

COLLAPSING GLOMERULOPATHY

Tubular Lesions

(Left) Collapsing glomerulopathy typically is accompanied by tubulointerstitial disease, here shown at low power. Marked dilation of proximal tubules filled with PAS positive protein is evident as well as tubular atrophy and interstitial inflammation. **(Right)** This PAS stain shows a glomerulus that has undergone near total collapse with dilatation of Bowman space ➡. Tubules are markedly dilated and contain abundant proteinaceous material ➡.

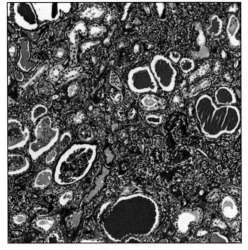
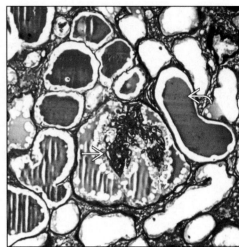

(Left) There is prominent interstitial inflammation amidst these atrophic tubules, many of which have proteinaceous casts ➡. **(Right)** Lymphoid interstitial infiltrates are often prominent in collapsing glomerulopathy and sometimes form lymphoepithelial structures with tubules, as shown here. The presence of tubulointerstitial disease indicates that CG is not exclusively a "podocytopathy."

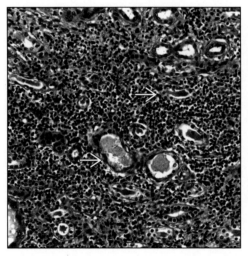
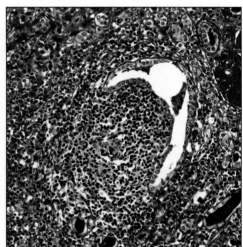

(Left) Just as proliferation of podocytes occurs in collapsing glomerulopathy, proliferation of proximal tubular cells also occurs, as shown here, with a Ki-67 stain. This indicates that proliferation is a more generalized phenomenon in CG. **(Right)** The reactive tubular cells in collapsing glomerulopathy are shed in the tubule, as shown here ➡. The sloughed cells may also include podocytes, which have been detected in the urine.

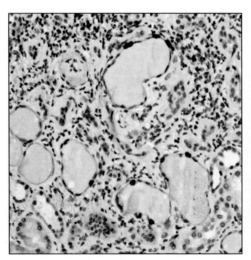
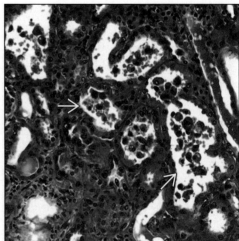

Transplants and Variants

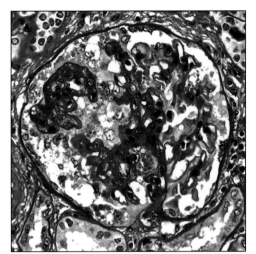

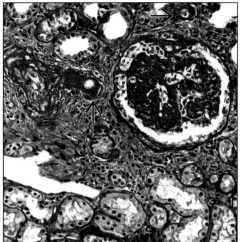

(Left) De novo CG developed in the native kidneys of this patient 10 years post heart-lung transplant. Severe arteriolar hyalinosis was also present. **(Right)** De novo CG developed 8 years post renal transplant while patient was on tacrolimus. The glomerulus shows collapse with prominent podocyte hypercellularity. The arterioles had severe hyalinosis ⮕, associated with de novo CG, and the vascular disease seen here may be a pathogenetic factor.

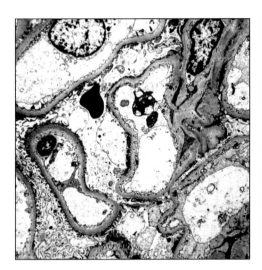

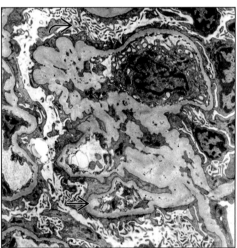

(Left) This biopsy was taken from a 7-year-old boy with recurrent CG 2 days post transplant and shows widespread effacement of foot processes but no collapse, resembling minimal change disease. **(Right)** In a nephrectomy performed for intractable protein loss in a 9-year-old boy with recurrent CG 2 years after transplant, collapse of glomerular capillaries ⮕ and prominent podocyte hypertrophy are shown with villous transformation ⮕. Recurrence began 2 days after transplant.

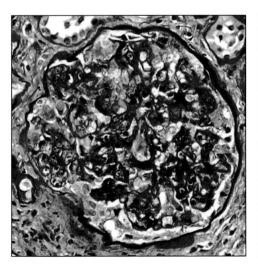

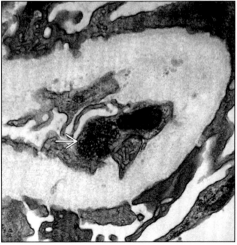

(Left) CG is shown in a woman who developed nephrotic syndrome while on interferon-β for treatment of multiple sclerosis. Collapse and prominent podocyte hyperplasia are present. Intracapillary leukocytes are also present, a feature of the cellular variant of FSGS. **(Right)** In CG present in a woman on interferon-β for treatment of multiple sclerosis, numerous tubuloreticular structures ⮕ were present in the glomerular endothelium, an effect of interferons-α and -β.

PAMIDRONATE-INDUCED COLLAPSING FSGS

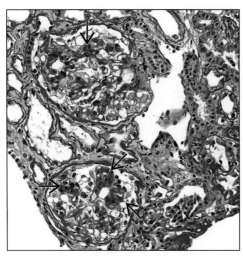

In a 67-year-old woman with multiple myeloma who received pamidronate and developed 50 g/d proteinuria requiring hemodialysis, glomerular capillary loops show segmental occlusion ➡.

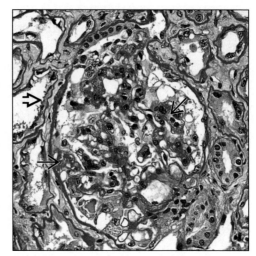

On high power, glomerular capillary loops are segmentally occluded ➡. Tubular injury was present with flattened tubular epithelium ➡.

TERMINOLOGY

Abbreviations
- Focal segmental glomerulosclerosis (FSGS)

Definitions
- Collapsing FSGS secondary to bisphosphonates such as pamidronate (Aredia) used in the treatment of osteolytic metastases, Paget disease, hypercalcemia of malignancy, and postmenopausal osteoporosis (PMO)

ETIOLOGY/PATHOGENESIS

Mechanism Uncertain
- Bisphosphonate binds calcium phosphate crystals within bone matrix, thus inhibiting osteoclast activity
- Podocyte dysfunction is thought to be cause of collapsing FSGS
  - Pamidronate is thought to interfere with podocyte function and metabolism, similar to its metabolic effects on osteoclasts
  - Hypothesis: Podocytes leave their terminally differentiated state and enter the cell cycle, acquiring a more immature phenotype
    - Evidenced by loss of podocyte synaptopodin and increased Ki-67 expression
- Tubular and podocyte mitochondrial injury may also be present
- No evidence of immunologic mechanism (scant infiltrate)

Drug Exposure
- Patients typically used higher than recommended doses
  - Disorder severity depend on dose and infusion time
  - Intravenous route of administration implicated
    - Oral bisphosphonates are mainly used for PMO and do not produce significant nephrotoxicity

- Zoledronate appears to mainly be associated with tubular injury, in contrast to pamidronate

CLINICAL ISSUES

Presentation
- Initial description by Markowitz et al was in older, white, HIV-negative patients
  - Cohort consisted of 5 women and 2 men, 6 with multiple myeloma and 1 with breast cancer with a mean serum creatinine of 3.6 mg/dL and mean urine protein of 12.4 g/d
  - Collapsing FSGS otherwise more common in blacks
- Nephrotic syndrome
- Renal dysfunction/severe renal insufficiency
- Fanconi syndrome

Treatment
- Cessation of pamidronate use
- Prevented by monitoring serum creatinine and adjusting dosage if renal insufficiency is present

Prognosis
- Renal function stabilizes with drug discontinuance
- Some have developed ESRD
- Protein excretion may increase when drug is restarted

MICROSCOPIC PATHOLOGY

Histologic Features
- Glomeruli
  - Collapsing or noncollapsing FSGS
    - Hyperplastic and hypertrophic visceral epithelial cells (podocytes)
    - Global wrinkling and retraction of glomerular basement membrane (GBM)
    - Swollen and contain protein resorption droplets
    - Increased Ki-67 positive cells in Bowman space
  - Minimal change disease has also been described

PAMIDRONATE-INDUCED COLLAPSING FSGS

Key Facts

Terminology
- Collapsing FSGS secondary to use of pamidronate, a bisphosphonate inhibitor of bone resorption

Clinical Issues
- HIV-negative patients with nephrotic syndrome and severe renal insufficiency, typically older and white
- Treatment: Cessation of pamidronate

Microscopic Pathology
- Collapsing FSGS
- Hyperplastic and hypertrophic glomerular epithelial cells
- Tubular injury and simplification
- IF: IgM and C3 segmentally stain glomerular tuft
- EM: GBM wrinkling and collapse
- Podocyte foot processes totally effaced

- Tubules and interstitium
  - Tubular injury and simplification, attributable to toxic acute tubular necrosis
    - Regenerative nuclear atypia
  - Tubular microcyst formation
  - Interstitial edema
  - Interstitial fibrosis eventually occurs
  - Interstitial inflammation is only sparse, without tubulitis or interstitial eosinophils

ANCILLARY TESTS

Immunofluorescence
- Segmental IgM and C3 in glomeruli

Electron Microscopy
- Transmission
  - Global GBM wrinkling and collapse of glomerular capillaries
  - Podocyte foot processes totally effaced
  - Podocyte hypertrophy

DIFFERENTIAL DIAGNOSIS

Collapsing Glomerulopathy of Other Causes
- Careful history is needed since there are no distinguishing features

DIAGNOSTIC CHECKLIST

Pathologic Interpretation Pearls
- Collapsing FSGS has many specific causes, and etiologic diagnosis should be sought

SELECTED REFERENCES
1. Ten Dam MA et al: Nephrotic syndrome induced by pamidronate. Med Oncol. Epub ahead of print, 2010
2. Nagahama M et al: Pamidronate-induced kidney injury in a patient with metastatic breast cancer. Am J Med Sci. 338(3):225-8, 2009
3. Perazella MA et al: Bisphosphonate nephrotoxicity. Kidney Int. 74(11):1385-93, 2008
4. Dijkman HB et al: Proliferating cells in HIV and pamidronate-associated collapsing focal segmental glomerulosclerosis are parietal epithelial cells. Kidney Int. 70(2):338-44, 2006
5. Desikan R et al: Nephrotic proteinuria associated with high-dose pamidronate in multiple myeloma. Br J Haematol. 119(2):496-9, 2002
6. Markowitz GS et al: Nephrotic syndrome after treatment with pamidronate. Am J Kidney Dis. 39(5):1118-22, 2002
7. Markowitz GS et al: Collapsing focal segmental glomerulosclerosis following treatment with high-dose pamidronate. J Am Soc Nephrol. 12(6):1164-72, 2001

IMAGE GALLERY

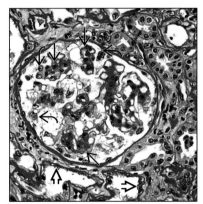 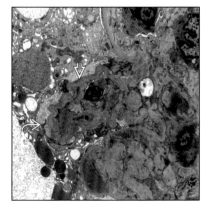 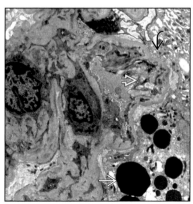

(Left) Glomerular capillary loops show segmental collapse ➡ with overlying podocyte hyperplasia ➡. Tubular injury can be observed with flattening of the tubular epithelium ➡. *(Center)* EM shows extensive foot process effacement (FPE) ➡, and glomerular capillary loops show nearly complete collapse ➡. *(Right)* EM shows extensive FPE ➡, glomerular capillary loop collapse ➡, and resorption droplets within podocytes ➡.

IgM NEPHROPATHY

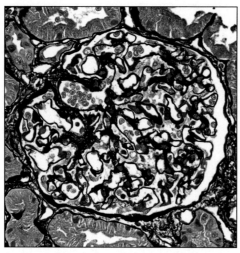

Most cases of IgM nephropathy have normal glomeruli by light microscopy. This biopsy from a child with nephrotic syndrome had 3+ IgM staining on immunofluorescence microscopy.

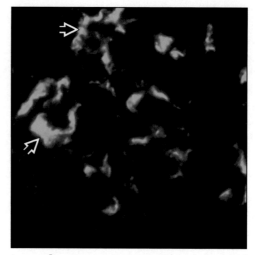

Immunofluorescence microscopy with antisera to IgM shows 3+ intensity mesangial ➡ staining. The light microscopy was entirely normal in this biopsy with a diagnosis of IgM nephropathy.

TERMINOLOGY

Abbreviations
- IgM nephropathy (IgMN)

Definitions
- Idiopathic glomerular disease characterized by dominant diffuse mesangial IgM immune deposits (≥ 2+ intensity) in nonsclerotic glomeruli
  - Described independently in 1978 by Cohen, Bhasin, and colleagues
  - Relationship to minimal change disease (MCD) and focal segmental glomerulosclerosis (FSGS) debated

ETIOLOGY/PATHOGENESIS

Presumed Immunologic Pathogenesis
- Dysregulated T-lymphocyte response with altered proportions of T-cell subsets
- Impaired B lymphocyte IgM to IgG switch in vitro
  - Elevated IgM levels
  - Elevated IgM circulating immune complexes
- Defective clearance of immune deposits by mesangial cells postulated

CLINICAL ISSUES

Epidemiology
- Incidence
  - Difficult to assess due to lack of uniform diagnostic criteria and indication for biopsy
    - In 1 series, 5% of medical kidney biopsies
- Age
  - Occurs in both children and adults
    - 1-75 years old; mean = 29 years
- Gender
  - Men presented with NS while women presented predominantly with isolated hematuria

Presentation
- Nephrotic syndrome
  - Presentation similar to MCD but with greater frequency of hypertension and hematuria
- Microhematuria
  - Can be isolated with no significant proteinuria

Natural History
- A few cases demonstrate evolution to FSGS on repeat biopsies, suggesting pathogenic link

Treatment
- Drugs
  - Corticosteroids
    - Up to 50% steroid dependent or steroid resistant
  - Cyclosporine or cyclophosphamide in steroid-resistant cases
  - Isolated case reports of rituximab response
- Recurs in transplants

Prognosis
- Long-term prognosis of steroid-responsive cases is good
- ~ 17% progress to chronic kidney disease

MICROSCOPIC PATHOLOGY

Histologic Features
- Glomeruli
  - Normal by light microscopy (~ 35%)
  - Mild segmental mesangial hypercellularity (~ 32%)
  - Mild mesangial sclerosis (~ 35%)
  - Global sclerosis (~ 15%)
- Tubules
  - Tubular atrophy in minority (~ 20%)
  - Acute tubular injury can be present
- Interstitium
  - Fibrosis or inflammation in minority (~ 7%)
- Vessels
  - Hyalinosis (~ 20%), intimal fibrosis (~ 5%)

IgM NEPHROPATHY

Key Facts

Terminology
- Idiopathic glomerular disease with dominant IgM immune deposits (≥ 2+ intensity)

Clinical Issues
- Studies have not used uniform criteria for diagnosis
- Occurs in both children and adults
- Nephrotic syndrome most common presentation, often with steroid dependance or resistance

Microscopic Pathology
- Glomeruli may appear entirely normal
- Mild segmental mesangial hypercellularity observed in minority

Ancillary Tests
- Diffuse foot process effacement
- Amorphous, mesangial electron-dense deposits in ~ 50% of cases

ANCILLARY TESTS

Immunofluorescence
- IgM mesangial deposits of ≥ 2+ intensity
- C3 mesangial deposits are often identified
- Low intensity (trace to 1+) IgG, IgA, and C1q staining can be observed due to nonspecific entrapment

Electron Microscopy
- Diffuse foot process effacement
- Mesangial, electron-dense deposits in ~ 50%

DIFFERENTIAL DIAGNOSIS

Minimal Change Disease
- Segmental low-intensity mesangial IgM may be observed in MCD due to nonspecific entrapment
- IgMN reserved for cases with ≥ 2+ IgM

Focal Segmental Glomerulosclerosis
- Minority of FSGS have ≥ 2+ IgM staining
- FSGS diagnosis should supersede IgMN

Immune Complex-mediated Diseases
- IgA nephropathy
  - Dominant or codominant IgA deposits
- Mesangioproliferative lupus nephritis
  - IgG dominant with IgA, IgM, C3, C1q ("full house")

Diffuse Mesangial Hypercellularity
- > 4 cells/mesangial area involving > 80% of glomeruli

- Occasional cases have IgM and C3 deposits

DIAGNOSTIC CHECKLIST

Pathologic Interpretation Pearls
- FSGS must be excluded

SELECTED REFERENCES
1. Betjes MG et al: Resolution of IgM nephropathy after rituximab treatment. Am J Kidney Dis. 53(6):1059-62, 2009
2. Swartz SJ et al: Minimal change disease with IgM+ immunofluorescence: a subtype of nephrotic syndrome. Pediatr Nephrol. 24(6):1187-92, 2009
3. Silverstein DM et al: Mesangial hypercellularity in children: presenting features and outcomes. Pediatr Nephrol. 23(6):921-8, 2008
4. Myllymäki J et al: IgM nephropathy: clinical picture and long-term prognosis. Am J Kidney Dis. 41(2):343-50, 2003
5. O'Donoghue DJ et al: IgM-associated primary diffuse mesangial proliferative glomerulonephritis: natural history and prognostic indicators. Q J Med. 79(288):333-50, 1991
6. Lin CY et al: In vitro B-lymphocyte switch disturbance from IgM into IgG in IgM mesangial nephropathy. Pediatr Nephrol. 3(3):254-8, 1989
7. Helin H et al: IgM-associated glomerulonephritis. Nephron. 31(1):11-6, 1982
8. Bhasin HK et al: Mesangial proliferative glomerulonephritis. Lab Invest. 39(1):21-9, 1978
9. Cohen AH et al: Nehprotic syndrome with glomerular mesangial IgM deposits. Lab Invest. 38(5):610-9, 1978

IMAGE GALLERY

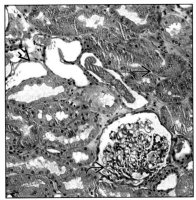 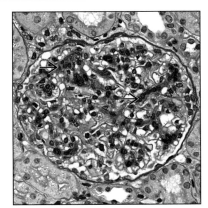 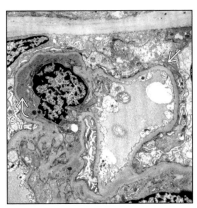

(Left) The renal biopsy with IgM nephropathy shows normal glomeruli ➡, but the proximal tubules demonstrate protein reabsorption droplets ➡, dilated lumens, and attenuated epithelium ➡. *(Center)* Mild segmental mesangial hypercellularity ➡ may be seen in IgMN, as demonstrated in this biopsy specimen with ~ 20% of glomeruli affected. *(Right)* The electron microscopy of IgMN reveals widespread foot process effacement ➡ and mesangial electron-dense deposits ➡.

MEMBRANOUS GLOMERULONEPHRITIS, PRIMARY

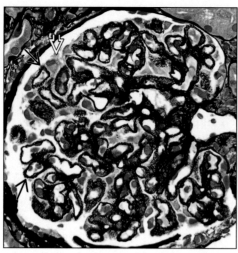

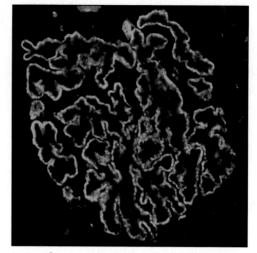

Jones methenamine silver stain shows focal subepithelial "spike" formation ⇨ and a prominent vacuolated appearance ⮞, which correlates with Ehrenreich-Churg stages III-IV.

Immunofluorescence microscopy for IgG shows intense granular to confluent staining of the capillary walls without definite mesangial staining, which is characteristic of primary MGN.

TERMINOLOGY

Abbreviations
- Membranous glomerulonephritis (MGN)

Synonyms
- Membranous nephropathy
- Membranous glomerulopathy
- Epimembranous nephropathy

Definitions
- Idiopathic chronic glomerular disease characterized by diffuse subepithelial immune complex deposits with intervening formation of matrix ("spikes") and nephrotic-range proteinuria

ETIOLOGY/PATHOGENESIS

Autoimmune Disease with In Situ Glomerular Immune Complex Formation
- Antigen is believed to be on podocyte surface
- IgG4 subclass autoantibodies predominant
- 4 autoantigens have been identified
  - M-type phospholipase A_2 receptor (PLA2R)
    - Expressed on podocytes and proximal tubules
    - IgG4 anti-PLA2R detected in ~ 70% of 1° MGN
    - Colocalized with IgG4 in glomeruli
    - Proteinuria can persist for months after therapy even when autoantibodies are undetectable
  - Aldose reductase (AR) and manganese superoxide dismutase 2 (SOD2)
    - Circulating and glomerular IgG4 recognizes these antigens and colocalizes to subepithelial deposits of MGN
    - AR and SOD2 are normally expressed in tubular epithelial cells, **not** glomeruli, and may be upregulated on podocytes in primary MGN
  - Membrane metalloendopeptidase (MME), also known as neutral endopeptidase or CD10

- Expressed on human podocytes and proximal tubular brush borders
- Rare cause of neonatal form of MGN in mothers with absent MME; unclear role in adult MGN
- Maternal anti-MME antibodies cross placenta and deposit on fetal podocytes
- 1st human antigenic target of MGN identified; subsequently, several other families reported
- Antigenic target(s) in secondary forms different from PLA2R but not yet identified

Genetic Factors
- 2 strongly linked loci in genome-wide SNP association studies
  - HLA-DQA1 allele
  - PLA2R allele
- May facilitate presentation of autoantigen

Other Mechanisms
- Planted antigen from circulation or deposition of circulating immune complexes were once postulated but have little supporting evidence in primary MGN

Animal Model of MGN
- Heymann nephritis in rats
  - Megalin is target antigen (Fx1A) on podocytes and proximal tubular brush borders
    - TBM deposits also present (vs. human MGN)
    - **Not** expressed on human podocytes, and no megalin antibodies described in humans

CLINICAL ISSUES

Epidemiology
- Incidence
  - 6-10% of native kidney biopsies in adults, ~ 3% in children (< 18 years old)
- Age
  - Peak: 30-50 years
- Gender

MEMBRANOUS GLOMERULONEPHRITIS, PRIMARY

Key Facts

Etiology/Pathogenesis
- Autoantibodies to PLA2R on podocyte
- Congenital form due to MME antibodies

Clinical Issues
- Nephrotic syndrome
- Insidious onset, ~ 33% progress to ESRD
- Peak age: 30-50 years

Microscopic Pathology
- Diffuse thickening of glomerular capillary wall
- Subepithelial "spikes" in PAS and Jones methenamine silver stains
- Immunofluorescence
  ○ Diffuse granular deposits along GBM that stain for IgG, usually C3
  ○ IgG4 usually dominant subclass

Electron microscopy
  ○ Subepithelial amorphous deposits
  ○ Intervening "spikes" of GBM
  ○ Deposits resurfaced by GBM and resorbed
  ○ Status of deposits is basis of staging

Top Differential Diagnoses
- Membranous lupus nephritis
- Postinfectious glomerulonephritis

Diagnostic Checklist
- Can occur with other diseases, such as diabetic nephropathy or crescentic GN
- Adverse pathologic prognostic features include interstitial fibrosis and tubular atrophy, FSGS, arteriosclerosis, and mixed stage deposits

---

  ○ M:F ratio = 2:1
- Ethnicity
  ○ Caucasian predilection

Presentation
- Nephrotic syndrome
- Proteinuria, asymptomatic
- Hematuria
  ○ Usually microscopic, rarely gross hematuria
- Renal vein thrombosis

Treatment
- Drugs
  ○ Variety of drugs used with limited success
    ▪ Prednisone
    ▪ Mycophenolate mofetil
    ▪ Rituximab
    ▪ Cyclophosphamide/chlorambucil

Prognosis
- 50% 10-year renal survival (90% in Japan)
- 33% spontaneously remit
- 33% stable with proteinuria with little progression
- 33% progress to end-stage renal disease (ESRD)
  ○ 10-30% recur after kidney transplantation
    ▪ 1 week to many years
    ▪ Graft loss occurs in 10-50% of recurrent MGN
  ○ Adverse clinical prognostic features: Nephrotic syndrome, azotemia, hypertension

MICROSCOPIC PATHOLOGY

Histologic Features
- Glomerulus
  ○ GBM thickened on H&E
  ○ Little or no increase in mesangial hypercellularity
  ○ Subepithelial "spike" formation or vacuolated appearance (when sectioned en face) on PAS or Jones silver stain
  ○ GBM may appear normal when only stage I deposits are seen by EM
  ○ Glomerulosclerosis

    ▪ Segmental
    ▪ Global
  ○ No inflammatory infiltrate in glomerulus
    ▪ Presence of leukocytes suggests renal vein thrombosis or other mechanisms superimposed (anti-GBM, ANCA)
- Tubules
  ○ Tubular protein resorption droplets
- Interstitium
  ○ Interstitial foam cells variably present
  ○ Interstitial fibrosis and tubular atrophy in later stages
- Vessels
  ○ Arteriosclerosis common
- Variants

Variants
- MGN and anti-GBM disease (rare)
  ○ Crescentic glomerular injury often diffuse
    ▪ Positive anti-GBM antibody titer
    ▪ Linear IgG staining of GBM along with granular staining of capillary walls
- MGN and antineutrophil cytoplasmic antibody (ANCA) disease (rare)
  ○ Necrotizing glomerular lesions with crescents
  ○ Positive ANCA titer
- MGN and anti-tubular basement membrane disease (rare)
  ○ Linear IgG staining of tubular basement membranes and prominent interstitial inflammation
  ○ Typically presents at < 5 years of age

ANCILLARY TESTS

Immunofluorescence
- Diffuse, fine deposits along GBM that stain for IgG and kappa and lambda light chains ± complement components; IgA and IgM usually not prominent
  ○ IgG4 is dominant subclass
  ○ Global (> 50% of single glomerulus) staining of capillary walls is typically seen, but segmental involvement may be present

○ Extent of complement deposition may correlate with renal function deterioration
- Little or no mesangial deposits
  ○ Tangential sections of GBM may be hard to distinguish from mesangial deposits
- No TBM immunoglobulin deposits

Electron Microscopy

- Subepithelial electron-dense deposits with intervening "spikes" of matrix
- 4 stages have been described by Ehrenreich and Churg
  ○ Stage I: Subepithelial deposits without significant basement membrane reaction between deposits
  ○ Stage II: Subepithelial basement membrane material ("spikes") present between subepithelial deposits
  ○ Stage III: Subepithelial (or intramembranous) deposits with basement membrane material between and surrounding deposits
  ○ Stage IV: Electron-lucent areas probably representing resorption of prior subepithelial immune complexes
- Location
  ○ Strictly subepithelial (and later, intramembranous)
  ○ Bowman capsular deposits occasionally reported
  ○ Mesangial deposits and subendothelial deposits suggest secondary forms (e.g., lupus nephritis)
  ○ TBM deposits generally suggest secondary MGN, such as lupus MGN
- Substructure
  ○ Usually amorphous
  ○ Microspherular substructural organization reported in primary MGN
    ▪ Neonatal form of MGN due to MME mutation shows microspherular substructure in subepithelial deposits
  ○ Substructural organization raises possibility of cryoglobulinemic glomerulonephritis or membranous lupus nephritis

DIFFERENTIAL DIAGNOSIS

Membranous Lupus Nephritis

- Favored by presence of mesangial deposits, full house (IgG, IgA, IgM, C3, C1q), tubuloreticular structures, and TBM deposits
- Deposits sometimes penetrate GBM and are associated with subendothelial deposits

Secondary Membranous Glomerulonephritis

- Mesangial deposits often present
- Usually no autoantibodies to PLA2R

Postinfectious Glomerulonephritis

- Lack of "spikes" around humps
- Deposits in mesangium and subendothelial space
- Intraglomerular inflammation and hypercellularity

DIAGNOSTIC CHECKLIST

Clinically Relevant Pathologic Features

- Adverse prognostic features
  ○ Interstitial fibrosis and tubular atrophy

▪ Inflammatory infiltrate of T cells and macrophages
○ Arteriosclerosis severity
○ Focal segmental glomerulosclerosis (FSGS)
  ▪ May be associated with decreased creatinine clearance at presentation
○ Homogeneous (single-stage) deposits may have better outcome
○ Heterogeneous (multistage) deposits
  ▪ Extent and stage of deposits not consistently correlated with outcome

Pathologic Interpretation Pearls

- MGN can occur concurrently with many renal diseases, such as diabetic nephropathy or crescentic GN

SELECTED REFERENCES

1. Cybulsky AV: Membranous nephropathy. Contrib Nephrol. 169:107-25, 2011
2. Stanescu HC et al: Risk HLA-DQA1 and PLA(2)R1 alleles in idiopathic membranous nephropathy. N Engl J Med. 364(7):616-26, 2011
3. Prunotto M et al: Autoimmunity in membranous nephropathy targets aldose reductase and SOD2. J Am Soc Nephrol. 21(3):507-19, 2010
4. Beck LH Jr et al: M-type phospholipase A2 receptor as target antigen in idiopathic membranous nephropathy. N Engl J Med. 361(1):11-21, 2009
5. Nasr SH et al: Membranous glomerulonephritis with ANCA-associated necrotizing and crescentic glomerulonephritis. Clin J Am Soc Nephrol. 4(2):299-308, 2009
6. Kowalewska J et al: Membranous glomerulopathy with spherules: an uncommon variant with obscure pathogenesis. Am J Kidney Dis. 47(6):983-92, 2006
7. Troxell ML et al: Concurrent anti-glomerular basement membrane disease and membranous glomerulonephritis: a case report and literature review. Clin Nephrol. 66(2):120-7, 2006
8. Troyanov S et al: Renal pathology in idiopathic membranous nephropathy: a new perspective. Kidney Int. 69(9):1641-8, 2006
9. Debiec H et al: Antenatal membranous glomerulonephritis due to anti-neutral endopeptidase antibodies. N Engl J Med. 346(26):2053-60, 2002
10. Beck L et al: Anti-PLA2R autoantibodies and response to Rituximab treatment in membranous nephropathy. J Am Soc Nephrol (in press)
11. Qin W et al: Antiphospholipase A2 receptor antibody in Chinese patients with membranous nephropathy. J Am Soc Nephrol (in press)

MEMBRANOUS GLOMERULONEPHRITIS, PRIMARY

Microscopic Features

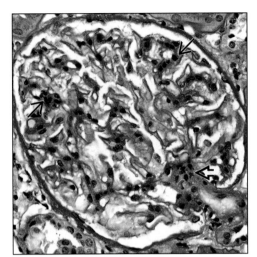
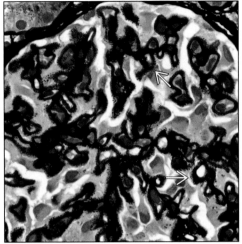

(Left) Periodic acid-Schiff may not demonstrate apparent GBM abnormalities when changes associated with MGN occur early. There is mild mesangial hypercellularity ➡, which should be assessed in areas removed from the vascular pole ➡. (Right) Jones methenamine silver reveals a "hair on end" pattern of subepithelial spikes of GBM in most capillaries ➡, best appreciated on well stained 2-3 μm silver or PAS stains under 100x oil.

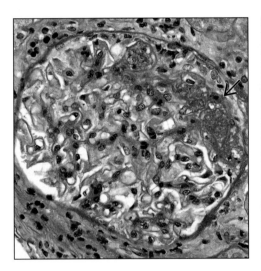
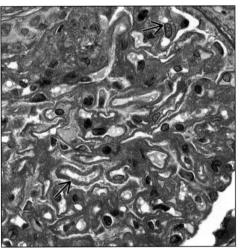

(Left) Periodic acid-Schiff demonstrates segmental sclerosis ➡ in a case of MGN. By light microscopy, the GBM abnormalities are not obvious, and the pathologic findings could be mistaken for focal segmental glomerulosclerosis in the absence of immunofluorescence or electron microscopy. (Right) Periodic acid-Schiff shows prominent thickening of the GBM with a hint of a vacuolated appearance ➡ that is not as distinct when compared with the Jones methenamine silver stain.

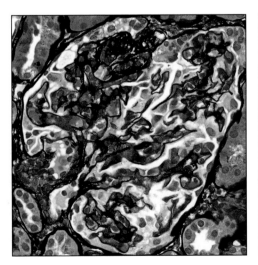
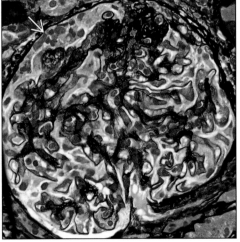

(Left) Jones methenamine silver shows some segmental sclerosis with a fibrous attachment to Bowman capsule and loss of the adjacent glomerular capillary lumina. The GBM shows a vacuolated appearance characteristic of MGN. (Right) Jones methenamine silver shows a small cellular crescent ➡ in this patient with a positive ANCA titer, which is consistent with a pauci-immune crescentic glomerulonephritis superimposed on MGN.

MEMBRANOUS GLOMERULONEPHRITIS, PRIMARY

Immunofluorescence

(Left) Immunofluorescence microscopy for IgG reveals strong and diffuse granular staining along the glomerular capillaries ➡ without mesangial staining in a case of MGN. This pattern of staining is characteristic of MGN.
(Right) Immunofluorescence microscopy for C3 reveals granular staining along the glomerular capillaries that is usually less intense and less extensive than IgG.

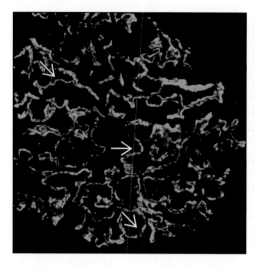 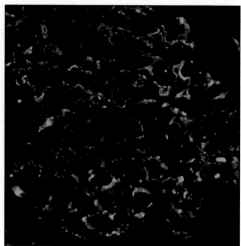

(Left) Immunofluorescence microscopy for kappa light chain demonstrates a granular staining pattern of the glomerular capillary walls similar to lambda, but the intensity is typically less than IgG. *(Right)* Immunofluorescence microscopy for lambda light chain shows a granular staining pattern of the capillary walls similar to kappa light chains. This finding excludes the consideration of a monoclonal immunoglobulin deposition disease.

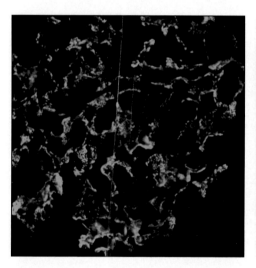 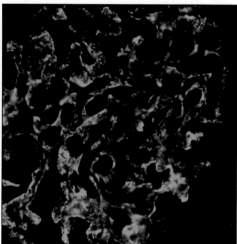

(Left) Immunofluorescence microscopy in MGN typically shows scanty IgA in the GBM deposits as shown by this case. Prominent IgA is more common in lupus membranous nephritis.
(Right) Immunofluorescence microscopy for C1q shows weak granular staining of the glomerular capillaries that is not always present. While this finding may raise the consideration of a secondary form of MGN, this can also be observed in primary cases of MGN. Here the deposits appear to be mainly mesangial.

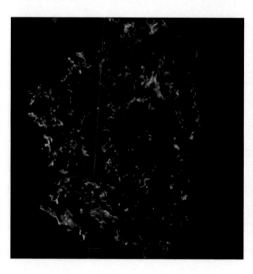 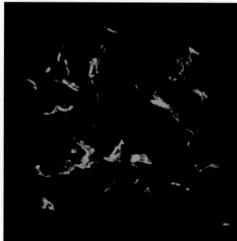

MEMBRANOUS GLOMERULONEPHRITIS, PRIMARY

Immunofluorescence: IgG Subclasses and PLA2R

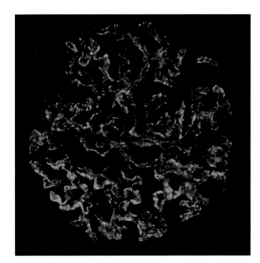 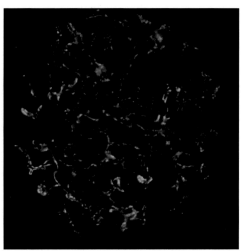

(Left) The granular deposits along the GBM stain moderately well with antibody to the IgG1 subclass in MGN. However, the most prominent subclass is usually IgG4. (Right) The granular deposits along the GBM stain only weakly with antibody to the IgG2 subclass in MGN. The most prominent subclass is usually IgG4, followed by IgG1.

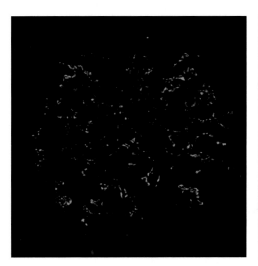 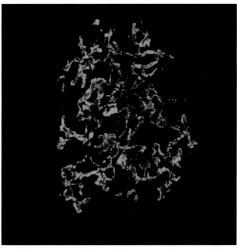

(Left) The granular deposits along the GBM stain only weakly with antibody to the IgG3 subclass in MGN. The most prominent subclass is usually IgG4, followed by IgG1. (Right) Immunofluorescence stain for IgG4 shows a similar granular pattern as the accompanying stain for phospholipase A2 receptor in a case of MGN. (Courtesy A.B. Collins, BS.)

 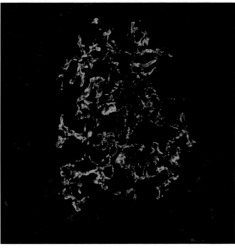

(Left) IF stain for PLA2R in a case of MGN. Granular staining in the GBM codistributes with IgG4 staining. Proximal tubules also stain for PLA2R. (Courtesy A.B. Collins, BS.) (Right) Merged image of IF photomicrographs in a case of MGN stained for PLA2R (red) and IgG4 (green) is shown. The GBM deposits stain yellow, indicating colocalization, consistent with the evidence that glomerular PLA2R is a target autoantigen in MGN. (Courtesy A.B. Collins, BS.)

MEMBRANOUS GLOMERULONEPHRITIS, PRIMARY

Electron Microscopy: Ehrenreich-Churg Stages

(Left) Electron microscopy reveals small discrete subepithelial electron-dense deposits ➡ without prominent basement membrane reaction to these MGN deposits, which is consistent with Ehrenreich-Churg stage I. There is diffuse effacement of the podocyte foot processes ➢. *(Right)* Electron microscopy shows small subepithelial deposits ➢ without significant basement membrane reaction to these deposits, which corresponds with minimal glomerular basement membrane alterations by light microscopy.

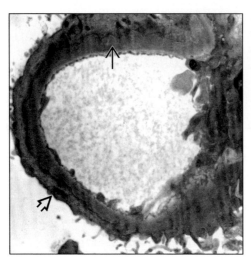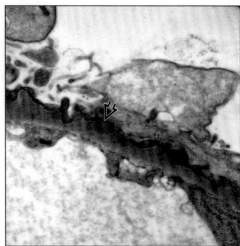

(Left) Electron microscopy shows discrete subepithelial deposits with variable basement membrane reaction, which corresponds to Ehrenreich-Churg stages I ➡ and II ➢ changes. Such minor alterations of the GBM may be difficult to identify by light microscopy. *(Right)* Electron microscopy reveals several subepithelial deposits consistent with Ehrenreich-Churg stages I ➢ and II ➡. The overlying podocyte foot processes are diffusely effaced.

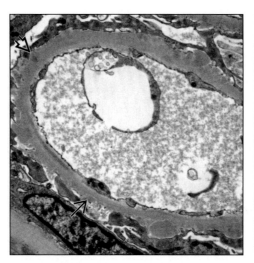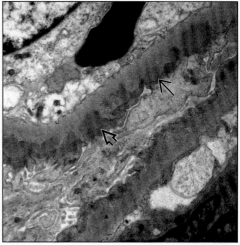

(Left) EM shows discrete subepithelial deposits with "spike" formation of basement membrane material (Ehrenreich-Churg stage II). *(Right)* EM shows variably sized subepithelial deposits completely surrounded by basement membrane material ➢ that correspond to Ehrenreich-Churg stage III. Variable reabsorption of these deposits is present, with 1 that is almost completely reabsorbed ➡. The podocyte foot processes show diffuse effacement ➡.

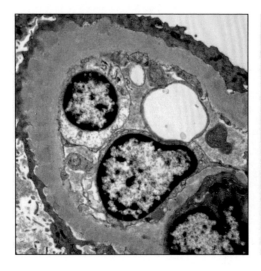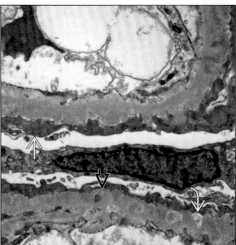

2

Electron Microscopy

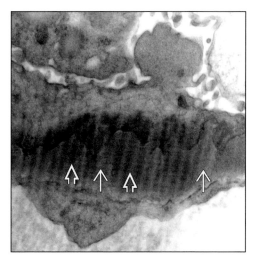

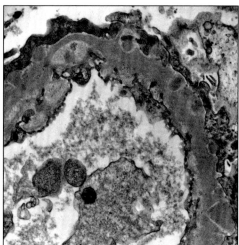

(Left) Electron microscopy at high magnification reveals several medium to large subepithelial electron-dense deposits ⮞ that are typical of the subepithelial deposits of MGN. Basement membrane material correlates with "spikes" ➔ that can be visualized by light microscopy in this MGN case with stage II Ehrenreich-Churg changes. (Right) EM shows small subepithelial deposits with electron-lucent areas consistent with stage II and IV changes.

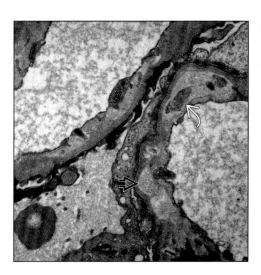

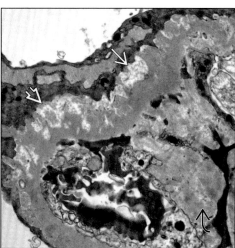

(Left) Electron microscopy demonstrates remodeling of the GBM with electron-lucent areas ⮞ that represent reabsorbed immune complexes. Some small deposits remain ➔. These findings are consistent with predominantly Ehrenreich-Churg stage IV changes. (Right) EM shows partially ⮞ to completely ➔ reabsorbed subepithelial deposits in an advanced MGN case. Increased mesangial matrix ⮞ is noted in this diabetic patient with early features of diabetic nephropathy.

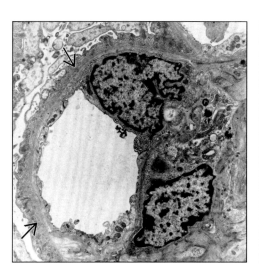

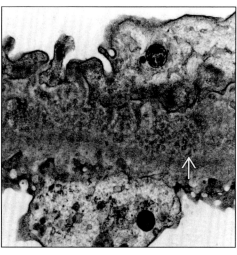

(Left) Electron microscopy shows an unusual case of MGN with microspherular subepithelial deposits ➔. This finding has been observed in both primary and secondary MGN cases, as well as in patients with the neonatal form of MGN due to neutral endopeptidase antibodies. (Courtesy J. Kowalewska, MD.) (Right) Electron microscopy reveals a microspherular substructure ➔ in the subepithelial deposits of this MGN case. (Courtesy J. Kowalewska, MD.)

MEMBRANOUS GLOMERULONEPHRITIS, PRIMARY

Variant Microscopic Features

(Left) Periodic acid-Schiff reveals a fibrocellular crescent ➡ in a glomerulus with prominent thickening of the GBM in a patient with positive ANCA titers. The constellation of findings is consistent with pauci-immune, ANCA-associated crescentic GN superimposed upon MGN. (Right) Jones methenamine silver confirms the fibrocellular nature of a crescent ➡ with focal disruption of Bowman capsule ⮞ and scarring of a portion of this glomerular tuft.

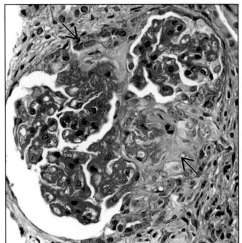
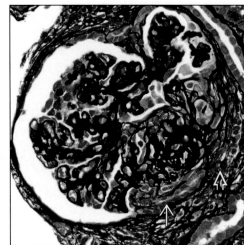

(Left) Jones methenamine silver shows an early crescent ➡ in a patient with positive ANCA titer. The presence of many glomerular crescents should raise the consideration of a superimposed pauci-immune crescentic injury even if the ANCA titers are negative. (Right) Hematoxylin & eosin shows a cellular crescent ➡ in the urinary space that compresses and obscures the residual glomerulus ⮞ and its tufts from a patient with both anti-GBM disease and MGN. (Courtesy M. Troxell, MD, PhD.)

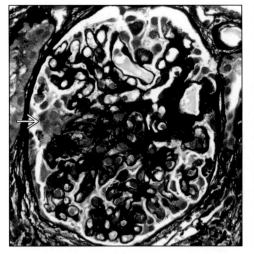
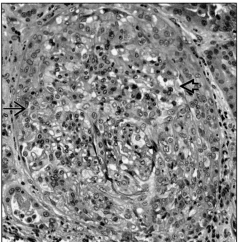

(Left) Periodic acid-Schiff shows a cellular crescent ⮞ filling up Bowman space from a glomerulus with anti-GBM disease superimposed upon MGN. The residual glomerular tufts show no evidence of endocapillary hypercellularity ➡. (Courtesy M. Troxell, MD, PhD.) (Right) Immunofluorescence microscopy for IgG shows both strong linear ➡ and granular ⮞ staining of the glomerular basement membranes consistent with anti-GBM disease and concurrent MGN. (Courtesy M. Troxell, MD, PhD.)

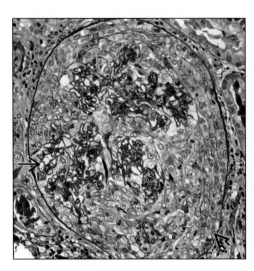
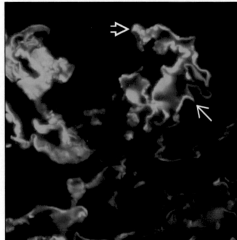

MEMBRANOUS GLOMERULONEPHRITIS, PRIMARY

Variant Microscopic Features

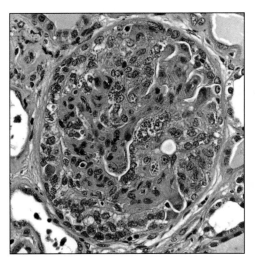

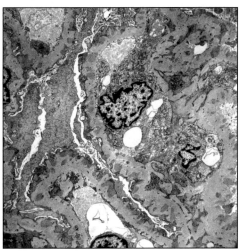

(Left) In a 24-year-old man on dialysis (nephrectomy for renal cell carcinoma) with a history of nephrotic syndrome, H&E shows MGN with collapsing glomerulopathy. The collapsing lesion is superimposed on end-stage MGN. *(Right)* EM shows still apparently recent (stage II) amorphous electron-dense deposits in MGN with end-stage renal disease. The 24-year-old man on dialysis (nephrectomy for renal cell carcinoma) with a history of nephrotic syndrome also had collapsing lesions.

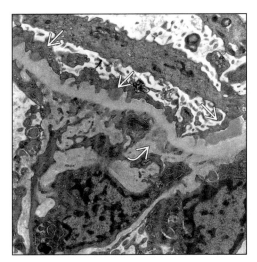

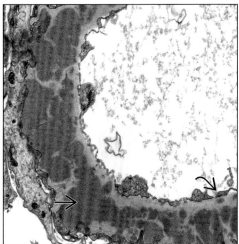

(Left) Recurrent MGN in an allograft 7 years after transplantation is shown. Subepithelial amorphous deposits are present ➡ with surrounding spikes, as well as mesangial deposits ➡, which are not uncommon in late allografts. *(Right)* Electron micrograph of a glomerular capillary loop in a patient with membranous lupus nephritis (Class V) is shown. Deposits that penetrate the GBM ➡ and lie under the endothelium ➡ are present. These features favor a diagnosis of lupus over primary MGN.

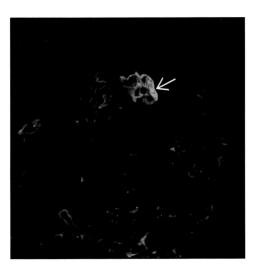

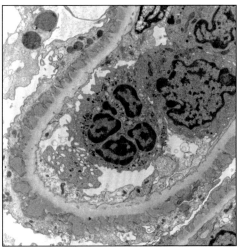

(Left) Immunofluorescence microscopy for fibrinogen stains a glomerular capillary thrombus ➡ in an MGN patient with nephrotic syndrome, renal vein thrombosis, and deep venous thromboses. *(Right)* Electron micrograph shows a glomerular capillary loop in MGN with luminal neutrophils and monocytes, which are associated with renal vein thrombosis. However, the finding is not highly specific or sensitive.

MEMBRANOUS GLOMERULONEPHRITIS, SECONDARY

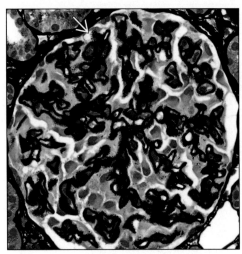

Jones methenamine silver reveals discrete subepithelial "spike" formation ➡ along all of the glomerular capillaries in this patient with both Sjögren syndrome and MGN.

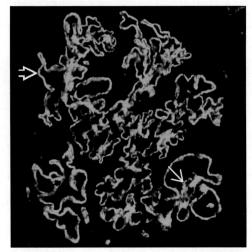

Immunofluorescence microscopy for IgG shows characteristic granular staining of the capillary walls ➡ in MGN. Additional granular mesangial staining ➡ is suggestive of secondary MGN.

TERMINOLOGY

Abbreviations
- Secondary membranous glomerulonephritis (2° MGN)

Synonyms
- Membranous nephropathy
- Membranous glomerulopathy
- Membranous glomerulonephropathy
- Epimembranous nephropathy

Definitions
- MGN in association with underlying disorder, infection, or administration of therapeutic agent

ETIOLOGY/PATHOGENESIS

Antibody Response
- Chronic response to organisms, self-antigens, or alloantigens that persist for months to years
  - Subepithelial deposits probably result from in situ immune complex formation (glomerular antigen)
  - Mesangial immune complexes probably are caused by circulating immune complexes
  - Mesangial immune complexes and subepithelial deposits may also be result of "planted" antigens from circulation

Conditions Associated with Secondary MGN
- Infectious agents
  - Hepatitis B
  - Hepatitis C
  - HIV
  - Epstein-Barr virus
  - Syphilis
- Autoimmune disorders
  - Systemic lupus erythematosus
  - Rheumatoid arthritis (RA)

- In the past, RA patients have been treated with gold or penicillamine, which are also associated with MGN
  - Sjögren syndrome
  - Mixed connective tissue disease
- Neoplasms
  - Carcinoma
    - Lung
    - Colon
    - Stomach
    - Breast
    - Bladder
    - Prostate
    - Kidney
    - Pancreas
  - Carcinoid
  - Lymphoma/leukemia
  - Melanoma
- Hematopoietic cell transplantation (HCT)
  - Most MGN cases associated with graft-vs.-host disease in allogeneic HCT
  - Rare in autologous HCT
- Pharmacologic agents
  - Gold
  - Penicillamine
  - α-glucosidase
    - Autoantibodies to recombinant α-glucosidase therapy associated with MGN in patients with Pompe disease
  - Bucillamine
  - Lithium
  - Mercury
  - Formaldehyde
  - Captopril
  - NSAIDs
  - Fluconazole
- Sarcoidosis
- Sickle cell disease
- Neurofibromatosis

MEMBRANOUS GLOMERULONEPHRITIS, SECONDARY

Key Facts

Terminology
- MGN in association with underlying disorder, infection, or administration of therapeutic agent

Etiology/Pathogenesis
- Common disease associations in secondary MGN include
  - Hepatitis B
  - Hepatitis C
  - Systemic lupus erythematosus
  - Rheumatoid arthritis
  - Carcinoma
  - Lymphoma/leukemia

Clinical Issues
- Nephrotic syndrome

Microscopic Pathology
- GBM thickening or subepithelial "spike" formation
- Mesangial hypercellularity may be present
- Glomerulitis, or increased circulating leukocytes within glomerular capillaries, reported in association with underlying malignancy

Ancillary Tests
- Electron microscopy
  - Subepithelial electron-dense deposits
  - Mesangial electron-dense deposits

Top Differential Diagnoses
- Primary (idiopathic) MGN
- Membranous (class V) lupus nephritis
- Combined MGN and IgA nephropathy

CLINICAL ISSUES

Presentation
- Proteinuria
- Nephrotic syndrome
- Edema

Laboratory Tests
- Urinalysis

Treatment
- Drugs
  - If primary cause is known, treatment may be directed at this process

Prognosis
- Dependent on underlying (or secondary) cause of MGN

MICROSCOPIC PATHOLOGY

Histologic Features
- GBM thickening or subepithelial "spike" formation
  - GBM may appear normal
- Mesangial hypercellularity may be present
- Glomerulitis, or increased circulating leukocytes within glomerular capillaries, reported in association with underlying malignancy
  - Glomerular capillary thrombi have been reported in subset of MGN associated with malignancies
- Tubules, interstitium, and vessels have no specific lesions

ANCILLARY TESTS

Immunofluorescence
- Granular capillary wall staining for IgG and kappa and lambda light chains ± complement components
  - IgG1 and IgG2 described in subepithelial deposits of MGN associated with carcinoma

- IgG3 is dominant subclass in membranous lupus nephritis
- Rare cases with carcinoembryonic antigen in deposits

Electron Microscopy
- Transmission
  - Subepithelial electron-dense deposits
  - Mesangial electron-dense deposits
  - Endothelial tubuloreticular inclusions may be observed in systemic lupus erythematosus or viral infections, such as hepatitis or HIV
  - Bowman capsular electron-dense deposits: Generally found in lupus nephritis, but a few idiopathic MGN cases have been reported
  - Tubular basement membrane electron-dense deposits: Generally associated with lupus nephritis

DIFFERENTIAL DIAGNOSIS

Primary (Idiopathic) MGN
- Subepithelial without mesangial immune complex deposition

Combined MGN and IgA Nephropathy
- Mesangial deposits with immunolocalization for immunoglobulin A
- Severe liver disease or cirrhosis often present

SELECTED REFERENCES

1. Chang A et al: Spectrum of renal pathology in hematopoietic cell transplantation: a series of 20 patients and review of the literature. Clin J Am Soc Nephrol. 2(5):1014-23, 2007
2. Lefaucheur C et al: Membranous nephropathy and cancer: Epidemiologic evidence and determinants of high-risk cancer association. Kidney Int. 70(8):1510-7, 2006
3. Markowitz GS: Membranous glomerulopathy: emphasis on secondary forms and disease variants. Adv Anat Pathol. 8(3):119-25, 2001

Microscopic Features

(Left) Jones methenamine silver stain shows a glomerulus without significant pathologic abnormalities. There is no significant mesangial or endocapillary hypercellularity. Early stages of MGN may resemble minimal change disease by light microscopy. *(Right)* Periodic acid-Schiff shows a glomerular thrombus ⇨ in this Sjögren syndrome patient with deep venous and renal vein thrombosis. Congestion by neutrophils ⇨ in glomerular capillaries may be seen but was not a prominent feature in this biopsy.

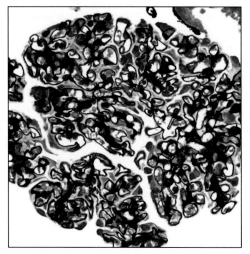
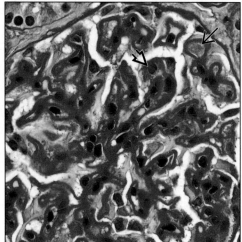

(Left) Hematoxylin & eosin shows prominent thickening of the glomerular basement membranes in this case of MGN. A glomerular thrombus ⇨ is noted in a capillary of this patient with renal vein thrombosis. *(Right)* Jones methenamine silver of MGN shows occasional circulating neutrophils within a few glomerular capillaries in this patient with an underlying malignancy. No apparent glomerular basement membrane abnormalities are noted.

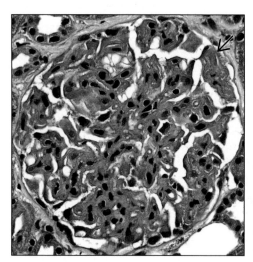
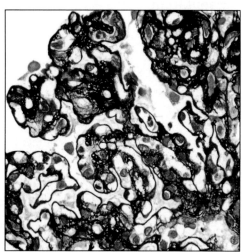

(Left) Hematoxylin & eosin shows several neutrophils ⇨ and small thrombi ⇨ within glomerular capillaries in MGN associated with colon carcinoma and renal vein thrombosis. Both features (neutrophils and thrombi) have been observed in both clinical settings of renal vein thrombosis and malignancy. *(Right)* Periodic acid-Schiff shows an interstitial germinal center ⇨, which can rarely be observed in lupus patients. This particular patient had lupus MGN.

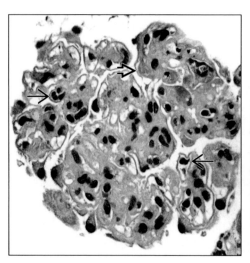
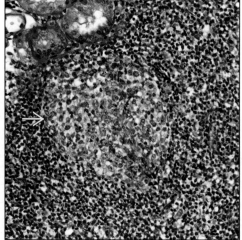

MEMBRANOUS GLOMERULONEPHRITIS, SECONDARY

Immunofluorescence and Electron Microscopy

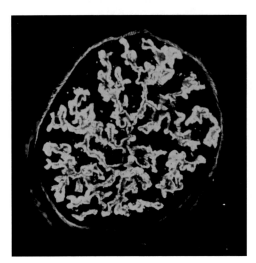
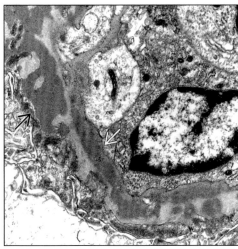

(Left) Immunofluorescence shows the widespread granular deposits of IgG typical of membranous glomerulonephritis in a patient with nephrotic syndrome 3 years after a bone marrow transplant. *(Right)* Electron micrograph in a patient with nephrotic syndrome 3 years after a bone marrow transplant shows subepithelial ⇒ and mesangial amorphous dense deposits ➥. This finding is believed to be due to an immune response to non-MHC alloantigens.

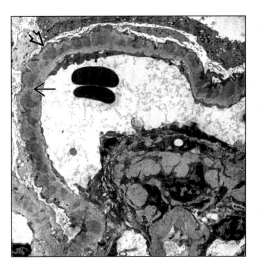
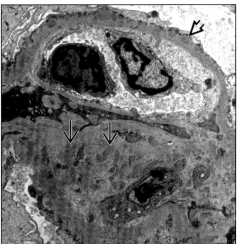

(Left) Electron microscopy reveals numerous subepithelial deposits with basement membrane material either between ⇒ or surrounding ⇒ some of the deposits. *(Right)* Electron microscopy reveals many subepithelial ⇒ electron-dense deposits, a finding that is diagnostic of MGN. The additional finding of mesangial ⇒ electron-dense deposits in this patient is consistent with a secondary form of MGN.

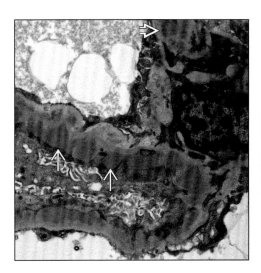
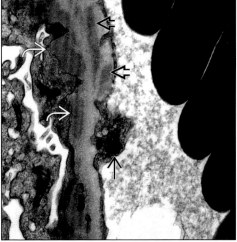

(Left) Electron microscopy shows many subepithelial ➥ and occasional mesangial ⇒ electron-dense deposits in this 49-year-old man with MGN. Mesangial deposits are characteristic of secondary MGN. *(Right)* Electron microscopy shows subepithelial ➥ and mesangial deposits extending to adjacent subendothelial areas ⇒. An endothelial tubuloreticular inclusion ⇒ confirms a secondary form of MGN and could also be seen in lupus nephritis, viral infection, or interferon therapy.

MEMBRANOUS GLOMERULONEPHRITIS WITH ANTI-TBM ANTIBODIES

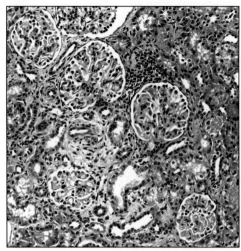

Glomeruli have focal, segmental proliferation and increased matrix in a child who has MGN with anti-TBM antibodies. The interstitium has foci of periglomerular lymphocytic infiltrate. (Courtesy B. Ivanyi, MD.)

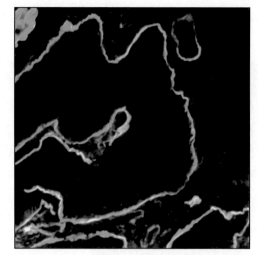

Linear staining of the proximal tubular basement membrane for IgG is shown in a child who has MGN with anti-TBM antibodies. C3 may also be present. (Courtesy B. Ivanyi, MD.)

TERMINOLOGY

Abbreviations
- Membranous glomerulonephritis (MGN)

Definitions
- Autoimmune disease characterized by MGN and autoantibodies to tubular basement membrane (TBM)

ETIOLOGY/PATHOGENESIS

Autoantibodies to TBM
- Noncollagenous 48-58 kd TBM autoantigen in TBM of proximal tubules
- Does not cross-react with GBM by indirect immunofluorescence
- May be a later complication since a younger sibling of an affected boy had MGN without anti-TBM

Autoantibodies Form Immune Complexes in Glomerulus
- Antigen in GBM deposits unknown
- MGN occurs without anti-TBM

Animal Models
- Anti-TBM disease in guinea pigs
  - No MGN component
  - Marked giant cell response around TBM
  - Response linked to MHC (strain XIII susceptible, strain II not)
    - Restricted idiotypes of autoantibodies
- Anti-TBM disease in rats
  - Pathology same as in guinea pig
  - Antigen and disease restricted to Brown-Norway (BN) rats
    - Lewis rats lack antigen, develop disease in BN renal allografts
- Anti-TBM disease in mice

- T-cell reactivity in addition to anti-TBM antibodies necessary

CLINICAL ISSUES

Epidemiology
- Incidence
  - Rare; 11 cases reported (1998)
  - HLA-B7 (4/5) and HLA-DR8 (2/5) may be risk factors
- Age
  - < 5 years old

Presentation
- Nephrotic syndrome in childhood
- Microhematuria
- Hypertension
- Fanconi syndrome (glycosuria, aminoaciduria)
- Diarrhea
- Neurological and ocular symptoms

Treatment
- None effective
- Recurrence reported in 1 transplant followed 2 years

MICROSCOPIC PATHOLOGY

Histologic Features
- Typical features of MGN plus interstitial nephritis
- Glomeruli
  - Diffusely thickened GBM with "spikes" on PAS and silver stains
  - Mesangial hypercellularity
- Tubules
  - Thickened TBM
  - Atrophic tubules
  - Tubular resorption droplets
- Interstitium
  - Mononuclear inflammation

MEMBRANOUS GLOMERULONEPHRITIS WITH ANTI-TBM ANTIBODIES

Key Facts

Terminology
- Autoimmune disease characterized by MGN and autoantibodies to TBM

Etiology/Pathogenesis
- Noncollagenous 48-58 kd proximal TBM autoantigen
- Does not cross-react with GBM

Clinical Issues
- < 5 years old

- Fanconi syndrome
- Nephrotic syndrome

Microscopic Pathology
- Typical features of MGN plus interstitial nephritis
- Linear IgG staining of proximal TBM
- Finely granular deposits of IgG along GBM
- Anti-TBM antibodies may appear after MGN

ANCILLARY TESTS

Immunofluorescence
- Finely granular deposits of IgG along GBM
  - IgA, C3, C1q, and IgM variably present
- Linear staining of TBM of proximal tubules for IgG ± other components

Electron Microscopy
- Subepithelial amorphous deposits in GBM ± intervening membrane "spikes"
- Thickening of TBM without electron-dense deposits

DIFFERENTIAL DIAGNOSIS

MGN with TBM Immune Complex Deposits
- Granular vs. linear IgG along TBM

Idiopathic MGN
- No linear deposits

DIAGNOSTIC CHECKLIST

Pathologic Interpretation Pearls
- Anti-TBM antibodies may appear after MGN

SELECTED REFERENCES

1. Iványi B et al: Childhood membranous nephropathy, circulating antibodies to the 58-kD TIN antigen, and anti-tubular basement membrane nephritis: an 11-year follow-up. Am J Kidney Dis. 32(6):1068-74, 1998
2. Katz A et al: Role of antibodies to tubulointerstitial nephritis antigen in human anti-tubular basement membrane nephritis associated with membranous nephropathy. Am J Med. 93(6):691-8, 1992
3. Butkowski RJ et al: Characterization of a tubular basement membrane component reactive with autoantibodies associated with tubulointerstitial nephritis. J Biol Chem. 265(34):21091-8, 1990
4. Ueda S et al: Autoimmune interstitial nephritis induced in inbred mice. Analysis of mouse tubular basement membrane antigen and genetic control of immune response to it. Am J Pathol. 132(2):304-18, 1988
5. Clayman MD et al: Isolation and characterization of the nephritogenic antigen producing anti-tubular basement membrane disease. J Exp Med. 161(2):290-305, 1985
6. Dumas R et al: [Membranous glomerulonephritis in two brothers associated in one with tubulo-interstitial disease, Fanconi syndrome and anti-TBM antibodies (author's transl).] Arch Fr Pediatr. 39(2):75-8, 1982
7. Hall CL et al: Passive transfer of autoimmune disease with isologous IgG1 and IgG2 antibodies to the tubular basement membrane in strain XIII guinea pigs: loss of self-tolerance induced by autoantibodies. J Exp Med. 146(5):1246-60, 1977
8. Hyman LR et al: Immunopathogenesis of autoimmune tubulointerstitial nephritis. I. Demonstration of differential susceptibility in strain II and strain XIII guinea pigs. J Immunol. 116(2):327-35, 1976

IMAGE GALLERY

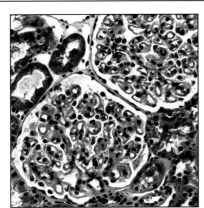 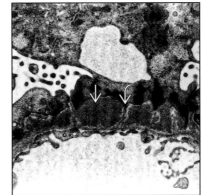 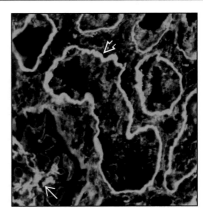

(Left) In a child with MGN with anti-TBM antibodies, glomeruli have diffusely thickened capillary walls and little hypercellularity. (Courtesy B. Ivanyi, MD.) (Center) Subepithelial deposits ➡ with intervening spikes ➡ are conspicuous in this sample from a 1-year-old child with MGN with anti-TBM antibodies. (Courtesy B. Ivanyi, MD.) (Right) Recurrent anti-TBM disease in a transplant shows linear immunostaining along the TBM ➡. Glomeruli have granular staining in the mesangium ➡. (Courtesy B. Ivanyi, MD.)

GRAFT-VS.-HOST GLOMERULOPATHIES

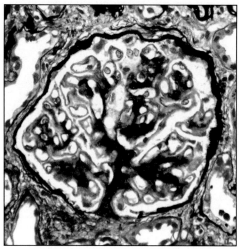

Jones methenamine silver demonstrates thick glomerular basement membrane with sparse silver staining due to the prominent extent of subepithelial immune complex deposition.

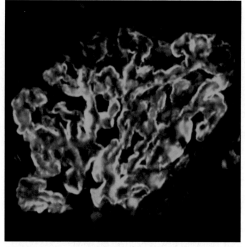

IgG demonstrates strong granular to confluent staining of the capillary walls in this hematopoietic cell transplant patient with MGN and GVHD.

TERMINOLOGY

Synonyms
- Graft-vs.-host disease (GVHD) glomerulopathy

Definitions
- Glomerular injury in setting of hematopoietic cell transplantation

ETIOLOGY/PATHOGENESIS

Hematopoietic Cell Transplantation (HCT)
- Mostly allogeneic (80-100%)
- 3 patterns
  o Membranous glomerulonephritis (MGN)
    ▪ Rare report in autologous HCT
  o Minimal change disease (MCD)
  o Focal segmental glomerulosclerosis
- Radiation &/or chemotherapy may be contributing factors

Experimental Model
- Chronic GVHD (parent to F1 bone marrow transplant) in mice leads to MGN due to antibodies to minor MHC antigens

CLINICAL ISSUES

Presentation
- Proteinuria, nephrotic range
  o Usual onset
    ▪ MCD ~ 8 months post transplant
    ▪ MGN ~ 14 months post transplant
  o Onset associated with decreased immunosuppression
- Associated with GVHD
  o Skin, mucous membranes, GI tract, lungs
  o Acute GVHD
    ▪ MCD ~ 40%

    ▪ MGN ~ 80%
  o Chronic GVHD
    ▪ MCD ~ 50%
    ▪ MGN ~ 90%

Treatment
- Drugs
  o Corticosteroids
  o Mycophenolate mofetil
  o Rituximab

Prognosis
- MCD ~ 90% complete remission
- MGN ~ 27% complete remission

MICROSCOPIC PATHOLOGY

Histologic Features
- 3 major patterns
  o Membranous glomerulonephritis (~ 60%)
    ▪ Glomerular basement membrane thickening
    ▪ Subepithelial "spike" formation by Jones silver stain
  o Minimal change lesion (~ 25%)
    ▪ Podocyte hypertrophy
    ▪ Tubular reabsorption droplets
    ▪ Otherwise normal
  o Focal segmental glomerulosclerosis (~ 15%)
    ▪ Segmental adhesions and sclerosis
    ▪ Tip lesions described
    ▪ Patchy tubular atrophy and fibrosis
- Other diseases may be present
  o Interstitial nephritis, acute tubular injury, polyomavirus nephropathy, thrombotic microangiopathy, recurrent amyloidosis, myeloma cast nephropathy

GRAFT-VS.-HOST GLOMERULOPATHIES

Key Facts

Terminology
- Graft-vs.-host disease (GVHD) glomerulopathy
- Glomerular injury in setting of hematopoietic cell transplantation and GVHD

Clinical Issues
- Proteinuria, nephrotic range

Microscopic Pathology
- 3 major patterns

- ○ Membranous glomerulonephritis
- ○ Minimal change lesions
- ○ Focal segmental glomerulosclerosis
- Concurrent interstitial nephritis, acute tubular injury, or thrombotic microangiopathy may be present

Top Differential Diagnoses
- MGN, primary
- Recurrent lymphoma

ANCILLARY TESTS

Immunofluorescence
- Membranous glomerulonephritis
  - ○ Fine granular deposits diffusely along GBM that stain for IgG and variably for other immunoglobulins and C3
  - ○ Kappa and lambda stain equally
- Minimal change lesion
  - ○ No deposits
- Focal segmental glomerulosclerosis
  - ○ Segmental IgM, C3

Electron Microscopy
- Membranous glomerulonephritis
  - ○ Subepithelial electron-dense deposits
    - ▪ Microspherule substructure may be present
  - ○ Mesangial electron-dense deposits
    - ▪ Variably present
- Minimal change lesion
  - ○ Podocyte foot process effacement
  - ○ No deposits
- Focal segmental glomerulosclerosis
  - ○ Same as MCD plus segmental adhesions
- Endothelial tubuloreticular inclusions (rare)

DIFFERENTIAL DIAGNOSIS

MGN, Primary
- Absence of mesangial immune complexes

Recurrent Lymphoma
- Manifested as MCD or MGN
- Lack of GVHD history

Thrombotic Microangiopathy
- Chronic phase shows double contours
- Fibrin and nonspecific trapping of IgM/C3

SELECTED REFERENCES

1. Sakai K et al: Secondary membranous glomerulonephritis associated with recipient residual lymphoma cells after allogeneic bone marrow transplantation. Clin Exp Nephrol. 13(2):174-8, 2009
2. Troxell ML et al: Renal pathology in hematopoietic cell transplantation recipients. Mod Pathol. 21(4):396-406, 2008
3. Chang A et al: Spectrum of renal pathology in hematopoietic cell transplantation: a series of 20 patients and review of the literature. Clin J Am Soc Nephrol. 2(5):1014-23, 2007
4. Brukamp K et al: Nephrotic syndrome after hematopoietic cell transplantation: do glomerular lesions represent renal graft-versus-host disease?. Clin J Am Soc Nephrol. 1(4):685-94, 2006
5. Reddy P et al: Nephrotic syndrome associated with chronic graft-versus-host disease after allogeneic hematopoietic stem cell transplantation. Bone Marrow Transplant. 38(5):351-7, 2006
6. Sutmuller M et al: Non-MHC genes determine the development of lupus nephritis in H-2 identical mouse strains. Clin Exp Immunol. 106(2):265-72, 1996

IMAGE GALLERY

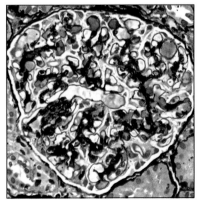 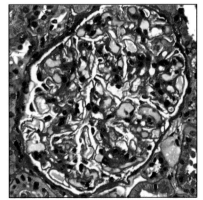 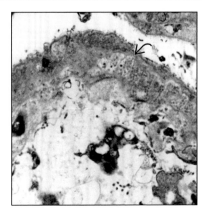

(Left) Jones methenamine silver reveals a normal-appearing glomerulus by light microscopy, but subepithelial immune complexes are noted by IF and EM. (Center) Periodic acid-Schiff shows mild thickening of the glomerular basement membranes in an HCT patient with MGN. (Right) Electron micrograph demonstrates subepithelial and intramembranous deposits with a microspherular substructure ⤢. A subset of MGN cases in the setting of GVHD may reveal this atypical finding.

CLASSIFICATION OF MPGN AND COMPLEMENT-RELATED DISEASES

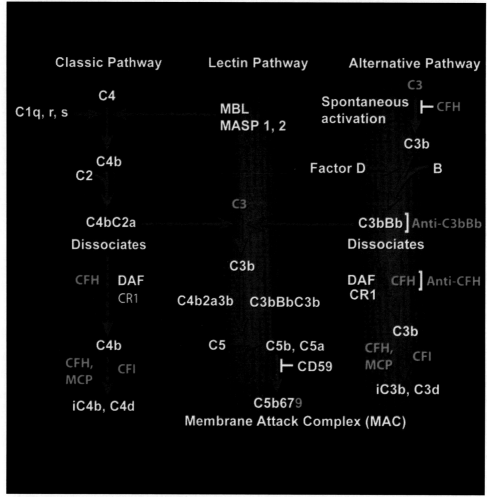

Schematic of the complement system is illustrated. Components known to be abnormal in C3-related glomerular diseases are indicated in green. Mutations involve loss of function of the complement inhibitors (CFH, CFI, MCP), lack of binding to inhibitors (C3), and autoantibodies that protect C3 convertase (C3bBb) from dissociation (C3NeF). CFH-related proteins have also been implicated. The alternate pathway "ticks over" spontaneously in the plasma by reaction with water and is activated by microbial surfaces. The classical pathway is activated by IgG or IgM complexes with antigen. The lectin pathway is triggered by carbohydrate structures on microbes.

TERMINOLOGY

Definitions
- Group of diseases caused or promoted by complement (C3) abnormalities

Background
- Membranoproliferative glomerulonephritis (MPGN)
  - Defined by presence of mesangial hypercellularity, subendothelial deposits, & duplication of GBM
    - Associated with prolonged or intermittent hypocomplementemia (C3, sometimes C4)
    - Some have immunoglobulin deposits & are probably a type of chronic immune complex disease
    - Now known as MPGN, type I
    - Similar pattern in chronic infections
  - Variant with prominent subepithelial deposits or diffuse intramembranous GBM deposits (MPGN, type III)

- Dense deposit disease
  - Defined originally by EM feature of hyperdense deposits
  - Has C3 deposition with little or no immunoglobulin
  - Sometimes termed MPGN, type II
  - Preferred term is dense deposit disease
- Problems recognized in classification
  - Same complement abnormality can lead to different glomerular pathologies
  - Same pathologic pattern can be caused by different complement abnormalities
- Complement abnormalities also associated with chronic immune complex GN of various types
  - Examples: MPGN type I/III, lupus nephritis
  - Complement abnormalities can cause
    - ↑ susceptibility to infection
    - ↓ clearance of immune complexes
    - ↑ complement activation

CLASSIFICATION OF MPGN AND COMPLEMENT-RELATED DISEASES

Classification of C3-related Glomerular Diseases

Category	Defining Features	Complement Abnormalities	Immunofluorescence
C3 Glomerulopathies			
Dense deposit disease (DDD)	Extremely dense GBM and mesangial deposits by EM; variable histologic patterns: MPGN, AGN, mesangial proliferative and crescentic GN	Autoantibody to C3bBb (> 80%) or C3 (rare); mutation in CFH (minority), C3 (rare), CFHR1 (rare), CFHR3 (rare)	C3(+), C1g(-), IgG(-), IgA(-), IgM(±)
C3 glomerulonephritis (primary GN with isolated C3 deposits)	C3 in mesangium without Ig; deposits not as dense as DDD; humps occasionally; 2 patterns: MPGN and epimembranous deposits	Autoantibody to C3bBb (~ 30%); mutation in CFH (minority), CFI (rare), MCP (rare)	C3(+), C1q(-), no Ig by definition
Familial MPGN III	MPGN type III (one family)	Linkage to chromosome 1 (factor H region)	C3(+), no Ig
CFHR5 nephropathy	MPGN I or III pattern, autosomal dominant	Mutation in CFHR5	C3(+), C1q(-), no Ig
Immune Complex Glomerulonephritis with C3 Abnormalities			
MPGN, type I	Mesangial proliferation + subendothelial and mesangial deposits, duplication of GBM; C3(+)Ig(+)	Autoantibody to C3bBb (20-50%); CFH mutation (minority); CFI mutation (minority); C9 (rare)	C3(+), C1q(±), C4(±), IgG, IgM(±), IgA(±)
MPGN, type III	Mesangial proliferation + subepithelial or intramembranous deposits; C3(+)Ig(+)	Autoantibody to C3bBb (C3NeF) (minority)	C3(+), C1q(±), C4(±), IgG(±), IgM(±)

CFH = complement factor H; CFI = complement factor I; MPGN = membranoproliferative glomerulonephritis; AGN = acute glomerulonephritis; CFHR = complement factor H-related proteins.

C3 Glomerulopathies
- Proposed new category
- Defined by presence of glomerular C3 deposits with little or no immunoglobulin
  - Dense deposit disease
  - C3 glomerulonephritis
  - CFHR5 nephropathy
  - Familial MPGN III

SELECTED PARTICIPANTS

Complement Factor H (CFH)
- Plasma protein inhibits activation of C3 to C3b

CFHR1-5
- 5 homologues of CFH with similar functions

C3bBb
- Combines with C3b to form alternate pathway C5 convertase, cleaves C5 to C5b; properdin stabilizes

Factor I (CFI)
- Inhibits active C3b by cleaving to iC3b & C3f

C3 Nephritic Factor (C3NeF)
- Autoantibody stabilizing/prolonging action of C3bBb

Membrane Cofactor Protein (MCP)
- Cell-bound protein that inactivates C3b & C4b

SELECTED REFERENCES
1. Alchi B et al: Membranoproliferative glomerulonephritis. Pediatr Nephrol. 25(8):1409-18, 2010
2. Fakhouri F et al: C3 glomerulopathy: a new classification. Nat Rev Nephrol. 6(8):494-9, 2010

IMAGE GALLERY

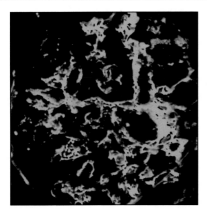  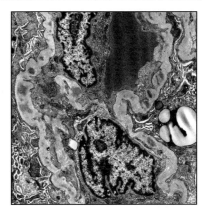

(Left) This group of disorders is characterized by a predominance of C3 deposition, as illustrated here. IgG is present in a subset (e.g., MPGN type I/III) but was absent in this case. *(Center)* Paucity of immunoglobulin defines the C3 nephropathy subgroup. There was little IgG (shown) but strong C3 staining in this 80-year-old man with acute increase in Cr to 5 mg/dL, low C3, and 3+ proteinuria. *(Right)* The pattern and density of deposits revealed by electron microscopy help define the categories.

MEMBRANOPROLIFERATIVE GLOMERULONEPHRITIS, TYPE I/III

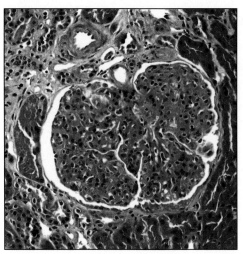

MPGN, type I shows exuberant mesangial hypercellularity, which gives a lobulated appearance and capillary wall thickening, as shown here in a 10-year-old boy with hematuria, proteinuria, and low C3.

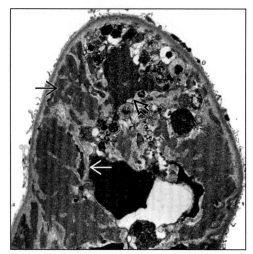

By EM, MPGN, type I shows numerous subendothelial electron-dense deposits ⟹ along the GBM ⟹ and new GBM layers ⟹, giving a "tram track" appearance in PAS or silver stains.

TERMINOLOGY

Abbreviations
- Membranoproliferative glomerulonephritis (MPGN)

Synonyms
- Hypocomplementemic glomerulonephritis (GN)
- Lobular GN
- Mesangiocapillary/mesangiopathic GN

Definitions
- Subendothelial electron-dense deposits with mesangial interposition between capillary wall and GBM with clinical finding of hypocomplementemia

ETIOLOGY/PATHOGENESIS

Infectious Agents
- May occur after infection, particularly upper respiratory tract infection

Autoimmune
- ± C3 nephritic factor, IgG autoantibody, or other autoantibodies, resulting in persistent activity of alternative complement pathway (~ 25% of MPGN type I patients)

Immune Complex Deposition
- Circulating immune complexes present in many MPGN, type I patients
- Activates classical & alternative complement pathways
- Chronic serum sickness caused by repeated injection of antigen resembles MPGN

Secondary Causes
- Many different etiologies can lead to 2° MPGN-type pattern
- Therefore, 1° MPGN is a diagnosis of exclusion

CLINICAL ISSUES

Epidemiology
- Incidence
  - ~ 5% of GN in children and adults
- Age
  - Primarily older children, adolescents, and young adults (~ 7-30 years old)
    - Rare in children < 2 years old or adults > 50 years old
- Gender
  - Approximately equal male:female ratio
- Ethnicity
  - Reportedly higher incidence in whites
  - Navajo Indians in USA may have high rates of nondiabetic ESRD due to GN of this type

Presentation
- Nephrotic syndrome
  - Occurs in > 50% of patients
  - Predominant feature in 2/3 of patients
- Proteinuria
  - May be subnephrotic
  - Syndrome often initially nephritic & eventually nephrotic
- Hypocomplementemia
  - Low C3 as in other types of MPGN
  - Low classic pathway components (C1, C2, and C4), Factor B, and properdin
  - ~ 80% of MPGN, type I; ~ 100% of MPGN, type II; & ~ 50% of MPGN, type III
- Hematuria
  - ± recurrent episodes of gross or microscopic hematuria
  - Acute nephritic syndrome in 10-20%
- Hypertension
  - Usually mild but may be malignant
  - ~ 1/3 of patients
- Renal vein thrombosis may be present

MEMBRANOPROLIFERATIVE GLOMERULONEPHRITIS, TYPE I/III

Key Facts

Terminology
- Subendothelial electron-dense deposits with mesangial interposition

Clinical Issues
- Older children, adolescents, & young adults (~ 7-30 years old)
- Nephrotic syndrome: > 50% of patients
- Hematuria: 10-20% with acute nephritic syndrome
- Hypocomplementemia

Microscopic Pathology
- Lobular, hypercellular glomerulus with thickened capillary walls & increased mesangial substance
- "Tram tracks" or duplication of GBM (best seen on PAS & silver stains)
- Crescents in ~ 20% of cases

- ± neutrophils and monocytes
- Hyaline aggregates of immune complexes in capillary lumina
- IF: Classic feature is C3 in capillary walls & mesangium, "railroad track," "lumpy-bumpy" granular C3, IgG, & early complement (C1q & C4)
- EM: Large, amorphous dense subendothelial and mesangial deposits in glomerulus
  - Type III (Burkholder): MPGN, type I + membranous GN (subendothelial + subepithelial deposits)
  - Type III (Anders and Strife): MPGN, type II (also known as dense deposit disease) + MPGN, type I

Top Differential Diagnoses
- Lupus erythematosus
- Cryoglobulinemia
- Chronic Infections

Laboratory Tests
- Complement often decreased, as above
  - In type I MPGN
    - ↓ C3 & total hemolytic complement (CH50) in 50%
    - C1q, C4, properdin, & factor B borderline/↓ in < 50%
  - In type III MPGN
    - ↓ C3, normal C4
    - ↓ C5, C6, C7, and C9 levels may be 2° to terminal pathway nephritic factor
- C3 nephritic factor (common in type II MPGN)
  - Present in ~ 25% of type I MPGN patients & absent in type III MPGN

Treatment
- Drugs
  - Steroids
    - Long-term, low-dose steroids used in children with 1° MPGN (lead to growth retardation & hypertension)
    - Repeat biopsy often performed within 5 years of therapy initiation to ascertain if continued therapy is needed
  - Antiplatelet agents (dipyridamole & aspirin) used alone or with steroids

Prognosis
- Variable but usually poor with persistent proteinuria
  - Classically a chronic, slowly progressive course
- 5-20% have clinical remission
- Survival has been measured at ~ 50% at ~ 10 years
  - Median renal survival time in MPGN, type I: 9-12 years, compared with MPGN, type II: 5-12 years
  - Prognosis of patients with MPGN, type III is similar to that of patients with MPGN, type I
  - Therapy improves survival to 60-85% at 10 years
- Prognostic features of poor outcome
  - Sclerotic glomeruli, crescents, interstitial fibrosis, & tubular atrophy (IF/TA)
- Clinical features of poor outcome

  - Severe nephrotic syndrome, ↑ creatinine, hypertension
- Features of good outcome
  - Focal/mild MPGN features on biopsy, asymptomatic hematuria, subnephrotic proteinuria
- ~ 30% of children with MPGN, type I have recurrence in 6 months to 1 year after transplant
  - ~ 40% of recurrences lead to graft failure

MACROSCOPIC FEATURES

General Features
- Nephrectomy, exam at transplant, or autopsy reveals pale kidneys
- ± cortical yellow flecks, representing tubular lipid & interstitial foam cells
- Advanced disease: Small granular kidneys ± prominent vessels

MICROSCOPIC PATHOLOGY

Histologic Features
- Glomeruli
  - Lobular, hypercellular glomeruli with thickened capillary walls & ↑ mesangial substance
  - Mesangial interposition: Mesangial cells migrate into peripheral capillary walls between GBM & endothelium
    - Partial if only capillary wall segment involved
    - Circumferential if involving entire circumference of individual capillary
    - Produces "tram tracks" or GBM reduplication (best seen on PAS & silver) 2° to GBM synthesis
    - ± subendothelial immune deposits (between duplicated GBMs) seen by light microscopy (PAS[+], nonargyrophilic on silver, & fuchsinophilic on trichrome)
  - ± sclerosis; ± sclerotic mesangial nodules
  - Crescents in ~ 20% of cases
  - ± neutrophils & monocytes

- ○ Hyaline aggregates of immune complexes in capillary lumina
- ○ **Type III: Burkholder variant**
  - ■ Combined features of type I MPGN & membranous GN
  - ■ Glomerular capillary loops markedly thickened due to subendothelial & subepithelial deposits & mesangial interposition
  - ■ Mesangial expansion with exudation of inflammatory cells
- ○ **Type III: Anders and Strife variant**
  - ■ Hybrid of type II (dense deposit disease) & type I MPGN
  - ■ Glomerular capillary walls have an irregular thickening that is eosinophilic, PAS(+), silver (JMS) (-)
  - ■ Silver stains show frayed GBM with disrupted, "moth-eaten" appearance
- • Tubulointerstitium
  - ○ Largely nonspecific with variable interstitial fibrosis and tubular atrophy, inflammation, & edema
  - ○ Tubular resorption droplets
  - ○ Interstitial foam cells
  - ○ Red cell casts
- • Vascular changes nonspecific

ANCILLARY TESTS

Immunofluorescence
- • MPGN, type I
  - ○ C3 in capillary walls & mesangium is classic feature
    - ■ To lesser extent, IgG present followed by IgM, IgA, & C1q
    - ■ Up to 25% have C3 only and would now be classified as C3 glomerulopathy
  - ○ Also "lumpy-bumpy" granular C3, IgG, & early complement (C1q & C4)
  - ○ "Railroad track" pattern may be seen on IF at high power
  - ○ Focal C3 deposits in the TBM
- • MPGN, type III subtypes have similar findings
  - ○ ~ 50% of cases have IgG & C3 (& less intense IgM, IgA, & C1q)
  - ○ ~ 50% stain only for C3
  - ○ Focal TBM C3 staining is present in ~ 1/3 of cases

Electron Microscopy
- • Transmission
  - ○ Large, dense deposits throughout glomerulus; primarily subendothelial but also mesangial
    - ■ Produces double GBMs with mesangial interposition
    - ■ GBM has a "sausage-string" or fusiform appearance
    - ■ Intramembranous dense deposits in GBM reflections
    - ■ Increased mesangial matrix
  - ○ "Mesangialization" of capillary loops
  - ○ Podocyte foot process effacement
  - ○ **Type III: Burkholder variant**
    - ■ Combined features of MPGN, type I & membranous glomerulonephritis
    - ■ Subendothelial deposits & mesangial interposition

- ○ **Type III: Anders and Strife variant**
  - ■ Hybrid of MPGN, type II (also known as dense deposit disease) & MPGN, type I
  - ■ Subendothelial & intramembranous deposits
  - ■ Deposits extend from GBM subendothelial to subepithelial portion, disrupting GBM lamina densa, giving a laminated, woven appearance
  - ■ TBM deposits present in ~ 1/3 of cases
  - ■ Initially described using silver impregnation techniques

DIFFERENTIAL DIAGNOSIS

Systemic Lupus Erythematosus (SLE)
- • IF shows "full house" staining pattern
- • Serology(+) in SLE: ANA(+), anti-ds DNA(+)

Mixed Cryoglobulinemia
- • Mixed cryoglobulinemia associated with chronic hepatitis C has been associated with number of cases of MPGN, type I
- • Characteristic PAS(+) "pseudothrombi" can be seen in glomerular capillary loops in cryoglobulinemic GN
- • Clinical laboratory can help identify cryoglobulin

Infectious Diseases
- • History, physical, & clinical laboratory data can help favor diagnosis of infectious disease
- • Bacterial
  - ○ Endocarditis & infected vascular shunts
  - ○ Post-streptococcal acute glomerulonephritis: Elevated antistreptolysin-O (ASLO) titers
- • Viral: Hepatitis B & C, HIV
- • Protozoal: Malarial & schistosomiasis
- • Other: Mycoplasma, mycobacteria

Sjögren Syndrome
- • Serology(+) in Sjögren syndrome: ANA(+), SSA/Ro(+) (less specific than SSB, also seen in other autoimmune conditions), SSB/La(+) (more specific)

Complement Deficiencies
- • MPGN-type pattern can be seen in a number of complement deficiencies (e.g., inherited C2, C3, C6, C7, & C8 deficiencies, etc.)
- • Subset with C3 and no immunoglobulin are now classified as "C3 glomerulonephritis"
- • Patients may also show signs of meningococcal infections & MPGN

α-1 Antitrypsin (A1AT) Deficiency
- • Protease inhibitor genotype ZZ (PiZZ) has abnormal phenotype usually accounting for most of these cases
  - ○ PiMM has the normal protease inhibitor (Pi) phenotype
- • Autosomal recessive
- • Severe liver disease or cirrhosis necessary prior to developing MPGN
- • Can present in early childhood
- • Severity worsens with increasing age
- • A1AT deposits and PiZ protein detected in subendothelial space

MEMBRANOPROLIFERATIVE GLOMERULONEPHRITIS, TYPE I/III

- Glomerular injury possibly reversible with liver transplantation

Transplant Glomerulopathy
- Usually C4d(+) peritubular capillaries (chronic humoral rejection)
- Minimal Ig and C3 deposits
- No electron dense deposits

Thrombotic Microangiopathy (TMA)
- GBM duplication lacking immunoglobulin deposits
  - Instead, subendothelial accumulation of electron-lucent, flocculent material
- Termed by some a "membranoproliferative glomerulopathy"

Chronic Liver Disease
- Such as from alcoholic cirrhosis
- May have MPGN pattern due to complement abnormalities, as mentioned previously
- Deposits are often electron-lucent, resembling lipid rather than immune deposits

Dysproteinemias
- Light chain deposition (due to kappa in ~ 80% of cases) may lead to GBM thickening, which may be confused with MPGN
  - Do not stain with complements since they are not immune complexes, unlike MPGN, which does typically stain for complement
- Heavy chain deposition disease
  - Single heavy chain stains (usually gamma, rarely alpha)
  - ± complement staining (e.g., C3 & C1) since complement can be activated on truncated, mutated heavy chain
- Fibrillary glomerulonephritis
  - Predominantly polyclonal IgG and complement
  - Randomly oriented fibrils 16-24 nm in diameter in mesangium & GBM
- Immunotactoid glomerulopathy
  - Polyclonal immunoglobulins
  - Tubulofibrillar structures 30-50 nm in diameter
- Amyloid not typically confused with MPGN since amorphous deposits are usually distinctive & Congo red(+)

IgA Nephropathy and Henoch-Schönlein Purpura
- Can have MPGN-type pattern
- Distinguished by dominant or codominant staining for IgA, C3(+), C1(-, or trace), and frequent lambda codominance

Neoplasms
- Leukemia & lymphomas (some with cryoglobulinemia)
- Carcinomas
- Melanoma
- Wilms tumor (*WT1* germline mutation)
- MPGN may remit after malignancy treated

Other Diseases
- Other diseases on broad differential diagnosis sometimes having an MPGN-type pattern include
  - Diabetes mellitus, drug abuse, sarcoidosis, sickle cell disease, pregnancy-associated disorders (e.g., eclampsia/preeclampsia), renal vein thrombosis, renal artery dysplasia, celiac sprue
- Typically have other characteristic clinicopathologic features suggesting proper etiology

DIAGNOSTIC CHECKLIST

Pathologic Interpretation Pearls
- Clinically, MPGN may initially mimic post-streptococcal GN since both often have preceding upper respiratory infection
  - Recommend biopsy if hematuria, proteinuria, & hypocomplementemia last ≥ 6 weeks since MPGN may be present
- Nosology of MPGN in transition
  - MPGN cases with C3 in absence of immunoglobulin now classified as "C3 glomerulonephritis," a member of "C3 glomerulopathies" category that includes dense deposit disease
  - Those with evidence of classical pathway activation (immunoglobulin &/or C1q) remain in MPGN I/III category
  - Some will have genetic abnormalities in complement system, others acquired abnormalities due to autoantibodies to components of complement system

SELECTED REFERENCES

1. Vernon KA et al: Experimental models of membranoproliferative glomerulonephritis, including dense deposit disease. Contrib Nephrol. 169:198-210, 2011
2. Alchi B et al: Membranoproliferative glomerulonephritis. Pediatr Nephrol. 25(8):1409-18, 2010
3. Fakhouri F et al: C3 glomerulopathy: a new classification. Nat Rev Nephrol. 6(8):494-9, 2010
4. Lorenz EC et al: Recurrent membranoproliferative glomerulonephritis after kidney transplantation. Kidney Int. 77(8):721-8, 2010
5. Benz K et al: Pathological aspects of membranoproliferative glomerulonephritis (MPGN) and haemolytic uraemic syndrome (HUS) / thrombocytic thrombopenic purpura (TTP). Thromb Haemost. 101(2):265-70, 2009
6. Bockenhauer D et al: Membranoproliferative glomerulonephritis associated with a mutation in Wilms' tumour suppressor gene 1. Pediatr Nephrol. 24(7):1399-401, 2009
7. Smith KD et al: Pathogenic mechanisms in membranoproliferative glomerulonephritis. Curr Opin Nephrol Hypertens. 14(4):396-403, 2005
8. Strife CF et al: Type III membranoproliferative glomerulonephritis: long-term clinical and morphologic evaluation. Clin Nephrol. 21(6):323-34, 1984
9. Burkholder PM et al: Mixed membranous and proliferative glomerulonephritis. A correlative light, immunofluorescence, and electron microscopic study. Lab Invest. 23(5):459-79, 1970

MEMBRANOPROLIFERATIVE GLOMERULONEPHRITIS, TYPE I/III

Microscopic Features

(Left) In a 41-year-old man with hematuria, proteinuria (~ 7 g/d), hypocomplementemia, and negative serologic work-up, hypercellular lobular glomeruli ➡ can be seen in a case of MPGN, type I. (Right) In a 53-year-old man with hematuria & proteinuria (3.6 g/d), low levels of complement proteins, & a negative serologic work-up, hypercellular glomeruli can be seen ➡ together with crescents ➡ in what was shown to be MPGN, type I by IF & EM.

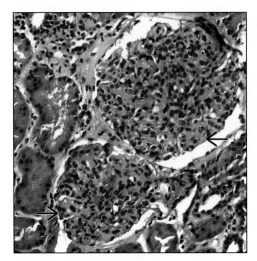
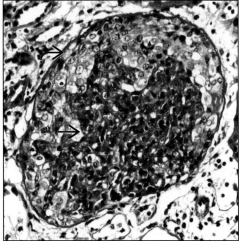

(Left) In the 41-year-old man with hematuria, proteinuria (~ 7 g/d), hypocomplementemia, and a negative serologic work-up, GBM duplication with cellular interposition can be seen ➡ in a silver stain in a case of MPGN, type I. (Right) Widespread duplication of the GBM ➡ can be seen in a PAS stain in this case of MPGN, type I, recurrent in an allograft 7 years after transplantation.

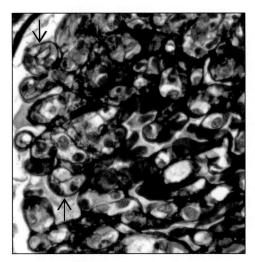
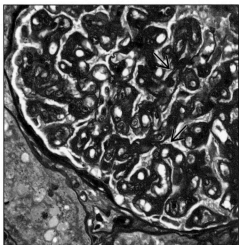

(Left) In a 9-year-old male with MPGN, type III-Burkholder variant, peripheral capillary loops showed GBM duplication ➡ with cellular interposition and increased mesangial cellularity ➡. (Right) In the 9-year-old male with MPGN, type III-Burkholder variant, peripheral capillary loops showed less argyrophilia ➡ than the hypercellular, lobular mesangium ➡.

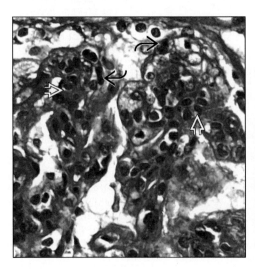
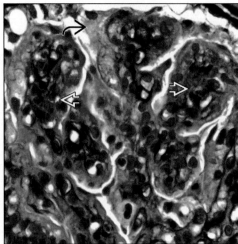

MEMBRANOPROLIFERATIVE GLOMERULONEPHRITIS, TYPE I/III

Immunofluorescence

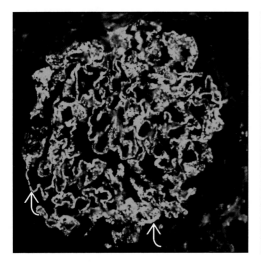
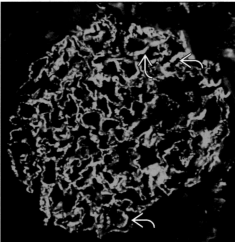

(Left) In a patient with MPGN, type I, staining for IgG by immunofluorescence shows a largely granular but also linear distribution along the GBM in some foci ➢, compatible with subendothelial deposits. (Right) Immunofluorescence staining for kappa shows a largely granular but also linear distribution along the GBM in some foci ➢, compatible with subendothelial deposits in a patient with MPGN, type I.

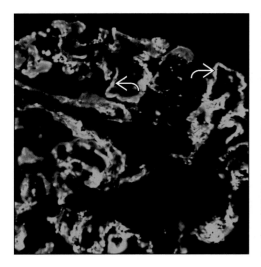
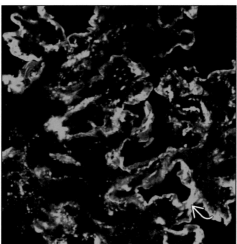

(Left) In a patient with MPGN, type I, there is staining for C1q by immunofluorescence, which can be appreciated in a vaguely linear pattern ➢ along the GBM, compatible with subendothelial deposits. (Right) There is staining for C1q by immunofluorescence, which can be appreciated in a vaguely linear pattern ➢ along the GBM, compatible with subendothelial deposits in a patient with MPGN, type I.

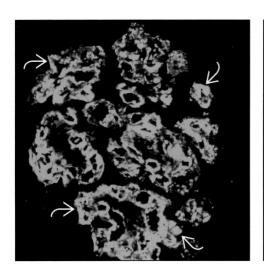
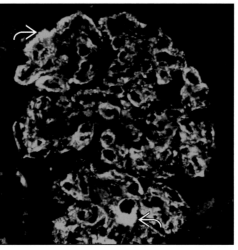

(Left) In a 14-year-old girl with MPGN, type III, there is bright C3 staining by IF ➢, appreciable as subendothelial deposits in the pattern of an expanded lobular glomerulus. She had hypocomplementemia, elevated ESR, hematuria, proteinuria (protein:creatinine ratio = 4), creatinine 0.4 mg/dL, cholesterol 278 mg/dL, and a negative serologic work-up. (Right) In the 14-year-old girl with MPGN, type III, there is bright IgM by IF ➢, appreciable as linear deposits along the GBM.

MEMBRANOPROLIFERATIVE GLOMERULONEPHRITIS, TYPE I/III

Electron Microscopy

(Left) In a 41-year-old man with MPGN, type I, subendothelial deposits ⊠ can be seen. *(Right)* In the 41-year-old man with MPGN, type I, large subendothelial deposits ⊠ can be seen together with cellular interposition into basement membrane material ⊠.

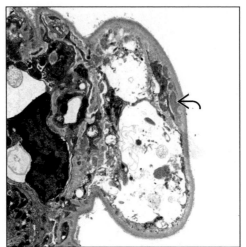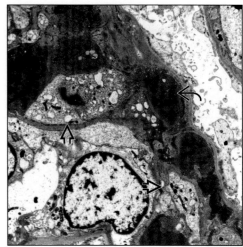

(Left) In the 41-year-old man with MPGN, type I, subendothelial deposits ⊠ can be seen. *(Right)* In a 14-year-old girl with hematuria, proteinuria, and a negative serologic work-up, frequent subepithelial deposits ⊠ could be seen as well as subendothelial deposits ⊠, compatible with a diagnosis of MPGN, type III-Burkholder variant.

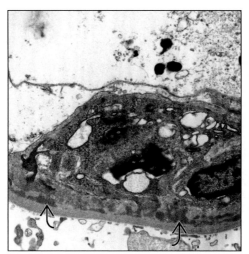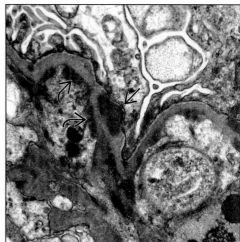

(Left) In the 14-year-old girl with hematuria, proteinuria, and a negative serologic work-up, frequent subepithelial deposits ⊠ could be seen as well as subendothelial deposits ⊠, compatible with a diagnosis of MPGN, type III-Burkholder variant. *(Right)* In the 14-year-old girl with MPGN, type III-Burkholder variant, subepithelial electron-dense deposits can be seen ⊠, some of which extend into the GBM. In addition, there is overlying podocyte foot process effacement ⊠.

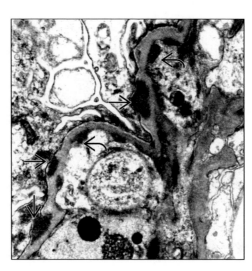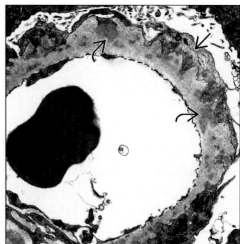

MEMBRANOPROLIFERATIVE GLOMERULONEPHRITIS, TYPE I/III

Electron Microscopy: Burkholder and Strife Variants

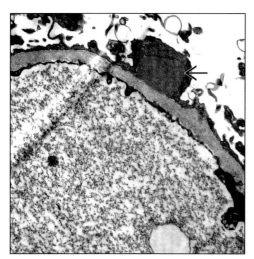
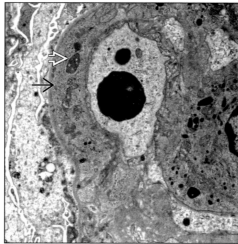

(Left) In the 14-year-old girl with MPGN, type III-Burkholder variant, a subepithelial deposit with a hump-like configuration can be appreciated ➡. (Right) A 66-year-old man with proteinuria (2 g/d), Cr 1.2 mg/dL, a history of non-Hodgkin lymphoma, and no κ/λ predominance or corresponding proteinemia has GBMs thickened by interposition of cellular material ➡ & faint deposits ➡ compared with the typical deposits, overall most compatible with MPGN, type III.

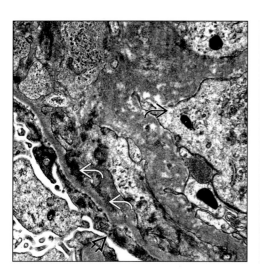
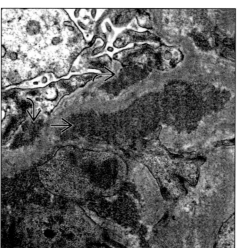

(Left) In the 66 year old with MPGN, type III, spreading apart of the GBM by cellular interposition was present ➡, together with scattered electron-dense deposits ➡ and podocyte foot process effacement ➡. (Right) In the 66-year-old man with MPGN, type III, some deposits ➡ were denser, and occasional subepithelial deposits ➡ were identified, although the substructure suggests the possibility of cryoglobulinemia.

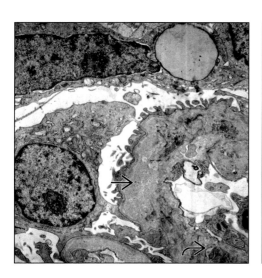
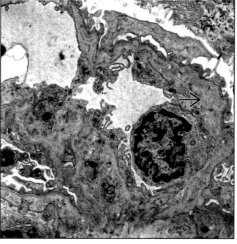

(Left) In a 12-year-old male with proteinuria, low albumin, and normal creatinine, GBMs were thickened by deposits ➡ that were less electron dense than the typical deposits and by cellular interposition ➡. These features are most compatible with MPGN, type III-Anders & Strife variant. (Right) In the 12-year-old male with MPGN, type III-Anders & Strife variant, GBMs are thickened by deposits ➡ that were less electron-dense than typical deposits.

DENSE DEPOSIT DISEASE

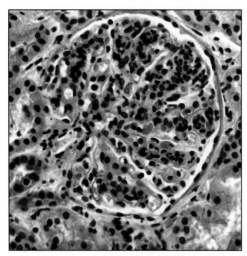

Dense deposit disease (DDD) often presents with an MPGN pattern, shown here in a biopsy from a 13-year-old boy with gross hematuria and proteinuria 3 days after a meningococcal septicemia. Serum C3 was undetectable.

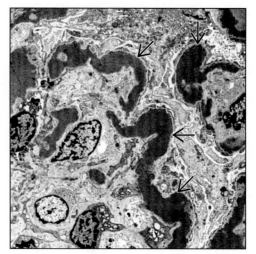

The diagnosis of DDD is made by electron microscopy, which reveals extremely dark, osmiophilic deposits along the GBM ➔. Deposits are found also in the mesangium, Bowman capsule, and TBM.

TERMINOLOGY

Abbreviations
- Dense deposit disease (DDD)

Synonyms
- Membranoproliferative glomerulonephritis (MPGN), type II

Definitions
- C3-related glomerulopathy manifested by broad, linear, extremely electron-dense deposits with C3 within GBM, mesangium, Bowman capsule, and TBM
  - Once classified as variant of MPGN, but MPGN pattern present in < 50%
  - Hyperdense deposits by EM are pathognomonic; therefore, DDD is preferred name
  - Initially reported by Galle and Berger in 1962

ETIOLOGY/PATHOGENESIS

Chronic Activation of Alternative Complement Pathway
- Autoantibodies to complement components
  - C3 nephritic factor (C3NeF): Autoantibody to C3 convertase of alternative pathway (C3bBb) prevents inactivation, resulting in continuous activation of complement alternative pathway
    - C3NeF present in > 80% of patients (~ 100% children, ~ 40% adults)
    - C3NeF may also be present in healthy individuals
    - Specificity of antibody affects functional consequences
  - Autoantibodies to CFH, factor B, or C3
- Mutations in complement component genes
  - Factor H mutations lead to low plasma levels or affect its C3bBb decay function
    - Tyrosine 402 to histidine common
  - C3 mutation resistant to factor H in fluid phase

Deposition of C3 in Lamina Densa of GBM
- Local activation of complement pathway
  - Recruitment of leukocytes
  - Inflammatory damage of glomerular components
  - Loss of heparan sulfate (principal negative charge barrier)

Precipitating Factors
- Infection, various (pneumonia, upper respiratory)
  - Group A streptococcal or meningococcal infections
- Post chemotherapy for breast cancer
- ~ 20% of adults with DDD have monoclonal gammopathy including myeloma
- ~ 70% of patients have monoclonal gammopathy of undetermined significance
- Some patients have multiple susceptibility factors

Animal Models
- CFH mutation in Norwegian Yorkshire pigs
- Mouse strain with CFH knockout
  - Prevented by combined factor B or factor I knockout
    - Proves necessity of alternative pathway convertase (C3bBb) and factor I-generated degradation products (iC3b, C3c, C3dg)

CLINICAL ISSUES

Epidemiology
- Incidence
  - Rare; estimated at 1-3 cases/million
    - Familial cases even rarer (~ 6 patients reported)
- Age
  - Primarily in children 5-15 years old
  - Increasingly appreciated in adults in recent series
    - ~ 55% are > 16 years old
    - 40% of adults are > 60 years old
- Gender
  - Female:male = 1.5:2

DENSE DEPOSIT DISEASE

Key Facts

Terminology
- C3 nephropathy with very electron-dense deposits within GBM and mesangium

Clinical Issues
- Rare (1-3 cases/million)
- Primarily children 5-15 years old, also adults
- Proteinuria/hematuria, nephritic or nephrotic syndrome
- C3NeF present in > 80%
- No effective treatment
- ~ 50% develop ESRD in 10-15 years
- Recurs in renal allografts
- Ocular drusen
- Acquired partial lipodystrophy (APL) (~ 5%)

Microscopic Pathology
- Varied glomerular pathology
  - Mesangial proliferation, acute exudative GN, MPGN, crescentic GN
- GBMs are thickened, eosinophilic, and refractile and stain strongly with PAS
- IF: "Garland" and granular mesangial pattern of C3 in 100%
  - IgM (35%), IgG (25%), IgA (15%), or C1q (10%)
- EM: Highly osmiophilic dense deposits within GBM, mesangium, Bowman capsule, and TBM
- Deposits in Bruch membrane and spleen

Top Differential Diagnoses
- AGN; MPGN, types I/III; MIDD

Presentation
- Hematuria (~ 90%)
  - Macrohematuria (~ 15%)/nephritic presentation
- Proteinuria (~ 95%)
  - Nephrotic range (~ 60%)
  - Proteinuria may undergo rapid fluctuation
- Renal insufficiency (~ 50%)
- Acquired partial lipodystrophy (APL) (3-5%)
  - Loss of subcutaneous fat in upper 1/2 of body may precede kidney disease onset by several years
  - ~ 83% of APL patients have low C3 levels and polyclonal C3NeF
  - ~ 20% go on to develop MPGN after median of 8 years after onset of lipodystrophy
- Ocular drusen common
  - ~ 10% develop decreased visual acuity

Laboratory Tests
- Decreased serum C3 in ~ 80% of patients
  - More common in children (100%) than adults (40%)
  - Increased C3dg and C3d
- C3NeF (antibody to C3bBb) present in > 80% of MPGN II patients
  - Persists in > 50% during disease course
  - C3NeF present in ~ 50% of MPGN, type I or III
- CFH mutations

Treatment
- Drugs
  - Steroids, immunosuppression not effective
  - Complement inhibition with eculizumab (anti-CD5 antibody) under study
  - Heparinoids may be used to protect GBM from complement activation
- Plasmapheresis and plasma exchange in patients with CFH mutations
  - Recombinant CFH

Prognosis
- Spontaneous remission rare
- ~ 50% develop ESRD within 10-15 years

- Mean time to ESRD is 5 years in adults, 20 years in children
- Recurs in almost all renal allografts
  - ~ 50% of allografts ultimately fail, typically in 1st 3 years

MICROSCOPIC PATHOLOGY

Histologic Features
- Glomerular patterns
  - Membranoproliferative glomerulonephritis (25-45%)
    - Mesangial proliferation, thickened GBM, duplication sometimes evident
    - Eosinophilic and refractile and stain brightly with PAS; fuchsinophilic on trichrome
    - DDD deposits stain poorly with Jones stain
  - Mild mesangial hypercellularity (30-50%)
    - Normal GBM by light microscopy
  - Crescentic glomerulonephritis (10-20%)
    - Focal crescents in > 50% of cases
  - Acute glomerulonephritis (10-20%)
    - Poly- or mononuclear cells, mesangial hypercellularity, normal thickness of GBM
  - Necrosis uncommon (~ 15%)
  - Focal, segmental, and global glomerulosclerosis, late
- Tubules and interstitium
  - Usually not affected early in disease
  - Thickened TBM sometimes evident due to deposits
  - Tubular atrophy and intersitial fibrosis develop late in disease
- Vessels
  - No specific changes
- Follow-up biopsies
  - Less acute glomerular inflammation
  - Increased glomerulosclerosis, tubular atrophy, fibrosis
  - Transitions
    - Progression from mesangial proliferative GN to MPGN pattern
    - Resolution of crescentic GN to mesangial proliferative GN

DENSE DEPOSIT DISEASE

ANCILLARY TESTS

Immunofluorescence
- Prominent C3 deposits (100%)
  - Ribbon-like ("garland") pattern in GBM
    - "Railroad track" or "double contour" pattern may be seen along GBM
  - Coarse spherules or ring-like deposits in mesangium
  - C3c appears to be main constituent of dense deposits
    - Some positive for C3d (absent from C3c), detects C3b, iC3b, and C3d
  - Tubular basement membrane (TBM) broad linear deposits (~ 60%)
  - Bowman capsule deposits (~ 30%)
  - C3 present before dense deposits are detectable in transplants
- Focal immunoglobulin deposits in minority
  - IgM (35%), IgG (25%), IgA (15%), C1q (10%)
    - IgM more common in children (~ 60%) than in adults (~ 20%)
  - Paucity of IgG indicates that dense deposits are not immune complexes

Electron Microscopy
- Highly osmiophilic dense deposits in lamina densa of GBM, resulting in very electron-dense appearance
  - Lack organized substructure and have dark homogeneous smudgy, hazy appearance
  - Segmental, discontinuous, or diffuse pattern of dense deposits along GBM
    - "Sausage-string" pattern
  - Sometimes deposits are subendothelial
  - Mesangium and small vessels may also contain same electron-dense deposits
  - Similar deposits in Bowman capsule (~ 45%) and TBM (~ 50%)
  - Reason for osmophilia is unknown; may be due to unsaturated lipids associated with ApoE accumulation
- Subepithelial "humps" sometimes present (~ 30%)
  - Less dense than intramembranous deposits
- Podocyte injury eventually occurs with actin cytoskeleton and slit diaphragm disruption resulting in podocyte hypertrophy, detachment, and death

Special Stains
- Deposits stain with fluorescent dye thioflavin T

Laser Capture-Mass Spectroscopy
- Deposits uniformly contain C3, C5, C8α, C9, CFH-related protein 1 (FHR1), clusterin, vitronectin, and apolipoprotein E (apoE)
- In contrast, immune complex GN usually had C4 and rarely had C9 or vitronectin; none had apoE

Other Organs
- Deposits may also be seen in choroidal blood vessels and splenic sinusoidal basement membrane
- Deposits along choriocapillaris-Bruch membrane-retinal pigment epithelial interface
  - Responsible for ocular drusen

- Detectable in 2nd decade of life
- Similar to age-related macular degeneration

DIFFERENTIAL DIAGNOSIS

MPGN, Types I/III
- Lack dense deposits
- Usually have immunoglobulin
- Duplication more prominent

Acute Glomerulonephritis (AGN)
- Lacks hyperdense deposits
- IgG present

Monoclonal Immunoglobulin Deposition Disease (MIDD)
- By definition has immunoglobulin deposition (single light chain &/or heavy chain)
- May have DDD and monoclonal gammopathy

DIAGNOSTIC CHECKLIST

Clinically Relevant Pathologic Features
- ESRD associated with older age and higher creatinine at presentation, "humps," possibly crescents

Pathologic Interpretation Pearls
- Most important findings are very dense, osmiophilic deposits on EM

SELECTED REFERENCES

1. Martínez-Barricarte R et al: Human C3 mutation reveals a mechanism of dense deposit disease pathogenesis and provides insights into complement activation and regulation. J Clin Invest. 120(10):3702-12, 2010
2. Sethi S et al: Dense deposit disease associated with monoclonal gammopathy of undetermined significance. Am J Kidney Dis. 56(5):977-82, 2010
3. Suga K et al: A case of dense deposit disease associated with a group A streptococcal infection without the involvement of C3NeF or complement factor H deficiency. Pediatr Nephrol. 25(8):1547-50, 2010
4. Nasr SH et al: Dense deposit disease: clinicopathologic study of 32 pediatric and adult patients. Clin J Am Soc Nephrol. 4(1):22-32, 2009
5. Sethi S et al: Glomeruli of dense deposit disease contain components of the alternative and terminal complement pathway. Kidney Int. 75(9):952-60, 2009
6. Smith RJ et al: New approaches to the treatment of dense deposit disease. J Am Soc Nephrol. 18(9):2447-56, 2007
7. Walker PD et al: Dense deposit disease is not a membranoproliferative glomerulonephritis. Mod Pathol. 20(6):605-16, 2007
8. Appel GB et al: Membranoproliferative glomerulonephritis type II (dense deposit disease): an update. J Am Soc Nephrol. 16(5):1392-403, 2005
9. Smith KD et al: Pathogenic mechanisms in membranoproliferative glomerulonephritis. Curr Opin Nephrol Hypertens. 14(4):396-403, 2005

DENSE DEPOSIT DISEASE

Light Microscopy

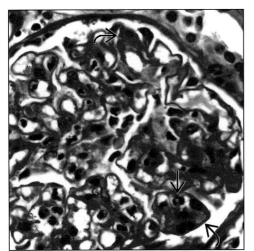

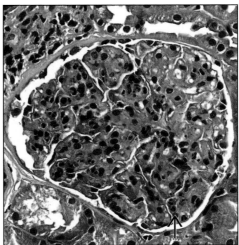

(Left) DDD is characterized by segmental PAS(+) thickening of the glomerular basement membrane ➡, visible by light microscopy and variable degrees of inflammation, seen here with neutrophils ➡. **(Right)** About 15% of DDD cases show an acute glomerulonephritis-type morphology with a vaguely lobular configuration of the glomerular tuft and numerous intracapillary neutrophils ➡.

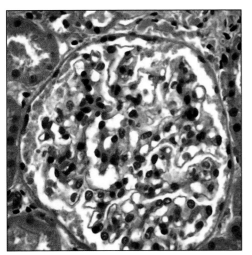

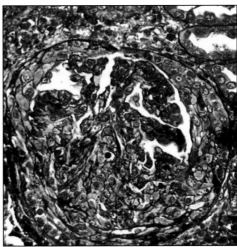

(Left) About 40% of DDD biopsies present with a mild mesangial hypercellularity and a normal GBM by light microscopy. This 8-year old boy had repeated microhematuria with strep infections. The diagnosis requires EM, which showed the characteristic dense deposits. **(Right)** Crescents, as seen in this biopsy from a 13-year-old girl, are common in DDD and extensive in about 15% of cases. Characteristic hyperdense deposits and subepithelial "humps" were evident by EM.

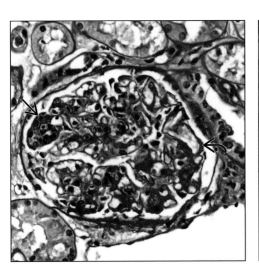

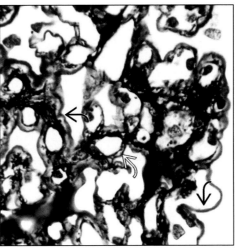

(Left) This case of DDD has PAS(+) thickening of the GBM ➡ and a mild acute glomerulonephritis-type morphology with increased numbers of inflammatory cells in glomerular capillaries ➡. **(Right)** The Jones stain in DDD shows decreased staining of the GBM ➡, which is normally argyrophilic. The loss is due to the dense deposits in the GBM. Double contours are segmentally present ➡ but uncommon, in contrast to MPGN, type I.

DENSE DEPOSIT DISEASE

Immunofluorescence

(Left) DDD classically has prominent bright granular deposits of C3 in the mesangium ➜ and segmentally linear ➜ deposits along the GBM. Immunoglobulins and C1q are typically absent or minimally present. *(Right)* The "garland" pattern of GBM staining ➜ for C3 in DDD is illustrated in a biopsy from a 9-year-old girl who developed end-stage renal disease 25 years later. Bowman capsule ➜ also stains, and the distinctive dark cores of mesangial deposits can be appreciated ➜.

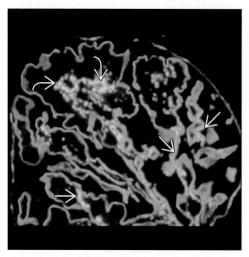 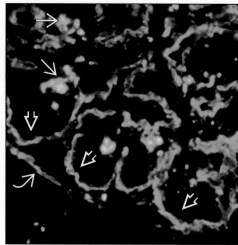

(Left) This case of DDD has prominent bright deposits of C3 in the mesangium ➜ and only segmental deposits in the GBM ➜. *(Right)* Scattered granular deposits of IgM are sometimes found in DDD, as illustrated in this case. IgG is almost always negative or minimally present.

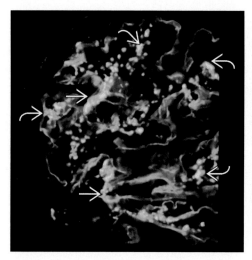 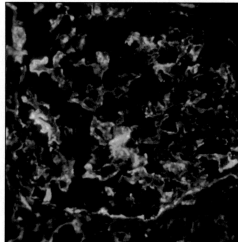

(Left) The tubular basement membranes in DDD focally contain dense deposits and stain for C3 in a broad segmental pattern ➜, as illustrated in this case of familial DDD in a 35-year-old man who received a renal transplant. His daughter also had DDD in a biopsy at age 6 years. *(Right)* Thioflavine T stain of a case of DDD viewed under fluorescence illumination (UV) is shown. The dense deposits ➜ characteristically have a blue autofluorescence, which is not seen in MPGN, type I.

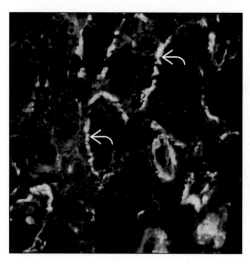 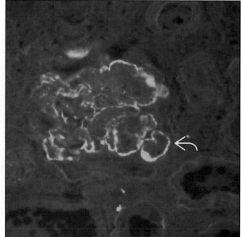

DENSE DEPOSIT DISEASE

Electron Microscopy

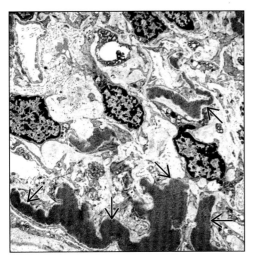

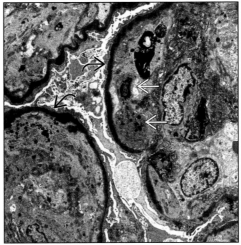

(Left) The diagnosis of DDD is based on EM, which reveals the extremely dark, osmiophilic deposits that replace and expand the GBM ➡. *(Right)* The classic lesions in DDD are extremely electron-dense deposits in the basement membrane (GBM) ➘ and mesangium of glomeruli. This biopsy from a 9-year-old girl also has prominent intracapillary inflammatory cells ➡. She developed renal failure over the next 25 years and received a transplant.

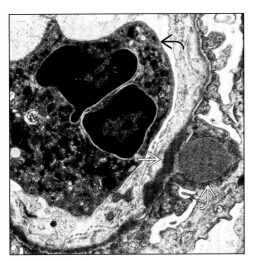

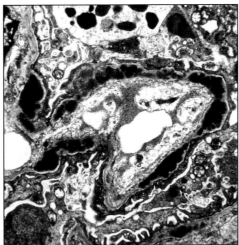

(Left) This case of DDD in a 13-year-old girl presented with acute glomerulonephritis clinically. In addition to the distinctive hyperdense deposits ➡ in the GBM, there is a subepithelial "hump" ➘, which has lower density. A neutrophil is in the capillary loop ➘. *(Right)* This case of DDD shows a variant pattern with interrupted, segmental deposition in the GBM. The 8-year-old boy had repeated episodes of gross hematuria associated with streptococcal infections.

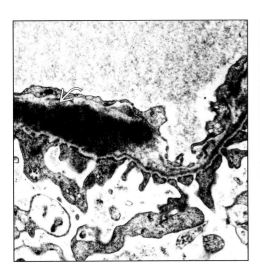

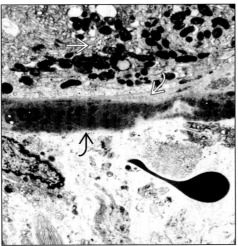

(Left) Sometimes the dense deposits in DDD are predominantly subendothelial, as in this case ➘. This may be an early stage of the disease. *(Right)* The dense deposits of DDD are found in the tubular basement membrane (TBM), as illustrated here ➘. A layer of uninvolved TBM can be seen ➘ between the tubular epithelial cells ➡ and the dense deposits. Other sites with deposits are the splenic sinusoids, the choroidal vessels, and the retina (ocular drusen).

C3 GLOMERULONEPHRITIS

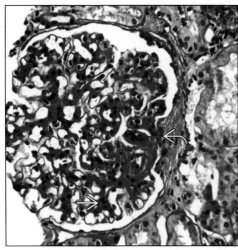

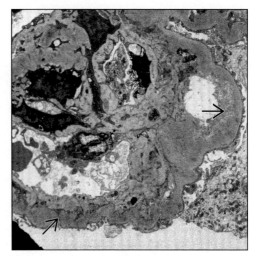

Mesangioproliferative pattern of C3 glomerulonephritis is shown. In this case, there is mild to moderate mesangial hypercellularity ➡ and a segmental adhesion ⇉ to Bowman capsule.

Intermediately electron-dense deposits ⊟→ are seen within glomerular capillary loops and within the mesangium by electron microscopy in this case with a membranoproliferative pattern.

TERMINOLOGY

Synonyms
- Primary glomerulonephritis with isolated C3 deposits
- Some entities previously classified as type I or III membranoproliferative glomerulonephritis (MPGN) belong in this category

Definitions
- Glomerulonephritis with isolated C3 deposits secondary to dysfunction of alternative complement pathway

ETIOLOGY/PATHOGENESIS

Dysregulation of Alternative Complement Pathway
- Initial activation of complement and complement amplification via alternative pathway amplification loop
- Defect in complement regulatory proteins or complement activators
  - Mutation in CFH, CFHR5, CFI, MCP, C3
  - Autoantibodies to C3bBb or C3

CLINICAL ISSUES

Epidemiology
- Age
  - Mean presentation: 30 years; range: 7 to > 70 years

Presentation
- Proteinuria, mild to nephrotic range
- Hematuria
- Hypertension
- Chronic renal failure

Laboratory Tests
- Serologic tests

- Serum C3 levels decreased in some patients
  - Associated with C3NeF
- Serum C4 level usually normal
- Specialized complement tests
  - Factor H, factor I, factor B
  - Serum soluble membrane attack complex
    - Increased levels in some patients
  - Alternative complement pathway functional and hemolytic assays
- Autoantibodies
  - C3 nephritic factor
  - Anti-C3 convertase and anti-factor H autoantibodies
- Genetic tests
  - Factor H, factor I, membrane cofactor protein (MCP; CD46)
    - H402 allele in cases with factor H mutation
  - Complement factor H-related protein family: CFHR1-5
    - CFHR5 mutation causing C3 glomerulonephritis identified in families of Cypriot origin
  - Complement factor B, C3

Treatment
- Surgical approaches
  - Low serum C3 level associated with presence of C3 nephritic factor
  - Renal transplantation (disease may recur in allograft)
- Drugs
  - Steroids
    - Response in some patients
  - Plasma infusions in patients with complement factor deficiencies
  - Plasmapheresis or rituximab in setting of acquired inhibitor (experimental)
  - C5 inhibition with eculizumab (experimental)

Prognosis
- Variable; subset of patients progress to end-stage renal disease while others retain normal renal function

C3 GLOMERULONEPHRITIS

Key Facts

Terminology
- Glomerulonephritis secondary to dysfunction of alternative complement pathway
  - Genetic or autoimmune
- Isolated C3 deposits by immunofluorescence with electron-dense deposits in glomeruli

Clinical Issues
- Proteinuria
- Hematuria
- Hypertension
- Hypocomplementemia (C3)
- Need to evaluate for complement system abnormalities

Microscopic Pathology
- Various glomerular patterns by LM
  - MPGN, type I
  - Mesangial and subepithelial to intramembranous deposits without MPGN
- C3 deposits in mesangium and GBM
- No significant immunoglobulin deposits
- Amorphous mesangial and subendothelial deposits by EM

Top Differential Diagnoses
- DDD
- MPGN of other causes
- Postinfectious glomerulonephritis

Diagnostic Checklist
- Key feature is C3 with little or no immunoglobulin and deposits less dense than those seen in DDD

MICROSCOPIC PATHOLOGY

Histologic Features
- Glomeruli
  - Mesangial and subepithelial to intramembranous deposits without MPGN pattern
    - No mesangial proliferation
    - No or minimal GBM duplication
  - Membranoproliferative glomerulonephritis (MPGN), type I
    - Mesangial hypercellularity
    - Mainly subendothelial and mesangial deposits; may have some subepithelial deposits
    - Diffuse glomerular basement membrane (GBM) duplication
    - Renal disease more severe in patients with MPGN pattern than non-MPGN pattern
- Tubules and interstitium
  - Interstitial fibrosis and tubular atrophy, usually mild to moderate

ANCILLARY TESTS

Immunofluorescence
- C3 deposits in mesangium and glomerular basement membranes
- No significant immunoglobulin deposits or C1q

Electron Microscopy
- Amorphous deposits in mesangium
- Subendothelial electron-dense deposits (MPGN pattern) &/or scattered subepithelial deposits
- Deposits may be electron dense or intermediately dense
  - Not as dense as dense deposit disease (DDD)
- Some cases may show overlapping features with DDD with intramembranous deposits

Mass Spectrometry
- Deposits composed of alternative and terminal complement pathway components, similar to DDD

DIFFERENTIAL DIAGNOSIS

MPGN, Type I/III
- Immunoglobulin deposition by IF along with C3

Dense Deposit Disease
- Deposits more electron dense
- DDD may be classified as a specific type of C3 glomerulonephritis

Immune Complex Glomerulonephritis
- Immunoglobulin deposition by IF along with C3

Postinfectious Glomerulonephritis
- Usually shows immunoglobulin deposits by IF
  - C3 can persist longer than immunoglobulin
- Clinical history of infection is helpful although C3 glomerulonephritis may manifest at time of infection

DIAGNOSTIC CHECKLIST

Pathologic Interpretation Pearls
- Key features are C3 with little or no immunoglobulin and deposits less dense by EM than DDD

SELECTED REFERENCES
1. Sethi S et al: Proliferative glomerulonephritis secondary to dysfunction of the alternative pathway of complement. Clin J Am Soc Nephrol. Epub ahead of print, 2011
2. Fakhouri F et al: C3 glomerulopathy: a new classification. Nat Rev Nephrol. 6(8):494-9, 2010
3. Gale DP et al: Identification of a mutation in complement factor H-related protein 5 in patients of Cypriot origin with glomerulonephritis. Lancet. 376(9743):794-801, 2010
4. Pickering MC et al: Translational mini-review series on complement factor H: renal diseases associated with complement factor H: novel insights from humans and animals. Clin Exp Immunol. 151(2):210-30, 2008
5. Servais A et al: Primary glomerulonephritis with isolated C3 deposits: a new entity which shares common genetic risk factors with haemolytic uraemic syndrome. J Med Genet. 44(3):193-9, 2007

C3 GLOMERULONEPHRITIS

Microscopic Features

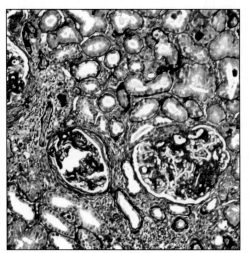
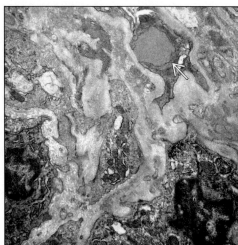

(Left) C3 glomerulonephritis with a mesangioproliferative and segmental sclerosing pattern is shown. The patient was a young man with nephrotic-range proteinuria and normal renal function. *(Right)* C3 glomerulonephritis with a membranoproliferative pattern in an older woman with a family history of glomerulonephritis is shown. A hump-shaped subepithelial deposit ➡ (nonspecific) is seen along with subendothelial deposits.

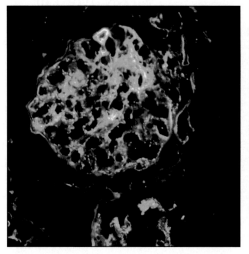
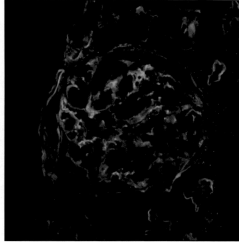

(Left) Granular mesangial and glomerular capillary loop staining is seen for C3 only by immunofluorescence. *(Right)* Immunofluorescence staining for IgG was negative in glomeruli. Negative staining for immunoglobulins (besides nonspecific staining for IgM in scars) is a requisite for the diagnosis of C3 glomerulonephritis.

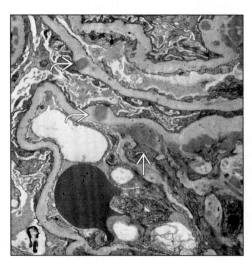
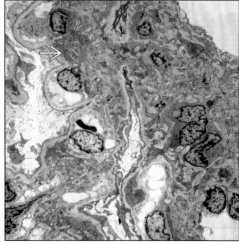

(Left) Mesangioproliferative glomerulonephritis pattern with C3 deposits shows mesangial electron-dense deposits ➡ and an occasional subepithelial to intramembranous deposit ➡. *(Right)* Mesangioproliferative glomerulonephritis pattern with C3 deposits shows mostly mesangial electron-dense deposits ➡ accompanied by mesangial expansion.

C3 GLOMERULONEPHRITIS

Microscopic Features

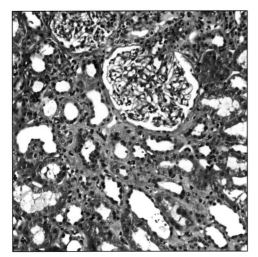 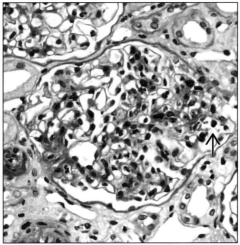

(Left) Recurrent C3 glomerulonephritis on a protocol biopsy from a 20-year-old woman 9 months post renal transplant is shown. The glomeruli show very mild mesangial hypercellularity. (Right) A glomerulus shows mild mesangial hypercellularity and mesangial matrix expansion. Neutrophils are present within segmental glomerular capillary loops ➡.

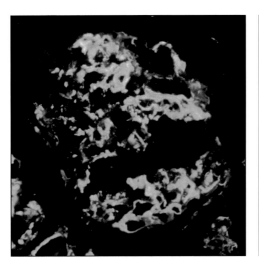 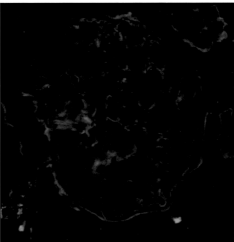

(Left) By IF, glomeruli show bright granular staining for C3 in mesangium and segmental glomerular capillary loops. Recurrence in allograft of "postinfectious glomerulonephritis" may represent C3 glomerulonephritis. (Right) IF is negative for IgG and for other immunoreactants. Negativity for immunoglobulins, with only staining for C3, raises the possibility of C3 glomerulonephritis, and evaluation for complement system abnormalities is warranted.

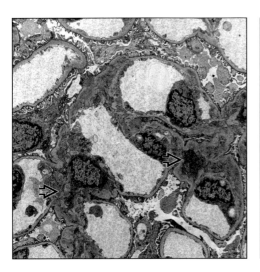 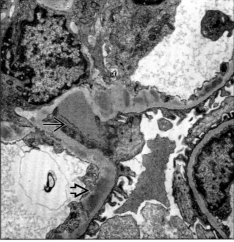

(Left) Amorphous electron-dense deposits, mostly within mesangium ➡, are seen by electron microscopy. Podocytes show largely preserved foot processes. (Right) Paramesangial to subendothelial ➡ and subepithelial ➡ amorphous electron-dense deposits are shown. Hump-shaped subepithelial deposits are reminiscent of postinfectious glomerulonephritis but are not specific. Findings are compatible with early recurrent C3 glomerulonephritis or early MPGN.

2

C1q NEPHROPATHY

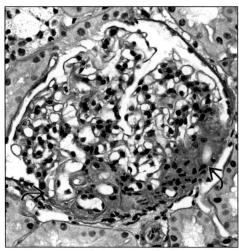

H&E from a 12-year-old girl with nephrotic syndrome due to C1q nephropathy is shown. Focal segmental glomerulosclerosis (FSGS) ⇗, a common histologic pattern in C1q nephropathy, is evident.

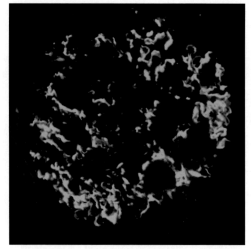

C1q nephropathy is characterized by dominant or codominant C1q deposits of ≥ 2+ intensity, seen in this 15-year-old boy with microhematuria & proteinuria. IgG staining was 2+, and lupus serologies were negative.

TERMINOLOGY

Definitions
- Idiopathic glomerular disease characterized by dominant or codominant C1q staining (≥ 2+ intensity) primarily in mesangium in patients with no evidence of systemic lupus erythematosus (SLE), membranoproliferative glomerulonephritis (MPGN), or infection
  - Originally described by Jennette and Hipp in 1985
  - Controversy remains whether it is a distinct entity

ETIOLOGY/PATHOGENESIS

Idiopathic
- No definitive single pathogenetic mechanism identified; speculation on 4 leading possibilities

Immune Complex Formation
- C1q is component of classical complement activation pathway and links innate immunity to IgG/IgM-mediated acquired immunity
  - Classical pathway is activated when C1q binds to Fc portion of immunoglobulin
    - C1q binding is strongest with IgM, IgG1, and IgG3
- Deposits may alter the course of minimal change disease (MCD) and focal segmental glomerulosclerosis (FSGS)

Direct Binding of C1q
- C1q receptors are expressed on monocytes, macrophages, platelets, neutrophils, lymphocytes, endothelial cells, and mesangial cells
  - C1q can thus directly bind to mesangial cells through C1q receptors
- C1q can also bind to polyanionic substances such as DNA, RNA, lipopolysaccharides, and viral and bacterial proteins

- C1q triggers phagocytosis of bacteria and neutralization of retroviruses
- C1q nephropathy has been reported in setting of BK polyoma nephritis and CMV infection

Increased Synthesis of C1q
- Macrophages and dendritic cells synthesize C1q
- Inflammatory cytokines upregulate C1q production

Nonspecific Entrapment of C1q
- Increased glomerular protein trafficking in severe proteinuria causes nonspecific entrapment of immunoglobulin in mesangium
- C1q fixes to entrapped immunoglobulin, and these changes may not represent "true" immune complexes
- This hypothesis may be best applicable to MCD/FSGS clinicopathological subset of C1q nephropathy

CLINICAL ISSUES

Epidemiology
- Incidence
  - Prevalence of C1q glomerulopathy ranges from 0.2-2.5% of renal biopsies from adults and children
    - Higher prevalence in biopsies from children (6%), especially those with nephrotic syndrome (16.5%)
  - Subclinical C1q ≥ 2+ in ~ 7% of asymptomatic donor kidneys
- Age
  - Often seen in older children and young adults
- Gender
  - No consistent gender predisposition
- Ethnicity
  - African-Americans have frequent nephrotic syndrome presentation with FSGS histology

Presentation
- Nephrotic syndrome (NS) (> 50%)
  - Abrupt onset is most frequent presentation
  - Often correlates with MCD/FSGS histology

C1q NEPHROPATHY

Key Facts

Terminology
- Dominant or codominant C1q staining (≥ 2+ intensity) in mesangium without evidence of SLE or MPGN

Etiology/Pathogenesis
- Possibilities include immune complex formation, direct binding of C1q, and nonspecific entrapment of C1q in glomeruli

Clinical Issues
- Prevalence: 0.2-2.5% of renal biopsies
- Some studies have documented higher rates of resistance to steroid therapy, but prognosis seems largely based on histology
- Nephrotic syndrome, asymptomatic hematuria &/or proteinuria, or chronic renal insufficiency

Microscopic Pathology
- Heterogeneity of glomerular changes
  - No glomerular abnormalities, resembling MCD
  - Mesangial proliferative glomerulonephritis
  - Focal segmental glomerulosclerosis
- Predominately mesangial C1q with C3, IgG, IgA, and IgM in various combinations
- Amorphous electron-dense deposits in mesangium
  - Occasionally subendothelial; rarely, subepithelial deposits

Diagnostic Checklist
- Glomerular pathology and degree of tubular atrophy and interstitial fibrosis have prognostic significance
- Strict adherence to threshold of ≥ 2+ intensity of C1q staining is important to prevent overdiagnosis

---

- Subnephrotic proteinuria (15-20%)
- Asymptomatic hematuria (10-15%)
  - Reports include incidental detection in Japanese children, who undergo routine urine screen
- Isolated hematuria and proteinuria (5-10%)
- Chronic renal insufficiency (15-20%)
  - Frequent presentation of mesangioproliferative GN
  - Hematuria and proteinuria may be present
- Gross hematuria (< 5%)
- Glomerulonephritis (< 5%)

Laboratory Tests
- Urinalysis shows variable proteinuria and hematuria based on clinical presentation
- Serum complements are normal, may be low C1q
- Serological studies supportive of lupus such as ANA, anti-ds DNA, and anti-C1q antibodies are negative
  - Serological studies remain negative even after several years of clinical follow-up
- HIV status is negative

Treatment
- Drugs
  - Corticosteroids
  - Cyclosporine in steroid-resistant NS
  - No treatment may be needed in setting of asymptomatic hematuria and proteinuria

Prognosis
- Some studies have documented higher rates of resistance to steroid therapy in NS due to C1q glomerulopathy, but prognosis seems largely based on histology
  - In MCD or mesangial proliferative GN histology, treatment response is better, and renal function is usually preserved
  - FSGS lesions are generally (but not always) associated with poorer outcomes and may progress to end-stage kidney disease
- Children diagnosed with C1q nephropathy after urine screen may normalize urinalysis even without corticosteroid therapy

MICROSCOPIC PATHOLOGY

Histologic Features
- Glomerular histology has 4 patterns
  - No glomerular abnormalities by light microscopy
    - ~ 40% of cases (range: 0-100%)
    - Biopsy resembles MCD
  - Mesangial proliferation
    - ~ 20% of cases (range: 0-75%)
    - Usually mild to moderate
    - Occasional cases show segmental endocapillary proliferation or focal crescents (~ 7%)
  - Focal segmental glomerulosclerosis
    - ~ 40% of cases (range: 0-90%)
    - ~ 50% associated with mesangial proliferation
    - FSGS lesions characterized by Bowman capsular adhesions and hyaline insudation
    - Other FSGS variants described include collapsing and cellular types
    - In a few instances, MCD histology in C1q nephropathy evolved into FSGS on follow-up biopsy
    - Some authors consider C1q nephropathy to be just a variant of FSGS
  - Incidental finding
    - Present in 7% of transplant donor kidneys
    - Occasionally with other diseases such as thin basement membrane disease, interstitial nephritis polycystic kidneys, global sclerosis
  - Relative frequency of histological findings varies based on study cited
  - Membranoproliferative histology is considered an exclusion criterion by most investigators
  - Some cases described have incidental or subclinical C1q deposition
- Features of acute tubular injury, such as loss of brush borders and simplified epithelium, seen in severe proteinuria
- Variable tubular atrophy and interstitial fibrosis
- Small vessel vasculitis is rare (~ 3%)

Glomerular Diseases

2

85

C1q NEPHROPATHY

ANCILLARY TESTS

Immunofluorescence

- Dominant or codominant C1q staining (≥ 2+ intensity) in mesangium and occasionally along glomerular capillary walls
  - Deposits in paramesangial location may have comma-shaped appearance
- Most cases have IgG (67%), IgM (81%), IgA (47%), and C3 (83%) deposits, but of lesser intensity than C1q staining
  - "Full house" (IgG, IgA, IgM, C1q, C3) in ~ 30%
  - C4 staining in 35%
- C1q deposits may disappear on follow-up biopsies, even in cases with FSGS histology
- De novo C1q deposits in renal allograft have no apparent clinical significance

Electron Microscopy

- Mesangial amorphous electron-dense deposits in ~ 90% (range: 45-100%)
  - Lack of electron-dense deposits in a few cases is probably due to segmental distribution of deposits
  - Usually paramesangial (near GBM reflection)
- Occasional subendothelial deposits (7-44%)
- Rare subepithelial deposits (0-17%)
- Podocyte foot process effacement ranges from mild to extensive and correlates with degree of proteinuria
- Tubuloreticular inclusions in endothelial cells uncommon (0-6%)

DIFFERENTIAL DIAGNOSIS

Lupus Nephritis

- Clinical and serological evidence of systemic lupus erythematosus
- More commonly subepithelial and subendothelial deposits
  - Deposits may have curvilinear substructure (thumbprints)
  - Tubuloreticular inclusions typically found in endothelial cells
- Deposits in tubular basement membrane common
- Glomerular inflammation, necrosis, crescents more common

IgA Nephropathy

- Dominant or codominant glomerular IgA staining on immunofluorescence
- C1q deposition typically scanty or absent

Focal Segmental Glomerulosclerosis (FSGS)

- Some believe C1q nephropathy is variant of FSGS
- Abundant mesangial deposits characteristic of C1q nephropathy

DIAGNOSTIC CHECKLIST

Clinically Relevant Pathologic Features

- Glomerular histologic lesion appears to predict outcome and treatment response

- Better with MCD than FSGS
- Degree of tubular atrophy and interstitial fibrosis has prognostic significance

Pathologic Interpretation Pearls

- Strict adherence to threshold of ≥ 2+ intensity of C1q staining is important to prevent overdiagnosis

SELECTED REFERENCES

1. Said SM et al: C1q deposition in the renal allograft: a report of 24 cases. Mod Pathol. 23(8):1080-8, 2010
2. Wenderfer SE et al: C1q nephropathy in the pediatric population: pathology and pathogenesis. Pediatr Nephrol. 25(8):1385-96, 2010
3. Kaneko K et al: Change in C1q deposition in C1q nephropathy. Pediatr Nephrol. 24(9):1775, 2009
4. Lim BJ et al: IgG nephropathy - confusion and overlap with C1q nephropathy. Clin Nephrol. 72(5):360-5, 2009
5. Mii A et al: Current status and issues of C1q nephropathy. Clin Exp Nephrol. 13(4):263-74, 2009
6. Roberti I et al: A single-center study of C1q nephropathy in children. Pediatr Nephrol. 24(1):77-82, 2009
7. Hisano S et al: Clinicopathologic correlation and outcome of C1q nephropathy. Clin J Am Soc Nephrol. 3(6):1637-43, 2008
8. Vizjak A et al: Pathology, clinical presentations, and outcomes of C1q nephropathy. J Am Soc Nephrol. 19(11):2237-44, 2008
9. Fukuma Y et al: Clinicopathologic correlation of C1q nephropathy in children. Am J Kidney Dis. 47(3):412-8, 2006
10. Krinsky CS et al: An 18-year-old woman with proteinuria and renal insufficiency. C1q nephropathy. Arch Pathol Lab Med. 130(4):e53-5, 2006
11. Lau KK et al: Pediatric C1q nephropathy and incidental proteinuria. Pediatr Nephrol. 21(6):883; author reply 884, 2006
12. Kersnik Levart T et al: C1Q nephropathy in children. Pediatr Nephrol. 20(12):1756-61, 2005
13. Nishida M et al: C1q nephropathy with asymptomatic urine abnormalities. Pediatr Nephrol. 20(11):1669-70, 2005
14. Hashimoto S et al: Steroid-sensitive nephrotic syndrome associated with positive C1q immunofluorescence. Clin Exp Nephrol. 8(3):266-9, 2004
15. Sharman A et al: Distinguishing C1q nephropathy from lupus nephritis. Nephrol Dial Transplant. 19(6):1420-6, 2004
16. Markowitz GS et al: C1q nephropathy: a variant of focal segmental glomerulosclerosis. Kidney Int. 64(4):1232-40, 2003
17. Isaac J et al: De novo C1q nephropathy in the renal allograft of a kidney pancreas transplant recipient: BK virus-induced nephropathy? Nephron. 92(2):431-6, 2002
18. Jennette JC et al: C1q nephropathy: a distinct pathologic entity usually causing nephrotic syndrome. Am J Kidney Dis. 6(2):103-10, 1985
19. Jennette JC et al: Immunohistopathologic evaluation of C1q in 800 renal biopsy specimens. Am J Clin Pathol. 83(4):415-20, 1985

C1q NEPHROPATHY

Microscopic Features

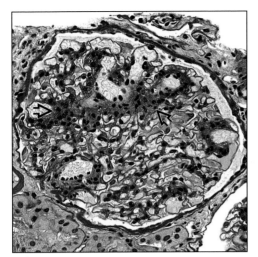

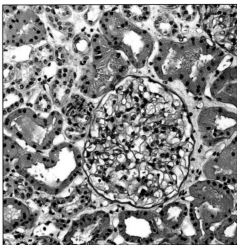

(Left) A 15-year-old boy with microscopic hematuria and non-nephrotic proteinuria was diagnosed with C1q nephropathy on immunofluorescence microscopy. Mild segmental mesangial proliferative glomerulonephritis ➡ is seen on light microscopy. (Right) A 26-year-old man with abrupt onset of nephrotic syndrome showed normal kidney on light microscopy. Immunofluorescence microscopy was compatible with C1q nephropathy.

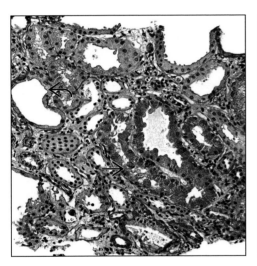

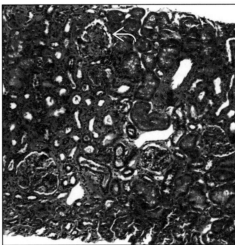

(Left) C1q nephropathy can present as an MCD phenotype with abrupt onset of nephrotic syndrome. Prominent protein resorption droplets ➡ are seen in the proximal tubules. Mild acute tubular injury is evident with simplified epithelium ➡. (Right) C1q nephropathy has a variety of light microscopic patterns. One of the most common is focal segmental glomerulosclerosis ➡, illustrated in this biopsy from a 14-year-old boy with nephrotic syndrome and negative lupus serologies.

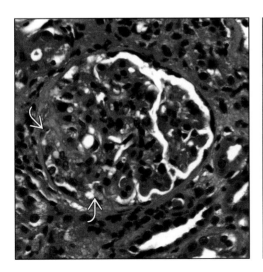

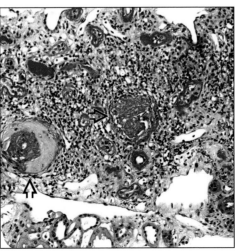

(Left) C1q nephropathy often shows segmental sclerosis and adhesions (FSGS) ➡. The glomeruli in this case, from a 14 year old with nephrotic syndrome, had a "full house" pattern by immunofluorescence, resembling lupus; however, ANA and anti-dsDNA antibodies were negative. (Right) Globally sclerotic glomeruli ➡ are seen in this case of NS and C1q nephropathy with FSGS in a 9-year-old African-American boy. Cases with extensive tubular atrophy have a poorer prognosis.

C1q NEPHROPATHY

Immunofluorescence

(Left) This is the 1st of 6 images from a 14-year-old boy with C1q nephropathy. This sample displays 2+ granular C1q staining, primarily in the mesangium. The IF pattern resembles lupus in that IgG, IgA, IgM, C3, and C1q are present ("full house"). C1q nephropathy is defined as dominant or codominant C1q in glomeruli of ≥ 2+ intensity in a patient without SLE. *(Right)* IgG is similar to C1q in intensity (2+) and distribution in this case of C1q nephropathy.

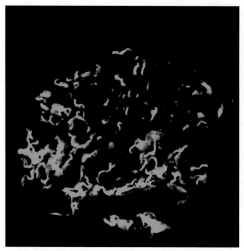 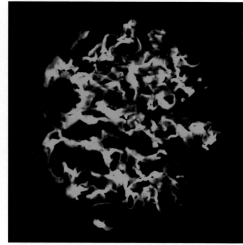

(Left) IgM is present primarily in the mesangium in a similar distribution to C1q although not as intense (1+). This distribution corresponds to the location of the amorphous electron-dense deposits seen by electron microscopy. *(Right)* IgA is present in the deposits in the mesangium in this case of C1q nephropathy, similar to C1q, although of lesser intensity (1+). Kappa and lambda stains were similar (1-2+) and equal.

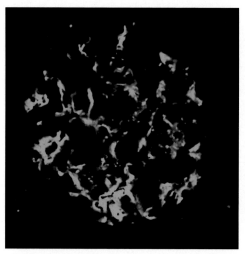 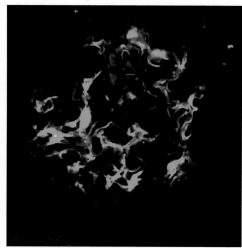

(Left) C3 is present in this case at a level similar to C1q (1-2+). *(Right)* Glomerular segments with sclerosis commonly stain for C3 ➡ and IgM, as shown in this case of C1q nephropathy. This universal pattern in focal segmental glomerulosclerosis is presumed to be nonspecific. It is also possible that IgM &/or C3 is reacting with products released from damaged cells.

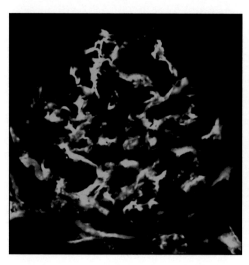 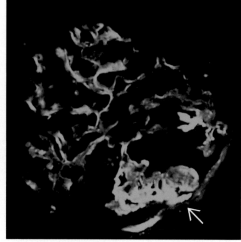

C1q NEPHROPATHY

Electron Microscopy

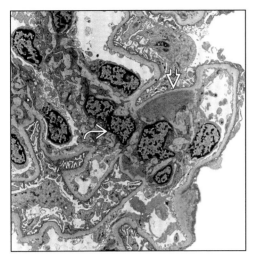
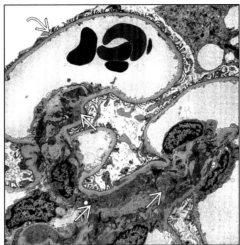

(Left) Electron-dense deposits in C1q nephropathy are typically paramesangial ⮞ in location. This biopsy from a 10-year-old boy with 2 g/d of proteinuria shows mild mesangial hypercellularity ⮞. *(Right)* Low-power view of C1q nephropathy shows the normal GBM ⮞ and amorphous electron-dense deposits primarily in the mesangium ⮞.

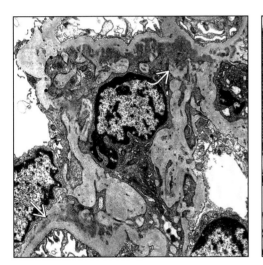
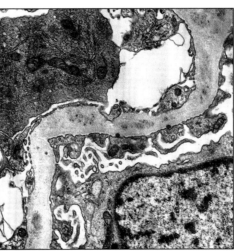

(Left) Abundant mesangial ⮞ and paramesangial ⮞ deposits in a case of C1q nephropathy are shown. The deposits "hug" the mesangial cells, similar to those in IgA nephropathy. No substructure is evident, in contrast to some cases of lupus nephritis. *(Right)* Deposits in C1q nephropathy are sometime found in the GBM and as subendothelial deposits, similar to lupus. Rare subepithelial deposits have also been reported.

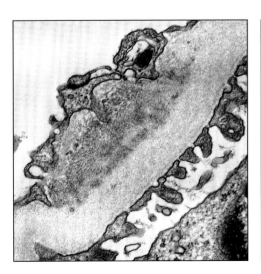
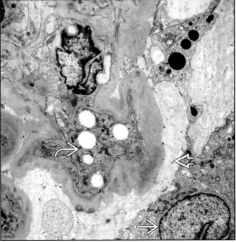

(Left) Subendothelial deposits in a 14-year-old boy with nephrotic syndrome due to C1q nephropathy are shown. No substructure is evident, and no tubuloreticular structures were found, which help distinguish this from lupus nephritis. *(Right)* A 9-year-old African-American boy with NS has dominant C1q deposits on IF, consistent with C1q nephropathy. Segmental glomerulosclerosis ⮞ is seen with overlying detached podocyte ⮞ and neobasement membrane layers ⮞.

ACUTE POSTSTREPTOCOCCAL GLOMERULONEPHRITIS

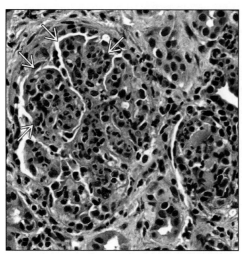

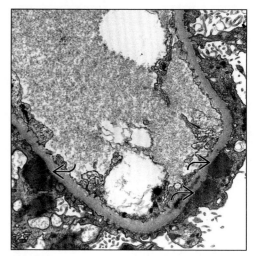

Acute poststreptococcal GN is often characterized by glomeruli with accentuated lobularity ➡ containing abundant neutrophils in what is termed an "exudative proliferative pattern."

EM shows a classic feature of PSAGN: Subepithelial deposits of immune complexes along the glomerular basement membrane, known as "humps" ⟶.

TERMINOLOGY

Abbreviations
- Acute poststreptococcal glomerulonephritis (PSAGN)

Synonyms
- Acute hemorrhagic Bright disease
- Diffuse proliferative and exudative glomerulonephritis

Definitions
- Acute glomerulonephritis related to recent streptococcal infection

ETIOLOGY/PATHOGENESIS

Infectious Agents
- *Streptococcus pyogenes*, group A, β-hemolytic (*Strep*)
  - Usually pharyngitis or skin infection (pyoderma)
    - Other sites include mastoiditis & otitis media
    - Pyoderma common in tropical countries
- Only certain strains are nephritogenic
  - Typed by surface M protein, a virulence factor
    - Pharyngitis strains: 1, 2, 25, & some 12
    - Pyoderma strains: 49 (Red Lake), 2, 42, 56-7, & 60
  - Different M-type strains cause rheumatic fever
- Other virulence factors
  - Provoke antibodies, useful for diagnosis, but not relevant to formation of immune complexes
    - DNase, hyaluronidase, streptokinase, NADase, proteinases, and hemolysins streptolysin-O (oxygen labile) & streptolysin-S (oxygen stable)
- Kidney is not infected
- PSAGN rarely recurs, in contrast to rheumatic fever

Acute Immune Complex Disease
- Target antigen(s) responsible for PSAGN still uncertain
- Leading candidates for target antigen(s)
  - Cationic cysteine proteinase exotoxin B (SPE B), a secreted protein that can bind plasmin
    - Colocalizes with IgG and C3 present in "humps"
  - Glyceraldehyde phosphate dehydrogenase (GAPDH), also a plasmin receptor
- Deposition of antibody-antigen complexes
  - Complement fixed in glomerular capillaries
    - Alternate pathway dominates
  - Attracts neutrophils & monocytes
  - Digestion of GBM components
    - Leakage of red cells & protein

History
- In 1812, W. C. Wells noted scarlet fever followed by "dropsy" & urine-containing red cells & coagulable substances
- In 1836, Richard Bright related renal failure to appearance of kidney at autopsy

Animal Models
- Administration of foreign serum protein (e.g., bovine serum albumin in rabbits)
  - "One shot" serum sickness
  - Mimics all features, including GN, "humps," & hypocomplementemia

CLINICAL ISSUES

Epidemiology
- Incidence
  - ~ 500,000 cases/year worldwide, 85% children
    - ↓ incidence in developed countries: Better hygiene decreases pyoderma
  - ~ 1:1,000 develop PSAGN after *Strep* pharyngitis has been treated
    - Higher in epidemics of nephritogenic strains
  - Familial risk factor noted by Wells, still undefined
    - No consistent HLA risk factors
- Age
  - Peak at age 6-8 years; rare < 2 years
  - Up to 33% are > 40 years old
- Gender
  - Male:female ≈ 2:1

ACUTE POSTSTREPTOCOCCAL GLOMERULONEPHRITIS

Key Facts

Terminology
- Acute diffuse proliferative ("exudative") GN with clinical history of streptococcal infection

Clinical Issues
- Gross hematuria in 30-60%; smoky, Coca-Cola urine
- Nephrotic syndrome in 5-10%
- Positive ASO anti-DNAse B, low C3
- Majority of children spontaneously resolve

Microscopic Pathology
- Diffuse hypercellularity
- Numerous neutrophils within capillary tufts
- Mesangial hypercellularity
- Glomerular capillaries are not thickened or duplicated
- Typically no necrosis

- Crescents, if present, are a poor prognostic feature
- Interstitial inflammation and edema, red cell casts

Ancillary Tests
- IF shows "starry sky," "garland," or mesangial pattern of IgG and C3, usually no C1q or IgA
- Amorphous, electron-dense "humps" without surrounding BM reaction
  - Occasional subendothelial, intramembranous, and mesangial deposits

Top Differential Diagnoses
- Nonstreptococcal postinfectious GN
- Proliferative GN with monoclonal immunoglobulin deposits
- MPGN, type I

Presentation
- Abrupt onset 1-4 weeks after *Strep* infection (average ~ 10 days)
- Hematuria
  - Almost all patients
  - Gross hematuria (~ 60% children, 30% adults)
    - "Smoky," Coca-Cola-, tea-, or coffee-colored urine
- Proteinuria
  - Nephrotic syndrome in 5-10%
- Edema
  - Sudden onset of periorbital edema
- Acute renal failure
  - ~ 60% elevated BUN
  - Oliguria/anuria
- Hypertension
  - Seen in ~ 85% of patients, largely due to sodium & fluid retention
- Anemia
- Subclinical in ~ 20%

Laboratory Tests
- Evidence of preceding *Strep* group A infection required for diagnosis
  - β-hemolytic organisms detected on sheep blood agar
- Serologic assays
  - Streptozyme® kit detects Ab to streptolysin, streptokinase, hyaluronidase, DNase, & NADase
  - Antistreptolysin O (ASO) titer best for pharyngitis, anti-DNase-B for pyoderma
    - 2 together are 95% sensitive
    - False positive due to ubiquity of Strep infections
- Low C3 (90%)
  - Precedes onset of hematuria
- Normal C4
  - Some low C1q, C4 early

Treatment
- Drugs
  - Post-infection sequelae rare with antibiotics

Prognosis
- Usually, spontaneous resolution in children

  - Overall, ~ 5% have decreased glomerular filtration rate (GFR) after 2 years
- Renal abnormalities persist in 1/3 adults > 60 years old
- C3 returns to normal within 8 weeks
- Microscopic hematuria may persist up to 5 years
- Repeated attacks extremely rare

MACROSCOPIC FEATURES

General Features
- Soft, pale with scattered petechiae
- Surface bulges due to edema
- Sometimes 25-50% > normal weight

MICROSCOPIC PATHOLOGY

Histologic Features
- Glomeruli
  - Diffuse hypercellularity with numerous neutrophils in capillary tufts
    - Hypercellularity mostly due to leukocytes, suggesting **intracapillary** GN rather than **proliferative** GN
    - Lymphocytes prominent, sometimes eosinophils, particularly in tropical cases
    - Mesangial hypercellularity and increased mesangial area/matrix
  - Accentuated glomerular lobularity with "clubbed" appearance
    - Glomerular capillaries variably patent
    - No GBM thickening
    - Duplication of the GBM, if present, suggests other diagnosis
  - Subepithelial "humps" visible in trichrome stain
    - Tiny nodules on epithelial side of GBM
  - Cellular, but not fibrous, crescents may be present
    - > 50% of glomeruli present in up to 40% of recent biopsied cases
    - Associated with poorer outcome
  - Necrosis rare
- Interstitium

ACUTE POSTSTREPTOCOCCAL GLOMERULONEPHRITIS

- o Monocytes, lymphocytes, neutrophils, eosinophils
  - ▪ May be prominent without glomerular disease
- o Edema
- o Little or no fibrosis
- Tubules
  - o Red cell casts in distal nephron
    - ▪ Compacted, hemolyzed, fragmented
    - ▪ Later in the course, pigmented casts appear
  - o Protein resorption droplets
  - o Acute tubular injury
  - o Atrophy may be present in late cases
- Vessels
  - o Vasculitis rare; requires excluding other diagnoses
- Late biopsies
  - o Resolving PSAGN not well defined
  - o Mesangial hypercellularity, loss of inflammatory component
  - o 86% healed (of 147 biopsies in 4 series)

ANCILLARY TESTS

Immunofluorescence

- 3 deposition patterns
  - o "Starry sky" or "lumpy-bumpy": Fine, irregular, granular (IgG and C3) in capillary walls & mesangium; seen early in disease course
  - o "Garland": Densely packed, thick, elongated, and confluent capillary wall deposits; seen in patients with crescents and nephrotic-range proteinuria; seen early in disease course; may have worse prognosis
  - o Mesangial: Granular, with sparing of capillary loops (C3 more common than IgG) noted later
- IgM seen in > 50% in some series
- IgA rarely seen
  - o Prompts consideration of other diseases
- IgE not usually evaluated but seen in ~ 50%
- C3 present without IgG in ~ 30%
- Properdin, C5b-9, factor B present in GBM & mesangium
  - o C1q and C4 usually lacking, supporting role of alternative complement pathway
  - o Factor H absent
- Fibrin in mesangium & crescents
- Variably reported *Strep* antigens (e.g., SPE B)

Electron Microscopy

- Amorphous, electron-dense "humps"
  - o Subepithelial (external) deposits on surface of GBMs
    - ▪ Without surrounding BM reaction ("spikes")
    - ▪ Deposits may become confluent
  - o Foot process effacement over "humps"
- Deposits in other locations may occur
  - o Mesangial subepithelial deposits common
  - o Intramembranous deposits may resemble dense deposit disease
  - o Subendothelial deposits uncommon
- Swollen endothelial cells
  - o Endothelium may be disrupted

Immunohistochemistry

- Infiltrating cells positive for CD4, CD8, Ki-67

DIFFERENTIAL DIAGNOSIS

Nonstreptococcal Postinfectious GN

- More common than PSAGN in some series
- Pathology similar if not identical
- IgA by IF prompts consideration of *Staph* infection

Membranoproliferative GN (MPGN), Type I

- Duplication of GBM favors MPGN
  - o Subendothelial deposits more prominent in MPGN

Proliferative GN with Monoclonal Immunoglobulin Deposits

- Predominance of 1 light chain type

Dense Deposit Disease

- Prominent intramembranous deposits by EM
- Usually no IgG

Cryoglobulinemic GN

- "Humps" rare, usually subendothelial & mesangial
- Organized EM deposits, "pseudothrombi"

Lupus Nephritis

- Usually IgA & C1q in glomeruli
- Subepithelial deposits typically have "spikes"
- TBM deposits present in ~ 30%

IgA Nephropathy

- Prominent mesangial IgA deposits
- Nephritis begins at time of respiratory infection ("synpharyngetic nephritis")

DIAGNOSTIC CHECKLIST

Clinically Relevant Pathologic Features

- Crescents increase risk of ESRD

Pathologic Interpretation Pearls

- PSAGN can be superimposed on other diseases
- Biopsy series biased for atypical or severe course

SELECTED REFERENCES

1. Eison TM et al: Post-streptococcal acute glomerulonephritis in children: clinical features and pathogenesis. Pediatr Nephrol. 26(2):165-80, 2011
2. Nasr SH et al: Postinfectious glomerulonephritis in the elderly. J Am Soc Nephrol. 22(1):187-95, 2011
3. Wong W et al: Outcome of severe acute post-streptococcal glomerulonephritis in New Zealand children. Pediatr Nephrol. 24(5):1021-6, 2009
4. Nadasdy T et al: Acute postinfectious glomerulonephritis and glomerulonephritis caused by persistent bacterial infection. In Jennette JC et al: Heptinstall's Pathology of the Kidney. 6th ed. Philadelphia: Lippincott Williams & Wilkins, 321-96, 2007
5. Batsford SR et al: Is the nephritogenic antigen in post-streptococcal glomerulonephritis pyrogenic exotoxin B (SPE B) or GAPDH? Kidney Int. 68(3):1120-9, 2005
6. Haas M: Incidental healed postinfectious glomerulonephritis: a study of 1012 renal biopsy specimens examined by electron microscopy. Hum Pathol. 34(1):3-10, 2003

ACUTE POSTSTREPTOCOCCAL GLOMERULONEPHRITIS

Microscopic Features

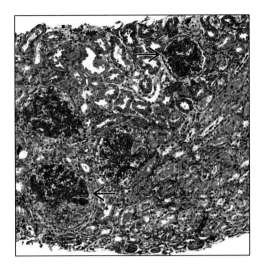

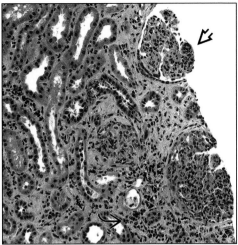

(Left) Low-power view of the cortex in PSAGN reveals that glomeruli ➡ are most prominently affected. In PSAGN, all glomeruli are typically involved (diffuse) and entire glomerular tufts are affected (global). (Right) Low-power light microscopy shows hypercellular glomeruli with a lobular architecture ➡ (sometimes referred to as "club-shaped") and an interstitial inflammatory infiltrate ➡ in a case of PSAGN.

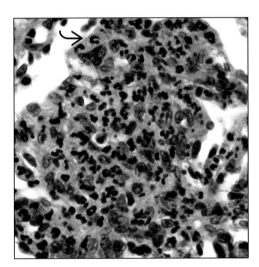

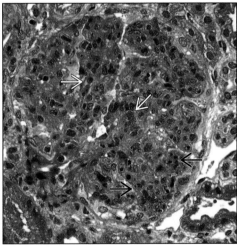

(Left) High-power view of a glomerulus in a case of poststreptococcal GN reveals striking hypercellularity with numerous neutrophils ➡, the presence of which makes this an "exudative" GN. (Right) PSAGN characteristically has endocapillary hypercellularity with a loss of open capillary loops. Neutrophils ➡, as well as an occasional eosinophil ➡, can be seen in a few capillaries.

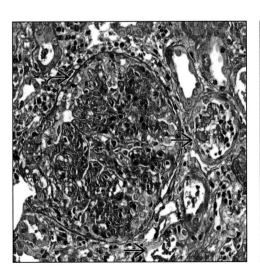

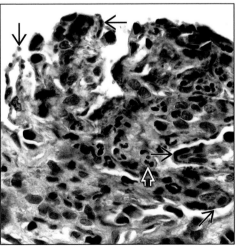

(Left) In a 9-year-old girl with acute poststreptococcal GN, high power of a PAS stain shows a lobular hypercellular glomerulus with crescent formation ➡ and adjacent tubules ➡ containing cast material, including red blood cells. (Right) A trichrome stain of a case of acute poststreptococcal GN shows fuchsinophilic subepithelial deposits ➡ along the glomerular basement membrane. Neutrophils ➡ can also be seen in glomerular capillary loops.

ACUTE POSTSTREPTOCOCCAL GLOMERULONEPHRITIS

Microscopic Features

(Left) *Periodic acid-Schiff shows prominent cellular crescents* ⮕ *in a 7-year-old boy with PSAGN. Patient presented with sudden onset of gross hematuria, hypertension, low C3 (25 mg/dL), normal C4, pneumonia, 10 g/d proteinuria, and positive anti-DNAse B antibodies.* **(Right)** *Light microscopy shows a hypercellular, lobulated glomerulus with numerous neutrophils* ⮕ *and a crescent in Bowman space* ⮕ *in a 7-year-old girl with acute poststreptococcal GN.*

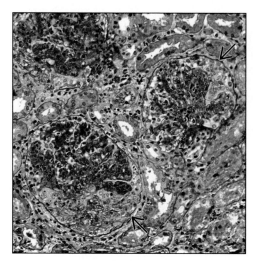
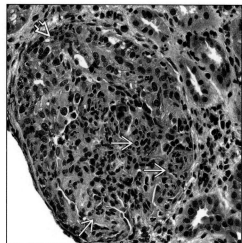

(Left) *In a case of acute poststreptococcal GN, a toluidine blue-stained, semi-thin "scout" section prepared for electron microscopy shows subepithelial, hump-like deposits* ⮕ *along the glomerular capillary loops. Glomerular capillary loops are hypercellular.* **(Right)** *H&E shows red cell casts* ⮕ *in the medulla. These can be distinguished from artifactual bleeding from the biopsy procedure by their compaction and mixing with proteinaceous material. Another useful feature is hemolysis and fragmentation.*

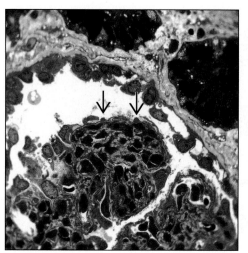
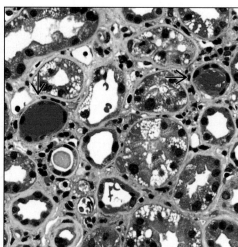

(Left) *Light microscopy shows prominent interstitial inflammation, fibrosis, & tubular atrophy with a mixed inflammatory infiltrate of mononuclear cells & neutrophils in a case of acute poststreptococcal GN.* **(Right)** *In a 9-year-old girl with acute poststreptococcal GN, there is an expansion of the interstitium by edema & an inflammatory infiltrate, including occasional eosinophils* ⮕. *A portion of a hypercellular glomerulus* ⮕ *can be seen.*

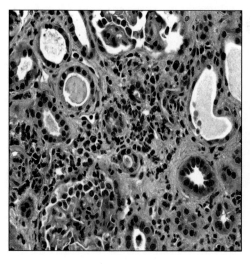
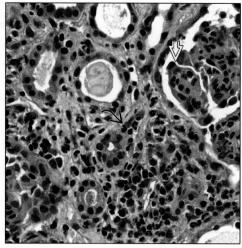

ACUTE POSTSTREPTOCOCCAL GLOMERULONEPHRITIS

Immunofluorescence

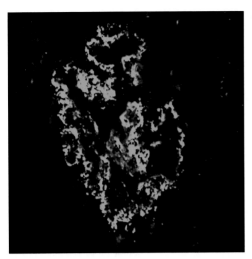
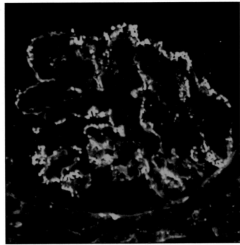

(Left) Positive immunofluorescence for IgG shows granular staining in a continuous band (or "garland" pattern) along the glomerular basement membrane in acute poststreptococcal GN. (Right) Positive immunofluorescence for IgG shows coarsely granular, "lumpy-bumpy" staining of the glomerular basement membrane in acute poststreptococcal GN.

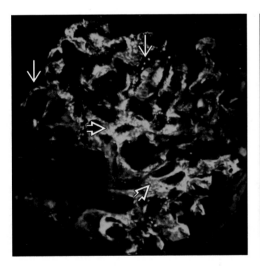
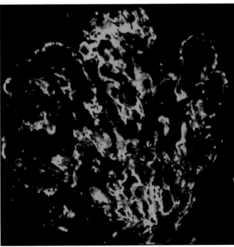

(Left) PSAGN with a mesangial dominant pattern ➡ of IgG deposition is shown in a 62-year-old man presenting with Cr 1.6, hypertension, 5 g/d proteinuria, low C3 & C4, positive ASO, and anti-DNAse. Scattered granular deposits along the GBM can also be seen ➡. (Right) Positive immunofluorescence for C3 shows a diffusely scattered, granular pattern (resembling a "starry sky") of staining of the glomerular basement membrane in acute poststreptococcal GN.

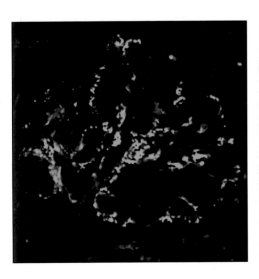
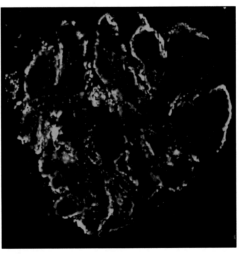

(Left) Immunofluorescence shows a coarsely granular, "lumpy-bumpy" pattern of staining along the glomerular basement membrane for kappa (kappa was equal to lambda) in acute poststreptococcal GN. (Right) Immunofluorescence shows a band-like pattern of staining ("garland") along the glomerular basement membrane for kappa in acute poststreptococcal GN. Kappa was equal to lambda.

2

ACUTE POSTSTREPTOCOCCAL GLOMERULONEPHRITIS

Electron Microscopy

(Left) In a 7-year-old girl with PSAGN, there are numerous subepithelial deposits ➡ along the GBM, some of which are confluent ➡. A number of the confluent deposits produce the "garland" pattern visible on immunofluorescence. *(Right)* EM shows PSAGN with neutrophil ➡ in the glomerular capillary loop infiltrating under the endothelium ➡ near subepithelial humps ➡ and in direct contact with the GBM ➡. Neutrophils are attracted by C5a and other chemokines and cause injury by digesting the GBM.

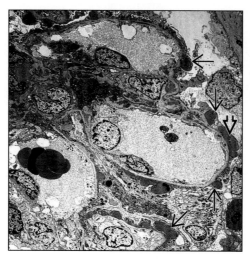
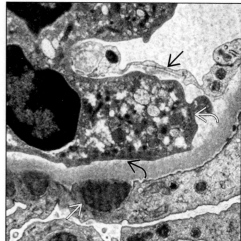

(Left) EM shows subepithelial "hump" ➡ on the GBM ➡ with little or no surrounding basement membrane reaction in a case of PSAGN. Intramembranous dense deposits are present ➡. *(Right)* Sometimes "humps" erode into the GBM continuity with intramembranous deposits. Loss of GBM integrity is probably the basis of hematuria. This biopsy is from 3-year-old girl with hypertension, Coca-Cola-colored urine, 3+ protein & blood on urinalysis, Cr 2.1 mg/dL, anti-DNase B 240, & Strep culture(-).

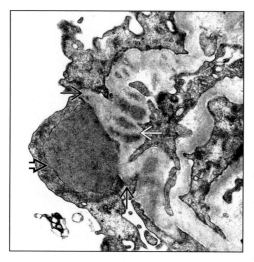
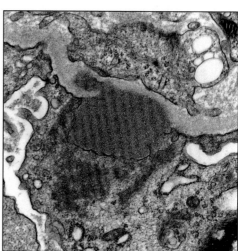

(Left) PSAGN can have prominent mesangial deposits ➡ in addition to the characteristic "humps," as in this child with acute renal failure, hypocomplementemia, and elevated anti-DNAse B. *(Right)* Subendothelial deposits ➡ are also focally present in PSAGN.

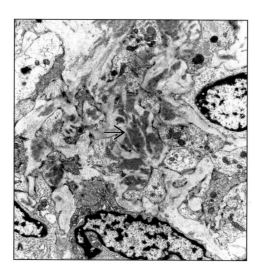
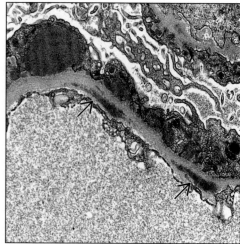

ACUTE POSTSTREPTOCOCCAL GLOMERULONEPHRITIS

Variant Microscopic Features

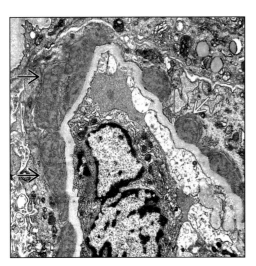 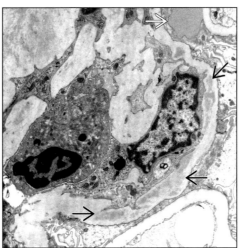

(Left) EM shows confluent subepithelial deposits ➡ in a 3 year old with PSAGN. Typical "humps" with the same texture are also seen ➡. These deposits have a variegated appearance and are of uncertain significance, which is not unusual. (Right) Intramembranous dense deposits ➡ are sometimes conspicuous in PSAGN and raise the question of dense deposit disease (DDD). Typically, they are less dense than in DDD. A subepithelial "hump" is present ➡.

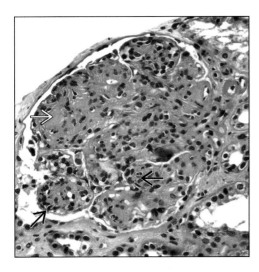 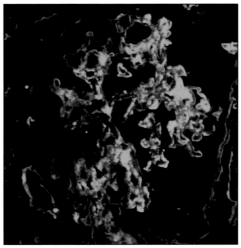

(Left) H&E shows acute postinfectious glomerulonephritis superimposed on diabetic glomerulopathy in a 55 year old. Nodules are evident ➡, but the neutrophils ➡ in capillaries indicate an additional process. This pattern can be associated with staphylococcal or streptococcal infections. (Right) Sparse granular deposits of IgG along the GBM are shown in a patient with postinfectious AGN superimposed on nodular diabetic glomerulosclerosis. IgA was negative.

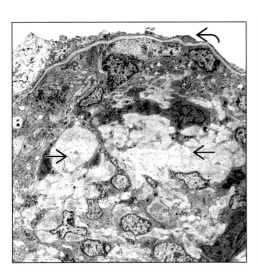 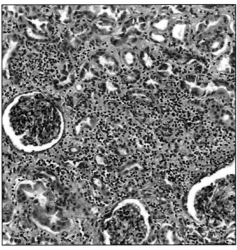

(Left) Nodular mesangial expansion ➡ and rare "humps" ➡ are present in this diabetic patient with acute glomerulonephritis after a toe infection. The organism in this case was not proved. (Right) Acute interstitial nephritis (AIN) without significant glomerulonephritis was described in the pre-antibiotic era. This child died after a streptococcal infection and was reported as a clinicopathologic case in 1929 by Cabot and Mallory. This cannot be distinguished from drug-induced AIN.

ACUTE POSTINFECTIOUS GLOMERULONEPHRITIS, NONSTREPTOCOCCAL

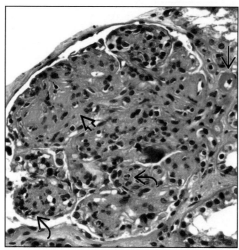

In a diabetic with postinfectious GN & a recently infected toe amputation, there is glomerular intracapillary ↑ cellularity, including neutrophils ➡, ↑ mesangium ⇨, & arteriolar hyalinosis ➡.

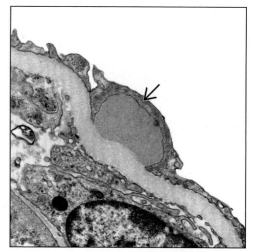

Electron microscopy shows subepithelial electron-dense deposits ➡ scattered along the glomerular basement membrane in postinfectious GN affecting a diabetic patient.

TERMINOLOGY

Synonyms
- Acute diffuse intracapillary proliferative (exudative) glomerulonephritis (GN)

Definitions
- GN occurring after exposure to an infectious agent other than β-hemolytic group A *Streptococcus*
- These disorders are called "postinfectious" even though they may occur concurrently with infection

ETIOLOGY/PATHOGENESIS

Infectious Agents
- Bacteria
  - *Staphylococcus* (coagulase positive and negative)
    - Most common cause in elderly (~ 50%)
    - Associated with diabetes mellitus and malignancy
  - *Streptococcus pneumoniae* (pneumococcus)
  - Group D streptococcus
  - Gram-negative bacilli
    - *E. coli, Pseudomonas, Salmonella, Proteus, Klebsiella*
  - Others
    - *T. pallidum, Brucella, Campylobacter, Nocardia, Legionella, Actinobacillus actinomycetem-comitans, Yersinia, Borrelia burgdorferi, Bartonella henselae, Propionibacterium acnes, Mycobacterium*
- Viruses
  - Adenovirus, measles, mumps, Coxsackievirus, varicella, Cytomegalovirus, Epstein-Barr, influenza, hepatitis B & C, ECHO, Parvovirus B19, vaccina virus, herpes
- Rickettsiae
  - Q fever (*Coxiella burnetii*)
- Fungi
  - *Candida*
- Parasites
  - Malaria, *Schistosoma*

Sites of Infection
- Infective endocarditis, lung infections, deep-seated visceral abscesses, infected shunts (e.g., ventriculoatrial), wound infections, appendix abscesses, osteomyelitis (including mastoiditis), valvular & vascular Dacron® prostheses

Pathogenesis
- Microbial antigens have been demonstrated in glomeruli of affected patients
- Believed to be circulating immune complexes that deposit in glomeruli
- Alternatively, antigens may traverse GBM and bind to glomerular sites
- Immunologic activation is thought to ensue, stimulating antibody and complement activation

Host Factors
- Alcoholism, diabetes, and intravenous drug use
- HLA class II allelic variation may lead to increased susceptibility to GN after exposure to "nephritogenic" strains of bacteria

CLINICAL ISSUES

Epidemiology
- Age
  - Children and young adults are most often affected classically (particularly in poststreptococcal GN), but recent literature has focused on these disorders in elderly individuals
    - Most common cause in elderly is *Staphylococcus* (~ 50%)
    - Associated with diabetes and malignancy
- Gender
  - M:F ≈ 2:1

Presentation
- Hematuria
  - Acute nephritic syndrome

ACUTE POSTINFECTIOUS GLOMERULONEPHRITIS, NONSTREPTOCOCCAL

Key Facts

Terminology

- GN typically occurring after exposure to an infectious agent

Etiology/Pathogenesis

- Usually called "postinfectious" but may occur concurrently with infection
- Variety of infections (bacterial, viral, parasitic, mycotic, etc.)
- Infectious Ag/Ab interactions & circulating immune complexes likely play a role

Clinical Issues

- Hematuria, hypocomplementemia, ± RF, ± cryoglobulins

Microscopic Pathology

- Diffuse proliferative, mesangial proliferative, focally proliferative, & MPGN
- Diffuse proliferative form most common & often exudative, with neutrophils
- May be superimposed on diabetic nephropathy

Ancillary Tests

- EM: Deposits in subepithelial location, having hump-shaped configuration, overlying basement membrane without surrounding GBM reaction
- IF: Scattered fine, large, or chunky deposits along GBM; typically stain with IgG & stain even more prominently with C3
  - IgM & IgA absent or minimal except in recently identified cases of IgA-dominant postinfectious GN

- Hypertension
- Oliguria
- Hypocomplementemia
  - Described in some patients, including all 5 patients with staphylococcal GN superimposed on diabetic nephropathy in series by Nasr et al

Laboratory Tests

- Circulating immune complexes
  - Disappear when infection is cured
- Cryoglobulins, usually type 3 (mixed)
- Rheumatoid factor (RF) may be positive

Treatment

- Surgical approaches
  - Abscesses and other deep-seated infections must sometimes be surgically treated
- Drugs
  - Antibiotics typically considered to be most effective therapy

Prognosis

- Around 90% of cases resolve in weeks
  - Persistent microhematuria or proteinuria may be found in those who appeared to recover normal renal function
- Adults have less favorable prognosis with only ~ 2/3 of patients recovering
  - If infections cannot be controlled (about 1/3 of patients), then GN persists and renal failure requiring dialysis may occur

MICROSCOPIC PATHOLOGY

Histologic Features

- Many cases are not biopsied; therefore, biopsy findings may overrepresent severe lesions
- Mesangial proliferative, focally proliferative, diffuse proliferative, and membranoproliferative GN
  - Diffuse, exudative, proliferative GN is most classic
    - Endocapillary proliferation
    - Numerous neutrophils

- Membranoproliferative pattern present in ~ 10%
- Hump-shaped deposits may sometimes be seen on silver, trichrome, and toluidine blue stains
- Crescents are present in severe cases (up to 1/3 of cases) and may predict worse prognosis
- Chronically, there is less exudation and endocapillary proliferation
- In large series of predominantly adult patients, most patients had glomerulosclerosis 3-15 years from onset on rebiopsy
  - Some mesangial hypercellularity and capillary wall thickening may also remain
- Concurrent diabetes may make it difficult to appreciate postinfectious GN since mesangial hypercellularity occurs in diabetes
  - Intracapillary inflammatory cells may provide a clue to presence of postinfectious GN

ANCILLARY TESTS

Immunofluorescence

- Scattered deposits having fine, large, or chunky appearance along GBM; typically stain with IgG and stain even more prominently with C3
  - Patterns described in streptococcal GN apply, including "starry sky," "garland," and mesangial
    - "Starry sky" and "garland" patterns are reportedly seen early in course of disease
    - Mesangial deposits are seen later
- IgM and IgA staining are absent or minimal except in recently identified cases of IgA-dominant postinfectious GN
- Concurrent diabetic nephropathy may be present with linear staining for IgG & albumin along GBMs & TBMs

Electron Microscopy

- Transmission
  - Deposits in subepithelial location having hump-shaped configuration and overlying basement membrane without a surrounding GBM reaction
    - These deposits or "humps" are numerous in acute phase and may be variegated

- Occasional mesangial and subendothelial deposits are present
- Hump-shaped deposits may be present in subepithelial area overlying mesangium between folds of GBM (a.k.a. "notch" or "waist" area)
- Mesangial notch deposits notably described by Haas in diabetic patients with postinfectious GN
  ○ Chronically, mesangial deposits predominate
  ○ Rare, hump-like, subepithelial deposits suggest infectious etiology of immune complex GN
    - Helps suggest possible etiology when biopsy is done in more chronic phase where only mesangial proliferation or focal membranoproliferative changes are present by light microscopy
  ○ Study by Haas suggests that clinically silent postinfectious GN results in healed, "incidental" postinfectious lesions, indicated by presence of subepithelial deposits by EM

DIFFERENTIAL DIAGNOSIS

Systemic Lupus Erythematosus (SLE)
- Systemic lupus erythematosus (SLE)
  ○ Positive clinical physical & laboratory findings are useful in making diagnosis of SLE
    - Physical findings characteristic of SLE (e.g., rashes and arthralgias)
    - Serologic and other assays showing, for example, ANA(+), double-stranded DNA(+), etc.
  ○ "Full house" immunofluorescence staining pattern (IgG, IgM, IgA, C1q/C4, and C3) is useful in identifying cases of SLE
  ○ Subendothelial deposits or numerous tubuloreticular structures on EM favor lupus

IgA Nephropathy
- IgA nephropathy typically has predominance of mesangial deposits and does not usually have well-formed subepithelial hump-like deposits
- Can be difficult to distinguish IgA nephropathy from cases of postinfectious GN if appearance is that of diffuse proliferative GN and history of preceding infection is unknown

Membranoproliferative GN (MPGN)
- MPGN, types I and III may have overlapping morphologic features with postinfectious GN
  ○ MPGN, type I typically has more GBM duplication than postinfectious GN
- Clinical history of infection (such as preceding pharyngitis or skin infection) helps favor a diagnosis of postinfectious GN
- Laboratory evidence may also help suggest postinfectious process

Cryoglobulinemic GN (Cryo GN)
- Cryo GN and postinfectious GN both may have nephritis, hypocomplementemia, type 3 cryoglobulins, and a RF(+)
- Both may have diffuse global endocapillary hypercellularity and numerous neutrophils

- Cryo GN can be favored if there are numerous glomerular capillary hyaline "thrombi"/"pseudothrombi"

Dense Deposit Disease (DDD)
- DDD, a form of C3 glomerulopathy, often does not have prominent GBM duplication like most MPGN and can be mistaken for proliferative GN-like postinfectious GN
- DDD often has predominance of C3 deposition whereas postinfectious GN typically has some immunoglobulin
- Deposits are typically intramembranous in DDD and very electron-dense as opposed to subepithelial deposits in postinfectious GN

C3 Glomerulonephritis
- Stain only for C3 without immunoglobulin (except for faint IgM) or C1q
- Deposits typically subendothelial &/or mesangial whereas in postinfectious GN, there are usually some subepithelial deposits

DIAGNOSTIC CHECKLIST

Pathologic Interpretation Pearls
- Clinical or laboratory evidence of infection preceding GN can help in favoring postinfectious GN
  ○ In postinfectious GN, clinical, laboratory, or pathologic evidence of systemic cause of GN is absent

SELECTED REFERENCES

1. Nasr SH et al: Postinfectious glomerulonephritis in the elderly. J Am Soc Nephrol. 22(1):187-95, 2011
2. Kanjanabuch T et al: An update on acute postinfectious glomerulonephritis worldwide. Nat Rev Nephrol. 5(5):259-69, 2009
3. Haas M et al: IgA-dominant postinfectious glomerulonephritis: a report of 13 cases with common ultrastructural features. Hum Pathol. 39(9):1309-16, 2008
4. Nadasdy T et al: Acute postinfectious glomerulonephritis and glomerulonephritis caused by persistent bacterial infection. Philadelphia: Lippincott Williams & Wilkins. 321-96, 2007
5. Nasr SH et al: Acute poststaphylococcal glomerulonephritis superimposed on diabetic glomerulosclerosis. Kidney Int. 71(12):1317-21, 2007
6. Haas M: Incidental healed postinfectious glomerulonephritis: a study of 1012 renal biopsy specimens examined by electron microscopy. Hum Pathol. 34(1):3-10, 2003
7. Haas M: Postinfectious glomerulonephritis complicating diabetic nephropathy: a frequent association, but how clinically important? Hum Pathol. 34(12):1225-7, 2003
8. Nasr SH et al: IgA-dominant acute poststaphylococcal glomerulonephritis complicating diabetic nephropathy. Hum Pathol. 34(12):1235-41, 2003

ACUTE POSTINFECTIOUS GLOMERULONEPHRITIS, NONSTREPTOCOCCAL

Microscopic Features

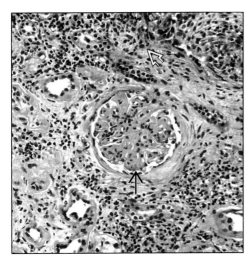

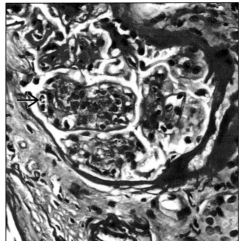

(Left) A glomerulus displays a nodule ⇒ in diabetic glomerulosclerosis concurrently affected by postinfectious GN in a 55-year-old diabetic patient with a history of the recent amputation of an infected toe. The interstitium contains an inflammatory infiltrate, including scattered eosinophils ⇒. *(Right)* In a case of diabetic glomerulosclerosis and concurrent postinfectious GN, scattered neutrophils ⇒ can be seen within glomerular capillary loops.

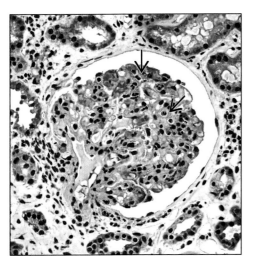

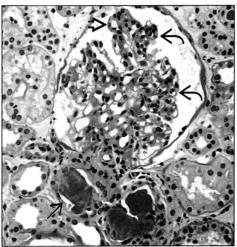

(Left) This glomerulus in a case of postinfectious GN shows hypercellularity, including intracapillary neutrophils ⇒. *(Right)* In this case of postinfectious GN, the glomerulus appears hypercellular and has vague lobules with glomerular basement membrane thickening ⇒ and occasional increases in endocapillary cellularity ⇒. Proteinaceous casts are present in the renal tubules ⇒.

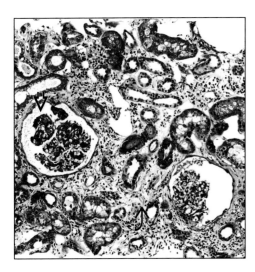

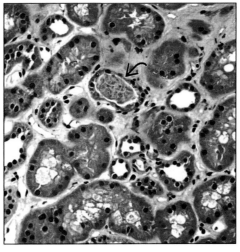

(Left) In a case of postinfectious GN, the glomeruli appear hypercellular and have vague lobules ⇒. The interstitium is expanded by inflammation, loose fibrosis, and admixed edema ⇒. *(Right)* In this case of postinfectious GN, the tubules are injured with tubular epithelial cell flattening ⇒ and contain pigmented cast material.

ACUTE POSTINFECTIOUS GLOMERULONEPHRITIS, NONSTREPTOCOCCAL

Immunofluorescence

(Left) In this case of postinfectious GN, there is prominent granular staining for C3 ➡ in a "starry sky" pattern. *(Right)* In this case of postinfectious GN, there is prominent granular staining for C3 in a "lumpy-bumpy" pattern ➡.

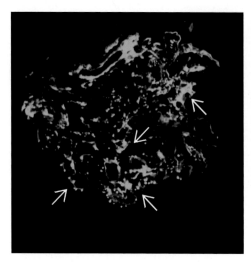
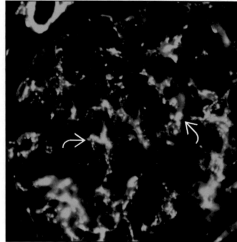

(Left) In this case of postinfectious GN and concurrent diabetes mellitus, there is staining for IgG along the periphery of glomerular capillary loops ➡ with an absence of staining in the center of glomerular nodules ➡. *(Right)* There is staining for C3 along the periphery of glomerular capillary loops ➡ with an absence of staining in the center of glomerular nodules ➡ in postinfectious GN with concurrent diabetes mellitus.

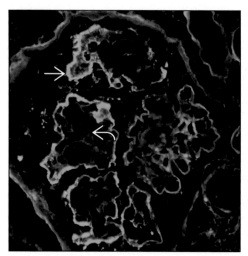
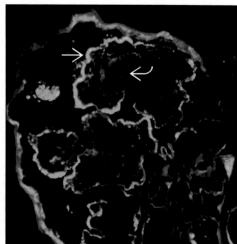

(Left) In this case of diabetes mellitus with concurrent postinfectious GN, there is broad mesangial staining for fibrin, including in well-formed nodules ➡ with focal intense staining ➡, a finding not associated with nodular type diabetic glomerulosclerosis. *(Right)* In diabetes mellitus with concurrent postinfectious GN, there is broad mesangial staining for C3 ➡, which is focally brighter than what would typically be seen in nodular-type diabetic glomerulosclerosis ➡.

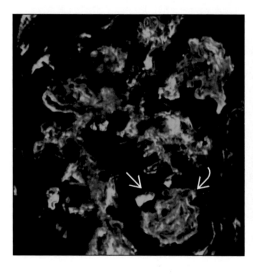
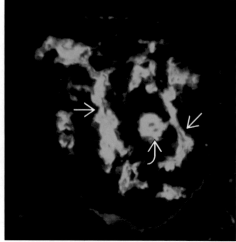

ACUTE POSTINFECTIOUS GLOMERULONEPHRITIS, NONSTREPTOCOCCAL

Electron Microscopy

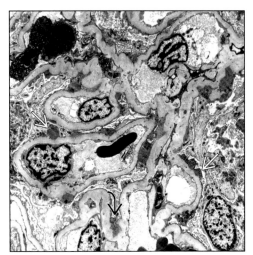

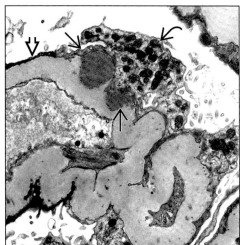

(Left) By electron microscopy (EM), there are well-formed, subepithelial, hump-like, electron-dense deposits ➡ in a case of postinfectious GN as well as electron-dense deposits ➡ at the reflection (or "notch") of the glomerular basement membrane. *(Right)* In this case of postinfectious GN, there are frequent subepithelial, hump-like, electron-dense deposits ➡. Overlying podocytes ▷ that are effaced and reactive contain increased numbers of cytoplasmic organelles ➡.

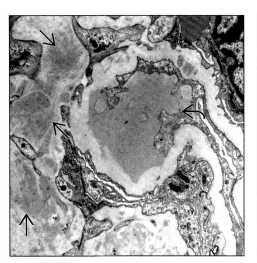

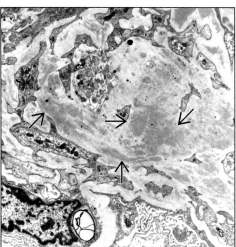

(Left) In this case of postinfectious GN in a diabetic patient, there are scattered, mesangial, electron-dense deposits ➡ as well as electron-dense subepithelial deposits overlying the mesangium ➡ at a GBM fold in what is referred to as the "notch" region. *(Right)* In this case of postinfectious GN and concurrent diabetic glomerulosclerosis, a mesangial nodule of the type in diabetes can be observed, containing scattered, electron-dense, mesangial deposits ➡.

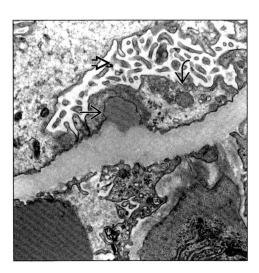

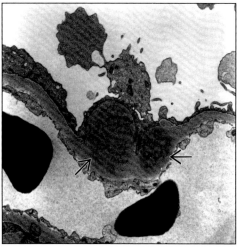

(Left) In this case of postinfectious GN, there are hump-like, subepithelial, electron-dense, immune-type deposits ➡. Podocytes show effacement ➡ and foci of microvillous change ▷. *(Right)* In this case of postinfectious GN, there are a couple of subepithelial electron-dense deposits with a vaguely variegated appearance ➡ but without a clear substructure.

GLOMERULONEPHRITIS OF CHRONIC INFECTION INCLUDING SHUNT NEPHRITIS

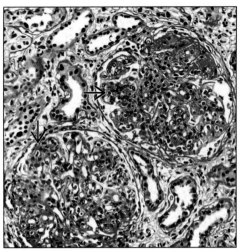

Membranoproliferative glomerulonephritis (MPGN) is the usual pattern seen in shunt nephritis with lobular expansion of the mesangium ➡. Crescents and acute proliferative GN are common in visceral abscess.

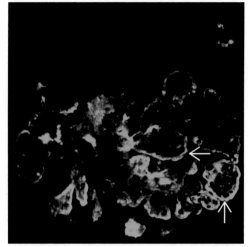

Finely granular IgM deposits are seen along glomerular capillaries that are often confluent ➡ in shunt nephritis. Visceral abscess GN is similar but typically expresses more C3 than immunoglobulin.

TERMINOLOGY

Abbreviations
- Shunt nephritis (SN)

Definitions
- Glomerulonephritis from chronic bacterial infection of cerebrospinal fluid (CSF) shunt or visceral abscess

ETIOLOGY/PATHOGENESIS

Infectious Agents
- Shunt nephritis (ventricular)
  - Ventriculoatrial (VA) and ventriculojugular (VJ) and less common ventriculoperitoneal (VP) shunts
  - Bacteria adhere to plastic shunt and form biofilm, protecting bacteria from antibiotics and immune system
    - 6-27% of VA shunts have bacterial colonization
    - Low-grade bacteremia in 4-5% of patients
  - Typically low virulence bacteria
    - *Staphylococcal epidermidis* (75% of all cases)
    - *S. albus*
    - Less often: *Acinetobacter, Bacillus, Corynebacterium, Listeria, Propionibacterium, Pseudomonas, Peptococcus,* and *Micrococcus*
- Chronic visceral infection (abscess)
  - Sites
    - Visceral abscesses: Lung, rectum, appendix, and septic abortion
    - Bone (osteomyelitis) and soft tissue: Subcutaneous and periodontal abscesses
    - Prostheses: Valvular, vascular, and other (e.g., Dacron)
    - Vascular device-associated infection (e.g., injection reservoirs and indwelling catheters)
  - *S. aureus* most common pathogen
- Portosystemic shunt immune complex GN not technically "shunt nephritis"

Chronic Immune Complex Glomerulonephritis
- Shedding of bacterial antigens, not bacteria
  - Blood cultures often negative
- Antigens and antibody lodge in glomeruli
- Trigger low-grade, persistent inflammation

CLINICAL ISSUES

Presentation
- Proteinuria, hematuria seen in virtually all cases
  - Nephrotic syndrome ~ 25%
- Acute or chronic renal failure
- Usually signs of infection: Fever, malaise, arthralgias, anemia, hepatosplenomegaly
- May have purpura, if cryoglobulinemia
- Symptoms related to increased intracranial pressure (SN) or visceral abscess

Laboratory Tests
- Often hypocomplementemia, cryoglobulinemia, rheumatoid factor
  - ↓ C3 and C4
- Hypergammaglobulinemia
  - IgM and variably IgG
- ↑ C-reactive protein (CRP)
- Occasional cases with positive ANCA or ANA
- Negative blood cultures do not exclude diagnosis

Treatment
- Removal of shunt, drainage of abscess, antibiotics

Prognosis
- Most recover with treatment of shunt infection
  - ~ 25% develop ESRD or die from complications
  - ~ 25% have persistent proteinuria and azotemia
  - ~ 5 years for GN to progress
- Recovery with prompt and effective treatment of visceral abscess, otherwise fatal or ESRD

GLOMERULONEPHRITIS OF CHRONIC INFECTION INCLUDING SHUNT NEPHRITIS

Key Facts

Terminology
- GN from bacterial infection of cerebrospinal shunts or visceral abscess

Etiology/Pathogenesis
- SN: Mostly *S. epidermidis* (75% of cases) and *S. albus*
- Visceral abscess: *S. aureus, Pseudomonas*

Clinical Issues
- Proteinuria/hematuria, acute or chronic renal failure
- Fever, malaise, arthralgias, purpura

Microscopic Pathology
- 3 major glomerular patterns
  - MPGN, type 1
  - Focal/diffuse proliferative GN &/or mesangial proliferation
  - Crescentic GN (visceral abscess)

Ancillary Tests
- SN: C3 in > 90%; IgM and IgG in > 60%
- Visceral abscess: C3 in 100%; IgM and IgG negative in 67%
- EM: Electron-dense, immune complex-type deposits, mostly mesangial and subendothelial, mesangial interposition

Top Differential Diagnoses
- Cryoglobulinemic GN (HCV)
- MPGN, type I

Diagnostic Checklist
- Crescents and necrosis common in visceral abscess

MICROSCOPIC PATHOLOGY

Histologic Features
- Shunt nephritis
  - 3 patterns
  - Membranoproliferative glomerulonephritis (MPGN), type I (> 60%)
    - Lobular mesangial expansion
    - Capillary wall thickening from subendothelial deposits and GBM duplication
  - Global glomerular endocapillary hypercellularity (~ 33%)
    - Resembles postinfectious GN
  - < 10% exclusively mesangial proliferation without GBM thickening
  - Crescents and necrosis uncommon
- Visceral abscess
  - Crescents common (~ 75%)
    - Glomerular necrosis common (~ 65%)
  - 3 patterns
    - Diffuse, MPGN-like in ~ 33%
    - Pure extracapillary proliferation (crescents) in ~ 33%
    - Focal or isolated mesangial proliferation in ~ 33%
- Biopsy after infection resolution
  - Mild residual hypercellularity
  - Deposits disappear by EM and IF
  - Fibrous crescents, global sclerosis

ANCILLARY TESTS

Immunofluorescence
- Band-like or granular along GBM ± mesangium
  - Broad granular pattern if subendothelial deposits
  - Mesangial associated with mesangial proliferation
- Immunoglobulins more prominent in SN than in visceral infections
  - SN: IgM (> 80%) > IgG (~ 67%) > IgA
  - Visceral abscess: IgM, IgG, IgA negative in ~ 67%
- C3 prominent in > 90% of visceral abscess cases and SN

- SN has C1q and C4 (25-33%)

Electron Microscopy
- Amorphous, electron-dense deposits widely distributed
  - Mesangial and subendothelial most common
  - Hump-like deposits in minority
    - Particularly those with acute diffuse proliferative GN features
- Mesangial interposition with new GBM formation
- Mesangial and endocapillary hypercellularity with occasional intracapillary leukocytes
- Focal podocyte foot process effacement

DIFFERENTIAL DIAGNOSIS

MPGN, Type I
- Pathologically similar
- Distinguished by presence of chronic infection

Cryoglobulinemic GN
- Can have morphologic pattern similar to SN
- Intraluminal "pseudothrombi" (PAS[+])

Portosystemic Shunt-associated GN
- IgA-dominant MPGN vs. IgM dominance in SN

DIAGNOSTIC CHECKLIST

Pathologic Interpretation Pearls
- Immunoglobulin usually negative in visceral abscess
- Crescents common in visceral abscess

SELECTED REFERENCES

1. Nadasdy T et al: Acute postinfectious GN and GN caused by persistent bacterial infection. In Jennette JC et al: Heptinstall's Pathology of the Kidney. 6th ed. Philadelphia: Lippincott Williams & Wilkins, 2007

GLOMERULONEPHRITIS OF CHRONIC INFECTION INCLUDING SHUNT NEPHRITIS

Microscopic Features

(Left) Shunt nephritis shows markedly expanded, lobular mesangial areas with increased mesangial cellularity and matrix, resembling MPGN, type I. One mesangial area ➡ in a normal glomerulus contains no more than 3 cells in a 2-3 micron section; however, this glomerulus contains many more. *(Right)* At high-power view, GBM duplication can be appreciated ➡ in shunt nephritis as well as mesangial hypercellularity.

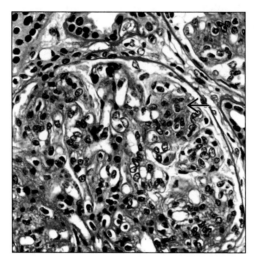 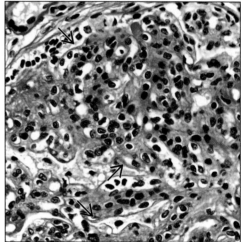

(Left) In shunt nephritis, glomeruli show hypercellular, lobular mesangial areas ➡. This pattern can be seen in MPGN, type I, mixed cryoglobulinemia, lupus nephritis, and C3 nephropathy. *(Right)* This trichrome stain shows the markedly expanded, lobular mesangial areas ➡ in shunt nephritis. The trichrome stain distinguishes collagen matrix material (blue/green) from deposits (red/purple).

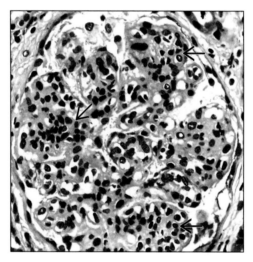 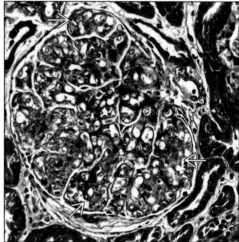

(Left) This Jones methenamine silver stain shows lobular areas of mesangial expansion ➡ in shunt nephritis. *(Right)* This Jones methenamine silver stain shows areas of glomerular basement membrane duplication ➡ in shunt nephritis. Duplication of the GBM is a feature of glomerular diseases that have subendothelial deposits (e.g., class IV lupus glomerulonephritis) or endothelial injury (e.g., thrombotic microangiopathy).

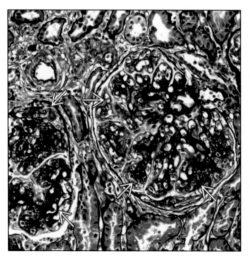 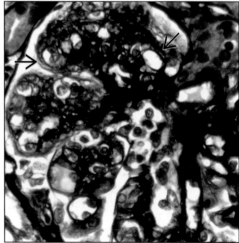

GLOMERULONEPHRITIS OF CHRONIC INFECTION INCLUDING SHUNT NEPHRITIS

Immunofluorescence and Electron Microscopy

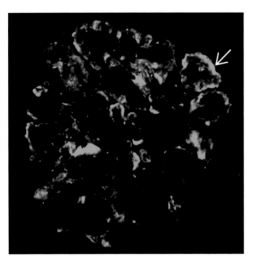
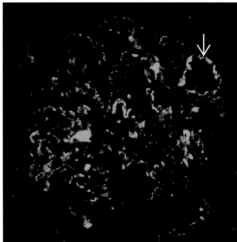

(Left) Immunofluorescence shows IgM deposition in a finely granular pattern, with areas of confluent peripheral accentuation ➡ in shunt nephritis. *(Right)* Immunofluorescence shows C3 deposition in a finely granular pattern, with areas of confluent peripheral accentuation ➡ in shunt nephritis. C3 is typically more extensive in GN associated with visceral abscess.

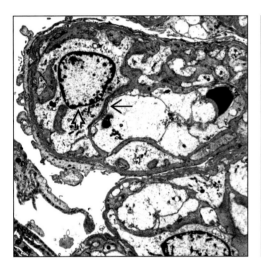
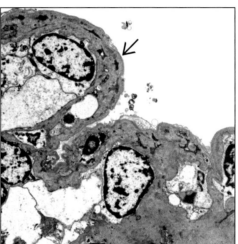

(Left) EM shows new basement membrane formation ➡ and mesangial cell interposition ➡ in shunt nephritis. *(Right)* This EM shows prominent glomerular basement membrane duplication and interposition of mesangial cells ➡ in shunt nephritis. Deposits are inconspicuous, suggesting that the clearance system almost compensates for the deposition.

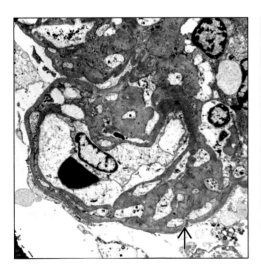
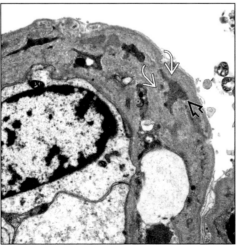

(Left) Areas of prominent glomerular basement membrane thickening and new basement membrane formation ➡ are typical of shunt nephritis. *(Right)* Electron-dense immune-type deposits ➡ can be seen with glomerular basement membrane duplication around the deposits ➡ in shunt nephritis. These deposits have been shown to disappear within several months after removal of the shunt.

ENDOCARDITIS

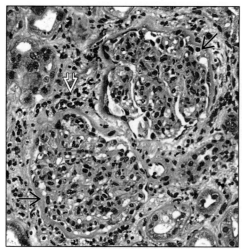

This slide from a 68-year-old African-American man with a history of staphylococcal endocarditis shows hypercellular glomeruli ⇒ and interstitial inflammation ⇒.

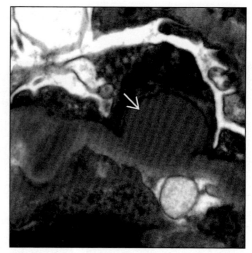

Electron microscopy of the renal biopsy from a 68-year-old man with a history of staphylococcal endocarditis shows a well-formed, subepithelial, electron-dense deposit ("hump") ⇒.

TERMINOLOGY

Abbreviations
- Subacute bacterial endocarditis (SBE)
- Acute bacterial endocarditis (ABE)

Synonyms
- Embolic nonsuppurative focal nephritis
- Focal embolic nephritis
- Focal and segmental proliferative, necrotizing, or sclerosing glomerulonephritis (GN)

Definitions
- GN following infection of heart valves (i.e., endocarditis)

ETIOLOGY/PATHOGENESIS

Infectious Agents
- SBE: Classic example is *Streptococcus viridans* group bacteria infecting a rheumatic heart
  - Coagulase-negative staphylococci, including *S. epidermis,* have also been observed
  - Others observed
    - *Actinobacillus actinomycetemcomitans, Enterococcus, Streptococcus mitis, Haemophilus influenzae, Neisseria gonorrhea, Chlamydia psittaci, Bartonella henselae, Coxiella burnetii*
    - Subacute endocarditis due to *Streptococcus bovis* and *N. subflava* bacteremia has been reported in a case with concurrent high antineutrophil cytoplasmic antibody (ANCA) (anti-proteinase-3) titer
    - Of note, positive ANCA has also been reported in another series of GN associated with endocarditis
- ABE: Classic example is *Staphylococcus aureus* infecting previously normal heart (e.g., as in an intravenous drug abuser)

  - Proportion of bacterial endocarditis-associated GN caused by *S. aureus* appears to be increasing, causing > 50% of all cases and > 1/3 of fatal cases
  - 40-70% of intravenous drug abusers with acute endocarditis from *S. aureus* have GN
- Immunologic injury is thought to be primary mechanism of endocarditis-associated GN
  - Presence of glomerular immune complexes is evidence of this process
  - Serum complement is depressed, also indicative of process involving immune system
  - Circulating immune complexes have been demonstrated in patients with infectious endocarditis
  - Eluates from kidney with focal GN associated with endocarditis have been shown to react with bacterial antigens derived from bacteria cultured from patient's blood
- Earlier investigators thought that direct action of bacterial emboli lead to endocarditis-associated GN when they observed emboli in glomeruli
  - Called "focal embolic GN" or "embolic nonsuppurative focal nephritis" before pathogenesis was attributed to mechanisms other than embolization
  - Focal GN in patients involving only right side of heart suggest that embolization is not major mechanism

CLINICAL ISSUES

Epidemiology
- Incidence
  - Antibiotic therapy has decreased incidence of GN due to endocarditis
  - Studies of endocarditis have indicated an incidence of GN in patients with infectious endocarditis of 2-60%

ENDOCARDITIS

Key Facts

Terminology
- GN following infection of heart valves

Etiology/Pathogenesis
- Subacute bacterial endocarditis (SBE)
  - e.g., *Streptococcus viridans* infecting a rheumatic heart
- Acute bacterial endocarditis (ABE)
  - e.g., *Staphylococcus aureus* infecting previously normal heart, as in an intravenous drug abuser

Clinical Issues
- Hematuria and proteinuria
- Renal dysfunction: ↑ BUN & creatinine (mostly with diffuse GN)
- Hypocomplementemia

Microscopic Pathology
- Diffuse or focal proliferative GN ~ 50%
  - Neutrophils and nuclear fragments in glomeruli
  - Focal crescents
- MPGN, type I pattern ~ 50%
  - Lobular mesangial hypercellularity, duplicated GBM
- IF: Usually IgG, IgM, and C3 (subendothelial & mesangial); sometimes IgA
- EM: Mesangial & subendothelial amorphous deposits

Top Differential Diagnoses
- Postinfectious GN, other site
- MPGN, type I
- Lupus nephritis
- ANCA-related GN

- Indicates that it is difficult to provide accurate measure of this incidence
  - Of endocarditis cases, renal disease is presenting feature in 20% of patients

Presentation
- Hematuria
  - Macroscopic hematuria
    - May be associated with the GN or renal infarction from "septic" emboli
  - May persist or resolve and may be intermittent
- Proteinuria
  - Usually mild; nephrotic syndrome rare
- Urinary casts
- Hypocomplementemia
  - Frequently seen (but not always) and not specific to renal involvement
  - Seen in 70-90% of patients with diffuse GN and 60% of patients with focal GN before advent of antibiotic therapy
  - Associated with activation of classical complement pathway
- Renal dysfunction
  - Variable to severe
    - BUN and creatinine elevations are typically associated with diffuse form of GN
  - Uremia seen in 5-10% of patients before epoch of antibiotics and in 3-4% after advent of antibiotics
- Roth spots
- Anemia
- Hepatosplenomegaly
- Purpura
- Pulmonary hemorrhage has been reported as initial symptom (& initially confused with Goodpasture syndrome)

Laboratory Tests
- Rheumatoid factor may be positive
- Circulating immune complexes may be present
- Cryoglobulins (mixed [type III]) have been reported

Treatment
- Surgical approaches

- Valve vegetation removal or valve replacement may be required
- Drugs
  - Antibiotic therapy may achieve resolution of milder endocarditis-associated GN
  - Antibiotic prophylaxis in patients at risk for endocarditis may reduce incidence of endocarditis-associated GN
  - Corticosteroids may be used in brief course
    - May help in resolution of nephritis without exacerbating the endocarditis
  - Plasmapheresis has been uncommonly used in aggressive cases

Prognosis
- Partial to total resolution of renal disease occurs after antibiotic therapy
  - Proteinuria, circulating immune complexes, cryoglobulinemia, and elevation of rheumatoid factor (if present) resolve with effective treatment

MACROSCOPIC FEATURES

General Features
- Abscesses may occur in severe cases
- Renal infarction (in up to 50-57% of cases according to some early studies, including autopsy data) may occur in severe cases
  - Single or multiple and grossly appreciable, of size associated with arcuate or large interlobular arteries
  - Infarcts are typically due to embolism of valve vegetations and not by 2° immune-mediated vasculitis
- Petechial hemorrhages ("flea-bitten") in 2/3 of patients classically studied by Heptinstall

Size
- Enlarged kidneys have been observed with widespread or diffuse GN; however, kidneys may have normal size

MICROSCOPIC PATHOLOGY

Histologic Features
- Glomerulonephritis
  - Focal and segmental GN (in 50-85% of patients)
    - Segmental or lobular hypercellularity or sclerosis
    - Focal segmental proliferative or necrotizing GN sometimes present
    - Lesions sometimes contain intracapillary thrombi in addition to fibrinoid necrosis
    - Chronic sclerotic lesions are seen at periphery of 1 or several lobules with adhesion or synechia between Bowman capsule & sclerotic lesion, sometimes with crescent formation
    - Advanced or scarred lesions are more commonly found in chronic cases such as the Libman healed, bacteria-free stage
    - Crescents are not typically present to extent that would warrant diagnosis of crescentic glomerulonephritis
  - Diffuse proliferation (~ 50-65% of patients)
    - Acute diffuse endocapillary proliferative GN may be present, referred to by some as a "glomerulitis"
    - Mild mesangial hypercellularity
    - Little increase in mesangial matrix
    - Little or no narrowing of glomerular capillary lumina in most
    - Severe acute diffuse endocapillary hypercellularity is sometimes present, narrowing or occluding glomerular capillaries
  - Membranoproliferative pattern
    - Resembles type I MPGN or shunt nephritis
    - Diffuse endocapillary hypercellularity, duplicated GBM, and lobular mesangial expansion
    - Trichrome may demonstrate subendothelial fuchsinophilic deposits
  - Polymorphonuclear leukocytes and nuclear fragments in glomeruli
    - Acute or fresh lesions consist of fibrinoid necrosis or intracapillary thrombosis in 1 or 2 glomerular lobules
    - Segmental hypercellularity
  - Organisms can rarely be found
- Interstitium
  - Interstitial inflammation typically present even in treated patients with quiescent disease
- Tubules
  - Red cell casts
  - Tubular atrophy
- Arteries
  - Intimal thickening (nonspecific)
  - Vasculitis rare

Other Diseases
- Secondary amyloidosis is rare complication of longstanding endocarditis
- Interstitial nephritis may be induced by antibiotic and other drug therapy

ANCILLARY TESTS

Immunofluorescence
- Immunoglobulin and complement show widespread granular deposition
  - IgG, IgM, and C3 are described in most reports (typically IgM > IgG & IgA), along glomerular capillaries and sometimes mesangium
  - IgA has also been reported less commonly
  - Linear pattern has been described but is not indicative of anti-GBM Ab formation
  - IgG and IgM may be seen in large subendothelial deposits
  - Bacterial antigens have been demonstrated with corresponding antisera
- Even though lesions may be focal by light microscopy, deposits are diffuse by immunofluorescence

Electron Microscopy
- Subendothelial, subepithelial, and mesangial deposits may be seen
  - Subepithelial dense deposits ("humps") are most often seen in acute diffuse proliferative GN (around 1/3 of patients with endocarditis GN)
  - MPGN-type cases typically have prominent subendothelial dense deposits
  - Discrete electron-dense deposits in mesangial regions, typically near endothelium of glomerular capillary
  - Capillary wall deposits are lost 1st after effective treatment; mesangial dense deposits may persist for ≥ 6 months
- Pure necrotizing cases may have no dense deposits

DIFFERENTIAL DIAGNOSIS

Postinfectious Glomerulonephritis, Other Site
- Variety of infections can give similar biopsy findings (e.g., osteomyelitis, abscesses, shunts, and infected catheters in contact with arteries, veins, or cardiac chambers)
- Findings may be similar to poststreptococcal GN
- Clinical correlation helps determine source of infection

Membranoproliferative Glomerulonephritis
- MPGN, type I caused by infectious endocarditis can be indistinguishable from MPGN of other causes
- Endocarditis-induced MPGN more often has dominant staining for IgM compared with idiopathic membranoproliferative MPGN
- Hyaline thrombi/"pseudothrombi" by light microscopy help to raise suspicion of hepatitis C infection
- Conspicuous necrosis in proliferative GN or MPGN often indicates possibility of endocarditis GN

Lupus Nephritis
- Clinical correlation (ANA[+], double-stranded DNA assay[+]) helps in attributing GN to lupus

ANCA-associated Pauci-immune Necrotizing Glomerulonephritis
• Endocarditis-associated focal necrotizing GN may have little or no immunostaining for complement or immunoglobulins, making them indistinguishable from ANCA-associated pauci-immune necrotizing GN
• It has been reported that ANCA-associated pauci-immune GN associated with infectious endocarditis is less aggressive than ANCA not associated with endocarditis

DIAGNOSTIC CHECKLIST

Pathologic Interpretation Pearls
• Proper clinical history of endocarditis is critical in raising suspicion of GN mediated by endocarditis
• Presence of necrotizing and crescentic GN indicates a worse prognosis

SELECTED REFERENCES

1. Nadasdy T et al: Acute postinfectious glomerulonephritis and glomerulonephritis caused by persistent bacterial infection. In Jennette JC et al: Heptinstall's Pathology of the Kidney. 6th ed. Philadelphia: Lippincott Williams & Wilkins, 2007
2. D'Agati VD et al: Atlas of Nontumor Pathology: Non-neoplastic Kidney Diseases. Washington, DC: American Registry of Pathology, 2005
3. Bauer A et al: Vasculitic purpura with antineutrophil cytoplasmic antibody-positive acute renal failure in a patient with Streptococcus bovis case and Neisseria subflava bacteremia and subacute endocarditis. Clin Nephrol. 62(2):144-8, 2004
4. Choi HK et al: Subacute bacterial endocarditis with positive cytoplasmic antineutrophil cytoplasmic antibodies and anti-proteinase 3 antibodies. Arthritis Rheum. 43(1):226-31, 2000
5. Majumdar A et al: Renal pathological findings in infective endocarditis. Nephrol Dial Transplant. 15(11):1782-7, 2000
6. Orfila C et al: Rapidly progressive glomerulonephritis associated with bacterial endocarditis: efficacy of antibiotic therapy alone. Am J Nephrol. 13(3):218-22, 1993
7. Iida H et al: Membranous glomerulonephritis associated with enterococcal endocarditis. Nephron. 40(1):88-90, 1985
8. Heptinstall RH. Pathology of the Kidney. 3rd ed. Boston: Little, Brown and Company, 1983
9. Perez GO et al: Immune-complex nephritis in bacterial endocarditis. Arch Intern Med. 136(3):334-6, 1976
10. Levy RL et al: The immune nature of subacute bacterial endocarditis (SBE) nephritis. Am J Med. 54(5):645-52, 1973
11. Gutman RA et al: The immune complex glomerulonephritis of bacterial endocarditis. Medicine (Baltimore). 51(1):1-25, 1972
12. Jennings RB et al: Post-streptococcal glomerulo-nephritis: histopathologic and clinical studies of the acute, subsiding acute and early chronic latent phases. J Clin Invest. 40:1525-95, 1961
13. Heptinstall RH et al: Focal glomerulonephritis. A study based on renal biopsies. Q J Med. 28:329-46, 1959
14. Libman E: A study of the endocardial lesions of subacute bacterial endocarditis; with particular reference to healing or healed lesions; with clinical notes. Am J Med. 13(5):544-9, 1952
15. Spain DM et al: The effect of penicillin on the renal lesions of subacute bacterial endocarditis. Ann Intern Med. 36(4):1086-9, 1952
16. Gorlin R et al: Long-term follow-up study of penicillin-treated subacute bacterial endocarditis. N Engl J Med. 242(26):995-1001, 1950
17. Baehr G et al: Glomerulonephritis as a complication of subacute streptococcus endocarditis. JAMA. 75(12):789-90, 1920
18. Baehr G: Glomerular lesions of subacute bacterial endocarditis. J Exp Med. 15(4):330-47, 1912

Microscopic Features

(Left) Low-power view of a renal biopsy from a 68-year-old man with a history of staphylococcal endocarditis shows hypercellular glomeruli ➡️ with a diffuse pattern of proliferation and renal tubules with injury and necrotic cellular debris ➡️. *(Right)* Higher power view of a renal biopsy from the 68-year-old man with staphylococcal endocarditis shows necrotic cellular debris ➡️ and hypercellular glomeruli ➡️.

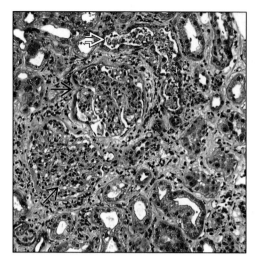
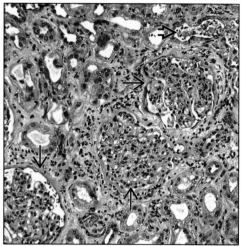

(Left) A glomerulus has ↑ cellularity in a 78-year-old man with serum Cr 3.7 mg/dL, 3.7 g/d proteinuria, hematuria, petechial rash, gastrointestinal ulcers, & S. aureus on blood culture secondary to endocarditis. *(Right)* Higher power of a glomerulus in the 68-year-old man with staphylococcal endocarditis shows intracapillary neutrophils ➡️, endocapillary hypercellularity ➡️, and mesangial hypercellularity ➡️.

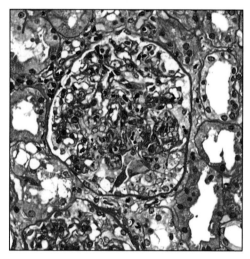
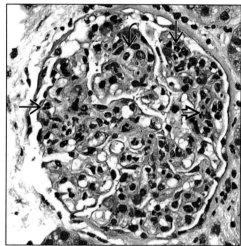

(Left) In the case of GN due to endocarditis in the 78-year-old man, a glomerulus has endocapillary hypercellularity in glomerular capillary loops with infiltrating neutrophils ➡️. *(Right)* Higher power of a PAS stain in the 68-year-old man with staphylococcal endocarditis shows a hypercellular glomerulus ➡️ and adjacent renal tubules with sloughing of the tubular epithelial cells ➡️.

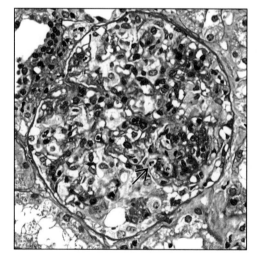
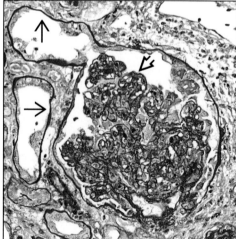

ENDOCARDITIS

Immunofluorescence and Electron Microscopy

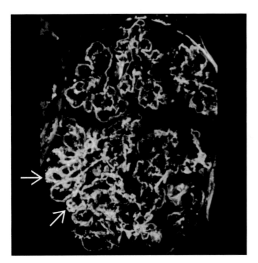
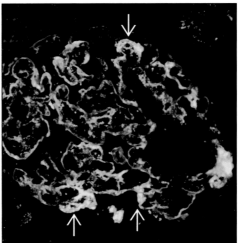

(Left) In the case of GN due to endocarditis in a 78-year-old man, a glomerulus has prominent granular and amorphous staining for C3, much of which can be appreciated along glomerular capillary loops ➡. *(Right)* In the case of GN due to endocarditis in a 78-year-old man with S. aureus bacteremia, a glomerulus has prominent granular and amorphous staining for IgA, much of which can be appreciated along glomerular capillary loops ➡.

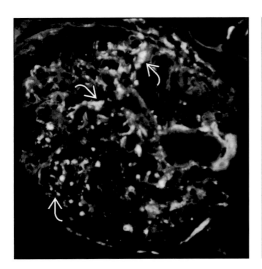
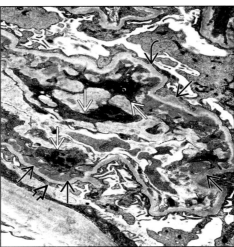

(Left) Immunofluorescence of C3 shows granular positivity ➡ in a 68-year-old man with staphylococcal endocarditis. *(Right)* In the case of GN due to endocarditis in a 78-year-old man, glomerular capillary loops are wrinkled ➡ and have cellular interposition ➡ with numerous adjacent subendothelial, electron-dense, immune-type deposits ➡. Podocytes are segmentally effaced ➡.

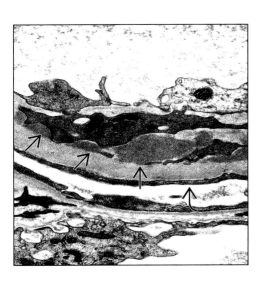
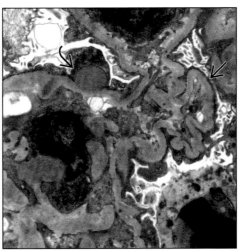

(Left) In the case of GN due to endocarditis in a 78-year-old man, there are electron-dense immune-type deposits ➡ in a subendothelial location. There is also extensive foot process effacement ➡. *(Right)* Electron microscopy in the 68-year-old man with staphylococcal endocarditis shows a well-formed, subepithelial, electron-dense deposit (also called a "hump") ➡ with extensive foot process effacement ➡.

HEPATITIS B VIRUS

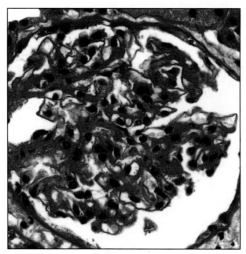

Periodic acid-Schiff reveals a normal glomerulus from a patient with membranous glomerulonephritis associated with HBV infection.

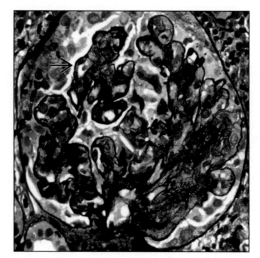

Jones methenamine silver stain reveals focal duplication of the glomerular basement membranes ➜ in this patient with features of membranoproliferative GN associated with hepatitis B infection.

TERMINOLOGY

Abbreviations
- Hepatitis B virus (HBV)

Definitions
- Immune complex-mediated glomerular injury associated with HBV infection

ETIOLOGY/PATHOGENESIS

Infectious Agents
- Hepatitis B virus
  - Hepadnavirus family
    - Strong preference for infection of liver cells
    - DNA also detectable in kidney, pancreas, and mononuclear cells
  - Modes of transmission include percutaneous, sexual, and perinatal or vertical (mother to child)

CLINICAL ISSUES

Epidemiology
- Incidence
  - High prevalence in Asia and Africa
    - Perinatal transmission results in > 90% chronic infection without acute response
  - Low prevalence in Western countries
    - Acquired during adolescence or early adulthood
    - Acute hepatitis with rare chronic progression
    - 1.5 per 100,000 people in United States infected with hepatitis B
- Gender
  - Males have slightly higher risk of death from liver disease than females

Laboratory Tests
- HBV serology
  - HBV surface antigen (HBsAg)

- Marker of active viral replication
    - Hepatitis B surface Ab (Anti-HBs)
  - HBe antigen
    - Loss or seroconversion in inactive carriers
  - HB core antigen
- HBV PCR test

Natural History
- Asymptomatic
  - Majority of HBV infections
- Chronic HBV infection
  - < 5%
- Cirrhosis
  - Develops in 20% of chronic HBV infections
    - 100x risk for hepatocellular carcinoma compared with noncarriers of HBV
  - 40% lifetime risk of death

Treatment
- Drugs
  - Antiviral agents
    - Lamivudine
    - Interferon-α
- Hepatitis B vaccine
  - Not useful when active infection is present

Prognosis
- HBV genotype A more responsive to interferon

MICROSCOPIC PATHOLOGY

Histologic Features
- Glomerular patterns of injury
  - Membranous glomerulonephritis (MGN)
    - Normal to thick glomerular basement membranes depending on stage of subepithelial immune complex deposition
    - Mesangial hypercellularity may be present
  - Membranoproliferative GN (MPGN)
    - Lobular accentuation of glomerular tufts

HEPATITIS B VIRUS

Key Facts

Etiology/Pathogenesis
- Hepatitis B virus

Clinical Issues
- High prevalence in Asia and Africa
  - Perinatal transmission results in > 90% chronic infection without acute response
- Low prevalence in Western countries
  - Acquired during adolescence or early adulthood
  - Acute hepatitis with rare chronic progression
- Antiviral agents
  - Lamivudine
  - Interferon-α

Microscopic Pathology
- Membranous glomerulonephritis (MGN)

- Normal to thick glomerular basement membranes, depending on stage
- ± "spikes" on PAS or silver stain
- Membranoproliferative GN (MPGN)
  - Lobular accentuation of glomerular tufts
  - Duplication of glomerular basement membranes ("tram track" appearance)
- Cryoglobulinemic GN
  - Lobular accentuation of glomerular tufts with "wire loop" or hyaline "thrombi" deposits

Top Differential Diagnoses
- Primary MGN
- Primary MPGN
- IgA nephropathy

- Duplication of glomerular basement membranes ("tram track" appearance)
- Interposition of cells between duplicated basement membranes
  - Cryoglobulinemic GN
    - MPGN pattern common
    - Prominent immune complex deposition in form of "wire loop" or hyaline "thrombi" deposits (intraluminal cryoglobulins)

ANCILLARY TESTS

Immunohistochemistry
- HBcAg stains subepithelial immune complexes along glomerular capillaries

Immunofluorescence
- MGN
  - Granular glomerular capillary wall staining for IgG, C3 (variable), and kappa and lambda
  - Mesangial staining also present
- MPGN
  - Coarse to granular glomerular capillary wall staining for IgG, C3 (variable), and kappa and lambda
- Cryoglobulinemic GN
  - Coarse to granular glomerular capillary wall staining for IgG &/or IgM, kappa and lambda

Electron Microscopy
- Transmission
  - MGN
    - Subepithelial immune deposits
    - Mesangial immune deposits
  - MPGN
    - Subendothelial and mesangial immune deposits
    - Duplication of GBMs
    - Subepithelial deposits variably present
  - Cryoglobulinemic GN
    - Subendothelial and mesangial immune deposits
    - Substructural organization of deposits may be present

- Tuboloreticular inclusions in endothelial cell cytoplasm may be present

DIFFERENTIAL DIAGNOSIS

Primary MGN
- Subepithelial without mesangial immune deposits

Primary MPGN
- Similar pathologic features to HBV-associated MPGN

IgA Nephropathy
- Concurrent IgA nephropathy with hepatitis B-associated MGN reported
  - May be secondary to hepatobiliary disease

DIAGNOSTIC CHECKLIST

Pathologic Interpretation Pearls
- Clinical correlation is necessary to establish HBV-associated immune complex disease

SELECTED REFERENCES

1. Dienstag JL: Hepatitis B virus infection. N Engl J Med. 359(14):1486-500, 2008
2. Passarino G et al: Histopathological findings in 851 autopsies of drug addicts, with toxicologic and virologic correlations. Am J Forensic Med Pathol. 26(2):106-16, 2005
3. Bhimma R et al: Hepatitis B virus-associated nephropathy. Am J Nephrol. 24(2):198-211, 2004
4. Ganem D et al: Hepatitis B virus infection--natural history and clinical consequences. N Engl J Med. 350(11):1118-29, 2004
5. Ozdamar SO et al: Hepatitis-B virus associated nephropathies: a clinicopathological study in 14 children. Pediatr Nephrol. 18(1):23-8, 2003

HBV-associated MGN

(Left) Jones methenamine silver stain reveals a prominent, vacuolated appearance ⇗ with "spike" formation ⇘ involving the glomerular basement membranes in the glomeruli of a patient with HBV-associated MGN. *(Right)* Immunofluorescence microscopy shows strong granular staining of the glomerular capillary walls ⇘ for IgG, which is diagnostic of MGN in this 51-year-old man with cirrhosis due to hepatitis B infection.

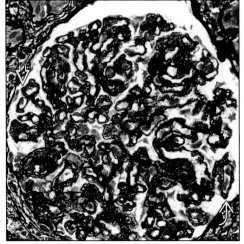
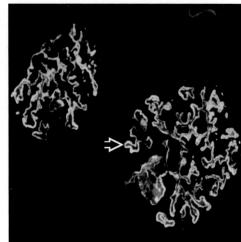

(Left) Immunohistochemistry for HBcAg shows strong and diffuse granular staining along the glomerular capillaries where subepithelial immune complexes are located in this patient with MGN associated with hepatitis B infection. *(Right)* Immunofluorescence microscopy for HBV surface antigen reveals granular staining ⇘ along the glomerular capillaries in locations where there are subepithelial immune complexes in an HBV-associated case of MGN.

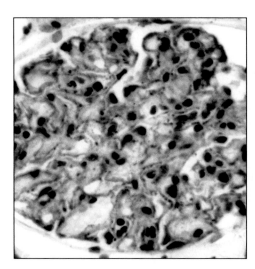
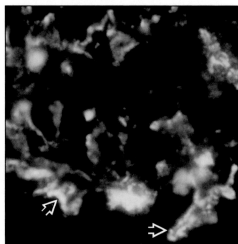

(Left) Electron microscopy reveals many variably sized, subepithelial, electron-dense deposits ⇘ with intervening basement membrane "spikes" ➡ between and surrounding most deposits. Extensive effacement of the podocyte foot processes correlates with the presence of nephrotic-range proteinuria. *(Right)* Small, discrete, electron-dense deposits in a few mesangial areas ⇘ are noted in another case of MGN with segmental distribution of subepithelial immune complex deposition.

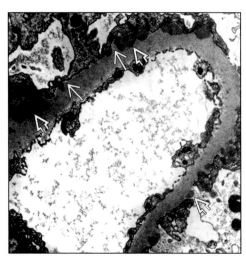
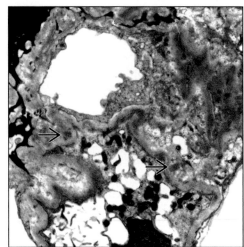

HEPATITIS B VIRUS

HBV-associated MPGN

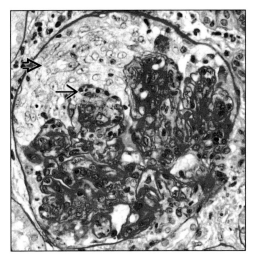 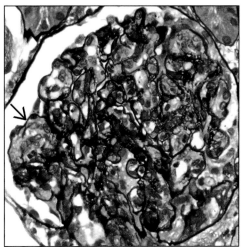

(Left) Endocapillary hypercellularity with increased inflammatory cells ➡ is present in the glomerular tufts in this patient with MPGN associated with HBV infection, but the cellular crescent ⮞ occupying and compressing the residual glomerulus obscures some of these alterations. (Right) Increased endocapillary cellularity in this glomerulus is noted. Focal duplication of the GBMs ➡ is also present, which is characteristic of MPGN associated with HBV infection.

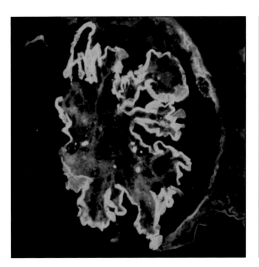 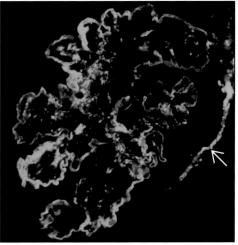

(Left) IgG reveals granular to confluent staining of glomerular capillaries, more suggestive of a membranous pattern. However, C3 staining along with light & electron microscopic findings were more consistent with a membranoproliferative pattern of injury. (Right) Granular C3 staining along the glomerular capillaries and mesangial areas is prominent in this glomerulus with MPGN associated with hepatitis B infection. Note focal Bowman capsule ➡ staining.

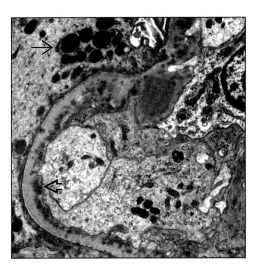 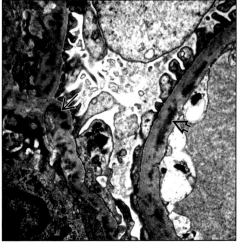

(Left) Numerous small, electron-dense deposits accumulate in a subendothelial region ⮞ along and within the GBM. Similar deposits in other cases have contained HBe antigens. Protein reabsorption droplets ➡ are noted in an adjacent podocyte with extensive foot process effacement. (Right) Many subendothelial ⮞ & mesangial ➡ electron-dense deposits are observed in this glomerulus showing membranoproliferative changes associated with HBV infection.

HEPATITIS C VIRUS

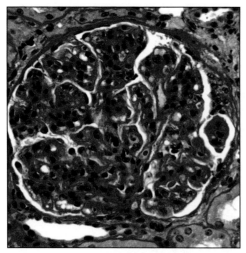
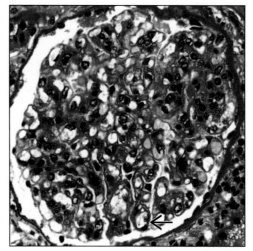

Periodic acid-Schiff reveals increased cellularity that highlights the lobularity of the glomerular tufts, which is characteristic of a membranoproliferative injury pattern.

Many double contours of the GBMs ➡ are noted in this patient with cryoglobulins (not shown) and hepatitis C infection.

TERMINOLOGY

Abbreviations
- Hepatitis C virus (HCV)

Definitions
- Wide spectrum of immune complex-mediated glomerular injuries in association with HCV infection

ETIOLOGY/PATHOGENESIS

Infectious Agents
- HCV
  - RNA virus: Single-stranded, positive sense
  - Infects hepatocytes and B lymphocytes
  - Blood-to-blood with rare sexual transmission
- Unknown pathogenic mechanism of kidney diseases
  - Possible contributing factors include
    - Circulating immune complexes of HCV antigen and antibodies
    - Cryoglobulins

CLINICAL ISSUES

Epidemiology
- Incidence
  - Over 200 million people worldwide are infected
- Age
  - Infected children have high rate of spontaneous resolution
- Gender
  - Young females may spontaneously resolve and are less likely than males to develop cirrhosis or hepatocellular carcinoma (HCC)

Presentation
- Proteinuria
- Hematuria

Laboratory Tests
- Serologic test
  - HCV antibodies
- PCR
  - HCV viral load
- HCV genotyping

Natural History
- 17-55% of HCV-infected patients progress to cirrhosis
- 2-23% develop HCC

Treatment
- Drugs
  - Ribavirin
  - Pegylated interferon-α
- Kidney &/or liver transplantation

Prognosis
- HCV genotype 2A and 3A have high cure rates

MICROSCOPIC PATHOLOGY

Histologic Features
- Membranoproliferative glomerulonephritis (MPGN)
  - Accentuation of glomerular tuft/lobules
  - Duplication of glomerular basement membranes or "tram track"
- Cryoglobulinemic GN
  - Endocapillary hypercellularity
  - "Wire loop" or hyaline "thrombi" deposits
    - PAS positive
- Membranous glomerulonephritis (MGN)
  - Thickened glomerular basement membranes with subepithelial "spike" formation
- Fibrillary GN
  - Mesangial expansion
- Immunotactoid glomerulopathy
  - Mesangial expansion
- IgA nephropathy
  - Variable mesangial hypercellularity

HEPATITIS C VIRUS

Key Facts

Terminology
- Hepatitis C virus (HCV)
- Wide spectrum of immune complex-mediated glomerular injuries in association with HCV infection

Clinical Issues
- Over 200 million people worldwide are infected
- Infected children have high rate of spontaneous resolution
- 17-55% of HCV-infected patients progress to cirrhosis
- 2-23% develop HCC

Microscopic Pathology
- Spectrum of glomerular injury
  - Membranoproliferative glomerulonephritis (MPGN)
  - Cryoglobulinemic GN
  - Membranous glomerulonephritis (MGN)
  - Fibrillary GN
  - Immunotactoid glomerulopathy
  - IgA nephropathy

Top Differential Diagnoses
- HCV-associated focal segmental glomerulosclerosis
- Hepatitis B virus-associated immune complex disease
- Lupus nephritis
- HIV-associated immune complex disease

Diagnostic Checklist
- No pathognomonic features for HCV infection
- Coinfection with HIV is common

ANCILLARY TESTS

Immunofluorescence
- MPGN
  - IgG and C3 granular staining of glomerular capillary walls and mesangial regions
- Cryoglobulinemic GN
  - IgG &/or IgM staining along glomerular capillaries and mesangial areas
  - Polyclonal or rare monoclonal light chain staining
- MGN
  - IgG granular staining of the capillary walls and some mesangial areas
- Fibrillary GN
  - IgG granular staining of capillary walls and mesangial areas
  - Polyclonal staining for kappa and lambda light chains
- Immunotactoid glomerulopathy
  - IgG granular staining of mesangial areas and capillary walls
  - Monoclonal light chain staining is typical
- IgA nephropathy
  - IgA granular mesangial staining with variable involvement of capillary walls

Electron Microscopy
- MPGN
  - Subendothelial & mesangial electron-dense deposits
  - Duplication of GBM
- Cryoglobulinemic GN
  - Subendothelial & mesangial electron-dense deposits
  - Substructural organization of deposits may be present
- MGN
  - Subepithelial & mesangial electron-dense deposits
- Fibrillary GN
  - Randomly arranged fibrils ~ 20 nm in diameter
- Immunotactoid glomerulopathy
  - Microtubules with hollow centers arranged in parallel arrays measuring > 30 nm in diameter
- IgA nephropathy
  - Mesangial electron-dense deposits with variable subendothelial or subepithelial involvement

DIFFERENTIAL DIAGNOSIS

HCV-associated Focal Segmental Glomerulosclerosis
- Segmental sclerosis of glomeruli
- Absence of immune complex deposition

Hepatitis B Virus-associated Immune Complex Disease
- Pathologically identical to HCV-associated immune complex disease

Lupus Nephritis
- Spectrum of glomerular injury mimics HCV-associated immune complex disease

DIAGNOSTIC CHECKLIST

Pathologic Interpretation Pearls
- No pathognomonic features for HCV infection
- Coinfection with HIV is common

SELECTED REFERENCES

1. Perico N et al: Hepatitis C infection and chronic renal diseases. Clin J Am Soc Nephrol. 4(1):207-20, 2009
2. Kamar N et al: Hepatitis C virus-related kidney disease: an overview. Clin Nephrol. 69(3):149-60, 2008
3. Barsoum RS: Hepatitis C virus: from entry to renal injury--facts and potentials. Nephrol Dial Transplant. 22(7):1840-8, 2007
4. Markowitz GS et al: Hepatitis C viral infection is associated with fibrillary glomerulonephritis and immunotactoid glomerulopathy. J Am Soc Nephrol. 9(12):2244-52, 1998

HCV-associated MPGN

(Left) A cellular crescent occupies the urinary space and surrounds the remaining glomerulus, which has a membranoproliferative pattern of injury characterized by endocapillary proliferation and a lobular appearance of the glomerular tufts. *(Right)* Duplication of the GBMs ➡ is characteristic of MPGN in this patient with HCV infection and is best observed with the Jones methenamine silver stain.

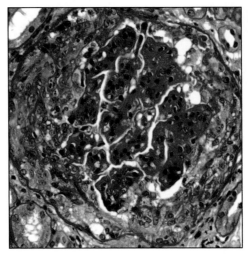
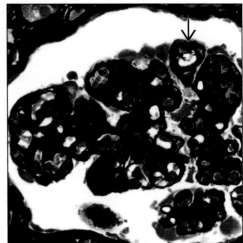

(Left) IgG staining of the glomerular capillaries and mesangial areas is characteristic for membranoproliferative GN. This staining pattern is not specific for HCV-associated MPGN and is identical to that seen in idiopathic MPGN. *(Right)* Strong granular to focally confluent C3 is prominent along the glomerular capillary walls with a similar pattern to IgG, which is characteristic of membranoproliferative GN.

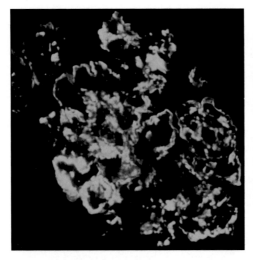
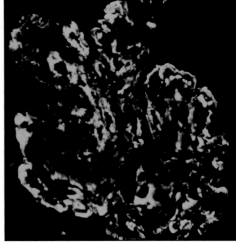

(Left) A large electron-dense deposit ➡ in this glomerular capillary is surrounded by the original GBM ➡ and a 2nd layer ➡, which would correspond with the double contours as seen by light microscopy. *(Right)* Interposition of cells ➡ between the duplicated GBMs is a characteristic finding of MPGN as identified in this patient with hepatitis C infection. Occasional subepithelial deposits ➡ are seen in this case with features of type III MPGN.

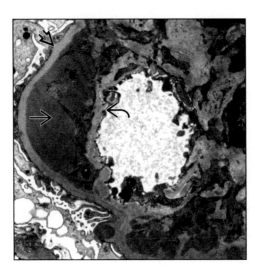
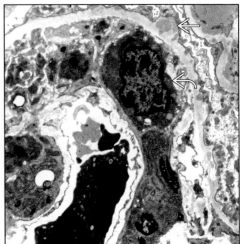

HEPATITIS C VIRUS

HCV-associated Cryoglobulinemic GN

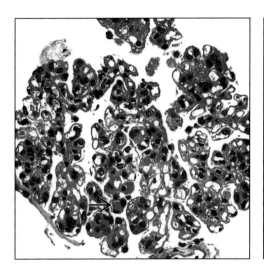 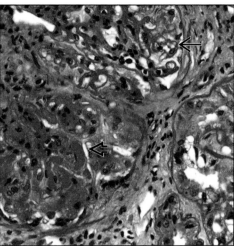

(Left) Several hyaline thrombi ➡ are present in this glomerulus from a patient with cryoglobulinemic GN associated with hepatitis C infection. Focusing up and down on the microscope reveals a characteristic refractile appearance due to the staining quality of the prominent accumulation of immune complexes. *(Right)* Numerous hyaline "thrombi" ➡ are present in the glomerular capillaries. The alterations in an adjacent glomerulus ➡ are not as noticeable.

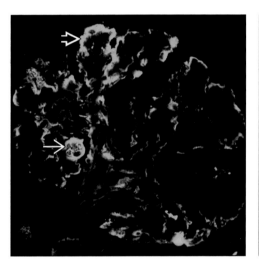 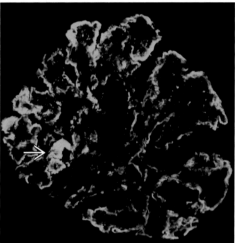

(Left) Strong peripheral capillary wall ➡ IgG staining and a probable hyaline "thrombus" ➡ in a glomerular capillary are present. *(Right)* IgM demonstrates strong staining of the peripheral glomerular capillaries with a hyaline "thrombus" ➡ in 1 glomerular capillary. HCV should be considered as a potential etiologic agent in almost any form of immune complex glomerulonephritis.

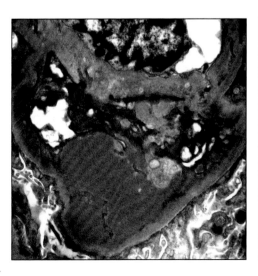 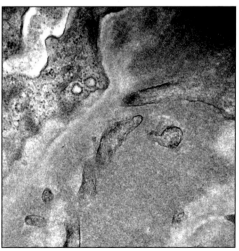

(Left) Large electron-dense deposits along the subendothelial aspect of this glomerular capillary would correspond with a "wire loop" deposit by light microscopy, which can also be observed in some cases of proliferative lupus nephritis. *(Right)* At high magnification, a vague substructure of the electron-dense deposits can be seen, but the presence or absence of this finding is not diagnostic for cryoglobulinemic GN.

HEPATITIS C VIRUS

HCV-associated Membranous GN

(Left) Periodic acid-Schiff reveals thick GBMs with increased mesangial matrix ➡, which is suggestive of a secondary form of membranous GN. *(Right)* Jones methenamine silver demonstrates prominent subepithelial "spikes" and vacuoles ➡ along all of the glomerular capillary basement membranes that are diagnostic of membranous GN. Correlation with clinical and laboratory data is necessary to confirm the association with hepatitis C infection.

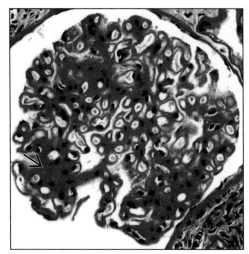
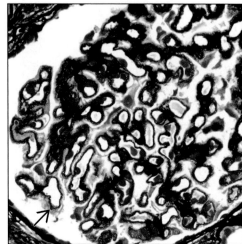

(Left) Immunofluorescence microscopy for IgG reveals strong granular staining of the glomerular capillaries ➡ with faint granular staining of the mesangial areas ➡. Mesangial staining suggests a secondary form of membranous GN, but establishing the presence of hepatitis C infection requires other lab tests. *(Right)* Immunofluorescence microscopy for kappa light chains reveals a similar but less intense staining pattern as IgG. Lambda light chain (not shown) had a similar staining pattern.

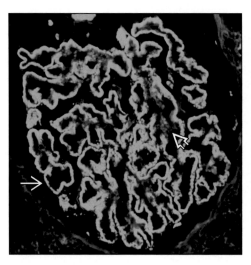
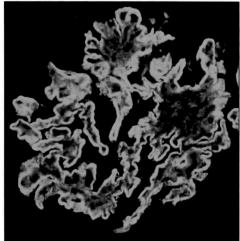

(Left) Electron microscopy demonstrates many subepithelial electron-dense deposits ➡ surrounded by basement membrane material ➡ consistent with Ehrenreich-Churg stage III changes. *(Right)* Electron microscopy reveals numerous subepithelial electron-dense deposits ➡ with basement membrane reaction between and surrounding some of the deposits. The podocyte foot processes show extensive effacement.

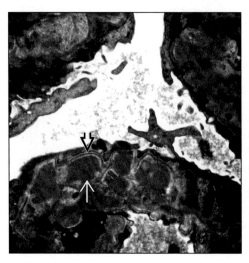
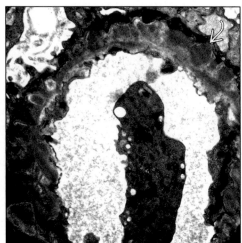

HEPATITIS C VIRUS

HCV-associated Fibrillary GN

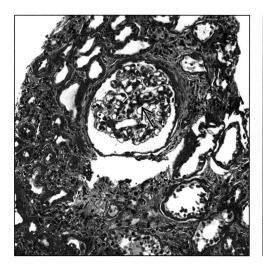

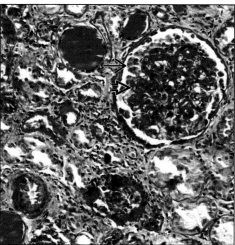

(Left) This case of fibrillary GN in a 50-year-old woman with a history of chronic kidney disease, hypertension, and hepatitis C infection reveals extensive global glomerulosclerosis (not shown), interstitial fibrosis, and tubular atrophy. A rare intact glomerulus shows very mild mesangial hypercellularity and mesangial matrix expansion ➡. *(Right)* Periodic acid-Schiff shows segmental sclerosis ⊳ with prominence of adjacent podocytes ➡.

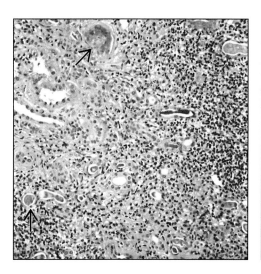

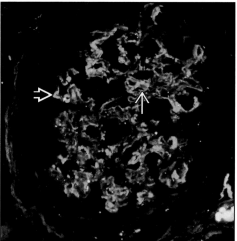

(Left) Hematoxylin and eosin shows marked and diffuse interstitial inflammation with atrophic tubules in an advanced case of fibrillary GN. A tubule contains a red blood cell cast ➡. *(Right)* Immunofluorescence reveals smudgy mesangial ➡ and glomerular capillary loop ⊳ staining for IgG. Polyclonal staining for kappa and lambda light chains (not shown) helps support the diagnostic consideration of fibrillary GN.

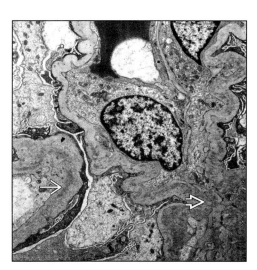

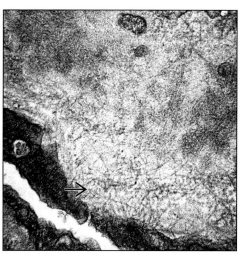

(Left) Electron-dense material with a fibrillar substructure is seen along the glomerular basement membranes ➡ and within the mesangial regions ⊳. A negative Congo red stain and the wider thickness of the fibrils support the diagnosis of fibrillary GN. *(Right)* Electron microscopy at high magnification reveals many randomly arranged fibrils ➡ that each measure approximately 17 nm in diameter.

HIV-ASSOCIATED COLLAPSING GLOMERULOPATHY

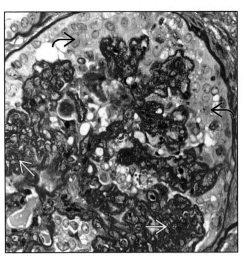

Classic appearance of HIVAN with glomerular collapse ⇒ and proliferation of overlying podocytes ⇾ is well demonstrated by PAS stains in this HIV(+) man. The podocyte hypercellularity mimics a crescent.

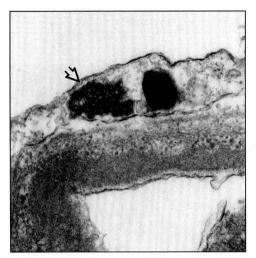

Tubuloreticular inclusions (TRIs) ⇾ are almost always detectable in the endothelium in HIVAN, in contrast to idiopathic collapsing glomerulopathy. This sample is from an HIV(+) black man with 29 g/d proteinuria.

TERMINOLOGY

Synonyms
- HIV-associated nephropathy (HIVAN)
- HIV-associated collapsing glomerulopathy

Definitions
- Characteristic renal disease developing in setting of HIV infection

ETIOLOGY/PATHOGENESIS

Infectious Agents
- HIV
  - Some suggest kidney is "reservoir" for HIV
    - HIV genome demonstrated in glomerular visceral and tubular epithelial cells in HIVAN
  - Abnormal maturation and differentiation of podocytes demonstrated (Barisoni et al)
  - Cytokines may have role
    - Abnormalities shown in transforming growth factor-β (TGF-β), basic fibroblast growth factor (bFGF), interleukin, and others
- AIDS not required for condition to occur

Genetic Factors
- Higher risk with African ancestry (except Ethiopian)
- *APOL1* polymorphism associated with HIVAN

Animal Models
- Mice transgenic for HIV regulatory genes develop collapsing glomerulopathy
  - Renal HIV gene expression necessary for transgenic HIVAN
    - Normal kidneys fail to develop nephropathy when transplanted into HIV transgenic mice
    - Transplantation of transgenic kidneys into nontransgenic litter mates shows the renal HIVAN phenotype

CLINICAL ISSUES

Epidemiology
- Incidence
  - Average incidence of acute kidney injury is 2.7 episodes per 100 person-years
    - Higher within 1st 3 months of disease recognition: 19.3 episodes per 100 person-years
- Gender
  - Majority (~ 70%) male, particularly according to original descriptions
- Ethnicity
  - Historically, up to 90% of African American blacks
  - Rare in whites

Presentation
- Proteinuria, nephrotic range
  - Severe, averaging 6-7 g/d
  - Edema, hypoalbuminemia, and hypercholesterolemia (nephrotic syndrome) uncommon
- Renal dysfunction
  - Creatinine at diagnosis typically ~ 5 mg/dL
- Hypertension
  - Uncommon (in < 50%)
- Microhematuria

Laboratory Tests
- CD4 count does not correlate with HIVAN development
- Hypercholesterolemia uncommon, possibly due to ↓ hepatic lipoprotein synthesis in AIDS patients

Treatment
- Drugs
  - Highly active antiretroviral therapy (HAART)
    - May reverse tubular microcysts and slow HIVAN progression
    - HAART reduction in viral load can ↑ renal survival
  - Angiotensin-converting enzyme (ACE) inhibitors

HIV-ASSOCIATED COLLAPSING GLOMERULOPATHY

Key Facts

Clinical Issues

- Up to 90% of cases occur in African-American blacks, mostly male
- Rapid progression to ESRD
- Hypertension uncommon (in < 50%)
- Nephrotic-range proteinuria and ↑ creatinine
- Treatment: HAART, ACE inhibitors

Macroscopic Features

- Enlarged with cysts

Microscopic Pathology

- Collapsing GS
- Microcystic tubular dilatation (30-40% of cases)
- Mononuclear cells (including lymphocytes and monocytes) and plasma cells
- Interstitial inflammation and edema

Ancillary Tests

- IF: IgM, C3, and C1q in capillary walls in segmental distribution
- EM
  - Podocyte foot process effacement and multilamination of subepithelial GBM
  - Tubuloreticular inclusions (TRIs) in endothelial cells, lymphocytes, and monocytes
  - Granular and, less commonly, granulofibrillar transformation of tubulointerstitial nuclei

Top Differential Diagnoses

- Idiopathic collapsing glomerulopathy and FSGS
- Diffuse mesangial hypercellularity and minimal change disease

---

- May slow HIVAN progression
- Hemodialysis
- Renal transplantation

Prognosis

- Rapidly progressive, with ESRD often developing within months in most
  - Early in AIDS epidemic, mean time to dialysis < 2 months and median survival time of renal disease to death is 4.5 months

IMAGE FINDINGS

Ultrasonographic Findings

- Enlarged, highly echogenic kidneys

MACROSCOPIC FEATURES

General Features

- Pale cortex
- 0.5-1.0 mm cysts in cortex or at corticomedullary junction

Size

- Enlarged, mean combined weight up to 500 g in adults
- 1.2-1.3x normal weight in children

MICROSCOPIC PATHOLOGY

Histologic Features

- Glomeruli
  - Collapsing glomerulopathy
    - Capillary loops globally or segmentally collapsed without corresponding mesangial matrix ↑
    - Shrunken down, global glomerulosclerosis (GS) ± cystic Bowman space dilatation, which contains proteinaceous material
    - ± marked podocyte hyperplasia, protein resorption droplets, and mitoses (contrary to prior thought that podocytes could not undergo mitosis)
    - ± enlarged glomeruli

- Global GS reduces glomerulus to acellular sclerotic ball
  - Podocytes prominent
    - May simulate a crescent
    - Starts with hypertrophy and hyperplasia of visceral epithelial cells
- Tubules
  - Microcystic tubular dilatation (30-40% of cases)
    - ± scalloped tubular outline
    - ± PAS(+) proteinaceous casts (fuchsin[+] on trichrome) in renal tubules
    - Autopsy studies have shown near-complete replacement of renal cortical parenchyma by microcysts
  - Patchy epithelial injury, regeneration, degeneration, and necrosis, and eventual tubular atrophy
    - Flattened tubular epithelium and mitotic figures
    - Tubular resorption droplets prominent
- Interstitium
  - Interstitial inflammation and edema
    - Mononuclear cells (including lymphocytes and monocytes) and plasma cells
  - Interstitial fibrosis typically present
- Vessels
  - Typically unremarkable
  - Rare cases of thrombotic microangiopathy

ANCILLARY TESTS

Immunofluorescence

- Segmental IgM, C3, and C1q
  - ± IgM and C3 granular positivity
  - Resorption droplets in podocytes and proximal tubules stain for multiple plasma proteins
- Prominent immune complex deposit would be indicative of additional diagnosis
  - Hepatitis C virus (HCV), lupus-like GN, IgA nephropathy can all be seen in HIV

Electron Microscopy

- Glomeruli

HIV-ASSOCIATED COLLAPSING GLOMERULOPATHY

○ Podocytes enlarged with ≥ 1 dense, round 2° lysosome and enlarged vacuoles
   ▪ Podocyte foot processes usually completely effaced
   ▪ Cell separated from original GBM by new basement membrane (BM) material
   ▪ BM-type material may eventually occlude capillary loops in a segmental sclerosing/collapsing-type process
   ▪ Nuclear bodies: Nuclear inclusions with broad morphologic variety
○ Foam cells in lumina
○ ± small nonspecific deposits in mesangium, correlating to mesangial IgM and C3
○ Tubuloreticular inclusions (TRIs) in endothelial cells, lymphocytes, and monocytes
   ▪ Measure ~ 25 nm and found in dilated endoplasmic reticulum cisternae as anastomosed tubular structures
   ▪ May be large and multiple per cell
   ▪ Most easily identified in glomerular endothelium but also in infiltrating leukocytes or arterial, peritubular capillary, or interstitial capillary endothelium
   ▪ Less common than in HIVAN initial description due to ↓ with HAART therapy, likely due to ↓ viral burden
   ▪ Also referred to as "interferon (IFN) footprints" or "myxovirus-like inclusions"; seen in other states, e.g., systemic lupus erythematosus (SLE), multiple sclerosis (MS), and IFN-α therapy
   ▪ HAART ↓ TRIs
   ▪ Cylindrical confronting cisternae: Fused membranous lamellae forming long cylinders (known as "test tube" and "ring-shaped" forms) occur in cells with TRIs (monocytes and lymphocytes) (also seen in SLE, MS, and IFN-α therapy)
○ Tubules
   ▪ Granular: Coarsely granular material disrupting nuclear membrane
   ▪ Granulofibrillar: Chromatin replaced by material with coarse or fine granularity, primarily seen postmortem
• HIV itself has not been definitively demonstrated in renal cells by standard EM methods

Immunohistochemistry
• IHC shows CD4(+) and CD8(+) cells and ↓ CD4/CD8 ratio
• HLA-DR on inflammatory and parenchymal cells (endothelial, glomerular mesangial, and visceral epithelial)
• Minor B-cell and macrophage component

DIFFERENTIAL DIAGNOSIS

Idiopathic Collapsing Nephropathy
• Patients typically HIV negative
• TRIs seen more often in HIVAN

Idiopathic/Primary FSGS
• Glomerular hyalinosis a common feature in idiopathic FSGS but not in HIVAN
• Collapsing FSGS with prominent hyperplastic podocytes more typical of HIVAN
• TRIs seen much more commonly in HIVAN
• HIV serology needed to attribute an FSGS to HIV

Heroin-associated Nephropathy (HAN)
• Difficult to distinguish HIVAN from HAN since patients may have both risk factors
• Prominent collapsing GS with microcystic tubular dilatation more commonly seen in HIVAN
• GS in HAN more typical of idiopathic form of FSGS, displaying hyalinosis

Diffuse Mesangial Hypercellularity (DMH) and Minimal Change Disease (MCD)
• Disorders usually milder than HIVAN and present with nephrotic syndrome and normal renal function (i.e., normal GFR)
• Typical HIVAN accounts for ≤ 50% of HIV-related glomerulopathies in children
   ○ DMH almost as common as HIVAN
      ▪ DMH often produces proteinuria in the nephrotic range
   ○ Minimal change disease also quite common
• Rapid renal failure course favors HIVAN

DIAGNOSTIC CHECKLIST

Pathologic Interpretation Pearls
• Although there are characteristic features, history of HIV infection is crucial to proper clinicopathologic diagnosis

SELECTED REFERENCES

1. Winston J et al: Kidney disease in patients with HIV infection and AIDS. Clin Infect Dis. 47(11):1449-57, 2008
2. Cohen AH et al: Renal injury associated with human immunodeficiency virus infection. In Jennette JC et al: Heptinstall's Pathology of the Kidney. 6th ed. Philadelphia: Lippincott Williams & Wilkins. 397-422, 2007
3. Winston JA et al: Nephropathy and establishment of a renal reservoir of HIV type 1 during primary infection. N Engl J Med. 344(26):1979-84, 2001
4. Barisoni L et al: The dysregulated podocyte phenotype: a novel concept in the pathogenesis of collapsing idiopathic focal segmental glomerulosclerosis and HIV-associated nephropathy. J Am Soc Nephrol. 10(1):51-61, 1999
5. Cohen AH et al: Demonstration of human immunodeficiency virus in renal epithelium in HIV-associated nephropathy. Mod Pathol. 2(2):125-8, 1989
6. Rao TK et al: Associated focal and segmental glomerulosclerosis in the acquired immunodeficiency syndrome. N Engl J Med. 310(11):669-73, 1984

HIV-ASSOCIATED COLLAPSING GLOMERULOPATHY

Microscopic Features

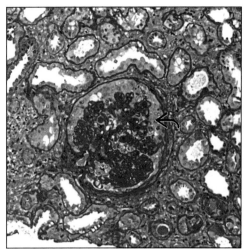

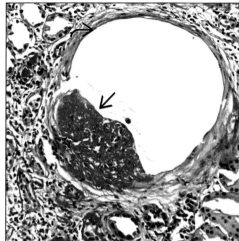

(Left) Collapsing glomerulopathy is the defining feature of HIVAN, as shown here in a glomerulus with marked epithelial hypercellularity ➡ resembling a crescent. The interstitium is also characteristically involved with diffuse mononuclear infiltrates, and tubules are dilated and proliferative. *(Right)* Collapsed glomerulus ➡ with a dilated Bowman space ➡ is shown in a case of HIVAN in a 58-year-old man not on HAART with CD4 count < 200, Cr 3.7, and > 3 g/d proteinuria.

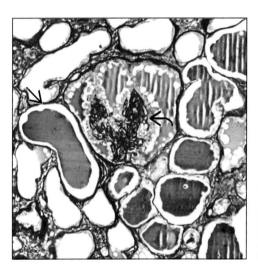

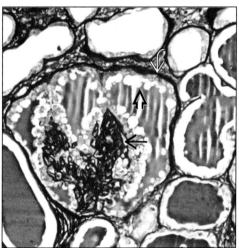

(Left) A collapsed glomerulus in a case of HIVAN ➡ is shown along with adjacent, markedly dilated tubules ➡ with marked epithelial cell flattening and abundant proteinaceous cast material. *(Right)* Higher power shows that the collapsed glomerulus in a case of HIVAN ➡ is surrounded by a dilated Bowman space ➡ with scalloping of proteinaceous cast material at the periphery ➡.

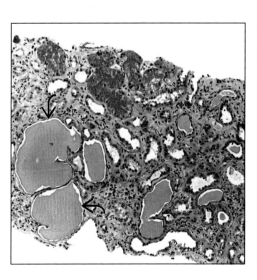

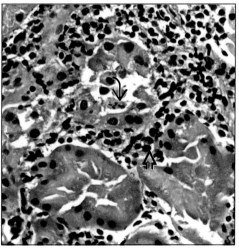

(Left) Massively dilated tubules ➡ are a characteristic of collapsing glomerulopathy in HIVAN as well as in other causes. Interstitial inflammation is also a typical feature. *(Right)* In the tubulointerstitium of a 58-year-old man with HIVAN, CD4 count < 200, Cr 3.7, and > 3 g/d proteinuria, there is tubular injury with evident mitotic activity ➡ and an inflammatory infiltrate composed of mononuclear cells and plasma cells ➡.

HIV-ASSOCIATED COLLAPSING GLOMERULOPATHY

Light Microscopy and Immunofluorescence

(Left) Jones silver stain of an early case of HIVAN in a 24-year-old man not on HAART with 6 g/d proteinuria, CD4 count of 629, Cr 1.9, and albumin 1.4 mg/dL shows peripheral glomerular capillary loop occlusion ⇨ and abundant tubular resorption droplets ➡. *(Right)* In the early case of HIVAN in a 24-year-old man, at high power (60x), one can observe peripheral glomerular capillary loop occlusion ➡ and fuchsinophilic podocyte resorption droplets ➳ on a trichrome stain.

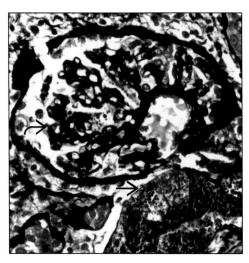 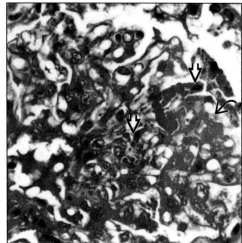

(Left) Proliferation of visceral ➡ & parietal ➡ epithelial cells, as well as tubular epithelium ➡, is characteristic of collapsing glomerulopathy regardless of cause and persists even at the end stage, as shown in this Ki-67 stain. *(Right)* In a 46-year-old man with HIV, 11 g/d proteinuria, & Cr 4.5, recently started on HAART, there is peripheral glomerular capillary loop staining for C3 by immunofluorescence along glomerular basement membranes ➡ & in collapsed glomerular capillary loops ➳.

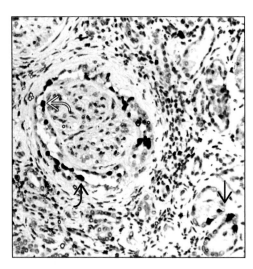 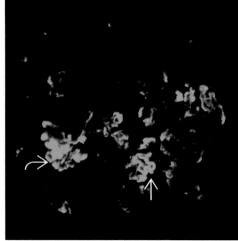

(Left) In a 46-year-old man with HIV, 11 g/day proteinuria, and creatinine 4.5, who recently started on HAART, there is peripheral glomerular capillary loop staining for IgM ➡ by immunofluorescence. *(Right)* HIV-infected patients have glomerular diseases other than collapsing glomerulopathy, such as IgA nephropathy, illustrated here with a stain for IgA in a 38-year-old HIV(+) Haitian woman. A lupus-like glomerulonephritis (GN) and fibrillary GN are also associated with HIV.

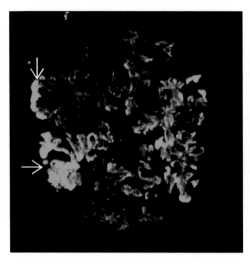 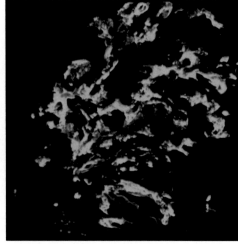

HIV-ASSOCIATED COLLAPSING GLOMERULOPATHY

Electron Microscopy

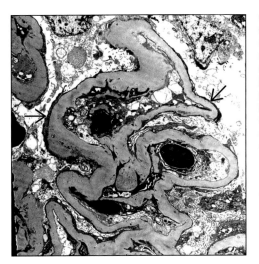

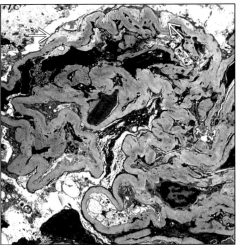

(Left) In a case of HIVAN in a 46-year-old man with HIV, 11 g/d proteinuria, and Cr 4.5, who recently started on HAART, EM shows collapsed glomerular capillary loops with completely effaced podocyte foot processes ➡. (Right) One of the characteristic features of collapsing glomerulopathy, whether due to HIV or other causes, is the separation of podocytes from the GBM by multilaminated new basement membrane ➡, originally described in heroin nephropathy.

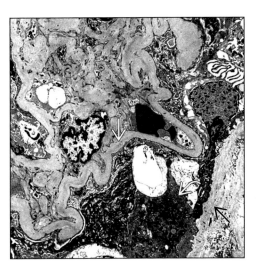

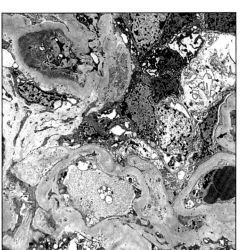

(Left) One of the debates in collapsing glomerulopathy is the nature of the proliferating epithelial cells. This image from a case of HIVAN shows a cell ➡ bridging between Bowman capsule ➡ and the GBM ➡, consistent with replacement of podocytes by parietal epithelium. (Right) In HIVAN, the podocytes are hyperplastic and have complete loss of foot processes. The podocytes lose expression of many markers of differentiation, such as WT1 and synaptopodin.

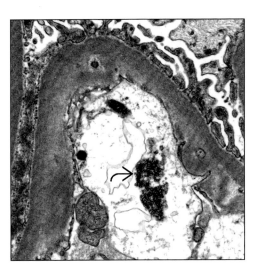

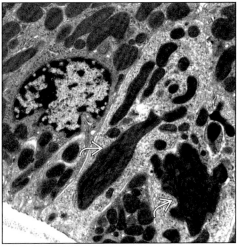

(Left) In this biopsy from a 58-year-old HIV(+) man not on HAART with a CD4 count < 200, Cr 3.7, and > 3 g/d proteinuria, there are TRIs in glomerular endothelium ➡. (Right) HAART has reduced HIVAN incidence considerably; however, the inhibitory effects of anti-reverse transcriptase on mtDNA can cause a mitochondriopathy, diagnosed by abnormally shaped and enlarged mitochondria by EM ➡ and manifested by LM by leading to interstitial fibrosis and tubular atrophy.

MISCELLANEOUS HIV-ASSOCIATED RENAL DISEASES

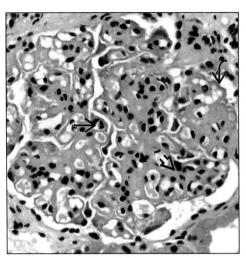

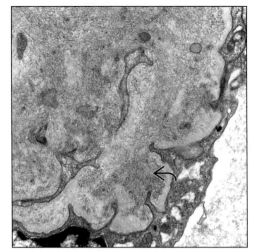

Lupus-like GN is one of the more frequent diseases associated with HIV, typically showing a markedly expanded mesangium ⊟, thickened capillary walls ⇗, and inflammatory cells in glomerular capillary loops ⇘.

Fibrillary GN is one glomerular disease associated with HIV infection. Fibrils ⇗ are evident in the GBM in an electron micrograph from a 50-year-old HIV(+), HCV(+) man with 11 g/d proteinuria. Congo red stain was (-).

TERMINOLOGY

Abbreviations
- HIV-associated renal diseases (HIV-ARD)

Definitions
- Renal diseases other than collapsing glomerulopathy (HIVAN) that occur particularly in patients infected with HIV, due to direct effect on kidney, altered immune system, or drug toxicity

HIV-ASSOCIATED LUPUS-LIKE GLOMERULONEPHRITIS

Terminology
- Chronic immune complex disease in HIV-infected patients that has LM, IF, and EM features of lupus nephritis, but patients have no other evidence of lupus nephritis
- Described by Haas et al and Nochy et al

Pathogenesis
- Probably related to immune dysregulation
- Loss of CD4(+) T regulatory cells causes autoimmune disease
- Role of infectious agent not excluded

Incidence
- Possibly 2nd most common form of glomerular lesions (after HIVAN) in HIV patients undergoing biopsy
- Many (13/14 in the Haas Baltimore study) were African-American
- Nochy's study in Europe showed equal proportions of whites and blacks having lupus-like GN
- In series of > 100 biopsies for glomerular disease in HIV(+) patients, 3% had lupus-like GN

Presentation
- Hematuria and proteinuria/nephrotic syndrome
- Share other features such as anemia, leukopenia, multiorgan involvement, and serositis

Laboratory Tests
- ± ANA and anti-double-stranded (ds) DNA and ↓ complements
  - Assessment somewhat complicated because some HIV patients have low-titer ANAs
    - Screening of > 150 patients with AIDS found 19 to be ANA(+) but only 2 at high titer and none anti-dsDNA Ab(+)

Treatment
- Corticosteroids, ACE inhibitors, highly active antiretroviral therapy (HAART) have all been used

Prognosis
- Outcome can be poor, because many patients present with advanced disease

Microscopic Pathology
- Focal/diffuse proliferative GN or membranous nephropathy

Immunofluorescence
- "Full house" pattern of IgG, IgA, IgM, C3, and C1q

Electron Microscopy
- Essentially all have tubuloreticular inclusions
- Most common pattern appears to be combination of mesangial, subendothelial, subepithelial, and intramembranous deposits

Differential Diagnosis
- Lupus nephritis
  - HIV-associated lupus-like GN lacks positive lupus serologies (ANA, dsDNA) and nonrenal manifestations

- o "Full house" immunofluorescence staining pattern is more commonly seen in lupus than in HIVAN
- o Tubuloreticular inclusions may be seen in both lupus nephritis and HIVAN

IgA NEPHROPATHY

Terminology
- IgA(+) glomerular disease arising in HIV(+) patients that has clinical and pathologic aspects similar to idiopathic IgA nephropathy
- Reports have also included Henoch-Schönlein purpura with nephritis

Pathogenesis
- Deposits eluted from glomeruli have shown specificity for HIV envelope (e.g., gp41, gp120, gp160) or core proteins (e.g., p24) (Kimmel et al)

Incidence
- Series (many of which are from Europe) indicate higher incidence of IgA nephropathy in white patients with HIV infection
- Data conflicts regarding prevalence of IgA deposits in patients dying from AIDS
  - o Some series indicate high prevalence of IgA deposits in AIDS patients, but this does not necessarily correlate with increased IgA nephropathy rate

Presentation
- Hematuria and low-grade proteinuria are common
- May present with Henoch-Schönlein purpura (HSP)-type picture (rash [leukocytoclastic angiitis of the skin], etc.)

Laboratory Tests
- Associated with IgA-containing cryoglobulins
- ↑ IgA levels, IgA-containing circulating immune complexes, and IgA-rheumatoid factor

Treatment
- ACE inhibitors may be useful

Prognosis
- Thought to be same as IgA nephropathy in non-HIV-infected patients

Microscopic Pathology
- Does not differ drastically from conventional IgA nephropathy seen in absence of HIV
  - o Mesangial proliferation ± collapsing glomerulosclerosis (coexisting HIVAN)

Immunofluorescence
- Shows mesangial IgA deposits like conventional IgA nephropathy seen in absence of HIV

Electron Microscopy
- In contrast with idiopathic IgA nephropathy, there are also numerous tubuloreticular structures that provide a clue to presence of HIV

THROMBOTIC MICROANGIOPATHY (TMA)

Terminology
- TMA associated with HIV infection
- Both syndromes resembling thrombotic thrombocytopenic purpura (TTP) and hemolytic uremic syndrome (HUS) can occur in HIV-infected patients

Pathogenesis
- Etiology not known
  - o HIV injury to endothelium or infection of megakaryocytes may be involved
  - o *Escherichia coli* 0157:H7 appears not to be involved
  - o Appears that ADAMTS13 level is not ↓ in HIV-associated TMA as it is in TTP
  - o Etiology role has been attributed to CMV infection, cryptosporidiosis, AIDS-related neoplasia, drugs, and antiphospholipid antibodies

Incidence
- Human data are lacking
  - o Multicenter autopsy study showed 15 of 214 patients (7%) with deaths attributable to AIDS had evidence of TMA
  - o French study (Peraldi et al) attributed rapid decline in renal function to HUS-type syndrome in 32 of 92 patients
  - o 6/27 (22.2%) pigtailed macaques (*Macaca nemestrina*) acutely infected with HIV-2 developed histological and EM features of renal TMA such as glomerular capillary platelet thrombi and mesangiolysis

Presentation
- Acute renal failure ± proteinuria and hematuria
- Microangiopathic hemolytic anemia and thrombocytopenia
- Presentations may be classified as either HUS or TTP (neurologic symptoms and fever)

Laboratory Tests
- ± thrombocytopenia ± schistocytosis

Treatment
- Treatment of underlying HIV may be best approach
- Plasmapheresis and fresh frozen plasma have been used
- Rituximab and corticosteroids have been used
- Hemodialysis may be needed at presentation

Prognosis
- High mortality: More severe in HIV-infected patients than in non-HIV-infected patients

Microscopic Pathology
- Pathologic findings are similar to those of TMA in non-HIV-infected patients
  - o Mucoid arterial intimal hyperplasia and intraluminal thrombi may be observed
  - o Fragmented intramural RBCs in vessels
- May coexist with HIVAN

MISCELLANEOUS HIV-ASSOCIATED RENAL DISEASES

Immunofluorescence
- As in other TMA, fibrinogen/fibrin may be found in glomerular capillary walls, in mesangium, and in arteriolar/arterial walls, corresponding to intravascular thrombi
- Glomerular capillary walls may show IgM, C3, IgG, and rarely IgA
- IgM may be seen in arteriolar/arterial walls

Electron Microscopy
- Tubuloreticular structures or other ultrastructural features may be identified, providing only clue to presence of HIV

Differential Diagnosis
- Hypertensive nephrosclerosis
  - If vascular changes are mild, then disease may actually not be TMA but rather a milder hypertension-related nephrosclerosis
  - Since HAART, patients with RNA levels of HIV-1 < 400 copies/mL are more likely to have hypertensive nephrosclerosis than HIVAN

OTHER IMMUNE COMPLEX DISEASES

Membranoproliferative GN (MPGN)
- Can be seen in HIV patients coinfected with hepatitis C virus (HCV)
- Type I or III MPGN or cryoglobulinemic-type GN can be seen
- Mainly Caucasian but also African patients
- In a series of > 100 biopsies for glomerular disease in HIV(+) patients, 10% had MPGN

Membranous GN
- May be present in HIV-infected patients, particularly those also infected with HCV
- In a study of those infected with HCV and HIV, 80% had MPGN and 20% had membranous nephropathy
  - Clinical course in this study was associated with rapid progression to renal failure or death (median: 5.8 months)

Infection-related Immune Complex GN
- HIVAN may have concurrent immune complex GN or acute postinfectious GN since HIVAN patients have infectious risks

Hepatitis C Virus (HCV)
- HCV-associated immune complex glomerulonephritis is common in HIV(+) patients
- HCV and HIV have common risk factors such as intravenous drug use

Fibrillary and Immunotactoid GN
- Fibrillary GN: Glomerular deposition of fibrils 15-25 nm long
  - Fibrillary GN is rarely reported in HIV, except in those coinfected with HCV
- Immunotactoid GN: Electron-dense microtubules in glomeruli, having hollow core, arranged in parallel arrays
  - Microtubules can be as small as 20 nm but average 40 nm and are usually > 30 nm in diameter
  - Has been reported in patients with HIV infection in absence of HCV

TUBULOINTERSTITIAL DISEASE

Drug-induced Mitochondriopathy
- Not uncommon in patients on HAART
  - Nucleotide reverse transcriptase inhibitors impair mitochondrial replication through DNA polymerase-γ inhibition
- May present with markedly elevated creatinine, subnephrotic proteinuria, and normoglycemic glycosuria
- Eosinophilic inclusions of tubular epithelial cells can be seen, which EM shows to be giant mitochondria
- EM of tubular cells shows enlarged mitochondria with abnormal shapes and small number of broken, distorted cristae
  - Enlarged mitochondria may be totally devoid of cristae
  - Changes resemble mitochondrial DNA (mtDNA) depletion syndromes

Other Drug Toxicity
- ATN and myoglobulinuria are associated with pentamidine and zidovudine
- Indinavir therapy can produce characteristic intratubular crystals, yielding resultant tubular injury

Acute Interstitial Nephritis
- "Diffuse infiltrative lymphocytosis syndrome"
- May occur in the absence of HIVAN
- May involve multiple organs
- Unknown whether this is directly related to HIV infection or secondary viral infection

Viral Infections
- Epstein-Barr virus (EBV) has been shown to cause some cases of acute interstitial nephritis
- Cytomegalovirus (CMV) is most common viral infection (up 30% of renal infections)
  - May produce hematuria and proteinuria
- Systemic candidiasis and cryptococcosis in 5-10% of patients at autopsy
- Mucormycosis may be aggressive and mass-forming
- Disseminated *Pneumocystis jirovecii* (*carinii*)
- Mycobacterial infections may produce ill-defined granulomatous inflammation

Bacterial Infections
- Syphilis
  - Often overlooked since recent resurgence after progressive decline in 1990s
  - Presents with proteinuria, nephrotic syndrome, acute nephritic syndrome, acute renal failure, and chronic progressive renal failure
  - Serology positive for syphilis

MISCELLANEOUS HIV-ASSOCIATED RENAL DISEASES

○ Manifests as proliferative GN, crescentic GN, membranous glomerulopathy, minimal change disease, interstitial nephritis, amyloidosis, and gumma formation
○ Treated with penicillin therapy
• Mycobacterial infections can cause renal disease

Fungal Infections

• *Histoplasma capsulatum*
○ Southern and midwestern parts of USA along Mississippi and Ohio River valleys
• Acute kidney injury or nephrotic syndrome with preserved renal function
• Diagnosis confirmed by blood or urine culture or by biopsy
○ Biopsy shows noncaseating granulomas, interstitial inflammation, and acute tubular injury
○ GMS(+) or PAS(+) yeast forms

RENAL NEOPLASMS

Lymphomas

• Usually B-cell origin (i.e., diffuse large B-cell lymphoma and Burkitt lymphoma)
• Angiocentric and intravascular lymphoma may occur (both are usually T cell in origin)
• Usually whitish or white-gray grossly as opposed to renal cell carcinoma, which is yellow
• Commonly composed of large immunoblast-type lymphoid cells with prominent nucleoli having a B-cell or Burkitt phenotype
• Some of the lymphomas are EBV-associated, which can be detected through such methods as EBV-encoded RNA (EBER) in situ hybridization (ISH)

Kaposi Sarcoma

• Purple-red lesion(s) in cortex
• Malignant spindle cells with slit-like endothelial spaces and extravasated red blood cells
• Immunohistochemistry can identify presence of human herpesvirus-8 (HHV-8) (which is diagnostic)

Renal Cell Carcinoma

• Not frequent
• Displays the usual renal cell carcinoma subtypes seen in non-HIV-infected individuals

Angiosarcoma

• Not frequent
• Highly malignant vascular proliferation
• Positive for vascular markers (CD31, CD34) but negative for HHV-8

DIAGNOSTIC CHECKLIST

Pathologic Interpretation Pearls

• HIV-associated immune complex glomerulonephritis with "lupus-like" features is possibly 2nd most common glomerulopathy in adults with HIV
• In addition, HIV leads to variety of other glomerular, tubulointerstitial, and vascular disorders

SELECTED REFERENCES

1. Bani-Hani S et al: Renal disease in AIDS: it is not always HIVAN. Clin Exp Nephrol. 14(3):263-7, 2010
2. Herlitz LC et al: Tenofovir nephrotoxicity: acute tubular necrosis with distinctive clinical, pathological, and mitochondrial abnormalities. Kidney Int. 78(11):1171-7, 2010
3. Radhakrishnan J et al: Case records of the Massachusetts General Hospital. Case 5-2010. A 51-year-old man with HIV infection, proteinuria, and edema. N Engl J Med. 362(7):636-46, 2010
4. Park YA et al: ADAMTS13 activity levels in patients with human immunodeficiency virus-associated thrombotic microangiopathy and profound CD4 deficiency. J Clin Apher. 24(1):32-6, 2009
5. Ross CL et al: HIV, thrombotic thrombocytopaenic purpura and rituximab in a violent noncompliant patient. Blood Coagul Fibrinolysis. 20(2):157-60, 2009
6. Brecher ME et al: Is it HIV TTP or HIV-associated thrombotic microangiopathy? J Clin Apher. 23(6):186-90, 2008
7. Cohen SD et al: Immune complex renal disease and human immunodeficiency virus infection. Semin Nephrol. 28(6):535-44, 2008
8. Fine DM et al: Thrombotic microangiopathy and other glomerular disorders in the HIV-infected patient. Semin Nephrol. 28(6):545-55, 2008
9. Winston J et al: Kidney disease in patients with HIV infection and AIDS. Clin Infect Dis. 47(11):1449-57, 2008
10. Cohen AH et al: Renal injury associated with human immunodeficiency virus infection. In Jennette JC et al: Heptinstall's Pathology of the Kidney. 6th ed. Philadelphia: Lippincott Williams & Wilkins, 2007
11. Estrella M et al: HIV type 1 RNA level as a clinical indicator of renal pathology in HIV-infected patients. Clin Infect Dis. 43(3):377-80, 2006
12. Haas M et al: HIV-associated immune complex glomerulonephritis with "lupus-like" features: a clinicopathologic study of 14 cases. Kidney Int. 67(4):1381-90, 2005
13. Alpers CE: Light at the end of the TUNEL: HIV-associated thrombotic microangiopathy. Kidney Int. 63(1):385-96, 2003
14. Haas M et al: Fibrillary/immunotactoid glomerulonephritis in HIV-positive patients: a report of three cases. Nephrol Dial Transplant. 15(10):1679-83, 2000
15. Kimmel PL: The nephropathies of HIV infection: pathogenesis and treatment. Curr Opin Nephrol Hypertens. 9(2):117-22, 2000
16. Cheng JT et al: Hepatitis C virus-associated glomerular disease in patients with human immunodeficiency virus coinfection. J Am Soc Nephrol. 10(7):1566-74, 1999
17. Peraldi MN et al: Acute renal failure in the course of HIV infection: a single-institution retrospective study of ninety-two patients anad sixty renal biopsies. Nephrol Dial Transplant. 14(6):1578-85, 1999
18. D'Agati V et al: Renal pathology of human immunodeficiency virus infection. Semin Nephrol. 18(4):406-21, 1998
19. Hall TN et al: Henoch-Schönlein purpura associated with human immunodeficiency virus infection. Nephrol Dial Transplant. 13(4):988-90, 1998
20. Górriz JL et al: IgA nephropathy associated with human immuno deficiency virus infection: antiproteinuric effect of captopril. Nephrol Dial Transplant. 12(12):2796-7, 1997
21. Gadallah MF et al: Disparate prognosis of thrombotic microangiopathy in HIV-infected patients with and without AIDS. Am J Nephrol. 16(5):446-50, 1996

Microscopic Features

(Left) In a 37-year-old man with HIV, 4+ proteinuria, creatinine 2.36 mg/dL, and a lupus-like GN, there is an interstitial inflammatory infiltrate with tubular atrophy ⮕, and glomeruli have prominent mesangial matrix expansion ⮔. *(Right)* In a 37-year-old man with HIV, 4+ proteinuria, creatinine 2.36 mg/dL, and a lupus-like GN, there is a marked expansion of mesangial matrix and cellularity ⮕.

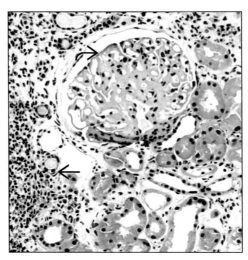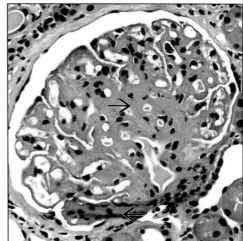

(Left) In a 37-year-old man with HIV, 4+ proteinuria, creatinine 2.36 mg/dL, and lupus-like GN, there is marked expansion of mesangial matrix and cellularity ⮔, as well as thick GBMs. *(Right)* Higher power view of a glomerulus in an HIV(+) 37-year-old man with 4+ proteinuria, creatinine 2.36 mg/dL, and lupus-like GN shows marked expansion of mesangial matrix and cellularity ⮔.

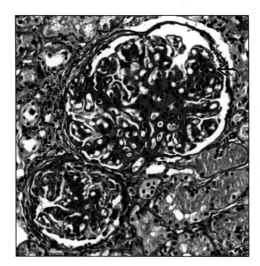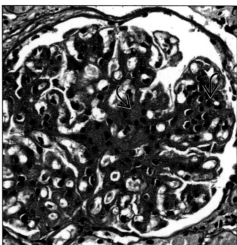

(Left) In a 56-year-old woman with HIV, hepatitis C, decreased C3, low normal C4, and hypertension, there is a marked increase in glomerular cellularity ⮕ in a lupus-like GN. The glomerulus also appears enlarged with vague lobules ⮔. *(Right)* A 56-year-old woman with HIV, hepatitis C, decreased C3, low normal C4, and hypertension shows a marked increase in glomerular cellularity ⮕ in a lupus-like GN.

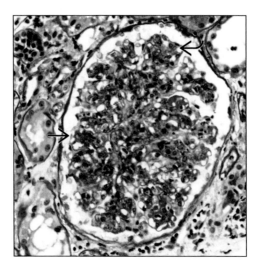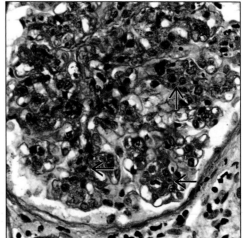

Immunofluorescence and Electron Microscopy

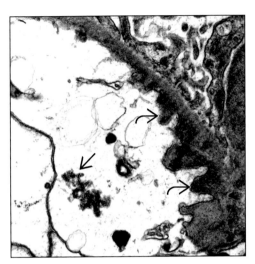
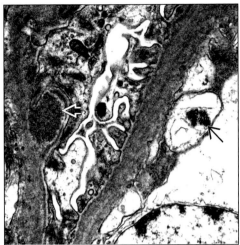

(Left) In a 56-year-old woman with HIV, hepatitis C, decreased C3, low normal C4, hypertension, & a lupus-like GN, tubuloreticular inclusions can be seen ⇨ along with occasional subendothelial electron-dense deposits ⇗. (Right) In a 15-year-old HIV(+) patient with microscopic hematuria, low-grade proteinuria, low albumin, and decreased C3 & C4, subepithelial deposits can be seen ⇨ along with tubuloreticular inclusions ⇨, altogether compatible with lupus-like GN.

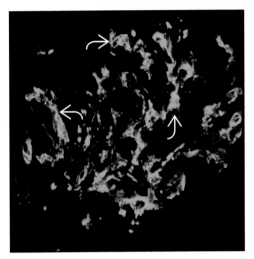
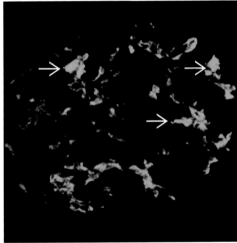

(Left) In a 38-year-old woman with a history of HIV and hepatitis C virus, bright IgA deposits can be seen in the mesangium in a dendritic pattern ⇗, which together with light and electron microscopic findings of typical IgA nephropathy justified the diagnosis of HIV-associated IgA nephropathy. (Right) In a 38-year-old woman with a history of HIV, hepatitis C virus, and HIV-associated IgA nephropathy, mesangial C3 deposits can be seen in the same location as the IgA deposits ⇨.

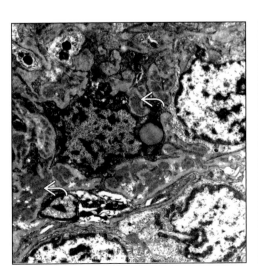
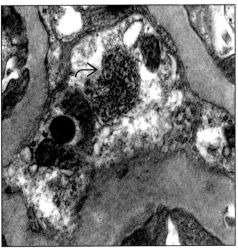

(Left) In a 38-year-old woman with a history of HIV, hepatitis C virus, and bright mesangial IgA deposits, EM shows mesangial deposits closely associated with reactive-appearing mesangial cells ⇗, compatible with the diagnosis of HIV-associated IgA nephropathy. (Right) In a 38-year-old woman with HIV-associated IgA nephropathy, there are tubuloreticular structures ⇗, which otherwise would have made this case virtually indistinguishable from IgA nephropathy not associated with HIV.

SYPHILIS

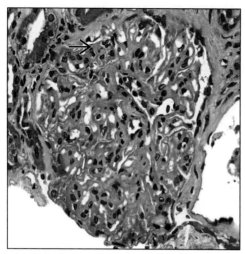

Global thickening of the glomerular capillaries and segmental endocapillary hypercellularity ➔ is seen in a case of immune complex glomerulonephritis in a 74 year old with tertiary syphilis.

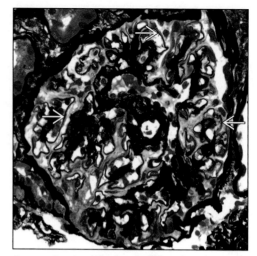

Segmental eosinophilic deposits ➔ on the subepithelial aspect of the GBM are associated with prominent swollen podocytes. "Spike" formation is not apparent.

TERMINOLOGY

Synonyms
- Lues, luetic infection, syphilitic nephrosis or nephritis

Definitions
- Chronic infection with tissue invasion and immunopathology caused by *Treponema pallidum* subspecies *pallidum*

ETIOLOGY/PATHOGENESIS

Infectious Agents
- *T. pallidum* subspecies *pallidum* is a microaerophilic spirochete that is venereally or vertically transmitted
- Kidney disease in syphilis arises in 3 ways
  - Direct infection by spirochetes
  - Immune complex-mediated nephritis in untreated disease
    - Circulating immune complexes and immune complex deposits contain treponemal antigens and IgG with antitreponemal specificity; renal lesions resolve with antibiotic therapy
    - Usually manifests in tertiary or less frequently in secondary stages of disease
  - Immune complex nephritis in response to antibiotic therapy
    - Destruction of *T. pallidum* releases bacterial antigens and incites immune complex formation and deposition (Jarisch-Herxheimer reaction)

CLINICAL ISSUES

Epidemiology
- Incidence
  - Congenital syphilis is rare in developed countries
    - Renal involvement occurs in up to 46% of cases
  - Acquired adult syphilis: 2.4-3.7 per 100,000
    - Prevalence: 7.7-12 per 100,000
    - Renal disease is rare, and prevalence is estimated at 0.3% of cases
- Age
  - Congenital infection is seen in infants from 2 weeks to 18 months, with median of 3 months
  - Acquired infection can present at any age

Presentation
- Primary syphilis is characterized by painless genital ulcer (chancre) with regional lymphadenopathy
- 25% of untreated primary disease progresses to secondary syphilis in weeks to months
  - Characterized by a mucocutaneous papular, scaling, or pustular rash and condylomata lata
- 20-40% of untreated secondary syphilis progresses to tertiary syphilis in 1-30 years after primary infection
  - Involves CNS (neurosyphilis) and cardiovascular systems (aortitis), and gummatous disease involving skin and bones
- Diagnosis of syphilis requires demonstration of organism or detection of specific antibodies
  - Condyloma lata and mucous membrane lesions have abundant organisms
    - Organisms are detected by dark field microscopy, immunofluorescence, or PCR
  - Treponemal antibody tests: *T. pallidum* hemagglutination assay (TPHA) and fluorescent treponemal antibody absorption test (FTA-Abs)
- Nephropathy in syphilis
  - Congenital syphilis: Nephrotic syndrome, nephritic syndrome or hematuria
  - Acquired syphilis: Secondary or tertiary stages may have nephrotic syndrome; nephritic syndrome is uncommon
  - Treatment-related nephropathy: Nephrotic syndrome or azotemia with hematuria after antisyphilitic therapy

SYPHILIS

Key Facts

Terminology
- Chronic infection with tissue invasion and immunopathology caused by *Treponema pallidum* subspecies *pallidum*

Etiology/Pathogenesis
- Direct infection of kidney
- Immunologic reaction to treponemal antigens giving rise to immune complex-mediated nephritis

Microscopic Pathology
- Congenital and acquired syphilis have similar lesions
  - Membranous nephropathy ± mesangial hypercellularity
  - Diffuse proliferative glomerulonephritis ± crescents
- Tubulointerstitial nephritis ± gumma formation
- Secondary amyloidosis (AA)

Treatment
- Drugs
  - Benzathine penicillin G or ceftriaxone

Prognosis
- Typically, disease is eliminated within 3-6 weeks of therapy
- Histologic resolution of renal lesions has been demonstrated 1-6 months after treatment

MICROSCOPIC PATHOLOGY

Histologic Features
- Congenital syphilis
  - Membranous nephropathy ± mesangial hypercellularity
  - Proliferative glomerulonephritis ± crescents is uncommon
  - Glomerulopathies are associated with interstitial mononuclear inflammation and edema
    - IF reveals IgG and C3 in capillary walls and mesangium
    - EM reveals subepithelial electron-dense deposits with "spike" and dome pattern in membranous nephropathy or with "humps" in proliferative (postinfectious-like) glomerulonephritis
- Acquired syphilis
  - Membranous nephropathy ± mesangial hypercellularity
  - Diffuse proliferative glomerulonephritis ± crescents

- Granular IgG and C3 by IF and electron-dense deposits in mesangium and capillary walls by EM
  - Treponemal antigen and antibody may be demonstrable in immune complexes
  - Tubulointerstitial nephritis ± gumma formation
  - Secondary amyloidosis (AA)

DIFFERENTIAL DIAGNOSIS

Membranous and Postinfectious Glomerulonephritis from Other Causes
- Resolved by serology and history

DIAGNOSTIC CHECKLIST

Pathologic Interpretation Pearls
- Immune complex glomerulonephritis is the principal cause of syphilitic nephritis and nephrosis

SELECTED REFERENCES
1. O'Regan S et al: Treponemal antigens in congenital and acquired syphilitic nephritis: demonstration by immunofluorescence studies. Ann Intern Med. 85(3):325-7, 1976

IMAGE GALLERY

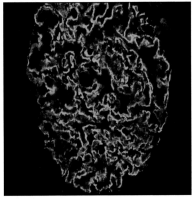 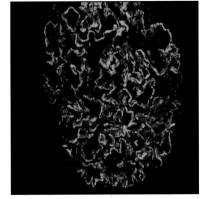 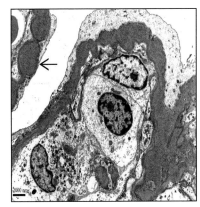

(Left) Granular and band-like staining of the glomerular capillary walls for IgG by IF is seen in a case of glomerulonephritis associated with tertiary syphilis. *(Center)* Global fine granular staining of the glomerular capillary walls for C3 is seen in glomerulonephritis associated with tertiary syphilis. *(Right)* Confluent and discrete ➡ subepithelial electron-dense deposits in immune complex glomerulonephritis associated with tertiary syphilis are shown. The pattern of deposits is atypical for both membranous and postinfectious glomerulonephritis.

LYME DISEASE MEMBRANOPROLIFERATIVE GLOMERULONEPHRITIS

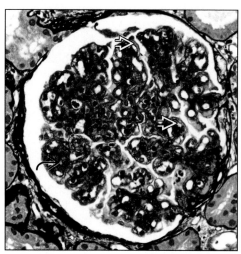

The renal biopsy from a 13-year-old girl demonstrates mesangial proliferation ➔ with extensive basement membrane double contours ➔. Extensive work-up revealed positive Lyme disease screen.

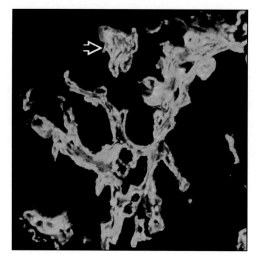

Immunofluorescence with antisera to C3 shows granular deposits in the mesangium and capillary walls ➔. The renal biopsy findings of MPGN, type 1 were associated with B. Burgdorferi infection.

TERMINOLOGY

Definitions
- Glomerulonephritis, typically with a membranoproliferative glomerulonephritis (MPGN) pattern, associated with *Borrelia burgdorferi* infection

ETIOLOGY/PATHOGENESIS

Infectious Agents
- Lyme disease is caused by a spirochete, *B. burgdorferi*, transmitted by ticks of genus *Ixodes*

Immune-complex Formation
- *B. burgdorferi* infection causes chronic antigenemia and immune complex formation
- Circulating immune complexes are deposited in glomeruli, with resultant glomerulonephritis

Autoimmunity
- Immunity against self-antigens may be precipitated by molecular mimicry of *Borrelia* organisms

Animal Studies
- MPGN associated with *B. burgdorferi* infection widely reported in dogs, especially Bernese mountain dogs

CLINICAL ISSUES

Epidemiology
- Incidence
  - Lyme disease is most common tick-borne infection in USA
    - Endemic in Northern Hemisphere
    - Highest incidence in USA is in Northeast and Wisconsin
  - Lyme disease MPGN rarely documented in humans (5 case reports to date)

Presentation
- Early symptoms after tick bite include fever, fatigue, and characteristic skin rash, erythema migrans
- Manifestations of untreated disease include arthritis and neurological and cardiac abnormalities
- Microscopic hematuria and proteinuria if renal involvement
  - Nephrotic syndrome
- Typically has remissions and exacerbations with variable organ involvement

Laboratory Tests
- Serological tests
  - ELISA for detection of IgM and IgG anti-*B. burgdorferi* antibodies is sensitive
    - False-positive rate for ELISA is high, and careful clinical evaluation is needed to determine validity
    - May be negative early in the infection due to slow development of immune response
    - May continue to be positive even after antibiotic therapy
  - Confirmatory serological test is Western blotting
- PCR
  - *B. burgdorferi* DNA can be detected in blood, urine, joint fluid, or CSF
  - Not clinically validated; susceptible to false-positive/false-negative results
- Low C3 level (may be normal)

Treatment
- Drugs
  - Oral doxycycline is usual
    - Specific drug and route depends on stage of disease
    - Duration of therapy ranges from 14-28 days and is longer for chronic disease
  - Corticosteroids, IVIG, and plasmapheresis have been used for MPGN

LYME DISEASE MEMBRANOPROLIFERATIVE GLOMERULONEPHRITIS

Key Facts

Terminology
- Immunological renal manifestation of MPGN, type 1 due to *Borrelia burgdorferi* infection

Clinical Issues
- High level of clinical suspicion is needed for diagnosis of MPGN due to Lyme disease
- Antibiotic therapy directed against spirochete
- Immunosuppressive therapy directed against host immunological response causing MPGN

Microscopic Pathology
- Diffuse and global glomerular hypercellularity is seen with lobular accentuation
- Dominant C3 staining and electron-dense deposits in mesangium and subendothelium
- Serological tests include ELISA and confirmatory Western blotting

Top Differential Diagnoses
- MPGN due to other causes

Prognosis
- With adequate therapy, complete resolution of MPGN manifestations has been documented in the literature

MICROSCOPIC PATHOLOGY

Histologic Features
- Diffuse and global glomerular hypercellularity is seen with lobular accentuation typical of MPGN, type I
  - Mesangial and endocapillary proliferation is seen with infiltrating lymphocytes and monocytes
- Several capillary loops demonstrate double contours with mesangial cell interposition
- Deposits on trichrome stain
- Varying degrees of interstitial inflammation, tubular atrophy, and interstitial fibrosis are seen
- In setting of chronic nephrotic-range proteinuria, interstitial foam cells may be observed

ANCILLARY TESTS

Immunofluorescence
- Dominant C3 staining in mesangium and peripheral capillary walls
- IgG in similar distribution in most cases
- Weak staining with IgM, IgA, and C1q
- 1 case with prominent IgA
- No evidence of light chain restriction with kappa and lambda

Electron Microscopy
- Amorphous, electron-dense deposits in predominantly subendothelial but also mesangial distribution
- Few subepithelial deposits may be seen
- GBM duplication is identified
- Mesangial cell interposition

DIFFERENTIAL DIAGNOSIS

MPGN Due to Other Causes
- Need high level of clinical suspicion to diagnose Lyme disease MPGN
- Other infectious and autoimmune causes should be clinically and serologically ruled out
- May be underreported cause of idiopathic MPGN

SELECTED REFERENCES

1. Aguero-Rosenfeld ME: Lyme disease: laboratory issues. Infect Dis Clin North Am. 22(2):301-13, vii, 2008
2. Bratton RL et al: Diagnosis and treatment of Lyme disease. Mayo Clin Proc. 83(5):566-71, 2008
3. Kirmizis D et al: MPGN secondary to Lyme disease. Am J Kidney Dis. 43(3):544-51, 2004
4. Kelly B et al: Lyme disease and glomerulonephritis. Ir Med J. 92(5):372, 1999
5. Pahl A et al: Quantitative detection of Borrelia burgdorferi by real-time PCR. J Clin Microbiol. 37(6):1958-63, 1999
6. Steere AC: Lyme disease. N Engl J Med. 321(9):586-96, 1989

IMAGE GALLERY

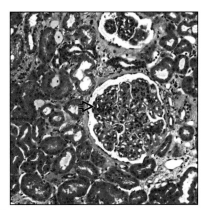 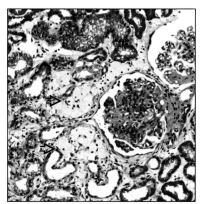 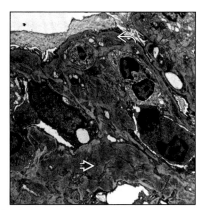

(Left) The findings of MPGN, type 1 due to Lyme disease include glomerular hypercellularity with lobular accentuation ➡. *(Center)* The biopsy shows scattered collections of interstitial foam cells ➡. The patient is a young girl with MPGN due to a Borrelia burgdorferi spirochete infection. The patient presented with nephrotic-range proteinuria and hematuria. *(Right)* Electron micrograph reveals mesangial ➡ and subendothelial ➡ deposits seen in MPGN due to Lyme disease.

SCHISTOSOMIASIS

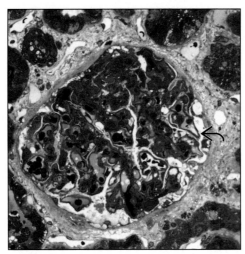

A Middle Eastern man with schistosomiasis presented with nephrotic syndrome. The glomerular basement membranes ➔ are thickened, and IF had a membranous pattern of IgG staining.

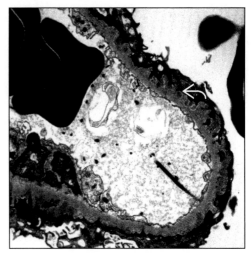

Electron micrograph reveals diffuse subepithelial deposits ➔ compatible with membranous glomerulonephritis in a kidney biopsy from a Middle Eastern man with schistosomiasis.

TERMINOLOGY

Definitions
- *Schistosoma* parasitic infection-related renal disease

ETIOLOGY/PATHOGENESIS

Infectious Agents
- *S. mansoni*
  - Parasite migrates to mesenteric vessels
  - Causes gastrointestinal symptoms and manifestations of portal hypertension
  - Causes glomerulonephritis
    - Circulating anodic antigen within gut epithelium of adult worm may be antigenic moiety of immune complexes
    - Immune complexes due to humoral host response
- *S. hematobium*
  - Migrates to perivesical venous plexus and causes genitourinary tract and colonic symptoms
  - Fibrosis and calcification of tissue-trapped ova in lower urinary tract lead to obstruction, reflux, infection, and stone formation
  - Glomerulonephritis less common
- *S. japonicum*
  - Causes hepatosplenomegaly and cirrhosis
  - Glomerulonephritis described only in animals

Source of Infection
- Intermediate host is freshwater snail
- Human infection occurs when cercariae in water penetrate skin

Role of Coinfection
- Concomitant *Salmonella* infection causes exuberant glomerulonephritis
- Hepatitis C virus infection may cause increased disease manifestations in endemic areas

CLINICAL ISSUES

Epidemiology
- Incidence
  - Affects 200,000,000 people worldwide
  - Endemic in Africa, Middle East (*S. mansoni, S. hematobium*), South America (*S. mansoni*), and Asia (*S. japonicum*)
  - Glomerulonephritis uncommon
- Age
  - Children and young adults in endemic areas

Presentation
- Hematuria
- Proteinuria
- Dysuria and polyuria in presence of hydronephrosis or chronic pyelonephritis
- Nephrotic syndrome may be seen

Treatment
- Drugs
  - Praziquantel is antiparasitic drug

Prognosis
- Antiparasitic drugs and immunosuppressive therapy have no effect on glomerulonephritis
- Antiparasitic therapy for several years may reduce urinary tract morbidity

MICROSCOPIC PATHOLOGY

Histologic Features
- Membranoproliferative glomerulonephritis (MPGN)
  - Mesangial and endocapillary proliferation, thickening of glomerular capillary walls with double contours
  - Early disease may only have mild mesangial proliferation
  - Focal segmental glomerulosclerosis may be seen
- Membranous nephropathy (MGN)

SCHISTOSOMIASIS

Key Facts

Etiology/Pathogenesis
- *Schistosoma mansoni* can cause glomerulonephritis
- *S. hematobium* can cause reflux nephropathy due to calcification of tissue-trapped ova
- Cercariae in water penetrate human skin

Clinical Issues
- Endemic in Africa, Middle East, South America, and Asia

Microscopic Pathology
- Membranoproliferative glomerulonephritis
- Membranous nephropathy
- Cortical scar in reflux nephropathy
- Amyloid AA deposition in glomeruli and arterial walls

Ancillary Tests
- Characteristic ova may be seen in urine (*S. hematobium* with terminal spine), stools (*S. mansoni* with lateral spine), or tissues

---

o Thickened glomerular basement membranes with "spikes"
- Cortical scar with chronic inflammation may suggest reflux nephropathy due to *S. hematobium* infection
  o Neutrophil casts suggest acute pyelonephritis
- Amyloid deposition composed of AA amyloid in glomeruli and arterial walls

ANCILLARY TESTS

Immunofluorescence
- Mesangial and capillary wall C3-dominant deposits in MPGN
  o IgM and IgG deposits can also be seen
  o Mesangial IgA may be present in membranoproliferative and focal segmental sclerosis forms
  o Schistosomal circulating anodic antigen has been demonstrated in immune complexes
- Glomerular capillary wall IgG staining in MGN

Electron Microscopy
- Electron-dense deposits in mesangium and subendothelium in MPGN
- Subepithelial deposits in MGN
- Randomly oriented fibrils (8-11 nm thick) in amyloidosis

Identification of Ova
- In urine (*S. hematobium* with terminal spine) or stools (*S. mansoni* with lateral spine), or tissues

DIFFERENTIAL DIAGNOSIS

Nonschistosomal Glomerulonephritis
- Clinical and travel history may be helpful

SELECTED REFERENCES

1. Gryseels B et al: Human schistosomiasis. Lancet. 368(9541):1106-18, 2006
2. Barsoum R: The changing face of schistosomal glomerulopathy. Kidney Int. 66(6):2472-84, 2004
3. Barsoum R et al: Immunoglobulin-A and the pathogenesis of schistosomal glomerulopathy. Kidney Int. 50(3):920-8, 1996
4. Abensur H et al: Nephrotic syndrome associated with hepatointestinal schistosomiasis. Rev Inst Med Trop Sao Paulo. 34(4):273-6, 1992
5. Martinelli R et al: Schistosoma mansoni-induced mesangiocapillary glomerulonephritis: influence of therapy. Kidney Int. 35(5):1227-33, 1989
6. Lambertucci JR et al: Glomerulonephritis in Salmonella-Schistosoma mansoni association. Am J Trop Med Hyg. 38(1):97-102, 1988
7. Sobh MA et al: Characterisation of kidney lesions in early schistosomal-specific nephropathy. Nephrol Dial Transplant. 3(4):392-8, 1988
8. Andrade ZA et al: Schistosomal glomerular disease (a review). Mem Inst Oswaldo Cruz. 79(4):499-506, 1984

IMAGE GALLERY

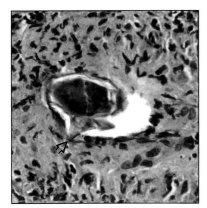 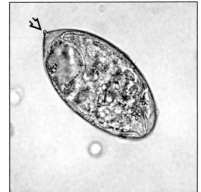 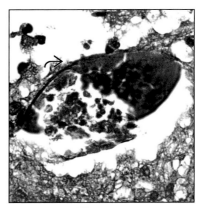

(Left) A 35-year-old African emigrant with rectal bleeding had an *S. mansoni* egg with characteristic lateral spine ⊡ on biopsy. *(Courtesy N. Banaei, MD.)* *(Center)* Urine microscopic examination shows an *S. hematobium* egg with a characteristic terminal spine ⊡. *(Courtesy N. Banaei, MD.)* *(Right)* A vulvar biopsy shows a Schistosoma egg ⊡ with adjacent tissue necrosis. The patient had traveled to Africa and presented with vulvar swelling and pain. *(Courtesy N. Banaei, MD.)*

IgA NEPHROPATHY

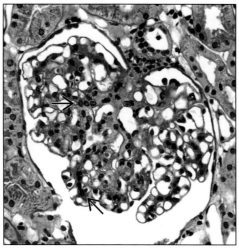

This glomerulus in IgA nephropathy (IgAN) shows mesangial hypercellularity ⊟ and expanded mesangial matrix. Most cases show this feature, but the additional pathology is quite variable.

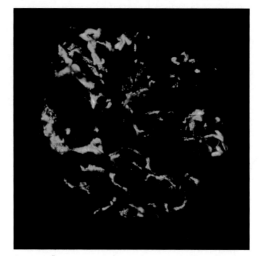

Immunofluorescence shows prominent IgA deposits, typical of IgAN. Indeed, IgAN was initially defined by immunofluorescence, due to characteristic deposition in the mesangium with a "tree trunk and branches pattern."

TERMINOLOGY

Abbreviations
- IgA nephropathy (IgAN)

Synonyms
- Berger disease

Definitions
- Glomerulonephritis with predominantly IgA deposits in mesangium in absence of systemic disease
- Initially described by Berger and Hinglais in 1968

ETIOLOGY/PATHOGENESIS

Genetic Factors
- HLA strongest genetic association in genome wide analysis
  - HLA-DQ and possibly HLA-B
- Abnormally glycosylated IgA1 in 25% of relatives
- Family history of nephritis in ~ 10%
  - 15-50% of cases in Northern Italy and Eastern Kentucky

Abnormal IgA Response
- Increased IgA response to intranasal antigens
- Elevated serum IgA levels in ~ 50%

Abnormal Glycosylation of IgA
- 5 O-glycosylation sites in IgA1 hinge region
  - N-acetylgalactosamine (GalNAc) attaches to Ser or Thr
  - Normally followed by attachment of galactose and sialic acid
- IgAN patients have IgA1 deficient in galactose (GD-IgA)
  - ↓ galactose attached to GalNAc
  - Detectable with *Helix aspera* lectin
    - Binds to terminal GalNAc
- Intrinsic property of IgAN B cells

Autoantibodies to Galactose Deficient-IgA1
- IgG or IgA1 autoantibodies bind to GalNAc neoepitopes on GD-IgA
  - Progression involves interaction between IgA and mesangial cells and ↑ cytokines
  - IgA/anti-IgA complexes stimulate mesangial cell proliferation
- GD-IgA antigen may be planted in mesangium
  - GD-IgA binds to transferrin receptor
  - Immune complexes may also form in blood
- Other antigens not excluded

Progression/Precipitating Factors
- Asymptomatic individuals can have mesangial IgA
- 2nd hit thought necessary to precipitate disease
  - Often exacerbated by upper respiratory infections
- Complement fixation by lectin pathway may contribute

CLINICAL ISSUES

Epidemiology
- Incidence
  - Most common cause of glomerulonephritis worldwide
    - 10 cases per 1,000,000 person-years in USA
    - Accounts for 1-3% of patients with end-stage renal disease in USA and Europe
    - Renal biopsy prevalence: USA (5%), Europe (15%), Japan (30%)
  - Lanthanic IgA
    - 6-16% of donor biopsies have IgA (usually no C3 or IgG)
    - Not clear whether this is precursor or incidental
- Age
  - Wide spectrum (1 to > 65 years)
  - Peak age: 20-30 years
- Gender
  - M:F = 2:1

IgA NEPHROPATHY

Key Facts

Etiology/Pathogenesis
- Abnormal glycosylation of IgA1
- Autoantibodies to galactose deficient IgA1
- Abnormally active IgA response

Clinical Issues
- Most common cause of glomerulonephritis worldwide
- Often asymptomatic hematuria ± proteinuria
- ↑ circulating serum IgA
- Recurs in transplants (30%)

Microscopic Pathology
- Usual: Mesangial hypercellularity and ↑ matrix
- Common: Focal, segmental inflammation of glomeruli
- Less common: Crescents ± necrosis

- Interstitial inflammation with eosinophils
- May be histologically normal (10%)

Ancillary Tests
- IF: IgA mesangial deposits (100%)
  - C3 (90%), IgG, IgM (50%), C1q (10%)
- EM: Amorphous electron-dense deposits in mesangium (100%)
  - Subepithelial or subendothelial deposits occasionally

Top Differential Diagnoses
- Henoch-Schönlein purpura
- Lupus nephritis
- Postinfectious glomerulonephritis (IgA-dominant)
- IgA nephropathy in cirrhosis of liver

- Ethnicity
  - Asians > whites > blacks

Presentation
- Microhematuria (88%)
- Macrohematuria (43%)
- Hypertension (25%)
- Proteinuria
  - Nephrotic-range proteinuria (10%)
  - > 1 g/d proteinuria (47%)
- Asymptomatic urinary abnormalities (40%)
- Loin or abdominal pain (30%)
- Acute renal failure (7%)
- Chronic renal failure
- Thrombotic microangiopathy

Laboratory Tests
- Elevated circulating IgA (50%)
- Normal complement levels

Treatment
- Angiotensin converting enzyme inhibitors or angiotensin receptor blockers are 1st line of drugs
- Steroids recommended if no response in 6 months
- Cyclophosphamide for crescentic disease
- No proven value of azathioprine, mycophenolate mofetil, or tonsillectomy
- Fish oil has debated benefit on renal function

Prognosis
- 10-year renal survival (80%)
  - Prognosis varies by pathologic and clinical features
  - Haas grade I+II (90%)
  - Haas grade III (55%)
  - Haas grade IV+V (20%)
  - Better survival in children
- Independent predictors of progression to ESRD
  - Reduced glomerular filtration rate (GFR)
  - Severe proteinuria
  - Hypertension
- Recurs in transplants in 30%
  - Graft loss due to recurrence in 5%

MICROSCOPIC PATHOLOGY

Histologic Features
- Highly variable glomerular pathology
- Glomeruli
  - Mesangial hypercellularity and increased matrix usual
    - > 3 mesangial cell nuclei per mesangial area not adjacent to vascular pole, in 3 micron thick section
    - PAS(+) mesangial deposits in adults
  - Focal, segmental inflammation of glomeruli common
  - Endocapillary hypercellularity
  - Necrotizing glomerulonephritis (10%)
  - Crescentic glomerulonephritis (5% have > 50% glomeruli involved)
  - Focal segmental glomerulosclerosis
    - Broken glomerular basement membrane (GBM) sometimes seen in scarred areas
  - Podocyte loss
  - Global glomerulosclerosis
  - Minor GBM thickening or duplication
  - Histologically normal in 10%
- Interstitium and tubules
  - Interstitial inflammation with eosinophils, mononuclear cells, plasma cells, and mast cells
  - Red blood cell (RBC) casts
    - Sometimes tubules are packed with RBCs, suggesting brisk bleeding from glomerulus
    - Pigmented casts indicative of prior red cell leakage
- Vessels
  - Rarely vasculitis

ANCILLARY TESTS

Immunofluorescence
- IgA-dominant staining of glomeruli
  - Mesangial deposits predominant; segmental GBM deposits may be present

o Capillary wall deposits correlate with mesangial and endocapillary cellularity
- IgA deposits usually accompanied by IgG (~ 50%), IgM (~ 50%), C3 (~ 90%)
  o Fibrinogen/fibrin usually present in mesangium
  o Lambda often more prominent than kappa (64%)
    ▪ Occasionally only lambda (3%)
  o C4d present in a subset (~ 30%)
    ▪ Thought to be lectin pathway
  o C1q uncommon (~ 10%)

Electron Microscopy
- Transmission
  o Electron-dense mesangial deposits
    ▪ Mesangium and paramesangium (100%)
    ▪ Subendothelial deposits (11%)
    ▪ Subepithelial deposits (6%)
    ▪ Intramembranous deposits (2%)
    ▪ Hump-like subepithelial deposits rare (vs. acute postinfectious glomerulonephritis)
    ▪ Immune deposits do not show substructure
  o GBM abnormalities often present
    ▪ Laminations of GBM may be segmentally severe, with particles reminiscent of Alport syndrome
    ▪ Thinning of GBM in 40%
    ▪ May be coincidental (or synergistic) thin basement membrane disease
  o Podocytes
    ▪ Extensive foot process effacement when proteinuria is present
  o Mesangium
    ▪ Hypercellularity
    ▪ Increased matrix

DIFFERENTIAL DIAGNOSIS

Nephritis of Henoch-Schönlein Purpura (HSP)
- Clinical evidence crucial in diagnosis: Skin rash on legs, buttocks; lower extremity arthritis; abdominal pain or GI bleeding
- Usually cannot be distinguished by renal biopsy
- Rarely observe vasculitis in kidney (~ 1%): Necrotizing arteritis or medullary capillaritis
- IgA deposits typically transient
- Capillary wall deposits can be more prominent

Familial IgA Nephropathy
- Indistinguishable by biopsy
- Has poorer prognosis (36% 15-year renal survival)

Lupus Nephritis
- IgA accompanied by "full house" staining pattern by immunofluorescence (IgG, IgM, C3, C1q)
- Nearly all cases of lupus nephritis will show brighter IgG staining than IgA by immunofluorescence

Postinfectious Glomerulonephritis (IgA-Dominant)
- Subepithelial hump-shaped deposits prominent by electron microscopy
- Deposits do not persist

IgA Deposits in HIV Infection
- IgA antibodies to HIV p24, gp41, gp120, gp160
- Prominent tubuloreticular structures in endothelial cells
- Mesangial proliferation ± collapsing glomerulopathy

IgA Nephropathy in Cirrhosis of Liver
- > 60% of cirrhotics have mesangial IgA at autopsy
- Rarely causes clinical renal disease or severe glomerular pathology

Incidental Mesangial IgA Deposits
- Commonly present (~ 10%) without symptoms
- Typically, little mesangial proliferation, no IgA or C3
- May be incidental finding in minimal change disease, membranous glomerulonephritis, thin basement membrane disease, or ANCA-related glomerulonephritis

Focal Segmental Glomerulosclerosis (FSGS)
- IgAN may have histologic pattern of FSGS
- FSGS lacks IgA predominant deposits

DIAGNOSTIC CHECKLIST

Clinically Relevant Pathologic Features
- Histologic grades correlate with prognosis
- Oxford Classification
  o Tubular atrophy/interstitial fibrosis most robust prognostic feature
  o Segmental glomerulosclerosis
- Other proposed prognostic features
  o Crescents
  o GBM deposits by EM or IF
  o C4d in mesangium

Pathologic Interpretation Pearls
- Acute renal failure may be caused by severe hematuria due to red cell casts
- Broken GBM fragments in scarred areas distinguish from focal, segmental glomerulosclerosis
- PAS(+) mesangial deposits are histologic clue for IgA nephropathy
- IgA nephropathy may be entirely normal by light microscopy
- Histologic lesions focal but IgA deposition diffuse
  o 1 nonsclerotic glomerulus is adequate to make or exclude diagnosis by immunofluorescence
- C1q stain usually negative in IgA nephropathy vs. lupus nephritis
- IgA deposits persistent in IgA nephropathy vs. HSP

GRADING

Lee Histologic Classification System (1982)
- I: Focal mesangial expansion
- II: Moderate focal proliferative
- III: Mild diffuse proliferative
- IV: Moderate diffuse proliferative; crescents in ≤ 45% of glomeruli
- V: Severe diffuse proliferative; crescents in > 45% of glomeruli

IgA NEPHROPATHY

Immunofluorescence

Antibody	Reactivity	Staining Pattern	Comment
IgA	Positive, granular	Mesangial	Predominant immunoglobulin, sometimes also GBM
IgG	Variable	Mesangial	Less than IgA, may be negative
IgM	Variable	Mesangial	Less than IgA, may be negative
C3	Positive, granular	Mesangial	Less than IgA, usually present
C1q	Negative	Mesangial	May be trace or focal
Fibrin	Positive, granular	Mesangial	Often present
Kappa	Positive, granular	Mesangial	Kappa often < lambda
Lambda	Positive, granular	Mesangial	Lambda often > kappa

Electron Microscopy

Compartment/Cell	Pattern/Finding	Comment
Mesangium	Amorphous	Predominant location also typically paramesangial
GBM	Normal	Occasional subepithelial or subendothelial deposits
Deposits	Amorphous	Predominantly in mesangium
TBM	No deposits	
Podocytes	Foot processes	Variable effacement, often normal

Haas Histologic Classification System (1997)

- I: Minimal or no mesangial hypercellularity
- II: Focal and segmental glomerulosclerosis without active cellular proliferation
- III: Focal proliferative glomerulonephritis
- IV: Diffuse proliferative glomerulonephritis
- V: ≥ 40% globally sclerotic glomeruli or area of cortical tubular atrophy

Oxford Classification System (2009)

- Clinicopathologic classification with pathologic features predictive of disease progression
- Key pathologic features to be reported on renal biopsy
  o Mesangial hypercellularity
    ▪ Mean < 4 mesangial cells/mesangial area (M0 score)
    ▪ Mean 4 or more mesangial cells/mesangial area (M1 score)
  o Segmental glomerulosclerosis or adhesions present (S1 score) or absent (S0 score)
  o Endocapillary hypercellularity present (E0 score) or absent (E1 score)
  o Cortical interstitial fibrosis and tubular atrophy
    ▪ 0-25% (T0 score)
    ▪ 26-50% (T1 score)
    ▪ > 50% (T2 score)
  o Total number of glomeruli with changes
    ▪ Endocapillary hypercellularity, extracapillary proliferation, global glomerulosclerosis, and segmental glomerulosclerosis

SELECTED REFERENCES

1. Bellur SS et al: Immunostaining findings in IgA nephropathy: correlation with histology and clinical outcome in the Oxford classification patient cohort. Nephrol Dial Transplant. Epub ahead of print, 2011
2. Kiryluk K et al: Aberrant glycosylation of IgA1 is inherited in both pediatric IgA nephropathy and Henoch-Schönlein purpura nephritis. Kidney Int. Epub ahead of print, 2011
3. Feehally J et al: HLA has strongest association with IgA nephropathy in genome-wide analysis. J Am Soc Nephrol. 21(10):1791-7, 2010
4. Espinosa M et al: Mesangial C4d deposition: a new prognostic factor in IgA nephropathy. Nephrol Dial Transplant. 24(3):886-91, 2009
5. Pankhurst T et al: Vasculitic IgA nephropathy: prognosis and outcome. Nephron Clin Pract. 112(1):c16-24, 2009
6. Roufosse CA et al: Pathological predictors of prognosis in immunoglobulin A nephropathy: a review. Curr Opin Nephrol Hypertens. 18(3):212-9, 2009
7. Working Group of the International IgA Nephropathy Network and the Renal Pathology Society et al: The Oxford classification of IgA nephropathy: rationale, clinicopathological correlations, and classification. Kidney Int. 76(5):534-45, 2009
8. Gharavi AG et al: Aberrant IgA1 glycosylation is inherited in familial and sporadic IgA nephropathy. J Am Soc Nephrol. 19(5):1008-14, 2008
9. Novak J et al: IgA glycosylation and IgA immune complexes in the pathogenesis of IgA nephropathy. Semin Nephrol. 28(1):78-87, 2008
10. Suzuki H et al: IgA1-secreting cell lines from patients with IgA nephropathy produce aberrantly glycosylated IgA1. J Clin Invest. 118(2):629-39, 2008
11. Novak J et al: IgA nephropathy and Henoch-Schoenlein purpura nephritis: aberrant glycosylation of IgA1, formation of IgA1-containing immune complexes, and activation of mesangial cells. Contrib Nephrol. 157:134-8, 2007
12. Donadio JV et al: IgA nephropathy. N Engl J Med. 347(10):738-48, 2002
13. Haas M: Histologic subclassification of IgA nephropathy: a clinicopathologic study of 244 cases. Am J Kidney Dis. 29(6):829-42, 1997
14. Lee SM et al: IgA nephropathy: morphologic predictors of progressive renal disease. Hum Pathol. 13(4):314-22, 1982
15. Berger J et al: [Intercapillary deposits of IgA-IgG] J Urol Nephrol (Paris). 74(9):694-5, 1968

IgA Nephropathy, Typical Case

(Left) H&E of the cortex shows focal minimal mesangial hypercellularity and normal tubules and interstitium. *(Right)* At higher magnification, a glomerulus shows very mild mesangial hypercellularity ➡. This was a focal finding (involving a minority of the glomeruli). Mesangial hypercellularity is defined as > 3 mesangial cells per mesangial region in a 2-3 micron thick section, best judged in a PAS-stained slide.

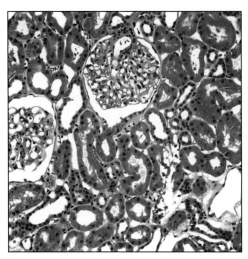
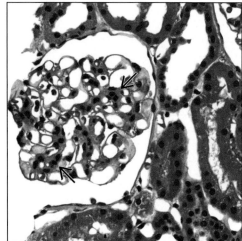

(Left) Rare red blood cell casts ➡ were identified in the medulla, indicating a glomerular origin of the hematuria. Massive red blood cell casts may be seen in patients who present with acute renal failure. *(Right)* Immunofluorescence stain for IgA shows bright granular staining, predominantly mesangial ➡. IgA is the dominant immunoglobulin. Segmental deposits are present along the glomerular basement membrane ➡.

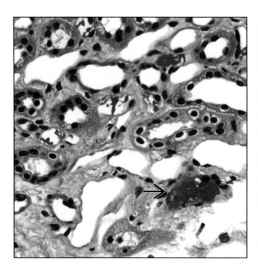
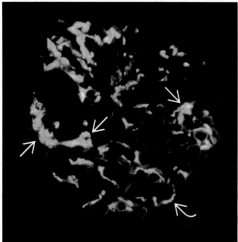

(Left) An immunofluorescence stain for kappa light chains shows granular mesangial staining similar to that for IgA. *(Right)* Immunofluorescence stain for lambda light chains shows granular mesangial staining that is more intense than for kappa. In most cases of IgA nephropathy, staining for lambda is brighter than that for kappa.

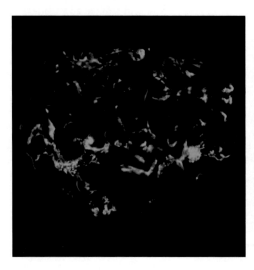
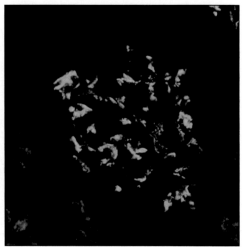

IgA Nephropathy, Microscopic Features

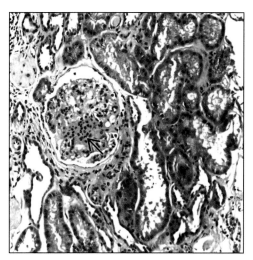

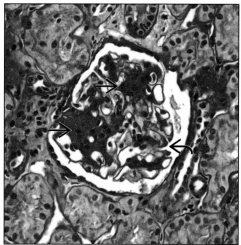

(Left) A glomerulus shows segmental marked mesangial hypercellularity ➡ in this 56-year-old woman with proteinuria, hematuria, hypertension, and slowly rising Cr (1.8 mg/dL). (Right) This section shows irregular, marked mesangial hypercellularity ➡ and a normal GBM. Podocytes are basophilic and enlarged, which correlates with proteinuria ➡ in this 19-year-old man with a 3-year history of proteinuria and episodes of gross hematuria. Serum IgA is 397 mg/dL (normal: 68-309).

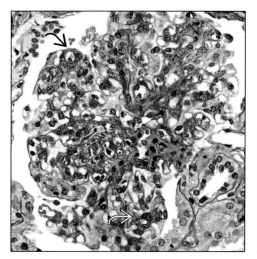

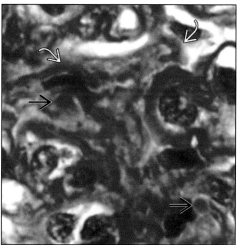

(Left) In a 68-year-old man with microhematuria, proteinuria, Cr 1.2, and elevated serum IgA, periodic acid-Schiff shows an increased mesangial matrix with PAS(+) deposits ➡, a diagnostically helpful feature sometimes found in IgA nephropathy. The GBM is segmentally duplicated ➡. (Right) A high-power section from a 16-year-old male with 2.3 g/d proteinuria and normal Cr shows PAS(+) deposits in the mesangium ➡ and ribbons of fragmented GBM ➡.

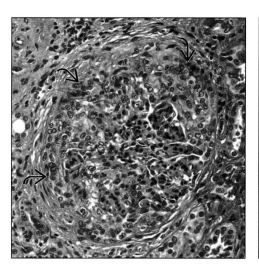

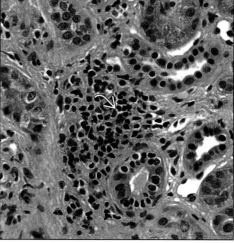

(Left) 16-year-old male with 2.3 g/d proteinuria and normal Cr. This high power section shows PAS(+) deposits in the mesangium ➡ and ribbons of fragmented GBM. (Right) This case shows a mononuclear infiltrate with eosinophils ➡, typical of IgA nephropathy. Prominent interstitial infiltrates in IgA nephropathy may be confused with acute interstitial nephritis.

IgA Nephropathy, Incidental

(Left) Light microscopy of a minimally involved kidney at low magnification shows normal glomeruli and a lack of interstitial fibrosis. Two red blood cell casts can be seen ➡. (Right) Red blood cell casts within tubules ➡ are shown. In this case, the red blood cell casts were the only light microscopic evidence of glomerular disease.

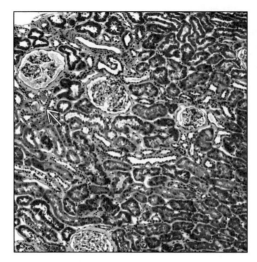
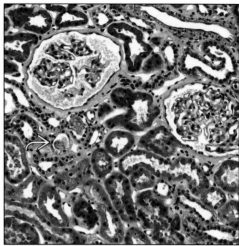

(Left) PAS-stained section show a normal glomerulus without mesangial expansion or glomerular basement membrane abnormalities. (Right) Immunofluorescence for IgA shows distinct granular mesangial deposits, 1-2+ in intensity, that affected all of the glomeruli despite their normal appearance by light microscopy. C3 was also present but less intense (1+). The IgA deposits by IF and the presence of electron-dense deposits on electron microscopy made the diagnosis.

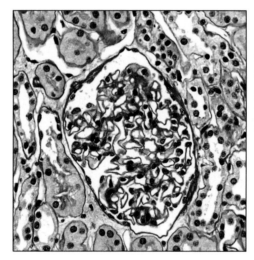
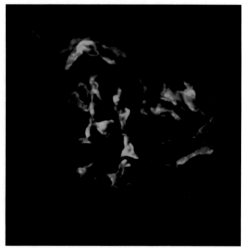

(Left) Electron microscopy of a glomerulus shows rare scattered electron-dense deposits in the mesangium ➡ in this example. (Right) This section shows a PAS(+) immunoglobulin "pseudothrombus" ➡ in a glomerular capillary in a 33-year-old man with proteinuria (1.2 g/d), normal Cr (1.1 mg/dL), and recurrent episodes of macrohematuria associated with exercise. A minority of cases of IgA nephropathy have cryoglobulins.

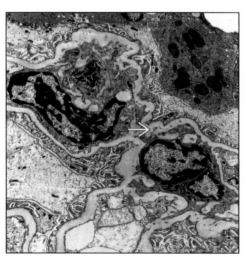
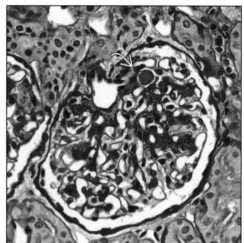

IgA Nephropathy, Typical Immunofluorescence

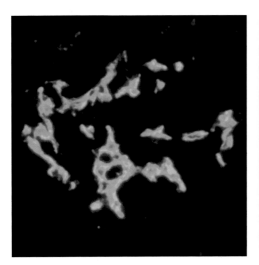 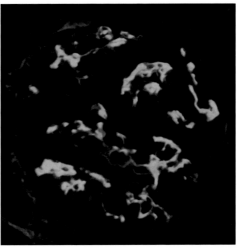

(Left) Immunofluorescence for IgA shows 4+ granular deposition that is strictly mesangial in location in this 19-year-old man with a 3-year history of micro- and macrohematuria. (Right) Immunofluorescence for IgG shows strictly mesangial deposition, somewhat less intense than IgA.

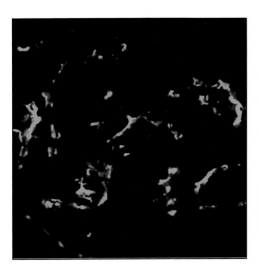 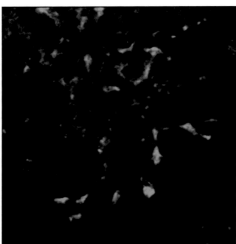

(Left) Immunofluorescence for C3 shows a sparse, more discrete deposition in the mesangium in this 23-year-old man with IgAN and a 3-year history of episodic gross hematuria, minimal proteinuria (0.7 g/d), and a normal Cr (0.9 mg/dL). (Right) Immunofluorescence of a glomerulus stained for C1q is trace positive. The paucity of C1q commonly observed in IgAN helps distinguish the disease from lupus nephritis, which usually has prominent C1q in glomeruli.

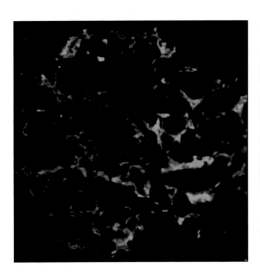 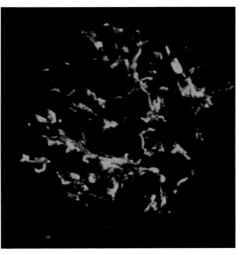

(Left) Immunofluorescence for kappa light chain shows segmental deposition in the mesangium (1+), noticeably less than the same case stained for lambda. (Right) Immunofluorescence for lambda light chain shows segmental deposition in the mesangium (1+), noticeably more than when stained for kappa.

Other Immunofluorescence Patterns

(Left) A stain for IgA shows mostly mesangial deposits; a few capillaries have peripheral loop deposits ➡. It is often difficult to be certain that the deposits are in the capillary wall, as the mesangial deposits typically line up along the GBM bordering the mesangium ➡. A parallel pattern helps distinguish the latter site. *(Right)* Immunofluorescence for IgA shows mostly mesangial and possibly GBM deposits ➡. Isolated granules cannot be localized without a capillary marker.

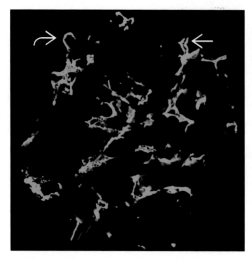 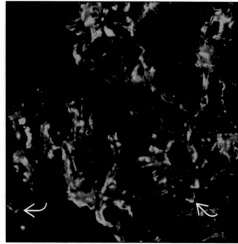

(Left) Immunofluorescence for fibrin or fibrinogen shows 3+ granular deposition that is strictly mesangial in location. Fibrin is commonly present in IgAN; whether it has pathogenetic significance is unknown. *(Right)* Immunofluorescence microscopy shows deposition of fibrin in a crescent ➡, which should be contrasted to the mesangial pattern. Fibrin is present in active (cellular or fibrocellular) crescents in all types of glomerulonephritis.

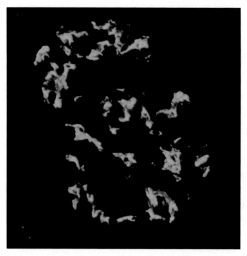 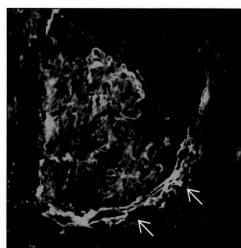

(Left) Immunofluorescence for IgA in a living related donor biopsy at the time of transplantation shows 1-2+ mesangial deposition. The donor was asymptomatic, and the recipient had end-stage renal disease due to reflux nephropathy. This case represents an asymptomatic IgA nephropathy. *(Right)* Immunofluorescence for IgA in a protocol biopsy 3 months after transplantation shows complete resolution of the IgA deposits seen in the donor biopsy.

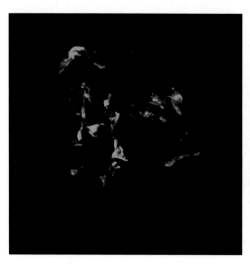 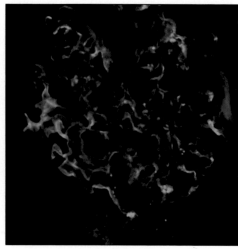

IgA NEPHROPATHY

Electron Microscopy

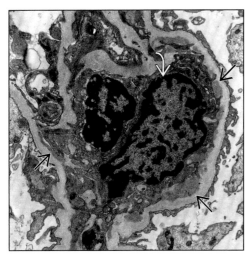

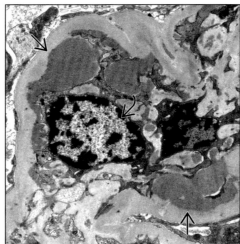

(Left) EM of a typical case shows amorphous electron-dense mesangial deposits ⇒ in close contact with a mesangial cell ⇒. *(Right)* On higher magnification, the electron-dense mesangial deposits ⇒ do not show substructure. The deposits are in close association with a mesangial cell ⇒.

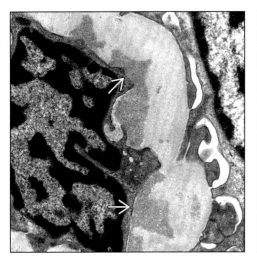

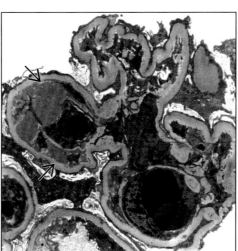

(Left) Higher magnification shows the finely granular texture and lack of substructure in the mesangial deposits and the close contact with the mesangial cell membrane ⇒. Interaction of the deposits with the mesangial cell is thought to be important in the pathogenesis of IgAN. *(Right)* EM of a glomerulus shows prominent subendothelial deposits ⇒ segmentally, a pattern less commonly seen in IgAN that is sometimes associated with a worse prognosis.

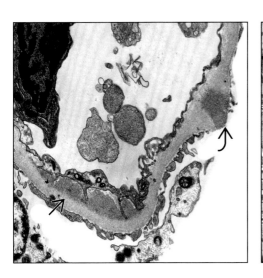

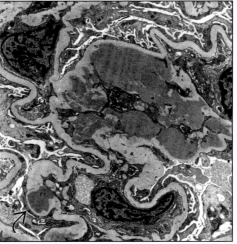

(Left) EM of a glomerular capillary loop shows subendothelial ⇒ and subepithelial ⇒ deposits. Deposits along the GBM, although less commonly seen, may be important in causing GBM injury and consequent hematuria and proteinuria. *(Right)* EM of a mesangial region shows large mesangial deposits, one of which appears to push through the GBM ⇒. This may be a mechanism of GBM disruption in IgAN.

Electron Microscopy

(Left) EM of a mesangial region shows large mesangial deposits, several of which are in a region of GBM disruption and in contact with a podocyte ➤. This may be a mechanism of GBM disruption in IgAN. *(Right)* EM shows a fragmented portion of GBM ➡ that has been partially repaired with new matrix formation. For hematuria to arise from an injured glomerulus, the GBM has to be disrupted; however, it is uncommon to observe the disruption in histologic or EM preparations.

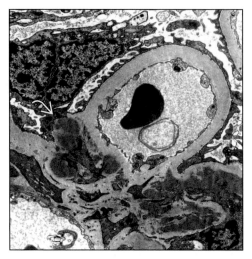
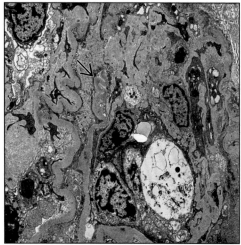

(Left) EM shows a segment of GBM with extreme thinning ➡. Overlying this segment is a podocyte with effaced foot processes. This is believed to be a site of previous disruption/injury and the beginning of a repair. *(Right)* EM shows a multilaminated segment of GBM ➡ with irregular layers of matrix. This repair process resembles the GBM lesions of Alport syndrome from which it is distinguished, primarily, by the segmental nature and preservation of GBM type 4 collagens.

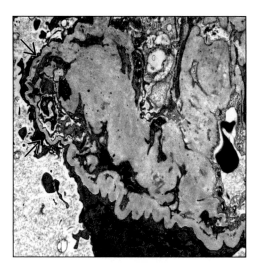
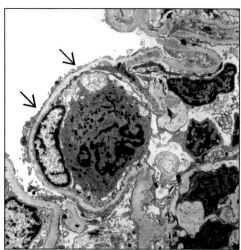

(Left) EM at high power shows a segment of laminated GBM with intervening particles that closely resembles Alport syndrome. In contrast to Alport syndrome, IgAN typically has only a few capillaries with this pattern and stains normally for the α 3, 4, and 5 chains of type 4 collagen. *(Right)* EM shows a thin but normal-appearing GBM in a patient with IgAN. This provides evidence of a 2nd disease, thin basement membrane disease, which may be synergistic with IgAN in causing hematuria.

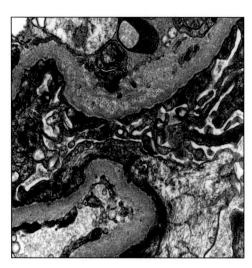
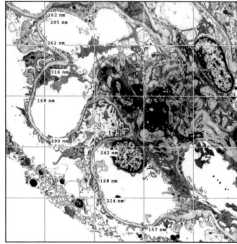

IgA NEPHROPATHY

Renal Failure Due to Severe Hematuria

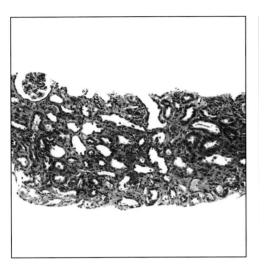

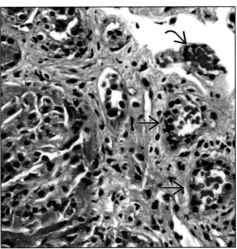

(Left) The cortex shows tubular dilation and loss of cytoplasm, indicative of acute tubular injury and obstruction. This patient presented with acute renal failure (creatinine 2.8 to 7 mg/dL in 1 month) associated with gross hematuria and RBC casts. The creatinine rapidly declined as the gross hematuria resolved. *(Right)* Here, red cells appear free in tubules ➡ and compacted in casts ➡. The glomerulus is hypercellular.

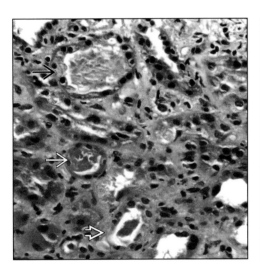

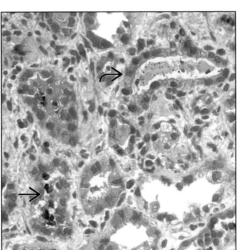

(Left) Various types of casts are seen, including pigmented with red cell ghosts ➡, red cells mixed with proteinaceous material ➡, and compacted red cells ➡. *(Right)* Immunoperoxidase staining for hemoglobin shows staining of red cells ➡ and red cell fragments ➡ in tubules.

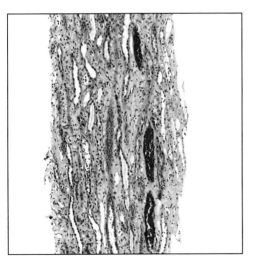

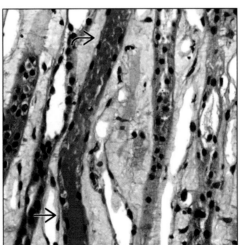

(Left) Hematoxylin & eosin of the medulla shows collecting ducts packed with red cells. These casts can obstruct the tubule, contributing to renal failure in heavy hematuria. *(Right)* At higher magnification, the medulla shows loose red cells in a tubule at the top ➡, embedded in a proteinaceous matrix, with the red cells becoming more compacted distally ➡.

Late Stages of IgA Nephropathy

(Left) PAS shows subtotal segmental glomerulosclerosis with adhesions to Bowman capsule over most of the surface in this 27-year-old man with elevated serum creatinine (5.6 mg/dL), hematuria, and urine protein to creatinine ratio of 7. Fragmentation of Bowman capsule ⊅ is suggestive of past crescent formation. (Right) Hematoxylin & eosin of the interstitium shows a cluster of foam cells, a feature associated with heavy proteinuria but not with any specific cause.

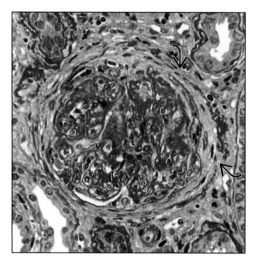 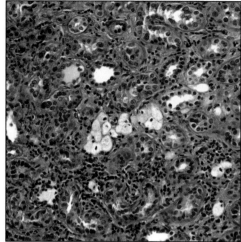

(Left) H&E of a glomerulus shows segmental glomerulosclerosis, adhesion to Bowman capsule, and hyaline deposits in this 51-year-old man with an 11-year history of IgA nephropathy, now end-stage. (Right) Gross pathology of an end-stage kidney with IgA nephropathy shows diffuse loss of cortical thickness without segmental scars or notable medullary abnormalities. This small but otherwise normal appearance is typical of end-stage kidneys with either glomerular disease or diffuse interstitial disease.

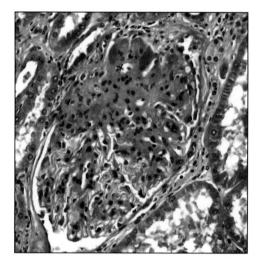 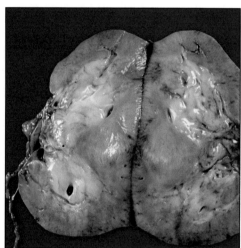

(Left) H&E of an end-stage kidney removed during transplantation shows persistence of mesangial hypercellularity ➡ even at this late stage. (Right) Immunofluorescence of an end-stage case of IgAN shows persistence of the IgA deposits in the mesangium. This finding is typical of IgAN, in contrast to Henoch-Schönlein purpura, in which the IgA deposits are usually transient.

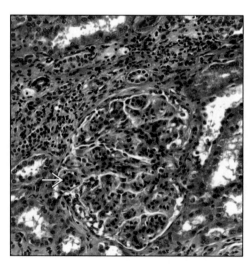 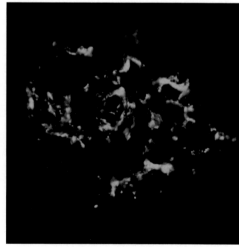

IgA NEPHROPATHY

Recurrent IgA Nephropathy in Allograft

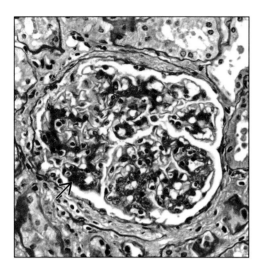

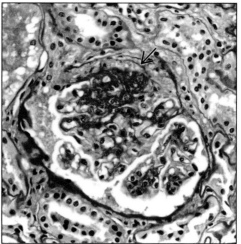

(Left) PAS shows mesangial hypercellularity ➡ and a generally normal GBM in a 43-year-old woman with recurrent IgAN 8 years after living unrelated renal transplantation. *(Right)* Biopsy from a 43-year-old woman who is status post living unrelated renal transplantation with elevated serum creatinine. PAS shows a segmental scar and adhesion to the Bowman capsule ➡ in a case with recurrent IgA nephropathy 8 years after transplantation.

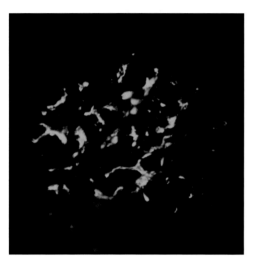

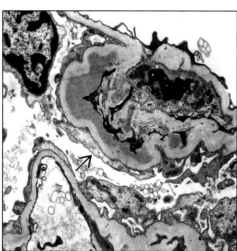

(Left) Biopsy from a 43-year-old woman with a living unrelated renal transplant and elevated serum Cr is shown. Immunofluorescence displays prominent IgA deposition in the mesangium (4+) in recurrent IgAN 8 years post transplant. *(Right)* EM shows amorphous electron-dense deposits closely applied to the mesangial cell. Segmental podocyte foot process effacement ➡ is also present in this case of recurrent IgAN 8 years after living unrelated renal transplantation in a 43-year-old woman.

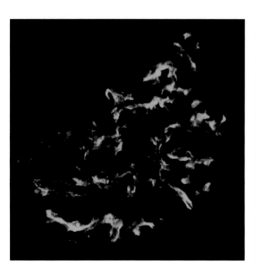

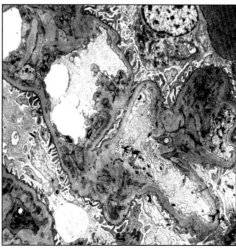

(Left) Immunofluorescence shows prominent IgA mesangial deposits in recurrent IgA nephropathy 4 months after transplantation. A biopsy at 15 days post transplant previously had only a trace IgA in this 22-year-old man. *(Right)* EM shows mesangial amorphous electron-dense deposits 4 months after transplantation in this 22-year-old man with recurrent IgA nephropathy.

HENOCH-SCHÖNLEIN PURPURA

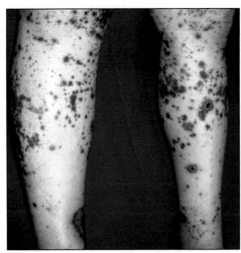

In this Henoch-Schönlein purpura (HSP) patient, purpura is diffusely present on the lower extremities, which is a common site for skin manifestations. (Courtesy V. Petronic-Rosic, MD.)

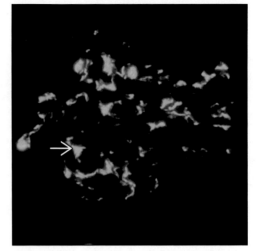

Glomerular IgA deposition in primarily mesangial areas ➡ is the characteristic pathologic finding for the diagnosis of HSP along with the presence of extrarenal manifestations.

TERMINOLOGY

Abbreviations
- Henoch-Schönlein purpura (HSP)
  - Johann Schönlein (1793-1864)
    - Described entity in 1837
  - Eduard Henoch (1820-1910)
    - German pediatrician; described patient with bloody diarrhea, joint pain, and rash in 1868
    - Student of Johann Schönlein

Synonyms
- HSP nephritis
- Anaphylactoid purpura
- Purpura rheumatica
- Heberden-Willan disease
  - William Heberden (1710-1801) and Robert Willan (1757-1812) described 1st cases in 1802 and 1808, respectively

Definitions
- Glomerular IgA immune complex deposition with extrarenal manifestations, such as purpura

ETIOLOGY/PATHOGENESIS

Infectious Agents
- Upper respiratory infection often precedes onset of HSP
  - HSP more common in winter months
- No definitive infectious agent identified as cause of HSP
  - IgA binding streptococcal M binding proteins identified in glomerular immune complexes of subset of HSP patients
  - Nephritis-associated plasmin receptor, group A streptococcal antigen, detected in mesangium of 30% of HSP patients

Abnormal Glycosylation of IgA1
- Galactose deficient or decreased galactosylation at hinge region of IgA molecule
  - HSP patients without renal involvement lack abnormal glycosylation of IgA1
- Increased binding of abnormal IgA1 to mesangial cells in vitro
- IgA1 bound with IgG specific for galactose-deficient IgA1 stimulates cultured mesangial cell proliferation
- Hepatic clearance of abnormal IgA1 is decreased in IgA nephropathy and possibly in HSP patients

Genetic Factors
- Complement deficiency
  - C2 deficiency or complete C4 deficiency increases likelihood of HSP development
  - C4B deficiency increases likelihood of nephritis in HSP patients
  - C4A deficiency worsens HSP nephritis severity

Possible Relationship with IgA Nephropathy
- IgA nephropathy precedes development of HSP in some patients
- Many similarities with clinical and pathologic features of HSP and IgA nephropathy
  - HSP may represent systemic form of IgA nephropathy
  - Systemic immune complexes also consist of IgA1 subclass

CLINICAL ISSUES

Epidemiology
- Incidence
  - 20 cases per 100,000 children
    - Most common childhood vasculitis
- Age
  - 90% of cases occur before age of 10 years
  - Can occur at any age

HENOCH-SCHÖNLEIN PURPURA

Key Facts

Etiology/Pathogenesis
- Unknown, abnormal glycosylation of IgA1

Clinical Issues
- Most common childhood vasculitis
- 90% of cases occur before age of 10 years
- Purpura
  - Often involves lower extremities and buttocks
  - Skin biopsy demonstrates leukocytoclastic vasculitis with IgA deposition in acute lesions
- Abdominal pain
- Arthritis
- Hematuria
  - More renal involvement in adults (50-80%) than in children (20-50%)
- Prognosis depends on extent of renal involvement
  - Often worse in adults vs. children

Microscopic Pathology
- Variable mesangial hypercellularity
- Cellular crescents variable extent
- IF: Prominent IgA deposits, primarily in mesangium
- EM: Amorphous deposits in mesangium
  - Also subendothelial and sometimes subepithelial deposits

Top Differential Diagnoses
- IgA nephropathy
- IgA-dominant postinfectious GN
- Mesangial proliferative lupus nephritis

Diagnostic Checklist
- Use International Study of Kidney Disease in Children (ISKDC) Histologic Classification (1977)

- Gender
  - Male > female
- Ethnicity
  - Caucasian > African descent

Site
- Kidney

Presentation
- Purpura usual initial sign
  - Often involves lower extremities and buttocks
  - May also involve face, trunk, and arms
- Hematuria and proteinuria
  - 40% of pediatric patients develop nephritis within 4-6 weeks after purpura
    - More renal involvement in adults (50-80%) than in children (20-50%)
- Gastrointestinal tract
  - Abdominal pain
  - Bleeding
  - Obstruction
- Arthritis

Laboratory Tests
- Serum IgA levels may be elevated
  - Not useful to distinguish HSP patients ± renal involvement
- Plasma IgE levels may be elevated
- Serum complement levels may be normal or low

Natural History
- Spontaneous regression common when no renal involvement is present

Treatment
- Options, risks, complications
  - No treatment may be necessary in mild cases
- Surgical approaches
  - Tonsillectomy
    - Combination with steroid therapy may be useful
    - Many clinical studies of tonsillectomy alone show mixed outcomes
- Drugs

  - High-dose corticosteroids
- Kidney transplantation
  - Recurrence rate of 15-20%
    - Recurrence possibly higher in related vs. unrelated donors
    - HSP patients with necrotizing and crescentic glomerulonephritis (GN) had recurrence after transplantation compared to 12% with mesangial proliferation
    - 10% graft loss due to recurrence
  - 10-year graft survival is approximately 90% in children and 75% in adults

Prognosis
- Dependent on extent of renal involvement
  - Often worse in adults vs. children

MICROSCOPIC PATHOLOGY

Histologic Features
- Glomerular alterations
  - May be normal
  - Variable mesangial hypercellularity
    - Mesangial hypercellularity defined as > 2 mesangial cell nuclei (per 2 μm thick section) or > 3 mesangial cell nuclei (per 3 μm thick section)
    - Mesangial PAS(+) granules representing IgA immune complexes may be present
  - Cellular crescent formation
    - Focal to diffuse
- Necrotizing vasculitis (rare)
  - Rare necrotizing capillaritis of peritubular capillaries of renal medulla
- Acute tubular injury
- Interstitial inflammation
  - May be prominent with significant crescentic glomerular injury
- Interstitial fibrosis and tubular atrophy

Other Sites
- Skin
  - Leukocytoclastic vasculitis

HENOCH-SCHÖNLEIN PURPURA

- IgA deposition in vessels may be patchy and present primarily in acute lesions
- GI tract
  - Leukocytoclastic vasculitis with IgA deposits

ANCILLARY TESTS

Immunofluorescence
- IgA dominant, primarily mesangial, and focally along GBM
  - Other reactants usually present: C3, IgG
  - Variable IgM, fibrin; little C1q
- Late in disease course, IgA disappears vs. persistence of IgA in IgA nephropathy

Electron Microscopy
- Amorphous deposits in mesangium
  - May be absent in some cases despite strong IgA staining
- Often subendothelial deposits
  - May correlate with crescent formation and necrosis
- Segmental subepithelial "humps" sometimes present

DIFFERENTIAL DIAGNOSIS

IgA Nephropathy
- Identical pathologic features as HSP
- Absence of extrarenal manifestations
- IgA deposits persist in contrast to HSP

Mesangial Proliferative Lupus Nephritis
- Requires clinical diagnosis of systemic lupus erythematosus
- IgA not dominant or codominant immunoglobulin

IgA-dominant Postinfectious GN
- May be associated with staphylococcal infection
- Large subepithelial electron-dense deposits ("humps")

Pauci-immune Crescentic GN
- 85% are positive for antineutrophil cytoplasmic antibodies, either antimyeloperoxidase or anti-proteinase-3
- Mesangial IgA deposits may be present, typically 1+ staining or less
- No significant mesangial or endocapillary hypercellularity should be present

DIAGNOSTIC CHECKLIST

Pathologic Interpretation Pearls
- Renal biopsy findings cannot distinguish between HSP and IgA nephropathy

Grading
- Meadow Histologic Classification System (1972)
  - Class I: Focal mesangial expansion
  - Class II: Moderate focal proliferative
  - Class III: Mild diffuse proliferative
  - Class IV: Moderate diffuse proliferative; crescents ≤ 50%
  - Class V: Severe diffuse proliferative; crescents > 50%
- International Study of Kidney Disease in Children (ISKDC) Histologic Classification (1977)
  - Class I: Minimal alterations
  - Class II: Pure mesangial proliferation
  - Class III: Focal (IIIa) or diffuse (IIIb) mesangial proliferation with < 50% crescents
  - Class IV: Focal (IVa) or diffuse (IVb) mesangial proliferation with 50-75% crescents
  - Class V: Focal (Va) or diffuse (Vb) mesangial proliferation with > 75% crescents
  - Class VI: Membranoproliferative-like GN

SELECTED REFERENCES

1. Edström Halling S et al: Predictors of outcome in Henoch-Schönlein nephritis. Pediatr Nephrol. 25(6):1101-8, 2010
2. Han SS et al: Outcome of renal allograft in patients with Henoch-Schönlein nephritis: single-center experience and systematic review. Transplantation. 89(6):721-6, 2010
3. Lau KK et al: Pathogenesis of Henoch-Schönlein purpura nephritis. Pediatr Nephrol. 25(1):19-26, 2010
4. Schmitt R et al: Tissue deposits of IgA-binding streptococcal M proteins in IgA nephropathy and Henoch-Schonlein purpura. Am J Pathol. 176(2):608-18, 2010
5. Hung SP et al: Clinical manifestations and outcomes of Henoch-Schönlein purpura: comparison between adults and children. Pediatr Neonatol. 50(4):162-8, 2009
6. Denton MD et al: Case records of the Massachusetts General Hospital. Case 20-2006. An 84-year-old man with staphylococcal bacteremia and renal failure. N Engl J Med. 354(26):2803-13, 2006
7. Counahan R et al: Prognosis of Henoch-Schönlein nephritis in children. Br Med J. 2(6078):11-4, 1977
8. Meadow SR et al: Schönlein-Henoch nephritis. Q J Med. 41(163):241-58, 1972

HENOCH-SCHÖNLEIN PURPURA

Skin Manifestations

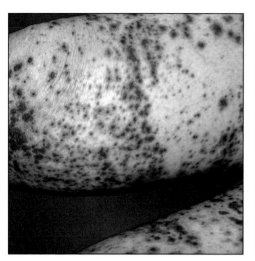
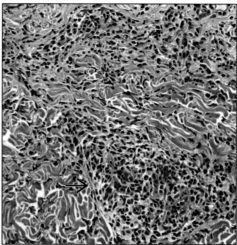

(Left) Purpuric macules, papules, patches, and plaques are diffusely present on the lower extremities of this patient with HSP. (Courtesy V. Petronic-Rosic, MD.) *(Right)* Leukocytoclastic vasculitis with prominent perivascular infiltration by leukocytes ⇲ is a result of vascular immune complex deposition. Some prefer the term hypersensitivity vasculitis because leukocytoclasis or degeneration of neutrophils may not always be present. (Courtesy J. Song, MD.)

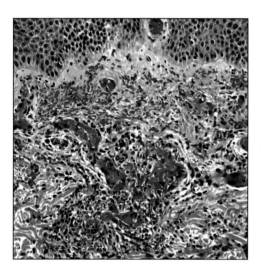
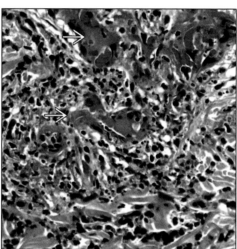

(Left) Leukocytoclastic vasculitis is the typical skin biopsy finding for HSP. Prominent inflammation is present in the dermal capillaries, and there are marked, extravasated red blood cells in the dermis. (Courtesy J. Song, MD.) *(Right)* Prominent fibrin deposition ⇲ is present along with perivascular inflammation and degeneration of neutrophils in this florid example of leukocytoclastic vasculitis. (Courtesy J. Song, MD.)

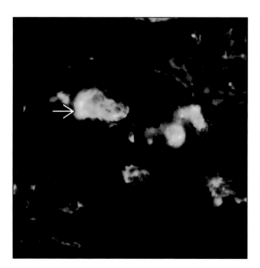
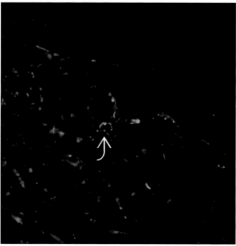

(Left) Granular IgA deposition in the dermal capillaries ⇲ is identified in the skin biopsy from an HSP patient with leukocytoclastic vasculitis early in the disease course. The absence of IgA deposition does not necessarily exclude HSP and may be due to the patchy distribution of immune complexes. (Courtesy K. Soltani, MD.) *(Right)* The granular deposits of IgA in the dermal vessels ⇲ in HSP can be very focal and subtle, as in this case, which was initially missed.

Microscopic Features

(Left) This glomerulus from a 4-year-old girl with HSP appears normal, but a necrotizing and crescentic injury (not shown) involved 20% of her glomeruli. Antineutrophil cytoplasmic antibodies were also present and may have contributed to the crescentic injury. *(Right)* Marked segmental mesangial hypercellularity ➡ is present in this glomerulus from an 8-year-old girl with HSP.

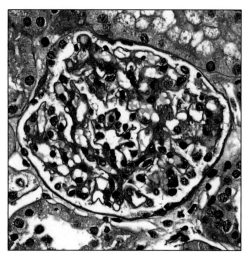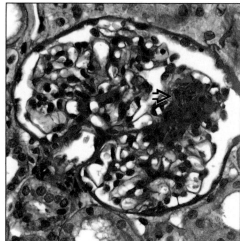

(Left) Many PAS(+) granules are present in the mesangium ➡ in an 84-year-old man with HSP. Similar PAS(+) mesangial deposits are sometimes found in IgA nephropathy. *(Right)* Segmental fibrinoid necrosis ➡ with the prominence of adjacent epithelial cells is a common finding in HSP patients. Marked accumulation of red blood cells within the adjacent tubular lumina ➡ correlates with the presence of gross hematuria.

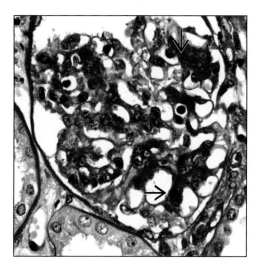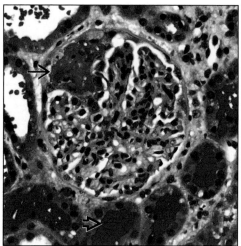

(Left) A small cellular crescent ➡ with fibrinoid necrosis occupies the upper portion of the urinary space and compresses the remaining glomerular tufts, which reveal mild mesangial hypercellularity in an HSP patient. *(Right)* Segmental fibrinoid necrosis with karyorrhexis ➡ is present in a glomerular tuft of a young patient with HSP. These histologic changes are identical to those seen in the spectrum of IgA nephropathy.

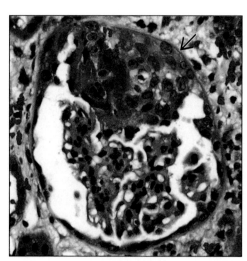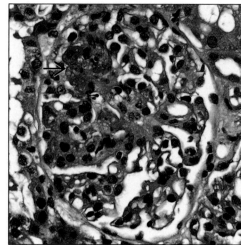

HENOCH-SCHÖNLEIN PURPURA

Immunofluorescence

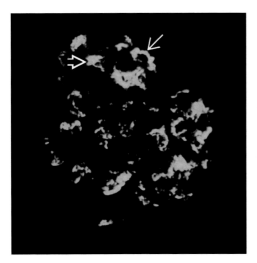

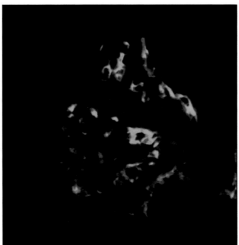

(Left) Strong granular IgA immunofluorescence staining of primarily mesangial regions ➡ and some capillary walls ➡ is consistent with IgA nephropathy or Henoch-Schönlein purpura. *(Right)* IgG immunofluorescence staining of glomeruli may be similar in intensity and distribution to IgA for HSP. The higher background staining for the IgG antibody can occasionally give the appearance of increased staining intensity compared to IgA.

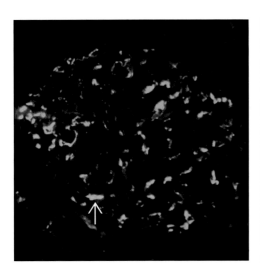

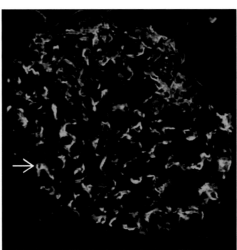

(Left) Granular C3 immunofluorescence staining can be observed in some of the mesangial areas ➡ in a glomerulus from a patient with HSP. This is a variable finding and may be negative in a significant subset of cases. *(Right)* Immunofluorescence microscopy for fibrinogen can highlight the mesangial ➡ immune complexes of HSP in a subset of cases, which is due to the glomerular deposition of cross-linked fibrin degradation products.

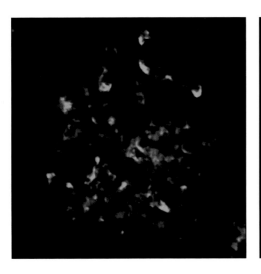

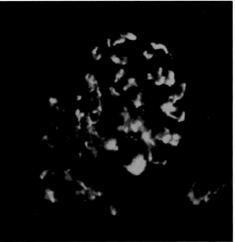

(Left) Kappa light chain immunofluorescence staining of the glomerular immune complexes often appears less intense compared with the lambda light chain staining (not shown) that is characteristic of HSP. *(Right)* Lambda light chain shows strong staining intensity of the glomerular immune complexes, which can be a useful finding to help support the diagnosis of HSP.

HENOCH-SCHÖNLEIN PURPURA

Electron Microscopy

(Left) Electron-dense deposits consistent with immune complexes are present in the mesangial region ➡ of this glomerulus from a patient with HSP, which appears identical to IgA nephropathy. *(Right)* Many subendothelial immune complexes ➡ are present within this glomerular capillary, which is a finding that may correlate with the presence of crescents. There is also extensive effacement of the overlying podocyte foot processes ➡ that correlates with the presence of proteinuria.

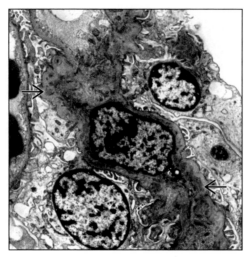 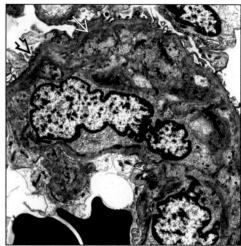

(Left) Small discrete deposits ➡ in the mesangial areas may be difficult to identify, and occasionally such deposits cannot be identified by electron microscopy despite strong IgA immunofluorescence glomerular staining. *(Right)* Large aggregates of electron-dense deposits ➡ may accumulate in mesangial regions, which are characteristic of HSP and appear identical to IgA nephropathy or mesangial proliferative lupus nephritis.

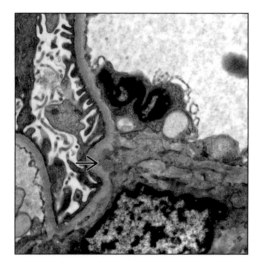 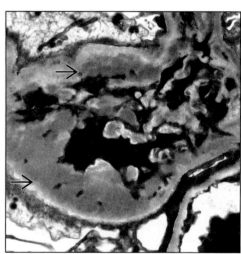

(Left) Rare subepithelial deposits ➡ along with the typical mesangial deposits ➡ may be present. Segmental thinning of the glomerular basement membranes ➡ was also present, but this was not diffuse and did not warrant the additional diagnosis of thin basement membrane disease. *(Right)* Prominent subendothelial electron-dense deposits ➡ may be present, and this finding often correlates with the presence of cellular crescent formation.

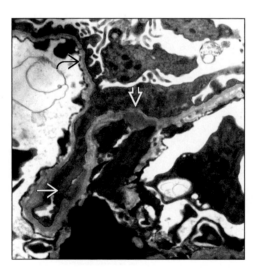 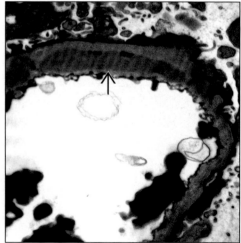

HENOCH-SCHÖNLEIN PURPURA

Other Features

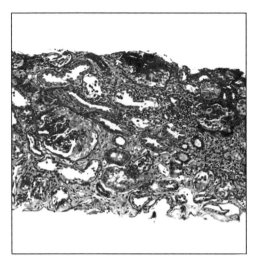
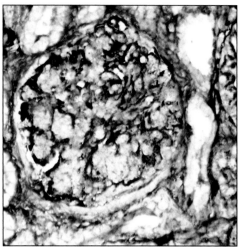

(Left) Crescents are evident in this low-power view of a case of HSP. If crescents are > 50% of glomeruli, the prognosis is worse. However, HSP with crescents still has a good prognosis. (Right) If frozen tissue is not available, immunohistochemistry for IgA can still be useful to make the diagnosis of HSP, as in this case. In paraffin sections, a high background in the tissue makes interpretation difficult; however, the mesangium is normally negative.

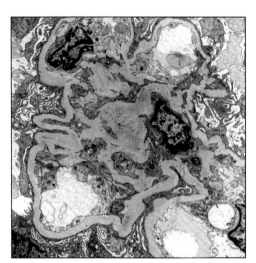
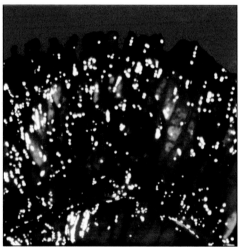

(Left) This patient with acute renal failure due to red cell casts had strong staining for IgA in the mesangial, but relatively few mesangial, electron-dense deposits in the 3 glomeruli were examined. The relative paucity of deposits may favor HSP over IgA nephropathy although this has not been formally tested. (Right) Small bowel in a patient with HSP shows submucosal petechial hemorrhages due to vasculitis. Intussusception can result from the intramural hemorrhage.

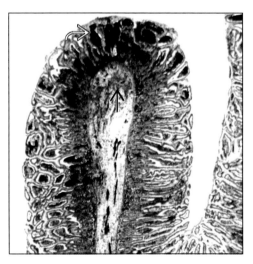
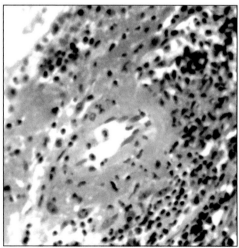

(Left) Small bowel in HSP shows focal hemorrhage ⇗ in a fold of mucosa, the cause of which is vasculitis in the lamina propria ⇒. (Right) H&E shows vasculitis in the small bowel lamina propria in HSP. The wall of this small artery has fibrinoid necrosis with neutrophils, nuclear dust, and local hemorrhage.

IgA ACUTE GLOMERULONEPHRITIS ASSOCIATED WITH *S. AUREUS*

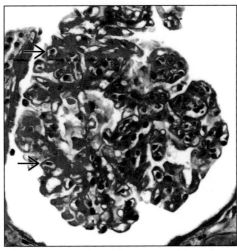

Glomerulitis may be mild in cases of IgA positive acute glomerulitis associated with Staphylococcus aureus infection. Many mononuclear and a few polymorphonuclear leukocytes are present ➡️.

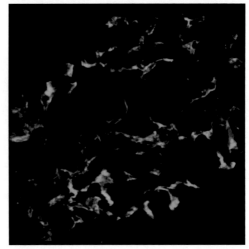

Acute glomerulonephritis associated with Staphylococcal aureus infection typically has prominent mesangial IgA deposits, which resemble IgA nephropathy or HSP.

TERMINOLOGY

Definitions
- Acute glomerulonephritis (GN) associated with *Staphylococcus aureus* infection with predominance of IgA deposition

ETIOLOGY/PATHOGENESIS

Infectious Agents
- *S. aureus*, coagulase positive, often methicillin resistant (MRSA)
  - Osteomyelitis, pneumonia, septic arthritis, discitis, soft tissue abscess, empyema, sinusitis, endocarditis
  - Septicemia
  - Not usually postinfectious GN but occurs during chronic infection
    - Average duration of infection is 5 weeks

Host Factors
- Diabetes mellitus, neoplasia, old age, alcoholism

Immune Response
- IgA antibodies to *S. aureus* cell membrane antigen (GenBank BAB41819.1)
- *S. aureus* enterotoxins may act as superantigens, stimulating T cells and leading to polyclonal B-cell activation
- 1 superantigen-like protein (SSL7) binds to Fc of IgA, blocking FcR activity

CLINICAL ISSUES

Presentation
- Persistent infection, septicemia
- Acute renal failure
- Hematuria
- Proteinuria, nephrotic range (20-80%)
- Hypertension

- Hypocomplementemia (minority)
- Purpura

Treatment
- Antibiotics and renal support
- Anecdotal reports of steroids/immunosuppression

Prognosis
- Data limited
  - Range of outcomes from complete recovery to ESRD
  - Recovery possible if infection successfully treated
- Underlying disease and age are important factors

Prevalence
- ~ 25% of renal biopsies with acute postinfectious glomerulonephritis

MICROSCOPIC PATHOLOGY

Histologic Features
- Glomerulus
  - Varies from mild mesangial hypercellularity to marked acute inflammation with crescents
  - Leukocytes in capillaries
    - Neutrophils and mononuclear cells
    - Usually not prominent
  - Mesangial hypercellularity
  - Normal GBM
  - Rare "pseudothrombi" due to cryoglobulins
- Tubules
  - Red cell casts common
  - May be active inflammation and tubular damage
- Interstitium
  - Focal interstitial mononuclear cells and scattered neutrophils and eosinophils
- Vessels: No vasculitis

IgA ACUTE GLOMERULONEPHRITIS ASSOCIATED WITH *S. AUREUS*

Key Facts

Etiology/Pathogenesis
- *Staphylococcus aureus*, coagulase positive, often MRSA
- Increased risk with diabetes mellitus, neoplasia, old age

Clinical Issues
- Infection, septicemia
- Acute renal failure
- Proteinuria, nephrotic range (20-80%)
- Purpura
- ~ 25% of biopsies with acute postinfectious glomerulonephritis

Microscopic Pathology
- Glomerular involvement varies from mild mesangial hypercellularity to marked acute inflammation with crescents

- Red cell casts common
- Focal interstitial nephritis

Ancillary Tests
- IgA dominant or codominant immunoglobulin, mostly mesangial
- EM deposits primarily mesangial and paramesangial
  - Occasional subepithelial "humps"
  - "Humps" sometimes have "cups" in contrast to poststreptococcal GN
  - Occasional subendothelial deposits

Top Differential Diagnoses
- IgA nephropathy
- Henoch-Schönlein purpura
- Acute glomurelonephritis from other causes

ANCILLARY TESTS

Immunofluorescence
- IgA dominant or codominant immunoglobulin, mostly mesangial
- Usually similar distribution of IgG and C3
- C1q variable
- IgM usually not conspicuous
- Lambda > kappa in majority
- *S. aureus* cell envelope antigen detected in 68%
- Rarely has pauci-immune staining

Electron Microscopy
- Amorphous, electron-dense deposits
  - Primarily mesangial and paramesangial
  - Occasional subepithelial deposits
    - In contrast to postinfectious GN, "humps" may have "cupping" reaction
  - Occasional subendothelial deposits
- Foot process effacement

DIFFERENTIAL DIAGNOSIS

IgA Nephropathy
- Typically less inflammation
- Chronic disease
- Absence of visceral staphylococcal infection

Henoch-Schönlein Purpura (HSP)
- Strong resemblance with acute inflammation, purpura
- Absence of visceral staphylococcal infection and vasculitis

Acute Glomerulonephritis from Other Causes
- No IgA predominance
- Evidence of non-*S. aureus* infection

DIAGNOSTIC CHECKLIST

Pathologic Interpretation Pearls
- Outcome does not correlate well with pathologic features
- "Humps" sometimes have "cups" in contrast to poststreptococcal GN

SELECTED REFERENCES

1. Riley AM et al: Favorable outcome after aggressive treatment of infection in a diabetic patient with MRSA-related IgA nephropathy. Am J Med Sci. 337(3):221-3, 2009
2. Nasr SH et al: Acute postinfectious glomerulonephritis in the modern era: experience with 86 adults and review of the literature. Medicine (Baltimore). 87(1):21-32, 2008
3. Nasr SH et al: Acute poststaphylococcal glomerulonephritis superimposed on diabetic glomerulosclerosis. Kidney Int. 71(12):1317-21, 2007
4. Ramsland PA et al: Structural basis for evasion of IgA immunity by Staphylococcus aureus revealed in the complex of SSL7 with Fc of human IgA1. Proc Natl Acad Sci U S A. 104(38):15051-6, 2007
5. Denton MD et al: Case records of the Massachusetts General Hospital. Case 20-2006. An 84-year-old man with staphylococcal bacteremia and renal failure. N Engl J Med. 354(26):2803-13, 2006
6. Kai H et al: Post-MRSA infection glomerulonephritis with marked Staphylococcus aureus cell envelope antigen deposition in glomeruli. J Nephrol. 19(2):215-9, 2006
7. Long JA et al: IgA deposits and acute glomerulonephritis in a patient with staphylococcal infection. Am J Kidney Dis. 48(5):851-5, 2006
8. Satoskar AA et al: Staphylococcus infection-associated glomerulonephritis mimicking IgA nephropathy. Clin J Am Soc Nephrol. 1(6):1179-86, 2006
9. Shimizu Y et al: Staphylococcal cell membrane antigen, a possible antigen in post-methicillin resistant Staphylococcus aureus (MRSA) infection nephritis and IgA nephropathy, exhibits high immunogenic activity that is enhanced by superantigen. J Nephrol. 18(3):249-56, 2005

IgA ACUTE GLOMERULONEPHRITIS ASSOCIATED WITH *S. AUREUS*

Light Microscopy and Immunofluorescence

(Left) Glomerular mesangial hypercellularity is prominent in this case of S. aureus-associated IgA glomerulonephritis. Red cell casts ➡ are frequent. *(Right)* Glomerulitis and mesangial hypercellularity are present in S. aureus glomerulonephritis associated with IgA deposits. A mild interstitial nephritis is also evident with occasional neutrophils and eosinophils.

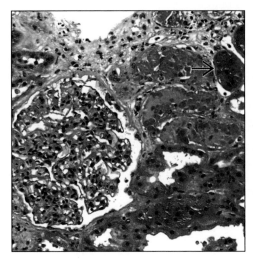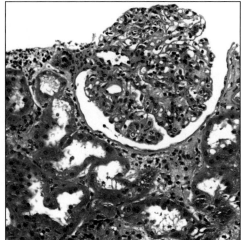

(Left) Staphylococcus aureus-associated acute glomerulonephritis (AGN) has pathologic features ranging from mild glomerulitis with occasional neutrophils to proliferative glomerulonephritis with crescents (PAS stain). *(Right)* IgG with a predominately mesangial pattern commonly accompanies IgA in S. aureus-associated AGN. The differential diagnosis includes idiopathic IgA nephropathy, HSP, and lupus nephritis.

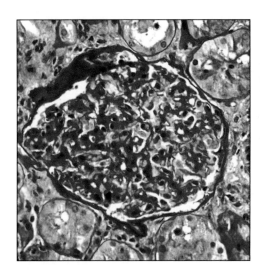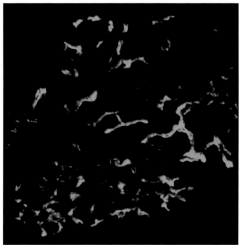

(Left) Acute glomerulonephritis associated with S. aureus septicemia and probably vertebral osteomyelitis is shown. Prominent C3 is present primarily in the mesangium and was accompanied by IgA and IgG. *(Right)* C1q can occasionally be present in S. aureus-associated AGN, as in this case. If C1q is prominent, a diagnosis of lupus should be considered.

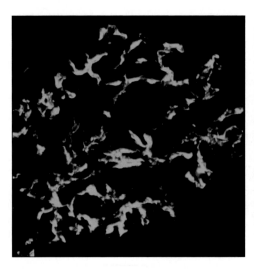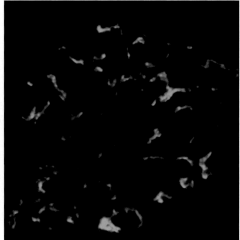

IgA ACUTE GLOMERULONEPHRITIS ASSOCIATED WITH *S. AUREUS*

Immunofluorescence and Electron Microscopy

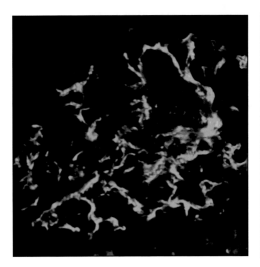 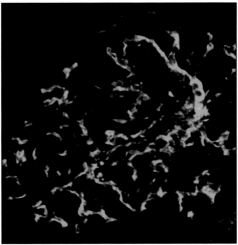

(Left) Lambda and kappa may show predominance of lambda in S. aureus-associated acute glomerulonephritis, as in this case, similar to the findings in IgA nephropathy and nephritis associated with Henoch-Schönlein purpura (HSP). (Right) Kappa is less extensive than lambda in the majority of cases of S. aureus-associated acute glomerulonephritis, a feature shared with IgA nephropathy and HSP which is in contrast to other forms of acute glomerulonephritis.

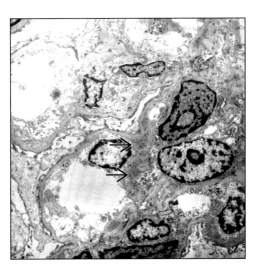 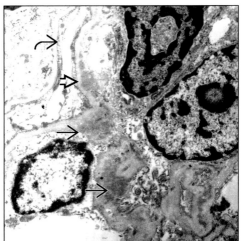

(Left) Deposits are primarily in the mesangium ⇨ in S. aureus-associated AGN. The GBM is normal, and no subendothelial or subepithelial deposits are present. (Right) The amorphous, electron-dense deposits are primarily in the mesangium ⇨ in S. aureus-associated AGN. Some are paramesangial ⇨, as in idiopathic IgA nephropathy. Podocyte foot processes show extensive effacement ⇨.

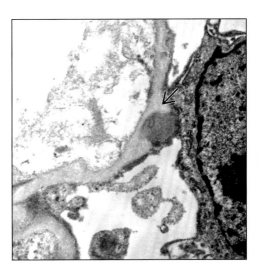 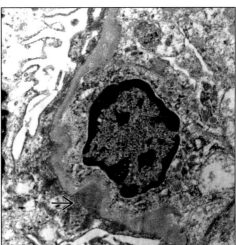

(Left) Subepithelial deposits can be sometimes found in S. aureus-associated AGN, but they may not form typical "humps." "Humps" in poststreptococcal GN do not have surrounding "spikes" or "cups" of basement membrane as this case does ⇨. (Right) Subepithelial deposits are found in S. aureus-associated AGN, but they may not form typical "humps" ⇨. Subepithelial deposits also occur sporadically in idiopathic IgA nephropathy.

HEPATIC GLOMERULOSCLEROSIS

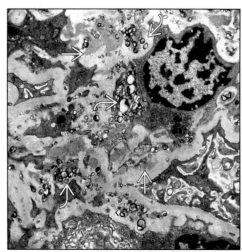

Hepatic glomerulosclerosis (HGS) characteristically has lipid debris in the mesangium ⇲, evident by electron microscopy. Amorphous electron-dense deposits typical of immune complexes are also present ➡.

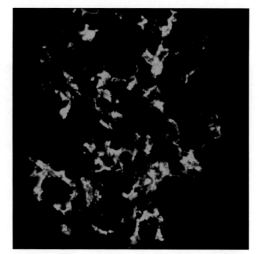

By immunofluorescence, prominent IgA deposits are present in the expanded mesangium in HGS. The pattern resembles IgA nephropathy although inflammatory changes are absent.

TERMINOLOGY

Abbreviations
- Hepatic glomerulosclerosis (HGS)

Synonyms
- Cirrhotic glomerulosclerosis

Definitions
- Glomerular disease related to cirrhosis or portal hypertension, manifested by accumulation of IgA and lipid debris in mesangium; excludes HCV immune complex diseases

ETIOLOGY/PATHOGENESIS

Failure of Normal Liver Clearance
Mechanisms
- Systemic shunting of blood bypasses liver Kupffer cells
  - HGS occurs with portal hypertension in absence of cirrhosis
- Accumulation of IgA immune complexes
- Lipid cell debris

Animal Models
- HGS with IgA deposition develops in rats with CCl4-induced cirrhosis

CLINICAL ISSUES

Epidemiology
- Incidence
  - ~ 60% prevalence of glomerular IgA deposits in cirrhotics at autopsy
  - ~ 35% at time of liver transplantation

Presentation
- End-stage liver disease or portal hypertension of any etiology

- Highest in alcoholic cirrhosis (~ 70%)
- Usually asymptomatic
- Hematuria (~ 9%) and proteinuria
  - Rarely, nephrotic-range proteinuria (~ 2%)

Prognosis
- Remission of nephrotic proteinuria and hematuria with correction of portal hypertension reported
- Reversibility after liver transplantation may be possible but not documented

MICROSCOPIC PATHOLOGY

Histologic Features
- Glomeruli show varied patterns
  - Normal
  - Mild to moderate mesangial expansion
    - Typical in asymptomatic patients
  - Prominent mesangial expansion, duplication of GBM and mesangial interposition
    - More common in biopsies for cause
    - Probably related to HCV and cryoglobulinemia
  - Crescents rarely reported
- Tubules
  - May show acute injury (hepatorenal syndrome)
  - Bile-stained casts
- Interstitium
  - No specific features
- Arteries
  - Intimal fibrosis common

ANCILLARY TESTS

Immunofluorescence
- Prominent IgA deposits, primarily in mesangium
  - Segmentally along GBM
  - Rarely monoclonal (4 cases)
  - IgA1 subclass

HEPATIC GLOMERULOSCLEROSIS

Key Facts

Terminology
- Glomerular disease caused by portal hypertension

Clinical Issues
- Present in ~ 60% of cirrhotics
- Asymptomatic hematuria, proteinuria
- Remission with correction of portal hypertension

Microscopic Pathology
- Glomeruli usually show mild mesangial expansion

- Other patterns: MPGN type I, normal

Ancillary Tests
- Mesangial deposits
  - Prominent IgA; lesser IgG, IgM, C3; often C1q
  - Electron-dense lipid granules, lucencies
  - Amorphous electron-dense deposits

Top Differential Diagnoses
- IgA nephropathy; MPGN, type I; HCV glomerulonephritis

- IgA usually accompanied by less intense deposits of IgG, IgM, C3, C1q, and, occasionally, fibrin
  - C3 in 50-80%
  - C1q in 50-70%

Electron Microscopy
- Electron-dense lipid granules in mesangium
  - Uncertain provenance
  - Sometimes seen as dense granules in rounded lucencies, 50-110 nm
- Amorphous electron-dense deposits in mesangium
  - Typical of immune complex deposits in other diseases
- Subendothelial deposits segmentally
  - Mesangial cell interposition

DIFFERENTIAL DIAGNOSIS

IgA Nephropathy
- Lacks characteristic lipid debris in mesangium
- C1q less commonly present (0-14%)
- C3 more commonly present (83-100%)

Membranoproliferative Glomerulonephritis, Type I
- Lacks characteristic lipid debris in mesangium
- IgA usually negative (~ 65%)

Hepatis C Virus-associated Immune Complex Glomerulonephritis
- More striking subendothelial IgG and IgM deposits
- Glomerular macrophage accumulation in mixed cryoglobulinemia
  - "Pseudothrombi"
- Lacks characteristic lipid debris in mesangium

SELECTED REFERENCES

1. Trawalé JM et al: The spectrum of renal lesions in patients with cirrhosis: a clinicopathological study. Liver Int. 30(5):725-32, 2010
2. Wadei HM et al: Kidney allocation to liver transplant candidates with renal failure of undetermined etiology: role of percutaneous renal biopsy. Am J Transplant. 8(12):2618-26, 2008
3. Axelsen RA et al: Renal glomerular lesions in unselected patients with cirrhosis undergoing orthotopic liver transplantation. Pathology. 27(3):237-46, 1995
4. Babbs C et al: IgA nephropathy in non-cirrhotic portal hypertension. Gut. 32(2):225-6, 1991
5. Gormly AA et al: IgA glomerular deposits in experimental cirrhosis. Am J Pathol. 104(1):50-4, 1981
6. Nakamoto Y et al: Hepatic glomerulonephritis. Characteristics of hepatic IgA glomerulonephritis as the major part. Virchows Arch A Pathol Anat Histol. 392(1):45-54, 1981
7. Sakaguchi H et al: Hepatic glomerulosclerosis. An electron microscopic study of renal biopsies in liver diseases. Lab Invest. 14:533-45, 1965

IMAGE GALLERY

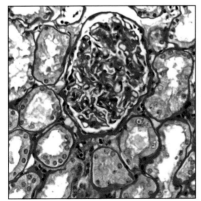 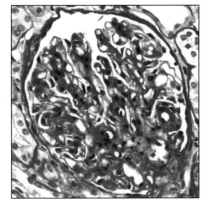 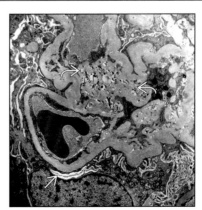

(Left) In hepatic glomerulosclerosis (HGS), the mesangial matrix is usually mildly expanded, as in this liver transplant candidate with end-stage cryptogenic cirrhosis (PAS stain). *(Center)* Mesangial matrix expansion with minimal GBM changes and no glomerular inflammation is the usual pattern of HGS (PAS stain). *(Right)* Biopsy from a liver transplant candidate with heavy proteinuria (> 10 g/d) and HGS shows mesangial lipid debris ➡ in lucent areas; podocyte foot process effacement was also prominent ➡ (EM).

SYSTEMIC LUPUS ERYTHEMATOSUS

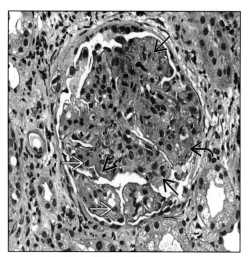

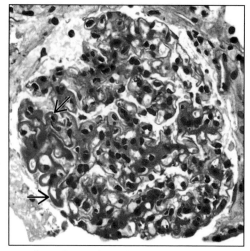

Endocapillary hypercellularity ➡, "wire loop" thickened capillary walls ➡, fibrinoid exudate ➡, and the rarely seen hematoxylin bodies ➡ are indicative of active lupus glomerulonephritis.

PAS shows lupus glomerulonephritis with prominent mesangial hypercellularity and segmental "wire loop" thickening of the capillary walls ➡. Lupus has a great spectrum of renal lesions.

TERMINOLOGY

Abbreviations
- Systemic lupus erythematosus (SLE); lupus nephritis (LN)

Synonyms
- Lupus nephritis; lupus glomerulonephritis (GN)

Definitions
- Systemic autoimmune disease manifested by inflammation of skin, joints, kidneys, and central nervous system, and with pathogenic IgG autoantibodies targeting nuclear, cell surface, and plasma protein self-antigens

ETIOLOGY/PATHOGENESIS

Autoimmune Disease
- Autoantibodies to nuclear antigens in 95%: Double-stranded (ds) DNA (nucleosomes), Ro (a ribonucleoprotein), La (an RNA binding protein), Sm (a ribonucleoprotein)
  - Other autoantigens
    - C1q and membrane phospholipids such as phosphatidylserine
    - Laminin, heparan sulfate proteoglycans, and podocyte antigens
    - Some autoantibodies promote coagulation: Lupus anticoagulant, antiphospholipid antibodies, and ADAMTS13
- Autoantibodies may be detectable years before disease onset
- Breakdown of tolerance to self-antigens, trigger unknown
  - "Waste disposal" hypothesis
    - Defective phagocytosis of apoptotic cells leads to abnormal pathways of disposal of these cells
    - Abnormal disposal allows exposure of immune system to intracellular sequestered antigens
    - Exposure to these self-antigens activates self-reactive T and B cells and development of autoantibodies

Environmental Triggers and Aggravating Factors
- Sunlight (UV)
- Drugs: Hydralazine, procainamide, quinidine

Genetic Factors
- 10% have relatives with SLE
- Higher concordance for monozygotic twins (25-69%) than dizygotic twins (1-2%)
- Polymorphisms/mutations of > 25 genes increase risk in genome-wide association studies
  - C1, C2, or C4 deficiency, probably causing defective clearance of immune complexes and apoptotic cells
  - Fcγ receptor IIB (inhibitory receptor on B cells)
  - Toll-like receptors (TLR 7 and 9)
  - Interferon (IFN) and tumor necrosis factor (TNF) signaling
  - HLA-DR2 and 3
  - TREX1, a DNA-degrading enzyme

Pathogenesis
- Immune complex (IC) formation and deposition in the kidney
  - Circulating IC trapped in capillaries and mesangium
    - Histone-rich nucleosomal antigens are trapped in glomeruli, possibly initiating immune complex (IC) deposition
  - In situ formation of IC due to planted or intrinsic antigen
  - Complement fixation
    - C3a and C5a attract neutrophils and macrophages
    - Endothelial activation by cytokines and complement

SYSTEMIC LUPUS ERYTHEMATOSUS

Key Facts

Terminology
- Systemic autoimmune disease manifested by inflammation of skin, joints, kidneys and central nervous system
  - IgG autoantibodies to DNA, RNA, proteins, phospholipids

Etiology/Pathogenesis
- Autoantibodies cause immune complex deposition, vasculitis, thrombotic microangiopathy
- Multiple genetic risk factors

Microscopic Pathology
- Glomerular pathology quite varied and is basis of ISN/RPS classification
  - Mesangial proliferation
  - Thickened GBM (extreme is wire loop)
  - Endocapillary hypercellularity
  - Necrosis, crescents
  - Thrombotic microangiopathy may dominate
- IF: IgG deposits in glomeruli are essential for diagnosis
  - Usually accompanied by IgM, IgA, C1q, and C3 (full house)
  - TBM deposits in ~ 50%
- EM: Amorphous and structured deposits
  - Mesangial, subendothelial, and subepithelial deposits
- Tubulointerstitial inflammation common

Top Differential Diagnoses
- Cryoglobulinemia
- MPGN, type I/III
- Postinfectious GN

- Inflammatory cells bind IC via Fc and complement receptors and are activated
- Persistent or recurrent inflammation leads to changes in intrinsic glomerular cell numbers and function and matrix homeostasis
- Thrombotic microangiopathy
  - Associated with lupus anticoagulant, antiphospholipid antibodies, and, rarely, antibodies to ADAMTS13
  - Arises independently of glomerular inflammation and IC
- Vasculitic glomerulonephritis
  - Necrosis with little or no IC deposition
  - Endothelial damage by uncertain mechanism
- Podocytopathy
  - Minimal change lesion, FSGS, or collapsing glomerulopathy
- T-cell-mediated autoimmune reactivity may also play a role

Insights from Animal Models
- Several spontaneous inbred mouse strains develop lupus-like glomerulonephritis, shown to be multigenic
  - NZB/NZW F1, MRL/lpr, BSXB
- Many specific genetic deficiencies promote murine lupus in susceptible strains
  - C4, C3, FcγRIIB, CD19, fas, Ro

CLINICAL ISSUES

Epidemiology
- Incidence
  - 12-64/100,000 worldwide
  - ~ 80% have nephritis during the course of the disease
    - 20% of patients have nephritis at onset
    - > 90% have nephritis at autopsy
- Age
  - Peak incidence from 15-40 years
    - Also occurs in infants and the elderly
- Gender
  - Female:male = 9:1
- Ethnicity
  - Less frequent in Caucasians
    - 1:250 females of African ancestry in USA
    - 1:1,400 females of European ancestry in USA

Presentation
- Gradual or sudden onset
- Variable presentation, correlates with pathologic classification
  - Isolated hematuria: ISN/RPS class I, II, and III
  - Nephritic syndrome: Class III and IV
  - Isolated proteinuria: Class II and III
  - Nephrotic syndrome: Class IV and V
  - Acute renal failure: Class IV
  - Chronic renal failure: Class VI
- Other features: Serositis, skin rash (malar, butterfly), anemia, arthritis, lymphadenopathy, thrombotic manifestations

Laboratory Tests
- Autoantibodies
  - 95% have autoantibodies to nuclear components
    - > 95% ANA (speckled pattern)
    - 30-70% anti-dsDNA
    - 30-50% anti-Ro (SSA)
    - 30-40% anti-U1RNP
    - 20-40% anti-Sm (highly specific for SLE)
  - 40-50% anticardiolipin
    - 15% antiphospholipid
  - 30-50% anti-C1q
    - Associations with lupus nephritis strongest for antibodies to dsDNA and C1q
- Complement levels
  - ↓ C3 in 30-50%, ↓ C4 in 67-80%, more common in active disease

Treatment
- Drugs
  - Immunosuppressive therapy used to decrease or arrest IC deposits, inflammation, and necrosis
    - Glucocorticoids, mycophenolate mofetil, cyclophosphamide

- Chlorambucil and azathioprine
  o Anti-B-cell antibodies targeting CD20 (rituximab) under evaluation
- Transplantation
  o Clinically significant recurrence is rare (~ 2%)
    ▪ IF studies detect subclinical recurrence in ~ 40%

Prognosis
- Typically remitting and recurring course
- 25% develop end-stage renal failure
  o 10-year renal survival is ~ 75%
  o 10-year patient survival is 72-98%
- Common causes of death
  o Infection, especially pneumonia
  o Chronic renal failure
  o Neoplasms: B-cell lymphomas, lung carcinoma

General Approach
- Kidneys are biopsied in SLE to determine type of renal disease, acute inflammatory activity, and extent of glomerular and tubulointerstitial scarring
- Accurate assessment requires at least 20 glomeruli
- 2004 ISN/RPS classification is standard for lupus glomerulonephritis

MICROSCOPIC PATHOLOGY

Histologic Features
- Lupus nephritis affects glomeruli, peritubular capillaries, muscular blood vessels, tubules, and interstitium with a spectrum of lesions
- Glomeruli
  o Glomerular lesions determine ISN/RPS classification (classes I-VI)
    ▪ Lesions can be active (acute) or chronic (sclerosing)
    ▪ Focal (< 50% of glomeruli affected; III) or diffuse (≥ 50% of glomeruli affected; IV)
    ▪ Segmental (part of a glomerulus) or global (> 50% of a glomerulus)
    ▪ Distinction between III and IV is only by extent of these lesions (< or ≥ 50%, respectively)
  o Normal (I)
    ▪ Requires mesangial IgG to diagnose lupus class I
    ▪ Class I is seen in < 1% of biopsies for cause
  o Mesangial hypercellularity (II)
    ▪ By itself is not considered an active lesion
    ▪ Class II is seen in 10-15% of biopsies
  o Endocapillary hypercellularity (III, IV)
    ▪ Proliferation of intrinsic glomerular cells and accumulation of leukocytes with capillary luminal reduction
    ▪ Class III is seen in 15-25% of biopsies
    ▪ Class IV is seen in 40-60% of biopsies
  o Extracapillary hypercellularity (crescents) (III, IV)
    ▪ Proliferation of parietal epithelium, accumulation of leukocytes, especially macrophages
    ▪ Defined as > 2 cells thick, > 25% of circumference of capsule
    ▪ Cellular or fibrous
    ▪ GBM rupture associated with crescents
  o Karyorrhexis, fibrinoid necrosis (III, IV)

- Prominent subendothelial deposits ("wire loops") (III, IV)
  ▪ Trichrome stain useful
  o Hyaline "pseudothrombi" (III, IV)
  o Hematoxylin bodies specific but rare (III, IV)
    ▪ In vivo LE cell
  o Membranous lesions (V)
    ▪ Diffuse thickening of GBM with granular subepithelial deposits (trichrome) with silver-positive "spikes"
    ▪ Class V is seen in 10-15% of biopsies
  o Chronic glomerular lesions
    ▪ Included in count of involved glomeruli for III vs. IV, if believed to be due to LN
    ▪ Glomerular sclerosis, segmental or global
    ▪ Glomerular fibrous adhesions
    ▪ Fibrous crescents
    ▪ GBM duplication
  o Variants
    ▪ Some patients with minimal lupus (I-II) present with podocytopathy (minimal change disease and focal segmental glomerulosclerosis)
    ▪ Focal segmental glomerular sclerosis can be a late scarring phase of lupus nephritis or secondary to loss of nephrons
    ▪ Pathology may be dominated by lesions of thrombotic microangiopathy with little immune complex disease
- Tubules and interstitium
  o Tubulointerstitial lesions are most commonly seen in association with class III and IV glomerular lesions
    ▪ May be active or chronic
    ▪ Occur ± IgG and C3 positive immune deposits
  o Active lesions are composed of T cells, macrophages, B cells, plasma cells, and neutrophils; with edema and tubulitis
    ▪ Tubulointerstitial immune deposits may be associated with lymphoid aggregates
  o Chronic lesions are characterized by interstitial fibrosis and tubular atrophy
  o Occasional cases have predominately tubulointerstitial disease with only minimal glomerular disease (e.g., class II)
- Vessels: 6 patterns observed
  o Normal (negative IF)
  o Uncomplicated vascular immune deposits
    ▪ Normal-looking vessels with IgG, IgA, IgM, C3, and C1q by IF
  o Noninflammatory lupus vasculopathy
    ▪ Hyaline deposits with Ig and C by IF
  o Necrotizing lupus vasculitis
    ▪ Fibrinoid necrosis and leukocytoclasis ± immune deposits
  o Thrombotic microangiopathy
    ▪ ± class III or IV glomerular lesions
  o Arterial and arteriolar sclerosis
    ▪ Nonlupus vasculopathy without immune deposits

SYSTEMIC LUPUS ERYTHEMATOSUS

ANCILLARY TESTS

Immunofluorescence
- Detection of IgG deposits in glomeruli essential for diagnosis
  o Usually accompanied by IgA, IgM, C3, and C1q ("full house")
  o Kappa and lambda equal
  o IgG1 and IgG3 are predominate subclasses
  o Fibrin in necrotizing lesions and thrombi
- Glomerular patterns
  o Mesangial only (class I, II)
  o Capillary wall, focal or diffuse, coarse granular, elongated (class III, IV)
  o Capillary wall, diffuse, finely granular (class V)
- Tubules
  o Granular IgG with variable other components common in tubular basement membrane (~ 50% of cases)
- Vessels
  o IgG and other components sometimes seen in small arteries, arterioles, and peritubular capillaries

Electron Microscopy
- Amorphous electron-dense deposits present in glomeruli in varied locations and extent
  o Mesangium, subendothelium, subepithelium
  o Subepithelial deposits sometimes penetrate GBM
  o Substructure may be focally manifested as "thumbprint" pattern
- Extraglomerular deposits of similar nature
  o Tubular basement membrane, Bowman capsule, peritubular capillaries, interstitium, small arteries
- Glomerular endothelial cells have tubuloreticular structures
  o Clusters of vesicles and tubules of diameter 20-25 nm in endoplasmic reticulum
  o Consequence of elevated levels of interferon

DIFFERENTIAL DIAGNOSIS

Type II Mixed Cryoglobulinemia
- Fibrillary substructure of deposits
- Macrophage predominance in glomerular capillaries
- Deposits can be sparse, usually little subepithelial
  o IgM-predominant immunoglobulin
- "Pseudothrombi" do not distinguish
- Often associated with hepatitis C virus

Membranoproliferative GN, Type I/III
- C3-dominant deposits, IgG, and IgM in a band-like pattern along capillary walls
- Usually no C1q
- Lupus serologies negative

Postinfectious GN
- IgG and C3 in a characteristic coarse granular ("lumpy-bumpy") pattern, with hump-like deposits along subepithelium
- Usually little C1q
- Deposits in GBM ("humps") do not have "spikes"

Idiopathic Membranous GN
- Absence of subendothelial, mesangial, and extraglomerular deposits, and tubuloreticular inclusions
- Antibodies to phospholipase A2 receptors
- Deposits typically do not penetrate the GBM

Drug-induced LN
- Many drugs implicated, e.g., propylthiouracil, isoniazid, hydralazine, procainamide, chlorpromazine
- Few have anti-ds DNA antibodies or renal disease (5%)
  o High frequency of antihistone antibodies
- Proof requires improvement after drug withdrawal

Lupus-like GN in HIV
- Negative or low titer ANA and negative dsDNA antibodies by definition
- 50% diffuse, 45% focal, and 5% membranous pattern
- ~ 20% of renal biopsies in HIV-infected patients

IgA Nephropathy
- IgA-dominant deposits without tubuloreticular inclusions or extraglomerular immune deposits

C1q Nephropathy
- Abundant mesangial immune deposits, with predominance of C1q
- No clinical evidence of lupus

Pauci-immune Crescentic GN
- Little or no endocapillary hypercellularity with little Ig and C deposition

Sjögren Syndrome
- Distinction based on serology and clinical features

DIAGNOSTIC CHECKLIST

Clinically Relevant Pathologic Features
- Histologic predictors of poor renal outcome
  o Class of LN broadly correlates with outcome but is less of a predictor because of tendency for class changes in follow-up biopsies
    ▪ In general, mesangial and membranous lesions have better prognosis than focal or diffuse proliferative lesions
  o Amount of subendothelial deposits
  o Activity index
  o Chronicity index
- ISN/RPS class, activity and chronicity indices, and presence of tubulointerstitial or vascular disease are essential for clinical management

Pathologic Interpretation Pearls
- Lupus nephritis is in differential diagnosis of almost every renal biopsy
- Heterogeneity of glomerular lesions by LM, glomerular and extraglomerular IgG, and endothelial tubuloreticular inclusions are most important diagnostic clues to LN
- Hematoxylin bodies are pathognomonic but rare

SYSTEMIC LUPUS ERYTHEMATOSUS

ISN/RPS Classification of Lupus Glomerulonephritis (2004)

Class	Name	Definition	Comments
I	Minimal mesangial LN	Normal by LM with mesangial deposits by IF or EM	May have other features such as podocytopathy or tubulointerstitial disease
II	Mesangial proliferative LN	Purely mesangial hypercellularity by LM with mesangial deposits by IF; may be few subepithelial or subendothelial deposits by IF or EM	May have other features such as podocytopathy, tubulointerstitial disease, or TMA
III	Focal LN	Active or inactive segmental or global endocapillary &/or extracapillary GN by LM in < 50% of glomeruli; usually with subendothelial deposits; designate whether lesions are active (A) &/or chronic (C)	Active lesions include endocapillary hypercellularity, cellular crescents, neutrophils/karyorrhexis, necrosis, and "wire loops"; chronic lesions include segmental or global glomerulosclerosis considered to be due to LN, and fibrous crescents
IV	Diffuse segmental or global LN	Active or inactive endocapillary &/or extracapillary GN by LM in ≥ 50% of glomeruli; designate whether lesions are active (A) &/or chronic (C) and whether lesions are either segmental (S) or global (G)	Examples: Class IV-S(A), segmental lesions with active features; class IV-G(A/C), global lesions with both active and chronic features
V	Membranous LN	Global or segmental granular deposits along the GBM by LM and IF or EM; ± mesangial alterations	May occur with class III or IV, which are designated class III/V or class IV/V, respectively
VI	Advanced sclerosing LN	> 90% of glomerular sclerosis without activity	Need to attribute the sclerosis to LN rather than ischemia

GRADING

ISN/RPS Classification of Lupus Glomerulonephritis (2004)

- Based on light and immunofluorescence microscopy; electron microscopy not required
  - ≥ 20 glomeruli should be sampled for accurate classification
  - Tubulointerstitial disease and thrombotic microangiopathy scored separately
  - Classification requires distinction of active and chronic lesions and determination of extent of glomerular involvement by these injury processes
    - Single glomerulus may have both acute/active lesions and chronic/sclerosing lesions
    - Heterogeneity of interglomerular and intraglomerular changes makes classification of these lesions difficult
- Transformation of glomerular lesions in repeat biopsies over months to years
  - Class II lesions upgrade to class III, IV, and V lesions in 33%
  - Class III lesions upgrade to class IV and V in 50%
  - Class IV lesions may upgrade to class V and VI lesions in 15%
  - Class III and IV lesions rarely downgrade to class II
  - Class V lesions may develop proliferative (class III or IV) lesions in ~ 45% of cases
  - Majority of reported cases (78%) have no change of class in follow-up biopsies
- Classes broadly correlate with outcome
  - Class I and II: Best survival
  - Class IV: Worse survival than III
    - Debate whether segmental and diffuse forms of class IV are different
  - Class V: Good long-term survival
  - Class VI: End-stage disease

Activity and Chronicity Indices

- Histologic lesions scored 0, none; 1+, mild; 2+, moderate; 3+, severe and summed
- Activity index (AI) (0-24)
  - Components: Endocapillary hypercellularity, neutrophils, fibrinoid necrosis/karyorrhexis, cellular crescents, "pseudothrombi"/"wire loops"
    - Scores for necrosis, karyorrhexis, and cellular crescents are doubled
- Chronicity index (CI) (0-12)
  - Components: Glomerular sclerosis, fibrous crescents, interstitial fibrosis, and tubular atrophy
- Reproducibility suboptimal

SELECTED REFERENCES

1. Morel L: Genetics of SLE: evidence from mouse models. Nat Rev Rheumatol. 6(6):348-57, 2010
2. Harley IT et al: Genetic susceptibility to SLE: new insights from fine mapping and genome-wide association studies. Nat Rev Genet. 10(5):285-90, 2009
3. Seshan SV et al: Renal disease in systemic lupus erythematosus with emphasis on classification of lupus glomerulonephritis: advances and implications. Arch Pathol Lab Med. 133(2):233-48, 2009
4. Rahman A et al: Systemic lupus erythematosus. N Engl J Med. 358(9):929-39, 2008
5. Furness PN et al: Interobserver reproducibility and application of the ISN/RPS classification of lupus nephritis- a UK-wide study. Am J Surg Pathol. 30(8):1030-5, 2006
6. Hill GS et al: Class IV-S versus class IV-G lupus nephritis: clinical and morphologic differences suggesting different pathogenesis. Kidney Int. 68(5):2288-97, 2005
7. Weening JJ et al: The classification of glomerulonephritis in systemic lupus erythematosus revisited. J Am Soc Nephrol. 15(2):241-50, 2004
8. Austin HA 3rd et al: Prognostic factors in lupus nephritis. Contribution of renal histologic data. Am J Med. 75(3):382-91, 1983

SYSTEMIC LUPUS ERYTHEMATOSUS

ISN/RPS Classification

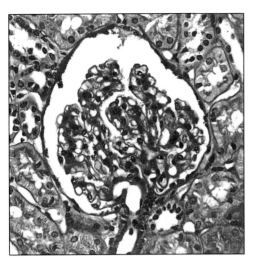
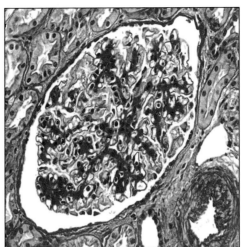

(Left) Class I lupus GN has normal glomeruli by light microscopy and mesangial immune deposits by immunofluorescence and electron microscopy. Class I is rarely seen in biopsies. *(Right)* Class II lupus GN shows mesangial hypercellularity and matrix expansion. Class II may not have subepithelial or subendothelial deposits by light microscopy or active inflammation. Mesangial hypercellularity is defined as ≥ 3 nuclei in 1 mesangial area in sections cut at 3 μm.

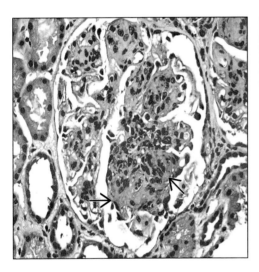
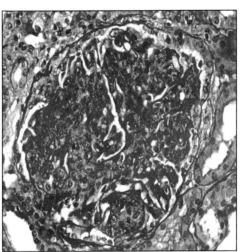

(Left) Class III lupus GN has < 50% of glomeruli involved with active or chronic lesions. A typical pattern is segmental capillary necrosis, with fibrinous ➡ and neutrophilic exudation. *(Right)* Class IV lupus GN has active or chronic lesions in ≥ 50% of glomeruli. One typical pattern shown here is global endocapillary hypercellularity with a homogeneous mononuclear cell population. The endocapillary cells are a combination of macrophages, mesangial cells, and endothelial cells.

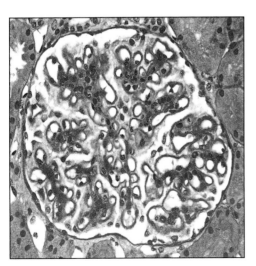
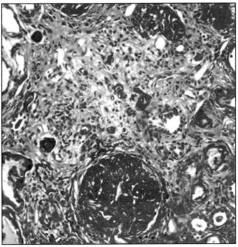

(Left) Class V lupus GN has diffuse and global thickening of the GBM and prominent podocytes, ± mesangial expansion and hypercellularity. *(Right)* Class VI lupus has predominately globally sclerotic glomeruli due to lupus GN (> 90%). Ischemic glomeruli do not count. Generally, ischemic glomeruli are collapsed and wrinkled with Bowman space filled in with fibrosis whereas lupus sclerotic glomeruli are larger and fill Bowman space.

SYSTEMIC LUPUS ERYTHEMATOSUS

Inflammatory Lesions

(Left) Marked endocapillary hypercellularity with a mixture of mononuclear and polymorphonuclear leukocytes is evident in this glomerulus. A small cellular crescent is evident ➡. Pericapsulitis is evident above the glomerulus. (Right) Global endocapillary hypercellularity with a mixture of neutrophils and mononuclear cells affects all the glomerular lobules. Pericapsulitis is also evident adjacent to Bowman capsule ➡.

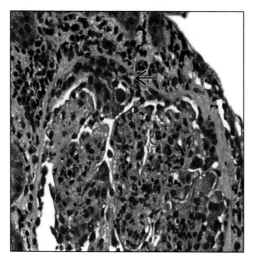
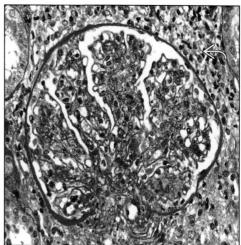

(Left) Segmental lobular expansion with marked hypercellularity ➡ is evident in this glomerulus with adhesion to Bowman capsule. Segmental GN is typical for ISN/RPS class III or class IV-S lupus nephritis. (Right) Diffuse lupus nephritis, ISN/RPS class IV-G (A) has endocapillary and extracapillary hypercellularity in this example. Karyorrhexis and segmental fibrinoid necrosis are also seen ➡.

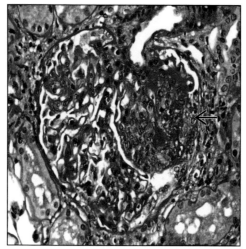
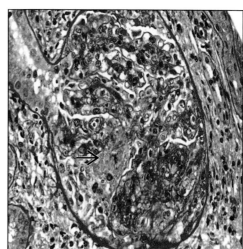

(Left) Segmental endocapillary and extracapillary hypercellularity ➡ is evident in a glomerulus with largely open capillaries and mesangial hypercellularity. These lesions are commonly seen in focal and diffuse segmental lupus nephritis. (Right) PAS shows global endocapillary hypercellularity with neutrophils, mononuclear cells, and numerous karyorrhectic fragments. Glomerular lesions like this are seen typically in diffuse global lupus nephritis, ISN/RPS class IV-G (A).

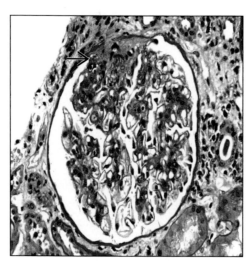
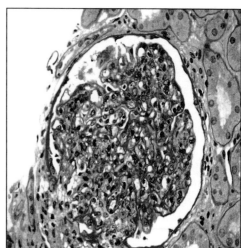

SYSTEMIC LUPUS ERYTHEMATOSUS

Inflammatory Lesions

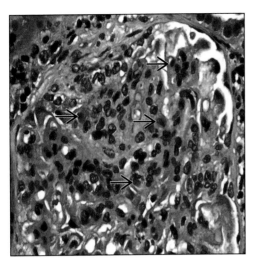 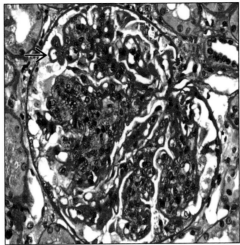

(Left) Marked endocapillary hypercellularity with a relatively uniform population of mononuclear cells and numerous hematoxylin bodies ➡ is shown. *(Right)* More than 50% of the glomerular cross-sectional area has endocapillary hypercellularity, and some capillaries have "wire loop" thickening ➡. Lesions like these are typical in ISN/RPS class IV-G lesions.

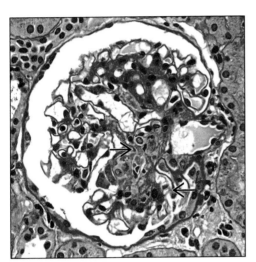 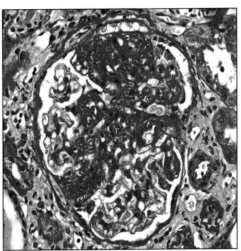

(Left) PAS shows segmental capillary basement membrane rupture with fibrinous and cellular exudation ➡. This was the only such lesion in a sample of 38 glomeruli and resulted in a change from mesangial (ISN/RPS class II) to focal (class III [A]) lupus nephritis. *(Right)* Broad segmental irregular scars with adhesions to Bowman capsule and endocapillary hypercellularity are features indicative of sclerosing GN. Such lesions can be seen in ISN/RPS class III (C) or IV-S (C) lupus nephritis.

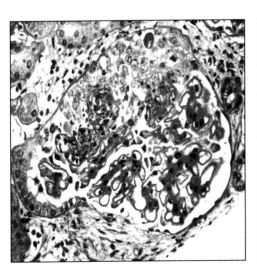 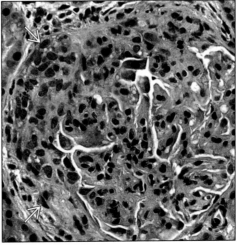

(Left) Membranous lupus GN may have segmental endocapillary and extracapillary hypercellularity, with karyorrhexis and a crescent. This is an example of mixed membranous and exudative/proliferative GN, ISN/RPS class III (A) and V lupus nephritis. *(Right)* Cellular crescents can be conspicuous in lupus nephritis (here in a class IV). A crescent is defined as a layer of 3 or more cells lining at least 25% of the circumference of Bowman capsule ➡.

SYSTEMIC LUPUS ERYTHEMATOSUS

GBM Lesions

(Left) *"Wire loop" thickening of the GBM in a patient with lupus GN (class IV) is shown. "Wire loops" are due to subendothelial deposits and were initially described in lupus by Baehr, Klemperer, and Shifrin in 1935.* *(Right) Segmental hyaline "wire loop" thickening* ⇒ *of the glomerular capillary walls may be evident without significant endocapillary hypercellularity.*

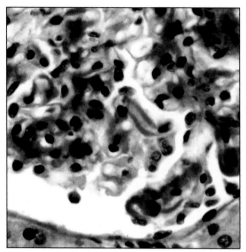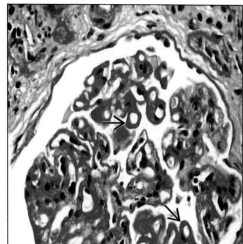

(Left) *"Wire loops"* ⇒ *and marked mesangial hypercellularity are evident in this glomerulus. Lesions like these may be class III or IV-S depending on the proportion of glomeruli with "wire loop" lesions.* *(Right) Duplication of the GBM can be marked* ⇒*, as in this case with lobular expansion with increased mesangial matrix, imparting a membranoproliferative glomerulonephritis-like appearance. Lesions like this are seen in ISN/RPS class IV-G lesions.*

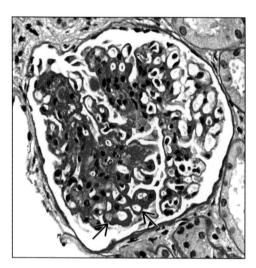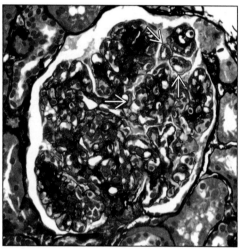

(Left) *Global subepithelial "spike" formation* ⇒ *is evident on Jones silver methenamine stain in an example of membranous lupus nephritis, ISN/RPS class V.* *(Right) Global subepithelial "spike" formation is barely evident* ⇒ *at this power in a glomerulus from a patient with SLE. There is little hypercellularity. Pure membranous glomerulopathy, ISN/RPS class V, is found in 10-15% of lupus nephritis biopsies.*

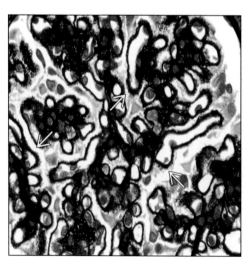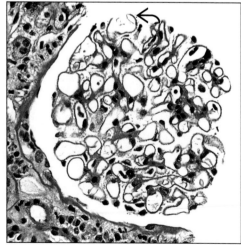

SYSTEMIC LUPUS ERYTHEMATOSUS

Variant Microscopic Features

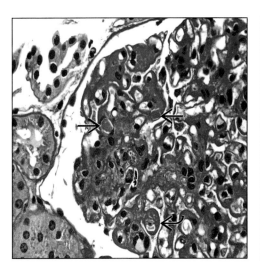
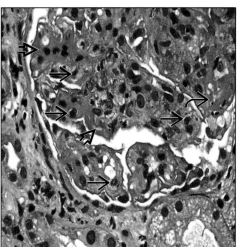

(Left) Hyaline "pseudothrombi" ➡ and "wire loop" thickening ➡ are evident in capillaries of this glomerulus. Such lesions may be associated with cryoglobulinemia in SLE. *(Right)* Abundant hematoxylin bodies ➡ are evident in a glomerulus with active lupus glomerulonephritis. Hyaline material corresponding to immune deposits is also evident ➡. Segmental fibrinoid exudate with nuclear karyorrhexis is also evident ➡.

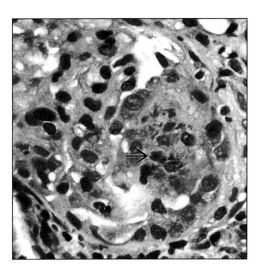
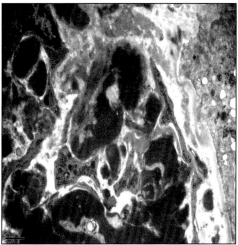

(Left) Hematoxylin bodies ➡ are pathognomonic of systemic lupus erythematosus. These are composed of large fragments of nuclear protein and nucleic acid with bound antinuclear antibody. *(Right)* Electron-dense nuclear fragments comprise the bulk of these hematoxylin bodies seen by electron microscopy. These are composed of nuclear histone proteins, nucleic acids, and bound antinuclear antibodies.

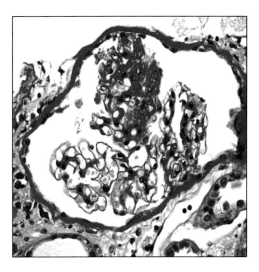
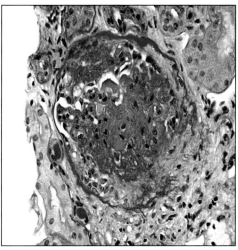

(Left) PAS shows segmental glomerular sclerosis in a biopsy with lupus nephritis. The distinction of segmental glomerular sclerosis due to prior inflammation from a lupus podocytopathy can be difficult. *(Right)* Diffuse glomerular sclerosis with fibrous crescent and disruption of Bowman capsule basement membrane is the type of lesion seen in sclerosing glomerulonephritis ISN/RPS class IV-G (C) or class VI lupus nephritis.

Variant Microscopic Features

(Left) Lupus podocytopathy with capillary collapse and visceral epithelial cell hyperplasia are features of collapsing glomerulopathy, arising in this case in a patient with SLE (silver stain). *(Right)* Segmental proliferative and exudative GN with neutrophils and karyorrhexis are evident in the lower 1/2 of this glomerulus. The upper lobules have mesangial hypercellularity ➡. This is an example of recurrent lupus nephritis in a renal allograft.

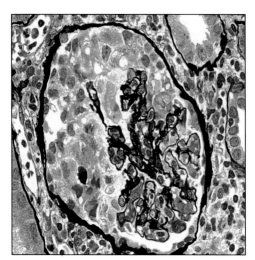 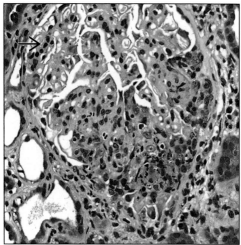

(Left) Segmental endocapillary hypercellularity and capillary basement membrane rupture ➡ may be subtle. In this case, 1 of 30 glomeruli had such a lesion. *(Right)* PAS shows a glomerulus with minimal mesangial thickening and hypercellularity ➡. Immune complexes were evident by IF (IgG and C3). This is an example of mild class II lupus nephritis. A few intracapillary leukocytes are present ➡.

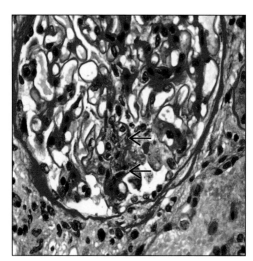 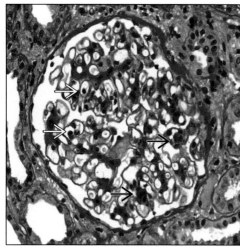

(Left) PAS shows thrombotic microangiopathy (TMA) ➡ involving the perihilar glomerular vessels and adjacent arteriole. This biopsy has mixed membranous and segmental sclerosing GN (ISN/ RPS class III [C] and V). *(Right)* Thrombotic microangiopathy in a 13-year-old girl with lupus anticoagulant is shown. Antiphospholipid syndrome occurs in about 1/3 of lupus patients with renal biopsies. TMA may be present in the absence of immune complex-mediated lesions of lupus.

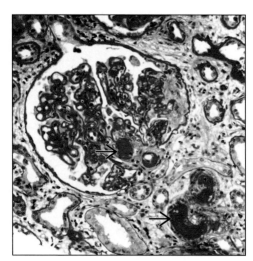 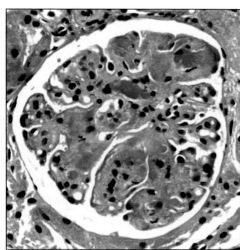

SYSTEMIC LUPUS ERYTHEMATOSUS

Immunofluorescence

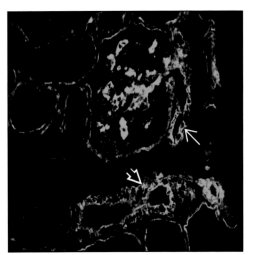 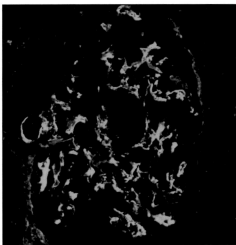

(Left) Immune complex deposits may affect any compartment of the kidney in lupus nephritis. IF demonstrates IgG in the glomerular mesangium, Bowman capsule, tubular basement membranes, and within the walls of arterioles ➡ adjacent to the glomerulus and in small arteries ⬀. (Right) In minimal mesangial and mesangial proliferative GN, ISN/RPS Classes I and II, there is typically global mesangial staining for IgG, as evident in this illustration.

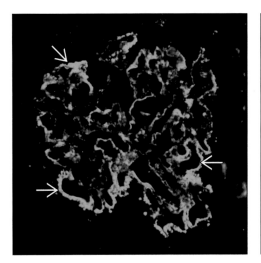 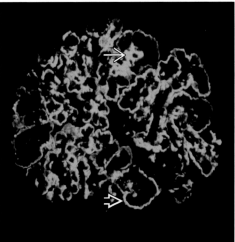

(Left) Segmental granular capillary wall staining for IgG ➡ is a feature of segmental lupus nephritis and a pattern frequently seen in ISN/RPS Classes III and IV-S. (Right) Bright granular mesangial ➡ and capillary wall ⬀ staining for IgG is evident in this example from a biopsy with diffuse global lupus glomerulonephritis, ISN/RPS class IV-G (A).

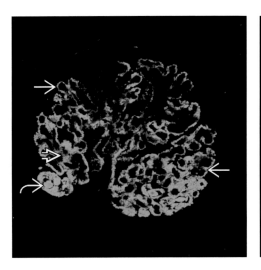 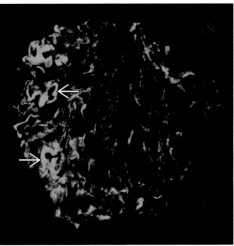

(Left) Immunofluorescence staining for IgG reveals global granular capillary wall staining ➡, with segmental mesangial staining ⬀. Hyaline "pseudothrombi" ⬂, which are large intracapillary immune complex deposits, have a globular staining pattern. (Right) Segmental band-like staining for IgG ➡ highlights subendothelial wire loop deposits in a biopsy with diffuse segmental lupus glomerulonephritis, ISN/RPS class IV-S (A).

SYSTEMIC LUPUS ERYTHEMATOSUS

Immunofluorescence

(Left) Global confluent granular staining of the glomerular capillary walls and segmental staining of the mesangium ➡ are seen in membranous lupus nephritis, ISN/RPS class V. *(Right)* Immunofluorescence staining for IgA shows widespread granular deposits predominately along the GBM. In contrast, IgA nephropathy shows predominantly mesangial IgA deposits and minor GBM deposits.

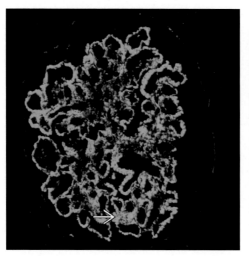
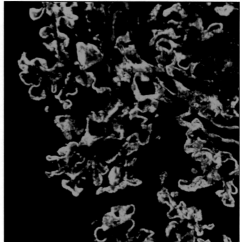

(Left) C1q is usually conspicuous in lupus nephritis. In this biopsy from a patient with class IV and V lupus glomerulonephritis, C1q is seen along the GBM in coarse granular deposits. *(Right)* The "wire loop" lesions of lupus are due to subendothelial deposits, which, like the mesangial deposits, typically stain for all of the usual reactants (IgG, IgM, IgA, C3, C1q), a "full house."

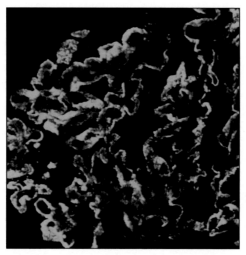
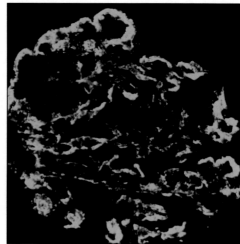

(Left) Fibrin is present in an arteriole in the vascular pole ➡ and segmentally in the glomerular tuft ➡ in a lupus patient with a high titer of IgG anticardiolipin antibodies. The dominant feature was thrombotic microangiopathy. *(Right)* Nuclear staining is sometimes detected in frozen sections of lupus nephritis. The IgG probably is from the plasma and binds to the nuclear antigens as a consequence of the permeabilization of the cells by freezing.

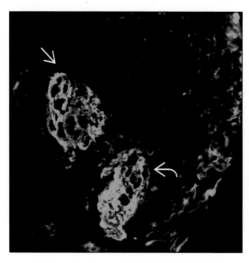
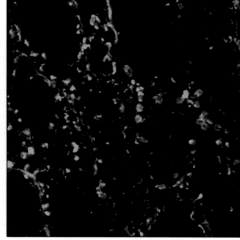

SYSTEMIC LUPUS ERYTHEMATOSUS

Electron Microscopy

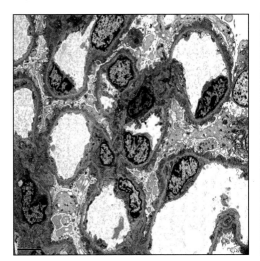

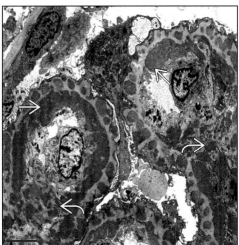

(Left) Mesangial and subepithelial electron-dense deposits are evident in this glomerulus with membranous (class V) and mesangial (class II) lupus nephritis. Podocytes have reactive changes with effacement of the foot processes. *(Right)* Subepithelial, intramembranous, subendothelial ➔, and mesangial ➹ dense deposits are evident in a biopsy with diffuse global lupus nephritis and membranous lupus nephritis, mixed class IV-G and V.

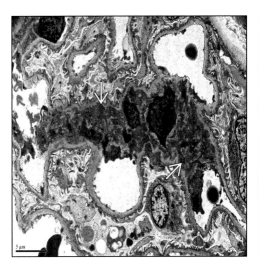

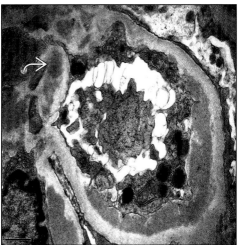

(Left) Mesangial proliferative lupus nephritis has abundant amorphous granular electron-dense deposits ➔. These are absent from the capillary walls. Podocyte foot processes are preserved. *(Right)* Subendothelial electron-dense deposit, the ultrastructural correlate of "wire loop" thickening, is evident in this capillary from a biopsy with diffuse lupus nephritis, ISN/RPS class IV-G. The endothelium is swollen, and there are numerous mesangial deposits ➹.

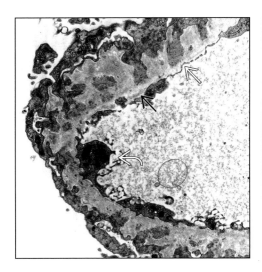

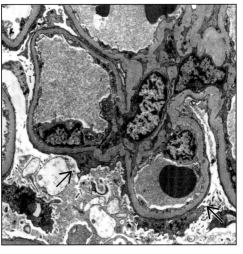

(Left) Deposits in class V lupus nephritis may penetrate the GBM ➔, in contrast to idiopathic membranous glomerulonephritis (MGN). Mesangial deposits, subendothelial deposits ➔, and tubuloreticular structures ➹ also favor lupus over idiopathic MGN. *(Right)* Minimal change disease in a patient with SLE for 15 years and heavy proteinuria. Foot processes are diffusely effaced ➔ without GBM deposits. Scant mesangial deposits were present (none in this field).

Electron Microscopy

(Left) Epimembranous and intramembranous electron-dense deposits are shown in an example of membranous lupus nephritis with mesangial immune complex deposits. **(Right)** Electron-dense deposits are seen along the subendothelium in this example from a biopsy with focal lupus nephritis. These deposits are associated with a well-formed tubuloreticular inclusion in the capillary endothelium.

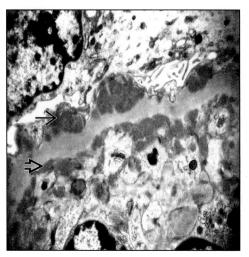 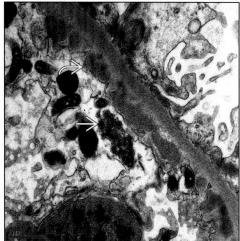

(Left) A swollen glomerular capillary endothelial cell has a tubuloreticular inclusion. There is subendothelial widening without electron-dense deposits at this site. Subepithelial deposits are evident. **(Right)** Tubuloreticular inclusions are most frequently observed in glomerular capillary endothelium; however, such lesions can also be seen in the peritubular capillary endothelium.

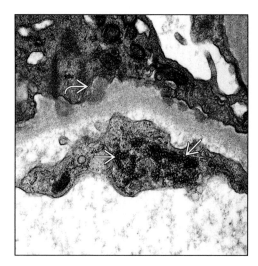 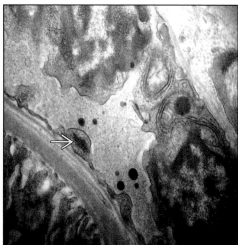

(Left) A large accumulation of mesangial electron-dense deposit seen in this illustration has a distinctive concentric tubular substructure, giving rise to the term "fingerprint deposits." **(Right)** A high-power electron micrograph of glomerular mesangium shows the parallel arrays of deposits with regular spacing, resembling fingerprints in lupus nephritis. These distinctive and probably pathognomonic deposits are unrelated to cryoglobulins and are found in about 6-20% of lupus biopsies.

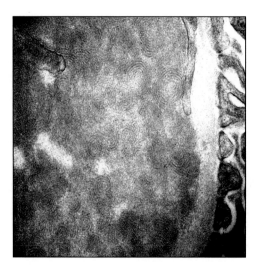 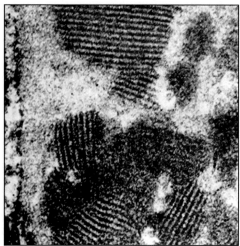

SYSTEMIC LUPUS ERYTHEMATOSUS

Tubulointerstitial Disease

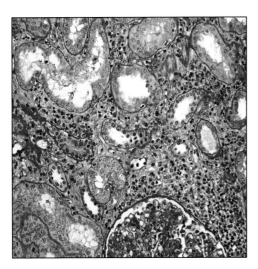
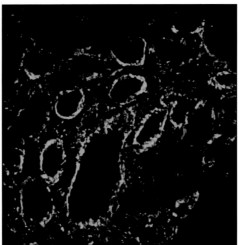

(Left) Tubulointerstitial nephritis shows a mononuclear inflammatory infiltrate composed of lymphocytes and numerous plasma cells in lupus nephritis. The glomerulus is hypercellular. *(Right)* Granular staining of the TBM and the interstitium by IF is evident in 30-60% of lupus nephritis with focal or diffuse GN. These deposits are often, but not always, accompanied by tubulointerstitial inflammation or fibrosis. C3, C1q, and light chains are commonly present with IgG.

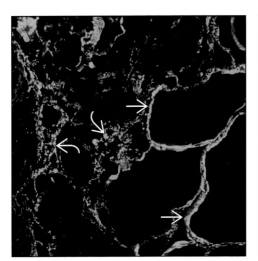
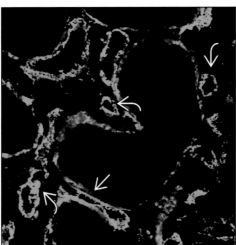

(Left) Prominent immunoglobulin deposits are present along the TBM ➡️ and in the interstitium ➡️, typical of lupus nephritis. Mixed cryoglobulinemia can have similar deposits in the interstitium. *(Right)* Deposits are found in occasional lupus cases in the peritubular capillaries, here detected with an antibody to C4d ➡️. The coarse granular pattern contrasts with the linear stain found in humoral rejection. TBM also contains C4d ➡️.

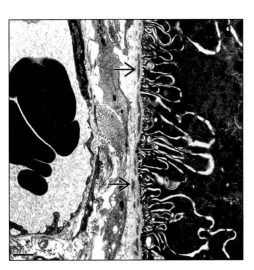
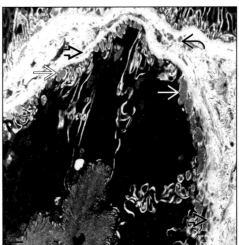

(Left) Tubulointerstitial and TBM electron-dense deposits ➡️ may be evident in the setting of lupus nephritis. There is an association between the presence of lymphoid aggregates and TBM immune deposits. *(Right)* Electron-dense deposits beneath the tubular epithelium ➡️, within the tubular basement ➡️, and on the outer aspect of the tubular basement membrane ➡️ are shown. Such deposits may or may not be associated with tubulointerstitial inflammation.

Glomerular Diseases

Lymphoid Aggregates

(Left) Prominent tubulointerstitial inflammation composed of mononuclear cells and numerous granulocytes ➡ may also be seen in LN. Interstitial fibrosis and early tubular atrophy are also evident in this section. Tubulointerstitial immune deposits may be seen with these findings. **(Right)** Lymphoid aggregates with germinal centers may sometimes be evident in tubulointerstitial nephritis of SLE. Immunohistochemical staining for T and B cells may be helpful in the exclusion of lymphoma in these instances.

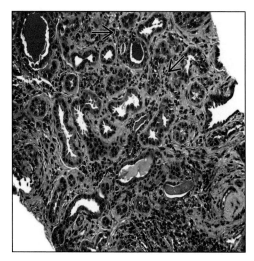
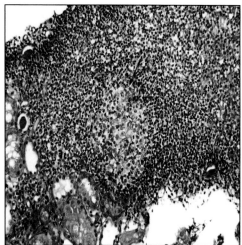

(Left) This tubulointerstitial lymphoid aggregate stained for B cells (anti-CD20) demonstrates prominent B-cell populations in the reactive germinal center with B cells scattered in the surrounding interstitium. **(Right)** This tubulointerstitial lymphoid aggregate stained for T cells by CD3 highlights scattered T cells in the germinal center and numerous cells in the marginal zone and surrounding interstitium.

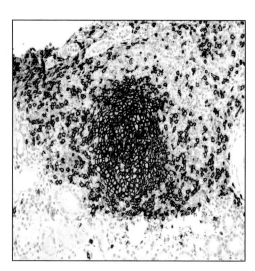
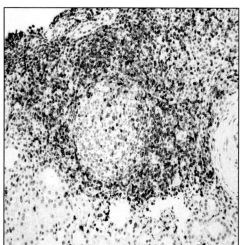

(Left) This tubulointerstitial lymphoid aggregate has a prominent network of follicular dendritic cells that stain for CD21 by immunohistochemistry. **(Right)** Lymphoid nodules are a common finding in LN, typically with chronic tubulointerstitial inflammation and class III or IV GN.

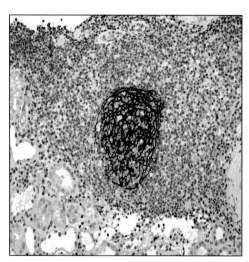
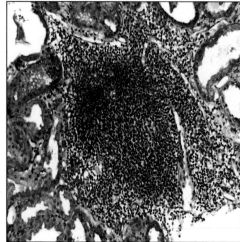

SYSTEMIC LUPUS ERYTHEMATOSUS

Vascular Lesions

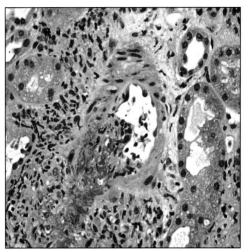
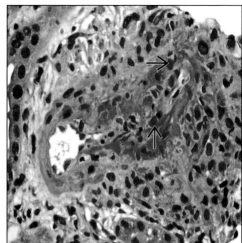

(Left) Necrotizing lupus arteritis with intimal inflammation, fibrin exudation, and medial necrosis with hematoxyphilic material is shown. *(Right)* Necrotizing lupus arteritis with transmural fibrinoid necrosis and numerous hematoxylin bodies ➡ is shown. Perivascular macrophages are also evident.

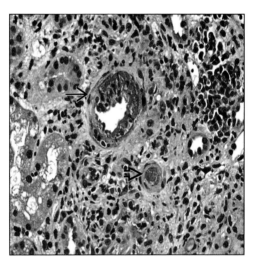
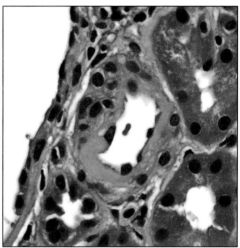

(Left) Necrotizing lupus arteritis ➡ has intimal and medial inflammation, leukocytoclasis, and fibrinoid necrosis. Thrombotic occlusion of a noninflamed arteriole is also evident ➡ in a biopsy with active lupus nephritis. *(Right)* Lupus vasculopathy with mural hyalinization is shown. The hyaline deposits lie just beneath the endothelium and stain for IgG, IgA, IgM, C3, and C1q by IF.

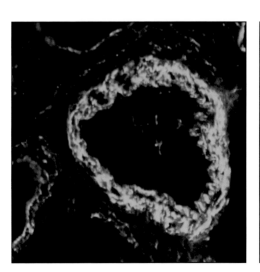
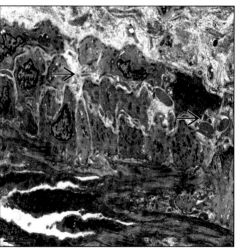

(Left) Granular IgG is often detectable by IF in the intima and media of arteries, frequently without morphologic abnormalities. *(Right)* Ultrastructural features of uncomplicated vascular wall immune deposits ➡ in a biopsy from a patient with lupus nephritis are shown. The deposits are located between the smooth muscle cells of the tunica media. The vessels were unremarkable by light microscopy.

MIXED CONNECTIVE TISSUE DISEASE

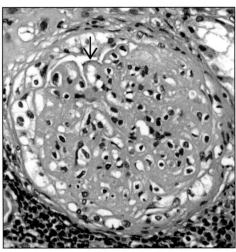

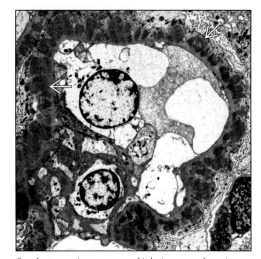

Glomerulus from a 58-year-old woman with a 20-year history of mixed connective tissue disease shows a markedly increased mesangial matrix and thick-ended glomerular basement membranes ➡.

By electron microscopy, multiple immune deposits are seen along the basement membrane ➡ in a case of membranous glomerulopathy due to mixed connective tissue disease.

TERMINOLOGY

Abbreviations
- Mixed connective tissue disease (MCTD)

Synonyms
- Undifferentiated autoimmune rheumatic and connective tissue disorder

Definitions
- Overlap syndrome with features of systemic lupus erythematosus (SLE), polymyositis, & systemic sclerosis (i.e., scleroderma)

ETIOLOGY/PATHOGENESIS

Autoimmune Disease of Unknown Etiology
- Autoantibodies may play pathogenetic role
- Those with antibody (Ab) to 70 kD U1-ribonucleoprotein (RNP) share common epitope with DR-molecule Ag-binding groove, suggesting Ag-driven anti-U1-RNP acquisition

CLINICAL ISSUES

Epidemiology
- Age
  - Usually 2nd to 3rd decades of life
- Gender
  - Female:male ≈ 16:1

Presentation
- Renal dysfunction of variable severity
  - Adults (10-26%) & children (33-50%)
- Proteinuria
  - ~ 20% at least mild (~ 500 mg/d)
  - Heavy proteinuria in ~ 1/3 ± nephrotic syndrome
- Microhematuria
- Hypocomplementemia

- Hypertension (HTN)
  - May be marked ± microangiopathic hemolytic anemia & renal failure, resembling "scleroderma kidney"
- Other organs
  - Mitral valve prolapse, esophageal & other dysmotility, hepatosplenomegaly, serositis, & lymphadenopathy
  - Restrictive lung disease
    - Impaired lung diffusion & pulmonary HTN
- Cutaneous lesions
  - Ulcers, digital & oral, including discoid, lupus-like disease
  - Digital gangrene, Raynaud phenomenon, swelling or sclerodermatous hand changes, or other vasculitis features
  - Alopecia, malar erythema, or photosensitivity
  - Edematous & puffy 1st & then tighter, "hide-bound"
- Arthritis/arthralgias, sometimes deforming
- Myositis

Laboratory Tests
- Anti-U1-small & heterogeneous nuclear RNP (U1-snRNP & hnRNP-A2) may be most characteristic of MCTD
  - U1-RNP Ab linked to SLE, scleroderma, and myositis overlap syndrome
  - Ab to Ku & U2-RNP seen with polymyositis & scleroderma
- Antinuclear antibody (ANA) often > 1:1,000 to 1:10,000
- Ab to ribonuclease-sensitive, saline-extractable nuclear antigen (ENA) (also termed RNP or Mo)
- Anti-Jo-1 seen with polymyositis & pulmonary fibrosis

Treatment
- Drugs
  - Steroids (i.e., corticosteroids)
    - Treats inflammatory & arthritic symptoms & crescentic lesions, leaving glomerulosclerosis

MIXED CONNECTIVE TISSUE DISEASE

Key Facts

Terminology
- Mixed connective tissue disease (MCTD)
- Overlap syndrome with features of systemic lupus erythematosus (SLE), polymyositis, & systemic sclerosis (i.e., scleroderma)

Clinical Issues
- Female:male ≈ 16:1
- 2nd to 3rd decades of life
- Renal dysfunction
- Proteinuria up to nephrotic range ± hematuria
- Systemic and pulmonary hypertension
- Cutaneous lesions: Ulcers, hand swelling, acrosclerosis, Raynaud, & vasculitis-like lesions
- Arthritis/arthralgias
- Myositis, synovitis, esophageal/other GI dysmotility, mitral valve prolapse

- ANA often > 1:1,000 to 1:10,000
- Various anti-ribonucleoproteins (RNPs)
- Steroid (i.e., corticosteroids) treatment used

Microscopic Pathology
- Glomerular lesions (membranous most common & also mesangial)
- ± crescents, fibrinoid necrosis
- Vascular disease, sometimes severe (22% of Bennett series)

Ancillary Tests
- Deposits on IF, IgG, & C3 most commonly ± others
- Deposits & tubuloreticular inclusions on EM

Top Differential Diagnoses
- Correlate pathology clinically to exclude other "collagen vascular" diseases (e.g., SLE)

- Sclerodermatous-type lesions or gastrointestinal dysmotility not typically alleviated

Prognosis
- Chronic renal failure in ~ 14%
- Morbidity (common) & mortality (10-20%)
  - Pulmonary HTN
  - Coronary or intrarenal artery vascular disease

MICROSCOPIC PATHOLOGY

Histologic Features
- Renal disease in 64%, Japanese autopsy series (Sawai)
- Glomeruli
  - Membranous nephropathy (35-40% of patients) most common (Bennett, Sawai)
  - Mesangial lesions in 35% (Bennett)
  - Membranoproliferative (7%) (Sawai)
  - Mesangial proliferative (7%) (Sawai)
  - 2° renal amyloidosis & minimal change nephrotic syndromes
  - ± glomerular fibrinoid necrosis & crescents
- Interstitial disease in 15% (Bennett)
- Vascular disease in 22% (Bennett)
  - Arterial intimal fibrosis ± mucoid intimal change
  - Medial hyperplasia
  - Fibrinoid necrosis & renal infarcts

ANCILLARY TESTS

Immunofluorescence
- Mesangial and GBM granular IgG & C3 (~ 30% of patients) ± IgA
  - May accompany diffuse mesangial & focal proliferative changes
- ± subendothelial IgG, IgA, IgM, & C3

Electron Microscopy
- Transmission
  - Amorphous deposits & tubuloreticular inclusions as in SLE

- "Fingerprint" lesions (± cryoglobulin)
- Tubular basement membrane deposits

DIFFERENTIAL DIAGNOSIS

Lupus Erythematosus
- Primarily excluded on basis of clinical features and autoantibodies

Membranous Glomerulonephritis (MGN)
- Mesangial and TBM deposits argue against idiopathic MGN

DIAGNOSTIC CHECKLIST

Pathologic Interpretation Pearls
- Membranous nephropathy is most common glomerular manifestation of MCTD

Diagnostic Criteria
- Anti-RNP > 1:600 and 3 of the following: Hand edema, synovitis, myositis, Raynaud phenomenon, & acrosclerosis (100% sensitive, 99.6% specific)

SELECTED REFERENCES

1. D'Agati VD: Renal disease in SLE, mixed connective tissue disease, Sjögren's syndrome, & rheumatoid arthritis. In Jennette JC et al: Heptinstall's Pathology of the Kidney. 6th ed. Philadelphia: Lippincott Williams & Wilkins, 2007
2. Venables PJ: Mixed connective tissue disease. Lupus. 15(3):132-7, 2006
3. Sawai T et al: Morphometric analysis of the kidney lesions in mixed connective tissue disease (MCTD). Tohoku J Exp Med. 174(2):141-54, 1994
4. Bennett R: Mixed connective tissue disease. In Grishman E et al: The Kidney in Collagen Vascular Diseases. New York: Raven Press. 167, 1993
5. Alarcón-Segovia D et al: Comparison between 3 diagnostic criteria for mixed connective tissue disease. Study of 593 patients. J Rheumatol. 16(3):328-34, 1989

MIXED CONNECTIVE TISSUE DISEASE

Microscopic Features

(Left) An enlarged glomerulus with an expanded mesangial matrix and thickened glomerular basement membrane ⧉ is seen in this 58-year-old woman with a 20-year history of mixed connective tissue disease (MCTD). *(Right)* In this case of MCTD with membranous glomerulopathy, there are areas of glomerular basement membrane thickening ⧉ appreciable on a PAS stain.

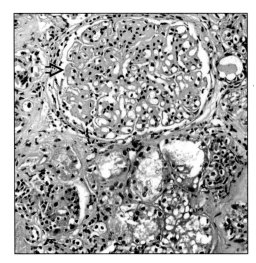
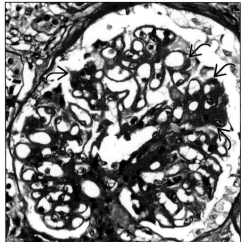

(Left) In this case of MCTD with membranous glomerulopathy, there are areas of basement membrane thickening ⧉ as well as mesangial expansion ⧉, culminating in segmental sclerosis. *(Right)* This trichrome stain of an MCTD case shows areas of glomerular basement membrane thickening ⧉ and mesangial expansion ⧉.

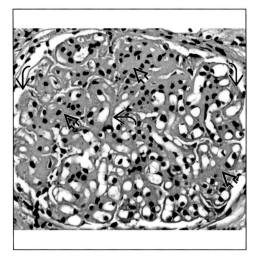
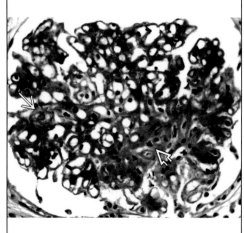

(Left) This PAS stain in a case of MCTD shows areas of glomerular basement membrane thickening ⧉. *(Right)* This trichrome stain of a case of MCTD shows areas of glomerular basement membrane thickening ⧉ and vague small red (fuchsinophilic) dots studding the glomerular basement membrane, which correspond to immune deposits seen on immunofluorescence and electron microscopy.

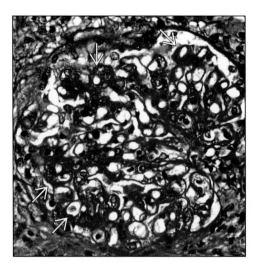
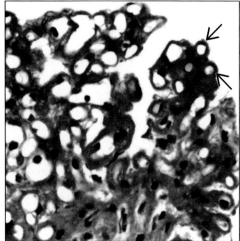

MIXED CONNECTIVE TISSUE DISEASE

Special Stains and Electron Microscopy

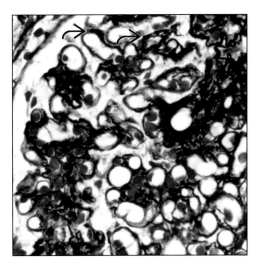
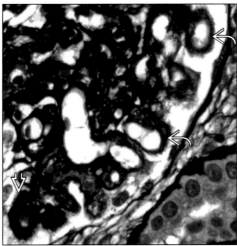

(Left) This silver stain of a case of MCTD shows areas of variable glomerular basement membrane thickening ➡. *(Right)* This high-power view of a silver stain in a case of MCTD shows areas of marked glomerular basement membrane thickening ➡, including an area of granular irregularity ➡, corresponding to immune complex deposition appreciable by immunofluorescence or electron microscopy.

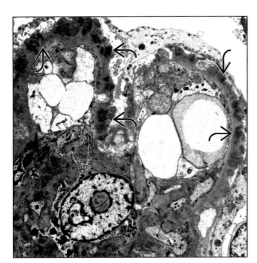
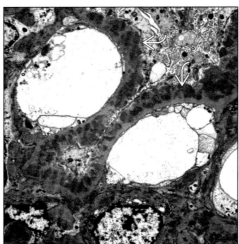

(Left) In this case of MCTD with membranous glomerulopathy, there are multiple immune-type deposits along the glomerular basement membrane ➡. *(Right)* In this case of MCTD with membranous glomerulopathy, there are multiple immune-type deposits ➡ along the glomerular basement membrane.

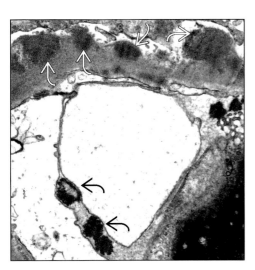
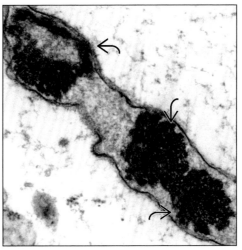

(Left) In this case of membranous glomerulopathy due to MCTD, there are multiple immune-type deposits along the glomerular basement membrane ➡, and there are also tubuloreticular-type inclusions ➡ in the glomerular capillary loop. *(Right)* In this case of MCTD with membranous glomerulopathy, tubuloreticular inclusions also known as "interferon footprints" ➡ are present, as are also seen in SLE and viral infections.

85um33344e44444444

Glomerular Diseases

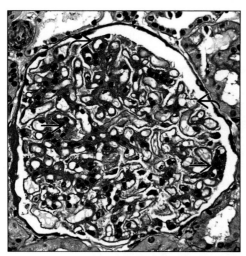 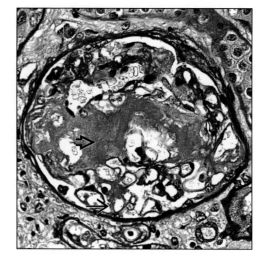

The GBM is diffusely thickened, and segmental increase in mesangial matrix and cellularity is observed in this biopsy specimen with membranous nephropathy. The patient received gold therapy for RA.

Amyloid deposits in the mesangium and capillary walls are weakly PAS positive. The patient has a longstanding history of RA, and chronic inflammation predisposes to AA amyloidosis.

TERMINOLOGY

Abbreviations
- Rheumatoid arthritis (RA)

Definitions
- Renal morphological findings observed in patient with RA, either directly related to RA or due to chronic inflammation and therapy

ETIOLOGY/PATHOGENESIS

Complications of Treatment
- Nonsteroidal anti-inflammatory drugs (NSAIDs) cause tubulointerstitial nephritis and acute renal failure
  - Often occurs after many months of NSAID use
  - Inhibition of cyclooxygenase and reduced synthesis of vasodilatory prostaglandins cause acute renal failure
    - Volume depletion, congestive heart failure, and ascites exacerbate the vasoconstrictor effects of NSAIDs
  - Some patients may also develop minimal change disease due to NSAIDs
- Gold salts and penicillamine therapy results in membranous nephropathy (MGN)
  - No correlation between cumulative dose administered and development of disease
- Cyclosporine nephrotoxicity
  - Related to vasoconstrictor effects or endothelial injury effects of cyclosporine
- Analgesic nephropathy due to use of combination drugs with phenacetin
  - Much less common in modern era, after withdrawal of phenacetin from market
  - Results in chronic interstitial nephritis, interstitial fibrosis, and papillary necrosis

- Penicillamine therapy linked to pauci-immune GN and pulmonary renal syndrome resembling Goodpasture syndrome
- Anti-tumor necrosis factor (TNF)-α can precipitate autoantibody formation
  - Causes proliferative or membranous lupus nephritis, pauci-immune glomerulonephritis (GN), or vasculitis

AA Amyloidosis
- Chronic inflammation in setting of RA can result in AA amyloidosis
- Duration of RA disease is often > 15 years

Renal Disease Directly Related to RA
- Quite rare but has been documented in absence of drug therapy
- Includes glomerular involvement by mesangial proliferative GN, MGN, and pauci-immune GN
- Vasculitis involving renal artery and its branches has been reported
- Thrombotic microangiopathy due to concomitant antiphospholipid antibody syndrome

CLINICAL ISSUES

Epidemiology
- Incidence
  - Renal involvement in RA is predominantly therapy related
    - MGN secondary to gold and penicillamine therapy occurs in 1-10% of RA patients
  - Based on autopsy series, prevalence of AA amyloidosis is approximately 15%
  - Direct kidney involvement as part of RA systemic disease is rare

Presentation
- Kidney involvement

RHEUMATOID ARTHRITIS

Key Facts

Etiology/Pathogenesis
- Predominantly therapy related
  - Tubulointerstitial nephritis and acute renal failure caused by NSAIDs
  - MGN caused by gold salts, penicillamine, and TNF-α antagonists
  - ANCA-related disease precipitated by penicillamine and TN-α antagonists
  - Arteriolar hyalinosis and interstitial fibrosis caused by calcineurin inhibitors
  - Papillary necrosis in analgesic nephropathy
- AA amyloidosis
  - Chronic inflammation in the setting of RA can result in AA amyloidosis
- RA renal diseases unrelated to therapy
  - Quite rare, but has been documented in absence of drug therapy
  - Mesangial proliferative GN, some cases of MGN, ANCA-related disease

Clinical Issues
- Clinical presentation varies based on type and extent of renal involvement
- Withdrawal of offending drug causes resolution of renal manifestations in most cases

Microscopic Pathology
- Varied patterns: MGN, amyloidosis, tubulointerstitial nephritis, pauci-immune GN

Diagnostic Checklist
- Mesangioproliferative GN, ANCA-related disease, and AA amyloidosis linked to RA

- Presentation varies based on type and extent of renal involvement
- Nephrotic syndrome is presenting feature in MGN, amyloidosis
- Rapidly progressive GN is seen with pauci-immune GN and vasculitis
- Acute renal failure with NSAID-related interstitial nephritis and acute tubular injury
- Isolated hematuria &/or proteinuria in mesangioproliferative GN related directly to RA
- Variable decline in renal function and mild proteinuria in most other instances
- Systemic manifestations of RA
  - Arthritis due to autoimmune inflammation of joints
  - Various extraarticular manifestations include pericarditis, pulmonary nodules, pulmonary interstitial fibrosis, mononeuritis multiplex, and systemic vasculitis
  - Diagnosis of RA is based on 2010 criteria established by collaborative efforts of American College of Rheumatology and European League Against Rheumatism

Laboratory Tests
- p-ANCA test positive in pauci-immune GN secondary to RA and treatment complication
- ANA, anti-DNA antibodies, and low serum complement levels in anti-TNF-α therapy-induced autoimmune disease

Treatment
- Drugs
  - Withdrawal of offending drug (NSAIDs; gold, penicillamine) causes resolution of tubulointerstitial nephritis and MGN, respectively, in most cases
    - If renal dysfunction persists, steroids can help accelerate recovery in NSAID interstitial nephritis
    - Resolution of disease after withdrawal of gold or penicillamine often takes up to a year
  - Corticosteroids and cyclophosphamide may be useful in treatment of AA amyloidosis
  - Immunosuppressive therapy for pauci-immune GN and mesangioproliferative GN

MICROSCOPIC PATHOLOGY

Histologic Features
- Tubulointerstitial nephritis
  - Tubulointerstitial inflammation due to NSAIDs is usually sparse
  - A few scattered eosinophils may be present
  - Interstitial edema and inflammation is present in nonatrophic parenchyma
  - Features of acute tubular injury may be evident with loss of proximal tubular brush borders and sloughed epithelial cells
- Membranous glomerulonephritis (MGN)
  - GBM may be thickened or show basement membrane "spikes," depending on stage of MGN
  - Subepithelial deposits can be highlighted by PAS and trichrome stains
  - Mild mesangial proliferation can be present, especially in therapy-induced membranous lupus nephritis
- Cyclosporine toxicity
  - Normal histology seen in vasoconstriction-induced acute nephrotoxicity
  - Tubular isometric cytoplasmic vacuoles in acute calcineurin inhibitor toxicity
  - Arteriolar hyaline insudation, particularly with medial or peripheral beaded appearance
  - Interstitial fibrosis with a striped pattern due to nonuniform involvement of arterioles
  - Acute thrombotic microangiopathy with endothelial swelling, fibrin thrombi, mesangiolysis, and fragmented RBCs
- Pauci-immune GN
  - Variable degree of glomerular fibrinoid necrosis and crescents
  - Small vessel vasculitis may be present
- Amyloidosis

- o Amyloid AA deposits in glomeruli, tubular basement membranes, interstitium, and blood vessels
  - ▪ Distribution of these amorphous deposits indistinguishable from other forms of amyloidosis
  - ▪ Amyloid deposits are weakly PAS and trichrome stain positive
  - ▪ Congo red stain is also positive with apple-green birefringence under polarized light
- Mesangioproliferative GN
  - o Mild to moderate mesangial proliferation
  - o No evidence of endocapillary proliferation, necrosis, or crescents
- Analgesic nephropathy
  - o Predominant tubular atrophy and interstitial fibrosis with relatively mild chronic interstitial inflammation
  - o Involvement of tubulointerstitial compartment disproportionately greater than extent of glomerulosclerosis
  - o Papillary necrosis may be identified on biopsy
- Minimal change disease
  - o Normal glomerular histology
  - o Acute tubular injury may be evident in setting of acute renal failure
- Other
  - o Extent of tubular atrophy and interstitial fibrosis is variable
  - o Arterio- and arteriolosclerosis present in setting of hypertensive nephrosclerosis
  - o Vasculitis of renal artery and its branches is rare and may not be sampled on renal biopsy

ANCILLARY TESTS

Immunohistochemistry

- Subtype of amyloid AA protein can be confirmed on immunohistochemistry

Immunofluorescence

- Diffuse or segmental capillary wall deposits identified in MGN with IgG and C3
  - o Therapy-induced membranous lupus nephritis can demonstrate mesangial and capillary wall deposits with "full house" staining
- Mesangial IgM immune deposits often dominant with weaker staining for other Ig and complement components in mesangioproliferative GN
- Subtyping of amyloid demonstrates AA protein with no evidence of immunoglobulin light or heavy chains
  - o Weak nonspecific entrapment of immunoglobulin light and heavy chains should not be misinterpreted as AL amyloid
- No immune complexes in NSAID interstitial nephritis, cyclosporine toxicity, analgesic nephropathy, pauci-immune GN, and minimal change disease

Electron Microscopy

- Subepithelial electron-dense deposits in MGN
  - o Proximal tubular lysosomal gold inclusions characterized by electron-dense filaments may be observed in gold-induced MGN

- Mesangial deposits in mesangioproliferative GN and membranous lupus nephritis
- Amyloid deposits are composed of nonbranching randomly oriented fibrils, 8-12 nm thick
- No deposits in interstitial nephritis, cyclosporine toxicity, analgesic nephropathy, and pauci-immune GN
- Extensive foot process effacement in NSAID-induced minimal change disease

DIAGNOSTIC CHECKLIST

Pathologic Interpretation Pearls

- Mesangioproliferative GN, ANCA-related disease, and AA amyloidosis linked to RA

SELECTED REFERENCES

1. Aletaha D et al: 2010 Rheumatoid arthritis classification criteria: an American College of Rheumatology/European League Against Rheumatism collaborative initiative. Arthritis Rheum. 62(9):2569-81, 2010
2. Pruzanski W: Renal amyloidosis in rheumatoid arthritis. J Rheumatol. 34(4):889; author reply 889, 2007
3. Stokes MB et al: Development of glomerulonephritis during anti-TNF-alpha therapy for rheumatoid arthritis. Nephrol Dial Transplant. 20(7):1400-6, 2005
4. Bruyn GA et al: Anti-glomerular basement membrane antibody-associated renal failure in a patient with leflunomide-treated rheumatoid arthritis. Arthritis Rheum. 48(4):1164-5, 2003
5. Chevrel G et al: Renal type AA amyloidosis associated with rheumatoid arthritis: a cohort study showing improved survival on treatment with pulse cyclophosphamide. Rheumatology (Oxford). 40(7):821-5, 2001
6. Murakami H et al: Rheumatoid arthritis associated with renal amyloidosis and crescentic glomerulonephritis. Intern Med. 37(1):94-7, 1998
7. Almirall J et al: Penicillamine-induced rapidly progressive glomerulonephritis in a patient with rheumatoid arthritis. Am J Nephrol. 13(4):286-8, 1993
8. Ludwin D et al: Cyclosporin A nephropathy in patients with rheumatoid arthritis. Br J Rheumatol. 32 Suppl 1:60-4, 1993
9. Boers M: Renal disorders in rheumatoid arthritis. Semin Arthritis Rheum. 20(1):57-68, 1990
10. Hall CL: The natural course of gold and penicillamine nephropathy: a longterm study of 54 patients. Adv Exp Med Biol. 252:247-56, 1989
11. Boers M et al: Renal findings in rheumatoid arthritis: clinical aspects of 132 necropsies. Ann Rheum Dis. 46(9):658-63, 1987
12. Honkanen E et al: Membranous glomerulonephritis in rheumatoid arthritis not related to gold or D-penicillamine therapy: a report of four cases and review of the literature. Clin Nephrol. 27(2):87-93, 1987
13. Barba L et al: Diagnostic immunopathology of the kidney biopsy in rheumatic diseases. Hum Pathol. 14(4):290-304, 1983
14. Antonovych TT: Gold nephropathy. Ann Clin Lab Sci. 11(5):386-91, 1981
15. Ramirez G et al: Renal pathology in patients with rheumatoid arthritis. Nephron. 28(3):124-6, 1981

RHEUMATOID ARTHRITIS

Rheumatoid Arthritis Treatment Complications

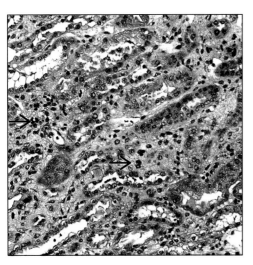 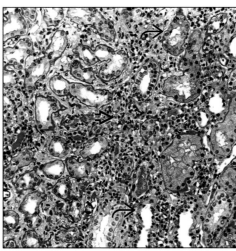

(Left) Mild interstitial edema is evident in this kidney biopsy from an RA patient with acute renal failure. Sparse interstitial infiltrate of lymphocytes and eosinophils is seen ➡ (H&E). The drug history is significant for NSAID use. *(Right)* Mild interstitial mononuclear inflammation ➡ and tubulitis ➡ are evident in this NSAID-induced acute tubulointerstitial nephritis (PAS stain). The patient has a long history of rheumatoid arthritis for which he received several medications including NSAIDs.

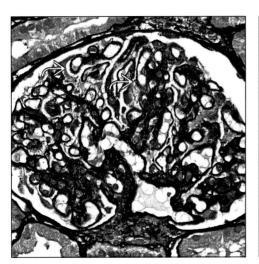 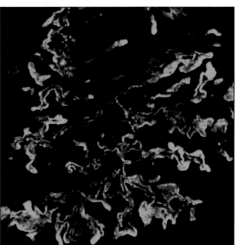

(Left) This 65-year-old woman with a 20-year history of RA has been treated with gold, penicillamine, steroids, and methotrexate over the years. The glomerulus shows MGN with thickened GBM with basement membrane "spikes" ➡, probably related to gold &/ or penicillamine therapy (silver stain). *(Right)* IgG immunofluorescence shows diffuse granular capillary wall deposits, typical of MGN. The patient received gold and penicillamine therapy for several years for RA.

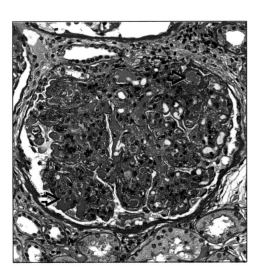 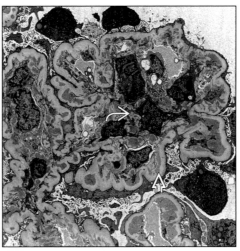

(Left) Membranoproliferative GN is seen in this RA patient treated with anti-TNF-α. The patient presented with nephrotic syndrome, positive ANA, and anti-ds DNA. Abundant deposits ➡ are seen in capillary lumens, and "full house" staining was evident on IF. *(Right)* Mesangial ➡ and subendothelial ➡ electron-dense deposits are seen in a patient with a several-year history of RA and recent treatment with anti-TNF-α. Patient developed lupus-like syndrome, including positive serologies.

RHEUMATOID ARTHRITIS

AA Amyloidosis in Rheumatoid Arthritis

(Left) Amyloid deposits ⇗ in the mesangium stain grayish blue on trichrome stain. The patient is a 71-year-old man with a several-year history of RA treated with steroids and methotrexate. The amyloid material is of AA subtype. *(Right)* The Congo red stain highlights the mesangial ⇨ and capillary wall ⇨ amyloid, which was further characterized as AA subtype. The patient presented with nephrotic syndrome, and prior history was significant for RA for many years.

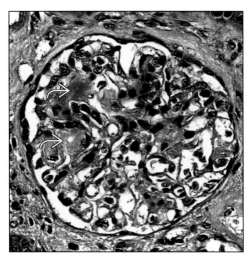
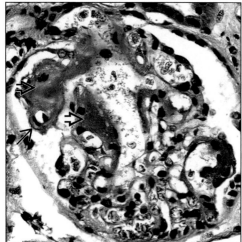

(Left) Apple-green birefringence ⇗ is observed on Congo red stain when examined under polarized light. The findings are characteristic of amyloid deposits, which were characterized as AA type in this patient with RA. *(Right)* Antibodies to amyloid A show positive staining ⇨ in glomeruli. The biopsy is from a patient with RA who presented with nephrotic syndrome. The prolonged chronic inflammation in RA predisposes to amyloid deposition.

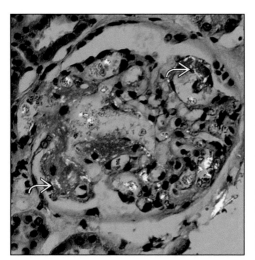
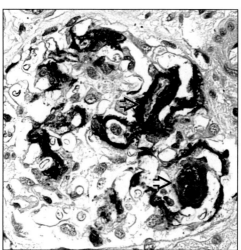

(Left) On ultrastructural examination, the amyloid deposits in this rheumatoid arthritis patient are composed of ill-defined electron-dense material in the mesangium ⇗ and lamina densa of the GBM ⇨. *(Right)* On high magnification, the amyloid deposits are composed of randomly oriented fibrils ⇨ that measure 8-12 nm in thickness. The AA amyloid in this patient with rheumatoid arthritis is indistinguishable from other forms of amyloid.

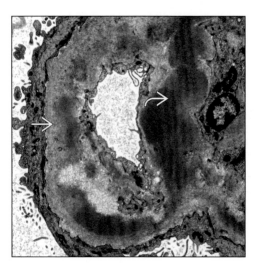
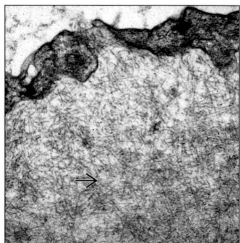

Glomerular Disease Directly Related to RA

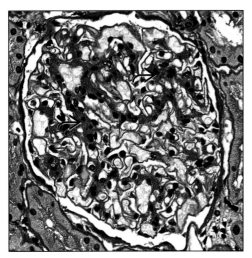
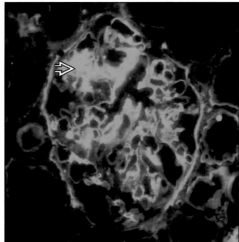

(Left) The renal biopsy is from a 29-year-old woman with RA, treated with steroids alone. She presented with mild proteinuria and hematuria, normal serum creatinine, ANA positive in low titers, but anti-ds DNA negative. Mild segmental mesangial proliferation is seen ➡ (PAS stain). (Right) IgG immunofluorescence staining demonstrates mesangial immune complexes ➡. The patient has RA treated with steroids alone, and biopsy showed mild segmental mesangial proliferation.

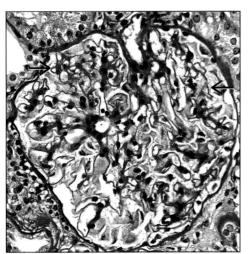
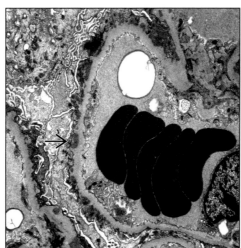

(Left) A 64-year-old man with RA, treated with methotrexate for several years until 9 months before the biopsy and no treatment with gold or penicillamine, presented with nephrotic syndrome. Biopsy shows minimally thickened GBM ➡, and IF showed diffuse granular capillary wall deposits with IgG and C3, typical of MGN. (Right) Subepithelial deposits ➡ are compatible with MGN in an RA patient. In absence of gold or penicillamine treatment, MGN is probably directly related to RA.

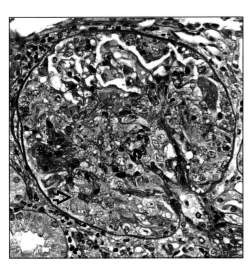
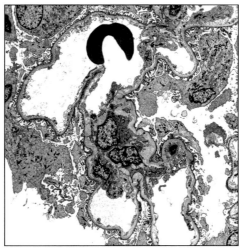

(Left) ANCA-related glomerular disease is seen in a 51-year-old RA patient with nephrotic proteinuria, hematuria, acute renal failure and hemoptysis; p-ANCA positive. Prior therapy was only steroids. The glomerulus shows capillary wall necrosis and a cellular crescent ➡. No immune complexes were identified on IF. (Right) Normal glomerulus with no deposits in an RA patient with pauci-immune GN is shown. Cellular crescents were seen elsewhere in this patient, who was treated with steroids alone.

MIXED CRYOGLOBULINEMIC GLOMERULONEPHRITIS

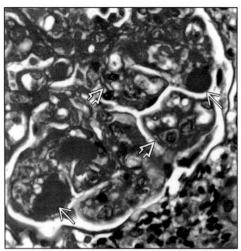

High-power view of a PAS stain shows hyaline, refractile "pseudothrombi" ➡ (also known as PAS-positive "coagulum"), and glomerular basement membrane duplication ➡ in a case of cryoglobulinemic GN.

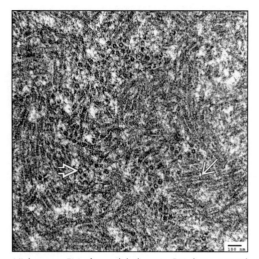

High-power EM of cryoglobulinemic GN shows curved microtubular structures ➡ and rings ➡. Without a history of cryoglobulinemia, this might be interpreted as immunotactoid glomerulopathy.

TERMINOLOGY

Abbreviations
- Cryoglobulinemic glomerulonephritis (CryoGN)

Synonyms
- Cryoglobulinemic GN
- Membranoproliferative GN
- Essential mixed cryoglobulinemic GN

Definitions
- GN due to specific proteins (immunoglobulins) that are soluble at 37°C and reversibly precipitate at cold temperatures
- Originally described by Meltzer, Franklin, McCluskey, and colleagues (1966)

ETIOLOGY/PATHOGENESIS

Infectious Agents
- Hepatitis C virus (HCV) comprises ≥ 30% of mixed cryoglobulinemias
  - It was once unknown that HCV caused these cases, & these cases were once termed "essential mixed cryoglobulinemias"

Type II Mixed Cryoglobulinemia
- Renal disease typically occurs with type II mixed cryoglobulinemia & not usually with type I or III
  - Monoclonal component is almost always IgM with kappa light chain (IgMκ)

CLINICAL ISSUES

Presentation
- "Essential mixed cryoglobulinemia syndrome"
  - Systemic vasculitis with cutaneous purpura, urticaria, weakness, & arthralgias
    - Biopsy shows leukocytoclastic vasculitis

  - 10-60% of cases have renal disease
- Proteinuria
  - 1/5 have nephrotic-range proteinuria or nephrotic syndrome
- Hematuria
  - Some have microscopic hematuria
  - ~ 25% of patients have acute nephritic syndrome with hypertension, increased serum creatinine, proteinuria, and macroscopic hematuria
  - < 5% of patients develop oliguric or anuric renal failure
- Renal dysfunction
  - Mild renal insufficiency may be present, but serum creatinine is typically normal
- Hypertension
  - Commonly occurs & may be rather severe
- Splenomegaly

Laboratory Tests
- Cryoglobulin precipitate, typically IgG and IgMκ, detectable as a "cryocrit" or percent of serum composed of precipitate
  - Best detected when blood specimen is maintained at 37°C until clotting is completed
- C4 (early complement component) low and C3 normal or slightly decreased
- Serum antibodies against HCV or HCV RNA in most patients

Treatment
- Surgical approaches
  - Renal transplantation uncommonly performed because of usual indolent nature
  - May recur in transplant
- Adjuvant therapy
  - Plasmapheresis for relief of acute exacerbation of renal disease
  - Cryofiltration, whereby patient's plasma is cooled, precipitating out cryoglobulins, and then rewarmed and reinfused

---

MIXED CRYOGLOBULINEMIC GLOMERULONEPHRITIS

Key Facts

Terminology
- GN due to immunoglobulins soluble at 37°C, reversibly precipitate with cooling

Etiology/Pathogenesis
- Renal disease usually type II mixed cryoglobulinemia & not type I or III
- Hepatitis C virus (HCV) comprises ≥ 30% of mixed cryoglobulinemias

Clinical Issues
- Proteinuria &/or hematuria
- Cryoglobulin serum precipitate, typically IgG and IgMκ
- "Essential mixed cryoglobulinemia syndrome" of vasculitis with cutaneous purpura, urticaria, weakness, & arthralgias

Microscopic Pathology
- Glomerular mesangial and capillary hypercellularity
- Glomerular basement membrane duplication
- Eosinophilic, refractile PAS(+) hyaline deposits fill capillary lumina

Ancillary Tests
- IgG, IgM, and C3 seen most often on IF
- Microtubules, rings, and annular structures on EM
- Many glomerular monocytes/macrophages may be CD68(+)

Top Differential Diagnoses
- Lupus nephritis, idiopathic MPGN, other GNs
- Immunotactoid glomerulopathy
- Thrombotic microangiopathy (TMA)

- Drugs
  - Corticosteroids
    - Aggressive immunosuppressive therapy (pulse methylprednisolone followed by oral steroids and cyclophosphamide) only used with caution to prevent hepatitis C reactivation; typically only used in patients with severe acute vasculitis and multisystem manifestations
  - Cytotoxic immunosuppressive drugs
    - Cyclophosphamide (Cytoxan)
  - Interferon-α
    - Used to treat hepatitis C virus-associated cryoglobulinemia
  - Ribavirin
  - Rituximab

Prognosis
- Typically more indolent than idiopathic MPGN
- Progression to ESRD uncommon, occurring in around 10% of cases (usually in 5-10 years)
- Death may result from infections, cardiovascular disease, and systemic effects of vasculitis

MICROSCOPIC PATHOLOGY

Histologic Features
- Glomeruli
  - Diffuse intracapillary hypercellularity with glomerular capillary loop occlusion
    - Leukocytes, particularly monocytes, compose the hypercellularity
  - Eosinophilic, refractile-appearing PAS(+) hyaline deposits fill capillary lumina
    - Known as "intraluminal thrombi" or perhaps more properly "pseudothrombi" since they are not actually composed of fibrin
    - Also called PAS(+) coagulum by some pathologists
  - Glomerular basement membrane (GBM) diffusely thickened, appreciated most readily on PAS or Jones stain
  - Reduplication or "tram tracking" of GBM

- Crescents (also known as extracapillary proliferation)
- Mild or marked mesangial proliferation associated with cases having heavy proteinuria and renal failure
- Tubulointerstitium
  - Interstitial fibrosis and tubular atrophy is usually mild/localized
  - Erythrocyte casts in tubular lumina, particularly during acute episodes
- Vessels
  - Vasculitis of small- and medium-sized arteries and arterioles (20-25% of cases)
  - Intimal and medial fibrinoid necrosis
  - Intraluminal glassy or refractile deposits in arterioles as they are in glomerular capillary loops
  - Intimal fibrosis eventually replaces areas of fibrinoid necrosis

ANCILLARY TESTS

Immunohistochemistry
- CD68 (KP-1) may stain numerous KP-1-positive monocyte/macrophages (also positive for esterase)

Immunofluorescence
- Granular IgM and IgG staining in glomerular capillaries in subendothelial location & often in mesangium
- IgM and C3 occur together in 92% of cases
- C4d is present in around 33% of cases, and C1q may be present
- Glomerular capillary lumina often with intense IgG and IgM in intraluminal thrombi
- IgG and IgM in arteriolar walls and intraluminal deposits in arterioles
- Fibrinogen in glomeruli and vasculature, particularly in cases with vasculitis

Electron Microscopy
- Transmission
  - Organized deposits

MIXED CRYOGLOBULINEMIC GLOMERULONEPHRITIS

Cryoglobulin Types

Type	Component(s)	Etiology
I	Single monoclonal immunoglobulin (usually IgM)	Multiple myeloma, monoclonal gammopathy of undetermined significance (MGUS), or Waldenström macroglobulinemia
II	2 immunoglobulins: Polyclonal IgG & monoclonal Ig (usually IgM) with reactivity against human IgG (also known as an anti-Ig rheumatoid factor)	> 30% hepatitis C virus (HCV)
III	Polyclonal IgG & polyclonal IgM	Various (systemic lupus erythematosus, infection, others)

"Mixed cryoglobulinemia," composed of either type II or type II cryoglobulins (together comprising 60-65% of cryoglobulins), is associated with rheumatologic conditions (e.g., connective tissue diseases), infectious diseases, lymphoproliferative disorders, and hepatobiliary disease. At least ~ 30% of cases are associated with hepatitis C virus (HCV), which was once termed "essential mixed cryoglobulinemia."

- Microtubular structures 10-25 nm wide, rings 30 nm wide, curved cylinders, and annular structures with spokes ~ 3 nm in diameter
- Tubular and annular pattern may be present in same case
- Usually in subendothelial location and within intraluminal thrombi in glomerular capillaries
- Intramembranous or subepithelial deposits ("humps") may be identified
- Deposits may also be fibrillar, may show "fingerprinting," or may show crystalloid substructure
- Rhomboid, membrane-bound osmiophilic cytoplasmic structures in mesangial and glomerular epithelial cells may be seen, resembling crystalloid structures seen in Fanconi lesion associated with plasma cell dyscrasias
- Some cases have amorphous electron-dense deposits (i.e., without clear organization)
  - Monocyte/macrophages are often associated with deposits, often in subendothelial location interposed between GBM and endothelial lining
    - Monocyte-type cells lead to GBM "reduplication" that is caused by mesangial cells in idiopathic MPGN
    - Neutrophils may be present

DIFFERENTIAL DIAGNOSIS

Idiopathic MPGN
- Cryoglobulinemic GN favored by
  - Large number of monocytes in glomerular capillary tuft
  - Glomerular capillary intraluminal thrombi
  - Vasculitis in small and medium-sized arterioles
  - EM with substructure characteristic of cryoglobulin
  - Positive cryoglobulin assay

Immunotactoid Glomerulopathy
- Microtubular structures in cryoglobulinemic GN are typically shorter and are against amorphous or granular, electron-dense background
- Cases otherwise classified as immunotactoid glomerulopathy are diagnosed as cryoglobulinemic GN if they fulfill clinical or laboratory criteria for cryoglobulinemia

Glomerulonephritis of Various Forms
- Cryoglobulins may be present in glomerulonephritis of various forms including
  - Systemic lupus erythematosus, postinfectious GN, Henoch-Schönlein purpura, and others
- Distinguishing clinical and pathologic features of those diseases are usually present, such as characteristic serologic findings

Thrombotic Microangiopathy (TMA)
- Presence of glomerular capillary "pseudothrombi" raises possibility of TMA
- Ultrastructural demonstration of immune-type deposits helps favor cryoglobulinemic GN

DIAGNOSTIC CHECKLIST

Pathologic Interpretation Pearls
- Though important in diagnosing cryoglobulinemic GN, intraluminal thrombi or "pseudothrombi" can be very focal and may be missed
- EM shows microtubular &/or annular deposits

SELECTED REFERENCES
1. Herrera GA et al: Renal diseases with organized deposits: an algorithmic approach to classification and clinicopathologic diagnosis. Arch Pathol Lab Med. 134(4):512-31, 2010
2. Jayne D: Role of rituximab therapy in glomerulonephritis. J Am Soc Nephrol. 21(1):14-7, 2010
3. Herrera GA et al: Renal diseases associated with plasma cell dyscrasias, amyloidoses, Waldenström's macroglobulinemia, and cryoglobulinemic nephropathies. In Jennette JC et al: Heptinstall's Pathology of the Kidney. 6th ed. Philadelphia: Lippincott Williams & Wilkins, 2007
4. Kay J et al: Case records of the Massachusetts General Hospital. Case 31-2005. A 60-year-old man with skin lesions and renal insufficiency. N Engl J Med. 353(15):1605-13, 2005
5. Kern WF et al: Atlas of Renal Pathology. Philadelphia: W.B. Saunders, 1999
6. Meltzer M et al: Cryoglobulinemia--a clinical and laboratory study. II. Cryoglobulins with rheumatoid factor activity. Am J Med. 40(6):837-56, 1966

Microscopic Features

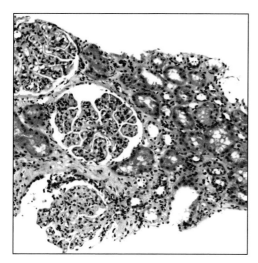

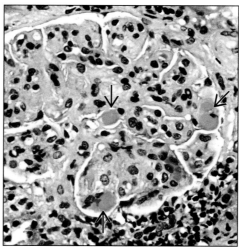

(Left) Low-power view of an H&E shows lobular hypercellular glomeruli in a case of cryoglobulinemic GN. This pattern can be seen in many diseases, including lupus and membranoproliferative glomerulonephritis. (Right) H&E stain shows an enlarged glomerulus with "pseudothrombi" ⇨ that are eosinophilic. Fibrin is typically brighter red and less PAS positive.

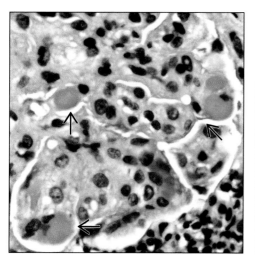

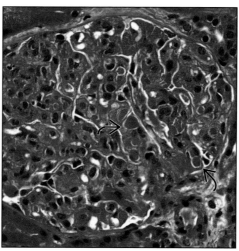

(Left) Higher-power view of an H&E shows a hypercellular glomerulus with "pseudothrombi" ⇨ in a case of cryoglobulinemic GN. (Right) Abundant "pseudothrombi" ⇨ are present in this patient who presented with acute renal failure, low C3, and no skin lesions. Macrophages and neutrophils occlude the capillaries. Her cryocrit was 5%. This case was idiopathic with negative HCV studies, even in the cryoprecipitate.

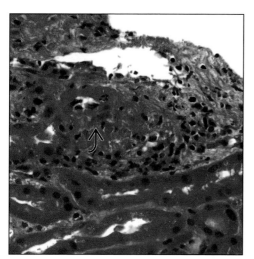

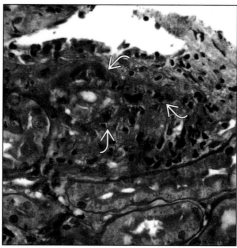

(Left) The vasculitis in mixed cryoglobulinemia looks similar in an H&E stained section to other forms of microscopic polyangiitis because the eosinophilic cryoglobulin deposits ⇨ resemble fibrin. (Right) Cryoglobulinemic vasculitis can be distinguished from other forms of microscopic polyangiitis because the rounded cryoglobulin deposits ⇨ are PAS(+) in contrast to the fibrin in fibrinoid necrosis. Careful search of multiple levels may reveal these changes on a renal biopsy.

MIXED CRYOGLOBULINEMIC GLOMERULONEPHRITIS

Immunofluorescence

(Left) IgG immunofluorescence shows patchy staining ➡, particularly within glomerular capillary loops. In mixed cryoglobulinemia, the deposits can be quite sparse, presumably because of degradation by the mononuclear cells. *(Right)* IgM immunofluorescence shows patchy staining, particularly along glomerular capillary loops ➡ and within glomerular capillary lumina ➡. IgM deposits are typically concentrated in the "pseudothrombi."

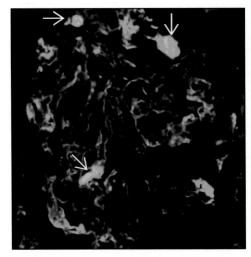
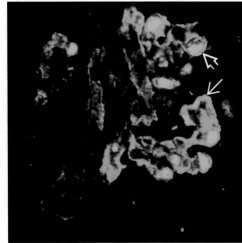

(Left) C3 immunofluorescence shows staining within glomerular capillary lumina ➡ and along glomerular capillary loops ➡. *(Right)* C1q immunofluorescence shows staining along glomerular capillary loops ➡ and within glomerular capillary lumina ➡.

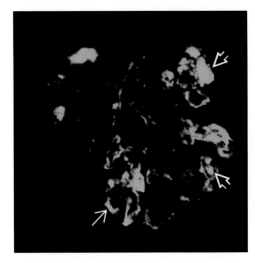
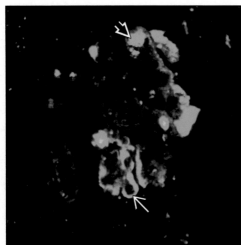

(Left) Kappa and lambda immunofluorescence show glomerular staining along capillary loops ➡ and in capillary lumens ➡ with slightly more kappa staining than lambda. *(Right)* An arteriole stains for the labeled immunoreactant, illustrating that this arteriole contains cryoglobulin. The arteriole is likely involved by vasculitis since it also contains fibrin, making this a "true" thrombus.

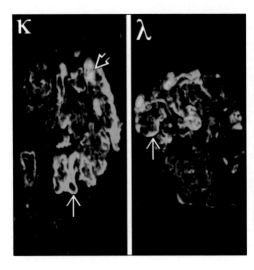
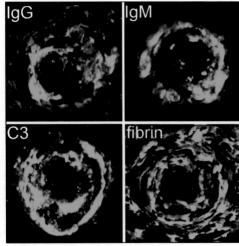

MIXED CRYOGLOBULINEMIC GLOMERULONEPHRITIS

Special Stains and Electron Microscopy

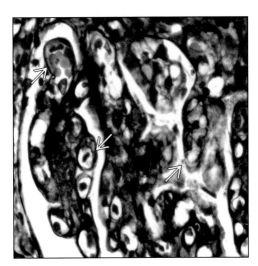

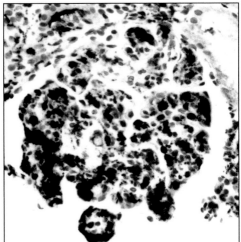

(Left) Jones silver stain shows "pseudothrombi" ➡ in a glomerular capillary loop in a case of cryoglobulinemic GN. Duplication of the GBM is also evident, which arises as a response to subendothelial deposits. *(Right)* A CD68 immunohistochemical stain is positive in many glomerular monocytes/ macrophages in a case of cryoglobulinemic GN. This positivity is commonly a prominent and characteristic feature.

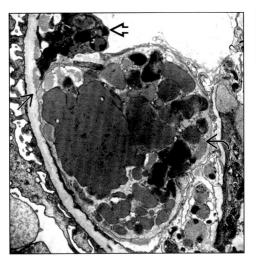

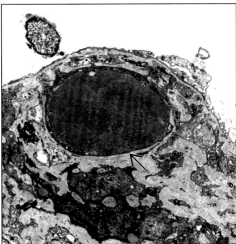

(Left) The cryoprecipitates in the glomerular capillaries are phagocytosed by macrophages ➡ and endothelial cells ➡. These may largely remove the immune complexes, leaving almost negative immunofluorescence findings. Subendothelial deposits are also present ➡. *(Right)* A "pseudothrombus" ➡ is present in a glomerular capillary loop in a case of cryoglobulinemic GN. It can be verified that this is not a true thrombus due to the lack of fibrin.

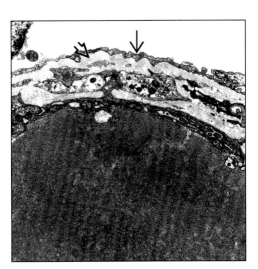

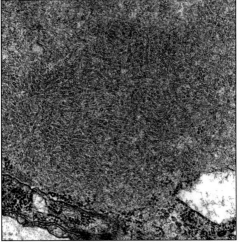

(Left) The glomerular basement membrane (GBM) is duplicated ➡ in this case of cryoglobulinemic GN, leading to "tram tracking" or "double contours." There is cellular interposition leading to GBM duplication, typically due to monocytes/ macrophages. In addition, podocytes are extensively effaced ➡. *(Right)* Higher power of the material in this case of cryoglobulinemic GN shows only a vague fibrillar/ microtubular substructure. The appearance and prominence of the fibrils is highly variable.

ANTI-GBM GLOMERULONEPHRITIS

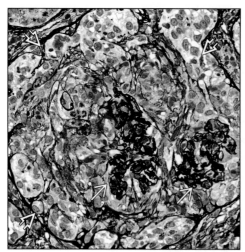

Jones silver stain from a patient with anti-GBM glomerulonephritis reveals a few the remnants of GBM ➡ surrounded by a cellular crescent ⇒ occupying all of Bowman space.

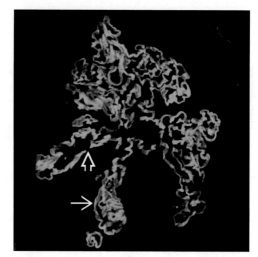

Strong linear IgG staining ➡ of the GBM is characteristic of anti-GBM disease. The glomerulus has a possible break in the GBM ⇒ and is compressed by a cellular crescent (not visible).

TERMINOLOGY

Abbreviations
- Anti-glomerular basement membrane glomerulonephritis (anti-GBM GN)

Synonyms
- Anti-GBM disease
- Goodpasture syndrome

Definitions
- Autoantibody deposition and targeting of the noncollagenous-1 domain of collagen IV leads to necrotizing and crescentic GN

ETIOLOGY/PATHOGENESIS

Autoantibody Deposition
- Autoantibody targets noncollagenous-1 (NC1) domain of α-3 chain of collagen IV (Goodpasture antigen)
- Autoantibody targeting noncollagenous-1 (NC1) domain of α-5 chain of collagen IV may also be present
  - Autoantibodies reactive to α-3 NC1 and α-5 NC1 are nonreactive to normal collagen
  - Conformational changes allow formation of neoepitopes for autoantibodies
  - Dissociation of α-3 chain of collagen IV in both kidney and lung increases binding affinity of autoantibodies

Genetic Predisposition
- Strong association with HLA-DR and DQ antigens

Precipitating Events
- Hydrocarbon exposure or cigarette smoking
  - Possible inhibition of putative enzyme that catalyzes formation of sulfilimine bonds between collagen hexamers

- May be triggering event to form neoepitopes for Goodpasture autoantibody formation
- Cigarette smoking may increase risk of pulmonary involvement
- Possible infectious agent
  - Flu-like symptoms prior to onset in some patients
  - Mini epidemics documented
    - 1971 (winter): 4 cases in Connecticut, USA
    - 1985 (June-October): 7 cases in Mersey region, England
    - 2005 (April-June): 7 cases in Chicago, Illinois, USA
  - Causative agent not identified
- Exposure to nonendogenous GBM antigens after kidney transplantation for Alport syndrome
  - Approximately 3-5% of Alport syndrome patients develop de novo anti-GBM disease after transplantation
  - Autoantibodies target epitopes on normal α-3 chain of collagen IV of renal allograft that are absent in native kidneys
    - Distinct mechanism from anti-GBM disease in Alport syndrome after kidney transplantation
    - Dissociation of α-3 chain of collagen IV in both kidney and lung decreases binding affinity of autoantibodies in post-transplant Alport syndrome patients

CLINICAL ISSUES

Epidemiology
- Incidence
  - Rare: 1 case per 1,000,000 per year in United States
- Age
  - Bimodal distribution with peaks in 2nd and 6th decades of age
- Gender
  - No overall gender predilection
  - Male predilection in 2nd decade
    - Pulmonary and renal involvement common

ANTI-GBM GLOMERULONEPHRITIS

Key Facts

Etiology/Pathogenesis
- Autoantibody targets noncollagenous-1 (NC1) domain of α-3 chain of collagen IV (Goodpasture antigen)
  - Conformational changes allow formation of neoepitopes for autoantibodies
  - Distinct antigenic target from anti-GBM GN in Alport syndrome patients after kidney transplantation
- Possible risk factors
  - Hydrocarbon exposure &/or cigarette smoking
  - Strong association with HLA-DR and DQ antigens

Clinical Issues
- Rare: 1 case per 1,000,000 per year in United States
- Bimodal distribution with peaks in 2nd and 6th decades of age

- Symptoms
  - Acute renal failure
  - Pulmonary hemorrhage
- Poor prognostic factors
  - Serum creatinine > 5 mg/dL at time of diagnosis
  - Anuria

Microscopic Pathology
- Cellular crescent formation ± segmental fibrinoid necrosis
  - Often involves > 80% of glomeruli
- Linear IgG and C3 staining of GBM

Top Differential Diagnoses
- Pauci-immune crescentic glomerulonephritis
- Immune complex-mediated GN

- Female predilection in 6th decade
  - Often crescentic GN alone without pulmonary involvement
- Ethnicity
  - Rare in African-Americans

Presentation
- Pulmonary hemorrhage
  - Hemoptysis
  - Dyspnea
  - Rales/rhonchi
  - Up to 2/3 of patients may not have overt pulmonary hemorrhage
- Acute renal failure
  - Rare cases with renal sparing
- Hematuria
- Proteinuria
  - Rarely nephrotic range

Laboratory Tests
- Anti-GBM titer
- Antineutrophil cytoplasmic antibodies (ANCA)
  - Present in 1/3 of anti-GBM disease patients

Treatment
- Drugs
  - Cyclophosphamide
  - High-dose corticosteroids
- Plasmapheresis/plasma exchange
- Renal transplantation
  - Recurrence is uncommon if anti-GBM antibodies are not present

Prognosis
- Poor prognostic factors
  - Serum creatinine > 5 mg/dL at time of diagnosis
  - Anuria
  - Dialysis requirement at presentation
- Patients with presence of antineutrophil cytoplasmic antibodies have intermediate prognosis

MACROSCOPIC FEATURES

General Features
- "Flea-bitten" appearance (or numerous red dots on cortical surface)
  - Corresponds to blood within tubular lumina or Bowman space
- Normal size to slightly enlarged kidneys

MICROSCOPIC PATHOLOGY

Histologic Features
- Cellular crescent formation ± segmental fibrinoid necrosis
  - Often involves > 80% of glomeruli
  - Rupture or breaks in GBM may be identified
  - Disruption of Bowman capsules
  - Periglomerular granulomatous inflammation or giant cell formation
    - Not specific for anti-GBM GN
  - Uninvolved glomerular tufts often without significant endocapillary hypercellularity
    - Neutrophils may be present adjacent to crescents or fibrinoid necrosis
    - Contrasts with immune complex-mediated GN with crescents
- Thrombotic microangiopathy involving glomerular capillaries
  - Present in subset of anti-GBM GN
- Interstitial inflammation
  - May be more prominent in patients with anti-tubular basement membrane (TBM) antibodies
  - Consists of lymphocytes, plasma cells, neutrophils, and macrophages
  - Prominent eosinophilic infiltrate may suggest Churg-Strauss syndrome
- Red blood cell casts
  - Aggregates of red blood cells in tubular lumina
- Necrotizing vasculitis rare
  - May be due to presence of antineutrophil cytoplasmic antibodies

ANTI-GBM GLOMERULONEPHRITIS

Immunofluorescence

Antibody	Reactivity	Staining Pattern	Comment
IgG	Positive, linear	GBM, linear	Bowman capsule and tubular basement membrane staining may be present; IgG > > > albumin; often predominantly IgG1
Kappa	Positive, linear	GBM, linear	Less intense than IgG
Lambda	Positive, linear	GBM, linear	Similar to but less intense than kappa
Albumin	Negative		Linear GBM staining may be present but significantly less intense than IgG

ANCILLARY TESTS

Immunofluorescence
- Strong linear IgG staining of glomerular basement membranes
  - Typically IgG1
    - Some female patients have high IgG4 titers
  - IgG4 staining reported in cases with mild or no renal involvement
    - May be due to inability of IgG4 to fix complement
  - Rare linear IgA staining reported
  - 10-20% reveal concurrent linear tubular basement membrane staining
    - May be limited to distal tubules where Goodpasture antigen is restricted
- Co-staining with IgM, IgA, C3, and C1q may be present

Electron Microscopy
- Break or disruption of GBM
- Neutrophils and monocytes in capillary loops
- Fibrin tactoids present where fibrinoid necrosis occurs
- Absence of immune complex deposition
- Crescents contain leukocytes, fibrin, parietal epithelium
- Ultrastructural findings not specific for anti-GBM GN

DIFFERENTIAL DIAGNOSIS

Pauci-immune Crescentic GN
- Lacks strong linear immunoglobulin deposition in GBM

Immune Complex-mediated GN
- Includes lupus nephritis, membranoproliferative GN, postinfectious GN, and IgA nephropathy
- Typically, glomeruli demonstrate significant endocapillary hypercellularity

Membranous GN and Anti-GBM GN
- Anti-GBM disease is superimposed upon very small subset of membranous GN patients
- Careful evaluation of immunofluorescence is necessary to establish diagnosis

Monoclonal Immunoglobulin Deposition Disease
- Strong confluent immunofluorescence staining of GBM, but tubular basement membranes and interstitium should also stain positively
- Monoclonal light chain staining is present
- Cellular crescents are rarely present

Diabetic Nephropathy
- Strong linear immunofluorescence of GBM for albumin as well as IgG
  - Segmental sclerosis or collapsed tufts with prominent overlying podocytes should not be misinterpreted as crescents
  - Superimposed pauci-immune crescentic GN can be observed in small subset of diabetic patients

DIAGNOSTIC CHECKLIST

Pathologic Interpretation Pearls
- Cellular crescent formation typically involves most glomeruli
  - Fibrocellular or fibrous crescents are not a generally prominent feature
- Uninvolved glomerular tufts should not reveal significant endocapillary hypercellularity, which excludes immune complex-mediated GN but not pauci-immune crescentic GN
- Anti-GBM autoantibodies may complicate other renal diseases, such as membranous GN, ANCA-related GN

SELECTED REFERENCES

1. Pedchenko V et al: Molecular architecture of the Goodpasture autoantigen in anti-GBM nephritis. N Engl J Med. 363(4):343-54, 2010
2. Sethi S et al: Linear anti-glomerular basement membrane IgG but no glomerular disease: Goodpasture's syndrome restricted to the lung. Nephrol Dial Transplant. 22(4):1233-5, 2007
3. Fischer EG et al: Anti-glomerular basement membrane glomerulonephritis: a morphologic study of 80 cases. Am J Clin Pathol. 125(3):445-50, 2006
4. Williams PS et al: Increased incidence of anti-glomerular basement membrane antibody (anti-GBM) nephritis in the Mersey Region, September 1984-October 1985. Q J Med. 68(257):727-33, 1988
5. Stave GM et al: Thrombotic microangiopathy in anti-glomerular basement membrane glomerulonephritis. Arch Pathol Lab Med. 108(9):747-51, 1984

ANTI-GBM GLOMERULONEPHRITIS

Microscopic Features

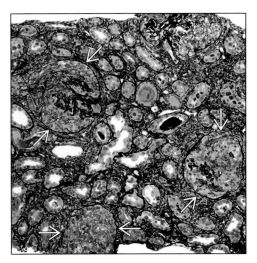
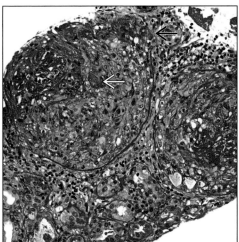

(Left) Diffuse crescentic and necrotizing injury of the glomeruli is characteristic of anti-GBM disease. No glomerulus in this biopsy was spared, which is a common feature. Crescents fill the space delineated by Bowman capsule ➡. *(Right)* Large cellular crescents occupy nearly every glomerulus in a biopsy with anti-GBM disease. Focal fibrinoid necrosis ➡ and disruption of Bowman capsule ➡ are associated with interstitial inflammation.

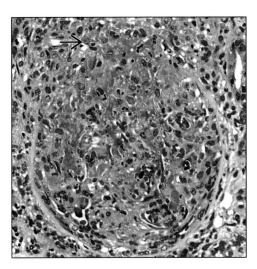
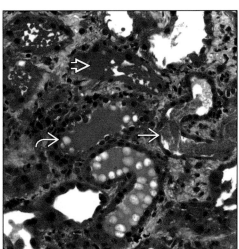

(Left) Fibrinoid necrosis permeates through the glomerulus and cellular crescent, with extension into the adjacent tubulointerstitium through a ruptured Bowman capsule ➡ in this specimen from a patient with anti-GBM disease. *(Right)* Numerous red blood cells ➡ and a red cell cast ➡ in the tubular lumina correlate with the urinalysis, which demonstrated hematuria. Nonspecific protein ➡ in adjacent tubules can be easily distinguished.

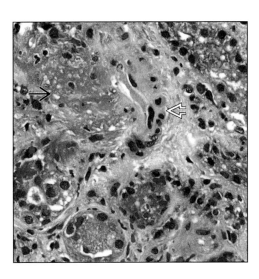
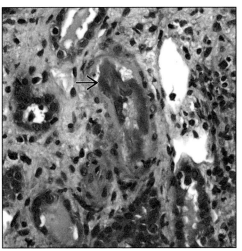

(Left) Fibrinoid necrosis ➡ with rupture of the vessel walls can be observed, as in this arteriole ➡. This patient had both positive anti-GBM and anti-myeloperoxidase titers, and the latter rather than the former may be the cause of the associated necrotizing vasculitis when present. *(Right)* Thrombotic microangiopathy involving vessels ➡ or glomerular capillaries (not shown) has been well described in a subset of anti-GBM GN patients.

Microscopic Features

(Left) Several multinucleated giant cells ⇥ are closely associated with this glomerulus with fibrinoid necrosis, which is a finding suggestive of anti-GBM disease. These giant cells are distinct from the perigranulomatous inflammation that is common in any crescentic injury with rupture of Bowman capsule. *(Right)* Multinucleated giant cells ⇥ associated with fibrinoid necrosis are specific but not pathognomonic for anti-GBM GN. The residual glomerulus is difficult to identify.

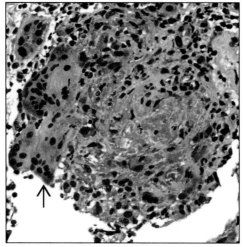 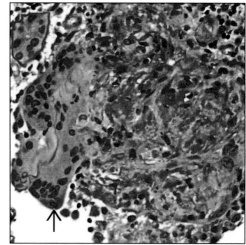

(Left) These multinucleated giant cells ⇥ are intimately associated with a severely injured glomerulus, which is distinct from the isolated interstitial granulomata that are suggestive of granulomatosis with polyangiitis (Wegener). *(Right)* CD68 immunohistochemistry confirms that the multinucleated giant cells ⇥ consist of macrophages, and many scattered macrophages are also present throughout the glomerular crescent as well as the adjacent tubules and interstitium.

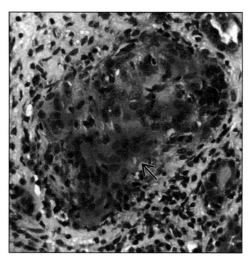 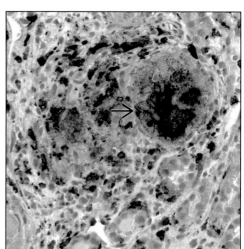

(Left) Fibrin ⇥ has spilled into the urinary space with inflammatory cells in this glomerulus from a patient with anti-GBM GN. A segment of Bowman capsule ⇥ is present. *(Right)* Fibrin tactoids ⇥ along with neutrophils ⇥ are present in glomerular capillaries in this case of anti-GBM disease. No immune complexes are present, and some glomeruli may lack any significant pathologic abnormalities. EM corroborates light microscopic features but is not useful to establish the diagnosis of anti-GBM disease.

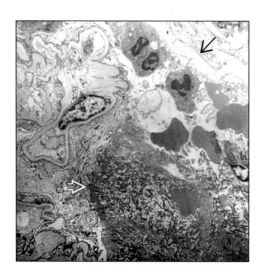 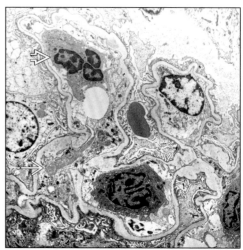

Variant Microscopic Features

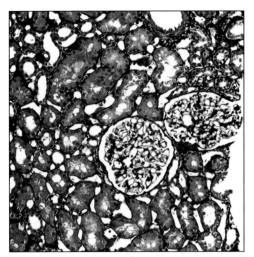

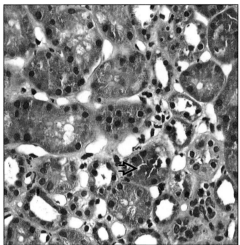

(Left) This is a "mild" case of anti-GBM nephritis from a patient with microscopic hematuria and mild proteinuria for several months. He had no evidence of lung involvement. This silver stain shows that most glomeruli appear normal, as do the vessels, tubules, and interstitium. *(Right)* Several red blood cells within a proximal tubular lumen ➡ correlate with the finding of microscopic hematuria in this specimen from a patient with a mild clinical course of anti-GBM disease.

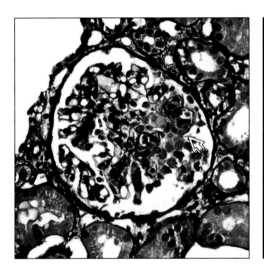

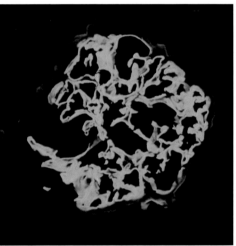

(Left) One of 25 glomeruli in this case of mild anti-GBM GN shows segmental necrosis with prominence of adjacent epithelial cells and rupture of the GBM ➡ (silver stain). A biopsy 2 months previously showed 1 cellular crescent of 18 glomeruli sampled. *(Right)* Immunofluorescence for IgG shows bright linear GBM staining typical of anti-GBM GN. Note the lack of staining in tubular basement membranes. Kappa and lambda light chains (not shown) should show similar but less intense staining.

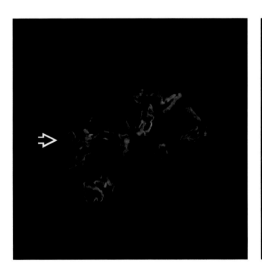

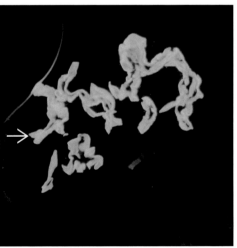

(Left) In contrast to typical cases of anti-GBM disease with diffuse crescents and necrosis that have strong linear IgG1 IF staining of the GBMs, this case shows relatively weak staining for IgG1 ➡. *(Right)* This case of anti-GBM disease shows bright linear GBM ➡ staining for IgG4 by IF. IgG4, in contrast to IgG1 and IgG3, does not fix complement nor bind to Fc receptors and may account for the milder disease phenotype in this case.

ANTI-GBM GLOMERULONEPHRITIS

Immunofluorescence

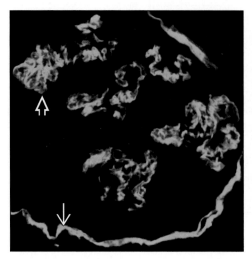 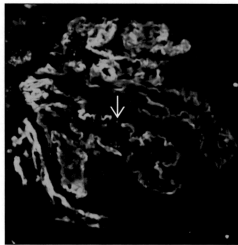

(Left) In anti-GBM GN, strong linear staining of the GBMs ➡ and Bowman capsule ➡ is identified by immunofluorescence microscopy. The glomerular tufts are compressed by a cellular crescent in Bowman space, which is inconspicuous. **(Right)** Kappa light chains reveal a similar linear staining pattern of the GBM. A break in the GBM ➡ is present. Lambda light chain staining was similar in intensity and distribution, which excludes monoclonal immunoglobulin deposition disease.

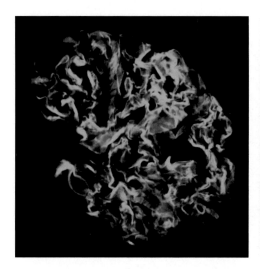 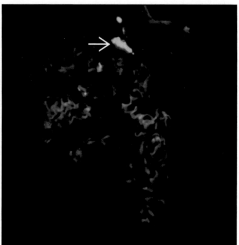

(Left) IgG1 typically shows strong linear staining of the GBM in an anti-GBM disease patient with no significant renal injury, but extensive pulmonary hemorrhage resulted in the death of this adolescent male. **(Right)** Immunofluorescence for albumin reveals no significant GBM staining with some protein reabsorption droplets present in a podocyte ➡. Comparison with albumin is useful to exclude nonspecific IgG GBM staining as observed in diabetic nephropathy.

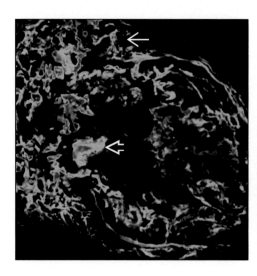 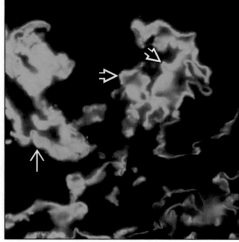

(Left) Fibrinoid necrosis is highlighted by strong fibrinogen staining ➡ in the crescent that has extended beyond Bowman capsule ➡ in this glomerulus. Fibrin is usually conspicuous in cellular crescents regardless of etiology. **(Right)** IgG immunofluorescence staining demonstrates both granular ➡ capillary wall staining, which indicates membranous GN, and linear staining of the GBM ➡ in this rare patient with concurrent anti-GBM GN. (Courtesy M. Troxell, MD, PhD.)

ANTI-GBM GLOMERULONEPHRITIS

Differential Diagnosis

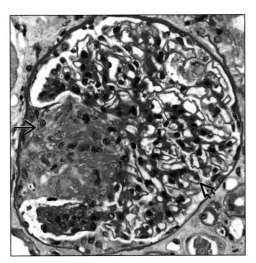 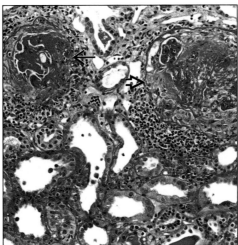

(Left) A cellular crescent with fibrinoid necrosis ⮕ occupies a part of the urinary space in a pauci-immune crescentic GN (ANCA related). The uninvolved glomerular tuft ⮕ appears normal, supporting the absence of immune complexes in this disease. **(Right)** Crescents in various temporal stages are characteristic of pauci-immune crescentic GN, such as this fibrous ⮕ and fibrocellular ⮕ crescent, but immunofluorescence is the definitive way to distinguish it from anti-GBM GN.

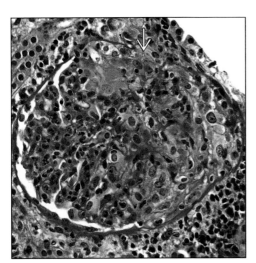 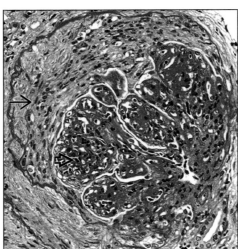

(Left) A cellular crescent and fibrinoid necrosis ⮕ are adjacent to a glomerulus with numerous neutrophils in the capillaries in a case of postinfectious GN. Some glomerular capillaries in anti-GBM may show many neutrophils. **(Right)** This cellular crescent ⮕ is associated with membranoproliferative GN. The glomerulus has increased lobularity, mesangial hypercellularity ⮕, and duplication of the GBM, features not typical of anti-GBM GN.

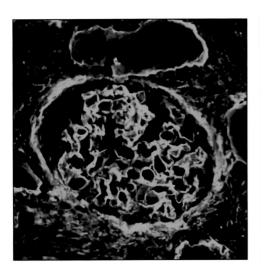 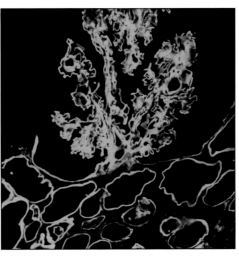

(Left) Confluent IgG staining of the glomerular and tubular basement membranes in this case of monoclonal immunoglobulin deposition disease mimics anti-GBM disease, but monoclonal lambda light chain staining was present. **(Right)** Linear staining of the glomerular and tubular basement membranes for albumin is present in this diabetic nephropathy case. IgG (not shown) had similar intensity, but the strong albumin staining along with the absence of crescents excludes anti-GBM GN.

INTRODUCTION TO DISEASES WITH MONOCLONAL IMMUNOGLOBULIN DEPOSITS

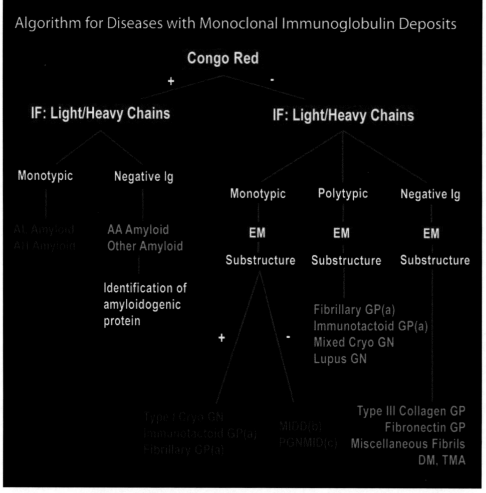

Diagnosis of diseases with monoclonal immunoglobulin deposits &/or substructure by EM is facilitated by following the path in this algorithm, which begins with whether the deposits are Congo red positive, followed by immunofluorescence (IF) for monotypic immunoglobulin chains (single light &/or heavy chain), equal staining of light chains (polyclonal) or no immunoglobulin staining. Electron microscopy is then used for assessment of the substructure. Immunotactoid and fibrillary GP sometimes have monotypic light chain (a). MIDD has either light chain, heavy chain, or both (b) and has no organized substructure. PGNMID usually, but not always, has amorphous deposits (c).

ETIOLOGY/PATHOGENESIS

Monoclonal Immunoglobulin
- May be produced by malignant lymphoid or plasma cell neoplasm

Reactive (Benign Monoclonal Proliferation)
- Some represent "monoclonal gammopathy of undetermined significance" (MGUS) without identifiable underlying neoplasm at time of renal biopsy
- Some cases never have an identified neoplastic proliferation
  - These appear to be clonal, but not malignant

APPROACH

Light Microscopy
- Quite variable appearances

- Mimic membranoproliferative GN, acute GN, membranous GN (MIDD, type I cryo, PGNMID)
- Mimic diabetes with nodular mesangial glomerulopathy (MIDD)
- Tubulointerstitial disease may predominate (MIDD, cast nephropathy, light chain proximal tubulopathy)

Special Stains
- Congo red stain essential to distinguish amyloidosis
  - Amyloidosis can be due to monoclonal immunoglobulin or other proteins
  - Thicker sections more sensitive
  - High-quality polarizing microscope more sensitive

Immunofluorescence
- Stains for light chains essential to distinguish this group of diseases
- Occasional forms show only heavy chain deposits
- Some monotypic light chains truncated & stain poorly

INTRODUCTION TO DISEASES WITH MONOCLONAL IMMUNOGLOBULIN DEPOSITS

Diseases with Monoclonal Immunoglobulin Deposits

Disease	Light Microscopy	Congo Red	IF	EM	Underlying Diseases
AL or AH amyloid	Amorphous eosinophilic material in GBM, mesangium; sometimes interstitium, vessels	+	Monotypic light (AL) or heavy (AH) chains	Fibrils, abundant, 8-12 nm, nonperiodic	Multiple myeloma in ~ 18%, MGUS in some cases, less commonly B-cell lymphoma
Monoclonal immunoglobulin deposition disease (MIDD)	Mesangial nodules, thickened GBM, TBM	-	Monotypic light chains &/or monotypic heavy chains	Amorphous, dense granular material GBM, TBM, mesangium	Dysproteinemia in > 70%, myeloma in ~ 40% of pure MIDD
Proliferative glomerulonephritis with monoclonal immunoglobulin deposits (PGNMID)	Acute, membranoproliferative or membranous glomerulonephritis	-	Monotypic light chains, gamma heavy chain; C3, ± C1q	Usually amorphous electron-dense "immune complex-type" deposits; subepithelial, subendothelial, mesangial	Dysproteinemia present in ~ 30%; myeloma rare
Type I cryoglobulinemia	MPGN, "pseudothrombi" in glomerular capillaries	-	Monotypic light chain and heavy chain	Fibrillary or tubular deposits, variable dimensions; occasionally amorphous	Chronic lymphocytic leukemia, Waldenström macroglobulinemia, other lymphoid-derived neoplasms
Light chain ("myeloma") cast nephropathy	Eosinophilic, PAS negative, fractured casts with giant cell reaction	-	Monotypic light/heavy chains	Granular, crystalline, or fibrillar casts	Multiple myeloma in ~ 90%
Light chain Fanconi syndrome (light chain proximal tubulopathy)	Crystalline structures within proximal tubular cytoplasm	-	Monotypic light chains in proximal tubular cytoplasm	Electron-dense crystalline structures within tubular epithelial cytoplasm	Multiple myeloma in ~ 50%, dysproteinemia in most
Diseases Sometimes Having Monotypic Immunoglobulin					
Immunotactoid glomerulopathy (GP)	Thickened GBM	-	Sometimes monotypic light chains	Tubular fibrils 20-80 nm	Monoclonal gammopathy in ~ 67%, myeloma in ~ 30%
Fibrillary GP	Thickened GBM, mesangial hypercellularity, crescents	-	Usually polyclonal; IgG4	Fibrils 10-30 nm	Monoclonal gammopathy in ~ 17%

Electron Microscopy

- Organized vs. amorphous deposits, location of deposits helps distinguish different types of diseases

Laboratory Tests

- Serum or urine immunoelectrophoresis does not always detect monoclonal immunoglobulin
- Serum or urine free light chain assay is more sensitive technique

SELECTED REFERENCES

1. Herrera GA et al: Renal diseases with organized deposits: an algorithmic approach to classification and clinicopathologic diagnosis. Arch Pathol Lab Med. 134(4):512-31, 2010
2. Markowitz GS: Dysproteinemia and the kidney. Adv Anat Pathol. 11(1):49-63, 2004
3. Lin J et al: Renal monoclonal immunoglobulin deposition disease: the disease spectrum. J Am Soc Nephrol. 12(7):1482-92, 2001

IMAGE GALLERY

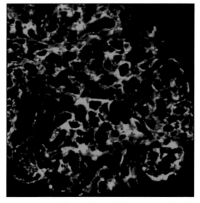  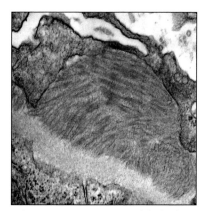

(Left) Routine analysis of renal biopsies includes immunofluorescence for light and heavy chains to detect monotypic immunoglobulin deposits. Here, deposits are positive for kappa light chain. *(Center)* The absence of one light chain (lambda in this case) in the presence of strong staining for the other light chain (kappa) is indicative of a monoclonal immunoglobulin deposit. *(Right)* EM is essential to determine whether the deposits have a substructure, the nature of which has diagnostic importance. Congo red staining is also crucial to detect amyloid.

MONOCLONAL IMMUNOGLOBULIN DEPOSITION DISEASE

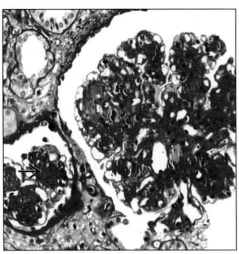

MIDD has many patterns. One classic pattern is nodular glomerulosclerosis, which shows PAS-positive mesangial nodules ➡ and can mimic diabetic glomerulosclerosis.

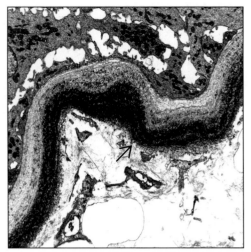

MIDD is often manifested in EM by finely granular electron-dense deposits along the tubular ➡ and glomerular basement membranes.

TERMINOLOGY

Abbreviations
- Monoclonal immunoglobulin deposition disease (MIDD)

Synonyms
- Systemic light chain disease
- Light chain deposition disease (LCDD)
- Heavy chain deposition disease (HCDD)
- Light and heavy chain deposition disease (LHCDD)
- Nonamyloidogenic light chain deposition
- Monoclonal immunoglobulin deposition disease, Randall type

Definitions
- Deposition of monoclonal immunoglobulin along glomerular and tubular basement membranes (GBMs/TBMs) and within mesangium
- Deposits are characterized by linear GBM and TBM staining by immunofluorescence (IF) and finely granular deposits by electron microscopy (EM)

ETIOLOGY/PATHOGENESIS

LCDD Deposits
- Differ from normal light chains in variable region, especially complementarity-determining regions and framework regions
- Composed of glycosylated light chains, resulting in larger molecule than normal light chain

HCDD Deposits
- Deletion of the CH1 constant domain of gamma heavy chain

CLINICAL ISSUES

Presentation
- Acute renal failure
- Chronic renal failure
- Nephrotic syndrome
- Proteinuria (58%; non-light chain)
- Multiple myeloma diagnosable in ~ 40% of patients with pure MIDD (without concurrent cast nephropathy or amyloidosis)
- Hypocomplementemia
  - Present in gamma-HCDD with complement-fixing IgG subclass deposited (gamma-1 or gamma-3)

Laboratory Tests
- Monoclonal protein in serum, urine, or both
  - M spike on serum or urine protein electrophoresis in ~ 50% of patients with pure MIDD
  - ~ 15-20% of patients do not have detectable serum or urine paraprotein at time of diagnosis, even by immunofixation
    - Serum or urine free light chain tests can increase sensitivity
- Elevated kappa or lambda free light chains in serum or urine
- Emerging test for free heavy chains in gamma heavy chain deposition disease
- Free light or heavy chain tests useful for monitoring response to therapy

Other Organ Involvement
- Cardiac disease (estimated ~ 19-80%)
- Peripheral neuropathy (20%)
- Other: Gastrointestinal, liver, pulmonary nodules, muscle, skin

MONOCLONAL IMMUNOGLOBULIN DEPOSITION DISEASE

Key Facts

Clinical Issues
- Nephrotic syndrome
- Acute or chronic renal failure
- Multiple myeloma diagnosable in ~ 40% of patients with pure MIDD
- Monoclonal protein in serum, urine, or both
- ~ 15-20% of patients do not have detectable serum or urine paraprotein at time of diagnosis, even by immunofixation

Microscopic Pathology
- Tubular basement membrane monoclonal immunoglobulin deposition
- Nodular glomerulopathy
- PAS positive nodules, nonargyrophilic

- By IF, linear basement membrane staining (glomerular, tubular, vascular) for kappa or lambda light chain (LCDD), plus a heavy chain (LHCDD), or heavy chain only (HCDD)
- Kappa light chain in ~ 80% of LCDD
- By EM, finely granular, punctate, "powdery" electron-dense deposits distributed along basement membranes; nonfibrillary

Top Differential Diagnoses
- Light chain deposition by immunofluorescence only
- Light chain tubulointerstitial nephritis
- Dense deposit disease (DDD)
- Nodular diabetic glomerulosclerosis
- Light chain Fanconi syndrome

MICROSCOPIC PATHOLOGY

Histologic Features
- Nodular glomerulopathy
  - PAS-positive nodules, nonargyrophilic
- Interstitial inflammation
- Interstitial edema
- Acute tubular injury
- TBM thickening may be present
- Congo red negative deposits
  - Concurrent amyloidosis may be present
- Rare cases may show thickened glomerular basement membranes with an associated membranoproliferative pattern
  - These cases must show linear GBM and TBM monoclonal immunoglobulin deposits to be diagnosed as MIDD
- Concurrent light chain cast nephropathy present in nearly 1/3 of renal biopsies with MIDD
- Concurrent amyloidosis in 13% of MIDD cases
- Necrotizing and crescentic glomerulonephritis (rare)
  - Seen more frequently in alpha-HCDD

ANCILLARY TESTS

Immunohistochemistry
- In absence of IF material, cases may show glomerular and TBM deposits for kappa or lambda light chain

Immunofluorescence
- Linear basement membrane staining (glomerular, tubular, vascular) for monoclonal immunoglobulin
  - Usually monotypic kappa light chain in LCDD (73-91% kappa)
  - Kappa or lambda light chain in LCDD
  - Heavy chain only in HCDD
    - Usually IgG
    - All IgG subclasses (1, 2, 3, and 4) have been reported to cause gamma-HCDD
    - Rare cases of IgA-HCDD
  - 1 heavy chain and 1 light chain in LHCDD

- Smudgy staining of mesangium for monoclonal protein
- Staining for IgG subclasses helps determine monoclonal nature of deposits in gamma-HCDD

Electron Microscopy
- Finely granular, punctate, "powdery" electron-dense deposits distributed along basement membranes; nonfibrillary
  - Similar appearing deposits in LCDD, LHCDD, and HCDD
- Monoclonal deposits may be seen by immunogold labeling

DIFFERENTIAL DIAGNOSIS

Light Chain Deposition by Immunofluorescence Only
- Monotypic light chain staining of GBM and TBM by IF, but no deposits detectable by EM and no changes by light microscopy
- Seen especially in cases of light chain cast nephropathy
- Uncertain significance
  - May be artifactual IF staining representative of monoclonal protein in urine

Light Chain Tubulointerstitial Nephritis
- Pattern of acute tubulointerstitial nephritis
- Absence of a glomerulopathy
- Negative IF and routine EM
- In some cases, light chain deposits seen in some TBMs by EM with immunogold labeling or by immunoperoxidase staining

Proliferative Glomerulonephritis with Monoclonal IgG Deposits
- Proliferative glomerulonephritis pattern by light microscopy
- Monotypic IgG kappa or IgG lambda staining by IF; IgG is restricted to 1 subclass

MONOCLONAL IMMUNOGLOBULIN DEPOSITION DISEASE

- Amorphous electron-dense deposits in glomeruli by EM
- Absence of TBM deposits by IF and EM
- Low incidence of associated multiple myeloma

Dense Deposit Disease (DDD)

- Some cases of DDD are associated with serum paraprotein, which may have C3 nephritic factor activity
- DDD shows staining by IF for C3 only, not monoclonal immunoglobulins
- Very electron-dense deposits along GBMs and in mesangium, distinct from finely granular deposits in GBMs and TBMs in MIDD

Nodular Diabetic Glomerulosclerosis

- Similar PAS positive nodular glomerulopathy to MIDD but without IF or EM findings of MIDD

Fibrillary or Immunotactoid Glomerulonephritis

- May show monotypic glomerular staining by IF, especially immunotactoid glomerulonephritis
  - Smudgy IgG kappa or IgG lambda mesangial staining and glomerular basement membrane staining
- Fibrillary substructure to deposits by EM
- Usual absence of TBM deposits

Type 1 Cryoglobulinemic Glomerulonephritis or Waldenström Macroglobulinemic Glomerulonephritis

- Deposition of a monoclonal immunoglobulin in glomeruli
- Membranoproliferative pattern of glomerular injury
- Absence of finely granular deposits along glomerular and TBMs

Light Chain Fanconi Syndrome (Light Chain Proximal Tubulopathy)

- Light chain deposits within tubular epithelial cells rather than within basement membranes
- Crystalline deposits within epithelial cytoplasm

Amyloidosis

- Congo red positive, amorphous, PAS negative deposits
- Fibrillary structure by EM
- Amyloid may be present in glomeruli, vessels, and interstitium

IgA Nephropathy

- Alpha-HCDD, in part due to its rarity, may be misdiagnosed as IgA nephropathy
- Like IgA nephropathy, alpha-HCDD may show necrotizing and crescentic glomerulonephritis
- By IF, alpha-HCDD shows linear TBM staining for IgA along with glomerular staining
- By EM, alpha-HCDD shows granular GBM and TBM deposits typical of MIDD
- Usual absence of TBM deposits in IgA nephropathy

Recurrent or De Novo MIDD in Allograft

- May be seen on protocol biopsies when clinically inapparent

DIAGNOSTIC CHECKLIST

Clinically Relevant Pathologic Features

- 31-45% of patients with pure MIDD have overt multiple myeloma at time of MIDD diagnosis
- 91% of patients with concurrent MIDD and cast nephropathy have multiple myeloma
- M spike on serum or urine protein electrophoresis in ~ 50% of patients with pure MIDD
- Hypocomplementemia
  - Present in gamma-HCDD with complement-fixing IgG subclass deposited (gamma-1 or gamma-3)

SELECTED REFERENCES

1. Herrera GA et al: Ultrastructural immunolabeling in the diagnosis of monoclonal light-and heavy-chain-related renal diseases. Ultrastruct Pathol. 34(3):161-73, 2010
2. Sethi S et al: Dense deposit disease associated with monoclonal gammopathy of undetermined significance. Am J Kidney Dis. 56(5):977-82, 2010
3. Alexander MP et al: Alpha heavy chain deposition disease: a comparison of its clinicopathological characteristics with gamma and mu heavy chain deposition disease. Mod Pathol. 20(Suppl. 2):270A, 2007
4. Salant DJ et al: A case of atypical light chain deposition disease--diagnosis and treatment. Clin J Am Soc Nephrol. 2(4):858-67, 2007
5. Gu X et al: Light-chain-mediated acute tubular interstitial nephritis: a poorly recognized pattern of renal disease in patients with plasma cell dyscrasia. Arch Pathol Lab Med. 130(2):165-9, 2006
6. Rosenstock JL et al: Fibrillary and immunotactoid glomerulonephritis: Distinct entities with different clinical and pathologic features. Kidney Int. 63(4):1450-61, 2003
7. Lin J et al: Renal monoclonal immunoglobulin deposition disease: the disease spectrum. J Am Soc Nephrol. 12(7):1482-92, 2001
8. Buxbaum J et al: Nonamyloidotic monoclonal immunoglobulin deposition disease. Light-chain, heavy-chain, and light- and heavy-chain deposition diseases. Hematol Oncol Clin North Am. 13(6):1235-48, 1999
9. Kambham N et al: Heavy chain deposition disease: the disease spectrum. Am J Kidney Dis. 33(5):954-62, 1999
10. Cheng IK et al: Crescentic nodular glomerulosclerosis secondary to truncated immunoglobulin alpha heavy chain deposition. Am J Kidney Dis. 28(2):283-8, 1996
11. Buxbaum J: Mechanisms of disease: monoclonal immunoglobulin deposition. Amyloidosis, light chain deposition disease, and light and heavy chain deposition disease. Hematol Oncol Clin North Am. 6(2):323-46, 1992
12. Randall RE et al: Manifestations of systemic light chain deposition. Am J Med. 60(2):293-9, 1976

MONOCLONAL IMMUNOGLOBULIN DEPOSITION DISEASE

Light Chain Deposition Disease

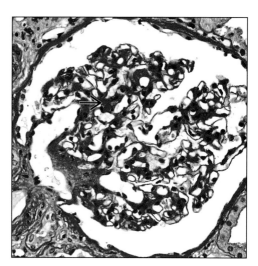
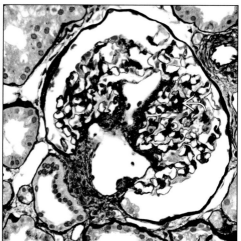

(Left) Light chain MIDD can show a variety of histologic patterns ranging from very mild mesangial expansion by PAS positive material, shown here ➡, to nodular glomerulosclerosis. *(Right)* A silver stain shows very mild mesangial expansion ➡ by nonargyrophilic material in a patient with light chain MIDD. The diagnosis would not be suspected without immunofluorescence demonstration of a single light chain and the electron-dense deposits by EM.

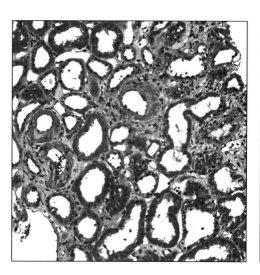
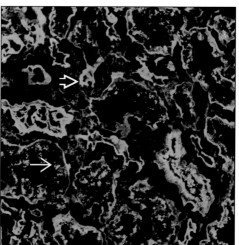

(Left) Tubules are dilatated and show flattening of the epithelium, both features of acute injury. This patient had proteinuria and acute renal failure. Tubular symptoms, such as polyuria, can dominate in light chain MIDD. *(Right)* IF staining reveals bright linear tubular basement membrane staining for kappa light chain ➡, the most common light chain in MIDD, with negative staining for lambda light chain (not shown). Tubular protein reabsorption droplets are also present and stain for kappa ➡.

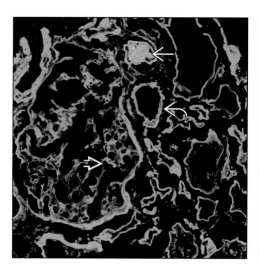
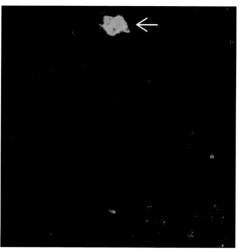

(Left) IF staining reveals bright linear glomerular ➡ and tubular ➡ basement membrane staining for kappa light chain. A cast ➡ is present, which also stained for kappa, but the casts were similarly stained for lambda. *(Right)* IF staining for lambda in a biopsy with a kappa light chain MIDD reveals negative glomerular and tubular basement membrane staining, but the cast does stain for lambda light chains ➡. Light chains are normally present in the urine in low concentrations.

MONOCLONAL IMMUNOGLOBULIN DEPOSITION DISEASE

Electron Microscopy

(Left) EM in light chain deposition disease shows finely granular electron-dense deposits along the glomerular basement membranes ➡. *(Right)* Higher magnification shows finely granular, "powdery" electron-dense deposits along the glomerular basement membranes ➡ in LCDD.

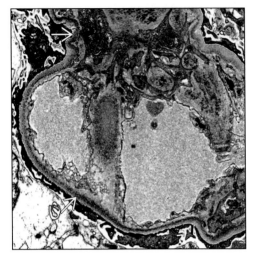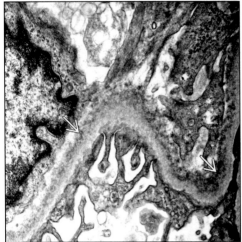

(Left) Granular electron-dense deposits are seen along the tubular basement membranes ⧩ in LCDD. *(Right)* Finely granular electron-dense deposits are shown along the tubular basement membranes ➡ in LCDD.

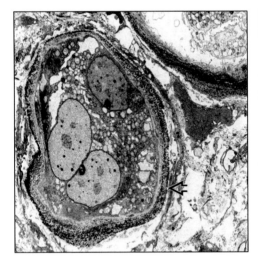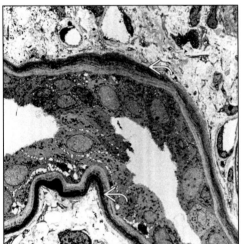

(Left) Gamma heavy chain deposition disease shows finely granular electron-dense deposits along the tubular basement membrane. The appearance of HCDD by electron microscopy is indistinguishable from LCDD. *(Right)* Gamma heavy chain deposition disease shows finely granular electron-dense deposits present along the glomerular basement membranes ➡ and within the mesangium ⧩, as in LCDD.

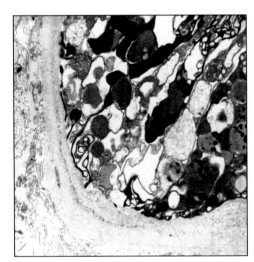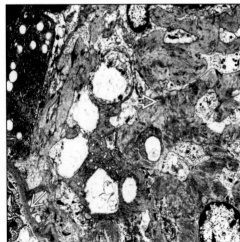

Gamma Heavy Chain Deposition Disease

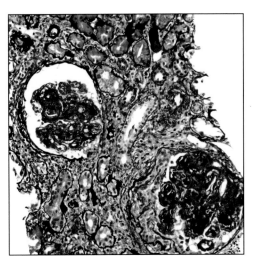
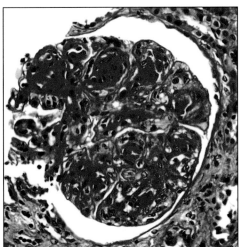

(Left) Nodular glomerulosclerosis is shown. Immunofluorescence showed bright linear glomerular and tubular basement membrane staining for IgG, without staining for light chains (silver stain). *(Right)* Nodular glomerulosclerosis with PAS-positive nodules is shown. This disease may be confused with nodular diabetic glomerulosclerosis.

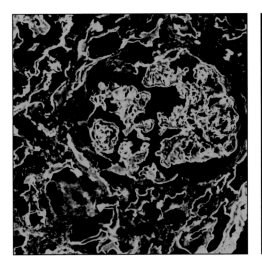
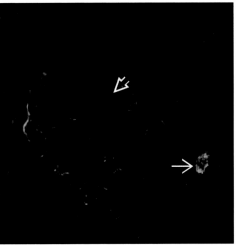

(Left) Immunofluorescence staining for IgG shows bright linear glomerular and tubular basement membrane staining and smudgy mesangial staining. This appearance may also resemble IgG staining in diabetes. *(Right)* Immunofluorescence staining for kappa light chain was negative ⇨, in contrast to the expected result in diabetes, as was staining for lambda light chain. Proteinaceous casts are positive ⇨, a useful internal control.

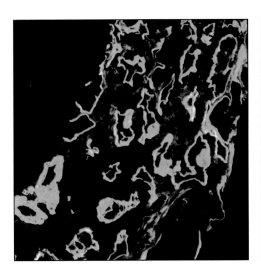
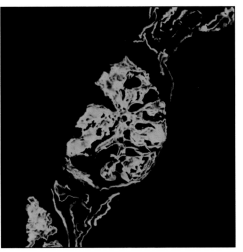

(Left) Immunofluorescence staining for the IgG3 subclass shows bright linear tubular basement membrane staining; glomeruli were also positive. Stains for IgG1, 2, and 4 were negative. The presence of staining for a single IgG subclass supports the diagnosis of heavy chain MIDD. *(Right)* Glomeruli were also positive for IgG3 and negative for other IgG subclasses as well as light chains.

MONOCLONAL IMMUNOGLOBULIN DEPOSITION DISEASE

Light and Heavy Chain Deposition Disease

(Left) A glomerulus shows a nodular expansion of the mesangium. This biopsy is from a 72-year-old woman with a history of multiple myeloma and an IgG kappa paraprotein. *(Right)* Higher magnification of a trichrome stain shows a glomerulus with nodular expansion of the mesangium ➡. Immunofluorescence showed bright linear staining of the glomerular and tubular basement membranes for IgG and kappa, without staining for lambda light chain.

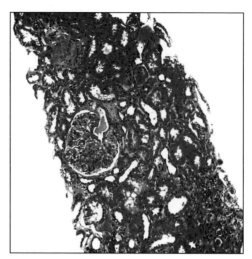 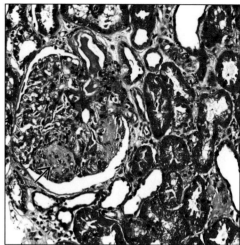

(Left) LHCDD shows linear glomerular basement membrane and mesangial staining for IgG; tubular basement membrane linear staining was present as well. Similar staining was seen for kappa light chain, with negative staining for lambda light chain. This case showed greater staining for IgG than the usual background linear IgG staining by immunofluorescence. *(Right)* LHCDD shows linear glomerular and tubular basement membrane staining for kappa light chain; similar staining for IgG was also seen.

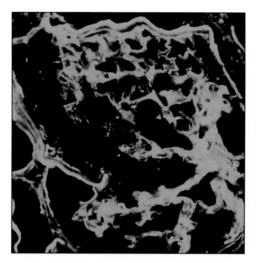 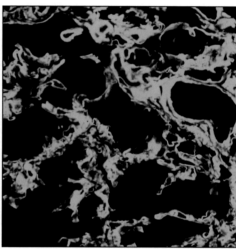

(Left) IgG kappa LHCDD shows negative glomerular and tubular basement staining for lambda light chain. The round yellow granules are autofluorescent lipids. *(Right)* Finely granular electron-dense deposits ➡ are present along the tubular basement membrane in this case of LHCDD.

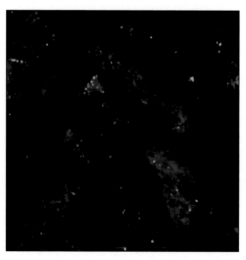 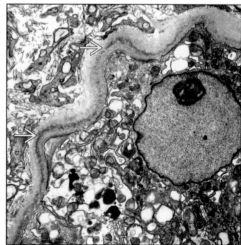

MONOCLONAL IMMUNOGLOBULIN DEPOSITION DISEASE

Alpha Heavy Chain Deposition Disease

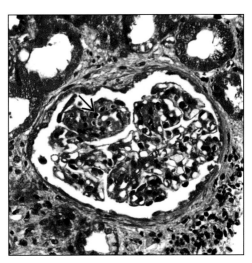 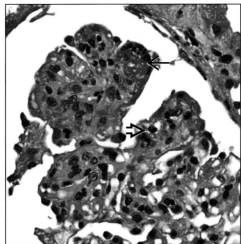

(Left) Trichrome stain shows nodular expansion of the glomerular mesangium ➡ in alpha-HCDD. (Courtesy S. Nasr, MD.) *(Right)* Segmental necrosis of the glomerular tuft ➡ is seen in alpha-HCDD. As opposed to gamma heavy chain or light chain deposition disease, it is not uncommon for alpha-HCDD to show glomerular necrosis or crescents. Segmental capillary loops contain neutrophils ➡. (Courtesy S. Nasr, MD.)

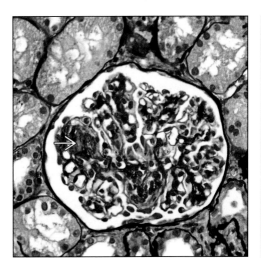 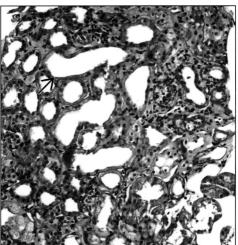

(Left) Most glomeruli show a nodular expansion of the mesangium by nonargyrophilic material ➡ and without crescents or necrosis (silver stain). (Courtesy S. Nasr, MD.) *(Right)* Focal tubules show features of acute injury ➡, including dilatation of the tubules, flattening of the epithelium, and loss of the tubular brush border. There is very focal interstitial inflammation. (Courtesy S. Nasr, MD.)

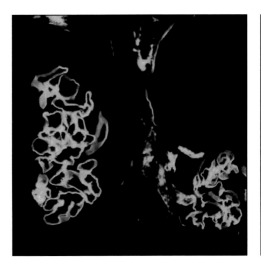 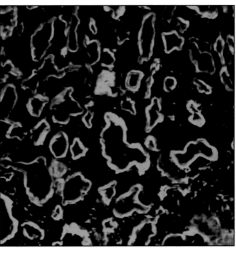

(Left) Immunofluorescence on pronase-digested paraffin sections shows linear GBM and smudgy mesangial staining for IgA. No glomeruli were present on the tissue originally submitted for immunofluorescence; pronase-digested paraffin sections reveal this glomerular staining. (Courtesy S. Nasr, MD.) *(Right)* Immunofluorescence reveals bright linear tubular basement staining for IgA. (Courtesy S. Nasr, MD.)

MONOCLONAL IMMUNOGLOBULIN DEPOSITION DISEASE

Differential Diagnosis

(Left) Dense deposit disease (DDD) in a 48-year-old woman with a serum monoclonal protein shows very electron-dense amorphous deposits within the mesangium and within the GBM ⇨, not to be confused with MIDD. Some cases of DDD are associated with paraproteins that show C3 nephritic factor activity. *(Right)* Dense deposit disease is seen in a woman with a paraprotein. Intramembranous very electron-dense deposits are seen within glomeruli ⇨, distinct from finely granular deposits of MIDD.

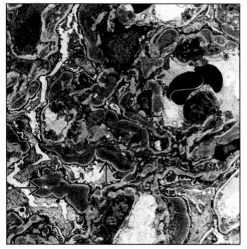 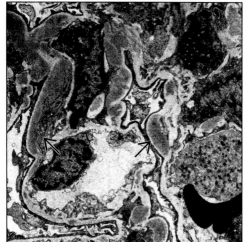

(Left) Dense deposit disease with very electron-dense tubular basement membrane deposits ⇨ is seen focally. In contrast to MIDD, these deposits do not have a granular substructure. *(Right)* In this case of dense deposit disease, focal tubular basement membrane deposits only stain for C3. Glomeruli also stained for C3.

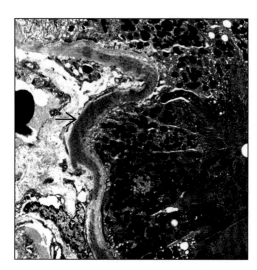 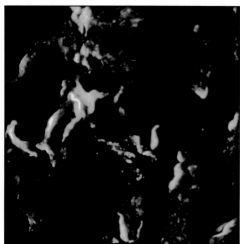

(Left) MIDD "by immunofluorescence only" with linear tubular basement membrane staining for IgG is seen on a protocol biopsy 5 years after kidney transplantation. Staining for kappa and lambda light chains was negative. The patient did not have evidence of a paraprotein by immunofixation. *(Right)* MIDD "by immunofluorescence only" does not show evidence of tubular basement membrane deposits, despite bright staining by IF for IgG. The findings are of uncertain significance.

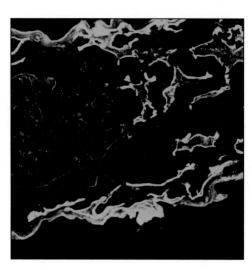 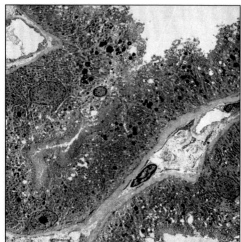

MONOCLONAL IMMUNOGLOBULIN DEPOSITION DISEASE

Variant Microscopic Features

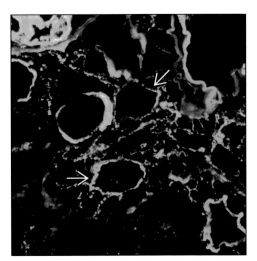
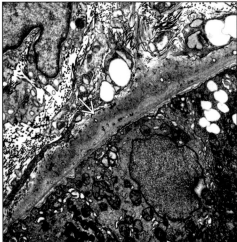

(Left) This case of LCDD has an unusual feature of granular ➡, rather than linear, tubular basement membrane staining for monoclonal kappa light chain. The lambda light chain stain was negative. (Right) Despite granular rather than linear tubular basement membrane staining by immunofluorescence, tubular basement membranes by EM show finely granular electron-dense deposits ➡.

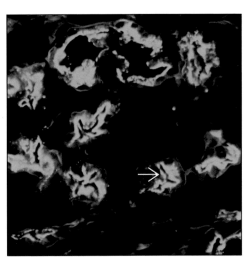
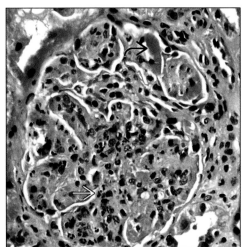

(Left) The apical surface of tubular epithelial cells shows unusual monotypic kappa light chain staining ➡. Tubular reabsorption droplets also showed monotypic staining for kappa. There is no TBM staining, so this does not represent light chain deposition disease. (Right) HL MIDD (IgG kappa) recurred 6 weeks post transplant with a pattern of acute glomerulonephritis. Neutrophils ➡ are seen in the capillaries, and the eosinophilic precipitates ➡ suggest cryoglobulinemia.

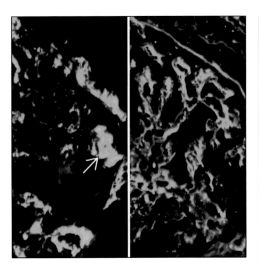
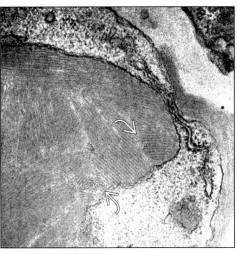

(Left) Recurrent HL MIDD 28 days post transplant shows striking intracapillary deposits of kappa ➡ (left) but not lambda (right) light chains. Gamma heavy chain was also present. The native kidney had nodular glomerulosclerosis but did not stain for light or heavy chains. (Right) EM shows recurrent HL chain MIDD (IgG kappa) that caused acute GN 6 weeks post transplant. The organized tubular substructure with a diameter of ~ 17 nm can be seen in the intracapillary precipitates ➡.

MONOCLONAL IMMUNOGLOBULIN DEPOSITION DISEASE

Variant Microscopic Features

(Left) A more proliferative glomerular pattern is seen in this case of HCDD, with endocapillary hypercellularity ➡ and segmental glomerular basement membrane duplication. *(Right)* Glomerular basement membrane duplication ⇉ is seen in this case of HCDD, along with finely granular glomerular basement membrane and mesangial deposits.

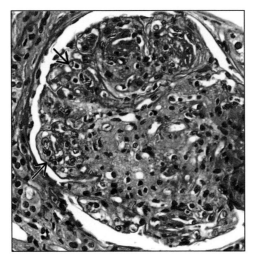
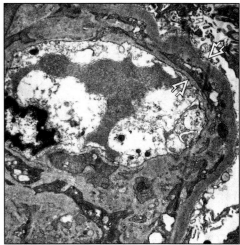

(Left) Segmental glomerular basement membrane duplication ➡, a membranoproliferative feature, can be seen on a silver stain in this case of LCDD. *(Right)* Immunofluorescence reveals linear glomerular ➡ and tubular ⇉ basement membrane staining and smudgy mesangial staining for kappa light chain.

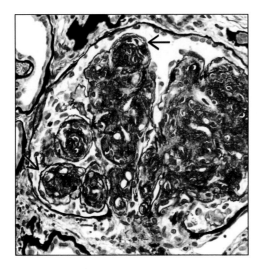
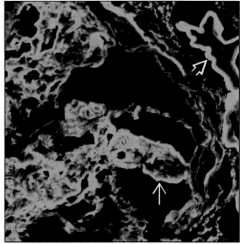

(Left) Finely granular electron-dense deposits are seen in the mesangium ➡ and in tubular glomerular basement membranes ⇉. *(Right)* Tubular basement membranes show finely granular electron-dense deposits ➡.

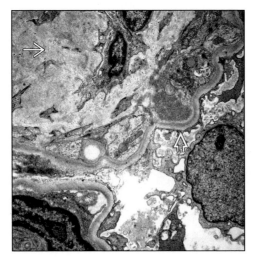
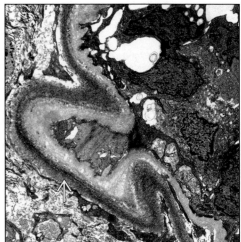

Differential Diagnosis

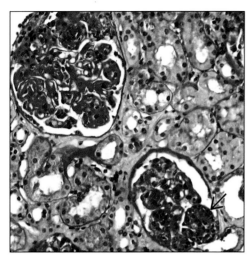

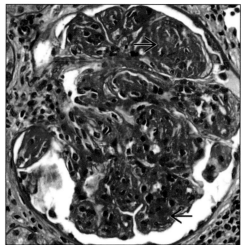

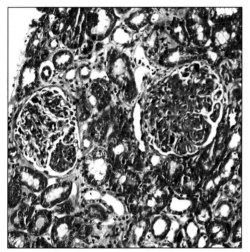

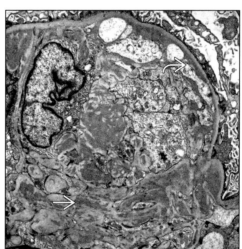

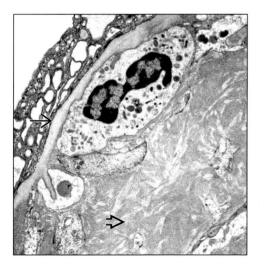

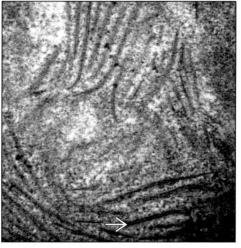

(Left) This case of immunotactoid glomerulonephritis shows a nodular expansion of the mesangium and endocapillary proliferation ➔. *(Right)* PAS positive nodular mesangial expansion ➔, similar to MIDD, is seen in this case of immunotactoid glomerulonephritis. This case showed monotypic glomerular staining for IgG lambda.

(Left) Trichrome stain shows variable mesangial expansion between glomeruli in this case of immunotactoid glomerulonephritis. This case showed monotypic glomerular staining for IgG lambda. *(Right)* This case of immunotactoid glomerulonephritis shows an expanded mesangium with mesangial ➔ and subendothelial ➔ immune deposits.

(Left) Note the absence ➔ of finely granular deposits along the glomerular basement membrane in this case of immunotactoid glomerulonephritis, which by light microscopy had a nodular appearance of the mesangium reminiscent of MIDD. The deposits show an organized substructure ➔. *(Right)* Fibrils with a hollow center are seen ➔. The differential diagnosis is type I cryoglobulinemic glomerulonephritis vs. immunotactoid glomerulonephritis, which may be a related entity.

PROLIFERATIVE GLOMERULONEPHRITIS WITH MONOCLONAL IgG DEPOSITS

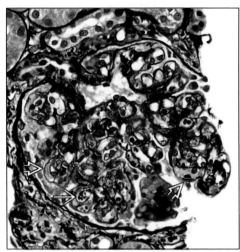

PGNMID with a membranoproliferative pattern shows mesangial and endocapillary ➡ hypercellularity with neutrophils and mononuclear cells. Glomerular basement membrane duplication ⟱ is also seen.

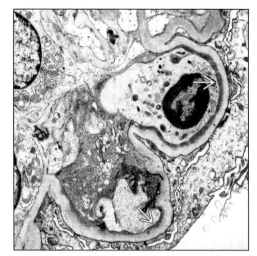

Electron micrograph from a case of PGNMID with a membranoproliferative pattern shows subendothelial electron-dense deposits ➡ that appear almost intramembranous.

TERMINOLOGY

Abbreviations
- Proliferative glomerulonephritis with monoclonal IgG deposits (PGNMID)

Synonyms
- Nasr glomerulopathy

ETIOLOGY/PATHOGENESIS

Monoclonal IgG Deposited in Glomeruli
- Usually IgG3; IgG3 highly complement-fixing and may be more "nephritogenic" than other IgG subclasses

CLINICAL ISSUES

Epidemiology
- Age
  - Average age is 55 years; range of 20-81
- Gender
  - Female predominance, 2:1

Presentation
- Nephrotic-range proteinuria in ~ 70%
- Nephrotic syndrome in ~ 50%
- Hematuria
- Renal dysfunction in ~ 65%
- Only rarely associated with multiple myeloma
- May recur in allograft
  - Recurrent disease presents as renal insufficiency, proteinuria, or hematuria

Laboratory Tests
- Low C3 (± C4) in ~ 25% of patients
- Negative tests for cryoglobulinemia
- Serum and urine monoclonal proteins in ~ 30% of patients

Treatment
- Drugs
  - Steroids alone or with other immunosuppressive agents
  - Angiotensin-converting enzyme inhibitor or angiotensin II receptor blocker

Prognosis
- Variable
  - ~ 40% show partial or complete recovery
  - ~ 20% progress to end-stage renal disease

MICROSCOPIC PATHOLOGY

Histologic Features
- Membranoproliferative pattern in 57%
  - Diffuse, global glomerular basement membrane (GBM) duplication
  - Mesangial hypercellularity and matrix expansion
  - May also have segmental membranous or endocapillary proliferative patterns
- Endocapillary proliferative pattern in 35%
  - May also have segmental membranoproliferative or membranous patterns
- Membranous pattern in 5%
  - Global subepithelial immune deposits
  - Cases usually show some proliferative features
- Mesangial proliferative pattern in 3%
- ~ 30% of cases show focal or diffuse crescents
- Focal segmental glomerulosclerosis may be present

ANCILLARY TESTS

Immunofluorescence
- Usual granular mesangial and GBM staining
- Monotypic IgG kappa or lambda staining
  - Most cases kappa light chain-restricted (73%)
- IgG subclass staining

PROLIFERATIVE GLOMERULONEPHRITIS WITH MONOCLONAL IgG DEPOSITS

Key Facts

Clinical Issues
- Nephrotic-range proteinuria in ~ 70%
- Renal dysfunction in ~ 65%

Microscopic Pathology
- Membranoproliferative pattern in 57%
- Endocapillary proliferative pattern in 35%
- Membranous or mesangial proliferative patterns less common
- ~ 30% of cases show focal or diffuse crescents
- Focal segmental glomerulosclerosis may be present

Ancillary Tests
- Restriction to a single IgG subclass, usually IgG3, by immunofluorescence
  - Light chain restricted, usually kappa

- Predominantly mesangial and subendothelial, electron-dense deposits by EM
- Serum or urine monoclonal protein found in ~ 30% of patients
- Negative staining for IgA and IgM

Top Differential Diagnoses
- Membranoproliferative glomerulonephritis (without monoclonal deposits)
- Membranous glomerulonephritis (without monoclonal deposits)
- Type I cryoglobulinemic glomerulonephritis
- Fibrillary or immunotactoid glomerulonephritis
- Proliferative glomerulonephritis secondary to monoclonal IgA
- Light and heavy chain deposition disease

- Restriction to a single IgG subclass required for diagnosis
  - Supportive of monoclonal nature of deposits
- IgG3 subclass restriction most common; IgG1 subclass next most common
  - No cases of IgG4 subclass restriction have been identified
- C3 almost always present; C1q present in most cases
- Negative staining for IgA and IgM
- No extraglomerular IgG deposits

Electron Microscopy
- Electron-dense deposits
  - Predominantly mesangial and subendothelial
  - Occasional subepithelial deposits with membranous pattern, at least segmentally
  - Deposits mostly amorphous
    - Rare areas of organized deposits may be present in some cases

DIFFERENTIAL DIAGNOSIS

Membranoproliferative Glomerulonephritis (MPGN)
- Typical MPGN shows polytypic staining of deposits for kappa and lambda light chains

Membranous Glomerulonephritis (MGN)
- Some cases of PGNMID have a predominantly membranous pattern
  - Usually some endocapillary proliferation
- Typical MGN shows polytypic staining of deposits for kappa and lambda light chains

Type I Cryoglobulinemic Glomerulonephritis
- Similar to PGNMID, type 1 cryoglobulin usually composed of IgG3
- Intraluminal immunoglobulin "pseudothrombi" in glomeruli by light microscopy
- Positive test for cryoglobulinemia

Fibrillary or Immunotactoid Glomerulonephritis
- May show monotypic IgG kappa or lambda staining by immunofluorescence (IF)
- Organized substructure (fibrils) of immune deposits by electron microscopy (EM)

Proliferative Glomerulonephritis Secondary to Monoclonal IgA
- Similar to PGNMID but with monoclonal IgA rather than IgG

Light and Heavy Chain Deposition Disease, Randall Type
- Linear glomerular and tubular basement membrane staining by IF
- Finely granular, electron-dense deposits along glomerular and tubular basement membranes and in mesangium

Amyloidosis
- Rare cases composed of both light and heavy chains
- Congo red(+) deposits, fibrils by EM

SELECTED REFERENCES

1. Nasr SH et al: Proliferative glomerulonephritis with monoclonal IgG deposits recurs in the allograft. Clin J Am Soc Nephrol. 6(1):122-32, 2011
2. Masai R et al: Characteristics of proliferative glomerulo-nephritis with monoclonal IgG deposits associated with membranoproliferative features. Clin Nephrol. 72(1):46-54, 2009
3. Nasr SH et al: Proliferative glomerulonephritis with monoclonal IgG deposits. J Am Soc Nephrol. 20(9):2055-64, 2009
4. Komatsuda A et al: Monoclonal immunoglobulin deposition disease associated with membranous features. Nephrol Dial Transplant. 23(12):3888-94, 2008
5. Soares SM et al: A proliferative glomerulonephritis secondary to a monoclonal IgA. Am J Kidney Dis. 47(2):342-9, 2006

2

PROLIFERATIVE GLOMERULONEPHRITIS WITH MONOCLONAL IgG DEPOSITS

Light Microscopy

(Left) PGNMID has a variable light microscopic appearance ranging from mild mesangial hypercellularity and inflammation (shown here) to full-blown acute glomerulonephritis. This case had IgG lambda deposits in subepithelial "humps." *(Right)* PGNMID may be unsuspected by light microscopy if the inflammatory change is mild, as in this case. Prominent "humps" were present that stained by immunofluorescence for IgG lambda (PAS-diastase).

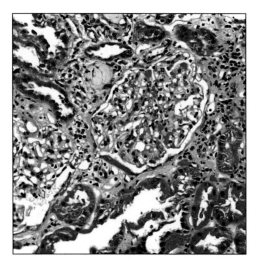 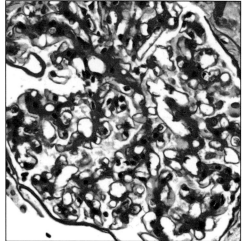

(Left) This case of PGNMID shows segmental endocapillary hypercellularity ⇨ and a small cellular crescent ⇨. IF and EM showed a predominantly membranous pattern. *(Right)* A silver stain shows focal endocapillary ⇨ proliferation, along with mesangial hypercellularity, seen in this case of PGNMID. By immunofluorescence, the glomeruli stained for IgG3 kappa.

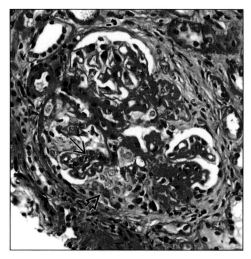 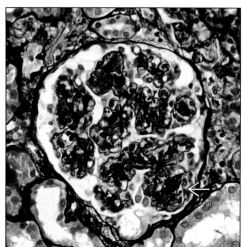

(Left) This case of PGNMID shows mostly a mesangioproliferative ⇨ pattern; a segmental membranous pattern was also seen. *(Right)* Segmental glomerular basement membrane "spikes" ⇨ can be seen in this case of PGNMID with a predominantly mesangioproliferative pattern (silver stain).

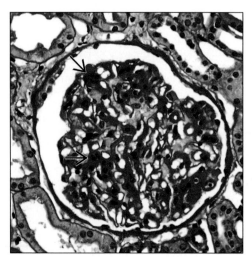 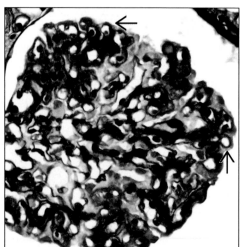

PROLIFERATIVE GLOMERULONEPHRITIS WITH MONOCLONAL IgG DEPOSITS

Immunofluorescence

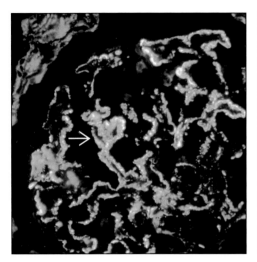
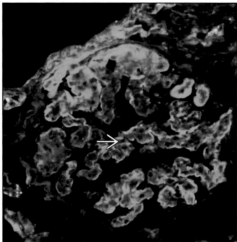

(Left) Immunofluorescence staining reveals predominantly glomerular basement membrane ➡ granular staining for IgG3, here with a membranous pattern in areas. Staining of glomeruli was negative for IgG1, IgG2, and IgG4. *(Right)* Immunofluorescence staining for IgG1 shows absence of staining of a glomerulus ➡. Glomeruli were also negative for IgG2 and IgG4 and showed staining only for IgG3, C1q, C3, and lambda light chain.

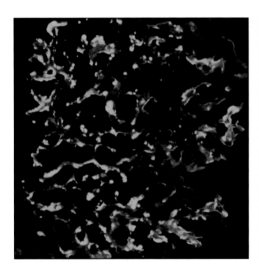
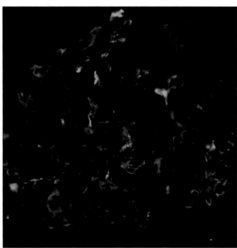

(Left) This case of PGNMID has widespread, rounded deposits along the GBM that stain for lambda (shown here) and gamma heavy chain, but not kappa light chain. These correspond to the "humps" seen by electron microscopy. *(Right)* This case of PGNMID would have been confused with acute glomerulonephritis if the light chain stains had not been done. This image shows little kappa in contrast to lambda and gamma heavy chain stains.

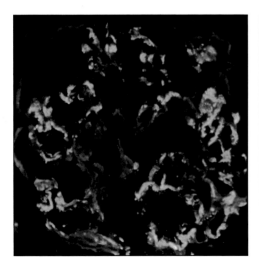
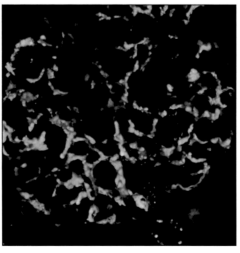

(Left) Immunofluorescence staining for IgG showed granular mesangial and segmental glomerular basement membrane staining. The same pattern was seen for IgG3 but with negative staining for IgG1, IgG2, or IgG4. *(Right)* Immunofluorescence staining for lambda light chain shows a similar staining pattern as IgG and IgG3 in this case, with mesangial and segmental glomerular basement membrane staining. Glomerular staining for kappa light chain was negative.

PROLIFERATIVE GLOMERULONEPHRITIS WITH MONOCLONAL IgG DEPOSITS

Electron Microscopy

(Left) Electron microscopy reveals linear subendothelial deposits ➡ in a case of PGNMID. *(Right)* This case of PGNMID showed a predominantly membranous pattern with regularly spaced subepithelial, electron-dense deposits ➡ with intervening basement membrane "spikes." By IF, the deposits showed monoclonal staining for IgG2 kappa. This case showed rare endocapillary proliferation and a rare, small, cellular crescent by light microscopy.

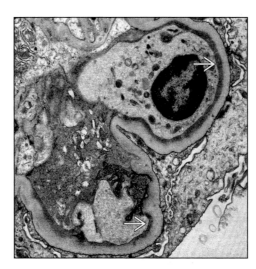
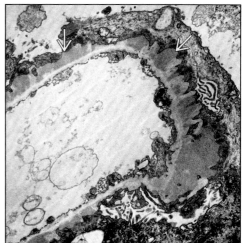

(Left) Low-power EM shows widespread, variegated deposits in the mesangium ➡ and subepithelial "humps" ➡ in a patient with PGNMID that stained for IgG lambda. *(Right)* PGNMID shows subepithelial deposits ➡ that resemble the "humps" of acute glomerulonephritis (GN) or sometimes have GBM "spikes" ➡, as shown here. No paracrystalline structure was evident although the deposits do have a heterogeneous density.

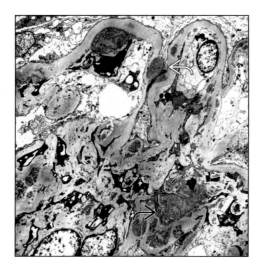
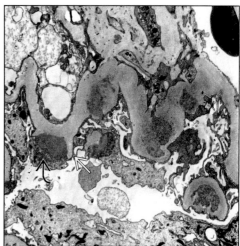

(Left) The deposits ➡ in PGNMID usually do not show substructure by electron microscopy. *(Right)* This case showed a segmental membranous pattern of immune complex deposition, with subepithelial deposits ➡ with intervening basement membrane "spikes." Subendothelial deposits ➡ are also present, in contrast to the usual idiopathic membranous glomerulonephritis (MGN). Monotypic light chains are also not a feature of MGN.

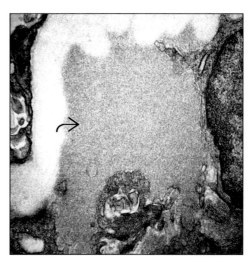
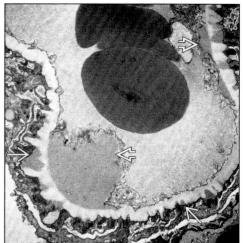

PROLIFERATIVE GLOMERULONEPHRITIS WITH MONOCLONAL IgG DEPOSITS

Recurrent PGNMID in Allografts

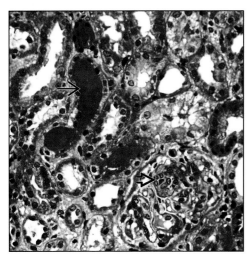
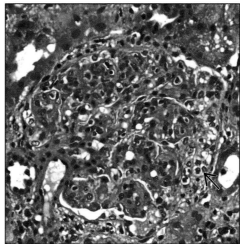

(Left) Recurrent PGNMID shows endocapillary and mesangial ⊟ hypercellularity in a glomerulus and red blood cell casts ⊟ at ~ 10 months post transplant (trichome). (Right) Diffuse endocapillary hypercellularity is seen in a case of recurrent PGNMID at ~ 10 months post transplant. Focal cellular crescents ⊟ were also present. IF showed monoclonal IgG kappa deposits in glomeruli.

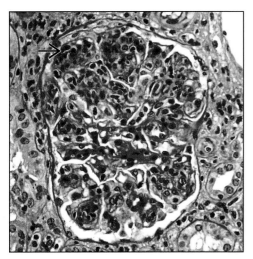
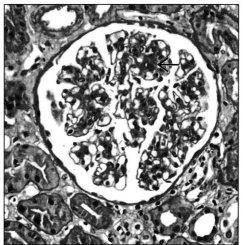

(Left) Recurrent PGNMID 10 months post transplant shows diffuse endocapillary hypercellularity ⊟, not to be confused with glomerulitis. The patient had proteinuria at 1.8 g/dL. (Right) Recurrent PGNMID 12 months post transplant shows progressively less endocapillary hypercellularity following treatment with cyclophosphamide; mesangial hypercellularity ⊟ is still present. The patient had only ~ 0.13 g/dL proteinuria.

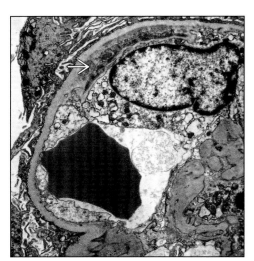
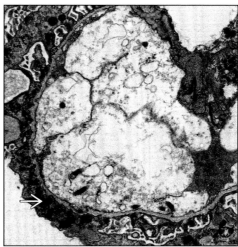

(Left) An occasional subendothelial electron-dense deposit ⊟ is seen, with early glomerular basement membrane duplication, in early recurrent PGNMID in a transplant. (Right) EM of early recurrent PGNMID in a renal allograft shows scattered subepithelial deposits ⊟. Recurrent PGNMID may show any glomerular disease pattern seen in the native kidney.

TYPE I CRYOGLOBULINEMIC GLOMERULONEPHRITIS

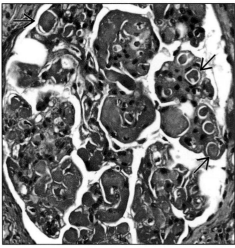

Type I cryoglobulinemic GN shows massive deposition of immune complexes, including immunoglobulin "pseudothrombi" ➔ within glomerular capillary lumens.

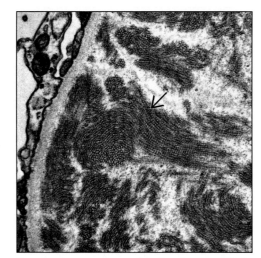

Deposits in type I cryoglobulinemia show fibrils, sometimes with a "curvilinear" pattern ➔, as shown in this patient with IgM kappa deposits.

TERMINOLOGY

Abbreviations
- Type I cryoglobulinemic glomerulonephritis (type I CryoGN)

Definitions
- Glomerulonephritis caused by cryoproteins derived from monoclonal immunoglobulins
- Cryoglobulins precipitate at low temperature (4°C) and redissolve at 37°C
- Cryoglobulinemia is categorized into 3 types based on the composition of the cryoprecipitate
  - Type I: Monoclonal Ig (single light chain species)
  - Type II: Monoclonal IgM rheumatoid factor and polyclonal Ig
  - Type III: Polyclonal immunoglobulin

ETIOLOGY/PATHOGENESIS

Monoclonal Immunoglobulin Deposition
- Physicochemical properties of monoclonal immunoglobulin
  - Promotes precipitation in plasma below 37°C
  - High level in plasma
- Precipitates probably form in skin (temperature related)
  - Fix complement (IgG3 most effective at this)
  - Lodge in glomeruli
  - Trigger inflammation locally in skin and kidney

Therapy Related
- Increased release of cytoplasmic or membrane Ig
  - Rituximab reported to precipitate severe type I cryoglobulinemia in Waldenström macroglobulinemia
  - After institution of melphalan for multiple myeloma

CLINICAL ISSUES

Epidemiology
- Incidence
  - Rare
  - 25-40% of patients with type I cryoglobulinemia develop renal disease
  - Only 18 biopsied cases reported as of 2002

Presentation
- Nephrotic syndrome
  - ~ 75%
- Hematuria
  - 100%
- Acute renal failure
- Purpura/cutaneous vasculitis
- Raynaud phenomenon
- History of lymphoproliferative disease
  - CLL
  - Lymphoma
  - Multiple myeloma
  - Waldenström macroglobulinemia
- Occasional cases without lymphoproliferative disease

Laboratory Tests
- Serum immunoelectrophoresis
- Cryoprecipitate assay
- Variable hypocomplementemia
- Negative for HCV

Treatment
- Partial remissions reported after treatment with cyclophosphamide or chlorambucil with corticosteroids

Prognosis
- Depends on underlying lymphoproliferative disease
- Remissions have been reported in myeloma (3 years)

TYPE I CRYOGLOBULINEMIC GLOMERULONEPHRITIS

Key Facts

Terminology
- GN caused by cryoproteins derived from monoclonal immunoglobulins

Etiology/Pathogenesis
- Precipitates probably form in skin and lodge in kidney
- Trigger inflammation locally

Clinical Issues
- 25-40% of patients with type I cryoglobulinemia develop renal disease
- Nephrotic syndrome
- Hematuria
- Purpura/cutaneous vasculitis
- History of lymphoproliferative disease

Microscopic Pathology
- Membranoproliferative GN
- Intracapillary "pseudothrombi" (hyaline thrombi)
- Congo red stain negative
- IF: Granular glomerular deposits stain for 1 light chain and 1 heavy chain
  - > 90% kappa light chain and ~ 85% IgG
- EM: Fibrillary (~ 50%) or microtubular (~ 25%) deposits

Top Differential Diagnoses
- Fibrillary or immunotactoid glomerulonephritis
- Monoclonal immunoglobulin deposition disease
- Membranoproliferative glomerulonephritis

Diagnostic Checklist
- Light chain stains essential in evaluation of GN

MICROSCOPIC PATHOLOGY

Histologic Features
- Glomeruli
  - Membranoproliferative GN
    - Mesangial hypercellularity, sometimes nodular
    - Duplication of the GBM
  - Intracapillary "pseudothrombi" (hyaline thrombi)
  - Endocapillary hypercellularity
    - Monocytes/macrophages (CD68[+]) prominent
    - Swollen endothelial cells
  - Sometimes crescents
  - Congo red stain is negative
- Interstitium and tubules
  - Variable inflammation, fibrosis
- Vessels
  - Vasculitis may be present

ANCILLARY TESTS

Immunofluorescence
- Granular GBM and mesangial deposits that stain for 1 light chain and 1 heavy chain
  - Most cases IgG (~ 85%), including IgG3; the rest are IgM (~ 15%); rare double heavy chain (IgA + IgG)
  - > 90% kappa light chain
- Similar pattern for C3 and sometimes C1q
- Intraglomerular capillary "pseudothrombi" have same pattern
- No tubular basement membrane deposits

Electron Microscopy
- Fibrillary (~ 50%) or microtubular (~ 25%) deposits
  - Intracapillary
  - Subendothelial, mesangial, subepithelial
  - Tend to be straight and aggregated in bundles
    - In contrast to curvilinear pattern in type II cryoglobulinemia
  - Intracytoplasmicolygonal crystals described in literature

Skin Biopsy
- Leukocytoclastic vasculitis
  - "Pseudothrombi"/monotypic Ig and C3

DIFFERENTIAL DIAGNOSIS

Fibrillary or Immunotactoid GN
- Some with monotypic light chains
- Lack circulating cryoglobulins

Monoclonal Immunoglobulin Deposition Disease
- Lacks organized deposits
- Lacks circulating cryoglobulins

Membranoproliferative Glomerulonephritis
- Lacks "pseudothrombi"
- Lacks monotypic light chains (single light chain)
- Lack of organized deposits

DIAGNOSTIC CHECKLIST

Pathologic Interpretation Pearls
- Light chain stains essential in evaluation of GN

SELECTED REFERENCES

1. Favre G et al: Membranoproliferative glomerulonephritis, chronic lymphocytic leukemia, and cryoglobulinemia. Am J Kidney Dis. 55(2):391-4, 2010
2. Shaikh A et al: Acute renal failure secondary to severe type I cryoglobulinemia following rituximab therapy for Waldenström's macroglobulinemia. Clin Exp Nephrol. 12(4):292-5, 2008
3. Karras A et al: Renal involvement in monoclonal (type I) cryoglobulinemia: two cases associated with IgG3 kappa cryoglobulin. Am J Kidney Dis. 40(5):1091-6, 2002
4. Gallo G et al: The spectrum of monoclonal immunoglobulin deposition disease associated with immunocytic dyscrasias. Semin Hematol. 26(3):234-45, 1989

TYPE I CRYOGLOBULINEMIC GLOMERULONEPHRITIS

Light Microscopy and Immunofluorescence

(Left) *"Pseudothrombi"* ➡ *in type I CryoGN stain red in trichrome, similar to fibrin thrombi, shown by immunofluorescence; however, they contain monotypic immunoglobulin.* *(Right)* *Type I CryoGN shows variable intracapillary hypercellularity, mostly due to mononuclear cells. Patient had chronic lymphocytic leukemia with an IgG kappa cryoprotein. Glomerulus does not contain "pseudothrombi." Macrophages phagocytose the deposits in cryoglobulinemia, and few may be evident in a biopsy.*

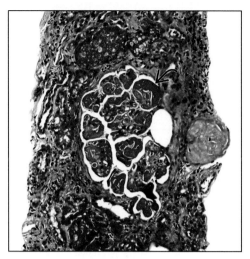 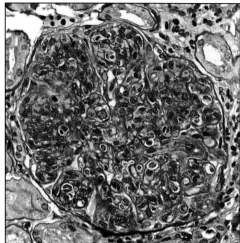

(Left) *The differential deposition of light chains is essential to demonstrate in the diagnosis of type I cryoglobulinemic GN. Shown here is kappa light chain staining with granular deposits ➡ along the GBM. Lambda was negative. The patient had CLL.* *(Right)* *In this case of type I cryoglobulinemic GN, the lambda light chain staining of glomeruli is negative except for rare speckles, but the deposits stained strongly for kappa light chain and gamma heavy chain (IgG).*

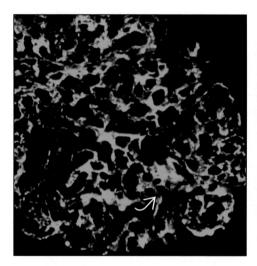 

(Left) *Type I cryoglobulinemia has a single heavy chain, in contrast to type II or III cryoglobulinemia. Shown here is a strongly positive granular stain for gamma heavy chain. Stains for mu (IgM) and alpha (IgA) heavy chains were negative.* *(Right)* *The deposits of type I cryoglobulinemia can fix complement and lead to prominent deposition of C1q (shown here) and C3 in a granular pattern along the GBM and in the mesangium. The glomeruli had an acute GN pattern by light microscopy.*

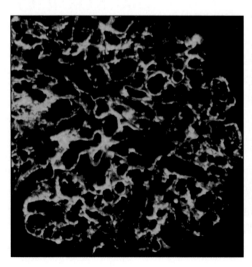 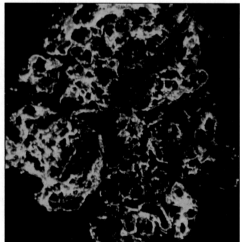

TYPE I CRYOGLOBULINEMIC GLOMERULONEPHRITIS

Immunofluorescence and Electron Microscopy

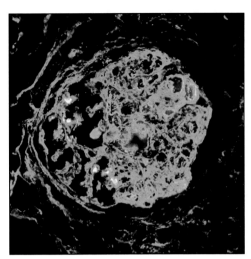
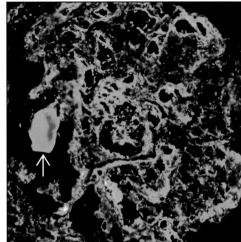

(Left) Immunofluorescence shows bright staining for IgM in the mesangium and in glomerular basement membranes in this case of type I cryoglobulinemic glomerulonephritis. There was monotypic staining for kappa light chain in this case. *(Right)* Immunofluorescence shows staining for kappa light chain in the mesangium and in glomerular basement membranes. Staining for lambda was negative. A typical proteinaceous cast ➡ stains for kappa.

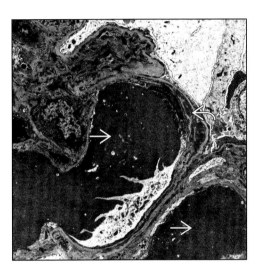
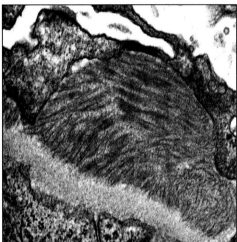

(Left) EM in type I cryoglobulinemic glomerulonephritis shows intraluminal "pseudothrombi" ➡ in a glomerulus. Subendothelial deposits ➡ are also present. *(Right)* This electron micrograph shows type I cryoglobulinemia exhibiting the typical finding of organized deposits. These have a varied appearance but are usually fibrillar, as in this case with subepithelial deposits due to IgG kappa deposition.

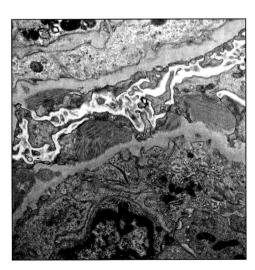
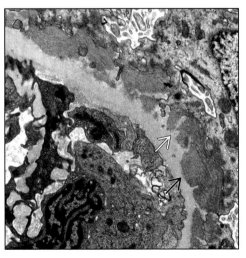

(Left) Type I cryoglobulinemic GN can have deposits that resemble the "humps" of acute glomerulonephritis, as illustrated in this electron micrograph from a patient with IgG kappa monoclonal cryoglobulins due to CLL. *(Right)* Type I cryoglobulinemia can resemble membranous glomerulonephritis (MGN), with subepithelial deposits ➡ and "spikes" ➡. The presence of a single light chain and organized deposits distinguish it from the usual MGN (EM).

WALDENSTRÖM MACROGLOBULINEMIA

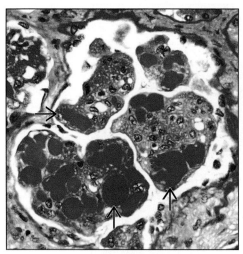

Numerous hyaline "thrombi" ➡, which represent prominent accumulations of IgM paraprotein, occupy the entire lumina of the glomerular capillaries from this patient with Waldenström macroglobulinemia.

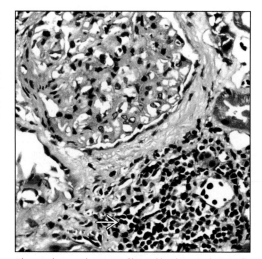

The renal parenchyma is infiltrated by the neoplastic cells ➡ of WM. In addition, immunoglobulin deposition of the glomerulus is not apparent but is detectable by IF (not shown). (Courtesy P. Lin, MD.)

TERMINOLOGY

Abbreviations
- Waldenström macroglobulinemia (WM)

Synonyms
- Lymphoplasmacytic lymphoma (LPL)
  - Not exactly a synonym for WM
  - WM comprises a subset of LPL

Definitions
- LPL with bone marrow involvement and any circulating IgM paraprotein

ETIOLOGY/PATHOGENESIS

Neoplastic B-Lymphocytes
- Postfollicular B cells may be cell of origin
  - Familial cases with younger age of onset reported

CLINICAL ISSUES

Epidemiology
- Incidence
  - Rare
- Age
  - Median age: > 60 years
- Gender
  - Male > female
- Ethnicity
  - Caucasian predilection

Presentation
- Proteinuria, nephrotic range
- Hyperviscosity syndrome in 10-30%
  - Reduced vision
  - Red blood cells with sludging and rouleaux formation
  - Increased risk of cerebrovascular accident

Laboratory Tests
- Serum or urine protein electrophoresis
  - Detection of any monoclonal IgM protein
- Bone marrow biopsy
- Cryoglobulins (8-18%), type I or II
- Cytogenetics
  - Deletion of chromosome 6q in majority of WM
    - Not specific for WM

Treatment
- Drugs
  - Rituximab
    - Can induce cryoglobulin flare and acute renal failure
- Plasmapheresis for hyperviscosity or cryoglobulins
- Hematopoietic cell transplantation, autologous or allogeneic
- Kidney transplantation if neoplasm controlled

Prognosis
- Median survival: 5-10 years

MICROSCOPIC PATHOLOGY

Histologic Features
- Glomeruli: Spectrum of injury
  - Rouleaux in capillaries
  - Cryoglobulinemia
    - Accumulation of "pseudothrombi" (hyaline thrombi) in capillaries
    - Proliferation, inflammation
  - Other manifestations of monoclonal protein
    - Amyloidosis
    - Monoclonal immunoglobulin deposition disease
  - Other pathology
    - Membranous glomerulonephritis (GN)
    - Membranoproliferative GN
    - Minimal change disease
- Tubules

WALDENSTRÖM MACROGLOBULINEMIA

Key Facts

Terminology
- Lymphoplasmacytic lymphoma (LPL) with bone marrow involvement and circulating IgM paraprotein

Clinical Issues
- Median age: > 60 years
- Proteinuria, nephrotic range
- Hyperviscosity syndrome

Microscopic Pathology
- Spectrum of glomerular disease
  - Cryoglobulinemic glomerulonephritis (GN)
  - Amyloidosis
  - Minimal change disease
  - Membranous GN

Top Differential Diagnoses
- Other hematologic malignancies, thrombotic microangiopathy

- Acute tubular injury
  - Associated with cryoglobulin flare
- Cast nephropathy rarely reported
- Interstitium
  - Interstitial infiltration by LPL may mimic renal or perirenal mass
  - T-cell lymphoma infiltrate in 1 case

ANCILLARY TESTS

Immunofluorescence
- "Pseudothrombi" stain for IgM, kappa or lambda

Electron Microscopy
- Transmission
  - Features according to glomerular involvement
  - "Pseudothrombi" and subendothelial deposits have microtubular/fibrillar substructure

Immunohistochemistry
- Neoplastic lymphoid infiltrate, if present
  - CD19(+), CD20(+), CD22(+), CD5(-), CD10(-)

DIFFERENTIAL DIAGNOSIS

Other Hematologic Malignancies
- Wide spectrum of B-cell malignancies can manifest with similar renal injuries, ranging from amyloidosis and cryoglobulinemic GN to cast nephropathy

Cryoglobulinemic GN
- May be identical to WM with circulating cryoglobulins
- Not all circulating cryoglobulins are due to an underlying hematopoietic malignancy

Thrombotic Microangiopathy
- Thrombi stain for fibrin rather than IgM

DIAGNOSTIC CHECKLIST

Pathologic Interpretation Pearls
- IgM paraproteins trigger work-up of monoclonal gammopathies
- Only the neoplastic infiltrate, if present, is specific for LPL
- WM diagnosis requires bone marrow biopsy and SPEP

SELECTED REFERENCES

1. Izzedine H et al: Immunoglobulin M 'Flare' after rituximab-associated acute tubular necrosis in Waldenström's macroglobulinemia. Int J Hematol. 89(2):218-22, 2009
2. Audard V et al: Renal lesions associated with IgM-secreting monoclonal proliferations: revisiting the disease spectrum. Clin J Am Soc Nephrol. 3(5):1339-49, 2008
3. Isaac J et al: Cast nephropathy in a case of Waldenström's macroglobulinemia. Nephron. 91(3):512-5, 2002
4. Veltman GA et al: Renal disease in Waldenström's macroglobulinaemia. Nephrol Dial Transplant. 12(6):1256-9, 1997

IMAGE GALLERY

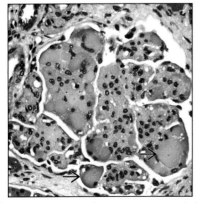
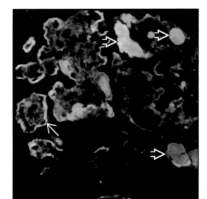
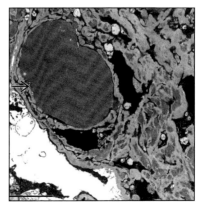

(Left) Large aggregates of paraprotein ("pseudothrombi") ➡ fill the glomerular capillaries in a patient with circulating cryoglobulins due to WM. *(Center)* IgM highlights prominent paraprotein deposition along capillary walls ➡ ("wire loop" deposits) and in the capillary lumina (hyaline thrombi) ➡. *(Right)* This large electron-dense deposit ➡ without substructure occupies the entire glomerular capillary lumen from a patient with WM.

MYELOMA CAST NEPHROPATHY

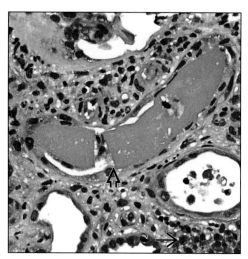

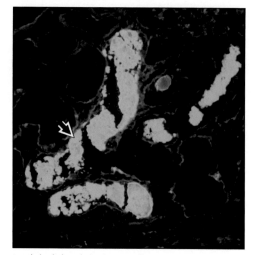

H&E demonstrates a tubular cast that appears broken into 2 fragments ⊵ (or a fractured appearance). Scattered interstitial inflammatory cells ➜ with plasma cells are present.

Lambda light chain immunofluorescence microscopy strongly stains tubular casts ⊵ in a patient with myeloma cast nephropathy. No kappa light chain staining was present (not shown).

TERMINOLOGY

Abbreviations
- Myeloma cast nephropathy (MCN)

Synonyms
- Light chain cast nephropathy
- Bence Jones cast nephropathy
- Myeloma kidney

ETIOLOGY/PATHOGENESIS

Plasma Cell Dyscrasia
- Monoclonal light chain overproduction
  - Light chains (Bence Jones proteins) freely filtered by glomeruli
  - Not all monoclonal light chains are nephrotoxic
  - Accumulation of Tamm-Horsfall protein and monoclonal light chains in distal nephron segments may lead to both obstruction and direct cytotoxicity
  - Precipitating factors for cast formation include
    - Dehydration
    - Diuretics
    - Hypercalcemia
    - Nonsteroidal anti-inflammatory drugs
    - Contrast media
    - Infections

CLINICAL ISSUES

Epidemiology
- Incidence
  - 30-50% among patients with multiple myeloma
- Age
  - Typically > 40 years
- Gender
  - Male > female

Presentation
- Acute renal failure & proteinuria

Laboratory Tests
- Serum &/or urine protein electrophoresis
  - Immunoelectrophoresis
  - Immunofixation electrophoresis

Treatment
- Drugs
  - Treatment for underlying plasma cell dyscrasia, if present
    - Colchicine, thalidomide, bortezomib
- Hematopoietic stem cell transplantation
- Plasmapheresis

Prognosis
- 5-year survival rate of 20-25%

MICROSCOPIC PATHOLOGY

Histologic Features
- Tubular casts
  - Usually involve distal nephron segments (distal tubules and collecting ducts)
  - PAS negative (vs. Tamm-Horsfall protein [THP])
  - Trichrome stains red (vs. blue THP)
  - Sharp-edged or fractured appearance
  - Lined by flattened to reactive tubular epithelial cells
  - Giant cell reaction to intratubular casts may be present
  - Prominent intratubular aggregates of neutrophils can be present
  - Rare crystal appearance may be present
- Interstitial inflammation
- Interstitial neoplastic plasma cell infiltrates may be present
  - Monoclonal staining by in situ hybridization or immunohistochemistry

MYELOMA CAST NEPHROPATHY

Key Facts

Terminology
- Synonyms
  - Light chain cast nephropathy
  - Myeloma kidney
- Accumulation of monoclonal light chains may form casts (both cytotoxic and obstructive) in distal nephron segments

Clinical Issues
- Acute renal failure
- 30-50% incidence among patients with multiple myeloma
- 5-year survival rate of 20-25%

Microscopic Pathology
- Tubular casts

- Usually involve distal nephron segments (distal tubules and collecting ducts)
- Sharp-edged or fractured appearance
- Giant cell reaction to intratubular casts
- Prominent intratubular aggregates of neutrophils can be present

Ancillary Tests
- Immunofluorescence or immunohistochemistry
  - Kappa is more common than lambda with ratio ranging from 2:1 to 4:1

Top Differential Diagnoses
- Rhabdomyolysis-associated acute tubular injury
- mTOR inhibitor toxicity
- Monoclonal immunoglobulin deposition disease
- Acute tubular injury

ANCILLARY TESTS

Immunofluorescence
- Kappa is more common than lambda with ratio ranging from 2:1 to 4:1
  - Can be performed on paraffin tissue sections with good results

Electron Microscopy
- Transmission
  - Monoclonal light chain tubular casts demonstrate a spectrum of substructural organization
    - Nonspecific appearance to crystalline, granular, or even fibrillar substructure
  - Immunogold labeling may be more sensitive than immunofluorescence or immunohistochemistry to demonstrate monoclonality in some cases

Immunohistochemistry
- κ and λ can be tested on paraffin tissue sections if tubular casts are not present in specimen submitted for immunofluorescence microscopy

DIFFERENTIAL DIAGNOSIS

Rhabdomyolysis-associated Acute Tubular Injury
- Tubular casts are pigmented with granular consistency
- Absence of monoclonal immunolocalization

mTOR Inhibitor Toxicity
- Reported in kidney transplant patients with delayed graft function after using an immunosuppressive regimen containing rapamycin
- Tubular casts with fractured appearance
  - Multinucleated giant cell reaction can be present
  - Casts may consist of myoglobin

Monoclonal Immunoglobulin Deposition Disease
- Often occurs concurrently with MCN

Amyloidosis
- Concurrent amyloidosis and MCN rarely occur

Acute Tubular Injury
- Proteinaceous casts are PAS positive
  - Absence of monoclonal staining in tubular casts

End-Stage Kidney
- Hyaline casts in atrophic tubules may be fractured
  - Lined by flattened or atrophic tubular epithelial cells
  - Absence of giant cell reaction, PAS positive
  - Absence of monoclonal immunofluorescence staining

Cryocrystalglobulinemia
- Resembles type I cryoglobulinemia but with crystalline deposits
- Crystalline structures in glomeruli and arterioles rather than tubular lumens in MCN

DIAGNOSTIC CHECKLIST

Pathologic Interpretation Pearls
- Careful evaluation of entire immunofluorescence specimen is necessary to exclude presence of monoclonal staining of tubular casts
  - Some proteinaceous casts in atrophic tubules may stain strongly for both kappa and lambda, but other casts may demonstrate monoclonal staining
- Absence of renal medulla in sample may result in missed diagnosis

SELECTED REFERENCES

1. Herrera GA: Renal lesions associated with plasma cell dyscrasias: practical approach to diagnosis, new concepts, and challenges. Arch Pathol Lab Med. 133(2):249-67, 2009
2. Markowitz GS: Dysproteinemia and the kidney. Adv Anat Pathol. 11(1):49-63, 2004
3. Hill GS et al: Renal lesions in multiple myeloma: their relationship to associated protein abnormalities. Am J Kidney Dis. 2(4):423-38, 1983

Microscopic Features

(Left) Light chain cast nephropathy in a 48-year-old woman who presented with acute renal failure is shown. Many tubules in the cortex are dilated and show flattening or vacuolization of the epithelium, which are features of acute tubular injury ➶. The glomeruli appear normal. *(Right)* These atypical casts ⊟ are PAS-negative and appear finely granular. These casts can be mistaken for intratubular cellular debris, which can be observed in the setting of acute tubular injury/ necrosis.

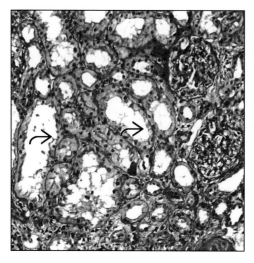
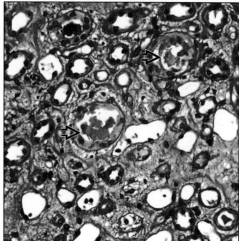

(Left) Hypereosinophilic casts in the distal nephron segments are admixed with a few inflammatory cells ➶. Prominent neutrophilic reaction surrounding casts can occasionally be present (not shown). *(Right)* The "myeloma" casts in the renal medulla can reveal a spectrum of appearances that range from a strong red ➶ to a variegated red-blue ➶ appearance, as shown in this Masson trichrome stain.

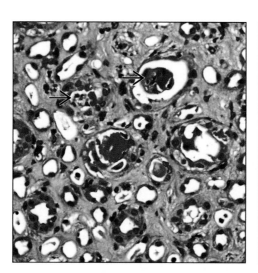
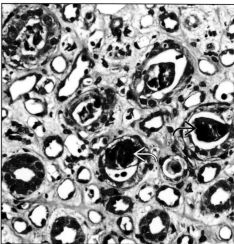

(Left) Atypical casts are strongly positive for kappa light chain ⊟. There is also confluent glomerular and tubular basement membrane staining (in this case dim) for kappa light chain but not for lambda light chain. This may be the earliest evidence of light chain deposition disease, which often occurs concurrently with myeloma cast nephropathy. *(Right)* These tubular casts are negative for lambda light chain ⊟ but stain strongly for kappa light chain (not shown).

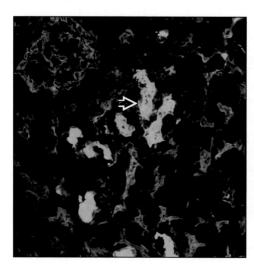
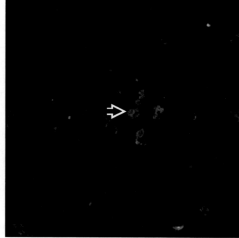

MYELOMA CAST NEPHROPATHY

Microscopic Features

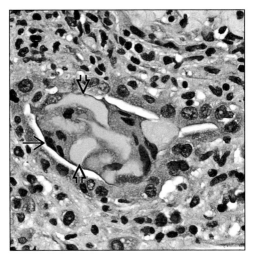

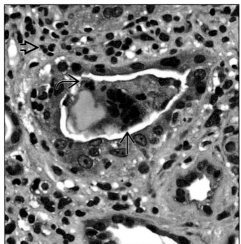

(Left) Several fragmented pieces ⊳ of this tubular cast are enveloped by macrophages forming a prominent giant cell reaction ⇥ that is characteristic of myeloma cast nephropathy. (Right) Prominent giant cell reaction ⇥ to the tubular cast is noted in the lumen on this tubule, and this feature alone is highly suggestive of myeloma cast nephropathy. Scattered inflammatory cells are noted in the interstitium ⊳ along with a few eosinophils ⇗ in the tubular lumen.

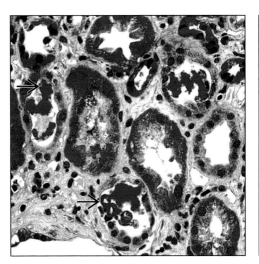

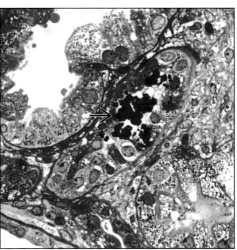

(Left) Strong fuchsinophilic staining highlights the light chain casts ⇥ in several tubules. The red intense staining may be diminished when the casts are admixed with cellular debris and variable amounts of Tamm-Horsfall protein (trichome). (Right) The light chain casts in the tubules stain strongly blue with a granular and coarse appearance ⇥ in the toluidine blue section submitted for electron microscopy.

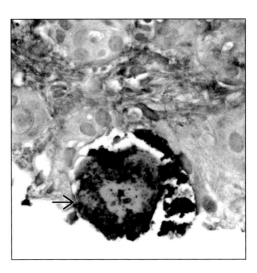

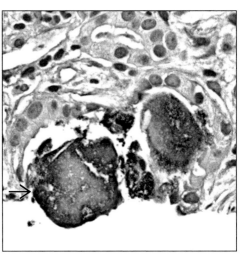

(Left) Immunohistochemistry on the paraffin section for kappa light chain shows strong staining in this tubular cast ⇥ and a blush of interstitial staining. (Right) Tubular casts were not prominent in the sample submitted for immunofluorescence microscopy. Lambda light chain immunohistochemistry reveals no significant staining of this intratubular cast ⇥. This finding, in conjunction with strong kappa light chain staining (not shown), supports the diagnosis of myeloma cast nephropathy.

MYELOMA CAST NEPHROPATHY

Variant Microscopic Features

(Left) Cast nephropathy and intratubular amyloid are present as a few tubules containing atypical, PAS-negative, or PAS-variable casts ⇊, some of which show a surrounding cellular reaction. (Right) These casts are atypical, but they do not have the hypereosinophilic appearance of usual light chain casts on H&E. By immunofluorescence, casts stained for lambda but not for kappa light chain.

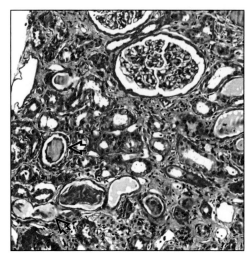
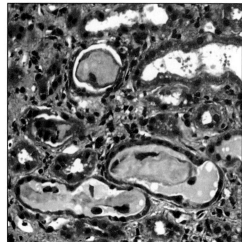

(Left) A Congo red stain was positive in tubular casts →, with apple green birefringence upon examination under polarized light. This is an unusual finding in myeloma cast nephropathy. No amyloid was present in other areas of the kidney biopsy, and the patient did not have systemic amyloidosis. (Right) Although amyloid was present in some tubular casts (not shown), there was no evidence of amyloid in the glomeruli, arterioles, or other areas of this biopsy.

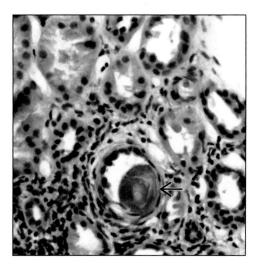
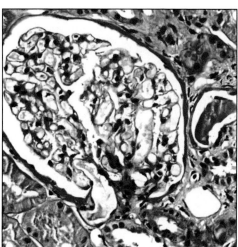

(Left) Electron micrograph of an atypical cast ➡ with an attached cell ⇊ from myeloma cast nephropathy has a granular appearance. Some casts have substructural organization with a lattice framework (not shown), but the absence of this finding is not unusual. (Right) At higher magnification, this tubular cast is composed of numerous randomly arranged fibrils, which can be observed in myeloma cast nephropathy whether or not the casts have amyloid.

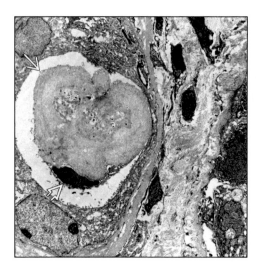
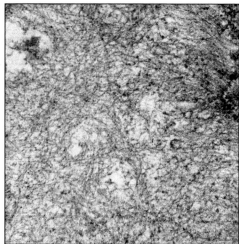

MYELOMA CAST NEPHROPATHY

Differential Diagnosis

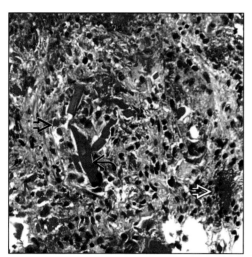

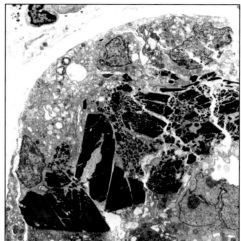

(Left) Unusual case with 3 diagnoses related to a lambda paraprotein shows light chain cast nephropathy ⇗, light chain proximal tubulopathy ⇗, and crystal-storing histiocytosis ⇗. *(Courtesy M. Fidler, MD.)* *(Right)* Crystalline structures formed from a lambda light chain paraprotein are shown within a tubule from myeloma cast nephropathy by electron microscopy.

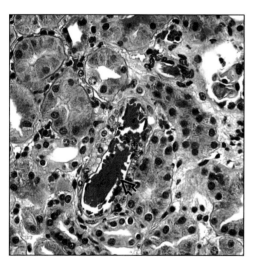

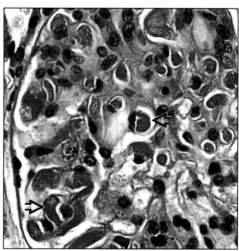

(Left) A specimen with cryocrystalglobulinemia shows a crystalline structure within an arteriole ⇗ rather than a tubule. Note surrounding red blood cells. By immunofluorescence, these structures stained for kappa but not lambda light chain. *(Courtesy A. Magil, MD.)* *(Right)* Cryocrystalglobulinemia is shown. Many immunoglobulin "pseudothrombi" ⇗, some of which show a crystalline structure, are within glomerular capillary loops.

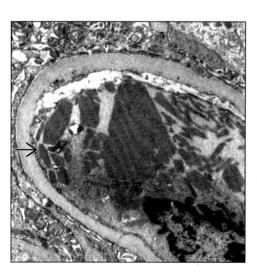

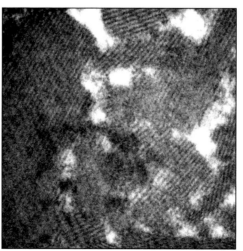

(Left) This glomerular capillary lumen contains cryoglobulin deposits ⇗ with crystalline substructure. "Myeloma" casts are never present within glomerular capillaries. *(Right)* The cryoglobulin deposits within the glomerular capillaries demonstrate crystalline substructure with a periodicity at higher magnification. "Myeloma" casts may demonstrate a similar substructural organization by electron microscopy but are always located within the tubular lumina and not capillaries.

LIGHT CHAIN FANCONI SYNDROME

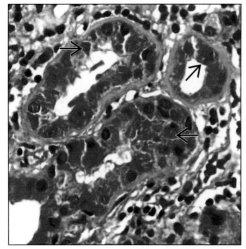

Intracytoplasmic crystalline material that stained for monotypic light chain can be seen in the proximal tubules in this patient who had light chain Fanconi syndrome ➡.

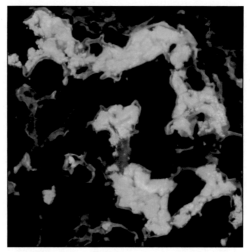

Immunofluorescence staining reveals monotypic staining of intracytoplasmic crystals for kappa light chain. The stain for lambda was much weaker.

TERMINOLOGY

Abbreviations
- Light chain Fanconi syndrome (LCFS)

Synonyms
- Light chain proximal tubulopathy
- Acute tubulopathy, light chain related
  ○ Related disorder with proximal tubular damage by toxic light chains

Definitions
- Chronic tubulointerstitial nephropathy caused by intracytoplasmic crystalline inclusions composed of monoclonal light chains present in proximal tubular epithelial cells

ETIOLOGY/PATHOGENESIS

Monoclonal Immunoglobulin Light Chains
- Produced by clonal proliferation of plasma cells
  ○ Most have multiple myeloma (may be smoldering) or monoclonal gammopathy of undetermined significance (MGUS)
  ○ Also associated with Waldenström macroglobulinemia and B-cell lymphomas
- Normal light chains reabsorbed by proximal tubule, where they are degraded
- In LCFS, abnormal light chain, usually kappa (VK1 subgroup), is resistant to enzymatic breakdown
  ○ Nephrotoxic light chains crystallize or precipitate within lysosomes in proximal tubules

CLINICAL ISSUES

Epidemiology
- Incidence
  ○ Rare (68 cases reported as of 2000)

Presentation
- Fanconi syndrome (acquired)
  ○ Normoglycemic glycosuria
  ○ Aminoaciduria
  ○ Uricosuria
  ○ Hyperphosphaturia with hypophosphatemia
  ○ Type II renal tubular acidosis
- Chronic renal failure, slowly progressive
- Monoclonal gammopathy
- Bence Jones proteinuria
- Plasma cell dyscrasia or lymphoma
- Adult-acquired Fanconi syndrome with monoclonal light chain raises suspicion of LCFS

Treatment
- Treatment of underlying plasma cell dyscrasia or lymphoma

MICROSCOPIC PATHOLOGY

Histologic Features
- Glomeruli
  ○ Normal
- Tubules
  ○ Intracellular crystalline inclusions within proximal tubular epithelial cells
    ■ Similar crystals in bone marrow plasma cells
  ○ Not all cases with Fanconi syndrome have crystals (10% in 1 series)
  ○ Acute and chronic tubular injury
- May show other manifestations of monoclonal protein deposition
  ○ Crystal-storing histiocytosis with monoclonal light chains
  ○ Myeloma cast nephropathy
  ○ Light chain deposition disease (in GBM and TBM)
- Interstitium
  ○ Commonly mononuclear inflammation, fibrosis

LIGHT CHAIN FANCONI SYNDROME

Key Facts

Terminology
- Chronic tubulointerstitial nephropathy caused by intracytoplasmic crystalline inclusions composed of monoclonal light chains present in proximal tubular epithelial cells

Etiology/Pathogenesis
- In LCFS, abnormal light chain, usually kappa (VK1 subgroup), is resistant to enzymatic breakdown

Clinical Issues
- Fanconi syndrome
  - Normoglycemic glycosuria
  - Aminoaciduria, uricosuria
  - Hyperphosphaturia with hypophosphatemia
- Chronic renal failure, slowly progressive
- Monoclonal gammopathy

Ancillary Tests
- Intracellular monotypic staining for kappa or lambda light chain
- Pronase-digested immunofluorescence sections may increase sensitivity of staining in LCFS

Top Differential Diagnoses
- Acute tubular injury due to other causes
  - No light chains present in proximal tubular epithelial cytoplasm
- Light chain cast nephropathy
- Inflammatory tubulointerstitial nephritis associated with light chains
- Protein reabsorption droplets with monotypic light chain staining
  - Absence of intracytoplasmic crystalline material

ANCILLARY TESTS

Immunohistochemistry
- Intracellular monotypic staining for κ or λ light chain
- Immunohistochemistry may increase sensitivity of staining in LCFS when routine immunofluorescence staining is negative

Immunofluorescence
- Intracellular monotypic staining for kappa or lambda light chain
  - Most cases positive for kappa
- Routine immunofluorescence may be negative
- Pronase-digested immunofluorescence sections may increase sensitivity of staining in LCFS

Serologic Testing
- Monoclonal protein in serum, usually IgG kappa
- Bence Jones proteinuria, usually kappa light chain

Electron Microscopy
- Electron-dense crystalline structures within cytoplasm of proximal tubular epithelial cells

DIFFERENTIAL DIAGNOSIS

Acute Tubular Injury Due to Other Causes
- No light chains present in proximal tubular epithelial cytoplasm
- Of note, light chains of LCFS are not always demonstrable by routine IF

Light Chain Cast Nephropathy
- Intratubular casts, rather than intracytoplasmic material, show monotypic staining for light chain
- Intratubular casts may have crystalline appearance and may show surrounding reactive tubular epithelial cells

Protein Reabsorption Droplets with Monotypic Light Chain Staining
- Absence of intracytoplasmic crystalline material

- Immunofluorescence staining pattern reflective of patient's urinary monoclonal protein that does not cause renal disease

Light Chain Deposition Disease
- Like LCFS, often shows tubular injury by light microscopy
- Linear glomerular and tubular basement membrane staining for monoclonal light chain by IF
- Finely granular, electron-dense deposits by EM along glomerular and tubular basement membranes
- May coexist with LCFS

Inflammatory Tubulointerstitial Nephritis Associated with Light Chains
- Pattern of acute interstitial nephritis

SELECTED REFERENCES

1. Herlitz LC et al: Light chain proximal tubulopathy. Kidney Int. 76(7):792-7, 2009
2. Stokes MB et al: Dysproteinemia-related nephropathy associated with crystal-storing histiocytosis. Kidney Int. 70(3):597-602, 2006
3. Bridoux F et al: Fanconi's syndrome induced by a monoclonal Vkappa3 light chain in Waldenstrom's macroglobulinemia. Am J Kidney Dis. 45(4):749-57, 2005
4. Decourt C et al: A monoclonal V kappa l light chain responsible for incomplete proximal tubulopathy. Am J Kidney Dis. 41(2):497-504, 2003
5. Déret S et al: Kappa light chain-associated Fanconi's syndrome: molecular analysis of monoclonal immunoglobulin light chains from patients with and without intracellular crystals. Protein Eng. 12(4):363-9, 1999
6. Aucouturier P et al: Monoclonal Ig L chain and L chain V domain fragment crystallization in myeloma-associated Fanconi's syndrome. J Immunol. 150(8 Pt 1):3561-8, 1993
7. Maldonado JE et al: Fanconi syndrome in adults. A manifestation of a latent form of myeloma. Am J Med. 58(3):354-64, 1975

LIGHT CHAIN FANCONI SYNDROME

Light Microscopy and Immunofluorescence

(Left) Trichome stain shows focal interstitial inflammation and early fibrosis and tubular atrophy in a case of LCFS. *(Right)* High magnification reveals intracytoplasmic structures ➡ that are fuchsinophilic on a trichrome stain. The trichrome stain is usually the best stain for visualizing crystalline structures in LCFS.

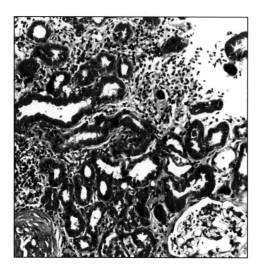
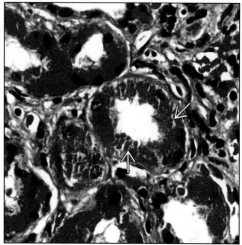

(Left) Intracytoplasmic crystals are seen on a silver stain ➡. *(Right)* This case has 3 diagnoses: Light chain cast nephropathy with crystalline-shaped atypical casts ➡, light chain Fanconi syndrome with crystalline structures within proximal tubular epithelial cells ➡, and crystal-storing histiocytosis seen within the interstitium ➡. By immunofluorescence, the crystals stained for lambda light chain. (Courtesy M. Fidler, MD.)

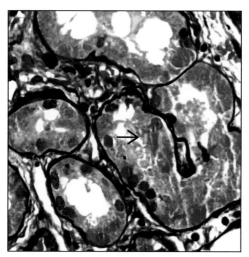
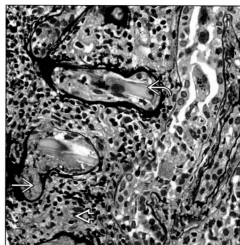

(Left) Immunofluorescence staining for kappa light chain reveals intracytoplasmic tubular epithelial cell staining ➡. A typical proteinaceous cast stains for kappa ➡; these casts also stained for IgA and lambda. Most cases of LCFS stain for kappa light chain. *(Right)* IF staining for lambda light chain reveals little staining of the tubular epithelial cell cytoplasm ➡ in a case of kappa light chain Fanconi syndrome. A few typical proteinaceous casts stained for lambda ➡.

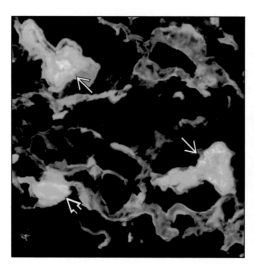
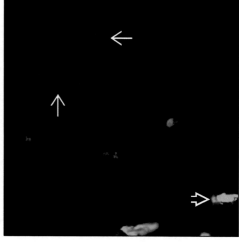

LIGHT CHAIN FANCONI SYNDROME

Electron Microscopy

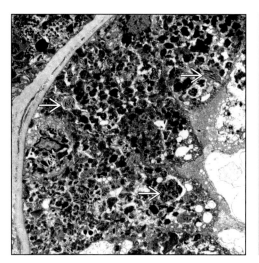

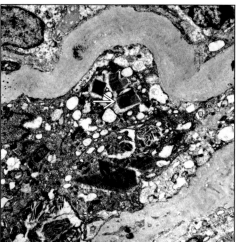

(Left) Electron micrograph shows a proximal tubule with crystalline structures within the cytoplasm ➡️. Lack of high-magnification electron micrographs of tubules may result in the diagnosis of light chain Fanconi syndrome being overlooked. *(Right)* EM shows crystalline structures ➡️ composed of light chains within the tubular cytoplasm. Note the absence of finely granular deposits along the basement membrane, which if present would indicate concurrent light chain deposition disease.

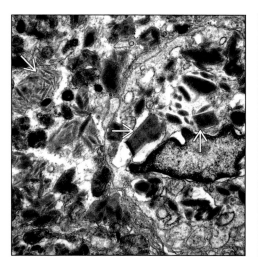

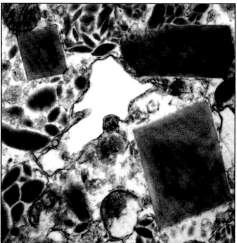

(Left) EM shows crystals of various sizes and shapes within the tubular epithelium ➡️. *(Right)* Electron-dense crystals are present within the tubular epithelial cytoplasm and are not apparently confined to lysosomes, as are normal reabsorbed proteins. Escape into the cytoplasm may be due to lysosomal rupture, which would be expected to injure the cell.

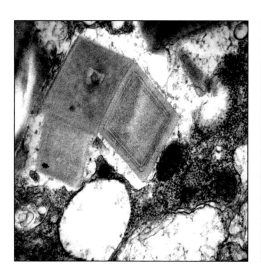

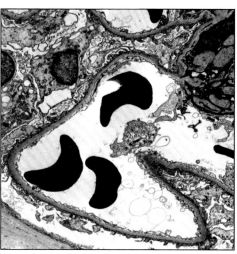

(Left) Crystals have a rhomboid shape here but may have other patterns, probably dependent on the primary sequence of the protein. *(Right)* The glomerulus is unaffected in this case of light chain Fanconi syndrome. Note the absence of glomerular deposits. Light chains can deposit in the GBM in systemic light chain disease. The difference is probably related to the physiochemic properties of the light chain.

AMYLOIDOSIS

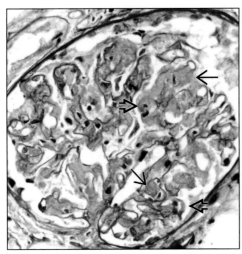

The classic appearance of amyloid deposits is a pale amorphous accumulation in the mesangium ⊋ and along the GBM ⊋ in PAS stains without cellular proliferation or inflammation.

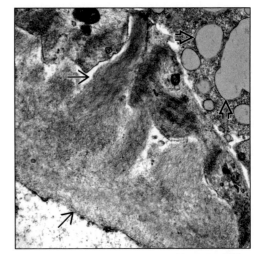

EM reveals subepithelial "spicular" amyloid fibrils ⊋ in the GBM. Fibrils are ~ 7-12 nm in diameter and are nonperiodic. Podocytes have effaced foot processes and reabsorption droplets ⊋.

TERMINOLOGY

Definitions
- Protein folding diseases characterized by accumulation of 7-12 nm diameter fibrils with a β-pleated sheet structure that confers birefringence after staining with Congo red

ETIOLOGY/PATHOGENESIS

Amyloidogenic Proteins
- > 20 different precursor proteins
  - Clonal proliferation of plasma cells (AL/AH types)
  - Chronic inflammation (AA type)
  - Genetic (multiple proteins)
  - Failure of excretion (β2-microglobulin)
  - Neoplasm (e.g., calcitonin)
- ~ 90% of renal amyloidosis cases are AL or AA

Pathogenesis
- Amyloidogenic proteins have an antiparallel, β-pleated sheet tertiary structure, accounting for Congo red staining and apple-green birefringence under polarized light
  - Resistance to metabolic processing leads to accumulation and interference with physiologic functioning
- Amyloid deposits composed of amyloidogenic protein and nonfibrillary glycoproteins serum amyloid P (SAP), apolipoprotein E, and glycosaminoglycans
  - SAP (also known as amyloid P component)
    - Normal plasma protein that binds all amyloid proteins
    - SAP present early and promotes deposits
    - Labeled SAP used to image amyloid in vivo

Renal Deposits
- Certain forms typically involve the kidney (AL, AA, fibrinogen, Apo AI and AII, Alys)

- Glomerular mesangial amyloid accumulation often occurs 1st as mesangial cells lose usual smooth muscle phenotype and acquire macrophage phenotype
  - Mesangial cells engage in endocytosis and deliver amyloidogenic light chains to lysosomal compartment, where fibril formation takes place
- Fibrils penetrate and aggregate in the GBM, suggesting that they may be locally formed

AL Amyloid
- Most common cause of renal amyloidosis in the USA/Western hemisphere
- Plasma cell dyscrasias or lymphoproliferative disorders
  - Only ~ 20% meet diagnostic criteria for multiple myeloma or B-cell leukemia/lymphoma when AL amyloidosis is diagnosed
    - Some B-cell neoplasms not identified until ≥ 15 years after AL amyloidosis diagnosis
- ~ 75% lambda light chains
  - Often from N-terminal fragment of variable light chain region
- 40% develop nephrotic syndrome
  - ~ 10% of AL patients lack glomerular deposits
- Formerly called primary amyloidosis

AH Amyloid
- Rare cases of AH amyloid composed of monoclonal Ig heavy chains
  - Can produce nephrotic syndrome

AA Amyloid
- Most common cause of amyloidosis in underdeveloped countries
  - Becoming less common in developed countries
- Derived from proteolytic cleavage of serum amyloid A (SAA) protein, an acute phase reactant
- Associated with chronic inflammatory conditions
  - Infections: Tuberculosis, osteomyelitis, bronchiectasis, decubitus ulcers, skin infections of drug abuse

AMYLOIDOSIS

Key Facts

Terminology
- Accumulation of any 1 of > 20 amyloid proteins, characterized by apple-green birefringence after Congo red stain due to β-pleated sheet structure

Clinical Issues
- Causes ~ 5% of nephrotic syndrome in adults
- Systemic disease (heart, GI, nerves)
- Most due to immunoglobulin light chain (AL amyloid)
- AA amyloid due to persistent/recurrent inflammation
- Many rare genetic forms
- Generally poor outcome

Microscopic Pathology
- Amorphous eosinophilic, PAS(+) material in glomerular mesangium and GBM

- Defining characteristic: Congo red stain confers apple-green birefringence in polarizing microscope
- Also variably present in vessels and interstitium
- EM: Straight, nonblanching fibrils, 7-12 nm in diameter
  - Randomly distributed in mesangium and penetrating GBM
- Amyloid protein should be identified by IF/IHC
  - Light chains (AL amyloid)
  - AA protein (AA amyloid)
  - Specific protein in genetic forms

Top Differential Diagnoses
- Other diseases with fibrils have no birefringence with Congo red

---

  - Autoimmune disease: Rheumatoid arthritis, inflammatory bowel disease
  - Genetic syndromes: Familial Mediterranean fever (FMF), *MEFV* gene (pyrin)
- 90% have nephrotic syndrome or renal insufficiency at diagnosis
- Formerly called secondary amyloidosis

ATTR (Transthyretin Amyloidosis)
- Composed of transthyretin, also known as prealbumin
- 85% of familial forms of amyloidosis

α-Fibrinogen
- Most common genetic form that affects glomerulus
- 5% of familial forms

β2-Microglobulin
- Associated with long-term dialysis
- May cause carpal tunnel syndrome, bone cysts, and joint disease

Leukocyte Chemotactic Factor 2 (LECT2)
- ~ 2.4% of renal amyloidosis cases
- No mutation identified

Other Amyloid Types Affecting Kidney
- Cystatin C, gelsolin, apolipoprotein AI or AII, lysozyme

CLINICAL ISSUES

Epidemiology
- Incidence
  - 1.4/100,000 per person-year; all types (France)
  - 0.6-1.0/100,000 per person-year; AL type (Minnesota)
  - About 10% of cases are familial
- Age
  - AL and AA amyloid: Typically 50-70 years old
  - Familial forms: < 40 years old; AFib older
- Gender
  - M:F = 2:1 overall

Presentation
- Proteinuria
  - Present in virtually all with renal involvement
  - ~ 5% of adult cases of nephrotic syndrome
- Hematuria
  - Rarely a presenting feature
- Extrarenal manifestations
  - Congestive heart failure, arrhythmias
  - Dysesthesias
    - Bladder dysfunction
  - Orthostatic hypotension
  - Hepatomegaly/splenomegaly
  - Macroglossia
  - Carpal tunnel syndrome

Laboratory Tests
- In > 90% of AL amyloidosis patients, monoclonal Ig can be found in blood or urine
  - Most remaining patients have abnormal monoclonal bone marrow plasma cell populations

Treatment
- Treat underlying disease
  - Myeloma
    - Alkylating agents (e.g., melphalan) may ↑ survival from 1 year to > 5 years
    - Bortezomib
    - Bone marrow transplantation
  - Inflammatory condition (e.g., immunosuppressive agents for rheumatoid arthritis)
    - Useful for AA amyloidosis
    - Colchicine useful for FMF but not as useful for other causes of AA amyloidosis
- Transplantation
  - Recurs post transplant (10-20%); graft failure in 33%
  - Outcome can be good in selected patients
    - AL in nonmyeloma patients without severe extrarenal disease

Prognosis
- Variable but generally poor
- Median survival: 2 years (Mayo series, 859 patients)

AMYLOIDOSIS

MACROSCOPIC FEATURES

General Features
- Enlarged, pale, firm, and with a "waxy" appearance
- Cut surfaces remain firm and flat in contrast to a normal kidney, which bulges after sectioning
- Lugol iodine stains glomeruli dark brown in cut surfaces (like starch)

MICROSCOPIC PATHOLOGY

Histologic Features
- Glomeruli
  - Expansion of mesangium and thickening of capillary walls by amorphous eosinophilic material
    - Amorphous deposits are acidophilic, "salmon orange"
    - Usually less acidophilic than collagen (i.e., mesangial sclerosis, interstitial fibrosis)
    - Normal mesangial matrix, presumably destroyed by activated metalloproteinases, is replaced by amyloid fibrils
    - Nodular mesangial expansion can often be seen
    - Amyloid is weakly PAS positive, less than GBM
  - Silver stains: Expanded mesangial areas but ↓ or no silver staining (i.e., "loss of argyrophilia")
    - GBMs also may be engulfed by the material, showing up as areas of complete GBM discontinuity
    - Subepithelial spikes in capillary loops ("cock's comb")
  - Amyloid deposition can 1st be seen in mesangium and blood vessel walls
    - Early mesangial deposits may be quite small and subject to being overlooked, resulting in erroneous diagnosis of minimal change disease/glomerulopathy
  - Little or no hypercellularity
  - Eventually, ESRD kidneys with glomerulosclerosis from amyloid can be suspected by pale staining on JMS or PAS stains
    - Mesangial and subendothelial deposits eventually obliterate glomeruli
  - Rare cases of AL and AA amyloid crescents
  - Trichrome stains blue in amyloid, usually paler than trichrome staining of collagen
- Tubulointerstitium
  - Congo red staining useful in identifying vascular and interstitial amyloid
    - Helps distinguish from interstitial fibrosis (IF)
  - Interstitial involvement often contiguous with involvement of TBMs and vessels
    - Eventually, IF and tubular atrophy (TA) may be extensive, admixed with interstitial inflammation
  - Tubular casts containing amyloid are sometimes present and, in rare case reports, are the only manifestation of amyloidosis
    - Material has fibrillar appearance characteristic of amyloid on EM
  - Interstitium may be expanded by amyloid material
    - Mast cells may lead to IF in AA type

- Blood vessels
  - Any vessel can be involved, including vasa recta of renal medulla
  - Blood vessel amyloid can look like hyalinosis
    - Congo red staining helps distinguish amyloid deposition from hyalinosis
  - Interlobular arteries and hilar arterioles are most commonly involved (> 95% of renal biopsies having glomerular involvement)

ANCILLARY TESTS

Immunofluorescence
- Pattern depends on type of amyloid
  - Deposits variably present in glomerular mesangium, GBM, interstitium, and vessels
  - AL: Single light chain predominates
  - AA: Neither or both light chains stain
  - Fibrinogen (Aα chain) only glomerular
- Kappa and lambda staining performed on all native renal biopsies, identifying most cases of AL amyloidosis
  - Positive stain is when 1 light chain clearly predominates
    - Light chains may be present in other forms of amyloidosis due to nonspecific trapping
  - Negative stains do not exclude AL amyloid
    - Staining may be negative if light chain is truncated
  - Variants
    - Rare cases stain for an immunoglobulin heavy chain but not for light chains (AH amyloidosis)
    - Rare cases have 1 heavy chain (typically gamma) and 1 light chain (AL/AH amyloid)

Electron Microscopy
- Fibrils
  - Nonbranching, nonperiodic, ~ 7-12 nm in diameter
    - Accurate measurement necessary
    - Internal references: Cell membrane 8.5 nm; actin: 5 nm
    - Amorphous "cottony" appearance at ~ 5,000x
    - Electron-lucent core at ~ 100,000x
  - Randomly distributed in mesangium and GBM
  - Fibrils sometimes extend transmurally, replacing entire glomerular basement membrane
    - In subepithelial zone, fibrils align roughly perpendicular to GBM, producing "spike" formation or "cock's comb" (also called "spicular amyloid")
- Podocyte foot processes often effaced, and cytoplasm has condensation of actin filaments

Detection of Amyloid
- Congo red
  - Apple-green birefringence with polarized light
    - In contrast to fibrillar collagen, amyloid fibrils are only birefringent after Congo red stain
    - Important to have simultaneous positive control
  - Red without polarization (called "congophilia")
    - Elastic fibers are congophilic but not birefringent

AMYLOIDOSIS

- o Small amyloid quantities may make it difficult to demonstrate apple-green birefringence
  - Higher quality polarizing microscope will have greater sensitivity
  - 9 μm sections recommended for Congo red staining to maximize detection of small quantities of amyloid
  - Placing Congo red stains under green fluorescent light makes amyloid deposits appear bright red; sensitive but not specific
- o Potassium permanganate treatment prior to Congo red staining used to discriminate between AL and AA amyloid
  - Birefringent Congo red staining retained by AL amyloid but lost by AA
- Thioflavine T and S
  - o Thioflavin T activated by blue light to emit yellow fluorescence; sensitive, not specific
  - o Reports of ↑ sensitivity vs. Congo red if small quantities of amyloid present
  - o Rarely used currently
- Crystal violet
  - o Metachromatic stain not usually used in routine diagnostic work

Identification of Amyloid Protein
- Immunohistochemistry
  - o AA protein
  - o Fibrinogen, transthyretin, lysozyme, lactoferrin, and β2-microglobulin
  - o SAP (does not discriminate between types)
    - Used to compare with stains for specific protein
- Immunofluorescence
  - o Light and heavy immunoglobulin chains
  - o Fibrinogen (Aα chain)
- Electron microscopy
  - o Immunogold labeling can identify κ or λ light chains
- Proteomics
  - o Laser microdissection (LMD) and tandem mass spectrometry (MS)-based proteomic analysis useful in typing of renal amyloidosis
    - Detect Ig heavy chain amyloid and rare cases where > 1 amyloid is present
  - o Microextraction followed by amino acid sequencing can be used in select cases

Abdominal Fat Pad Fine Needle Aspiration
- Sensitivity ~ 20-60%; specificity ~ 100%
- Core biopsy probably more sensitive

Rectal Biopsy
- Provides diagnosis in a substantial fraction (no recent studies on test performance)

DIFFERENTIAL DIAGNOSIS

Fibrillary Glomerulopathy
- No birefringence with Congo red
- Fibrils usually, but not always, larger (10-30 nm)
  - o If > 20 nm, rules out amyloidosis
- SAP may be present (false-positive)

Immunotactoid Glomerulopathy
- No birefringence with Congo red
- Fibrils always larger (> 20 nm)
- Often associated with underlying plasma cell dyscrasia

Type III Collagen (Collagenofibrotic) Glomerulopathy
- No birefringence with Congo red
- Fibrils have a periodicity of collagen, 65 nm
- Often arranged in parallel and usually have a curved pattern
- No staining for light chains or AA protein

Incidental Mesangial Matrix Fibrils
- No birefringence with Congo red
- Usual matrix fibrils ~ 6 nm diameter
- Fibrils not abundant
- No "spikes" through GBM
  - o Usually just in mesangium or under endothelium

Fibronectin Glomerulopathy
- No birefringence with Congo red
- Stain for fibronectin
- Red on trichrome (vs. blue for amyloid)

Cryoglobulinemic Glomerulonephritis
- No birefringence with Congo red
- Deposits have somewhat "tubular" pattern, ~ 10-20 nm in diameter
- Glomerular inflammation (macrophages)

Nonamyloid Monoclonal Ig Deposition Disease (MIDD)
- No birefringence with Congo red, by definition
- Most lack fibrils and have dense amorphous deposits
- Mesangium stains more densely eosinophilic than amyloid, which appears "softer"

Diabetic Glomerulosclerosis
- No birefringence with Congo red
- Mesangium stains more PAS(+) and eosinophilic than amyloid, which appears "softer"
- Fibrils in mesangium and subendothelium are sparse

DIAGNOSTIC CHECKLIST

Clinically Relevant Pathologic Features
- Interstitial fibrosis and renal function at presentation are predictors of survival

Pathologic Interpretation Pearls
- Quality of polarizing microscope is crucial determinant of sensitivity

SELECTED REFERENCES

1. Halloush RA et al: Diagnosis and typing of systemic amyloidosis: The role of abdominal fat pad fine needle aspiration biopsy. Cytojournal. 6:24, 2010
2. Herrera GA et al: Renal diseases with organized deposits: an algorithmic approach to classification and clinicopathologic diagnosis. Arch Pathol Lab Med. 134(4):512-31, 2010

AMYLOIDOSIS

Amyloid Types Affecting Kidney

Amyloid Protein	Clinical Features	Tissue/Organ Distribution	Renal Pathology
Neoplastic/Clonal B Cell/Plasma Cell			
AL/AH (Ig light/ heavy chain)	Most common cause of renal amyloidosis; nephrotic syndrome common (40%); fatigue, weight loss, neuropathy, GI symptoms, hepatosplenomegaly, carpal tunnel	Widespread: Kidney, heart, GI, liver, spleen, nerves	Glomerular, interstitial, and arterial deposits (~ 10% lack glomerular deposits)
Chronic Inflammation			
AA (serum amyloid A)	Chronic infection or inflammation; neoplasia, minority idiopathic (~ 10%); wide age range (~ 10-90); presents with nephrotic syndrome or renal insufficiency	Widespread: Almost always involves kidney; GI, liver, spleen, thyroid, adrenal; less commonly heart	Glomerular deposits usually predominate; some cases with only tubulointerstitial &/or vascular deposits
	Hereditary periodic fever syndromes (FMF, HIDS, FCU, and MWS); episodes of fevers, with pain with peritonitis, pleuritis; onset of amyloidosis < 40 years old; nephrotic syndrome or renal insufficiency	Widespread, as above	Glomerular deposits usually predominate; prominent peritubular rings; sometimes primarily in medulla
Genetic Mutation			
AFib (fibrinogen Aα chain)	Onset 20s-70s, then rapid kidney failure (1-5 years); often no family history; recurs in transplants; at least 4 different mutations	Kidney, not heart or nerves	Exclusively glomerular deposits; stain positive for fibrinogen
AApoAI (apolipoprotein A-I)	Hypertension and renal failure without nephrotic syndrome	Liver, kidney, heart	Arterial and interstitial deposits
AApoAII (apolipoprotein A-II)	Slowly progressive renal insufficiency	Kidney, heart	Glomerular, arterial, and interstitial deposits
Alys (lysozyme)	Dermal petechiae, GI bleeding	Kidney, liver, spleen, skin, GI tract	Glomerular and arterial deposits
AATR (transthyretin)	Congestive heart failure, peripheral neuropathy; > 100 different mutations; cardiac variant with wild-type AATR in elderly (senile systemic amyloidosis)	Heart and nerves; sometimes eye and kidney	Primarily glomerular deposits but sometimes limited to medullary interstitium
ACys (cystatin C)	Stroke, no renal disease	Cerebral vessels primarily	Arterial deposits
AGel (gelsolin)	Cranial nerves, cornea, cutis laxa (Finnish hereditary amyloidosis)	Nerves, cornea, skin, kidney	Glomerular deposits
Decreased Excretion			
Aβ2m (β2- microglobulin)	Osteoarthropathy and neuropathy in patients on chronic hemodialysis	Most organs, especially vascular deposits, juxtaarticular cysts	Deposits present but not clinically significant
Unclassified			
ALECT2 (leukocyte chemotactic factor 2)	Proteinuria, nephrotic syndrome; no mutation yet identified	Kidney only	Diffuse involvement of glomeruli, arteries, and interstitium

FMF = familial Mediterranean fever; HIDS = hyper-IgD syndrome; FCU = familial cold urticaria; MWS = Muckle-Wells syndrome. Adapted from Merlini G et al: Molecular mechanisms of amyloidosis. N Engl J Med. 349(6):583-96, 2003.

3. Larsen CP et al: Prevalence and morphology of leukocyte chemotactic factor 2-associated amyloid in renal biopsies. Kidney Int. 77(9):816-9, 2010
4. Sattianayagam PT et al: Solid organ transplantation in AL amyloidosis. Am J Transplant. 10(9):2124-31, 2010
5. Sethi S et al: Mass spectrometry-based proteomic diagnosis of renal immunoglobulin heavy chain amyloidosis. Clin J Am Soc Nephrol. 5(12):2180-7, 2010
6. Gillmore JD et al: Diagnosis, pathogenesis, treatment, and prognosis of hereditary fibrinogen A alpha-chain amyloidosis. J Am Soc Nephrol. 20(2):444-51, 2009
7. Herrera GA: Renal lesions associated with plasma cell dyscrasias: practical approach to diagnosis, new concepts, and challenges. Arch Pathol Lab Med. 133(2):249-67, 2009
8. Howie AJ et al: Physical basis of colors seen in Congo red-stained amyloid in polarized light. Lab Invest. 88(3):232-42, 2008

9. Osawa Y et al: Renal function at the time of renal biopsy as a predictor of prognosis in patients with primary AL-type amyloidosis. Clin Exp Nephrol. 8(2):127-33, 2004
10. Mai HL et al: Immunoglobulin heavy chain can be amyloidogenic: morphologic characterization including immunoelectron microscopy. Am J Surg Pathol. 27(4):541-5, 2003
11. Merlini G et al: Molecular mechanisms of amyloidosis. N Engl J Med. 349(6):583-96, 2003
12. Tóth T et al: Increased density of interstitial mast cells in amyloid A renal amyloidosis. Mod Pathol. 13(9):1020-8, 2000
13. Gertz MA et al: Amyloidosis: prognosis and treatment. Semin Arthritis Rheum. 24(2):124-38, 1994
14. Wright JR et al: Clinical-pathologic differentiation of common amyloid syndromes. Medicine (Baltimore). 60(6):429-48, 1981

2

AMYLOIDOSIS

Microscopic Features

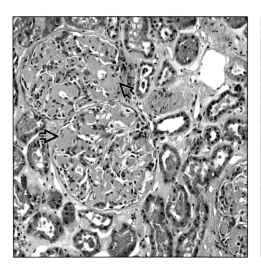

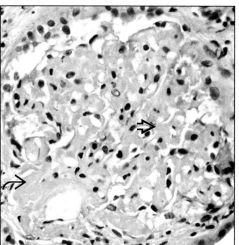

(Left) At medium power, light microscopy shows deposition of abnormal extracellular material in the glomerulus, primarily in the mesangium, shown in other studies to be amyloid ➡. *(Right)* Relatively high power in a 68 year old with amyloidosis, proteinuria of 5 g/d, and creatinine of 1.3 mg/dL shows that there is accumulation of amorphous extracellular material in the mesangium ➡ and in the arteriole entering the glomerulus ➡.

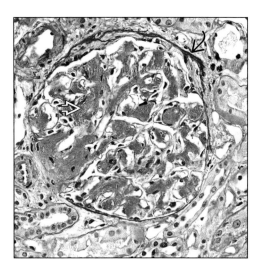

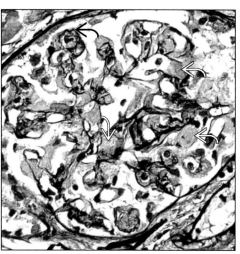

(Left) Light microscopy shows accumulation of material in the mesangium ➡, which stains less intensely by PAS stain than the basement membranes of the kidney (e.g., Bowman capsule) ➡. *(Right)* Silver stains can be used to advantage in amyloidosis, in which they reveal the location of the pale-staining amyloid ➡ that is less argyrophilic than the surrounding basement membranes ➡.

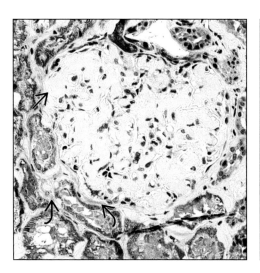

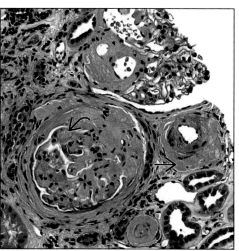

(Left) On a trichrome stain, this glomerulus with amyloidosis shows that the amyloid material is pale blue ➡, being less dark than the fibrous tissue "skeleton" ➡ of the surrounding kidney. Fibrillary GN, which has somewhat similar deposits by EM, is characteristically red on trichrome stain. *(Right)* By H&E, there is accumulation of amyloid in nearly sclerotic glomeruli ➡ and in vessels ➡.

AMYLOIDOSIS

Congo Red Stain and Immunofluorescence

(Left) In this early case of amyloidosis, a Congo red stain may show subtle focal accumulation of amyloid ⇉ along the glomerular basement membrane and mesangium that has a red tinge ("congophilia") under standard light microscopy without polarization.
(Right) By polarized light examination, a Congo red stain in this case of amyloidosis shows accumulation in the mesangium ⇉ and classic apple-green birefringence ⇉. Interstitial deposits are also revealed ⇉.

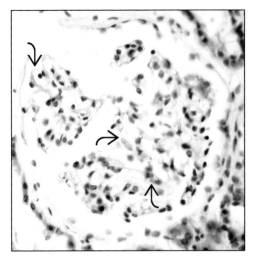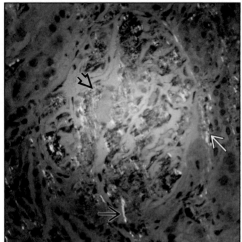

(Left) In this case of amyloidosis, Congo red shows accumulation of amyloid in the interstitium between tubules ⇉, staining red ("congophilic") under standard light microscopic examination without polarization. *(Right)* In this case of amyloidosis, Congo red shows accumulation of amyloid in the interstitium between tubules ⇉, having an apple-green birefringence by polarized light examination.

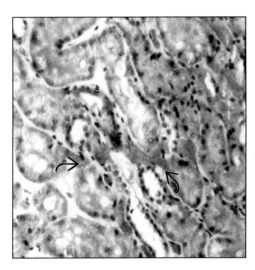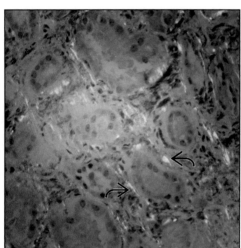

(Left) In a 48-year-old man with familial Mediterranean fever and ESRD, there is extensive interstitial accumulation of apple-green birefringent amyloid material ⇉ on polarized light examination of a Congo Red stain, shown in other studies to be AA amyloid. *(Right)* Thioflavin T fluorescence shows bright glomerular staining in the glomerular mesangium in a case of amyloidosis ⇉. Thioflavine T is not specific and stains nonamyloid deposits (e.g., dense deposit disease).

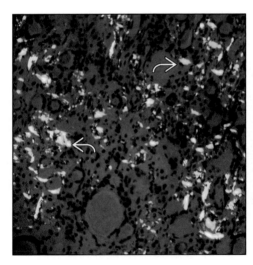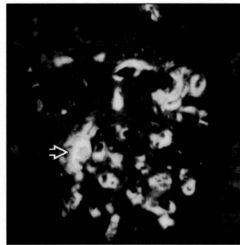

AMYLOIDOSIS

Immunofluorescence and Immunohistochemistry

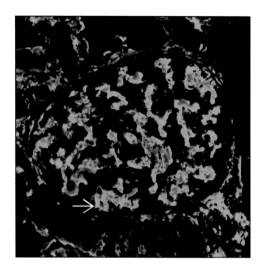

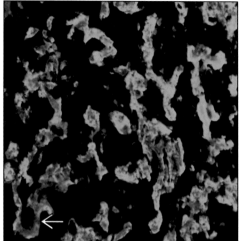

(Left) In a case of amyloidosis, extensive accumulation of lambda light chain can be appreciated in the glomerulus ➜ using immunofluorescence for lambda. *(Right)* Higher power examination of a case of amyloidosis shows accumulation of lambda light chain along glomerular capillary loops ➜. The kappa stain was much weaker, indicating that the diagnosis is AL amyloid (the most common type affecting the kidney).

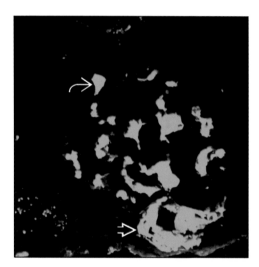

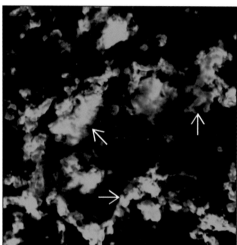

(Left) Examination of a case of amyloidosis using immunofluorescence for lambda shows extensive accumulation of lambda light chain in the glomerulus ➜, primarily in the mesangium, and also in the afferent arteriole ➜. *(Right)* Immunofluorescence for lambda in a case of amyloidosis shows extensive amorphous accumulation in the interstitium ➜.

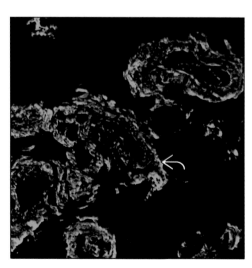

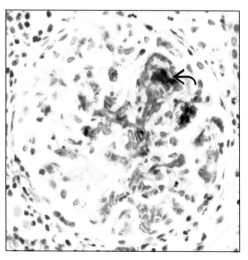

(Left) Identification of the amyloid protein is a necessary part of the pathology work-up. Immunofluorescence for AA amyloid shows extensive accumulation in vessels ➜ in this case of renal amyloidosis due to AA amyloid. *(Right)* Immunohistochemistry can be used to demonstrate serum amyloid A in paraffin sections, here shown in a glomerulus ➜, indicating AA amyloidosis. These cases typically have weak and equal staining for light chains.

2

Electron Microscopy

(Left) EM of a glomerular capillary loop in a patient with amyloidosis and nephrotic syndrome shows marked thickening of the GBM ⇗ due to accumulation of amyloid fibrils, which appear amorphous at this power. **(Right)** High power of glomerular capillary loops in a 68 year old with amyloidosis shows amyloid accumulation along the GBM ⇗ and extensive podocyte foot process effacement with microvillous transformation ➔ and resorption droplets ⇗.

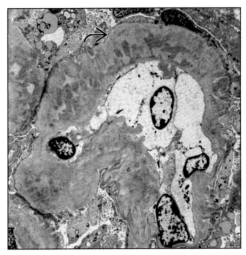
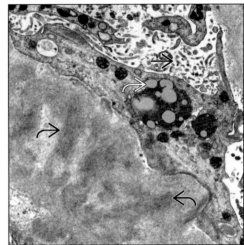

(Left) In this case of amyloidosis, amyloid accumulates along the GBM, having overlying podocyte foot process effacement ➔ and an early "spicular" or comb-like accumulation ⇗ of amyloid. **(Right)** High-power examination of this case of amyloidosis shows a random arrangement of fibrils ➔ with measurements in the range of 7-12 nm, which is compatible with amyloid.

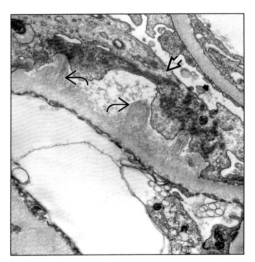
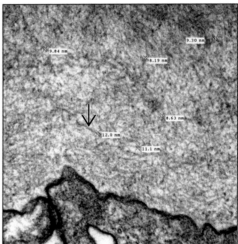

(Left) An unusual case of amyloidosis resembles dense deposit disease by electron microscopy, with electron-dense sausage-like deposits along the glomerular basement membranes ➔ and within the mesangium ➔. **(Right)** In this case of amyloidosis, there is accumulation of amyloid material in a small blood vessel underneath the endothelium ➔ and between smooth muscle cells.

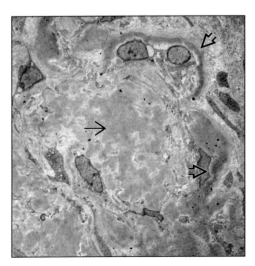
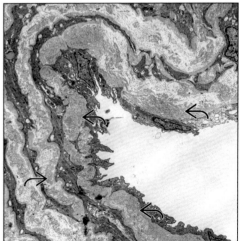

Unusual Forms of Amyloidosis

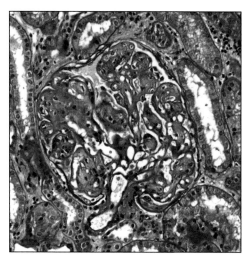 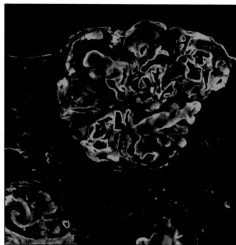

(Left) The mesangium is expanded by weakly PAS(+) material in 55-year-old woman of northern European ancestry with nephrotic syndrome and no family history of renal disease. The mesangial material stained for fibrinogen, indicating AFib amyloidosis. (Courtesy M. Picken, MD.) (Right) AFib amyloidosis is identified by IF, as shown here with antibodies to fibrinogen. κ and λ light chains may also be present at low levels, confusing the diagnosis. (Courtesy M. Picken, MD.)

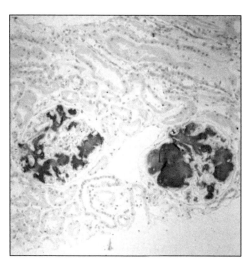 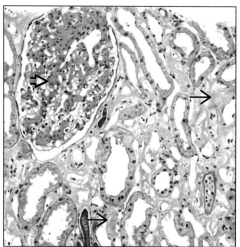

(Left) IHC with anti-fibrinogen is positive in AFib amyloidosis. These are exclusively in the glomerulus. AFib is the most common genetic form of amyloidosis in the kidney, caused by a mutation in the fibrinogen Aα chain. (Courtesy M. Picken, MD and R. Linke, MD.) (Right) Amorphous, PAS(-) material is present within glomeruli ⇨ and the interstitium ➡ in a patient with amyloidosis, shown to be LECT2 amyloidosis by antibody stains and mass spectroscopy. (Courtesy M. Fidler, MD.)

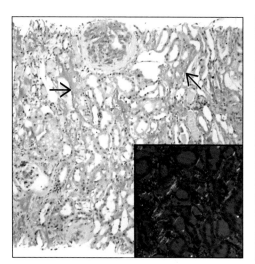 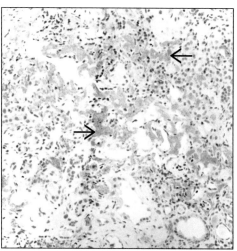

(Left) The interstitium stains positively by Congo red ➡. The Congo red-positive material shows apple green birefringence upon examination under polarized light (insert). IF and AA amyloid staining were negative. Mass spectrometry confirmed LECT2 amyloidosis. (Courtesy M. Fidler, MD.) (Right) An immunohistochemical stain for LECT2 shows pale but positive staining of the amyloid material ➡. Mass spectrometry on this case revealed LECT2 deposits. (Courtesy M. Fidler, MD.)

FIBRILLARY GLOMERULOPATHY

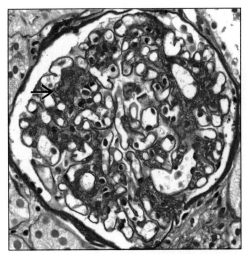

Periodic acid-Schiff shows diffuse expansion of mesangial areas ➡ by eosinophilic material with normal glomerular basement membranes in a young female with FGN.

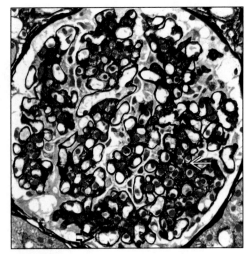

Jones methenamine silver reveals increased mesangial hypercellularity ➡ and focal duplication of the glomerular basement membrane ➡.

TERMINOLOGY

Synonyms
- Fibrillary glomerulonephritis (FGN)
- Nonamyloidotic fibrillary glomerulopathy
- Congo red negative amyloidosis-like glomerulopathy

Definitions
- Glomerular disease characterized by nonamyloid, nonperiodic fibrillar deposits of immunoglobulin, 10-30 nm in diameter

ETIOLOGY/PATHOGENESIS

Unknown
- Fibrils contain IgG, usually IgG4 ± IgG1, with both light chains (polyclonal)
  - Occasional cases monotypic light chains (10-20%)
  - Most cases idiopathic
- Associations
  - Malignancy (23%)
  - Dysproteinemia (17%)
  - Autoimmune disease (15%), including systemic lupus erythematosus
  - Infection, including hepatitis C virus (3%)

CLINICAL ISSUES

Epidemiology
- Incidence
  - < 1% of native kidney biopsies
- Age
  - Average: ~ 50 years; range: 19-81 years
- Gender
  - Slight female predilection
- Ethnicity
  - Caucasian predilection (> 90%)

Presentation
- Proteinuria (100%)
  - Nephrotic (38%)
- Hematuria (52%)
- Hypertension (70%)
- Renal insufficiency

Laboratory Tests
- Normocomplementemic (97%)

Treatment
- Drugs
  - None effective, corticosteroids if acute inflammation

Prognosis
- 40-50% progress to ESRD in 2-4 years
  - Occasional complete (5%) or partial (8%) remission
- Recurrence rate of 35-50% in kidney allografts

MICROSCOPIC PATHOLOGY

Histologic Features
- Glomeruli
  - Diffuse mesangial expansion by eosinophilic material
  - Mesangial sclerosis &/or hypercellularity pattern
    - Can manifest as nodular glomerulosclerosis
    - Segmental &/or global glomerular scarring
  - Membranoproliferative pattern
    - Focal GBM duplication
  - Marked subepithelial deposits may mimic membranous GN
  - Cellular crescents in ~ 25% of cases
    - Usually < 20% of glomeruli
  - Congo red stain negative
  - PAS and Jones silver stain negative (or weak)
- Tubules and interstitium
  - Interstitial fibrosis and tubular atrophy common
  - Interstitial inflammation may be prominent when tubular basement membrane deposits present

FIBRILLARY GLOMERULOPATHY

Key Facts

Clinical Issues
- Rare: < 1% of native kidney biopsies
- Associated with malignancy, dysproteinemia, and autoimmune disease
- Proteinuria (100%)
- Hematuria (~ 50%)
- 40-50% progress to ESRD within 2-4 years
- 35-50% recur in kidney allografts

Microscopic Pathology
- Diffuse mesangial expansion by eosinophilic material
  - Congo red negative
- Several histologic patterns
  - Mesangial proliferation
  - Membranoproliferative GN
  - Crescents ~ 25%
  - Segmental &/or global glomerular scarring

- IF: IgG and C3 in mesangium and along GBM
  - Usually IgG4, rarely IgM and IgA
  - Usually kappa = lambda
- EM: Nonbranching, randomly arranged fibrils
  - Thicker than amyloid
  - Average: 20 nm; range: 10-30 nm

Top Differential Diagnoses
- Amyloidosis
- Immunotactoid glomerulopathy
- Cryoglobulinemic glomerulonephritis
- Fibronectin glomerulopathy

Diagnostic Checklist
- IgG, kappa and lambda light chains strongly positive

ANCILLARY TESTS

Immunofluorescence
- Prominent IgG deposits in mesangium and along GBM
  - Often IgG4 (90%) with (80%) or without (10%) IgG1; rarely IgG1 alone (10%)
    - IgG4 heavy chains spontaneously reassociate, impairing detection of monotypic light chains
  - Kappa = lambda in most cases
    - 10-20% monotypic light chains (70% lambda)
  - May mimic anti-GBM disease or MGN
- C3 almost always strongly positive (92%), often lesser C1q (60%)
- May have IgM (47%) or IgA (28%) but at a lesser intensity than IgG
- TBM deposits of IgG in a subset

Electron Microscopy
- Randomly arranged fibrils deposited in mesangial areas and along GBM
  - Fibrils without hollow core or organized substructure
    - Average diameter: 18-20 nm; range: 10-30 nm
    - Resemble amyloid fibrils but usually larger diameter
  - Fibrils composed of immunoglobulins by immunogold labeling
- TBM has fibrillar deposits in subset of cases

DIFFERENTIAL DIAGNOSIS

Amyloidosis
- Congo red positive with apple-green birefringence under polarized light; 8-12 nm thick fibrils

Immunotactoid Glomerulopathy
- Microtubular substructure of deposits larger (30-50 nm thick fibrils)
- Often associated with underlying plasma cell dyscrasia
- Usually (~ 80%) monotypic

Cryoglobulinemic Glomerulonephritis
- Serum cryoglobulins present
- Membranoproliferative pattern of injury with "pseudothrombi" on light microscopy
- Strong IgM, not IgG4 dominant

Fibronectin Glomerulopathy
- Mesangial and subendothelial deposition of PAS(+) material
- Negative immunofluorescence staining

DIAGNOSTIC CHECKLIST

Pathologic Interpretation Pearls
- Pathologic predictor of poor outcome
  - Global glomerulosclerosis

SELECTED REFERENCES

1. Nasr SH et al: Fibrillary glomerulonephritis: a report of 66 cases from a single institution. Clin J Am Soc Nephrol. Epub ahead of print, 2011
2. Alpers CE et al: Fibrillary glomerulonephritis and immunotactoid glomerulopathy. J Am Soc Nephrol. 19(1):34-7, 2008
3. Rosenstock JL et al: Fibrillary and immunotactoid glomerulonephritis: Distinct entities with different clinical and pathologic features. Kidney Int. 63(4):1450-61, 2003
4. Markowitz GS et al: Hepatitis C viral infection is associated with fibrillary glomerulonephritis and immunotactoid glomerulopathy. J Am Soc Nephrol. 9(12):2244-52, 1998
5. Fogo A et al: Morphologic and clinical features of fibrillary glomerulonephritis versus immunotactoid glomerulopathy. Am J Kidney Dis. 22(3):367-77, 1993
6. Iskandar SS et al: Clinical and pathologic features of fibrillary glomerulonephritis. Kidney Int. 42(6):1401-7, 1992
7. Devaney K et al: Nonamyloidotic fibrillary glomerulopathy, immunotactoid glomerulopathy, and the differential diagnosis of filamentous glomerulopathies. Mod Pathol. 4(1):36-45, 1991

2

FIBRILLARY GLOMERULOPATHY

Variant Microscopic Features

(Left) H&E shows a prominent increase in eosinophilic material in mesangial areas ⊋, which leads to an appearance of decreased patent glomerular capillaries. *(Right)* Periodic acid-Schiff shows mesangial expansion by eosinophilic material ⊋ that stains less pink than the glomerular basement membranes ⊋ and resembles amyloid but is distinct from diabetic nephropathy. The mesangial matrix in diabetic patients stains equally intense as the glomerular basement membranes.

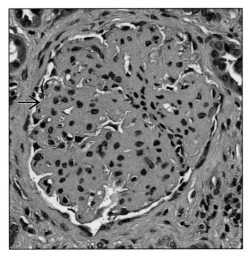
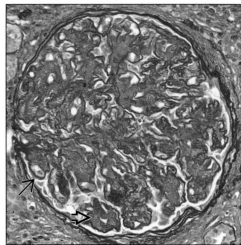

(Left) Jones methenamine silver may deemphasize the extent of deposition in mesangial areas in comparison to PAS and hematoxylin and eosin stains. *(Right)* H&E highlights a cellular crescent ⊋ that occupies the urinary space and compresses the glomerulus ⊋. The increased mesangial cellularity and intracapillary inflammatory cells is consistent with an inflammatory injury of the glomerulus.

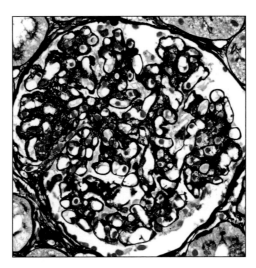
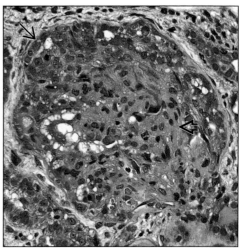

(Left) This glomerulus shows collapsing glomerulopathy with prominence of the glomerular epithelial cells, which mimics a cellular crescent. Definite fibrinoid necrosis or rupture of the GBM was not identified (periodic acid-Schiff). *(Right)* Periodic acid-Schiff reveals a florid cellular crescent ⊋ that is compressing the remaining glomerular tufts ⊋. The collapsed glomerular tufts somewhat resemble collapsing glomerulopathy. Cellular crescents are found in about 20% of FGN.

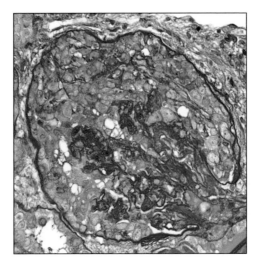
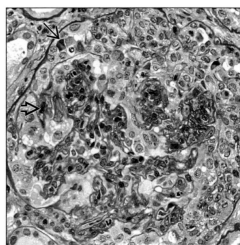

FIBRILLARY GLOMERULOPATHY

Microscopic Features

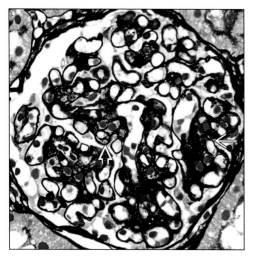 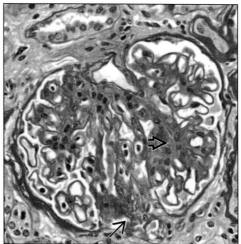

(Left) Jones methenamine silver reveals mild glomerular alterations in the form of segmental mesangial hypercellularity ⇒ and focal glomerular basement membrane alterations ⇒. (Right) Periodic acid-Schiff shows thickened capillary walls and segmental mesangial matrix expansion ⇒ and hypercellularity in this injured glomerulus from a patient with fibrillary glomerulonephritis. A fibrous attachment ⇒ to Bowman capsule is present at the glomerular tip.

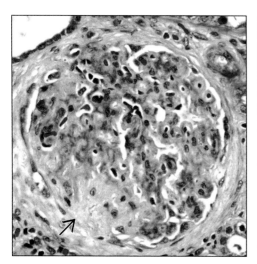 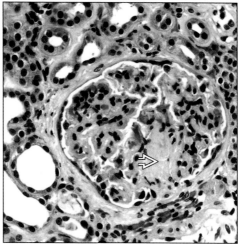

(Left) Masson trichrome shows segmental glomerular scarring ⇒ with loss of many glomerular capillary lumina and a fibrous attachment to Bowman capsule. This glomerular injury is common in advanced FGN as the glomerular scarring progresses toward global glomerulosclerosis. (Right) Hematoxylin and eosin shows eosinophilic material deposited segmentally in the mesangium ⇒. There is moderate interstitial fibrosis and tubular atrophy adjacent to the glomerulus.

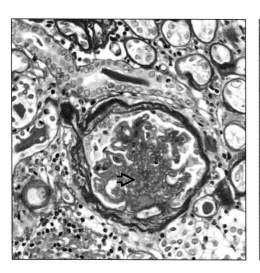 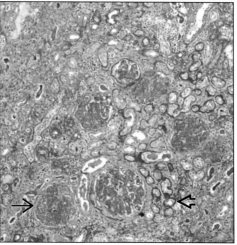

(Left) Periodic acid-Schiff shows prominent mesangial matrix expansion ⇒. There is frequent tubular atrophy with tubular casts, which is associated with interstitial fibrosis and mild interstitial inflammation. (Right) Periodic acid-Schiff highlights several globally sclerotic glomeruli ⇒ that are closely clustered together, which indicates substantial tubular loss. There is also diffuse interstitial fibrosis and tubular atrophy ⇒ in this advanced case of fibrillary glomerulonephritis.

Immunofluorescence

(Left) *Immunofluorescence microscopy for IgG shows strong mesangial* ⮞ *staining with focal staining of glomerular capillary walls* ➡, *which correlates with the light microscopic alterations of the glomeruli.* *(Right)* *Immunofluorescence for IgG of FGN with a crescent* ⮞ *shows strong confluent staining of the capillary walls ("pseudolinear" pattern)* ➡ *and mesangial regions. The confluent staining may resemble anti-GBM disease, but the mesangial staining* ⮞ *excludes this diagnosis.*

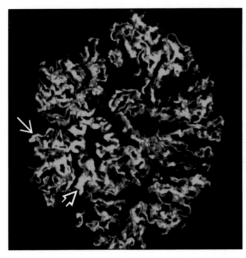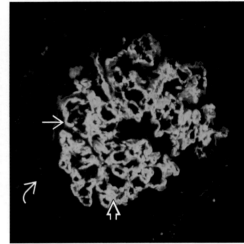

(Left) *Immunofluorescence shows C3 deposition in the glomerular mesangium* ➡ *and along the glomerular capillary walls* ⮞. *(Right)* *Immunofluorescence microscopy shows granular C1q deposition in the mesangial regions* ⮞, *which can be observed in a small subset of cases. The staining pattern is similar to IgG and kappa and lambda light chain staining (not shown).*

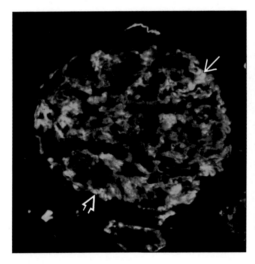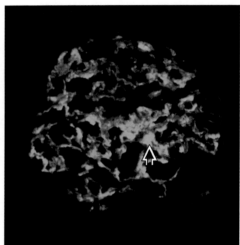

(Left) *Immunofluorescence microscopy for kappa light chain demonstrates a similar but less intense staining pattern to IgG and lambda light chains (not shown). Rare cases of monoclonal staining have been reported.* *(Right)* *Immunofluorescence microscopy shows that IgG staining of the tubular basement membranes* ➡ *can be observed in a subset of fibrillary glomerulonephritis. Prominent interstitial inflammation (not shown) was also noted by light microscopy.*

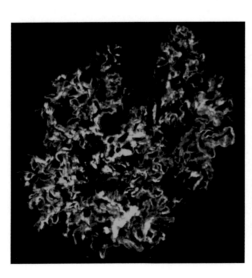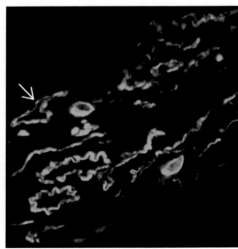

FIBRILLARY GLOMERULOPATHY

Electron Microscopy

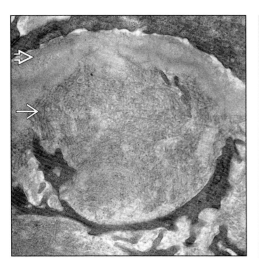
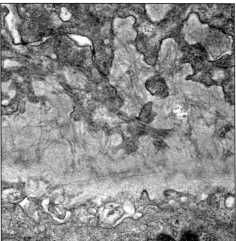

(Left) Electron micrograph shows numerous fibrillar deposits primarily limited to a subendothelial location ⇨ without involvement of the overlying glomerular basement membrane ⇨. *(Right)* Electron microscopy of fibrillary glomerulonephritis shows fibrils arranged in a haphazard pattern in the GBM and mesangial matrix. The Congo red stain was negative, and the diagnosis was further supported by the presence of characteristic polyclonal light chain IF staining.

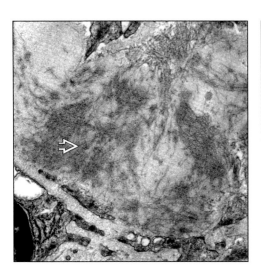
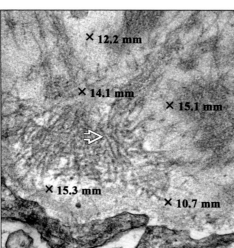

× 12.2 mm
× 14.1 mm
× 15.1 mm
× 15.3 mm
× 10.7 mm

(Left) Electron microscopy shows prominent accumulation of randomly arranged fibrils ⇨ in a subendothelial region. At low magnification, these aggregates of fibrils may resemble discrete immune complexes, but closer examination reveals their fibrillar substructure. *(Right)* Electron microscopy shows randomly arranged fibrils ⇨ with thicknesses that typically range from 12-30 nm (average of 20 nm). On occasion, discrete electron-dense deposits are intermixed with fibrils.

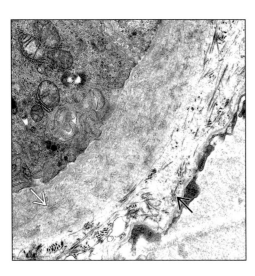
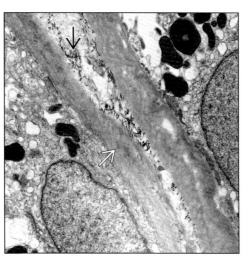

(Left) Electron microscopy demonstrates many fibrils ⇨ within the tubular basement membrane that are clearly thinner than adjacent collagen fibrils ⇨ in the interstitium. *(Right)* Electron microscopy reveals thick collagen fibrils ⇨ in the interstitium adjacent to the fibrils within the tubular basement membranes ⇨ of an advanced case of fibrillary glomerulonephritis. Deposition of fibrils in the tubular basement membranes is present in a small subset of fibrillary GN.

IMMUNOTACTOID GLOMERULOPATHY

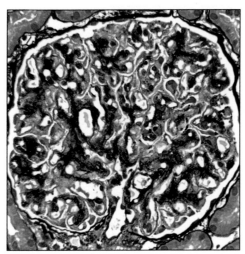

Jones methenamine silver reveals that the immune deposits along the glomerular capillaries are mostly negative for silver staining in this case of immunotactoid glomerulopathy. (Courtesy J. Kowalewska, MD.)

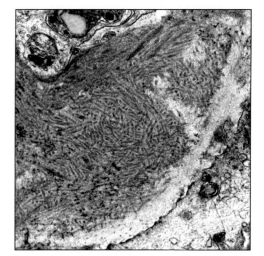

The characteristic microtubular pattern of deposits in immunotactoid glomerulopathy is evident even in this medium-power electron micrograph.

TERMINOLOGY

Abbreviations
- Immunotactoid glomerulopathy (ITG)

Synonyms
- Congo red negative organized glomerular immunoglobulin deposits

Definitions
- Congo red negative microtubular deposits typically > 30 nm in diameter and arranged in parallel arrays

ETIOLOGY/PATHOGENESIS

Unknown Mechanism
- Microtubular glomerular deposits usually represent monotypic immunoglobulins

CLINICAL ISSUES

Epidemiology
- Incidence
  - Rare
  - < 0.1% of adult native kidney biopsies
- Age
  - 5th to 6th decade
    - Older than patients with fibrillary glomerulonephritis
- Gender
  - Slight female predilection
- Ethnicity
  - Caucasian predilection

Site
- Typically limited to kidney

Presentation
- Nephrotic syndrome

- Hematuria
- Hypocomplementemia
- 67% of patients have an associated monoclonal gammopathy or hematologic malignancy

Laboratory Tests
- Serum or urine protein electrophoresis
- Immunofixation or immunoelectrophoresis

Treatment
- Drugs
  - Chemotherapy for underlying lymphoproliferative disorder or plasma cell dyscrasia, if present

Prognosis
- Data limited: Median time to end-stage renal disease is ~ 2 years
  - Clinical course depends on underlying lymphoproliferative disorder, if present
  - Occasional response to chemotherapy
    - Repeat biopsies show loss of deposits in a minority
- Recurrence after kidney transplantation (~ 50%), more benign course

MICROSCOPIC PATHOLOGY

Histologic Features
- Glomerulus
  - Varied patterns: Mesangioproliferative, membranoproliferative, nodular glomerular disease
    - Mesangial expansion by eosinophilic, PAS-positive material
    - GBM: Focal splitting and occasional "spikes"
    - Rare crescents (vs. fibrillary glomerulonephritis)
- Tubular atrophy
- Interstitial fibrosis
- Extrarenal deposits rarely reported (e.g., peripheral nerve)

IMMUNOTACTOID GLOMERULOPATHY

Key Facts

Terminology
- Congo red negative organized glomerular immunoglobulin deposits

Clinical Issues
- Caucasian predilection
- Nephrotic syndrome, hematuria, and hypocomplementemia
- Often associated with monoclonal gammopathy or hematologic malignancy

Microscopic Pathology
- Mesangial expansion with eosinophilic, PAS-positive material
- Mesangioproliferative or membranoproliferative pattern

- Focal splitting and occasional "spikes" of basement membrane
- Immunofluorescence with predominant IgG, with some cases showing IgA or IgM
- Electron microscopy shows microtubules organized in parallel arrays (> 30 nm) with hollow core

Top Differential Diagnoses
- Cryoglobulinemic glomerulonephritis
- Fibrillary glomerulopathy
- Fibronectin glomerulopathy
- Type III collagen glomerulopathy

Diagnostic Checklist
- Congo red negative deposits with microtubular appearance and diameter typically > 30 nm

ANCILLARY TESTS

Immunofluorescence
- Predominantly IgG, with rare cases showing IgA or IgM
  - IgG1 is most common subclass when monotypic deposits present
- Kappa &/or lambda light chain
  - Most cases are monoclonal, but polyclonal staining can be observed
- C3 usually positive, and C1q less frequently positive

Electron Microscopy
- Transmission
  - Microtubular deposits with hollow core or electron-lucent tubular lumen organized in parallel arrays
    - Typically > 30 nm in diameter (range: 20-90 nm)
  - Subendothelial location in irregular, chunky pattern along capillary loops and mesangium
  - Subepithelial and intramembranous deposits may also be seen

DIFFERENTIAL DIAGNOSIS

Cryoglobulinemic Glomerulonephritis
- Electron-dense deposits often with substructural organization
- Serum positive for cryoglobulins

Fibrillary Glomerulopathy
- Randomly arranged fibrils with average thickness of 20 nm without hollow core
- Polyclonal IF staining; commonly IgG4

Fibronectin Glomerulopathy
- Fibrillar deposits < 30 nm; IgG negative
- Positive immunohistochemistry for fibronectin

Type III Collagen Glomerulopathy
- Periodic banded collagen fibrils by EM and type III collagen by IHC

Nail-Patella Syndrome
- Rare disorder with nail hypoplasia &/or bone abnormalities
- Periodic, sparse collagen fibrils by EM in GBM

Lupus Nephritis
- "Full house" immunofluorescence staining pattern
- Electron-dense deposits may show rare microtubular pattern

DIAGNOSTIC CHECKLIST

Pathologic Interpretation Pearls
- Monoclonal immunoglobulin staining pattern
- Congo red negative deposits with microtubular appearance and diameter typically > 30 nm

SELECTED REFERENCES

1. Rosenstock JL et al: Fibrillary and immunotactoid glomerulonephritis: Distinct entities with different clinical and pathologic features. Kidney Int. 63(4):1450-61, 2003
2. Bridoux F et al: Fibrillary glomerulonephritis and immunotactoid (microtubular) glomerulopathy are associated with distinct immunologic features. Kidney Int. 62(5):1764-75, 2002
3. Fogo A et al: Morphologic and clinical features of fibrillary glomerulonephritis versus immunotactoid glomerulopathy. Am J Kidney Dis. 22(3):367-77, 1993
4. Alpers CE: Immunotactoid (microtubular) glomerulopathy: an entity distinct from fibrillary glomerulonephritis? Am J Kidney Dis. 19(2):185-91, 1992

IMMUNOTACTOID GLOMERULOPATHY

Microscopic Features

(Left) Periodic acid-Schiff shows mild diffuse expansion of mesangial areas with focal hypercellularity ⊅ and irregular and segmental thickening of the glomerular basement membranes ➡ due to the presence of immune deposits in this case of ITG. *(Courtesy J. Kowalewska, MD.)* *(Right)* Hematoxylin and eosin shows prominent deposition of refractile amorphous eosinophilic deposits along the capillary walls ➡ and some mesangial areas ⊅.

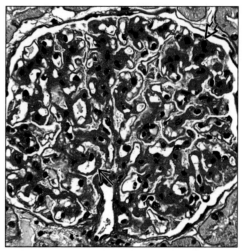
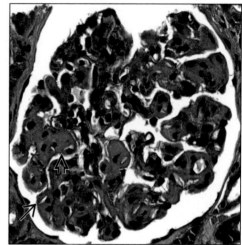

(Left) Increased eosinophilic material is present in mesangial areas and along glomerular capillaries on H&E. Focusing up and down on the slide shows a refractile quality to this material that resembles that of a "wire loop" deposit in lupus nephritis. *(Right)* Periodic acid-Schiff shows segmental increase of eosinophilic material in the mesangium with normal adjacent glomerular tufts, segmental sclerosis, and adhesion to Bowman capsule. The GBM is normal at this magnification.

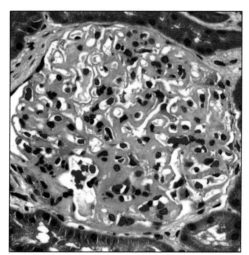
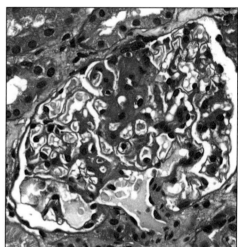

(Left) Periodic acid-Schiff shows mixed increase in mesangial extracellular material with little hypercellularity and variable increase in capillary wall thickness in a biopsy with immunotactoid glomerulopathy. *(Right)* H&E shows acute glomerulitis in immunotactoid glomerulopathy. Abundant neutrophils are present in the capillary loops ➡, resembling acute postinfectious glomerulonephritis. EM showed subepithelial "humps" containing microtubules.

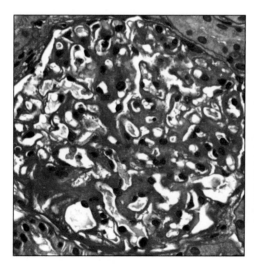
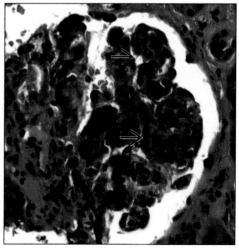

IMMUNOTACTOID GLOMERULOPATHY

Immunofluorescence

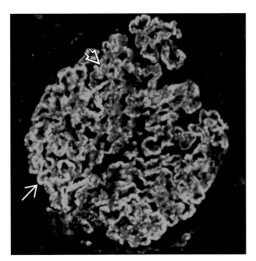
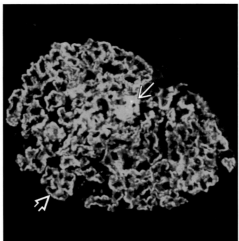

(Left) Immunofluorescence microscopy for IgG shows strong staining along glomerular capillaries ⇨ and mesangial areas ⇨. (Courtesy J. Kowalewska, MD.) *(Right)* Immunofluorescence microscopy for C3 shows strong staining of the glomerular capillaries ⇨ and mesangial areas ⇨ in a similar pattern as IgG. The location of the deposits correlates with the light microscopic findings. (Courtesy J. Kowalewska, MD.)

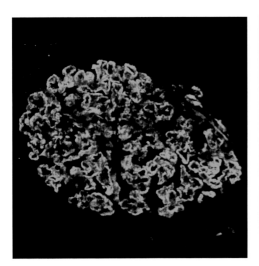
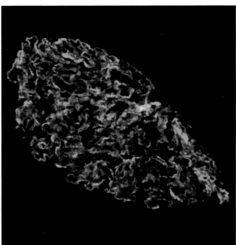

(Left) IF for kappa light chains in ITG shows strong granular staining along the glomerular capillaries with a similar pattern to IgG and slightly less intensity. (Courtesy J. Kowalewska, MD.) *(Right)* Lambda light chains are similar to kappa but less intense in this polyclonal staining of the immune deposits. Among 18 cases in 2 series, 84% have a single predominant light chain ("monoclonal"), with kappa more common than lambda. (Courtesy J. Kowalewska, MD.)

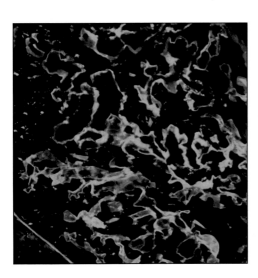
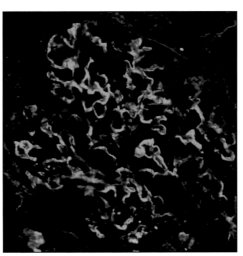

(Left) IgG is present diffusely but finely along the GBM and focally in the mesangium in this case of immunotactoid glomerulopathy. Stains for IgA and IgM were negative, as well as anti-IgG4, the isotype most common in fibrillary glomerulonephritis. *(Right)* This C3 stain is of a case with immunotactoid glomerulopathy with segmental increase along the GBM. Immunotactoid cases are uniformly IgG(+) and C3(+), and the majority are C1q(+).

IMMUNOTACTOID GLOMERULOPATHY

Electron Microscopy

(Left) Electron microscopy shows numerous electron-dense deposits throughout the glomerular capillary walls and mesangial regions. There is extensive podocyte foot process effacement. (Courtesy J. Kowalewska, MD.)
(Right) Electron microscopy shows prominent thickening of the glomerular capillary walls due to the presence of microtubular deposits ➡ that are randomly arranged and occasionally in parallel arrays. (Courtesy J. Kowalewska, MD.)

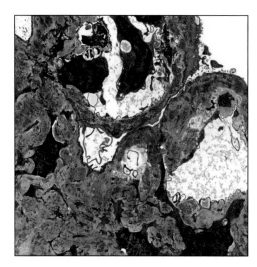
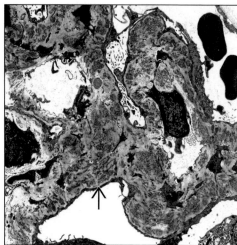

(Left) Large mesangial and subendothelial deposits ➡ are present with a substructure barely appreciable at this power (4,500x). Foot processes are extensively effaced. (Right) Electron microscopy shows numerous deposits ➡ without the usual parallel organization, but the characteristic hollow cores ➡ of the microtubules of ITG are present. The nature of the background amorphous material is unknown.

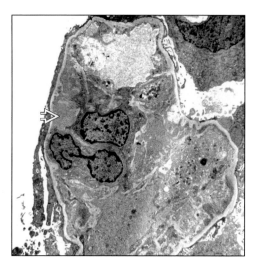
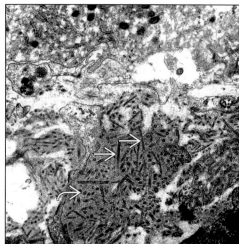

(Left) High-power electron micrograph shows immunotactoid tubules that are approximately 30 nm in diameter. (Right) Electron microscopy in this case of immunotactoid glomerulopathy shows electron-dense deposits consisting of characteristic microtubules ➡. The measurements of the microtubules are shown, which in this case range from 30-55 nm in diameter. Overall, the diameters in different cases range from ~ 30-90 nm, with the average being approximately 38 nm.

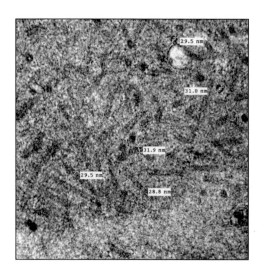
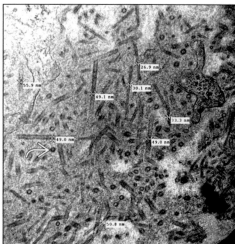

Electron Microscopy

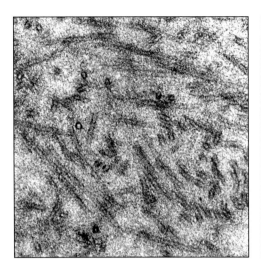

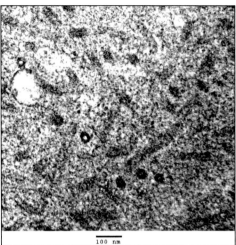

100 nm

(Left) The microtubules of ITG have a less dense core, best appreciated in the circular cross sections. (Courtesy J. Kowalewska, MD.) (Right) The 100 nm scale bar shows that the microtubules measure around 40 nm in diameter. Fibril diameter should be measured to help distinguish immunotactoid glomerulopathy (30-90 nm) from amyloidosis (8-12 nm), fibrillary glomerulonephritis (10-25 nm), and cryoglobulinemia (~ 20-35 nm).

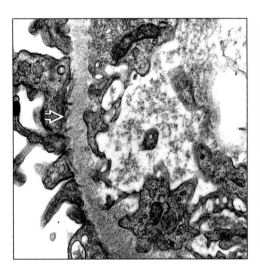

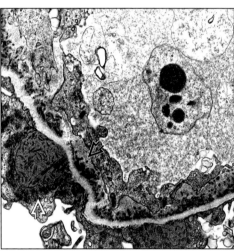

(Left) EM shows subtle deposition of tubular deposits underneath the otherwise normal podocytes ➤, which might be overlooked. The size & placement of the tubules suggest they are formed within the basement membrane by polymerization or aggregation of smaller, more soluble subcomponents. (Right) EM of ITG shows prominent subendothelial deposits ➤ and a subepithelial "hump" ➤. The endothelium is reactive with loss of fenestrations.

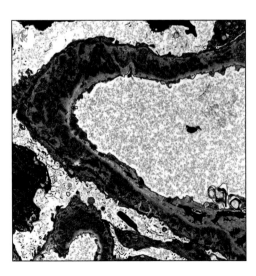

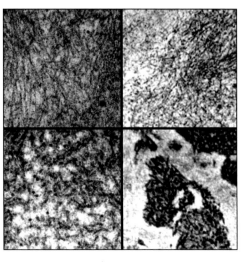

(Left) Electron microscopy illustrates an advanced case of ITG with marked thickening of the GBM containing numerous microtubular deposits in subepithelial and intramembranous locations. (Courtesy J. Kowalewska, MD.) (Right) Composite electron micrographs were printed at the same magnification to compare the appearance of amyloid fibrils (upper left), fibrillary glomerulonephritis (upper right), mixed cryoglobulinemia (lower left), and ITG (lower right).

FIBRONECTIN GLOMERULOPATHY

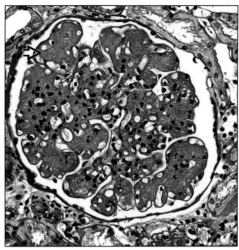

Renal biopsy in a patient with fibronectin glomerulopathy shows PAS-positive material ⊳ expanding the mesangium and subendothelium of an enlarged glomerulus.

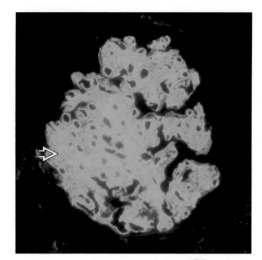

Intense immunofluorescence staining ⊳ is seen in glomerular deposits with antisera to fibronectin, consistent with FN glomerulopathy. Staining for immunoglobulins and complement is negative.

TERMINOLOGY

Abbreviations
- Fibronectin (FN) glomerulopathy

Definitions
- Nonimmune lobular glomerulopathy with massive mesangial and subendothelial deposits composed of fibronectin

ETIOLOGY/PATHOGENESIS

Autosomal Dominant Inheritance
- Mutations in fibronectin *FN1* gene documented recently in some patients
  - *FN1* gene mapped to region in chromosome 2q34
  - Abnormal FN may affect function of glomerular endothelial cells and podocytes
- No role of villin, desmin, or uteroglobin genes

Glomerular Fibronectin Deposition
- FN is an extracellular matrix glycoprotein involved in cellular adhesion, migration, and cytoskeleton maintenance
- Deposition of plasma FN rather than local synthesis by mesangial cells
- Plasma FN levels are not elevated
- Possible role of defective FN degradation by metalloproteinases

CLINICAL ISSUES

Epidemiology
- Age
  - Age at presentation ranges from 14-64 years

Presentation
- Proteinuria, may be in nephrotic range
- Microhematuria

- Hypertension
- Renal insufficiency
- History of affected 1st-degree relatives

Treatment
- No specific treatment

Prognosis
- Progression of renal insufficiency variable
- Some patients progress slowly to end-stage kidney
- Can recur in transplanted kidney

MICROSCOPIC PATHOLOGY

Histologic Features
- Glomeruli are diffusely enlarged with lobular accentuation and minimal hypercellularity
- Severe mesangial and variable subendothelial expansion by deposits
- Deposits stain intensely with periodic acid-Schiff and red with trichrome but fail to stain with methenamine silver or Congo red
- No disease-specific changes in tubulointerstitium or vascular structures

ANCILLARY TESTS

Immunohistochemistry
- FN immunostain is positive within deposits

Immunofluorescence
- Immunoglobulin and complement immunoreactivity is usually negative, but a few cases have weak staining
- Antisera to FN highlight mesangial and subendothelial deposits

Electron Microscopy
- Massive electron-dense deposits replacing mesangium and in subendothelial spaces

FIBRONECTIN GLOMERULOPATHY

Key Facts

Terminology
- Nonimmune lobular glomerulopathy with massive mesangial and subendothelial fibronectin deposits

Etiology/Pathogenesis
- Autosomal dominant inheritance
- Mutations in fibronectin *FN1* gene documented recently in some patients

Microscopic Pathology
- Glomeruli are diffusely enlarged with lobular accentuation and minimal hypercellularity
- Deposits stain with PAS and trichrome but not with methenamine silver or Congo red

Ancillary Tests
- Deposits stain for fibronectin but not for immunoglobulins, C3, or C1q
- Fibrillar and granular deposits by EM

- Mostly amorphous deposits with focal filamentous structures measuring 9-16 nm in diameter
- Glomerular basement membranes are uninvolved

DIFFERENTIAL DIAGNOSIS

Immune Complex-mediated Glomerulonephritis
- Characteristic immunofluorescence staining for immunoglobulins and complement as in IgA nephropathy, lupus nephritis
- Intense staining for FN is not identified

Amyloidosis
- Congo red stain positive
- Immunoglobulin light or heavy chain restriction on immunofluorescence or amyloid A staining based on subtype
- Ultrastructural features characteristic of randomly oriented fibrils that are 8-12 nm thick

Fibrillary Glomerulopathy
- Immunoglobulin and complement deposition seen on immunofluorescence microscopy
- Ultrastructural features of nonbranching fibrils, 10-30 nm thick in mesangium, lamina densa, and, occasionally, in subepithelial spaces

Monoclonal Immunoglobulin Deposition Disease
- Immunofluorescence microscopy shows immunoglobulin light or heavy chain restriction
- Granular electron-dense deposits in lamina rara interna in addition to mesangium

SELECTED REFERENCES

1. Herrera GA et al: Renal diseases with organized deposits: an algorithmic approach to classification and clinicopathologic diagnosis. Arch Pathol Lab Med. 134(4):512-31, 2010
2. Yong JL et al: Fibronectin non-amyloid glomerulopathy. Int J Clin Exp Pathol. 3(2):210-6, 2009
3. Castelletti F et al: Mutations in FN1 cause glomerulopathy with fibronectin deposits. Proc Natl Acad Sci U S A. 105(7):2538-43, 2008
4. Niimi K et al: Fibronectin glomerulopathy with nephrotic syndrome in a 3-year-old male. Pediatr Nephrol. 17(5):363-6, 2002
5. Gibson IW et al: Glomerular pathology: recent advances. J Pathol. 184(2):123-9, 1998
6. Gemperle O et al: Familial glomerulopathy with giant fibrillar (fibronectin-positive) deposits: 15-year follow-up in a large kindred. Am J Kidney Dis. 28(5):668-75, 1996
7. Hildebrandt F et al: Glomerulopathy associated with predominant fibronectin deposits: exclusion of the genes for fibronectin, villin and desmin as causative genes. Am J Med Genet. 63(1):323-7, 1996

IMAGE GALLERY

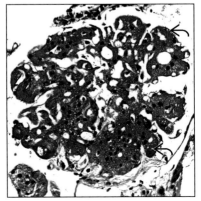 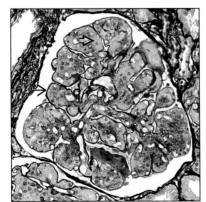 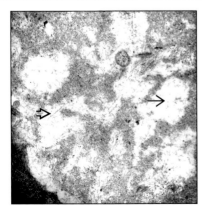

(Left) Fibronectin deposits ➡ in the mesangium and subendothelium stain red with trichrome stain. *(Center)* Fibronectin deposits ➡ in the glomerulus fail to stain with methenamine silver stain, but the glomerular basement membrane ➡ at the periphery is highlighted. *(Right)* On ultrastructural examination, fibronectin deposits in the mesangium are mostly granular with focal fibrillar structures ➡. Scattered electron-lucent areas ➡ are also seen.

DIABETIC NEPHROPATHY

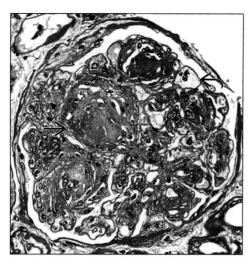

Prominent Kimmelstiel-Wilson nodules ⇒ are seen in a glomerulus affected by diabetic nephropathy. The glomerular capillary lumens are obliterated, and an occasional foam cell ⊇ is seen.

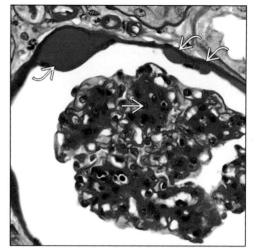

Deposits of hyaline material are present under the parietal epithelium of Bowman capsule, forming "capsular drops" ⊇ characteristic of diabetic nephropathy. Diffuse mesangial sclerosis is present ⇒.

TERMINOLOGY

Abbreviations
- Diabetic nephropathy (DN)

Synonyms
- Diabetic glomerulosclerosis

Definitions
- Renal disease caused by diabetes mellitus (DM) types 1 and 2, including thickening of GBM, expansion of mesangium, nodular diabetic glomerulosclerosis, arteriolar hyalinosis, and arteriosclerosis

ETIOLOGY/PATHOGENESIS

Diabetes Mellitus
- Type 1 DM: Autoimmune disease that destroys pancreatic islets
- Type 2 DM: Insulin resistance, related to obesity and other factors
- Both lead to insulin deficiency and hyperglycemia
- DN is a multifactorial process, but inadequate glycemic control is most important contributor
  - Both initiation and maintenance of DN require hyperglycemia
  - Removal of hyperglycemic state as in successful pancreas transplantation can cause regression of DN lesions

Hyperglycemia
- Causes accumulation of advanced glycosylated end products (AGE) due to nonenzymatic glycosylation of proteins
  - Many proteins affected including GBM collagen and other matrix proteins
  - AGE result in injury and remodeling
    - Promote protein crosslinking

- Stimulate synthesis of growth factors (TGF-β, IGF, VEGF) that cause increased extracellular matrix production
    - Binding of AGE to cell surface receptors (RAGE) increases intracellular oxidative stress
    - Podocytopenia via apoptosis
- Activates protein kinase C
  - Directly and via stimulation of aldol reductase, leading to increased sorbitol production, fructose, and diacylglycerol
  - Increases matrix production
- Induces defects in mitochondrial electron transport
  - Elevated nitric oxide and superoxide production results in vasodilatation and oxidation
  - Increased reactive oxygen species and oxidative stress

Genetic Factors
- Inherited factors may explain variable risk of developing DN regardless of glycemic control
  - Studies of siblings show high concordance rate of DN risk in both types 1 and 2 DM
  - Multiple genetic loci and gene polymorphisms have been implicated
    - Renin-angiotensin system, angiotensin-converting enzyme, angiotensinogen, angiotensin II type 1 receptor
    - Insulin resistance (ENPP1, PPARG2, glucose transporter 1, apolipoprotein E)
    - Superoxide dismutase 1 gene, CCR5, CNDP1 genes

Cardiovascular Factors
- Glomerular hyperfiltration observed in early DM promotes extracellular matrix accumulation and increased TGF-β1 expression
  - Loss of autoregulation in DM may predispose to hyperfiltration
  - Increased glomerular capillary pressure causes glomerulomegaly
  - Modulates progression of DN

DIABETIC NEPHROPATHY

Key Facts

Etiology/Pathogenesis

- Inadequate glycemic control is most important contributor to DN
- Hyperglycemia leads to advanced glycosylated end products (AGE), which are believed responsible for many DN features
- Glomerular hyperfiltration promotes extracellular matrix accumulation and increased TGF-β1 expression
- Multiple genetic loci and gene polymorphisms are implicated in DN susceptibility

Clinical Issues

- African-Americans and Native-Americans with type 2 DM are at higher risk of developing DN
- Microalbuminuria is earliest sign of DN and predicts loss of renal function

Microscopic Pathology

- Earliest change is diffusely thickened but otherwise normal GBM
- Mesangial hypercellularity and increased matrix
- Mesangial sclerosis becomes nodular (Kimmelstiel-Wilson nodules)
- Mesangiolysis contributes to microaneurysms
- Hyaline insudation in glomeruli (fibrin cap, capsular drops) and afferent and efferent arterioles
- Linear IgG in GBM
- Commonly complicated by other renal diseases in patients selected for biopsy

Top Differential Diagnoses

- Monoclonal immunoglobulin deposition disease, MPGN, idiopathic nodular glomerulosclerosis

---

- Systemic hypertension may aggravate progression of DN via angiotensin II
  - Angiotensin II increases glomerular capillary permeability via preferential constriction of efferent glomerular arteriole
  - Angiotensin II stimulates extracellular matrix proteins via TGF-β1 and increases AGE production
- Endothelial dysfunction
  - Probably due to oxidative and endoplasmic reticulum stress

Podocytopenia

- Causes include oxidative stress, AGE, fatty acids, peroxisome proliferator-activated receptors (PPARγ)
- Detected by WT-1 immunostain
- Correlates with proteinuria

Other Risk Factors

- Smoking, hyperlipidemia, obesity, and low vitamin D levels

Murine Models of DN

- Generally do not reproduce nodular glomerulosclerosis of human DN
- Type 1 DM: Islet cell destruction
  - Streptozotocin-induced diabetes (chemical)
  - NOD mouse (autoimmune)
- Type 2 DM: Insulin resistance
  - *db/db* mouse-leptin receptor deficient
  - BTBR-*ob/ob* mouse
    - Leptin deficient + other genetic predisposition
    - Full spectrum of pathology, including nodular DN

CLINICAL ISSUES

Epidemiology

- Incidence
  - 0.5% type 1, 5% type 2 DM in USA
  - Most common cause of end-stage renal disease (ESRD) in USA
  - Prevalence of DN increases with duration of DM

- ~ 15% of patients with type 1 DM develop DN after 20 years
- Prevalence is trending lower with improved treatment
- Ethnicity
  - Higher risk of DN in African Americans and Native Americans with type 2 DM

Presentation

- Microalbuminuria is earliest manifestation of DN
  - Defined as proteinuria of 30-300 mg/d (or μg/mg creatinine)
    - Not detected by standard urine dipstick method
  - Typically occurs ≥ 5 years after onset of DM
  - Predicts loss of renal function and is associated with progression to ESRD
- Proteinuria
  - Urine protein > 300 mg/d is detected by urine dipstick analysis
  - Indicates overt nephropathy that develops 20 years after onset of clinical DM although it may be much earlier in type 2 DM
  - Nephrotic-range proteinuria and nephrotic syndrome can develop
- Reduced renal function
  - Independent phenotype of early DN found in ~ 33% regardless of microalbuminuria
- Increased glomerular filtration rate (GFR)
  - Indicator of hyperfiltration and progressive DN
- Hypertension
- Retinopathy
  - Correlates with advanced DN
  - May be missed without fluorescein angiography
- Acute pyelonephritis and papillary necrosis may complicate DN
- Microhematuria
  - Associated with papillary necrosis or nephrocalcinosis

Laboratory Tests

- Hemoglobin A1C levels indicate long-term glycemic control

DIABETIC NEPHROPATHY

- Cystatin C to monitor early renal function decline

Treatment
- Drugs
  - Strict glycemic control
    - Oral hypoglycemic agents and insulin therapy
  - Renin-angiotensin system blockade
    - Direct renoprotective effects in DN
    - Angiotensin-converting enzyme inhibitors and angiotensin II receptor blockers
  - Treatment of hypertension and hyperlipidemia
- Weight loss if obese

Prognosis
- Rate of progression is variable and is modulated by complex genetic and environmental factors, therapeutic interventions
- DN is associated with hypertension and increased cardiovascular disease
- DN can recur in a transplanted kidney due to persistent hyperglycemic state

MACROSCOPIC FEATURES

General Features
- Kidneys are bilaterally enlarged
  - End-stage kidneys may be normal or slightly small
- Cortical scars may be present due to hypertensive renal disease or pyelonephritis
  - Loss of pyramids indicates papillary necrosis

MICROSCOPIC PATHOLOGY

Histologic Features
- Morphological changes in DN due to types 1 and 2 DN are similar
- Glomeruli
  - Earliest change is diffuse GBM thickening
    - Present even in absence of proteinuria
    - Detectable at light microscopy level only when ≥ 4x
  - Glomerulomegaly
    - Diameter > 50% of 400x field is a useful guide (220 µm)
  - Mesangial expansion and sclerosis
    - Diffuse mesangial hypercellularity in early phase
    - Accumulation of type IV and VI collagen, laminin, and fibronectin
  - Kimmelstiel-Wilson (KW) nodules
    - Round to oval mesangial lesions with acellular, matrix core with peripheral sparse crescent-shaped mesangial nuclei
    - Matrix may be less dense, especially at periphery of these nodules, and is termed "mesangiolysis"
    - Stains positive for periodic acid-Schiff (PAS) and Jones methenamine silver (JMS) stains, negative with Congo red
    - Often 1 or 2 per glomerular cross section and irregularly distributed
    - Progressive mesangial sclerosis results in obliterated capillary lumens

- Described in autopsies by Paul Kimmelstiel and Clifford Wilson in 1936 who noted that all 7 patients had a clinical history of DM
- Lesions seen in non-DM are related to hypertension and smoking
  - Microaneurysms
    - Mesangiolysis contributes to capillary lumen confluence and microaneurysms
    - Fragmented red cells are seen occasionally
    - Thrombi are rare
  - Hyaline insudation in glomerular capillary walls (fibrin cap)
  - Capsular drop observed between parietal epithelium and Bowman capsule
    - Probably represents tracking of plasma proteins from vascular pole to Bowman capsule
    - Reported in ~ 5% of biopsies from non-DM
  - Segmental glomerulosclerosis
    - Likely initiated by podocyte damage and exposed GBM
    - Capillary tuft adhesions to Bowman capsules
    - Lesions ("tip lesions") at tubular pole result in atubular glomeruli
  - Global glomerulosclerosis increases progressive DN
    - Sclerosed glomeruli are enlarged with abundant hyaline insudation
  - No inflammatory change (neutrophils, necrosis)
  - Rarely, crescents have been described
    - May be unusual response to heavy proteinuria
- Tubules
  - Prominent protein resorption and lipid droplets seen in proximal tubules in setting of severe proteinuria
  - Tubular atrophy and interstitial fibrosis progressively increase in advanced DN
  - Tubular basement membranes (TBM) are thickened due to excessive collagen deposition
    - Both atrophic and nonatrophic tubules demonstrate TBM thickening
  - In acute diabetic ketoacidosis, proximal tubules contain abundant clear vacuoles of glycogen
    - Armanni-Epstein lesion
- Interstitium
  - Interstitial inflammation is variable with lymphocytes, occasional eosinophils and neutrophils
    - Occasional interstitial neutrophils may not necessarily represent acute pyelonephritis
  - Prominent interstitial neutrophil infiltrates or neutrophil casts suggest acute pyelonephritis
- Arteries
  - Larger arteries, including proximal interlobular and arcuate arteries, show intimal fibrosis
  - Atherosclerosis with lipid deposits in smaller arteries typical of severe DN
- Arterioles
  - Arteriolar hyalinosis
    - Hyaline (plasma protein) insudation in terminal interlobular arteries and arterioles
    - Present in intima and media or can be transmural
    - Arteriolar hyaline causes luminal occlusion with ischemic collapse and sclerosis of downstream glomeruli

DIABETIC NEPHROPATHY

o Both afferent and efferent arterioles are affected
- Efferent arteriolar hyalinosis strongly favors DN but is not pathognomonic
- Afferent arterioles are thicker walled and more perpendicular to tuft
- Efferent arterioles typically are thinner walled and curve around tuft
o Nodular DN is rarely, if ever, observed in absence of prominent arteriolar hyalinosis

ANCILLARY TESTS

Immunofluorescence
- Diffuse linear staining (≥ 2+ intensity) of GBM and TBM for IgG and albumin
  o Due to nonimmunological trapping of proteins in thickened, abnormal basement membranes
  o No specific deposition of light chains in contrast to monoclonal immunoglobulin deposition disease
- Segmental scars and insudative lesions in glomeruli/arterioles show nonspecific entrapment of IgM and C3
- No specific immune complexes are observed unless superimposed glomerulonephritis is present
- Protein reabsorption droplets in tubules stain for albumin and other plasma proteins

Electron Microscopy
- Diffuse thickening of otherwise normal-appearing GBM lamina densa
  o Segmental thinning may be observed near site of microaneurysms
  o Typically > 600 nm
- Increased deposition of mesangial matrix
  o Fine fibrillar quality (fibrillosis; 10 nm thick) typical of collagen
  o Lucent foci may be identified at periphery of mesangial sclerosis (mesangiolysis)
  o Nodules contain cellular debris but no amorphous deposits suggestive of immune complexes
- Foot process effacement is variable
  o Typically less extensive than in other causes of severe proteinuria such as minimal change disease
- Lucent foci may be identified at periphery of mesangial sclerosis, compatible with mesangiolysis
- Insudative lesions in glomeruli and arterioles are electron dense and admixed with lucent areas and basement membrane-like particles
- TBM is thickened and laminated

Immunohistochemistry
- WT1 immunostain used to document podocytopenia

DIFFERENTIAL DIAGNOSIS

Monoclonal Immunoglobulin Deposition Disease (MIDD)
- Diffuse deposits of either kappa or lambda and, in rare cases, heavy chains on IF
- Ultrastructural examination reveals fine granular dense deposits in mesangium, GBM, and TBM

- Monoclonal protein sometimes detected in serum &/or urine
- Mesangial nodules in MIDD are often uniform in size and have less matrix on JMS stain

Membranoproliferative Glomerulonephritis (MPGN)
- Mesangial hypercellularity and duplicated basement membranes are prominent
  o GBM is not duplicated in uncomplicated DN
- Immunofluorescence and electron microscopy reveal immune complexes &/or C3 deposits
- Lobular accentuation in MPGN may resemble KW nodules

Amyloidosis
- Amyloid nodules are usually acellular, Congo red positive, weakly PAS positive, and Jones methenamine silver negative
- Immunofluorescence may demonstrate light chain restriction in primary amyloidosis or amyloid A deposits in AA amyloidosis
- Ultrastructurally, amyloid fibrils are randomly oriented, nonbranching, and measure 8-12 nm in diameter

Idiopathic Nodular Glomerulosclerosis
- Possible etiologies include prolonged subclinical type 2 DM, smoking, and hypertension
- Nodular glomerulosclerosis, mimicking DN, is seen in patient with no documented history of DM

Fibrillary and Immunotactoid Glomerulonephritis (GN)
- Rarely nodular, can have diffuse proliferative or membranoproliferative pattern
- Immunofluorescence shows deposition of polyclonal IgG and C3 in mesangium and capillary walls
- Electron microscopy shows randomly oriented fibrils (16-24 nm thick) in mesangium and GBM
- Immunotactoid glomerulopathy has thicker microtubular deposits (20-50 nm) that are monoclonal IgG with light chain restriction

Other Glomerular Diseases Superimposed on DN
- Approximately 33% of biopsies with DN have superimposed glomerular diseases
  o Membranous nephropathy
    - Thickened GBM and basement membrane "spikes"
    - Immunofluorescence reveals diffuse glomerular capillary wall deposits of IgG and C3
    - Subepithelial, electron-dense deposits on electron microscopy
  o IgA nephropathy
    - Mesangial proliferation can mimic early mesangial sclerosing DN
    - Immunofluorescence reveals dominant IgA deposits
    - Widespread, mesangial, electron-dense deposits
  o Postinfectious glomerulonephritis
    - Patient usually presents with nephritic syndrome and history of infection

2

- Diffuse endocapillary proliferative and exudative glomerulonephritis
- Immunofluorescence shows prominent granular GBM C3 and usually IgG deposits
- Mesangial deposits and subepithelial "humps" on ultrastructural examination
  - ANCA-mediated glomerulonephritis
    - Clinical presentation usually is rapidly progressive glomerulonephritis
    - Glomerular necrosis and crescents
    - No immune complexes or electron-dense deposits
  - Minimal change disease (MCD)
    - Abrupt onset of nephrotic syndrome favors MCD
    - No evidence of immune complexes or electron-dense deposits
    - Foot process effacement is diffuse in contrast to focal effacement usually seen in DN

DIAGNOSTIC CHECKLIST

Clinically Relevant Pathologic Features

- Severity of mesangial sclerosis, global glomerulosclerosis, and interstitial fibrosis correlates with progression of disease and reduced renal function
- Neutrophil casts and interstitial neutrophils should prompt evaluation of urine cultures

Pathologic Interpretation Pearls

- Diagnosis of DN unlikely unless there is prominent arteriolar hyalinosis
- Mesangial KW nodules in DN are often variably sized and paucicellular
- Capsular drop is characteristic but not specific for DN
- Pronounced hyaline insudation in globally sclerosed glomeruli suggests DN
- Biopsies from diabetic patients often show other renal diseases
  - It is uncommon to biopsy patients with typical presentation of DN
- Linear IgG may mimic anti-GBM nephritis

REPORTING CRITERIA

Classification of DN (Tervaert 2010)

- Class I: Isolated GBM thickening
  - GBM > 395 nm thick in females or > 430 nm thick in males; age ≥ 9 years
- Class II: Mesangial expansion
  - Width of mesangial matrix exceeds 2 mesangial cell nuclei in > 25% of mesangial areas
  - IIa: Mild, < mean area of capillary lumen
  - IIb: Severe, > mean area of capillary lumen
- Class III: Nodular sclerosis (Kimmelstiel-Wilson lesion)
  - ≥ 1 convincing KW lesion
- Class IV: Advanced diabetic glomerulosclerosis
  - Global glomerulosclerosis in > 50% of glomeruli
  - Lesions from class I-III
- Classes cannot have lesions of higher class (e.g., class III cannot have > 50% global sclerosis)
- Severity of interstitial fibrosis and vascular lesions scored

- Overlaps to some extent with clinical classification and corresponds to clinical stage of DN

SELECTED REFERENCES

1. D'Agati V et al: RAGE, glomerulosclerosis and proteinuria: roles in podocytes and endothelial cells. Trends Endocrinol Metab. 21(1):50-6, 2010
2. Hudkins KL et al: BTBR Ob/Ob mutant mice model progressive diabetic nephropathy. J Am Soc Nephrol. 21(9):1533-42, 2010
3. Su J et al: Evaluation of podocyte lesion in patients with diabetic nephropathy: Wilms' tumor-1 protein used as a podocyte marker. Diabetes Res Clin Pract. 87(2):167-75, 2010
4. Tervaert TW et al: Pathologic classification of diabetic nephropathy. J Am Soc Nephrol. 21(4):556-63, 2010
5. Perkins BA et al: Early nephropathy in type 1 diabetes: the importance of early renal function decline. Curr Opin Nephrol Hypertens. 18(3):233-40, 2009
6. Stitt-Cavanagh E et al: The podocyte in diabetic kidney disease. ScientificWorldJournal. 9:1127-39, 2009
7. Forbes JM et al: Oxidative stress as a major culprit in kidney disease in diabetes. Diabetes. 57(6):1446-54, 2008
8. Jefferson JA et al: Proteinuria in diabetic kidney disease: a mechanistic viewpoint. Kidney Int. 74(1):22-36, 2008
9. Alsaad KO et al: Distinguishing diabetic nephropathy from other causes of glomerulosclerosis: an update. J Clin Pathol. 60(1):18-26, 2007
10. Toyoda M et al: Podocyte detachment and reduced glomerular capillary endothelial fenestration in human type 1 diabetic nephropathy. Diabetes. 56(8):2155-60, 2007
11. Fioretto P et al: Reversal of lesions of diabetic nephropathy after pancreas transplantation. N Engl J Med. 339(2):69-75, 1998
12. Ibrahim HN et al: Diabetic nephropathy. J Am Soc Nephrol. 8(3):487-93, 1997
13. Pagtalunan ME et al: Podocyte loss and progressive glomerular injury in type II diabetes. J Clin Invest. 99(2):342-8, 1997
14. Mauer SM: Structural-functional correlations of diabetic nephropathy. Kidney Int. 45(2):612-22, 1994
15. Fioretto P et al: An overview of renal pathology in insulin-dependent diabetes mellitus in relationship to altered glomerular hemodynamics. Am J Kidney Dis. 20(6):549-58, 1992
16. Ziyadeh FN et al: The renal tubulointerstitium in diabetes mellitus. Kidney Int. 39(3):464-75, 1991
17. Alpers CE et al: Idiopathic lobular glomerulonephritis (nodular mesangial sclerosis): a distinct diagnostic entity. Clin Nephrol. 32(2):68-74, 1989
18. Monga G et al: Pattern of double glomerulopathies: a clinicopathologic study of superimposed glomerulonephritis on diabetic glomerulosclerosis. Mod Pathol. 2(4):407-14, 1989
19. Mogensen CE: Microalbuminuria predicts clinical proteinuria and early mortality in maturity-onset diabetes. N Engl J Med. 310(6):356-60, 1984
20. Kimmelstiel P et al: Intercapillary lesions in the glomeruli of the kidney. Am J Pathol. 12(1):83-98, 1936

DIABETIC NEPHROPATHY

Microscopic Features

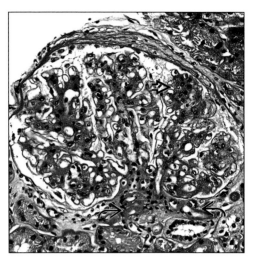

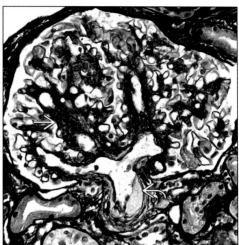

(Left) The glomerulus is enlarged with diffuse mesangial sclerosis and moderate proliferation ➡. Mild arteriolar hyaline insudation is seen, a feature characteristic of DN. It is likely in both afferent and efferent limbs ➡. (Right) Moderate mesangial sclerosis ➡ is highlighted by Jones methenamine silver stain. Also, the glomerular basement membranes are diffusely thickened, and arteriolar hyaline ➡ is seen at the vascular pole in a renal biopsy with DN.

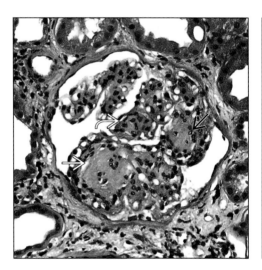

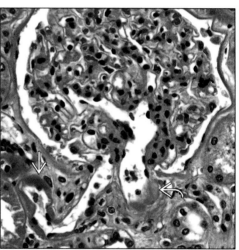

(Left) Classic Kimmelstiel-Wilson (KW) nodules ➡ in a biopsy from a patient with longstanding DM show a paucicellular center with peripheral elongated mesangial nuclei ➡ and a ring of capillaries. Foci of mesangial hypercellularity ➡ likely represent precursor lesions. (Right) Afferent ➡ and efferent ➡ arterioles show hyaline deposits characteristic of, but not absolutely specific for, DN. Efferent arterioles are thinner and typically curve around the glomerulus.

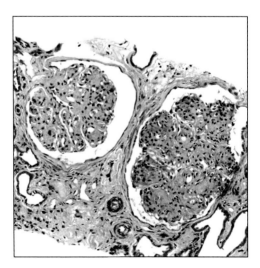

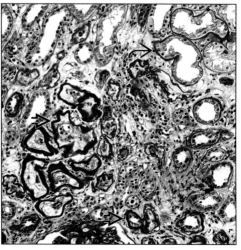

(Left) Mesangial nodules in DN stain for collagen on trichrome stain. In this 58-year-old woman with nephrotic syndrome, many KW nodules are present, resembling membranoproliferative glomerulonephritis. However, duplication of the GBM was not present. (Right) Excessive deposition of extracellular matrix results in thickened tubular basement membranes in both atrophic ➡ and nonatrophic ➡ tubules. Mild interstitial inflammation is also seen (PAS stain).

DIABETIC NEPHROPATHY

Microscopic Features

(Left) A large KW nodule ⮕ *in a glomerulus, along with diffuse mesangial sclerosis, is typical of advanced DN. Arteriolar hyalinosis* ➡ *is seen at the vascular pole, and synechia at the tubular pole* ➡ *probably results in an atubular glomerulus.* *(Right) Advanced DN is characterized by diffuse and nodular* ⮕ *glomerulosclerosis and thickened glomerular and tubular basement membranes. Mesangiolysis at the periphery of a KW nodule* ➡ *and segmental adhesion to Bowman capsule are also seen* ➡*.*

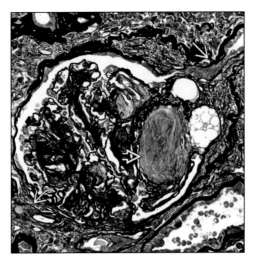 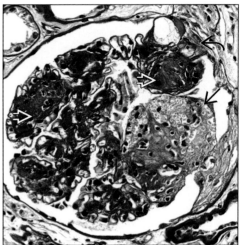

(Left) Mesangiolysis ⮕ *with entrapped red blood cells is seen at the periphery of a KW nodule in DN. This degradation of mesangial matrix results in microaneurysms. A foam cell is seen in the adjacent capillary lumen* ➡*. (Right) Capillaries form a microaneurysm* ➡ *capping one of the mesangial nodules* ➡*. It is possible that thrombosis and organization of the microaneurysm is responsible for the nodule. Alternatively, the nodular lesion predisposes to the microaneurysm.*

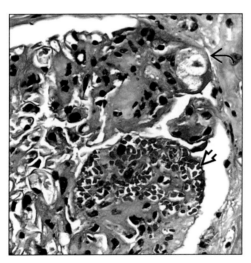 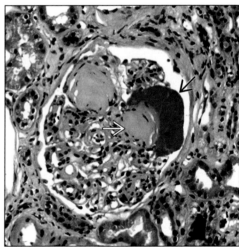

(Left) The nodules are becoming acellular, with loss of podocytes and endothelial and mesangial cells. Vague laminations are evident in the nodules, suggesting recurrent episodes of injury and organization ➡*. (Right) Abundant hyaline insudation* ➡ *is quite characteristic of DN and is often seen even in globally sclerosed glomeruli. Nodular mesangial sclerosis* ➡ *is also evident in this glomerulus affected by DN.*

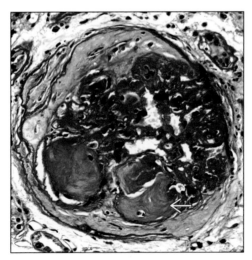 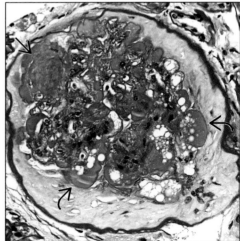

DIABETIC NEPHROPATHY

Immunofluorescence and Electron Microscopy

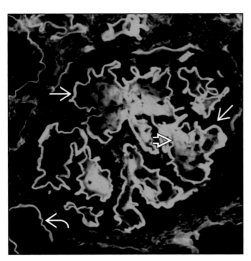

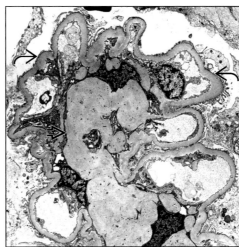

(Left) Diffuse linear IgG staining is seen along the GBM ➡ and TBM ➡ in diabetic nephropathy due to nonimmunological trapping of immunoglobulin in the altered basement membranes and should not be confused with anti-GBM nephritis. Nodules ⇥ can also be seen. *(Right)* The mesangium ⇥ is normocellular but expanded by increased mesangial matrix deposition. The glomerular basement membranes ➡ are also diffusely thickened (> 700 nm) in DN.

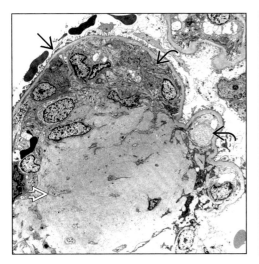

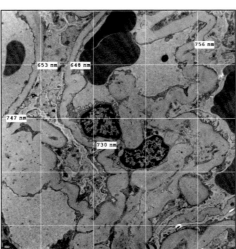

(Left) Nodular mesangial expansion is characteristic ⇥ of DN. The capillary lumens ➡ are obliterated by mesangial KW nodules and circulating inflammatory cells. The podocyte foot processes are extensively effaced ➡, indicative of severe proteinuria. *(Right)* Marked thickening of GBM and widespread foot process effacement are evident in a biopsy from a 52-year-old man with DM, 9 g/d proteinuria, and Cr 2.6 mg/dL. The effacement of foot processes is usually less extensive in DN.

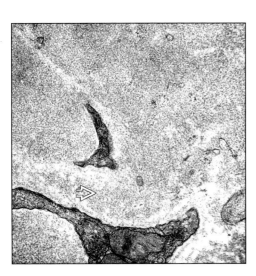

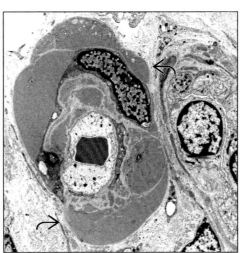

(Left) On higher magnification within the mesangium, accentuated mesangial matrix fibers ⇥ can be seen in some "diabetic fibrillosis" cases. These fibers measure approximately 10 nm in diameter and are not composed of immunoglobulin or amyloid. *(Right)* Arteriolar hyalinosis ➡ in DN is characterized by plasma protein insudation in the media and adventitia. If correctly identified, involvement of the efferent arteriole is considered specific for DN.

Classification of Diabetic Glomerulosclerosis

(Left) Class I: Normal mesangium is seen in a 23-year-old man with type 1 DM for 17 years. Arterioles ⮵ are normal, but GBM is thickened on electron microscopy. The patient had microalbuminuria, serum Cr 2.4 mg/dL, and no evidence of retinopathy. (Right) Class I: Thickened GBMs by electron microscopy measure 350-750 nm, averaging ~ 500 nm (upper limit of normal GBM is 430 nm in males and 395 nm in females). The podocytes are normal in this 23-year-old man with type 1 DM for 17 years.

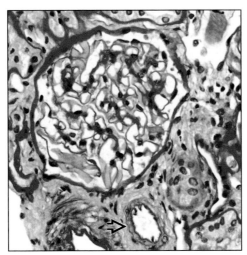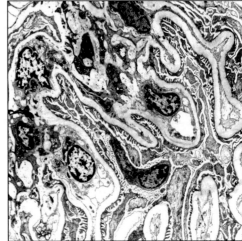

(Left) Class IIa: Mild mesangial sclerosis is seen in which the width of the mesangium is < the average diameter of the glomerular capillaries. The distinction between IIa and IIb is likely to be poorly reproducible among different observers. Class II requires that no nodules are present and < 50% of glomeruli are globally sclerotic. (Right) Class IIb: Severe mesangial sclerosis is seen in which the width of the mesangium is > the average diameter of the glomerular capillaries (PAS stain).

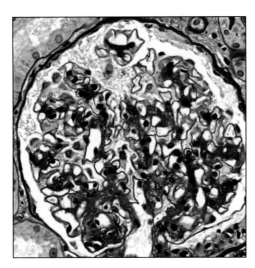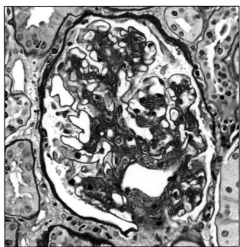

(Left) Class III nodular diabetic glomerulosclerosis (Kimmelstiel-Wilson lesion): Two mesangial nodules ⮵ are present containing peripherally disposed mesangial cells surrounded by a necklace of capillary loops. Class III may not have > 50% global glomerulosclerosis (which would be class IV). (Right) Class IV: Advanced diabetic glomerulosclerosis with > 50% of globally sclerotic glomeruli is seen in this 53-year-old man with type 2 DM for 15 years (PAS stain).

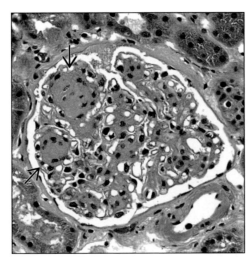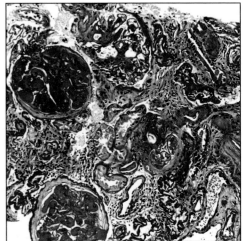

DIABETIC NEPHROPATHY

Superimposed Diseases on DN

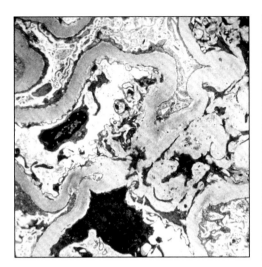 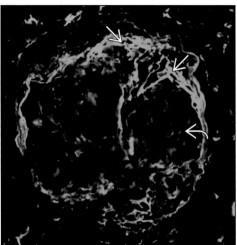

(Left) EM shows minimal change disease in a 51-year-old man with DM who was stung by a swarm of hornets and developed hemolytic anemia and nephrotic syndrome over 2 weeks. The GBM is diffusely thickened, and the podocytes show widespread effacement, the latter more extensive than in the usual DN. *(Right)* Fibrin ➡ stains the crescents around the KW nodules ➡ in a 69-year-old with DM & c-ANCA positivity. She has pauci-immune glomerulonephritis superimposed on DN.

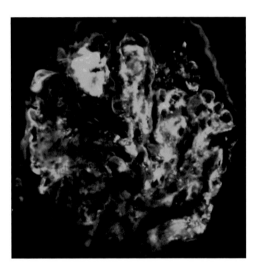 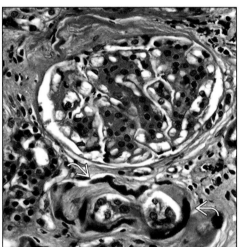

(Left) IgA nephropathy superimposed on nodular DN is seen with granular mesangial IgA deposits. Patient had a longstanding history of microhematuria, an uncommon finding in uncomplicated DN. *(Right)* Class IIb DN with superimposed nephrocalcinosis is seen, manifested by basophilic TBM deposits of calcium phosphate ➡. Nephrocalcinosis may be due to the use of gadolinium scans, which can be associated with nephrogenic systemic fibrosis.

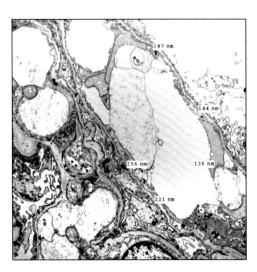 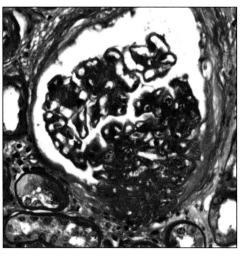

(Left) EM shows thin basement membrane disease (TBMD) in a 48-year-old woman with a 10-year history of type 2 DM, microhematuria, and mild proteinuria (400 mg/d) with Cr 0.7 mg/dL. Apparently, DM does not necessarily thicken the GBM in TBMD. *(Right)* Focal segmental glomerulosclerosis is a common finding in patients with DN. Common pathophysiological mechanisms include glomerular hypertension (hyperfiltration) and podocyte loss (PAS stain).

IDIOPATHIC NODULAR GLOMERULOPATHY

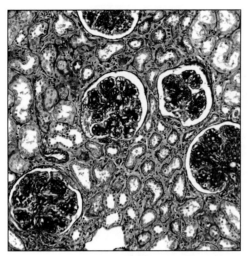

In ING, glomeruli have nodular mesangial expansion, hypertrophy, & hypercellularity incidentally found in a nephrectomy for tumor in a 63-year-old woman with no history of diabetes.

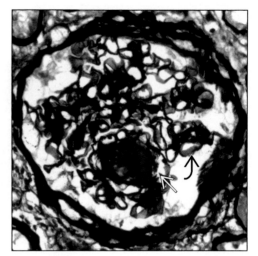

In a case of ING, there is a relatively acellular glomerular nodule ➡. Glomerular basement membranes ➔ are possibly only segmentally thickened with no duplication.

TERMINOLOGY

Abbreviations
- Idiopathic nodular glomerulopathy (ING)/ glomerulosclerosis (GS)

Synonyms
- Smoking-associated nodular GS
- Idiopathic lobular glomerulonephritis
- Nodular mesangial sclerosis

Definitions
- Nodular GS, associated with smoking &/or hypertension (HTN) without history of diabetes mellitus (DM)

ETIOLOGY/PATHOGENESIS

Environmental Exposure
- Smoking
  - Leads to microalbuminuria in healthy individuals
  - Risk factor for renal dysfunction
  - Advanced glycation end products (AGE) formation, oxidative stress, angiogenesis, & altered intrarenal hemodynamics
    - AGE alters extracellular matrix (ECM) by protein crosslinking and interaction with cell surface receptors such as receptor to AGE (RAGE)
    - Mediators include NF-κB, MAPK, JAK/STAT, Smad, TGF-β, IGF, VEGF, fibrogenic cytokines, PDGF, type IV collagen, laminin, heparan sulfate, & fibronectin
  - Chronic obstructive pulmonary disease (COPD)
    - Activates sympathetic & renin-angiotensin systems, leading to HTN & ECM production

Hypertension
- Smoking-induced renal injury probably more likely with preexisting sclerotic insult, such as hypertensive nephrosclerosis

- ING has been reported with only history of HTN in absence of smoking

CLINICAL ISSUES

Epidemiology
- Age
  - Elderly
- Gender
  - Male predominance a feature of most series
- Ethnicity
  - White predominance noted in larger series

Presentation
- Renal dysfunction (~ 80% of patients)
- Proteinuria, nephrotic range (~ 70% of patients)

Treatment
- Drugs
  - Angiotensin II blockade

Prognosis
- ESRD has been noted
  - 35.3% over 14.2-month period in 1 series

MICROSCOPIC PATHOLOGY

Histologic Features
- Glomeruli
  - Rounded/nodular acellular PAS(+) expansion of mesangium composed of lamellated matrix material
    - Nuclei often found at periphery of nodules
  - Minute endothelial-lined channels present in and around nodules
    - Capillaries compressed or collapsed
    - Increased capillary density compared with normal controls
  - Glomerulomegaly

IDIOPATHIC NODULAR GLOMERULOPATHY

Key Facts

Terminology
- Idiopathic nodular glomerulopathy (ING)/ glomerulosclerosis (GS)
- Nodular GS, associated with smoking &/or HTN without DM

Etiology/Pathogenesis
- Smoking leads to physiologic & molecular derangement (e.g., advanced glycation end product [AGE] production)

Clinical Issues
- Patients are typically elderly, male, & white
- Renal dysfunction
- Nephrotic-range proteinuria

Microscopic Pathology
- Rounded or nodular acellular PAS-positive areas

- Minute endothelial-lined channels
- Glomerulomegaly
- Moderate to severe arteriosclerosis and arteriolosclerosis with hyalinosis

Ancillary Tests
- No immune deposits by immunofluorescence or EM
- Segmental GBM thickening and mesangial matrix expansion by EM

Top Differential Diagnoses
- Diabetic glomerulosclerosis
- MPGN, lobular variant
- Monoclonal immunoglobulin deposition disease
- Thrombotic microangiopathy

- o Segmental glomerular basement membrane (GBM) thickening
- o Little or no GBM duplication
- Vessels
  - o Moderate to severe arteriosclerosis and arteriolar hyalinosis
- Tubules and interstitium
  - o Fibrosis and tubular atrophy common

ANCILLARY TESTS

Immunohistochemistry
- Endothelial markers (e.g., CD31/34) stain glomerular capillaries at periphery of nodules
- AGE demonstrable
  - o Common marker is fluorescent derivative of ribose, pentosidine
  - o Present in mesangial nodules and zones of interstitial fibrosis in ING and diabetic nephropathy

Immunofluorescence
- No immune deposits
- Linear IgG and albumin in GBM

Electron Microscopy
- Transmission
  - o No deposits
  - o GBM typically has moderate segmental thickening
  - o Mesangium segmentally expanded by increased matrix

DIFFERENTIAL DIAGNOSIS

Diabetic Glomerulosclerosis
- No certain way to distinguish except by history of DM
  - o GBM thickening more diffuse & dramatic in DM
  - o Vascular disease usually more severe in DM
  - o ING typically has more nodules in each glomerulus, and nodules are about the same size

Membranoproliferative Glomerulonephritis
- Lobular variant resembles ING

- May represent "healing" or progressive sclerosis of longstanding GN that previously had mesangial hypercellularity
- Immune-type deposits are usually found in MPGN (C3) but not ING

Monoclonal Immunoglobulin Deposition Disease (MIDD)
- Lobular pattern common
- Kappa/lambda light or heavy chain on IF & immune-type deposits on EM

Thrombotic Microangiopathy
- Nodules typically not prominent
- GBM not thickened but duplicated

SELECTED REFERENCES

1. Liang KV et al: Nodular glomerulosclerosis: renal lesions in chronic smokers mimic chronic thrombotic microangiopathy and hypertensive lesions. Am J Kidney Dis. 49(4):552-9, 2007
2. Nasr SH et al: Nodular glomerulosclerosis in the nondiabetic smoker. J Am Soc Nephrol. 18(7):2032-6, 2007
3. Zhou XJ et al: Membranoproliferative glomerulonephritis. In Jennette JC: Heptinstall's Pathology of the Kidney. 6th ed. Philadelphia: Lippincott, Williams & Wilkins, 2007
4. Kuppachi S et al: Idiopathic nodular glomerulosclerosis in a non-diabetic hypertensive smoker--case report and review of literature. Nephrol Dial Transplant. 21(12):3571-5, 2006
5. Markowitz GS et al: Idiopathic nodular glomerulosclerosis is a distinct clinicopathologic entity linked to hypertension and smoking. Hum Pathol. 33(8):826-35, 2002
6. Herzenberg AM et al: Idiopathic nodular glomerulosclerosis. Am J Kidney Dis. 34(3):560-4, 1999
7. Alpers CE et al: Idiopathic lobular glomerulonephritis (nodular mesangial sclerosis): a distinct diagnostic entity. Clin Nephrol. 32(2):68-74, 1989

IDIOPATHIC NODULAR GLOMERULOPATHY

Microscopic Features

(Left) In this case of ING, there is arteriolar hyalinosis ⮕, a feature also seen in diabetes and hypertension, but here there was no history of diabetes. Mesangial expansion ⮕ is also present, compatible with early glomerular nodule formation, and well-formed nodules were present in other glomeruli. In addition, there was proteinuria; proteinaceous casts ⮞ can be identified. *(Right)* This PAS stain in a case of ING shows a relatively acellular nodule ⮕ that stains PAS(+).

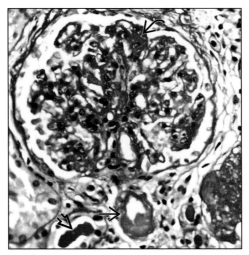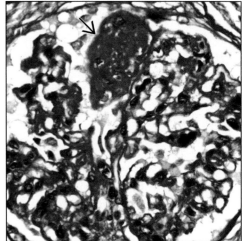

(Left) ING sometime shows features of thrombotic microangiopathy, as in this case with an apparent organizing occlusion of a glomerular capillary ⮕. This may be the origin of the mesangial nodules. *(Right)* This glomerulus from a patient with ING has hemorrhage and congestion in glomerular capillaries with loss of endothelial nuclei ⮕, suggestive of localized severe endothelial injury.

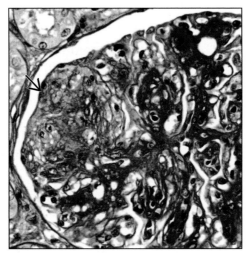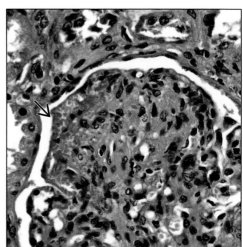

(Left) This glomerulus from a patient with ING shows segmental duplication of the GBM ⮕, a feature not common in diabetes, which is more typical of thrombotic microangiopathy. *(Right)* In this case of ING, trichrome staining reveals foci of arteriolar hyalinosis ⮕, a feature associated with diabetes and hypertension (and calcineurin inhibitor use in renal transplants); however, there was no diabetes history here.

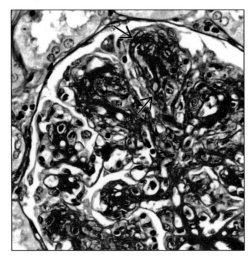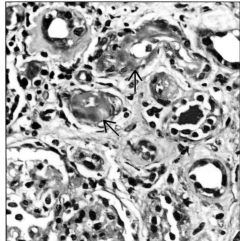

IDIOPATHIC NODULAR GLOMERULOPATHY

Immunohistochemistry and Electron Microscopy

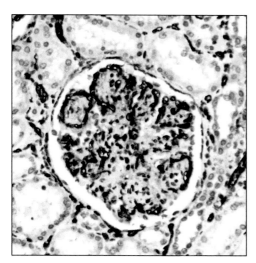

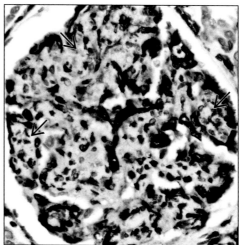

(Left) A ring of CD34 positive capillaries surround the mesangial nodules in ING, with an increase in the overall numbers of capillaries compared with normal glomeruli. *(Right)* CD31 immunohistochemistry stains the endothelium of increased numbers of small capillaries at the periphery of glomerular nodules ⇨ in a case of ING.

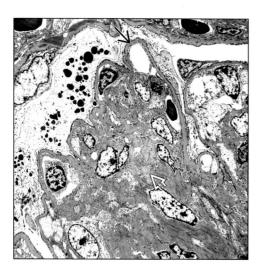

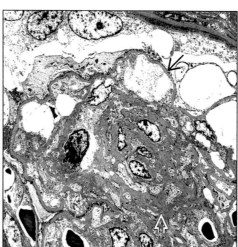

(Left) Electron microscopy shows glomerular basement membranes ⇨ with a relatively normal thickness and a mesangial nodule ⇨ at the center of the glomerular capillaries in a case of ING. *(Right)* Electron microscopy shows glomerular basement membranes ⇨ with a relatively normal thickness and a mesangial nodule ⇨ at the center of the glomerular capillaries in a case of ING.

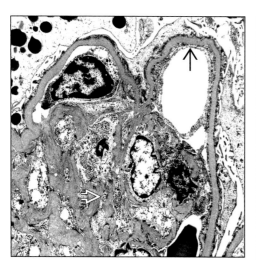

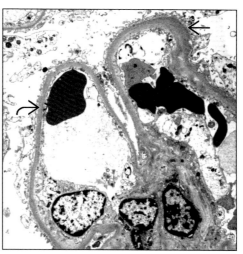

(Left) Electron microscopy shows glomerular basement membranes ⇨ with a relatively normal thickness and a mesangial nodule ⇨ at the center of the collection of glomerular capillaries in a case of ING. *(Right)* Segmental glomerular basement membrane thickening is present ⇨ in this case of ING; in general, however, the remainder of glomerular basement membranes ⇗ have a relatively normal thickness.

ALPORT SYNDROME

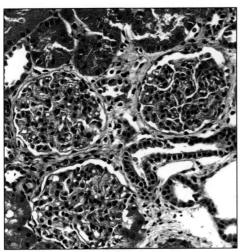

This kidney biopsy is from a 2-year-old boy who presented with proteinuria and a family history of X-linked Alport syndrome. The glomeruli show mild mesangial hypercellularity but are generally unremarkable.

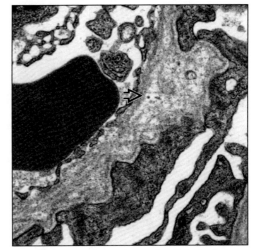

This GBM segment in a boy with X-linked AS shows classic splitting and multilamellation ("basket weaving"), diagnostic of AS. The GBM also contains microparticles ("bread crumbs") ⊵.

TERMINOLOGY

Abbreviations
- Alport syndrome (AS)

Synonyms
- Hereditary nephritis

Definitions
- Inherited glomerular disease secondary to mutations in the α3, α4, or α5 chains of type IV collagen, characterized by hematuria with hearing and eye abnormalities

ETIOLOGY/PATHOGENESIS

Genetics
- *COL4A5*
  - Encodes α5 type IV collagen chain
  - X-linked form
    - Maps to chromosome Xq26-48
  - 85% of patients
    - 10-15% are de novo mutations
    - Female carriers may show disease depending on degree of mosaicism following lyonization
  - Mutations in adjacent *COL4A6* gene result in diffuse leiomyomatosis
- *COL4A3*
  - Encodes α3 type IV collagen chain
  - Autosomal recessive inheritance
    - Maps to chromosome 2q35-37
  - Autosomal dominant inheritance has been described but is rare
  - Disease may result from compound heterozygous or homozygous mutations
- *COL4A4*
  - Encodes α4 type IV collagen chain
  - Autosomal recessive inheritance
    - Maps to chromosome 2q35-37

- Heterozygote phenotype in thin basement membrane disease
  - Autosomal dominant inheritance has been described but is rare
  - Disease may result from compound heterozygous or homozygous mutations
- Mutations of *COL4A3* and *COL4A4* account for 15% of AS patients

Pathogenesis
- Normal GBM and distal TBM composed primarily of α3α4α5 trimeric collagen IV molecules
  - Deficiency in any 1 of the 3 chains leads to failure of formation of trimer and lack of other 2 chains
  - Bowman capsule contains α5α5α6 trimers, so expression of α5 not dependent on α3 or α4
  - α1α1α2 collagen IV chains, minimally present in subendothelial side of normal GBM, increased in AS
- Mutations may result in protein misfolding, truncation, or absence of chain
  - Protein misfolding may lead to degradation of α3α4α5 type IV collagen
- Nature of mutation in X-linked form influences age of onset of ESRD
  - Earliest onset (mean: 25 years) with truncating mutation
  - Intermediate onset (mean: 28 years) with splice site mutations
  - Later onset (mean: 37 years) with missense mutations
  - Mutation at 5' end with earlier onset and more extrarenal manifestations

CLINICAL ISSUES

Epidemiology
- Incidence
  - 1:5,000-1:10,000 gene frequency in USA
  - Cause of 3% of ESRD in children

ALPORT SYNDROME

Key Facts

Etiology/Pathogenesis
- 85% X-linked inheritance of mutations in *COL4A5*
- 15% autosomal recessive *COL4A3, COL4A4*

Clinical Issues
- Presentation
  - Hematuria, proteinuria, sensorineural deafness, hypertension, eye abnormalities
- 90% of X-linked males and 12% of X-linked carrier females develop ESRD by age 40

Microscopic Pathology
- Early: Minimal glomerular changes, mesangial hypercellularity, interstitial foamy macrophages
- Late: Thick capillary loops, FSGS, global sclerosis, tubular atrophy, interstitial fibrosis
- Electron microscopy

- GBM multilamellation, microparticles, scalloping, and thin GBM
- Immunofluorescence: Decreased α3, α4, α5 (IV) collagen in GBM
  - X-linked male AS: Absent staining
  - X-linked female heterozygotes: Mosaic loss
  - Autosomal recessive: α5 (IV) present in BC

Ancillary Tests
- Skin biopsy
  - X-linked form has absent α5 (IV) collagen staining in men, mosaic in women

Diagnostic Checklist
- Lamination of GBM can also be seen in repair in other diseases

---

- Associated with 1-2% of ESRD in Western countries
- Age
  - X-linked males (hemizygotes)
    - Median: 33 years
  - X-linked female heterozygote carriers
    - Median: 37 years
  - Autosomal recessive
    - Median: 35 years
- Ethnicity
  - None specific

Presentation
- Hematuria
  - Males typically present with gross hematuria
  - Females typically present with microscopic hematuria
  - Tends to be persistent in males and intermittent in females
  - Exacerbated by exercise, infection
- Proteinuria, 1-2 g/d
  - Tends to develop later in disease course
  - Variable in X-linked AS
  - Common in autosomal recessive AS
    - Nephrotic syndrome in 30%
- Sensorineural deafness
  - 90% of X-linked hemizygotes by age 40
  - 10% of X-linked heterozygotes by age 40
  - 67% of AR homozygotes before age 20
- Hypertension
- Eye abnormalities
  - Anterior lenticonus in ~ 22% of patients < 25 years old
    - Pathognomonic of AS
    - Associated with rapid ESRD and hearing loss
  - Retinal flecks in ~ 37% of patients < 25 years old
- Leiomyomatosis (rare)
  - Mutations in *COL4A6* and *COL4A5*

Laboratory Tests
- Direct DNA sequencing or linkage analysis of *COL4A3/A4/A5*
- Sensitivity of linkage analysis reported to be ~ 60%

Treatment
- None available to reverse
- Transplantation for ESRD
  - Rarely, anti-GBM disease may develop post transplant

Prognosis
- X-linked males
  - 90% develop ESRD by age 40
- X-linked carrier females
  - 12% develop ESRD by age 40
  - 60% develop ESRD by age 60
- Autosomal recessive
  - Earlier and more rapid progression to ESRD
- Autosomal dominant
  - Slower progression to ESRD

MICROSCOPIC PATHOLOGY

Histologic Features
- Glomeruli
  - Early changes
    - Minimal changes
    - Mild mesangial hypercellularity
    - Small capillary diameter
    - Lamination of GBM hard to appreciate by light microscopy (LM)
  - Late changes
    - Focal segmental glomerulosclerosis (FSGS)
    - Global glomerulosclerosis
- Interstitium and tubules
  - Interstitial fibrosis and tubular atrophy
  - Interstitial foamy macrophages
- Vessels
  - Arteriosclerosis

ANCILLARY TESTS

Immunofluorescence
- No specific deposition of IgG, IgA, IgM, C3, C1q, kappa, or lambda

ALPORT SYNDROME

Collagen IV α1, α3, and α5 Staining Patterns

AS Variant	α1 (IV) Chain	α3 (IV) Chain	α5 (IV) Chain
Normal	GBM (±), BC, DT	GBM (+), DT (+)	GBM, BC, DT, CD
X-linked (male)	GBM (+), BC, DT	Absent GBM, DT	Absent GBM, DT, BC, EBM
X-linked heterozygote (female)	GBM (+), BC, DT	Decreased, mosaic GBM, DT	Decreased, mosaic GBM, DT, BC, EBM
Autosomal recessive	GBM (+), BC, DT	Absent or decreased GBM, DT	Absent GBM, DT, present BC only
Thin basement membrane disease	GBM (±), BC, DT	May be weaker than normal in GBM; normal in DT	May be weaker than normal in GBM; normal in BC, DT

GBM = glomerular basement membrane; BC = Bowman capsule; DT = distal tubule basement membrane; CD = collecting duct; EBM = epidermal basement membrane.

- Segmental IgM and C3 typical in FSGS lesions

Electron Microscopy
- Transmission
  - Multilamellation of the GBM lamina densa imparting a "basket weave" appearance
  - GBM microparticles or "bread crumbs" between laminations
  - Scalloping or "outpouching" of subepithelial surface of GBM
  - Irregular, variable GBM thickness, both thick and thin
  - Podocyte foot process effacement
  - Thin GBM measuring < 200 nm as only lesion
    - X-linked carrier females
    - Autosomal recessive carriers
    - Identical to thin basement membrane disease
    - Typically have milder clinical course

Demonstration of Collagen IV α Chains
- Normal distribution
  - α5 is present in GBM, Bowman capsule (BC), distal TBM, collecting duct, and EBM of skin
  - α3 and α4 are normally expressed in GBM and basement membrane of distal tubules
  - α1 is abundant in GBM during development; decreases with normal GBM maturation
- X-linked AS: Male
  - Absent α5(IV) staining in GBM, TBM, BC
  - Absent α3(IV) staining GBM, TBM
  - α1(IV) increased in GBM
- X-linked AS: Female (heterozygote)
  - α5 and α3 expression may be preserved, decreased, or may show mosaic pattern in GBM and TBM
- Autosomal recessive AS
  - Absent or severely decreased α3 and α5 staining in GBM and distal TBM
  - Preserved α5 staining in BC
- Skin biopsy
  - EBM shows absent α5(IV) in males with X-linked AS
  - EBM shows mosaic α5(IV) staining in X-linked female heterozygotes
  - Normal α5(IV) in autosomal recessive AS

DIFFERENTIAL DIAGNOSIS

Thin Basement Membrane Disease
- Normal collagen IV α3-5 staining pattern
- Generally no structural damage to glomeruli

IgA Nephropathy
- Mesangial IgA deposits
- May have laminations of GBM as part of repair

Nail-Patella Syndrome
- Type III collagen deposition in GBM by EM
  - Highlighted using phosphotungstic acid
- Lamina densa electron-lucent areas on EM

DIAGNOSTIC CHECKLIST

Clinically Relevant Pathologic Features
- Global GBM multilamellation/thickening has worse prognosis

Pathologic Interpretation Pearls
- Carriers of either X-linked or AR forms may show only GBM thinning
- Immunofluorescence of collagen IV α3 and α5 chains can distinguish AS from TBMD and autosomal recessive AS from X-linked AS
- Lamination of GBM can also be seen in repair in other diseases such as IgA nephropathy

SELECTED REFERENCES

1. Bekheirnia MR et al: Genotype-phenotype correlation in X-linked Alport syndrome. J Am Soc Nephrol. 21(5):876-83, 2010
2. Pedchenko V et al: Molecular architecture of the Goodpasture autoantigen in anti-GBM nephritis. N Engl J Med. 363(4):343-54, 2010
3. Haas M: Alport syndrome and thin glomerular basement membrane nephropathy: a practical approach to diagnosis. Arch Pathol Lab Med. 133(2):224-32, 2009
4. Heidet L et al: The renal lesions of Alport syndrome. J Am Soc Nephrol. 20(6):1210-5, 2009
5. Marcocci E et al: Autosomal dominant Alport syndrome: molecular analysis of the COL4A4 gene and clinical outcome. Nephrol Dial Transplant. 24(5):1464-71, 2009
6. White RH et al: The Alport nephropathy: clinicopathological correlations. Pediatr Nephrol. 20(7):897-903, 2005
7. Byrne MC et al: Renal transplant in patients with Alport's syndrome. Am J Kidney Dis. 39(4):769-75, 2002
8. Longo I et al: COL4A3/COL4A4 mutations: from familial hematuria to autosomal-dominant or recessive Alport syndrome. Kidney Int. 61(6):1947-56, 2002
9. Mothes H et al: Alport syndrome associated with diffuse leiomyomatosis: COL4A5-COL4A6 deletion associated with a mild form of Alport nephropathy. Nephrol Dial Transplant. 17(1):70-4, 2002

ALPORT SYNDROME

Microscopic Features

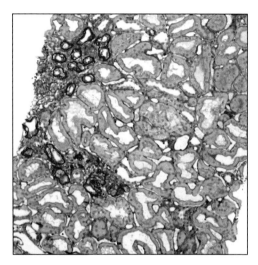

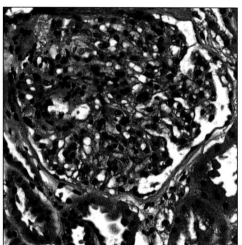

(Left) Light microscopy is often nondiagnostic in Alport syndrome (AS). This PAS stain shows focal tubular atrophy. Diagnosis of AS requires electron microscopy and immunofluorescence demonstration of the lack of α3, α4, or α5 (IV) collagen chains in glomeruli or α5 (IV) collagen in skin biopsies. (Right) Glomeruli in Alport syndrome sometimes show abnormally small capillary loops, as shown here in a 66-year-old woman with hematuria and proteinuria whose 2 brothers died of kidney disease.

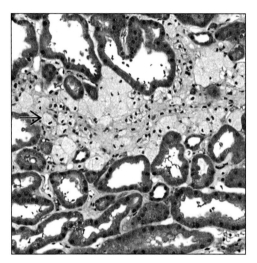

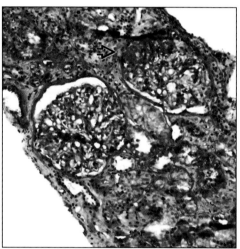

(Left) H&E shows interstitial foamy macrophages ⇥ in a biopsy from a 51-year-old woman with hematuria, recent & worsening proteinuria, & sensorineural deafness. Interstitial foamy macrophages, once thought specific for AS, are now seen in biopsies from patients with nephrotic syndrome of a variety of diagnoses. (Right) Focal segmental glomerulosclerosis (FSGS) ⇥ in this biopsy led to an initial diagnosis of FSGS. However, based on GBM abnormalities seen on EM, AS was suggested.

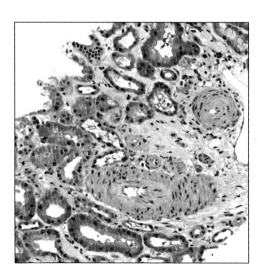

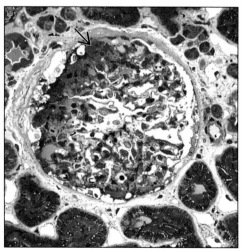

(Left) Arterial and arteriolar thickening associated with hypertension may be seen in some Alport patients. (Right) Alport syndrome may be mistaken for idiopathic focal, segmental glomerulosclerosis by LM. This glomerulus shows a segmental scar and adhesion ⇥ (toluidine blue stain). The diagnosis was made by EM and demonstration of diminished α3, α5 (IV) collagen staining.

Electron Microscopy

(Left) EM from a 41-year-old Brazilian man with recurrent hematuria, proteinuria, and mild renal insufficiency. The daughter and aunt also had hematuria and proteinuria. Diffuse, irregular thickening of the GBM is evident with effacement of foot processes. Stains for α3 and α5 (IV) collagen chains confirmed the diagnosis. (Right) A characteristic feature of AS is GBM outpouching ➡. This biopsy was from a middle-aged woman with hematuria and proteinuria. Collagen α3 and α5 (IV) chains were decreased.

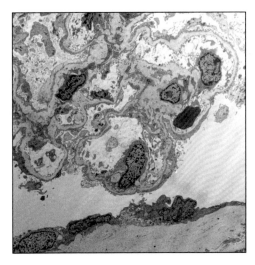
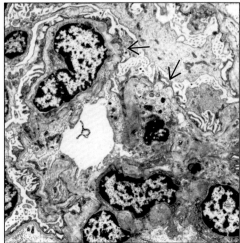

(Left) An 8-year-old girl, daughter of a woman with Alport syndrome, shows GBM "basket weaving" and "bread crumbs" ⬖. These are features of collagen IV α3-5 triplex degeneration. (Right) This electron micrograph of a kidney biopsy from a 35-year-old woman with a family history of AS shows segmental GBM thickening alternating with thin segments. Notably, GBM splitting is focal ➡. Her 8-year-old daughter also had typical Alport syndrome findings.

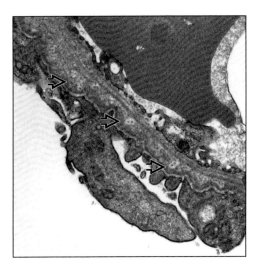
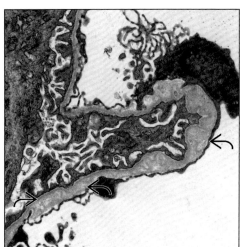

(Left) Scalloping of the subepithelial GBM is characteristic of AS ➡. Normally the GBM has a smooth subepithelial surface. (Right) The glomerulus in this case of AS shows segmental capillary loop thickening and GBM abnormalities with segmental GBM thinning ⬖ and ballooning expansion ➡. Thick GBM segments show lucent areas but no multilamellation.

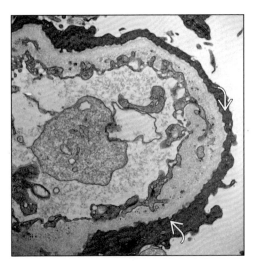
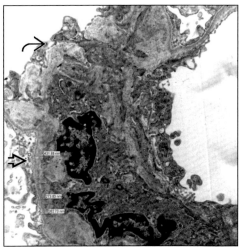

Electron Microscopy

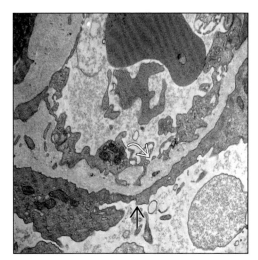
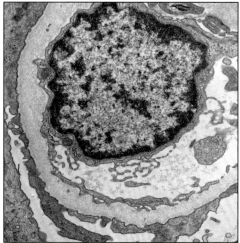

(Left) EM from a 41-year-old man shows markedly irregular subendothelial GBM surface ➔ with splitting & scalloping, typical of AS. Foot process effacement is prominent ➔. α3, α5 (IV) collagen chains were reduced by immunofluorescence. *(Right)* EM shows diffusely abnormal GBM, with loss of density and fine laminations in a man with X-linked AS. The particles are not conspicuous in this case, which had typical reduction of α3, α5 (IV) collagen chains reduced by IF.

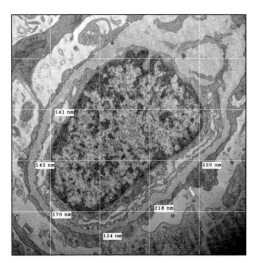
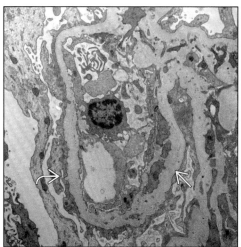

(Left) One manifestation of AS is a segmentally thin GBM, as illustrated here. AS might be confused with thin basement membrane disease (TBMD); however, other segments of GBM had typical reticulated laminated GBM, and α3, 5 (IV) collagen chains were markedly reduced by IF. *(Right)* This glomerular capillary in a 41-year-old man with X-linked AS shows irregular thickening of the GBM ➔ and scalloping on the subepithelial side of the GBM ➔, typical of AS.

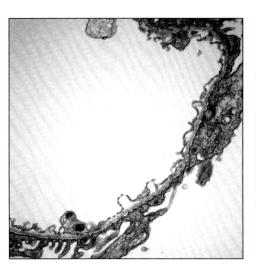
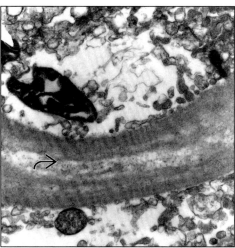

(Left) EM shows a thin GBM segment, without splitting, from a woman with AS. In other glomerular capillaries, the GBM was markedly thickened. Collagen IV α3-5 stains were severely decreased. Early AS may be manifested by thinning of the GBM before the characteristic "basket weave" pattern develops. *(Right)* Tubular basement membrane may also show "bread crumbs" ➔ &/or multilamellation in AS.

Male X-Linked AS (Hemizygous)

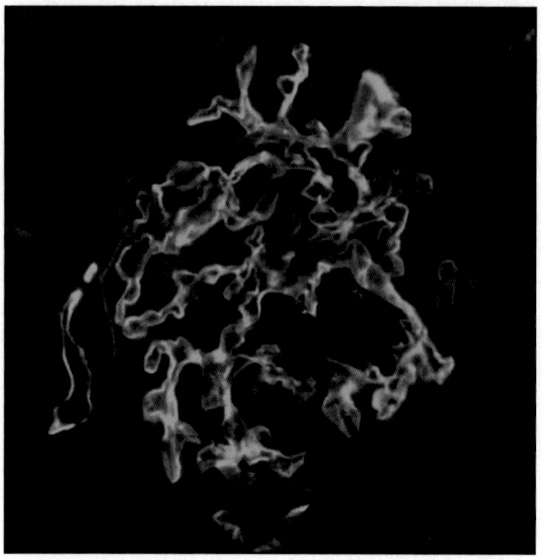

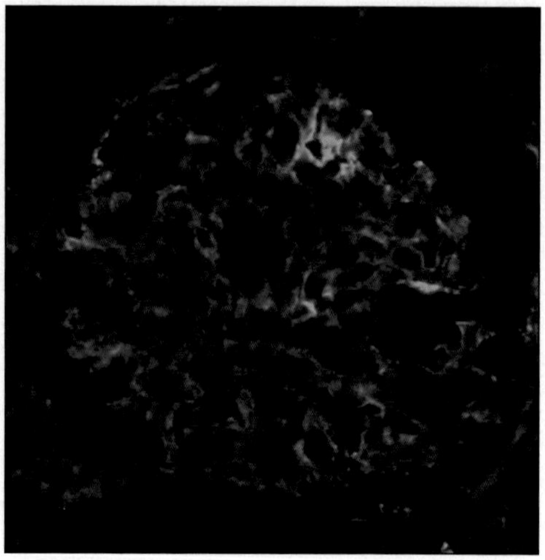

(Left) *Normal kidneys stained with a monoclonal antibody to α3 (IV) collagen show bright linear staining of the GBM and distal TBM, which contain α3, 4, 5 (IV) collagen chains. Bowman capsule is negative.* ***(Right)*** *Glomerulus from a 9-year-old boy with X-linked AS shows very weak, focal staining for α3 (IV) collagen in the GBM compared with the normal control. X-linked AS has a mutation in the α5 (IV) collagen gene, but α3 (IV) collagen requires α5 chain (and α4) to be deposited in the GBM.*

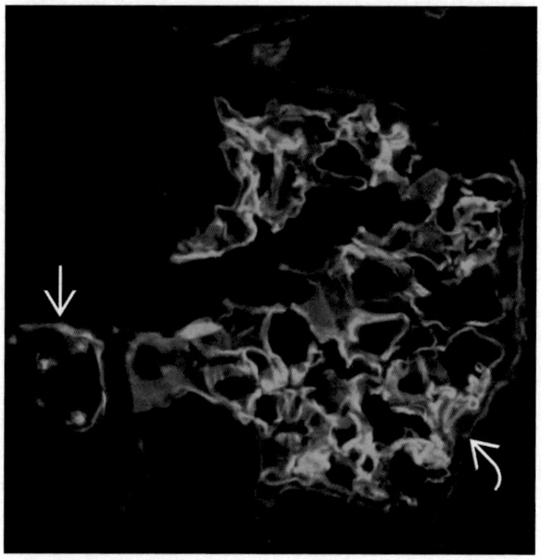

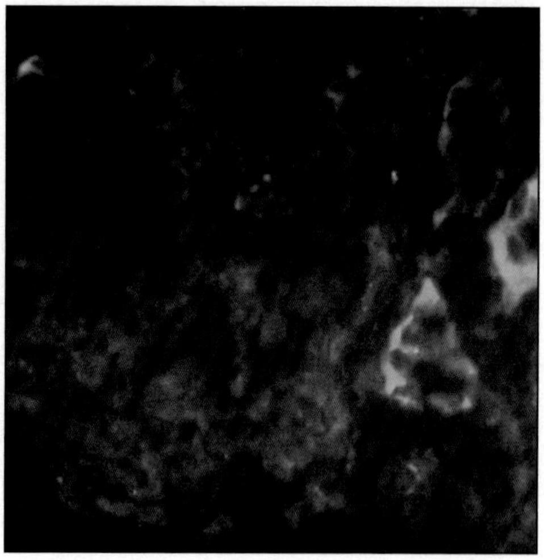

(Left) *The normal human kidney has α5 (IV) collagen in the GBM, distal TBM →, and Bowman capsule ↪. The bright linear staining pattern is typical.* ***(Right)*** *Glomeruli in X-linked AS have negative staining for α5 (IV) collagen in GBM, Bowman capsule, and distal TBM. Renal biopsy is from an 8-year-old boy with Alport syndrome; α3 (IV) was also negative. Absent α5 (IV) in Bowman capsule distinguishes X-linked from autosomal recessive AS.*

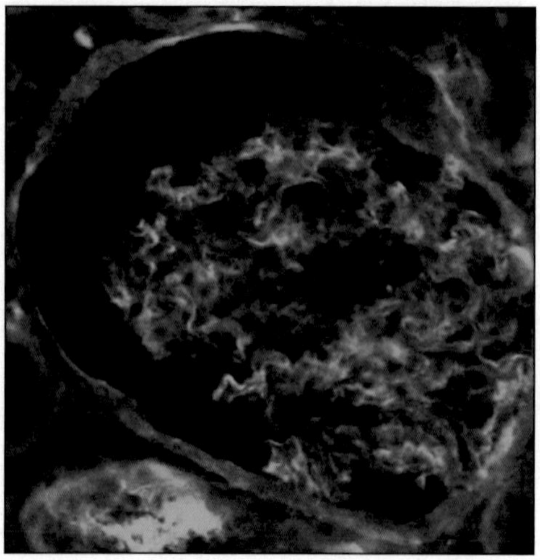

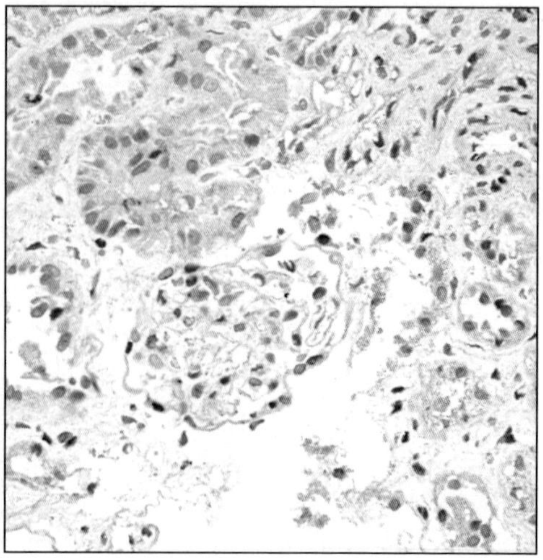

(Left) *Renal biopsy from a 9-year-old boy with microhematuria since age 4 and proteinuria shows that no staining for α5 (IV) collagen is evident in the GBM or Bowman capsule. Lack of staining in the Bowman capsule distinguishes X-linked from autosomal recessive AS.* ***(Right)*** *This biopsy from a male with X-linked AS is entirely negative for α5 (IV) collagen chains in glomeruli, Bowman capsule, and distal tubules by immunohistochemistry, structures that are normally α5 (IV) collagen positive.*

ALPORT SYNDROME

Female X-Linked AS (Heterozygous)

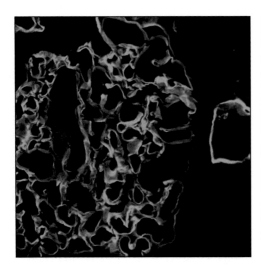
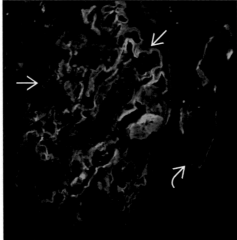

(Left) Normal control kidney stained with a monoclonal antibody to α3 (IV) collagen chain shows bright linear GBM and distal TBM staining but no staining of Bowman capsule. *(Right)* This biopsy is from a 64-year-old woman with hematuria. Her mother, brother, and sister also had hematuria. A stain for α3 (IV) collagen chains reveals decreased staining with segmental loss in the GBM ➡ and distal TBM ➡, which is highly suggestive of X-linked AS in a female heterozygote.

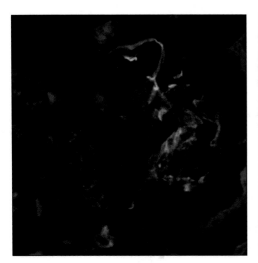
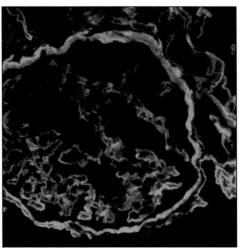

(Left) IF for α3 (IV) collagen shows interrupted (mosaic) GBM staining in a biopsy from a woman diagnosed with FSGS 5 years previously. She had marked GBM changes by EM (thick and thin areas). *(Right)* Positive collagen α1 (IV) in a woman with X-linked Alport syndrome shows increased accumulation of α1 (IV) in the glomerulus, where it is normally limited to the subendothelium and mesangium. This stain is useful to confirm that irregular staining for α3, 5 (IV) is not an artifact.

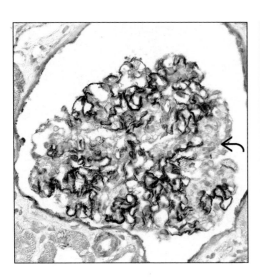
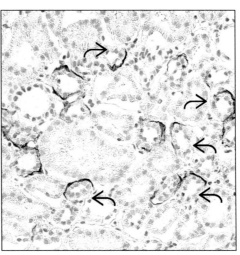

(Left) α5 (IV) collagen staining shows mosaic GBM in a woman with X-linked AS. Notice the focal negative staining in the capillary loops ➡. The pattern is characteristic of X-linked AS in female heterozygotes. *(Right)* Mosaic pattern of α3 (IV) in distal tubules ➡ is evident in heterozygotic women with X-linked Alport syndrome due to the random inactivation of the X chromosome. Expression of α3 requires α5 (IV) expression.

Autosomal Recessive AS and Skin Biopsies

(Left) α5 (IV) shows absent staining in the GBM and positive staining of Bowman capsule. This pattern is seen in autosomal recessive AS. Bowman capsule contains α5, α5, α6 (IV) collagen chains and does not require α3 or α4 collagen to express α5, in contrast to the GBM and distal TBM. **(Right)** In autosomal recessive AS, α3 (IV) collagen is entirely negative in the GBM and distal TBM, sites where α3 (IV) collagen is normally expressed. This pattern is similar to that in males with X-linked AS.

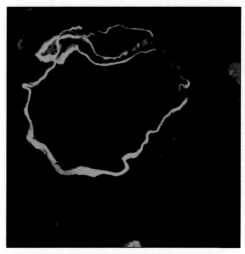
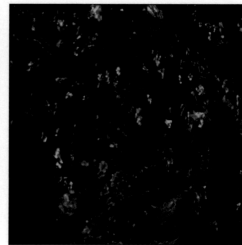

(Left) Immunofluorescence of normal skin shows bright linear staining for α1 (IV) collagen chains in the epidermal and vascular basement membranes. The EBM contains collagen α1 (IV), α2 (IV), α5 (IV), and α6 (IV) chains but no α3 (IV) or α4 (IV). **(Right)** Staining of skin with α5 (IV) is a screening test for X-linked AS. Shown here is normal skin in which the antibody to α5 (IV) collagen highlights the epidermal basement membrane (EBM).

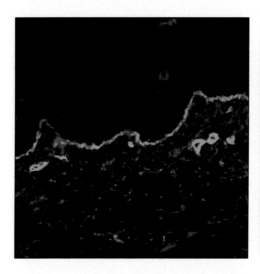
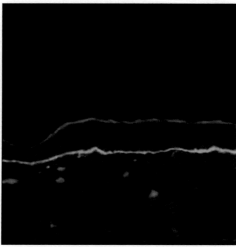

(Left) This skin biopsy is from a boy with proteinuria and a family history of AS. The skin shows absent α5 (IV) collagen chain ➡, diagnostic of X-linked AS. Patients with autosomal recessive AS have normal α5 (IV) staining in the skin since they have mutations in α3 or α4 (IV) collagen genes. **(Right)** This skin biopsy is from a woman with X-linked AS. The epidermal basement membrane shows interrupted (mosaic) α5 (IV) collagen staining ➡ due to random inactivation of the X chromosome.

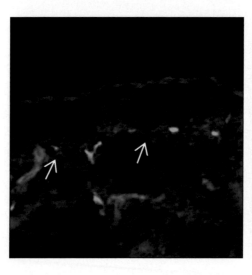
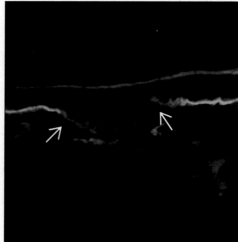

Differential Diagnosis

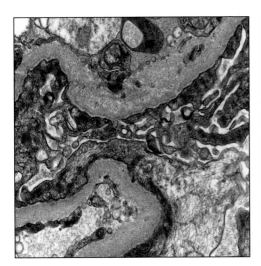
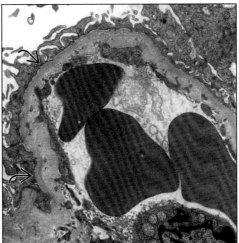

(Left) EM shows lamination and particles in the GBM in a patient with IgA nephropathy. Focal multilamination can be seen as a repair process in glomerulonephritis and without other evidence is not sufficient for the diagnosis of AS. (Right) Focal lamination and particles in the GBM in IgA nephropathy are shown. Other segments of the GBM were normal. A clue that is against AS is the presence of normal subepithelial GBM ➡. In AS, the entire thickness of the GBM is abnormal.

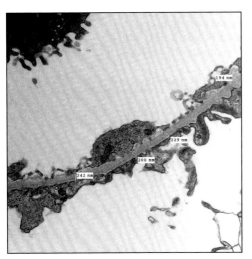
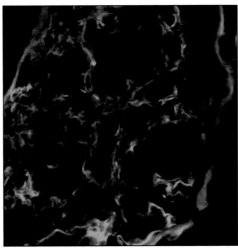

(Left) EM shows diffusely thin GBM in a female with X-linked AS. Ruling out TBMD without genetic analysis or IF for collagen chains is not possible in some patients, particularly if family history is unclear. (Right) TBMD can have reduced staining for collagen components due to the thin GBM, as shown here in a biopsy stained for α5 (IV) collagen from a woman with recurrent hematuria and normal renal function. Bowman capsule stains normally, which is a useful clue.

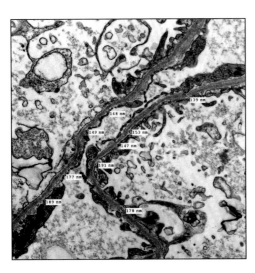
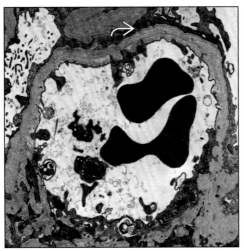

(Left) Apparent TBMD in a 49-year-old man with global glomerulosclerosis & chronic renal failure is shown. Though there was no GBM multilamellation, this may be AS masquerading as TBMD since TBMD typically does not cause significant glomerulosclerosis. (Right) This biopsy is from a 44-year-old woman with hematuria & proteinuria. The GBM is focally thickened with splitting ➡, strongly suggestive of AS. α3, α5(IV) chains were present by IF. Genetic analysis is required for confirmation.

THIN BASEMENT MEMBRANE DISEASE

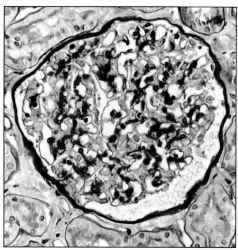

This PAS stained slide from a woman with thin basement membrane disease (TBMD) shows a normal glomerulus, typical of TBMD by light microscopy. The GBM averaged 230 nm by electron microscopy.

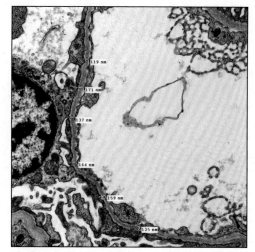

Electron microscopy in TBMD reveals a diffusely thin but otherwise normal GBM of < 200 nm (normal is 320 ± 50 nm in females, 370 ± 50 nm in males). Morphometry is recommended to assess the thickness of the GBM.

TERMINOLOGY

Abbreviations
- Thin basement membrane disease (TBMD)

Synonyms
- Benign familial hematuria (BFH)

Definitions
- Autosomal dominant disorder presenting with asymptomatic microscopic hematuria characterized by diffuse GBM thinning

ETIOLOGY/PATHOGENESIS

Genetics
- Autosomal dominant in majority of BFH
- Rare mutations in collagen α3 and α4 (IV)
- 40% of patients with GBM thinning have mutations in *COL4A3* or *COL4A4* genes
  - Encode α3 and α4 chains of type IV collagen, respectively
  - Heterozygotes, typically women
  - Autosomal recessive Alport syndrome (ARAS)

CLINICAL ISSUES

Epidemiology
- Incidence
  - Common
    - 1-5% of population
- Age
  - All ages
- Gender
  - Some studies indicate slight female predominance, but this is inconclusive
- Ethnicity
  - None specifically

Presentation
- Persistent microscopic hematuria
  - Dysmorphic RBCs and RBC casts
- Macroscopic hematuria (5-22%)
- Flank pain (7-31%)
- Proteinuria, subnephrotic (rare)

Laboratory Tests
- Gene sequencing *COL4A3*, *COL4A4*, *COL4A5*

Treatment
- No specific treatment
- Close monitoring for HTN, proteinuria, elevated creatinine

Prognosis
- Excellent

MICROSCOPIC PATHOLOGY

Histologic Features
- Generally within normal limits
- Mild mesangial hypercellularity
- Red cell and pigment casts
- Rare cases associated with FSGS

ANCILLARY TESTS

Immunofluorescence
- Nonspecific IgM, C3, and C1q occasionally seen
- No specific IF findings
- Preserved α3, α4, and α5 type IV collagen staining
  - Normal expression does not, however, definitively exclude AS

Electron Microscopy
- Transmission
  - Uniform (> 50%) thinning of glomerular basement membrane measuring < 200 nm in thickness

THIN BASEMENT MEMBRANE DISEASE

Key Facts

Clinical Issues
- Presents with persistent microscopic hematuria
- Autosomal dominant inheritance
- 1-5% of population

Microscopic Pathology
- Minimal changes

Ancillary Tests
- Immunofluorescence

- ○ Preserved α3, α4, and α5 (IV) collagen
- ○ Normal expression does not definitively exclude AS
- Electron microscopy
  - ○ Uniform GBM thinning (< 200 nm)
- Genetic testing
  - ○ Mutations in *COL4A3* or *COL4A4* genes

Top Differential Diagnoses
- Alport syndrome
- IgA nephropathy

Morphometry for GBM Thickness
- Normal GBM thickness
  - ○ Adult males: 370 ± 50 nm
  - ○ Adult females: 320 ± 50 nm
  - ○ 150 nm at birth, 200 nm at 1 year, gradually increases to adult thickness at 11 years of age
- Simple method
  - ○ Distance between base of podocyte foot processes and edge of endothelial cells
  - ○ Only measure peripheral capillaries
  - ○ Calculate mean and standard deviation
- Alternative method with harmonic mean and grid
  - ○ Measure wherever grid crosses GBM
  - ○ Normal male adult: 373 ± 84 nm (mean ± 2 standard deviations)
  - ○ Normal female adult: 326 ± 90 nm (mean ± 2 standard deviations)
  - ○ Harmonic mean reduces effect of nonperpendicular measurements

DIFFERENTIAL DIAGNOSIS

Alport Syndrome (AS)
- Sensorineural deafness and ocular abnormalities
- More likely to have proteinuria and hypertension
- Typically progresses to ESRD
- GBM multilamellation is classic
- X-linked AS may initially present with thin GBM
  - ○ Absent α3 and α5 (IV) collagen by IF

- Female carriers of X-linked AS may present with hematuria and GBM thinning
  - ○ Mosaic α3 and α5 (IV) collagen IF pattern
- ARAS may present with hematuria and GBM thinning
  - ○ IF shows absent or decreased GBM α3 and α5 (IV) collagen
  - ○ Preserved Bowman capsule α5 (IV) collagen
- Genetic testing for *COL4A3*, *COL4A4*, and *COLA5* gene mutations for complex cases

SELECTED REFERENCES

1. Haas M: Alport syndrome and thin glomerular basement membrane nephropathy: a practical approach to diagnosis. Arch Pathol Lab Med. 133(2):224-32, 2009
2. Tryggvason K et al: Thin basement membrane nephropathy. J Am Soc Nephrol. 17(3):813-22, 2006
3. Gregory MC: The clinical features of thin basement membrane nephropathy. Semin Nephrol. 25(3):140-5, 2005
4. Savige J et al: Thin basement membrane nephropathy. Kidney Int. 64(4):1169-78, 2003
5. Liapis H et al: Histopathology, ultrastructure, and clinical phenotypes in thin glomerular basement membrane disease variants. Hum Pathol. 33(8):836-45, 2002
6. Kashtan CE: Alport syndrome and thin glomerular basement membrane disease. J Am Soc Nephrol. 9(9):1736-50, 1998
7. Lemmink HH et al: Benign familial hematuria due to mutation of the type IV collagen alpha4 gene. J Clin Invest. 98(5):1114-8, 1996

IMAGE GALLERY

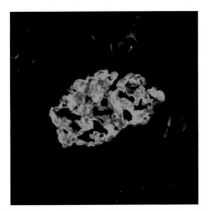 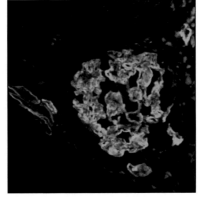 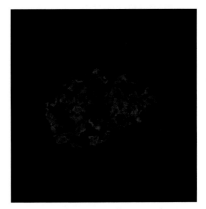

(Left) Stains for α3 collagen chain help distinguish TBMD from Alport syndrome. TBMD shows preservation of α3 (IV) collagen in the GBM, in contrast to Alport syndrome (FITC immunofluorescence). *(Center)* Immunofluorescence for α4 (IV) collagen chains shows preservation of α4 (IV) collagen in the GBM and distal TBM in TBMD. *(Right)* Antibody to collagen α5 (IV) also stains normally in TBMD, in contrast to Alport syndrome. Sometimes the stain is weaker due to the thin GBM.

PIERSON SYNDROME

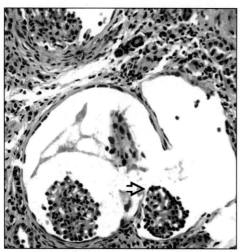

Glomeruli in Pierson syndrome show mesangial hypercellularity or prominent podocytes forming a corona over the capillary loops ➯, often called fetal glomeruli.

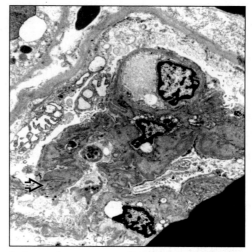

Podocyte foot processes show extensive effacement and degeneration in Pierson syndrome. The glomerular basement (GBM) is wrinkled ➯ due to collapse.

TERMINOLOGY

Definitions
- Congenital nephrotic syndrome, neurologic defects, and microcoria due to *LAMB2* mutations

ETIOLOGY/PATHOGENESIS

Mutations in LAMB2
- Encodes the laminin β2 subunit
  - Normal component of GBM, anterior eye, and neuromuscular junction
  - Important for maturation and function of GBM, nerve-terminal differentiation, and anterior eye development
  - Maps to chromosome 3p
- Laminins are family of 16 heterotrimeric glycoproteins
  - Major noncollagenous component of basement membranes
    - Organize and stabilize basement membranes
    - Promote cell adhesion
  - Composed of 3 different chains: α, β, γ
  - 3α, 6β, and 2γ chains are known and have different tissue distribution
- Autosomal recessive inheritance
  - Truncating mutations cause severe disease
  - Missense mutations have milder clinical course

CLINICAL ISSUES

Epidemiology
- Incidence
  - 2.5% of nephrotic syndrome cases present in 1st year of life
- Age
  - Truncating mutations: < 3 months
  - Missense mutations: 3 months to 10 years

Presentation
- Proteinuria
- Edema
- Neurodevelopmental abnormalities
- Ophthalmologic findings
  - Truncating mutations are associated with a severe phenotype
    - Microcoria: Narrow, nonreactive pupils
    - Posterior lenticonus
  - Missense mutations are associated with a milder phenotype
    - Retinal detachment
    - Posterior synechiae
    - Hypopigmented fundus
    - May present with isolated nephrotic syndrome without eye abnormalities
- Prenatal findings
  - Oligohydramnios
  - Enlarged placenta

Laboratory Tests
- Increased amniotic α-fetoprotein
- Mutational analysis for *LAMB2* on chromosome 3

Treatment
- None curative

Prognosis
- Patients with severe phenotype typically die within 1st year of life
- Milder phenotype progresses to ESRD from 1-10 years of age

IMAGE FINDINGS

Ultrasonographic Findings
- Large, hyperechogenic kidneys detectable by 15 weeks of gestation

PIERSON SYNDROME

Key Facts

Etiology/Pathogenesis
- Mutations in *LAMB2* resulting in decreased/absent expression of laminin β2
- Other laminins are intact

Clinical Issues
- Patients with severe phenotype have ocular abnormalities, characteristically microcoria
- Patients with milder phenotype may or may not have ocular abnormalities

Image Findings
- Ultrasound shows large, hyperechogenic kidneys at 15 weeks

Microscopic Pathology
- Diffuse mesangial sclerosis is associated with severe phenotype

- Fetal glomeruli are seen with milder phenotype

Ancillary Tests
- Molecular genetic testing for *LAMB2* mutations
- Immunofluorescence: Absent laminin β2 expression

Top Differential Diagnoses
- Diffuse mesangial sclerosis
- Frasier syndrome
- Denys-Drash syndrome
- Podocin deficiency
- Congenital nephrotic syndrome of the Finnish type

MICROSCOPIC PATHOLOGY

Histologic Features
- Truncating mutations → severe phenotype
  - Increased mesangial matrix identical to idiopathic diffuse mesangial sclerosis
  - Fetal glomeruli with obliteration of capillaries
  - Prominent podocytes appear in coronal pattern over the GBM
- Missense mutations → milder phenotype
  - Variable findings
    - Focal segmental glomerulosclerosis
    - Minimal glomerular changes

ANCILLARY TESTS

Immunofluorescence
- Negative staining for laminin β2
- Other laminins such as γ1 and α2 are intact

Electron Microscopy
- Transmission
  - Diffuse podocyte foot process effacement
  - Irregular lamellation and wrinkling of the GBM

DIFFERENTIAL DIAGNOSIS

Diffuse Mesangial Sclerosis
- Delayed progression to ESRD; takes ~ 3 years

Frasier Syndrome
- Focal segmental glomerulosclerosis
- Female external genitalia, streak gonads, XY karyotype
- Mutations in intron 9 of *WT1*
- Autosomal dominant inheritance

Denys-Drash Syndrome
- Diffuse mesangial sclerosis
- Male gonadal dysgenesis
- Mutations in exons 8 or 9 of *WT1*

Podocin Deficiency
- FSGS or minimal change on renal biopsy
- Mutations in *NPHS2*

Congenital Nephrotic Syndrome of the Finnish Type
- Minimal changes and cystic dilatation of tubules on light microscopy
- Absent slit diaphragms on electron microscopy
- Mutations in *NPHS1*

SELECTED REFERENCES

1. Matejas V et al: Mutations in the human laminin beta2 (LAMB2) gene and the associated phenotypic spectrum. Hum Mutat. 31(9):992-1002, 2010
2. Choi HJ et al: Variable phenotype of Pierson syndrome. Pediatr Nephrol. 23(6):995-1000, 2008
3. Liapis H: Molecular pathology of nephrotic syndrome in childhood: a contemporary approach to diagnosis. Pediatr Dev Pathol. 11(4):154-63, 2008
4. Hasselbacher K et al: Recessive missense mutations in LAMB2 expand the clinical spectrum of LAMB2-associated disorders. Kidney Int. 70(6):1008-12, 2006
5. Jarad G et al: Proteinuria precedes podocyte abnormalities in Lamb2-/- mice, implicating the glomerular basement membrane as an albumin barrier. J Clin Invest. 116(8):2272-9, 2006
6. Mark K et al: Prenatal findings in four consecutive pregnancies with fetal Pierson syndrome, a newly defined congenital nephrosis syndrome. Prenat Diagn. 26(3):262-6, 2006
7. VanDeVoorde R et al: Pierson syndrome: a novel cause of congenital nephrotic syndrome. Pediatrics. 118(2):e501-5, 2006
8. Zenker M et al: Congenital nephrosis, mesangial sclerosis, and distinct eye abnormalities with microcoria: an autosomal recessive syndrome. Am J Med Genet A. 130A(2):138-45, 2004
9. Zenker M et al: Human laminin beta2 deficiency causes congenital nephrosis with mesangial sclerosis and distinct eye abnormalities. Hum Mol Genet. 13(21):2625-32, 2004

Light Microscopy and Immunofluorescence

(Left) Early changes in a renal biopsy from an infant with Pierson syndrome reveal small, immature (fetal)-appearing glomeruli with prominent clustering podocyte nuclei. *(Right)* Chronic lesions in Pierson syndrome are shown. Glomeruli are globally or partially sclerosed, and some are fetal appearing ⊟. The interstitium has an extensive infiltrate of mononuclear cells. Periglomerular fibrosis is also evident ➡. The tubules are markedly atrophic.

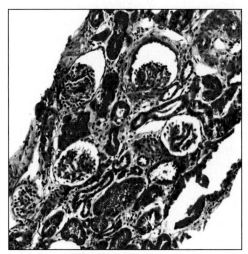
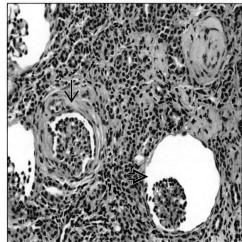

(Left) Normal human neonatal kidneys show prominent laminin β2 in glomeruli ➡. Tubular basement membranes and vessels are negative. *(Right)* On rhodamine immunofluorescence, this biopsy from a patient with Pierson syndrome demonstrates no staining with mouse anti-human laminin β2 antibody.

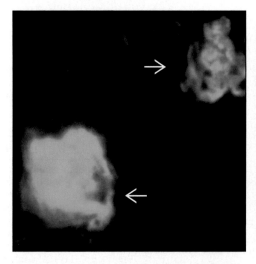

(Left) Normal synaptopodin expression in Pierson syndrome is shown (FITC immunofluorescence). *(Right)* Normal nephrin positivity in a patient with congenital nephrotic syndrome rules out Finnish nephropathy (rhodamine immunofluorescence).

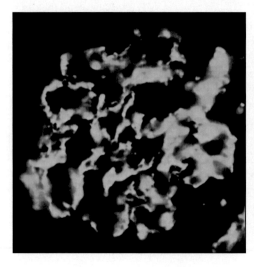
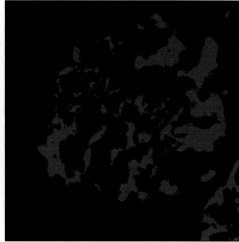

Immunofluorescence and Electron Microscopy

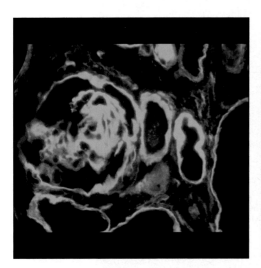
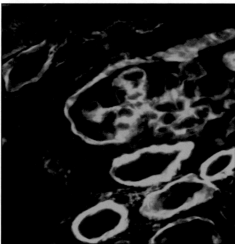

(Left) Laminin γ1 expression with rat anti-mouse antibody is normal in a biopsy from a patient with Pierson syndrome (FITC immunofluorescence). *(Right)* Laminin β1 highlights glomerular and tubular basement membranes in a biopsy from a patient with Pierson syndrome (FITC immunofluorescence).

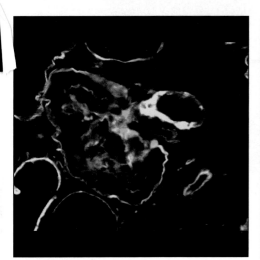
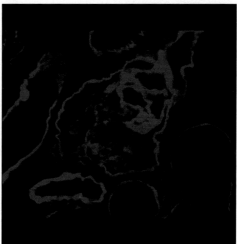

(Left) Double staining with overlay of γ1 and β1 laminin is shown. Yellow color indicates that both are positive. *(Right)* Normal laminin α2 expression in Pierson syndrome is shown (rhodamine immunofluorescence).

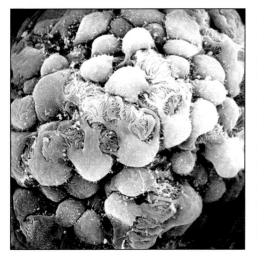
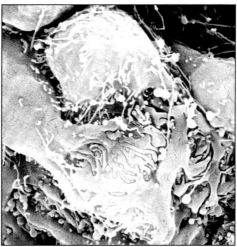

(Left) Normal mouse podocytes on EM show interdigitating foot processes. (Courtesy G. Jarad, MD.) *(Right)* Pierson mouse podocytes on EM show villiform transformation of the foot processes. (Courtesy G. Jarad, MD.)

CONGENITAL NEPHROTIC SYNDROME OF THE FINNISH TYPE

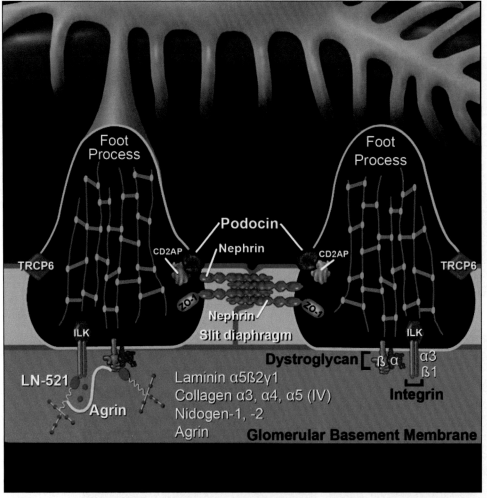

This schematic of the slit diaphragm demonstrates the interaction between various proteins known to be mutated in different types of inherited nephrotic syndromes. Nephrin, a key component of the slit diaphragm, is mutated in patients with FN. Given nephrin's role in slit diaphragm structure, it is not surprising that FN patients present with massive proteinuria. Podocin mutations present with similar clinical symptoms and pathologic findings of FSGS.

TERMINOLOGY

Abbreviations
- Finnish nephropathy (FN)

Synonyms
- Microcystic kidney disease

Definitions
- Steroid-resistant nephrotic syndrome in neonates up to 3 months of age due to mutations in nephrin (*NPHS1*) gene

ETIOLOGY/PATHOGENESIS

Genetics
- Autosomal recessive disease
- Homozygous mutation in *NPHS1*
  - Maps to chromosome 19q13.1
  - Encodes protein nephrin

- Transmembrane protein of immunoglobulin (Ig) superfamily with 8 extracellular immunoglobulin-like domains with N-glycosylated sites
- N-glycosylation is important for protein folding, formation of slit diaphragm, and localization in GBM
- Forms "zipper" structure of slit diaphragm described by Karnovsky
  - Over 70 mutations have been identified in Finland and elsewhere around the world
  - Fin-major
    - Frameshift mutation in chromosome 19q13.1 leading to absent slit diaphragms and no nephrin protein expression
  - Fin-minor
    - Nonsense mutations in exon 26 produce a truncated or nonfunctioning nephrin
- Compound heterozygous *NPHS1* mutations are rare
  - May present as adult onset focal segmental glomerulosclerosis (FSGS)

CONGENITAL NEPHROTIC SYNDROME OF THE FINNISH TYPE

Key Facts

Terminology
- Finnish nephropathy (FN)
  - Occurs in neonates up to 3 months of age and is due to mutations in nephrin (NPHS1) gene

Etiology/Pathogenesis
- Mutations in NPHS1 gene encoding nephrin
- Nephrin is major structural protein of slit diaphragm, important for its formation and maintenance
- Absent or mutant nephrin results in absent slit diaphragms and massive proteinuria

Clinical Issues
- Presents at birth or shortly after (< 3 months of age) with massive proteinuria and steroid-resistant nephrotic syndrome
- Prognosis depends on nature of NPHS1 mutation

- Autosomal recessive inheritance

Ancillary Tests
- Mutational analysis of NPHS1 on chromosome 19
- Staining for nephrin protein expression

Top Differential Diagnoses
- Podocin deficiency
- Early diffuse mesangial sclerosis (DMS)
  - Idiopathic or associated with Pierson syndrome or WT1 mutations (Denys-Drash)

- Heterozygotes with 1 normal NPHS1 allele (carriers) are normal post birth
  - In utero may have transient deficiency of nephrin during podocytogenesis
  - Can lead to false-positive α-fetoprotein (AFP) test in amniotic fluid and maternal serum

CLINICAL ISSUES

Epidemiology
- Incidence
  - Highest in Finland
    - 1:10,000-1:80,000 births (gene frequency 1:200)
    - Fin-major accounts for 78% of Finnish cases
    - Fin-minor accounts for 22% of Finnish cases
  - Occurs worldwide at lower frequency
    - 61% of nephrotic syndrome in first 3 months of life
  - Numerous other point mutations are described in non-Finnish patients, resulting in variable nephrin synthesis
- Age
  - Onset < 3 months: Homozygous mutation
  - Onset 6 months to 5 years: Compound heterozygous mutation
  - Rare cases of adult onset FSGS attributed to NPHS1 mutations

Presentation
- Massive proteinuria-nephrotic syndrome
- Elevated AFP in amniotic fluid and maternal serum

Laboratory Tests
- AFP elevated in maternal plasma and amniotic fluid (in utero nephrotic syndrome)
- Antinephrin antibodies post transplant

Treatment
- Supportive therapy
- Transplantation once patient weight is > 8 kg
  - Patients who are transplanted have 30% rate of recurrent nephrotic syndrome

- Not a recurrence but instead secondary to anti-nephrin antibodies
- Plasmapheresis, cyclophosphamide, and methylprednisolone prolongs graft survival in patients with antinephrin antibodies

Prognosis
- Mean time to ESRD = 32 months
  - Rate of progression is variable
    - Somewhat slower in females (40 months) than males (21 months)
    - Patients with Fin-major have earliest onset and most rapid course
    - Patients with Fin-minor have later onset and delayed progression
- Many severely affected infants with FN die from infection
- Compound heterozygotes develop ESRD later at 6-15 years of age
- Fetal carriers of NPHS1 mutations are normal post birth

IMAGE FINDINGS

Ultrasonographic Findings
- Echogenic kidneys with symmetric distribution of microcysts
- Nuchal translucency

MACROSCOPIC FEATURES

General Features
- Kidneys slightly enlarged, edematous
- Diffuse microcystic change on kidney cross sections

MICROSCOPIC PATHOLOGY

Histologic Features
- Glomerulus

- o Minimal glomerular changes resembling minimal change disease
- o Mesangial hypercellularity
- o Immature glomeruli
- o Focal and global glomerulosclerosis in advanced stages
- Tubules
  - o Reabsorption droplets
    - ▪ α-fetoprotein in reabsorption droplets in utero
  - o Microcystic dilation of proximal and distal tubules
  - o Tubular atrophy in progressive disease
- Interstitium
  - o Interstitial fibrosis in progressive disease
  - o Chronic interstitial inflammation, variable
- Vessels
  - o Arterial wall thickening
  - o May be normal

ANCILLARY TESTS

Immunofluorescence
- Routine immunoglobulin stains are negative; IgM and C3 highlight focal segmental glomerulosclerotic lesions
- Negative nephrin staining in classic cases with Fin-major or Fin-minor mutations
  - o Entirely absent nephrin is not seen in all patients, particularly those with point mutations

Molecular Genetics
- NPHS1 gene sequencing for known and novel mutations

Electron Microscopy
- Transmission
  - o Podocyte foot process effacement
    - ▪ Absent slit diaphragms
    - ▪ Variable villous transformation
  - o Mesangial expansion
  - o Endothelial blebs (endotheliosis)
    - ▪ Normal fenestrations and attachment to GBM
  - o Normal glomerular basement membrane

DIFFERENTIAL DIAGNOSIS

Podocin Deficiency
- Mutations in NPHS2, encodes podocin
- May be histologically indistinguishable from FN when it affects neonates
- Accounts for 15% of nephrotic syndrome in 1st 3 months of life

Early Diffuse Mesangial Sclerosis (DMS) Including Pierson Syndrome
- Early idiopathic DMS and Pierson syndrome may present with minimal changes, mimicking FN histologically
- Mutations in WT1, PCLE1, or LAMB2 account for ~ 5.6% of nephrotic syndrome in 1st 3 months

Minimal Change Disease (MCD)
- Even with widespread foot process effacement, occasional filtration slit diaphragms can be found (and some nephrin staining)

Focal Segmental Glomerulosclerosis (FSGS), Idiopathic
- Occasional cases of familial and sporadic childhood and adult onset FSGS have documented homozygous or compound heterozygous NPHS1 mutations

DIAGNOSTIC CHECKLIST

Clinically Relevant Pathologic Features
- Microcystic tubular dilatation
- Glomerulosclerosis and interstitial fibrosis in late stages

Pathologic Interpretation Pearls
- Minimal glomerular changes on light microscopy
- Absent slit diaphragms on electron microscopy
- Negative nephrin staining
- NPHS1 mutations occasionally in adults with FSGS

SELECTED REFERENCES
1. Machuca E et al: Genetics of nephrotic syndrome: connecting molecular genetics to podocyte physiology. Hum Mol Genet. 18(R2):R185-94, 2009
2. Santín S et al: Nephrin mutations cause childhood- and adult-onset focal segmental glomerulosclerosis. Kidney Int. 76(12):1268-76, 2009
3. Liapis H: Molecular pathology of nephrotic syndrome in childhood: a contemporary approach to diagnosis. Pediatr Dev Pathol. 11(4):154-63, 2008
4. Philippe A et al: Nephrin mutations can cause childhood-onset steroid-resistant nephrotic syndrome. J Am Soc Nephrol. 19(10):1871-8, 2008
5. Hinkes BG et al: Nephrotic syndrome in the first year of life: two thirds of cases are caused by mutations in 4 genes (NPHS1, NPHS2, WT1, and LAMB2). Pediatrics. 119(4):e907-19, 2007
6. Kuusniemi AM et al: Plasma exchange and retransplantation in recurrent nephrosis of patients with congenital nephrotic syndrome of the Finnish type (NPHS1). Transplantation. 83(10):1316-23, 2007
7. Patari-Sampo A et al: Molecular basis of the glomerular filtration: nephrin and the emerging protein complex at the podocyte slit diaphragm. Ann Med. 38(7):483-92, 2006
8. Northrup M et al: Congenital nephrotic syndrome, Finnish type: sonographic appearance and pathologic correlation. J Ultrasound Med. 22(10):1097-9; quiz 1100-1, 2003
9. Koziell A et al: Genotype/phenotype correlations of NPHS1 and NPHS2 mutations in nephrotic syndrome advocate a functional inter-relationship in glomerular filtration. Hum Mol Genet. 11(4):379-88, 2002
10. Patrakka J et al: Proteinuria and prenatal diagnosis of congenital nephrosis in fetal carriers of nephrin gene mutations. Lancet. 359(9317):1575-7, 2002
11. Ruotsalainen V et al: Nephrin is specifically located at the slit diaphragm of glomerular podocytes. Proc Natl Acad Sci U S A. 96(14):7962-7, 1999
12. Kestila M et al: Positionally cloned gene for a novel glomerular protein--nephrin--is mutated in congenital nephrotic syndrome. Mol Cell. 1(4):575-82, 1998

CONGENITAL NEPHROTIC SYNDROME OF THE FINNISH TYPE

Gross and Light Microscopic Features

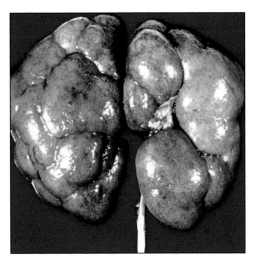

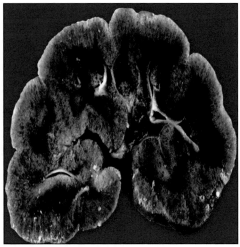

(Left) Gross kidney appearance from newborn with FN shows edematous kidneys with fetal lobulations. (Right) Bisected kidney from a patient with FN demonstrates diffuse minute cysts.

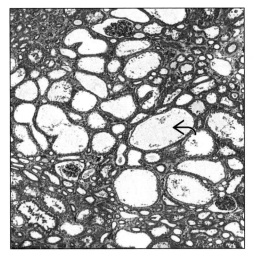

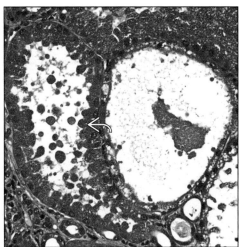

(Left) H&E shows nephrectomy specimen from a patient with FN. Sections show diffuse tubular microcystic dilatation ⇗ and mild interstitial fibrosis. (Right) High-power view shows cystic tubules. Tubular epithelial cell cytoplasm is edematous and fragmented due to massive proteinuria ⇗.

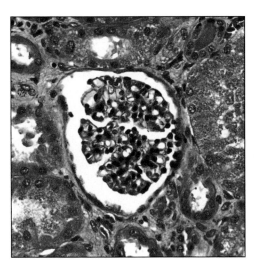

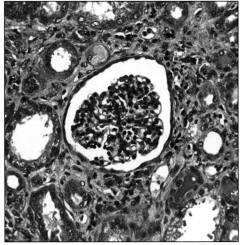

(Left) H&E shows glomerulus with minimal histopathological changes in a renal biopsy from a newborn baby with FN. (Right) Mild mesangial hypercellularity is among the light microscopic findings of FN.

CONGENITAL NEPHROTIC SYNDROME OF THE FINNISH TYPE

Light Microscopy and Immunofluorescence

(Left) Trichrome stain shows advanced FN with occasional globally sclerosed glomeruli and extensive microcystic tubular dilatation. *(Right)* This trichrome stained section from a patient with FN shows fetal (immature)-appearing glomeruli with prominent podocytes ➔. This feature is also seen in congenital nephrotic syndrome of other causes, including DMS and Pierson syndrome. Mild interstitial inflammation and moderate fibrosis are also present.

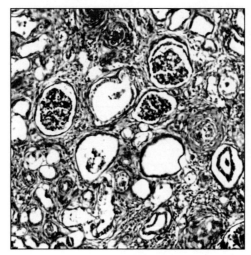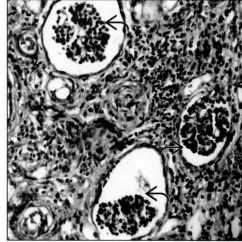

(Left) IF with antibody to synaptopodin highlights the GBM in this patient with congenital nephrotic syndrome of the Finnish type (FN). This stain is used here as a positive control. *(Right)* Double staining in the glomerulus in an infant with FN with antibody to nephrin is entirely negative. Absent nephrin expression is typical of severe mutations leading to abolished protein production (IF).

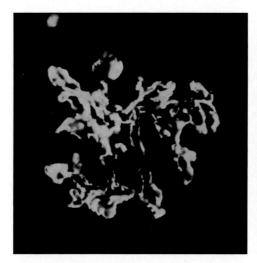

(Left) IF shows glomeruli from a 2-month-old baby with congenital nephrotic syndrome of the Finnish type. Synaptopodin highlights the GBM. *(Right)* In an atypical case of FN, double staining with antibody to nephrin (rhodamine label) in the glomerulus shows nephrin antigen is present. Some NPH1 mutations allow for nephrin antigen synthesis in spite of significant proteinuria and presumably defective slit diaphragms. Thus a positive nephrin stain does not rule out FN.

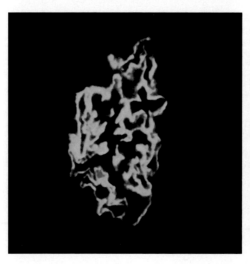

CONGENITAL NEPHROTIC SYNDROME OF THE FINNISH TYPE

Electron Microscopy

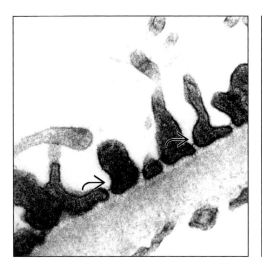

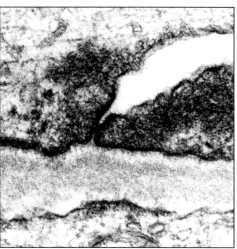

(Left) Slit diaphragms ⮕ in a normal human glomerulus consist of bridge-like structures extending between adjacent foot processes. *(Right)* High-magnification view of a pore between 2 podocyte foot processes shows that the slit diaphragm is absent in a patient with congenital nephrotic syndrome of the Finnish type.

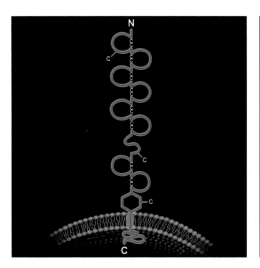

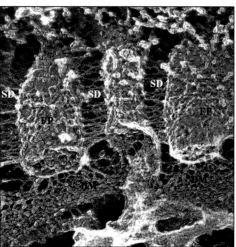

(Left) The nephrin molecule is a transmembrane protein with an extracellular domain that forms noncovalent bonds with a 2nd nephrin molecule extending from an adjacent podocyte foot process. Four nephrin molecules from adjacent podocytes are required for 1 slit diaphragm formation. *(Right)* This freeze fracture EM shows how interlacing nephrin molecules compose the slit diaphragm (SD). Thread-like connections extend from foot processes (FP) to GBM (BM). *(Courtesy G. Jarad, MD.)*

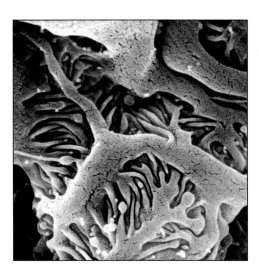

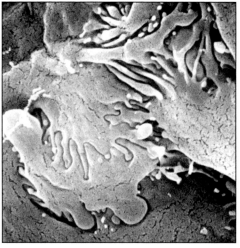

(Left) Scanning electron microscopy shows podocyte cell body and interdigitating foot processes from normal mouse kidney. *(Courtesy G. Jarad, MD)* *(Right)* Podocytes from a mouse with congential nephrotic syndrome show wide foot processes and loss of the interdigitating distribution pattern. *(Courtesy G. Jarad, MD.)*

PODOCIN DEFICIENCY

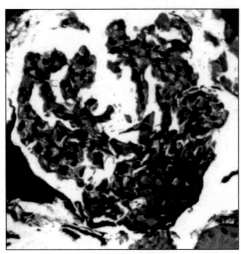

A 10-year-old boy previously diagnosed with minimal change disease had persistent proteinuria of 3 g/d. A repeat biopsy showed perihilar FSGS. Podocin was undetectable by immunofluorescence.

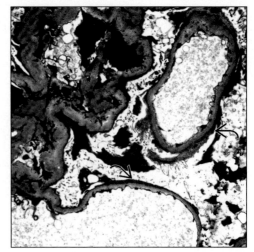

In this case of podocin deficiency, the glomerular capillary loops show diffuse foot process effacement ➔. (Courtesy L. Barisoni-Thomas, MD.)

TERMINOLOGY

Definitions
- Inherited or sporadic steroid-resistant nephrotic syndrome secondary to mutations in *NPHS2* gene

ETIOLOGY/PATHOGENESIS

Genetics
- Mutation in *NPHS2*
  - Encodes podocin
    - Important for maintaining podocyte foot process structure and signaling
    - Interacts with nephrin and CD2AP to form part of slit diaphragm
  - Autosomal recessive inheritance
    - Maps to chromosome 1q25-q31
    - > 50 mutations reported to date

CLINICAL ISSUES

Epidemiology
- Incidence
  - *NPHS2* mutations account for 10-30% of cases of pediatric steroid-resistant nephrotic syndrome
  - Rare cause of adult onset steroid resistant nephrotic syndrome
- Age
  - Truncation mutations onset at median of 1.7 years
  - Missense mutations onset at median of 4.7 years
  - R229Q mutation: Adult onset (> 18 years)
  - R138Q mutation: Very early onset (12 ± 3 months)
- Gender
  - M:F = 1:1

Presentation
- Proteinuria, may be nephrotic range
- Nephrotic syndrome

Treatment
- Drugs
  - Cyclosporine

Prognosis
- 90% of familial cases progress to ESRD within 73 months (median)
- 35% of sporadic cases progress to ESRD within 76 months (median)
- Recurrence post transplant
  - 7.7% of patients with homozygous or compound heterozygous mutations
  - 62.5% of patients with heterozygous mutations

MICROSCOPIC PATHOLOGY

Histologic Features
- Glomeruli: Various patterns
  - Focal and segmental glomerulosclerosis (50%)
  - Minimal changes (50%)
  - Mesangial hypercellularity
  - No distinctive feature described by light microscopy compared with nongenetic FSGS
- Tubules and interstitium
  - Variable fibrosis, tubular atrophy

ANCILLARY TESTS

Immunofluorescence
- C3 deposits are occasionally present
- Antipodocin antibodies show decreased, granular staining of capillary loops

Molecular Genetics
- Sequencing *NPHS2* gene

Electron Microscopy
- Transmission
  - Effacement of podocyte foot processes

PODOCIN DEFICIENCY

Key Facts

Clinical Issues
- Proteinuria, may be nephrotic range
- 90% of familial cases progress to ESRD within ~ 6 years
- 35% of sporadic cases progress to ESRD within ~ 6 years

Microscopic Pathology
- Focal and segmental glomerulosclerosis (50%)
- Minimal changes (50%)

- Mesangial hypercellularity

Ancillary Tests
- Sequencing *NPHS2* gene
- Immunohistochemistry with antibody to human podocin

Top Differential Diagnoses
- Idiopathic FSGS
- Other inherited forms of FSGS
- Minimal change disease

○ Segmental adhesion

DIFFERENTIAL DIAGNOSIS

Primary (Idiopathic, Nonhereditary) FSGS
- Diffuse podocyte foot process effacement
- Normal podocin immunoreactivity

Other Inherited Forms of FSGS
- Includes inherited mutations in *WT1, NPHS1, LAMB2, PLCE1, TRPC6,* and *CD2AP*
- Normal podocin immunoreactivity

Minimal Change Disease
- Normal podocin immunoreactivity
- Negative family history

DIAGNOSTIC CHECKLIST

Pathologic Interpretation Pearls
- Distinction among various genetic causes of FSGS depends on demonstration of lack of relevant protein or mutation in relevant gene

SELECTED REFERENCES

1. Hildebrandt F: Genetic kidney diseases. Lancet. 375(9722):1287-95, 2010
2. Caridi G et al: Clinical features and long-term outcome of nephrotic syndrome associated with heterozygous NPHS1 and NPHS2 mutations. Clin J Am Soc Nephrol. 4(6):1065-72, 2009
3. Machuca E et al: Clinical and epidemiological assessment of steroid-resistant nephrotic syndrome associated with the NPHS2 R229Q variant. Kidney Int. 75(7):727-35, 2009
4. Hinkes B et al: Specific podocin mutations correlate with age of onset in steroid-resistant nephrotic syndrome. J Am Soc Nephrol. 19(2):365-71, 2008
5. Liapis H: Molecular pathology of nephrotic syndrome in childhood: a contemporary approach to diagnosis. Pediatr Dev Pathol. 11(4):154-63, 2008
6. Tonna SJ et al: NPHS2 variation in focal and segmental glomerulosclerosis. BMC Nephrol. 9:13, 2008
7. Hinkes BG et al: Nephrotic syndrome in the first year of life: two thirds of cases are caused by mutations in 4 genes (NPHS1, NPHS2, WT1, and LAMB2). Pediatrics. 119(4):e907-19, 2007
8. Franceschini N et al: NPHS2 gene, nephrotic syndrome and focal segmental glomerulosclerosis: a HuGE review. Genet Med. 8(2):63-75, 2006
9. Caridi G et al: NPHS2 (Podocin) mutations in nephrotic syndrome. Clinical spectrum and fine mechanisms. Pediatr Res. 57(5 Pt 2):54R-61R, 2005
10. Ruf RG et al: Patients with mutations in NPHS2 (podocin) do not respond to standard steroid treatment of nephrotic syndrome. J Am Soc Nephrol. 15(3):722-32, 2004
11. Tsukaguchi H et al: NPHS2 mutations in late-onset focal segmental glomerulosclerosis: R229Q is a common disease-associated allele. J Clin Invest. 110(11):1659-66, 2002
12. Boute N et al: NPHS2, encoding the glomerular protein podocin, is mutated in autosomal recessive steroid-resistant nephrotic syndrome. Nat Genet. 24(4):349-54, 2000

IMAGE GALLERY

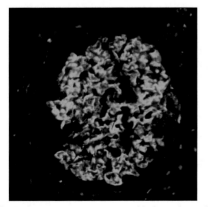 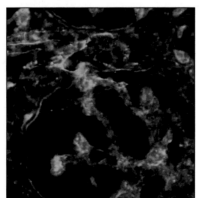 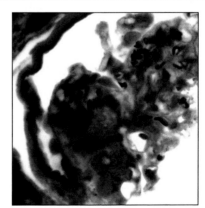

(Left) Podocin staining in a normal kidney shows linear capillary loop staining (FITC immunofluorescence). *(Center)* Decreased podocin staining in a biopsy specimen from a 10-year-old boy with persistent proteinuria is shown (FITC immunofluorescence). (Courtesy L. Barisoni-Thomas, MD.) *(Right)* Focal segmental glomerulosclerosis in 1 glomerulus is shown. (Courtesy L. Barisoni-Thomas, MD.)

ALPHA-ACTININ-4 DEFICIENCY

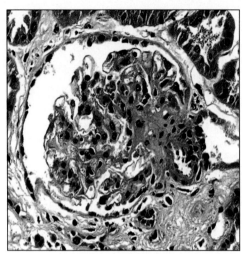

Renal biopsy from a 29-year-old woman with severe proteinuria, found to have an α-actinin-4 mutation, shows focal segmental glomerulosclerosis in the perihilar region. (Courtesy J. Henderson, MD, PhD.)

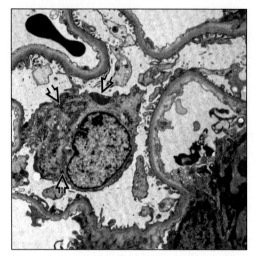

Segmental foot process effacement and podocyte lifting off the basement membrane are shown; note the electron densities in the podocyte cytoplasm ⊵.

TERMINOLOGY

Definitions
- Familial focal segmental glomerulosclerosis (FSGS) caused by *ACTN4* gene mutations

ETIOLOGY/PATHOGENESIS

Genetics
- *ACTN4*
  - Encodes α-actinin-4
    - Widely expressed actin binding protein
    - In kidney, α-actinin-4 is localized to podocyte, predominantly in foot processes
    - Mutations occur in exon 8
    - Mutations cause increased α-actinin-4 aggregation
    - Aggregates of α-actinin-4 may have direct toxic effects to podocytes, causing loss of α-actinin-4 function
  - Autosomal dominant inheritance
  - Maps to chromosome 19q13
  - Highly but not fully penetrant, thereby affecting disease severity

CLINICAL ISSUES

Epidemiology
- Incidence
  - Very rare
- Age
  - 16-56 years
  - Mild proteinuria may begin in teenage years
- Gender
  - M:F = 1:1

Presentation
- Subnephrotic-range proteinuria (most common)
- Nephrotic syndrome

- Hematuria (rare)

Prognosis
- Slowly progressive renal failure in some individuals

MICROSCOPIC PATHOLOGY

Histologic Features
- FSGS
- Perihilar segmental sclerosis is common
- Perihilar arteriolar hyalinosis
- Variable interstitial fibrosis and tubular atrophy
- Variable degrees of arteriosclerosis

Predominant Pattern/Injury Type
- Glomerulosclerosis, focal, segmental

Predominant Cell/Compartment Type
- Podocyte

ANCILLARY TESTS

Molecular Genetics
- Sequencing exon 8 of *ACTN4* gene

Electron Microscopy
- Transmission
  - Segmental podocyte foot process effacement
  - Microvillous degeneration of podocytes
  - Podocyte cytoplasmic vacuolization
  - Electron-dense aggregates within podocyte cytoplasm
  - Vague mesangial electron-dense deposits
  - Segmental GBM thickening
  - Focal GBM duplication
  - Subendothelial edema
  - Closure of endothelial fenestrae

ALPHA-ACTININ-4 DEFICIENCY

Key Facts

Etiology/Pathogenesis

- Mutations in *ACTN4* gene encoding α-actinin-4
- Mutations cause increased α-actinin-4 aggregation and loss of normal function

Clinical Issues

- Commonly present with subnephrotic proteinuria

Microscopic Pathology

- Perihilar segmental sclerosis is common

- Arteriolar hyalinosis of perihilar arteriole

Ancillary Tests

- Electron microscopy
  - Podocyte electron-dense aggregates and segmental foot process effacement are characteristic
- Antibodies to α-actinin-4 show decreased glomerular capillary staining

Top Differential Diagnoses

- Primary FSGS, secondary FSGS

DIFFERENTIAL DIAGNOSIS

Primary (Idiopathic Nonhereditary) FSGS

- Extensive podocyte foot process effacement
- Lack of podocyte electron-dense aggregates
- α-actinin-4 expression is normal

Other Inherited Forms of FSGS

- Includes inherited mutations in *WT1*, *NPHS1*, *NPHS2*, *LAMB2*, *PLCE1*, *TRPC6*, and *CD2AP*
- Segmental podocyte foot process effacement
- Lack of podocyte electron-dense aggregates
- α-actinin-4 expression is normal

FSGS Secondary to Hypertension

- Prominent arteriolar hyalinosis
- Prominent arteriosclerosis
- Segmental podocyte foot process effacement affecting < 50% of total glomerular surface area
- Lack of podocyte electron-dense aggregates
- α-actinin-4 expression is normal

SELECTED REFERENCES

1. Henderson JM et al: Patients with ACTN4 mutations demonstrate distinctive features of glomerular injury. J Am Soc Nephrol. 20(5):961-8, 2009
2. Choi HJ et al: Familial focal segmental glomerulosclerosis associated with an ACTN4 mutation and paternal germline mosaicism. Am J Kidney Dis. 51(5):834-8, 2008
3. Lee SH et al: Crystal structure of the actin-binding domain of alpha-actinin-4 Lys255Glu mutant implicated in focal segmental glomerulosclerosis. J Mol Biol. 376(2):317-24, 2008
4. Michaud JL et al: FSGS-associated alpha-actinin-4 (K256E) impairs cytoskeletal dynamics in podocytes. Kidney Int. 70(6):1054-61, 2006
5. Weins A et al: Mutational and Biological Analysis of alpha-actinin-4 in focal segmental glomerulosclerosis. J Am Soc Nephrol. 16(12):3694-701, 2005
6. Yao J et al: Alpha-actinin-4-mediated FSGS: an inherited kidney disease caused by an aggregated and rapidly degraded cytoskeletal protein. PLoS Biol. 2(6):e167, 2004
7. Kos CH et al: Mice deficient in alpha-actinin-4 have severe glomerular disease. J Clin Invest. 111(11):1683-90, 2003
8. Michaud JL et al: Focal and segmental glomerulosclerosis in mice with podocyte-specific expression of mutant alpha-actinin-4. J Am Soc Nephrol. 14(5):1200-11, 2003
9. Kaplan JM et al: Mutations in ACTN4, encoding alpha-actinin-4, cause familial focal segmental glomerulosclerosis. Nat Genet. 24(3):251-6, 2000

IMAGE GALLERY

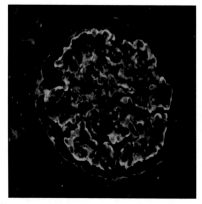 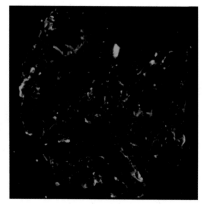 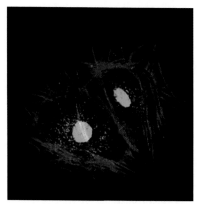

(Left) Actinin-4 staining in a normal glomerulus is shown. (Courtesy J. Henderson, MD, PhD.) *(Center)* Biopsy from a patient with ACTN4 gene mutation shows decreased, irregular, granular staining of the glomerular capillaries. (Courtesy J. Henderson, MD, PhD.) *(Right)* Cytoplasmic actin (red) in normal cultured podocytes demonstrates the actin cytoskeleton. WT1 staining (green) highlights podocyte nuclei. (Courtesy S. Akilesh, MD.)

DIFFUSE MESANGIAL SCLEROSIS

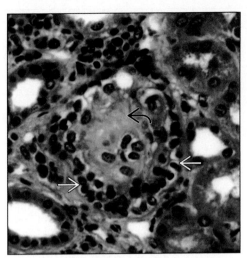

Classic late diffuse mesangial sclerosis (DMS) shows replacement of the mesangium with matrix ➡ and podocyte proliferation forming a pseudocrescent ➡.

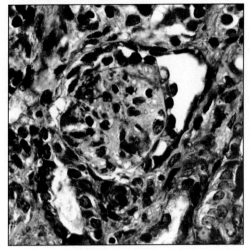

In DMS, the trichrome stain highlights mesangial collagen deposition and reveals the absence of capillary loops.

TERMINOLOGY

Abbreviations
- Diffuse mesangial sclerosis (DMS)

Definitions
- Glomerular disease early in life with characteristic mesangial accumulation of extracellular matrix and podocyte proliferation
  - Although most cases are idiopathic, a subset are caused by a variety of genetic and other factors

ETIOLOGY/PATHOGENESIS

Genetic Factors
- *WT1*
  - Encodes Wilms tumor-1
    - Zinc finger transcription factor involved in regulating cellular proliferation and gonad and podocyte differentiation
  - Maps to chromosome 11p13
  - Mutations in exons 8 and 9 are occasionally associated with sporadic DMS
  - Exon 9 mutations typical of Denys-Drash syndrome
    - Hotspot in exon 9 R394W/Q/L
  - Intron 9 mutations typical of Frasier syndrome
- *PLCE-1*
  - Encodes phospholipase C enzyme (PLCϵ1) on chromosome 10q
  - Truncating mutations are associated with DMS
  - Nontruncating missense mutations are associated with FSGS
  - Inherited in autosomal recessive pattern
- Gallaway-Mowat syndrome
- Type 1 carbohydrate-deficient glycoprotein syndrome
- Laminin-β2 mutations (Pierson syndrome)

Infectious Agents
- Cytomegalovirus

  - DMS associated with cytomegalic inclusion bodies described in newborn with congenital nephrotic syndrome

CLINICAL ISSUES

Presentation
- Nephrotic syndrome
  - Steroid resistant
  - < 2 years of age but may be as late as 4 years

Laboratory Tests
- α-fetoprotein may be elevated

Treatment
- Surgical approaches
  - Bilateral nephrectomy may be required to prevent massive protein loss or in the event of poorly controlled hypertension
  - Renal transplantation is considered once patient's weight is > 8 kg
- Drugs
  - IVIG, ACE inhibitors, corticosteroids, cyclosporine
  - Ganciclovir has proven effective in DMS associated with Cytomegalovirus

Prognosis
- Typically progresses to ESRD within 3 years
- Children without identified mutations have milder clinical course
- Post-transplant recurrence of DMS has not been described

MICROSCOPIC PATHOLOGY

Histologic Features
- Early glomerular changes

DIFFUSE MESANGIAL SCLEROSIS

Key Facts

Terminology
- Diffuse mesangial sclerosis

Etiology/Pathogenesis
- *WT1* mutations (Denys-Drash or Frasier syndromes)
- Laminin β2 mutations (Pierson syndrome)
- Idiopathic

Clinical Issues
- Progression to ESRD in 3 years
- Presents early in life, usually under 2 years of age
- Slower progression to ESRD if no mutation is identified

Microscopic Pathology
- Early glomerular changes resemble fetal glomeruli

- Late glomerular changes consist of replacement of mesangium by fibrillar matrix and mesangial consolidation
- Pseudocrescents
- Tubules dilated with hyaline casts

Ancillary Tests
- Gene sequencing of *WT1*, *PLCE1*, and *LAMB2* genes
- Karyotyping to rule out male pseudohermaphroditism (Frasier syndrome)

Top Differential Diagnoses
- Denys-Drash syndrome
- Frasier syndrome
- Pierson syndrome

- o Prominent, closely spaced podocytes that create fetal (immature)-looking glomeruli without mesangial sclerosis
- o Pseudocrescents composed of proliferating visceral podocytes and parietal epithelial cells
- Early tubular changes
  - o May be dilated with hyaline casts secondary to heavy proteinuria
- Late glomerular changes
  - o Mesangial consolidation
  - o Fibrillar mesangial matrix increase

ANCILLARY TESTS

Immunofluorescence
- IgM, C1, and C3 may all stain sclerotic mesangial areas

Cytogenetics
- Karyotyping to rule out male pseudohermaphroditism

Molecular Genetics
- *WT1*, *PLCE1*, and *LAMB2* gene mutation analysis

Electron Microscopy
- Transmission
  - o Podocyte proliferation
  - o Increased mesangial matrix
  - o Wide, lamellated GBM

DIFFERENTIAL DIAGNOSIS

Denys-Drash Syndrome
- Patients with male gonad dysgenesis
- Autosomal dominant mutations in *WT1* exon 9
- Association with Wilms tumor and gonadoblastoma

Frasier Syndrome
- DMS or FSGS associated with *WT1* intron 9 mutations
- Male pseudohermaphroditism

Pierson Syndrome
- Patients have ocular abnormalities (microcoria)

- DMS associated with *LAMB2* mutations
- Autosomal recessive

DIAGNOSTIC CHECKLIST

Pathologic Interpretation Pearls
- Fetal-appearing glomeruli
- Solidified glomerular mesangium

SELECTED REFERENCES

1. Nso Roca AP et al: Evolutive study of children with diffuse mesangial sclerosis. Pediatr Nephrol. 24(5):1013-9, 2009
2. Gbadegesin R et al: Mutations in PLCE1 are a major cause of isolated diffuse mesangial sclerosis (IDMS). Nephrol Dial Transplant. 23(4):1291-7, 2008
3. Liapis H: Molecular pathology of nephrotic syndrome in childhood: a contemporary approach to diagnosis. Pediatr Dev Pathol. 11(4):154-63, 2008
4. Hinkes BG et al: Nephrotic syndrome in the first year of life: two thirds of cases are caused by mutations in 4 genes (NPHS1, NPHS2, WT1, and LAMB2). Pediatrics. 119(4):e907-19, 2007
5. Besbas N et al: Cytomegalovirus-related congenital nephrotic syndrome with diffuse mesangial sclerosis. Pediatr Nephrol. 21(5):740-2, 2006
6. Hinkes B et al: Positional cloning uncovers mutations in PLCE1 responsible for a nephrotic syndrome variant that may be reversible. Nat Genet. 38(12):1397-405, 2006
7. Niaudet P et al: WT1 and glomerular diseases. Pediatr Nephrol. 21(11):1653-60, 2006
8. Jeanpierre C et al: Identification of constitutional WT1 mutations, in patients with isolated diffuse mesangial sclerosis, and analysis of genotype/phenotype correlations by use of a computerized mutation database. Am J Hum Genet. 62(4):824-33, 1998
9. Habib R et al: Diffuse mesangial sclerosis: a congenital glomerulopathy with nephrotic syndrome. Adv Nephrol Necker Hosp. 22:43-57, 1993

DIFFUSE MESANGIAL SCLEROSIS

Microscopic Features

(Left) H&E shows early DMS with mesangial hypercellularity and closure of capillary lumens (ball-like glomeruli). Podocyte proliferation is also apparent. The pattern has some resemblance to collapsing glomerulopathy. *(Right)* WT1 stains podocyte nuclei ➢ in a case of early stage DMS, in contrast to collapsing glomerulopathy, which is WT1 negative.

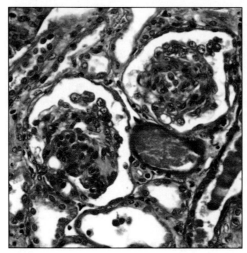
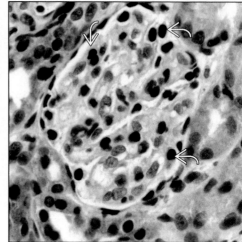

(Left) Occasionally, DMS is mistaken for crescentic glomerulonephritis. In this example, the majority of glomeruli contained pseudocrescents composed of proliferating podocytes. Unlike true crescents, pseudocrescents do not contain fibrin or inflammatory cells. *(Right)* WT1 stain of a case of DMS demonstrates that the majority of proliferating cells in this pseudocrescent are podocytes, in contrast to the crescents of parietal epithelium in glomerulonephritis.

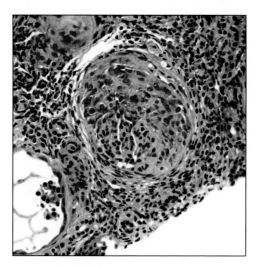
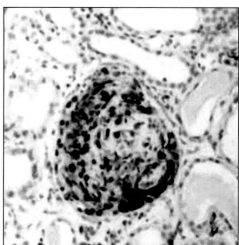

(Left) Advanced DMS with lobular-appearing glomeruli is shown. Note the increased fibrillar mesangial matrix and closure of the capillary lumens. *(Right)* The collagenous nature of the mesangial sclerosis is revealed with trichrome stain, as well as the hypercellular crowded podocytes ➢ and loss of glomerular capillaries.

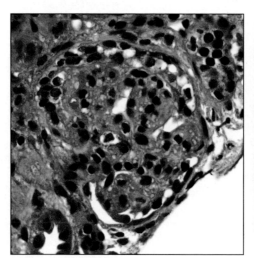
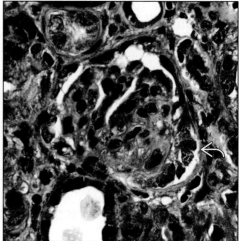

DIFFUSE MESANGIAL SCLEROSIS

Ancillary Techniques

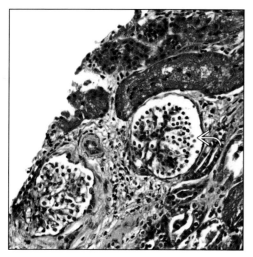
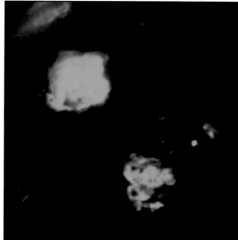

(Left) Early DMS is characterized by prominent podocytes, giving the glomeruli a fetal appearance ➡. *(Right)* Immunofluorescence for laminin β2 shows diffuse glomerular capillary loop staining in a biopsy from a patient with DMS. These findings rule out typical Pierson syndrome in which laminin β2 is absent.

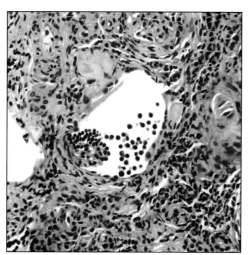
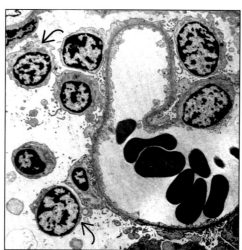

(Left) Advanced DMS demonstrates podocyte proliferation with detachment of podocytes into Bowman space and retraction of the capillary tuft. *(Right)* This electron micrograph is from a case that showed podocyte proliferation with detachment of podocytes into Bowman space ➡ and retraction of the capillary tuft. The closely spaced proliferating podocytes can be seen detached from the GBM, which is a sign of heavy proteinuria.

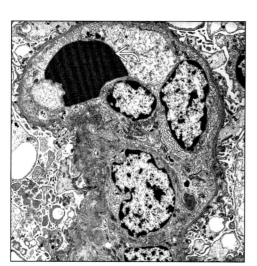
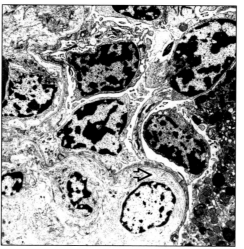

(Left) Electron microscopy shows DMS glomeruli with mesangial matrix increase, foot process effacement, and GBM multilamination. The latter resembles Alport syndrome, which must be excluded. A red blood cell is in a glomerular capillary ➡, which is bounded by reactive endothelial cells. *(Right)* Podocytes appear crowded. Segmental GBM multilamination is a constant feature of DMS ➡. The glomerular capillaries are not evident.

DENYS-DRASH SYNDROME

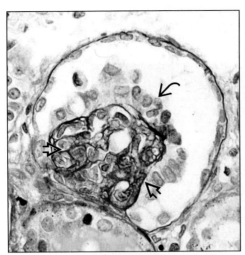

This glomerulus in a 3-month-old with DDS and DMS shows an abnormally developed glomerulus with expanded mesangial matrix ➢, capillary loop obliteration, and epithelial cell hyperplasia ➢.

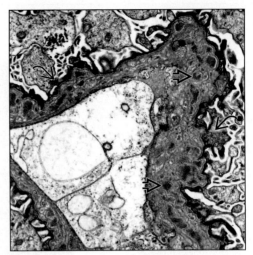

Electron microscopy in Denys-Drash syndrome reveals podocyte foot process effacement ➢. The GBM is markedly thickened and multilayered with deposition of electron-dense ➢ material.

TERMINOLOGY

Abbreviations
- Denys-Drash syndrome (DDS)

Definitions
- Triad syndrome due to *WT1* mutation
  - Male pseudohermaphroditism
  - Progressive nephropathy due to diffuse mesangial sclerosis (DMS)
  - Risk of Wilms tumor (WT)
- Incomplete forms occur
  - Nephropathy is the 1 constant component
    - Nephropathy and Wilms tumor
    - Nephropathy and male pseudohermaphroditism

ETIOLOGY/PATHOGENESIS

Genetic Factors
- Autosomal dominant
- *WT1* mutation
  - Encodes for WT1 protein
    - Transcription factor involved in regulating podocyte proliferation and differentiation
  - Maps to chromosome 11p13
  - Mutations in exon 9
    - Hotspot in exon 9 common in DDS R394W/Q/L

CLINICAL ISSUES

Presentation
- Steroid-resistant nephrotic syndrome
  - Onset usually before age 2
- Ambiguous genitalia with XY karyotype
  - Up to 40% phenotypically female
- Wilms tumor
  - Age at diagnosis less than in sporadic WT
    - Mean: 13.5 months; median: 9 months
  - More often bilateral than in sporadic WT
    - 30% in DDS compared with 5% in sporadic WT
  - Nephrogenic rests more common than in sporadic WT
    - 80% in DDS compared with 25% in sporadic WT

Laboratory Tests
- Gene sequencing of *WT1* gene

Treatment
- Wilms tumor associated with DDS
  - Chemotherapy
  - Bilateral nephrectomy with unilateral WT and end-stage renal disease (ESRD)
  - Nephron-sparing surgery with bilateral disease
- Renal transplantation for ESRD or bilateral nephrectomy

Prognosis
- DMS rapid progression to ESRD in 2-3 years
- WT outcomes similar to sporadic WT

MICROSCOPIC PATHOLOGY

Histologic Features
- Glomeruli: Diffuse mesangial sclerosis
  - Early glomerular changes
    - Immature glomerulus with closely spaced podocytes
    - Hyperplastic podocytes and parietal epithelial cells
    - Mesangial matrix increase
    - Mesangial hypercellularity
  - Late glomerular changes
    - Glomerulosclerosis
    - Thickened capillary loops
    - Mesangial matrix increase with hypercellularity
    - Hyperplastic podocytes and parietal epithelial cells
    - Segmental capsular adhesions
- Tubules
  - Early tubular changes

DENYS-DRASH SYNDROME

Key Facts

Terminology
- Triad syndrome
  - Male pseudohermaphroditism
  - Steroid-resistant nephrotic syndrome due to DMS
  - Risk of Wilms tumor (WT)

Etiology/Pathogenesis
- *WT1* exon 9 mutations

Clinical Issues
- Rapid progression to ESRD in 2-3 years
- Wilms tumor at early age, often bilateral

Microscopic Pathology
- Diffuse mesangial sclerosis

Ancillary Tests
- Gene sequencing for *WT1* mutation

- Distinctive GBM ultrastructural abnormalities
  - Thickened and multilayered GBM
  - Electron-dense and lucent foci

Top Differential Diagnoses
- Sporadic DMS
  - Consider incomplete DDS
  - Risk of WT
- Sporadic Wilms tumor
  - Consider incomplete form of DDS
  - Examine nonneoplastic cortex
- Frasier syndrome
  - Develop FSGS rather than DMS
  - Risk of gonadoblastoma rather than WT
- Pierson syndrome
  - Diffuse mesangial sclerosis or fetal-appearing glomeruli

- Tubular ectasia
  - Late tubular changes
    - Tubular atrophy and interstitial fibrosis

ANCILLARY TESTS

Electron Microscopy
- GBM irregularly thickened and multilayered
- GBM lucent foci &/or electron-dense material
- Diffuse podocyte foot process effacement
- Mesangial matrix increase with hypercellularity

DIFFERENTIAL DIAGNOSIS

Sporadic DMS
- Must always consider incomplete forms of DDS
  - Risk of Wilms tumor
- Resembles collapsing glomerulopathy
  - GBM is ultrastructurally normal

Sporadic Wilms Tumors
- Must always consider incomplete form of DDS
  - Examine nonneoplastic kidney for DMS

Frasier Syndrome
- Normal female external genitalia
  - Streak gonads and XY karyotype
- Focal segmental glomerulosclerosis on renal biopsy
- *WT1* mutations in donor splice site of intron 9
  - Rarely, mutation in exons 8 and 9, as in DDS
- Risk of gonadoblastoma
- Autosomal dominant

Pierson Syndrome
- Ocular abnormalities (microcoria)
- Diffuse mesangial sclerosis or fetal glomeruli on renal biopsy
- Mutations in the *LAMB2* gene
- Autosomal recessive

DIAGNOSTIC CHECKLIST

Pathologic Interpretation Pearls
- DMS on biopsy prompts consideration of syndromic diseases

SELECTED REFERENCES
1. Nso Roca AP et al: Evolutive study of children with diffuse mesangial sclerosis. Pediatr Nephrol. 24(5):1013-9, 2009
2. Ismaili K et al: WT1 gene mutations in three girls with nephrotic syndrome. Eur J Pediatr. 167(5):579-81, 2008
3. Aucella F et al: WT1 mutations in nephrotic syndrome revisited. High prevalence in young girls, associations and renal phenotypes. Pediatr Nephrol. 21(10):1393-8, 2006
4. Niaudet P et al: WT1 and glomerular diseases. Pediatr Nephrol. 21(11):1653-60, 2006
5. Yang AH et al: The dysregulated glomerular cell growth in Denys-Drash syndrome. Virchows Arch. 445(3):305-14, 2004
6. Fukuzawa R et al: A necropsy case of Denys-Drash syndrome with a WT1 mutation in exon 7. J Med Genet. 39(8):e48, 2002
7. Natoli TA et al: A mutant form of the Wilms' tumor suppressor gene WT1 observed in Denys-Drash syndrome interferes with glomerular capillary development. J Am Soc Nephrol. 13(8):2058-67, 2002
8. Cetinkaya E et al: Association of partial gonadal dysgenesis, nephropathy and WT1 gene mutation without Wilms' tumor: incomplete Denys-Drash syndrome. J Pediatr Endocrinol Metab. 14(5):561-4, 2001
9. McTaggart SJ et al: Clinical spectrum of Denys-Drash and Frasier syndrome. Pediatr Nephrol. 16(4):335-9, 2001
10. Breslow NE et al: Renal failure in the Denys-Drash and Wilms' tumor-aniridia syndromes. Cancer Res. 60(15):4030-2, 2000
11. Yang Y et al: WT1 and PAX-2 podocyte expression in Denys-Drash syndrome and isolated diffuse mesangial sclerosis. Am J Pathol. 154(1):181-92, 1999
12. Schumacher V et al: Spectrum of early onset nephrotic syndrome associated with WT1 missense mutations. Kidney Int. 53(6):1594-600, 1998
13. Mueller RF: The Denys-Drash syndrome. J Med Genet. 31(6):471-7, 1994

DENYS-DRASH SYNDROME

10 Day Old and 2 Week Old with DDS

(Left) Biopsy in a 10-day-old infant with DDS is shown. There is end-stage diffuse mesangial sclerosis with adjacent interstitial fibrosis. The entire glomerular tufts are consolidated with clusters of central mesangial cells ➡ and no discernible glomerular capillaries. *(Right)* This sclerotic glomerulus from the 10-day-old infant with DDS shows abundant mesangial matrix and mesangial cells ➡. Capsular adhesions are not present, distinguishing this from focal segmental glomerulosclerosis.

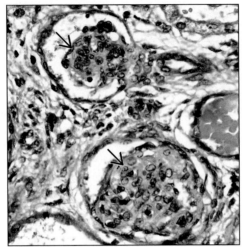
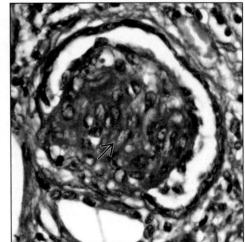

(Left) This glomerulus from the 10-day-old infant with DDS shows prominent epithelial proliferation ➡ in association with the glomerular obliteration from diffuse mesangial sclerosis. The pattern resembles collapsing glomerulopathy. *(Right)* Biopsy from a 2-week-old infant with Denys-Drash syndrome is shown. There is tubular cell attenuation imparting the impression of tubular ectasia ➡. In addition to glomerulosclerosis ➡, there is extensive interstitial fibrosis with mild nonspecific inflammation.

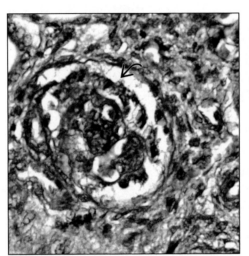
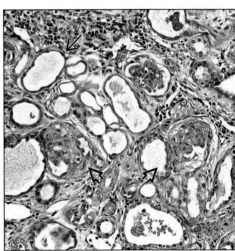

(Left) This glomerulus from the 2-week-old infant with DDS shows central mesangial hypercellularity ➡. The capillary loops are difficult to resolve, and mild epithelial cell proliferation and hypertrophy are present ➡. *(Right)* This last glomerulus from the 2-week-old infant with DDS shows capillary loop obliteration and prominent epithelial proliferation ➡. Despite the degree of sclerosis, capsular adhesions are not present, distinguishing this from focal segmental glomerulosclerosis.

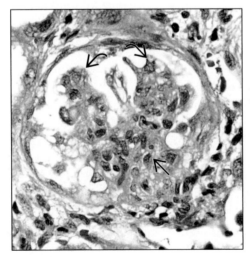
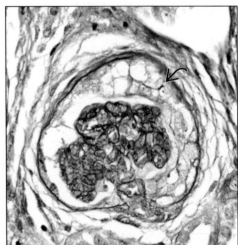

DENYS-DRASH SYNDROME

3 Month Old and 1 Year Old with DDS

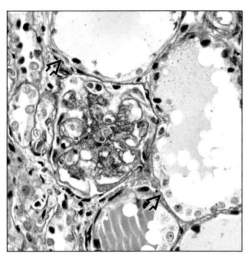
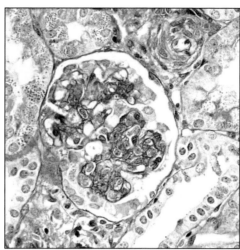

(Left) Biopsy from a 3-month-old infant with DDS is shown. This glomerulus is small and shows mesangial matrix increase with capillary loop irregularity. The adjacent tubules show ectasia ⇒ and cell attenuation. (Right) This glomerulus from a 3-month-old with DDS shows residual capillary loops associated with mesangial cell and matrix increase and epithelial cell proliferation. The cellularity could suggest immune complex disease, but immunofluorescence studies were negative.

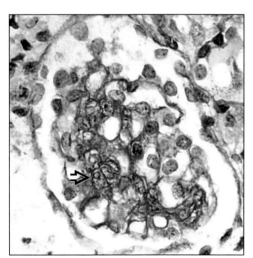
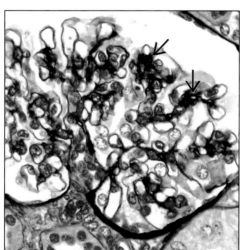

(Left) This glomerulus in DDS appears small with extensive mesangial matrix increase and mild hypercellularity ⇒. (Right) A range of glomerular changes can be seen in a single biopsy in DDS, as illustrated in a biopsy from a 1 year old. This glomerulus has only mild mesangial matrix increase ⇒ and would be regarded as minimal change disease (MCD) if the findings of diffuse mesangial sclerosis and podocyte hyperplasia were not also present in other glomeruli.

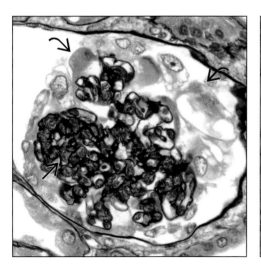
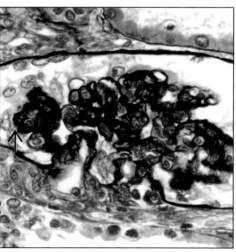

(Left) This glomerulus in a 1 year old with DDS has an impressive mesangial matrix increase ⇒ with numerous mesangial cells. There is also capillary loop obliteration and impressive large vacuolated epithelial cells ⇒ enveloping the glomerular tufts. Other glomeruli resembled MCD. (Right) A markedly abnormal glomerulus has extensive capillary loop obliteration ⇒. This section is from the same biopsy in a 1 year old with DDS that showed MCD-like changes in other glomeruli.

DENYS-DRASH SYNDROME

Biopsy at 2 Years and Nephrectomy at 7 Years

(Left) Biopsy from a 2 year old with DDS shows a dimorphic glomerular population. One glomerulus is small and immature appearing ➡. The 2 larger glomeruli appear more mature. *(Right)* Biopsy from a 2 year old with DDS shows ectatic tubules and that the glomerulus has epithelial cell hypertrophy with protein resorption droplets ➡. The immature glomeruli elsewhere in this biopsy and these tubular changes prompt consideration of Finnish-type congenital nephrotic syndrome.

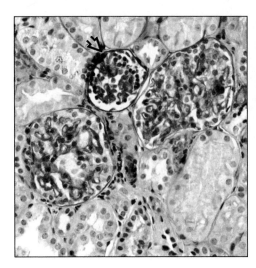
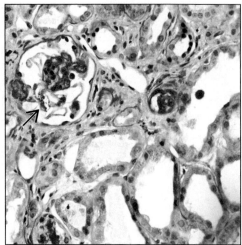

(Left) In a 2 year old with DDS, this glomerulus has mesangial matrix increase ➡, hypercellularity, and a capsular adhesion ➡. The GBM has widespread thickening ➡ and irregularity. Podocytes have protein resorption droplets ➡. *(Right)* In a 2 year old with DDS, this glomerulus shows segmental mesangial matrix increase ➡ and mild hypercellularity with exuberant epithelial proliferation ➡ overlying the sclerotic portion. The remainder of the glomerulus is minimally affected.

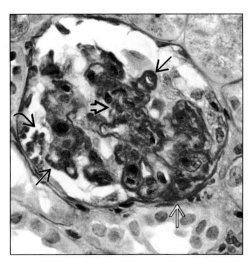
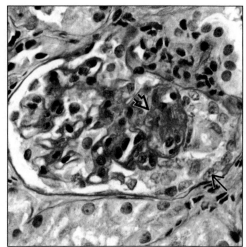

(Left) This section is from a nephrectomy performed for florid nephrotic syndrome prior to transplant in a 7 year old with DDS. There is advanced nephrosclerosis. Biopsy at age 2 showed DMS. *(Right)* This nephrectomy specimen performed prior to transplant in a 7 year old with DDS shows persistent mesangial hypercellularity. The advanced sclerosis with hyaline deposits ➡ and capsular adhesions make recognition of underlying diffuse mesangial sclerosis as the primary disease difficult to recognize.

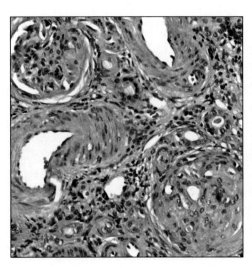
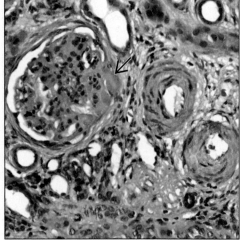

DENYS-DRASH SYNDROME

Electron Microscopy

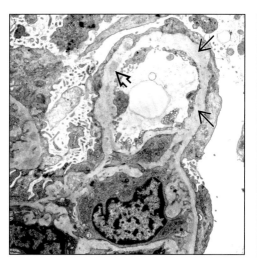

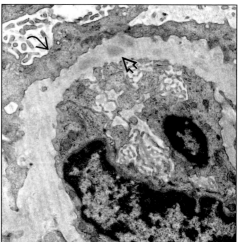

(Left) This electron micrograph from a 2 year old with Denys-Drash syndrome shows diffuse podocyte foot process effacement. There is prominent irregularity and thickening of the capillary loop basement membrane (GBM) ➡, which contains electron-dense deposits ➡. *(Right)* This glomerular capillary loop shows diffuse podocyte foot process effacement ➡. There is marked thickening and irregularity of the GBM with small deposition of electron-dense material ➡.

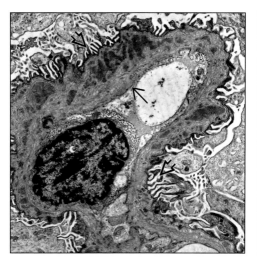

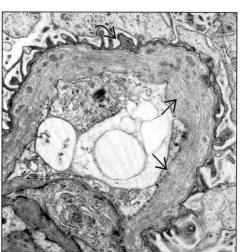

(Left) This electron micrograph shows marked GBM irregularity ➡. It is heavily embedded with electron-dense material not regarded as immune deposits. Although there is segmental effacement podocyte of foot processes, some foot processes are intact ➡. *(Right)* This electron micrograph shows podocyte foot process effacement ➡. The thickened capillary loop GBM is lamellated ➡ and strongly resembles alterations that occur in Alport hereditary nephritis.

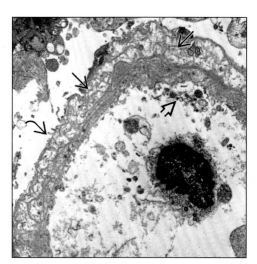

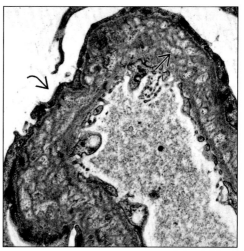

(Left) This electron micrograph shows a complex reticulated and multilayered ➡ alteration of the capillary loop basement membrane with numerous lucent foci. The endothelial ➡ and epithelial ➡ cells show marked artifactual autolysis. *(Right)* This electron micrograph from a case of DDS shows an extremely thickened and multilayered capillary loop basement membrane riddled with lucent foci ➡. There is complete podocyte foot process effacement ➡.

FRASIER SYNDROME

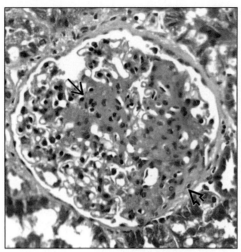

This is a renal biopsy from a 7-year-old patient with Frasier syndrome. It shows mesangial matrix expansion with mesangial hypercellularity ➔ and segmental sclerosis ➔. (Courtesy T. Cook, MD.)

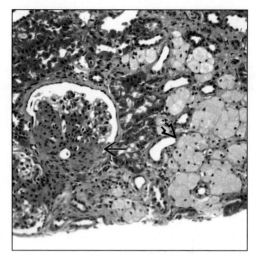

FS in a 13-year-old patient shows perihilar segmental sclerosis ➔ and generalized mesangial matrix increase. There are large collections of interstitial foam cells ➔. (Courtesy T. Cook, MD.)

TERMINOLOGY

Abbreviations
- Frasier syndrome (FS)

Definitions
- Triad syndrome due to mutations of *WT1* gene
  - Steroid-resistant nephrotic syndrome
  - Male pseudohermaphroditism
  - Risk of gonadoblastoma

ETIOLOGY/PATHOGENESIS

Genetic Factors
- Autosomal dominant
- *WT1* mutation 11p13
  - Encodes for Wilms tumor protein
    - Zinc transcription factor
    - Regulates cellular proliferation and podocyte differentiation
- Genotype-phenotype correlation
  - Mutations in donor splice site intron 9 (KTS)
    - Nephrotic syndrome, older, slower progression and no Wilms tumor compared to missense mutations
    - If XY, Frasier syndrome, risk of gonadoblastoma
    - If XX, isolated nephrotic syndrome
  - Rarely, mutation of exon 8 or 9
    - Typically seen in Denys-Drash syndrome
  - Missense mutations
    - Nephrotic syndrome, some Wilms tumors
  - Nonsense mutations
    - Wilms tumor

CLINICAL ISSUES

Presentation
- Infantile to young adult

- Usually from ages 2-6 years
- Steroid-resistant proteinuria or nephrotic syndrome
- Decreased renal function
- Male pseudohermaphroditism
  - Usually female with ambiguous phenotype
    - XY karyotype with streak gonads
    - Present with primary amenorrhea
  - FS may occur in phenotypic males
- XX karyotype patients have normal external genitalia
- Gonadoblastoma
- Rarely Wilms tumor, 2 reported cases

Laboratory Tests
- *WT1* gene sequencing
  - Mutations in donor splice site of intron 9
  - Rarely, DDS may present with intron 9 mutation
    - Clinical presentation distinguishes from DDS

Treatment
- Surgical approaches
  - Prophylactic gonadectomy to prevent gonadoblastoma
  - Nephron-sparing surgery in rare patients with Wilms tumor without ESRD
  - Renal transplant
    - Generally no recurrence; 1 case report of post-transplant proteinuria

Prognosis
- Slowly progressive renal disease
  - End-stage renal disease in 2nd to 3rd decade

MICROSCOPIC PATHOLOGY

Histologic Features
- Glomeruli
  - Normal, segmental or global sclerosis
  - Focal segmental glomerulosclerosis (FSGS)
    - Capillary loop collapse with capsular adhesion
    - Hyalinosis and lipid deposition

FRASIER SYNDROME

Key Facts

Terminology
- Triad syndrome
  - Steroid-resistant nephrotic syndrome
  - Male pseudohermaphroditism
  - Risk of gonadoblastoma

Etiology/Pathogenesis
- *WT1* mutations

Clinical Issues
- Autosomal dominant
- Steroid-resistant nephrotic syndrome
- Slow progression to ESRD
- Associated with gonadoblastoma
- Associated with male pseudohermaphroditism
  - Occurs in phenotypically normal males & females

Microscopic Pathology
- FSGS/minimal change disease

Ancillary Tests
- Sequencing of *WT1* gene
  - Intron 9 mutations

Top Differential Diagnoses
- Denys-Drash syndrome
  - Male pseudohermaphroditism
  - Risk of Wilms tumor
  - Diffuse mesangial sclerosis
- Pierson syndrome
  - Microcoria
  - Diffuse mesangial sclerosis
- Podocin deficiency
  - Focal segmental glomerulosclerosis

- Mesangial matrix increase
- Tubules and interstitium
  - Initially may appear normal
  - Tubular atrophy and interstitial fibrosis with progression
- Vessels
  - No specific features reported

ANCILLARY TESTS

Immunohistochemistry
- Decreased WT1 speckled staining reported, but limited experience

Immunofluorescence
- IgM, C3, light chains in segmental scars and hyalinosis
- IgG, IgA, C1q, and fibrinogen negative

Electron Microscopy
- Transmission
  - Glomerular basement membrane irregular thickening
  - Podocyte foot process effacement
  - Mesangial matrix expansion

DIFFERENTIAL DIAGNOSIS

Podocin Deficiency
- Autosomal recessive
- Mutations in podocin gene, *NPHS2*
  - Absent podocin by IHC
- Normal external genitalia and karyotype
- No neoplastic diathesis
- Variable age of onset depending upon mutation type
  - Ranges from < 3 months to 28 years

Pierson Syndrome
- Autosomal recessive
- Mutation of *LAMB2* encoding for laminin β2
- Normal karyotype and external genitalia
- Ocular abnormalities, usually microcoria

- No neoplastic diathesis
- Steroid-resistant nephrotic syndrome
  - Presents < 3 months to 10 years of age
  - Diffuse mesangial sclerosis on biopsy

Denys-Drash Syndrome
- Autosomal recessive
- Mutations in exons 8 and 9 of *WT1*
- Male pseudohermaphroditism
- Rapid clinical progression to ESRD
- Diffuse mesangial sclerosis on biopsy
- Risk of Wilms tumor

SELECTED REFERENCES

1. Benetti E et al: A novel WT1 gene mutation in a three-generation family with progressive isolated focal segmental glomerulosclerosis. Clin J Am Soc Nephrol. 5(4):698-702, 2010
2. Chernin G et al: Genotype/phenotype correlation in nephrotic syndrome caused by WT1 mutations. Clin J Am Soc Nephrol. 5(9):1655-62, 2010
3. Liapis H: Molecular pathology of nephrotic syndrome in childhood: a contemporary approach to diagnosis. Pediatr Dev Pathol. 11(4):154-63, 2008
4. Niaudet P et al: WT1 and glomerular diseases. Pediatr Nephrol. 21(11):1653-60, 2006
5. McTaggart SJ et al: Clinical spectrum of Denys-Drash and Frasier syndrome. Pediatr Nephrol. 16(4):335-9, 2001
6. Mrowka C et al: Wilms' tumor suppressor gene WT1: from structure to renal pathophysiologic features. J Am Soc Nephrol. 11 Suppl 16:S106-15, 2000
7. Koziell A et al: Frasier and Denys-Drash syndromes: different disorders or part of a spectrum? Arch Dis Child. 81(4):365-9, 1999
8. Klamt B et al: Frasier syndrome is caused by defective alternative splicing of WT1 leading to an altered ratio of WT1 +/-KTS splice isoforms. Hum Mol Genet. 7(4):709-14, 1998

Patient with 3 Sequential Biopsies

(Left) This biopsy of a 7-year-old patient with FS shows both normal ⇥ and segmentally sclerotic glomeruli ⇥. Focal tubular atrophy and interstitial fibrosis are also present ⇥. (Courtesy T. Cook, MD.) *(Right)* A 7 year old with podocyte foot process effacement ⇥ and segmental glomerular basement membrane attenuation ⇥ and thickening ⇥ is shown. The mesangium is normal ⇥. These changes are very similar to early stages of Alport syndrome. (Courtesy T. Cook, MD.)

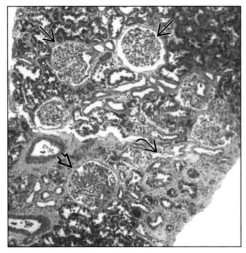
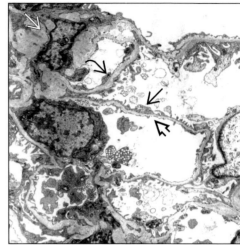

(Left) FS has diffuse podocyte foot process effacement with only a short segment of foot process preservation ⇥. The capillary loop basement membranes range from thin ⇥ to thickened ⇥ segments. (Courtesy T. Cook, MD.) *(Right)* This glomerulus in FS shows podocyte foot process effacement ⇥. The GBM is thin ⇥ in portions with other segments showing irregularity along the endothelial side ⇥. The mesangial matrix and mesangial cells ⇥ are normal. (Courtesy T. Cook, MD.)

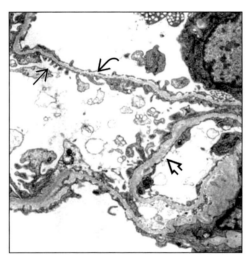
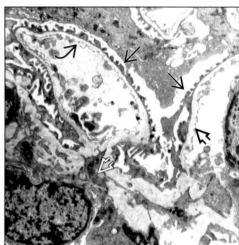

(Left) This 2nd biopsy was performed in an 11-year-old patient with FS. FSGS is evident ⇥. The sclerotic segment appears to be hilar in location. The 2nd glomerulus ⇥ appears normal. (Courtesy T. Cook, MD.) *(Right)* There is diffuse podocyte foot process effacement with a short segment of preservation ⇥. The mesangium is prominent. IF showed 1+ IgA, 2+ IgM and C1q deposition not typical of Frasier syndrome. Basement membrane irregularity is present ⇥. (Courtesy T. Cook, MD.)

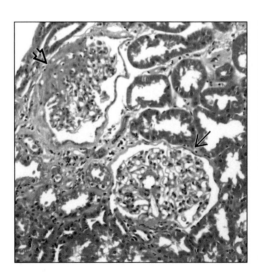
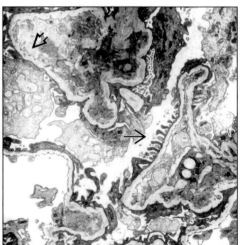

FRASIER SYNDROME

Patient with 3 Sequential Biopsies

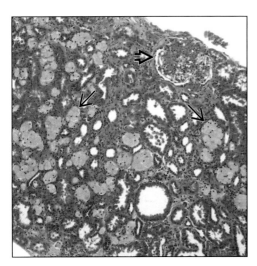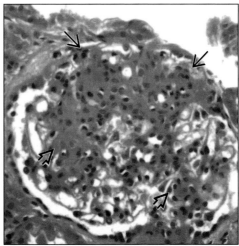

(Left) A biopsy obtained from a 13-year-old patient with FS shows persistent segmental sclerosis ➡. There are large numbers of interstitial foam cells ➡. Immunofluorescence showed no IgA, but IgM and C3 were present in areas of sclerosis. *(Courtesy T. Cook, MD.)* *(Right)* This glomerulus in FS shows prominent mesangial matrix increase ➡ with mild hypercellularity and segmental obliteration of capillary loops ➡. These are features typical of FSGS. *(Courtesy T. Cook, MD.)*

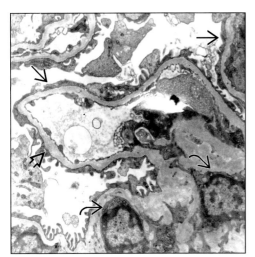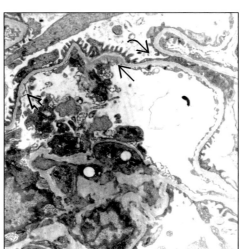

(Left) Note diffuse effacement of podocyte foot processes ➡. The mesangial matrix is increased, & 2 mesangial cells ➡ are visible in this portion of the mesangium. There is persistent mild irregularity in GBM thickness ➡. *(Courtesy T. Cook, MD.)* *(Right)* Note mild irregularity in capillary loop basement membrane thickness ➡ & loss of podocyte foot processes ➡. There is mild mesangial hypercellularity & a small amount of electron-dense hyaline ➡. *(Courtesy T. Cook, MD.)*

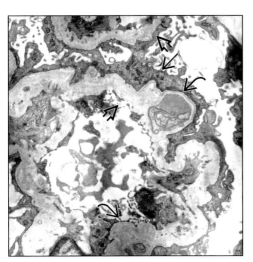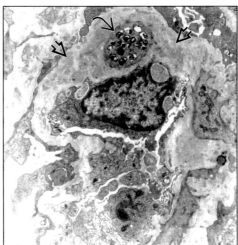

(Left) Note diffuse effacement of podocyte foot processes ➡ and marked irregular basement membrane thickening ➡. Electron-dense hyaline ➡ is also present within several paramesangial matrix areas. *(Courtesy T. Cook, MD.)* *(Right)* Diffuse effacement of podocyte foot processes is evident over mesangial areas. This portion of the glomerulus contains prominent mesangial hyaline deposition ➡. Mesangial cells contain intracellular lipochrome deposits ➡. *(Courtesy T. Cook, MD.)*

GLOMERULOPATHY OF HEREDITARY MULTIPLE EXOSTOSES

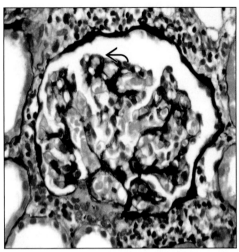

Renal biopsy from a 37-year-old woman with nephrotic-range proteinuria and hereditary multiple exostoses shows mild mesangial matrix increase and focal capillary loop thickening ➘. (Courtesy I. Roberts, MD.)

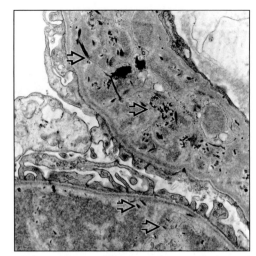

Fibrillar collagen deposits in lamina densa and subendothelial areas ➲ are characteristic of hereditary multiple exostoses involving the kidney. (Courtesy I. Roberts, MD.)

TERMINOLOGY

Abbreviations
- Hereditary multiple exostoses (HME)

Definitions
- Autosomal dominant inherited condition resulting in osteochondromas and abnormal glomerular collagen deposition secondary to mutations in *EXT1* gene

ETIOLOGY/PATHOGENESIS

Genetics
- 2 genes, *EXT1* and *EXT2*, account for 80% of cases of multiple exostoses
  - *EXT1* encodes protein exostosin-1
    - Localized to Golgi apparatus
    - Complex with gene product of EXT2 forms glycosyl transferase for heparin sulfate glycosaminoglycan synthesis
  - Frameshift mutation 238 del A in *EXT1*
  - Maps to chromosome 8q24.11-q24.13
- Autosomal dominant
- Exostoses deficient in heparan sulfate and perlecan and accumulate collagen I and X
  - Postulated to be a similar process in the glomerulus
- Response to steroids suggests that steroids facilitate alternative heparin sulfate synthesis

Pathophysiology
- Defective exostosin-1 results in deficient heparan sulfate glycosaminoglycans
- Heparan sulfate deficiency alters podocyte structure and function
- Mechanism leading to proteinuria and accumulation of collagen in glomerulus is unclear

CLINICAL ISSUES

Epidemiology
- Incidence
  - Very rare (5 cases, 1 family)
- Age
  - Hearing impairment in infancy
  - Osteochondromas develop in childhood
  - Renal symptoms develop in adulthood

Presentation
- Steroid-sensitive nephrotic syndrome
- Hearing abnormalities
- Multiple osteochondromas
  - Benign, metaphyseal, cartilage-capped bone tumors
  - Distal femur (90%)
  - Proximal tibia (84%)
  - Fibula (76%)
  - Humerus (72%)

Laboratory Tests
- Sequencing *EXT1* gene

Treatment
- Drugs
  - Steroids

Prognosis
- Steroids reported effective, but experience limited

MICROSCOPIC PATHOLOGY

Histologic Features
- Glomeruli
  - Mild mesangial hypercellularity
  - Mild increase in mesangial matrix
  - Focal capillary wall thickening
  - Pauci-immune pattern with crescents in 1 case
- Tubules, interstitium, and vessels
  - No specific changes described

GLOMERULOPATHY OF HEREDITARY MULTIPLE EXOSTOSES

Key Facts

Etiology/Pathogenesis
- *EXT1* gene mutations

Clinical Issues
- Steroid-sensitive nephrotic syndrome
- Osteochondromas

Microscopic Pathology
- Nonspecific changes

Ancillary Tests
- Electron microscopy
  - GBM and mesangial collagen fibril deposition
- Gene sequencing *EXT1* gene

Top Differential Diagnoses
- Nail-patella syndrome
- Collagen type III glomerulopathy
- Fibronectin glomerulopathy
- Fibrillary glomerulopathy

ANCILLARY TESTS

Immunofluorescence
- Negative IgG, IgA, IgM, C3, & C1q

Electron Microscopy
- Transmission
  - Diffuse mesangial fibrillar collagen deposition
  - GBM and mesangial collagen fibril deposition
    - Associated with focal GBM duplication and mesangial interposition
  - Moderate podocyte foot process effacement

DIFFERENTIAL DIAGNOSIS

Nail-Patella Syndrome
- Autosomal dominant inherited defect in *LMX1B* gene
- Presents with proteinuria ± hematuria
  - Nephrotic syndrome is atypical
- Mild glomerular changes
- Nail and bone abnormalities
- Irregular type III collagen within GBM
- Characteristic "moth-eaten" appearance of GBM

Collagen Type III Glomerulopathy
- Abundant subendothelial and mesangial collagen fibrils
- Collagen fibrils are curved, ~ 60 nm periodicity
- Autosomal recessive inheritance pattern

Fibronectin Glomerulopathy
- Lobular glomeruli, with expanded mesangial matrix
- 9-16 nm, granular, fibrillary electron-dense deposits

Fibrillary Glomerulopathy
- Random 10-30 nm fibrils in mesangium and GBM
- IgG and C3 in deposits

SELECTED REFERENCES

1. Jennes I et al: Multiple osteochondromas: mutation update and description of the multiple osteochondromas mutation database (MOdb). Hum Mutat. 30(12):1620-7, 2009
2. Chen S et al: Loss of heparan sulfate glycosaminoglycan assembly in podocytes does not lead to proteinuria. Kidney Int. 74(3):289-99, 2008
3. Nadanaka S et al: Heparan sulphate biosynthesis and disease. J Biochem. 144(1):7-14, 2008
4. Roberts IS et al: Familial nephropathy and multiple exostoses with exostosin-1 (EXT1) gene mutation. J Am Soc Nephrol. 19(3):450-3, 2008
5. McCormick C et al: The putative tumor suppressors EXT1 and EXT2 form a stable complex that accumulates in the Golgi apparatus and catalyzes the synthesis of heparan sulfate. Proc Natl Acad Sci U S A. 97(2):668-73, 2000
6. Kanwar YS et al: Increased permeability of the glomerular basement membrane to ferritin after removal of glycosaminoglycans (heparan sulfate) by enzyme digestion. J Cell Biol. 86(2):688-93, 1980

IMAGE GALLERY

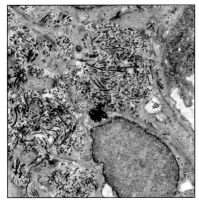 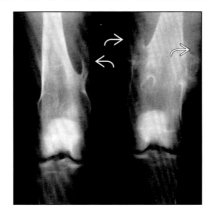 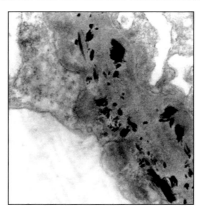

(Left) Mesangial and GBM fibrillar collagen deposits are shown from a biopsy of a 37-year-old woman with HME who presented with nephrotic syndrome. *(Courtesy I. Roberts, MD.)* *(Center)* Radiologic image shows multiple osteochondromas ➦ in the distal femurs of a 13-year-old girl with HME but no kidney manifestations. *(Courtesy M. Kyriakos, MD.)* *(Right)* This phosphotungstic acid stained section shows lamina densa collagen bundles characteristic of nail-patella syndrome.

TYPE III COLLAGEN GLOMERULOPATHY

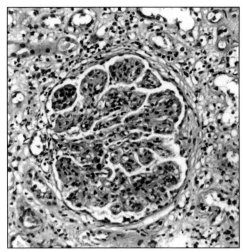

Type III collagen glomerulopathy has a varied glomerular pathology. In this particular case, the glomeruli are hypercellular with a lobular appearance. (Courtesy G. Herrera, MD.)

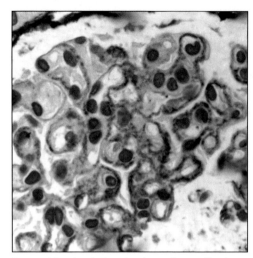

Immunohistochemical stain for collagen III shows deposits of collagen III in the GBM and mesangium in a case of type III collagen glomerulopathy. Normal glomeruli have no detectable collagen III.

TERMINOLOGY

Synonyms
- Collagenofibrotic glomerulopathy

Definitions
- Idiopathic glomerular disease defined by accumulation of mesangial and subendothelial type III collagen
- Initially described by Arakawa and colleagues in 1979

ETIOLOGY/PATHOGENESIS

Proposed Etiologies
- Probably systemic disease of collagen metabolism
  - Increased level of N-terminal procollagen type III in blood
    - Indicative of increased synthesis/catabolism
    - Deposit in glomeruli
    - Excreted in urine
- Occasional cases in siblings suggest a genetic component, as yet unidentified
- Some believe this is a primary disease of the glomerulus

CLINICAL ISSUES

Epidemiology
- Incidence
  - Rare (~ 0.1% of biopsies)
- Age
  - All ages
- Gender
  - M:F = 1:1
- Ethnicity
  - Majority of reported cases are Japanese
  - Cases also reported in USA, Europe, India, South America, China

Presentation
- Microhematuria
- Hypertension
- Edema
- Proteinuria, nephrotic range in 60%
- Anemia
  - Adults typically have anemia of chronic disease
  - Children occasionally present with thrombotic microangiopathy
- Hemolytic uremic syndrome, children

Laboratory Tests
- 10-100x increase in serum and urine N-terminal procollagen type III peptide (PIIINP)

Treatment
- Drugs
  - No specific treatment
  - Steroid therapy is reported to slow disease progression

Prognosis
- Variable disease course, limited data
  - ~ 35% of adults and ~ 90% of children progress to end-stage renal failure

MICROSCOPIC PATHOLOGY

Histologic Features
- Glomeruli
  - Lobular or mesangial hypercellularity, variable
    - Nodular pattern at times resembles diabetic glomerulopathy
  - Expansion of mesangium with eosinophilic, silver-positive material
  - Thickening of GBM
    - Occasional double contours
  - Closure of capillary loops
  - No inflammation
- No specific changes in tubules, interstitium, or vessels

TYPE III COLLAGEN GLOMERULOPATHY

Key Facts

Terminology
- Idiopathic glomerular disease defined by accumulation of mesangial and subendothelial type III collagen

Clinical Issues
- Rare (< 0.1% of biopsies)
- Presents with hematuria or proteinuria
- Hemolytic uremic syndrome, children
- Variable disease course
- Increased serum and urine procollagen III peptide

Microscopic Pathology
- Lobular glomeruli without inflammation
- Thickened capillary walls
- Mesangial and capillary wall expansion with eosinophilic, silver-positive material

Electron microscopy
- Mesangial and subendothelial curvilinear fibrils
- Fibers tend to be frayed and curved, ~ 60 nm periodicity
- Immunohistochemical staining for type III collagen positive in mesangium and GBM

Top Differential Diagnoses
- Nail-patella syndrome
- Hereditary multiple exostoses
- Fibronectin glomerulopathy
- Fibrillary glomerulopathy

Diagnostic Checklist
- Diagnosis made by demonstration of collagen III in glomeruli

---

ANCILLARY TESTS

Immunohistochemistry
- Staining for type III collagen identifies abnormal collagen in mesangium or GBM
  - Isolated case reports also had accumulation of collagen I or V
- Mesangial cells express α-smooth muscle actin

Immunofluorescence
- Focal segmental IgM and C3 along the GBM occasionally

Electron Microscopy
- Mesangial and subendothelial fibrillar deposits
  - Fibers tend to be frayed and curved
  - Best demonstrated using tannic acid-lead or phosphotungstic acid
  - Collagen fibers have characteristic periodicity (banded pattern) and measure 60 nm
  - Contrasts with fibrin, with 22 nm periodicity
- GBM lamina densa is of normal thickness
- Foot process effacement variable

DIFFERENTIAL DIAGNOSIS

Nail-Patella Syndrome
- Nail and bone abnormalities
- EM shows irregular type III collagen within GBM
- Characteristic "moth-eaten" appearance of GBM

Hereditary Multiple Exostoses
- Mesangial and subendothelial collagen deposition
- Multiple osteochondromas

Fibronectin Glomerulopathy
- Negative for collagen III in glomeruli
- Granular, fibrillary electron-dense deposits measuring 9-16 nm in diameter

Fibrillary Glomerulopathy
- Capillary wall and mesangium have smudgy to granular staining for IgG, C3, kappa, and lambda
- Random 10-30 nm fibrils in mesangium and capillary walls

DIAGNOSTIC CHECKLIST

Pathologic Interpretation Pearls
- Diagnosis made by demonstration of collagen III in glomeruli

SELECTED REFERENCES

1. Herrera GA et al: Renal diseases with organized deposits: an algorithmic approach to classification and clinicopathologic diagnosis. Arch Pathol Lab Med. 134(4):512-31, 2010
2. Khubchandani SR et al: Banded collagen in the kidney with special reference to collagenofibrotic glomerulopathy. Ultrastruct Pathol. 34(2):68-72, 2010
3. Ferreira RD et al: Collagenofibrotic glomerulopathy: three case reports in Brazil. Diagn Pathol. 4:33, 2009
4. Alchi B et al: Collagenofibrotic glomerulopathy: clinicopathologic overview of a rare glomerular disease. Am J Kidney Dis. 49(4):499-506, 2007
5. Iskandar SS et al: Glomerulopathies with organized deposits. Semin Diagn Pathol. 19(3):116-32, 2002
6. Yasuda T et al: Collagenofibrotic glomerulopathy: a systemic disease. Am J Kidney Dis. 33(1):123-7, 1999
7. Vogt BA et al: Inherited factor H deficiency and collagen type III glomerulopathy. Pediatr Nephrol. 9(1):11-5, 1995
8. Gubler MC et al: Collagen type III glomerulopathy: a new type of hereditary nephropathy. Pediatr Nephrol. 7(4):354-60, 1993
9. Imbasciati E et al: Collagen type III glomerulopathy: a new idiopathic glomerular disease. Am J Nephrol. 11(5):422-9, 1991
10. Arakawa M et al: [Idiopathic mesangio-degenerative glomerulopathy]. Jpn J Nephrol 21:914-5, 1979

TYPE III COLLAGEN GLOMERULOPATHY

Electron Microscopy

(Left) This example of type III collagen glomerulopathy demonstrates characteristic curvilinear fibrils of collagen in the mesangium ➡, GBM ➡, and the subendothelial space. *(Right)* Collagen fibrils are present in the glomerular capillary wall ➡ in this case of type III collagen glomerulopathy. There is also GBM duplication and mesangial cell interposition.

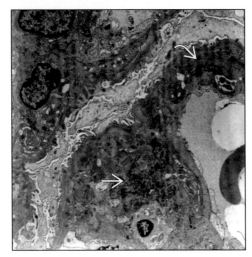 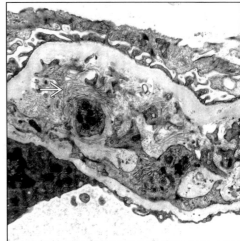

(Left) This specimen was stained with tannic acid-lead and processed for electron microscopy. The tannic acid highlights the randomly arranged, curved, and banded collagen fibers within the mesangium. *(Right)* Tannic acid-lead staining demonstrates subendothelial curved collagen fibers with banded cross striations measuring ~ 60 nm, typical of type III collagen glomerulopathy.

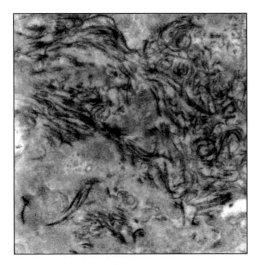 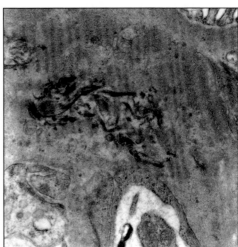

(Left) Patients with nail-patella syndrome, shown here, also have banded collagen III deposits in the GBM, but in contrast to type III collagen glomerulopathy, these are relatively focal and scarce and associated with a "moth-eaten" appearance of the GBM. *(Right)* In contrast to collagen III glomerulopathy, fibrillary glomerulopathy fibrils, illustrated here at high magnification, are randomly arranged and measure 15-25 nm in diameter.

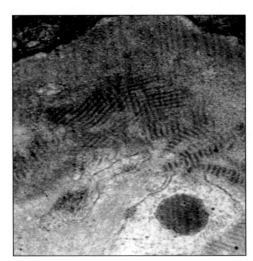 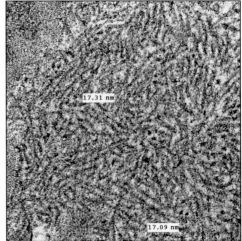

TYPE III COLLAGEN GLOMERULOPATHY

Immunohistochemistry and Special Stains

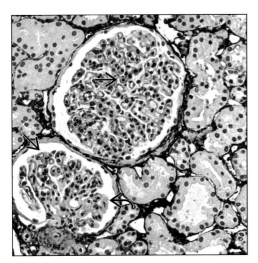
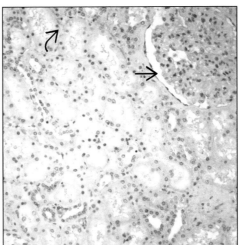

(Left) An immunohistochemical stain for collagen III (Biogenex MU167-UC) shows prominent GBM ➡ and mesangial deposits of collagen III. Some capillaries are negative ➡. The interstitium also stains, but this is a normal feature of interstitial fibrosis. *(Right)* In contrast, a normal kidney stained with antibody to collagen III shows no glomerular immunoreactivity ➡. Small amounts are, however, seen in the interstitium ➡.

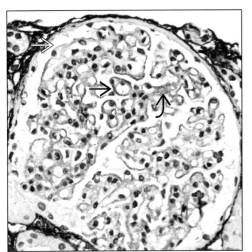
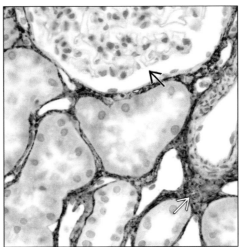

(Left) An immunohistochemical stain for collagen III shows prominent GBM ➡ and mesangial ➡ deposits of collagen III. Some capillaries are negative ➡. This case has little mesangial hypercellularity. *(Right)* This normal kidney (donor biopsy) was stained with an antibody to collagen III (Biogenex MU167-UC). No staining of the glomerulus ➡ is evident. Fine intertubular deposits are increased in the interstitium ➡.

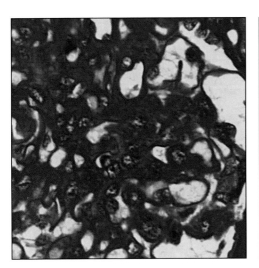
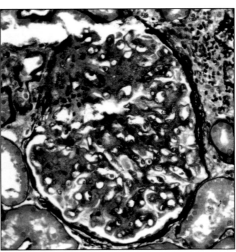

(Left) Picrosirius red, a fibrillar collagen stain, stains specifically collagen types I and III, which are birefringent when polarized. The increased mesangial matrix is highlighted in this case of type III collagen glomerulopathy. (Courtesy M. Antonia dos Reis, MD and R. Correa, MD.) *(Right)* Fibrillary GN, shown here, can resemble collagen III glomerulopathy by light microscopy but is readily distinguished by immunofluorescence since the deposits consist of IgG, not collagen (silver stain).

NAIL-PATELLA SYNDROME

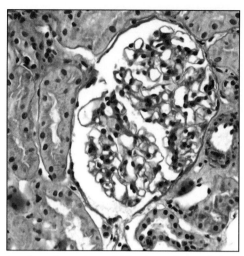

In nail-patella syndrome (NPS), glomeruli typically have minimal changes by light microscopy. The glomerulus illustrated has minimal mesangial hypercellularity.

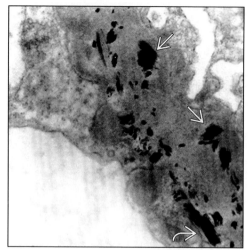

In NPS, phosphotungstic acid stain reveals electron-dense bundles of collagen fibrils ➡ in the GBM by electron microscopy. This stain helps visualize bundles and their ~ 60 nm periodicity ➡.

TERMINOLOGY

Abbreviations
- Nail-patella syndrome (NPS)

Synonyms
- Hereditary onychoosteodysplasia (HOOD) syndrome

Definitions
- Inherited syndrome presenting with nail, skeletal abnormalities, and proteinuria secondary to mutations in *LMX1B* gene

ETIOLOGY/PATHOGENESIS

Genetics
- Autosomal dominant inheritance
  - Variable phenotype
- *LMX1B* gene mutations
  - Maps to chromosome 9q34.1 (ABO linkage)
  - Encodes LIM homeodomain transcription factor critical for limb development
    - Expressed in podocytes
    - Regulates transcription of α3 and α4 type IV collagen, CD2AP, and podocin
    - Homeodomain region mutations associated with proteinuria

CLINICAL ISSUES

Epidemiology
- Incidence
  - Rare (~ 1/50,000)

Presentation
- Renal manifestations (30-60% of cases)
  - Proteinuria (~ 20%)
    - May develop nephrotic syndrome
  - Microscopic hematuria (~ 10%)

  - Hypertension
- Glaucoma, cataracts
- Hearing defects
- Renal artery aneurysms
- Hypoplastic, dystrophic, or absent nails (98% of cases)
- Small, irregularly shaped, or absent patella (74% of cases)
- Limited extension, pronation, and supination of elbow (70% of cases)
- Iliac horns (70% of cases)
  - Posterior, bilateral bony processes
  - Considered pathognomonic

Treatment
- No specific therapy
- Recurrent disease in transplant has not been reported
- Transplantation is not associated with anti-GBM disease

Prognosis
- ~ 10% of patients progress to end-stage renal disease

IMAGE FINDINGS

Radiographic Findings
- Absent or displaced patella
- Iliac horns
- Dysplasia of radial head

Ultrasonographic Findings
- Large iliac horns may be seen on fetal ultrasound in 3rd trimester

MICROSCOPIC PATHOLOGY

Histologic Features
- Glomeruli
  - May appear normal by light microscopy
  - May have focal thickening of capillary loops

NAIL-PATELLA SYNDROME

Key Facts

Etiology/Pathogenesis
- *LMX1B* mutations

Clinical Issues
- Iliac horns are pathognomonic (70% of cases)
- Absent, hypoplastic, or dystrophic nails
- Small, irregularly shaped, or absent patellae
- Proteinuria
- 10% progress to ESRD

Ancillary Tests
- Routine transmission electron microscopy sections stained with uranyl acetate show "moth-eaten" GBM
- Sequencing *LMX1B* gene

Top Differential Diagnoses
- Collagenofibrotic glomerulopathy
- Fibronectin glomerulopathy
- Fibrillary glomerulopathy
- Hereditary multiple exostoses

- Tubules, interstitium, vessels: No specific changes

ANCILLARY TESTS

Immunofluorescence
- No immunoglobulin or complement deposits
- IgM and C3 in sclerotic glomerular lesions
- Superimposed disease (IgA, anti-GBM) described

Molecular Genetics
- Sequencing *LMX1B* exons 2 through 6 and corresponding introns
  - 85% of mutations are in this region

Electron Microscopy
- "Moth-eaten" GBM in uranyl acetate stained sections
- Electron-dense collagen fibrils within GBM display characteristic periodicity in phosphotungstic, acid-stained sections
- Irregular thickening of GBM

DIFFERENTIAL DIAGNOSIS

Collagenofibrotic Glomerulopathy
- Abundant subendothelial and mesangial collagen fibers
- Collagen fibrils have curved appearance, ~ 60 nm periodicity

Fibronectin Glomerulopathy
- 14-16 nm, granular, fibrillary electron-dense deposits

Hereditary Multiple Exostoses
- Mesangial and subendothelial collagen
- Multiple osteochondromas

DIAGNOSTIC CHECKLIST

Pathologic Interpretation Pearls
- Intramembranous banded collagen fibrils on EM found on all patients

SELECTED REFERENCES

1. Joosten H et al: An aid to the diagnosis of genetic disorders underlying adult-onset renal failure: a literature review. Clin Nephrol. 73(6):454-72, 2010
2. Kamath S et al: Nail-patella syndrome with an emphasis on the risk of renal and ocular findings. Pediatr Dermatol. 27(1):95-7, 2010
3. Lemley KV: Kidney disease in nail-patella syndrome. Pediatr Nephrol. 24(12):2345-54, 2009
4. Sweeney E et al: Nail-patella syndrome. GeneReviews [Internet]. Seattle: University of Washington, 2003. Updated July 28, 2009
5. Miner JH et al: Transcriptional induction of slit diaphragm genes by Lmx1b is required in podocyte differentiation. J Clin Invest. 109(8):1065-72, 2002
6. Chapman JA et al: The collagen fibril--a model system for studying the staining and fixation of a protein. Electron Microsc Rev. 3(1):143-82, 1990

IMAGE GALLERY

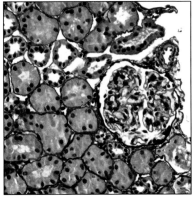 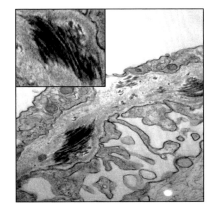 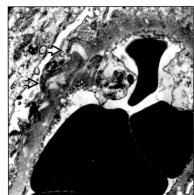

(Left) In this case of nail-patella syndrome, glomeruli, tubules, and interstitium are unremarkable. *(Center)* Characteristic fibrillar collagen bundles display the axial packing arrangement of positive and negative staining pattern known as periodicity, seen after phosphotungstic acid staining. *(Right)* "Moth-eaten" GBM appearance ⊵ in areas corresponding to fibrillar collagen deposits is the clue to the diagnosis by electron microscopy with uranyl nitrate staining.

LECITHIN-CHOLESTEROL ACYL TRANSFERASE DEFICIENCY

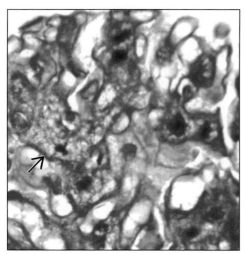

Lipids deposited in LCAT deficiency are extracted by solvents employed in tissue processing. This results in a vacuolated appearance to the mesangial matrix ⇨ and capillary loop basement membranes.

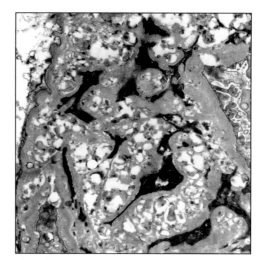

This electron micrograph shows the characteristic lipid deposits with a vacuolar appearance within the mesangial matrix. The accumulated material imparts a "honeycomb" appearance to the mesangium.

TERMINOLOGY

Abbreviations
- Lecithin-cholesterol acyltransferase (LCAT) deficiency

Synonyms
- Phosphatidylcholine-sterol o-acyltransferase deficiency

Definitions
- Diseases caused by complete or partial LCAT deficiency
  - Familial LCAT deficiency (FLD)
  - Fish eye disease (FED)

ETIOLOGY/PATHOGENESIS

Genetic Disorder
- Autosomal recessive
- Mutation of *LCAT* gene on chromosome 16q22
  - More than 36 mutations described
- Defect in LCAT-mediated cholesterol ester formation
- Failure to secrete active LCAT into plasma
  - Accumulation of unesterified cholesterol in cornea, kidneys, and erythrocytes
- LCAT normally carried in high-density lipoproteins (HDL) with ApoA1
  - Decreased HDL
- Increased free cholesterol-phospholipid vesicles (LpX)

Animal Model
- Murine LCAT deficiency (increased LpX)

CLINICAL ISSUES

Epidemiology
- Incidence
  - Rare cases reported worldwide
    - 60 with complete LCAT deficiency
    - 20 with partial LCAT deficiency

- Ethnicity
  - Initially reported in Norway
    - Now appears widely distributed

Presentation
- **Complete LCAT deficiency**
  - Familial LCAT deficiency
  - Corneal cataracts
  - Hemolytic anemia
  - Renal insufficiency by 4th decade
    - Proteinuria may begin in childhood
    - Progression of renal disease is variable
  - Atherosclerosis in rare cases
  - Hypertension
- **Partial LCAT deficiency**
  - Fish eye disease
  - Corneal opacities
    - Resemble eyes of a boiled fish
  - No overt renal disease

Laboratory Tests
- Reduced plasma total cholesterol
- Decreased HDL
- Low LCAT activity in plasma
- Urinalysis shows hematuria, leukocyturia, and casts

Treatment
- Medical treatment for anemia, renal insufficiency, and atherosclerosis
- Renal failure
  - Dialysis
  - Renal transplantation
- Corneal transplantation

Prognosis
- Renal transplantation
  - Moderately successful
  - Does not reverse serum lipoprotein abnormalities
  - Mesangial lipid deposits recur within weeks
    - Do not initially impair renal function

LECITHIN-CHOLESTEROL ACYL TRANSFERASE DEFICIENCY

Key Facts

Terminology
- Complete or partial LCAT deficiency
- Familial LCAT deficiency
- Fish eye disease

Etiology/Pathogenesis
- Defect in LCAT-mediated cholesterol ester-formation
- Mutation of *LCAT* gene on chromosome 16q22

Clinical Issues
- Corneal opacities and cataracts
- Hemolytic anemia
- Renal insufficiency with proteinuria
- Atherosclerosis in rare cases

Microscopic Pathology
- Glomerular mesangial expansion
  - Bubbly, vacuolated matrix
- Capillary loop thickening
  - GBM "spikes," vacuoles, duplication
- Tubular atrophy and interstitial fibrosis
  - Interstitial foam cells
- EM: Rounded granular and lamellar dense lipid deposits in GBM and mesangium
- Lipid deposits in liver, spleen, and bone marrow

Ancillary Tests
- Laboratory tests
  - Reduced plasma total cholesterol
  - Decreased high-density lipoprotein

Top Differential Diagnoses
- Hepatic glomerulopathy
- Alagille syndrome

MICROSCOPIC PATHOLOGY

Histologic Features
- Glomeruli
  - Mesangial expansion with occasional increased cellularity and foam cells
    - Mesangium appears bubbly or vacuolated
  - Capillary loop thickening
    - Silver stain shows GBM "spikes" and vacuoles
    - Subendothelial deposits can occlude capillaries
  - Progresses to segmental and global sclerosis
- Tubules and interstitium
  - Tubular atrophy and interstitial fibrosis
    - Interstitial foam cells

Other Organs
- Liver and spleen
- Bone marrow shows sea-blue histiocytes

ANCILLARY TESTS

Immunofluorescence
- Negative for immunoglobulin and complement

Electron Microscopy
- Transmission
  - Glomerular capillary loop lipid deposits
    - Intramembranous with GBM "spikes" and vacuolization
    - Subendothelial with GBM duplication
  - Mesangial matrix deposits
    - Expansion with densities and lucencies
  - Interstitial foam cells
  - Lipid deposits also in vascular endothelial and smooth muscle cells

Glomerular Lipid Characterization
- Contain ApoB and ApoE lipoproteins by immunohistochemistry
  - Positive acid-hematin staining for phospholipids
  - Positive for oxidized phosphocholine
- Little or no oil red O lipids, ApoA1, or malondialdehyde
  - Negative Nile blue stain (neutral and acid lipids, esterified cholesterol)

DIFFERENTIAL DIAGNOSIS

Hepatic Glomerulopathy
- IgA deposits usual
- Lipid, mostly mesangial

Alagille Syndrome
- Glomerular deposits oil red O positive
- Deficient bile ducts in liver

SELECTED REFERENCES

1. Joosten H et al: An aid to the diagnosis of genetic disorders underlying adult-onset renal failure: a literature review. Clin Nephrol. 73(6):454-72, 2010
2. Baass A et al: Characterization of a new LCAT mutation causing familial LCAT deficiency (FLD) and the role of APOE as a modifier gene of the FLD phenotype. Atherosclerosis. 207(2):452-7, 2009
3. Kettritz R et al: The case: the eyes have it. Kidney Int. 76(4):465-6, 2009
4. Vaziri ND: Causes of dysregulation of lipid metabolism in chronic renal failure. Semin Dial. 22(6):644-51, 2009
5. Jimi S et al: Possible induction of renal dysfunction in patients with lecithin:cholesterol acyltransferase deficiency by oxidized phosphatidylcholine in glomeruli. Arterioscler Thromb Vasc Biol. 19(3):794-801, 1999
6. Horina JH et al: Long-term follow-up of a patient with lecithin cholesterol acyltransferase deficiency syndrome after kidney transplantation. Transplantation. 56(1):233-6, 1993
7. Hovig T et al: Familial plasma lecithin: cholesterol acyltransferase (LCAT) deficiency. Ultrastructural aspects of a new syndrome with particular reference to lesions in the kidneys and the spleen. Acta Pathol Microbiol Scand A. 81(5):681-97, 1973

LECITHIN-CHOLESTEROL ACYL TRANSFERASE DEFICIENCY

Microscopic Features

(Left) This patient with familial LCAT deficiency shows mild glomerular involvement. There is mild mesangial matrix expansion ⮱ and a mild increase in mesangial hypercellularity. The capillary loops ⮱ are minimally thickened. *(Right)* This patient with LCAT deficiency shows severe glomerular involvement. This glomerulus shows prominent mesangial matrix expansion ⮱ with increased cellularity. There is marked thickening ⮱ of the glomerular capillary loop basement membranes.

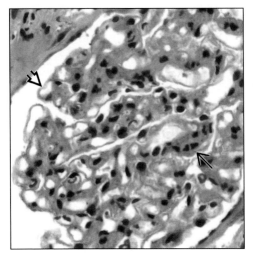
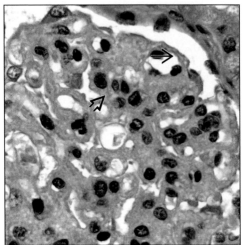

(Left) This silver stain in LCAT deficiency reveals detail of the basement membrane thickening. There are capillary loop basement membrane "spikes" ⮱ identical to changes seen in membranous glomerulonephritis. *(Right)* This silver stained glomerulus in LCAT deficiency shows vacuolated capillary loops ⮱ and "spikes" due to accumulation of lipid. This mimics membranous glomerulonephritis. However, in LCAT deficiency, the immunofluorescence studies would be negative for immune reactants.

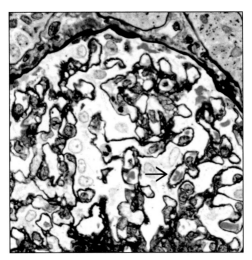
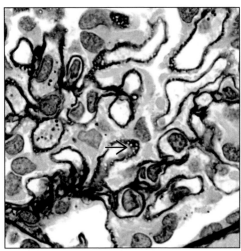

(Left) A silver stained glomerulus from a patient with LCAT deficiency shows massive intramembranous and subepithelial lipid deposition with occlusion of the capillary loops ⮱. This imparts an amyloid-like appearance. *(Right)* This silver stained glomerulus in LCAT deficiency shows massive lipid deposition in the capillary loops and mesangium. The mesangial matrix ⮱ is rarified, and many of the capillary loops are completely occluded ⮱. This imparts an amyloid-like appearance.

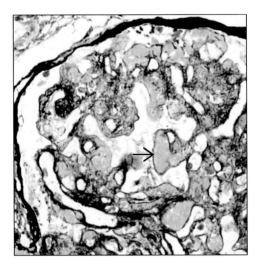
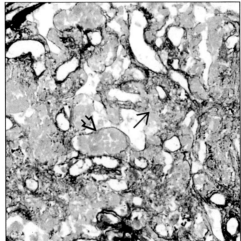

LECITHIN-CHOLESTEROL ACYL TRANSFERASE DEFICIENCY

Ultrastructural Features

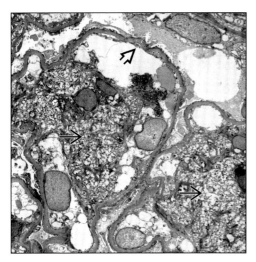

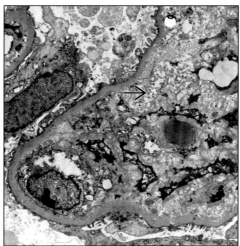

(Left) This is an electron micrograph of a glomerulus from a patient with mild LCAT deficiency. It shows electron-dense lamellar structures ➡ within the expanded mesangium. The capillary loops ➡ are not involved. *(Right)* This electron micrograph shows the characteristic lipid deposits ➡ diagnostic of LCAT deficiency. The mesangial matrix has a vacuolated appearance with lucent and lamellar material. The accumulated material imparts a "honeycomb" quality to the mesangium.

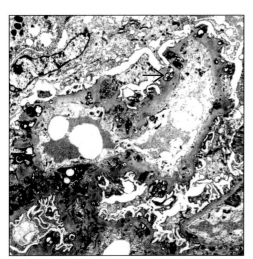

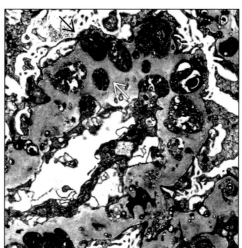

(Left) This electron micrograph shows marked irregularity of the glomerular capillary loop basement membrane due to intramembranous lipid material ➡ and basement membrane response. This accounts for the "spike" formation on silver stain by light microscopy. *(Right)* There is massive intramembranous ➡ and subepithelial ➡ lipid deposition in the capillary loops of this patient with LCAT deficiency. The rounded deposits are solid or have a lamellar substructure.

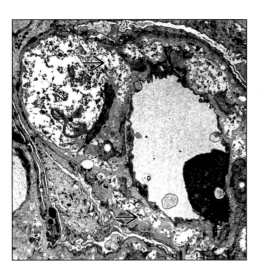

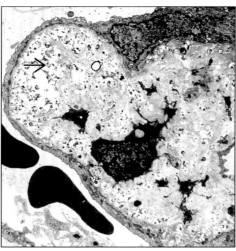

(Left) This is an example of severe glomerular involvement in LCAT deficiency. The glomerular capillary loops and mesangial matrix contain numerous subendothelial and intramembranous lipid ➡ of differing density, size, and shape. This produces the thickened foamy appearance of the capillary loops on silver stains by light microscopy. *(Right)* In this electron micrograph of LCAT deficiency, there is massive subendothelial lipid deposition ➡. The capillary loop is nearly occluded.

LIPOPROTEIN GLOMERULOPATHY

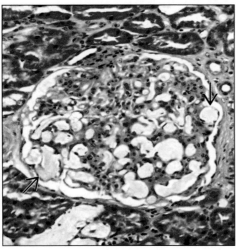

In lipoprotein glomerulopathy, glomeruli have segmentally dilated capillaries filled with pale-staining lipid material ⮕ that is not well preserved in routine paraffin sections.

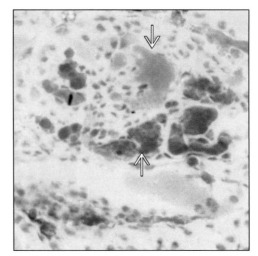

The lipid thrombi ⮕ distend glomerular capillaries in lipoprotein glomerulopathy and are well preserved in fresh frozen tissue and positive with oil red O.

TERMINOLOGY

Abbreviations
- Lipoprotein glomerulopathy (LPG)

Definitions
- Glomerular disease characterized by glomerular capillary lipoprotein thrombi, proteinuria, and progressive renal failure

ETIOLOGY/PATHOGENESIS

Genetics
- Mutation in *APOE* gene
  - Encodes apolipoprotein E (ApoE)
    - Major component of chylomicrons and intermediate density lipoprotein (IDL) particles that transport triglycerides
    - Cleared from circulation by receptor-mediated endocytosis in liver
  - Autosomal recessive trait
    - Chromosome 19
    - Mutation results in defective lipoprotein receptor binding
    - Hyperlipoproteinemia results (type III)
- 2 major loci of mutations
  - Exon 3
    - Kyoto mutation Cys25Arg
    - Gln3Lys
  - Exon 4 (LDL receptor binding site)
    - Tokyo Leu141-Lys143 del
    - Sendai Arg145Pro
    - Arg147Pro
    - Arg150Gly
    - Arg150Pro
    - Las Vegas Ala152Asp
    - Gln156-Lys173 del

CLINICAL ISSUES

Epidemiology
- Incidence
  - Rare; < 80 cases reported
- Age
  - 4-69 years; mean: 32 ± 2.2 years
- Gender
  - M:F = 3:2
- Ethnicity
  - Predominantly Japanese, Taiwanese, and Chinese
  - Occasionally reported in Caucasians/Europeans

Presentation
- Proteinuria, mild to severe
- Elevated serum apolipoprotein E to approximately 2x upper normal range
- Elevated very low-density lipoprotein
- Elevated intermediate-density lipoprotein
- May be associated with IgA, membranous, or lupus nephritis
- May be associated with psoriasis vulgaris

Laboratory Tests
- *APOE* gene sequence analysis

Treatment
- Drugs
  - Fibrates
  - Niceritrol
  - Probucol

Prognosis
- 50% of patients progress to renal failure
- Intensive lipid-lowering therapy has been shown to result in clinical and pathologic remission

LIPOPROTEIN GLOMERULOPATHY

Key Facts

Etiology/Pathogenesis
- *APOE* gene mutations

Clinical Issues
- Majority of cases reported in patients of Asian ancestry

Microscopic Pathology
- Glomerular intracapillary lipoprotein thrombi
- Oil red O positive thrombi

Ancillary Tests
- Apolipoprotein E serum concentration
- *APOE* gene sequencing
- Immunohistochemistry with antibodies to B or E apolipoproteins

Top Differential Diagnoses
- Fat emboli

MICROSCOPIC PATHOLOGY

Histologic Features
- Marked dilatation of glomerular capillary loops with pale substance
- Foam cells in glomeruli or interstitium

ANCILLARY TESTS

Frozen Sections
- Oil red O staining on frozen sections shows lipid thrombi in glomerular capillaries

Immunohistochemistry
- Antibodies to apolipoproteins B or E highlight intraglomerular thrombi

Immunofluorescence
- No specific deposition of immunoglobulin or complement

Electron Microscopy
- Glomerular capillaries contain variably sized granules and vacuoles forming lamellated structures
  - Clusters of circulating IDLs ~ 24-35 nm
- Lipid droplets in mesangial and endothelial cells

DIFFERENTIAL DIAGNOSIS

Fat Emboli
- Round globules of fat
- Little or no apolipoprotein component
- No finely vacuolated pattern on electron microscopy

SELECTED REFERENCES

1. Cheung CY et al: A rare cause of nephrotic syndrome: lipoprotein glomerulopathy. Hong Kong Med J. 15(1):57-60, 2009
2. Zhang B et al: Clinicopathological and genetic characteristics in Chinese patients with lipoprotein glomerulopathy. J Nephrol. 21(1):110-7, 2008
3. Rovin BH et al: APOE Kyoto mutation in European Americans with lipoprotein glomerulopathy. N Engl J Med. 357(24):2522-4, 2007
4. Ieiri N et al: Resolution of typical lipoprotein glomerulopathy by intensive lipid-lowering therapy. Am J Kidney Dis. 41(1):244-9, 2003
5. Miyata T et al: Apolipoprotein E2/E5 variants in lipoprotein glomerulopathy recurred in transplanted kidney. J Am Soc Nephrol. 10(7):1590-5, 1999
6. Saito T et al: Lipoprotein glomerulopathy: renal lipidosis induced by novel apolipoprotein E variants. Nephron. 83(3):193-201, 1999
7. Saito T et al: Lipoprotein glomerulopathy: glomerular lipoprotein thrombi in a patient with hyperlipoproteinemia. Am J Kidney Dis. 13(2):148-53, 1989

IMAGE GALLERY

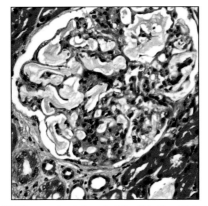
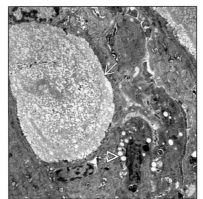
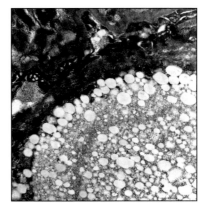

(Left) Wispy, pale pink material within the dilated glomerular capillary loops are a unique finding in LPG. *(Center)* In LPG, glomerular capillaries are filled with vacuolated lipoprotein thrombi ➡. Mesangial and subendothelial cells contain lipid vacuoles ➡. *(Right)* Higher magnification of intracapillary thrombi in LPG shows vacuolated lipoprotein particles.

TYPE III HYPERLIPOPROTEINEMIA

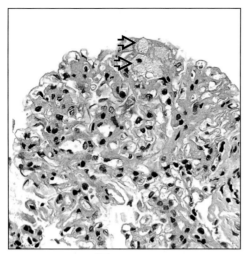

Foamy macrophages ⊳ are seen in this glomerulus from biopsy of a 55-year-old man with nephrotic syndrome and type III hyperlipoproteinemia (cholesterol 559 mg/dL and triglycerides 2169 mg/dL). (Courtesy J. Churg, MD.)

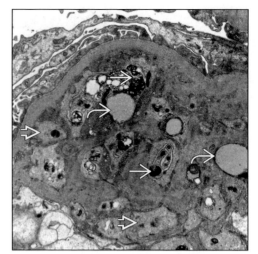

Glomerular capillary lumen is obliterated by a mixture of foamy cells ⊒, lipid vacuoles ↗, and dark-staining membrane-bound particles and lysosomes ➔. (Courtesy J. Churg, MD.)

TERMINOLOGY

Synonyms
- Type III hyperlipidemia

Definitions
- Hypercholesterolemia and hypertriglyceridemia associated with apolipoprotein-E2 allele

ETIOLOGY/PATHOGENESIS

Genetics
- *APOE*
  - Encodes apolipoprotein E
  - Maps to chromosome 19q13.2
  - 3 alleles: $\epsilon 2$, $\epsilon 3$, $\epsilon 4$
    - $\epsilon 2$ is least common (~ 5% frequency)
- Autosomal recessive
  - Approximately 5% of *APOE2* homozygotes develop type III hyperlipidemia
  - Secondary genetic &/or environmental factors implicated
- *APOE2* carriers also prone to developing type III hyperlipidemia
- Rare variant mutations result in autosomal dominant inheritance pattern

Pathogenesis
- ApoE2 proteins bind ineffectively to the low density lipoprotein (LDL) receptor, leading to ineffective clearance of lipoproteins and accumulation in plasma

CLINICAL ISSUES

Epidemiology
- Incidence
  - 0.02% of population
- Age
  - Children and adults affected
- Gender
  - Males more commonly affected

Presentation
- Nephrotic-range proteinuria
- Hyperlipidemia (turbid plasma)
- Nephrotic syndrome
- Palmar and tuberous xanthomas
- Hepatomegaly and splenomegaly
- Premature vascular disease
- Ascites

Laboratory Tests
- Lipid profile: Type III hyperlipidemia
  - Hypercholesterolemia (> 300 mg/dL)
    - Very low density lipoprotein (VLDL):triglyceride ratio > 0.3
    - Normal high density lipoprotein (HDL)
    - Decreased LDL
  - Hypertriglyceridemia (> 300 mg/dL)
- ApoE genotyping
  - *APOE2* homozygosity

Treatment
- Drugs
  - Lipid-lowering agents
  - ACE inhibitors
- Plasmapheresis
- Dietary modifications

MICROSCOPIC PATHOLOGY

Histologic Features
- Glomeruli
  - Endothelial and mesangial foamy macrophage aggregates
  - Segmental sclerosis
  - Mesangial hypercellularity
- Tubules
  - Atrophy as disease progresses

TYPE III HYPERLIPOPROTEINEMIA

Key Facts

Etiology/Pathogenesis
- *APOE2* homozygotes
- Autosomal recessive

Clinical Issues
- Males more commonly affected
- Nephrotic syndrome
- Premature vascular disease
- Palmar and tuberous xanthomas
- Hypercholesterolemia (> 300 mg/dL)

- VLDL/TG ratio > 0.3
- Hypertriglyceridemia (> 300 mg/dL)

Microscopic Pathology
- Glomeruli
  - Foam cells
  - Segmental sclerosis

Top Differential Diagnoses
- Lipoprotein glomerulopathy
- FSGS

- Interstitium
  - Foamy macrophages
  - Fibrosis as disease progresses
  - Lymphocytic infiltrates
- Vessels
  - Thickening

ANCILLARY TESTS

Electron Microscopy
- Transmission
  - Capillary loop foam cells
    - Lamellated electron-dense material
    - Cholesterol clefts
  - Mesangial, endothelial, and tubular lipid vacuoles
  - Extensive podocyte foot process effacement
  - Increased mesangial matrix

DIFFERENTIAL DIAGNOSIS

Lipoprotein Glomerulopathy
- Lipoprotein thrombi in glomerular capillary loops
  - Highlighted using fresh frozen tissue for oil red O staining
- Typically associated with unique *APOE* gene mutations
- Rarely associated with type III hyperlipidemia

Focal Segmental Glomerulosclerosis (FSGS)
- Glomerular capillary, tubular, and interstitial foam cells can be seen in FSGS and other diseases with nephrotic syndrome
  - Lack abundant aggregates of foam cells seen in type III hyperlipidemia
- Associated with type IIa, IIb, and IV hyperlipidemia

DIAGNOSTIC CHECKLIST

Pathologic Interpretation Pearls
- Aggregates of glomerular and interstitial foam cells with FSGS should prompt lipid analysis

SELECTED REFERENCES

1. Eichner JE et al: Apolipoprotein E polymorphism and cardiovascular disease: a HuGE review. Am J Epidemiol. 155(6):487-95, 2002
2. Mahley RW et al: Pathogenesis of type III hyperlipoproteinemia (dysbetalipoproteinemia). Questions, quandaries, and paradoxes. J Lipid Res. 40(11):1933-49, 1999
3. Saito T: Abnormal lipid metabolism and renal disorders. Tohoku J Exp Med. 181(3):321-37, 1997
4. Balson KR et al: Glomerular lipid deposition and proteinuria in a patient with familial dysbetalipoproteinaemia. J Intern Med. 240(3):157-9, 1996
5. Ellis D et al: Atypical hyperlipidemia and nephropathy associated with apolipoprotein E homozygosity. J Am Soc Nephrol. 6(4):1170-7, 1995

IMAGE GALLERY

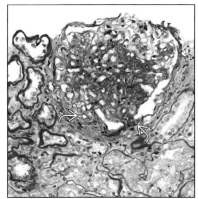 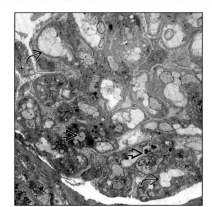 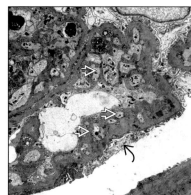

(Left) This case of type III hyperlipoproteinemia shows FSGS with adhesions to Bowman capsule ➡ and tubular atrophy. *(Center)* At this low magnification, the glomerulus shows diffuse capillary loop thickening and subendothelial lipid accumulation. Lumens are filled with lipid vacuoles ➡ and lysosomal particles ➡. *(Right)* High magnification of the glomerular capillary reveals foot process effacement ➡ and intramembranous foamy and membranous material ➡. *(Courtesy J. Churg, MD.)*

GALLOWAY-MOWAT SYNDROME

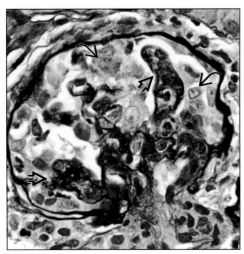

This glomerulus from a 3 year old with GMS shows diffuse mesangial sclerosis. There is capillary loop collapse ⇨, mesangial matrix increase, and prominent epithelial hyperplasia ⇗.

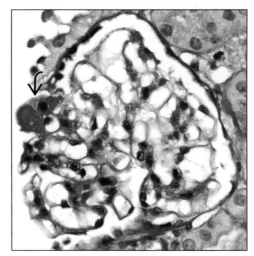

This glomerulus from a 2 year old with GMS shows focal segmental glomerulosclerosis. There is a segmental sclerosing lesion ➔ with hyaline accumulation. The remainder of the glomerulus is normal.

TERMINOLOGY

Abbreviations
- Galloway-Mowat syndrome (GMS) glomerulopathy

Synonyms
- Nephrosis-microcephaly syndrome

Definitions
- Early onset nephrotic syndrome and microcephaly with other central nervous system anomalies
  o Hiatal hernia included in early descriptions

ETIOLOGY/PATHOGENESIS

Developmental Anomaly
- Autosomal recessive
- Genetic basis unknown
  o May represent heterogeneous set of disorders

CLINICAL ISSUES

Presentation
- Wide spectrum of neurological manifestations
  o Microcephaly
  o Psychomotor delay
  o Seizures
- Steroid-resistant nephrotic syndrome in 1st months of life
  o Diffuse mesangial sclerosis (DMS)
  o Focal segmental glomerulosclerosis (FSGS)/minimal change disease
- May have dysmorphic facial features
  o Micrognathia
  o Ocular abnormalities
  o Receding forehead
  o Large floppy ears
- Hiatal hernia in some cases

Treatment
- No known treatment

Prognosis
- Fatal in childhood, usually by 6 years
- Nephrotic syndrome progresses to ESRD in 2-3 years

MACROSCOPIC FEATURES

General Features
- Dysmorphic craniofacial features
- Deformities of extremities
- Ocular abnormalities
- Abnormal gyri and sulci in brain
- Cerebellar atrophy

MICROSCOPIC PATHOLOGY

Histologic Features
- Diffuse mesangial sclerosis
  o Glomerular capillary loop collapse
  o Epithelial hyperplasia overlying collapsed loops
    ▪ Strongly resembles collapsing glomerulopathy
  o Mesangial matrix increase ± hypercellularity
  o Tubular ectasia and tubulointerstitial scarring
  o Immunofluorescence
    ▪ Negative for immune reactants
    ▪ IgM and C3 in areas of sclerosis
  o Electron microscopy
    ▪ Irregular glomerular basement membrane thickening
    ▪ Lucent foci and lamina densa splitting
    ▪ Diffuse podocyte foot process effacement
- Focal segmental glomerulosclerosis
  o Segmental sclerosing lesions
  o Immunofluorescence
    ▪ Negative for immune reactants
    ▪ IgM and C3 in areas of sclerosis

GALLOWAY-MOWAT SYNDROME

Key Facts

Terminology
- Early onset nephrotic syndrome and microcephaly

Etiology/Pathogenesis
- Genetic basis not known

Clinical Issues
- Diverse neurological symptoms
- Progressive nephrotic syndrome leading to ESRD
- Fatal in early childhood

Microscopic Pathology
- Diffuse mesangial sclerosis
  - Capillary loop collapse
  - Epithelial cell hyperplasia
  - Mesangial matrix increase ± hypercellularity
  - Podocyte foot process effacement
  - GBM irregularities

- Focal segmental glomerulosclerosis
  - Segmental sclerosing lesions
  - Podocyte foot process effacement abnormalities
  - No GBM abnormalities
- Minimal change disease
  - May be seen in early biopsies but evolve into FSGS or DMS

Top Differential Diagnoses
- Diffuse mesangial sclerosis
  - Denys-Drash syndrome
  - Pierson syndrome
  - Lowe syndrome
- Focal segmental glomerulosclerosis
  - Frasier syndrome
  - Nail-patella syndrome

- Electron microscopy
  - Glomerular basement membrane normal
  - Podocyte foot process effacement
- Minimal change disease
  - May subsequently evolve into diffuse mesangial sclerosis
  - May subsequently evolve into focal segmental glomerulosclerosis
- Other glomerular lesions described
  - Diffuse mesangial hypercellularity
    - May subsequently evolve into DMS or FSGS
    - GBM changes resembling DMS must be absent
  - Collapsing glomerulopathy
    - Likely misdiagnosed as DMS because no EM performed

DIFFERENTIAL DIAGNOSIS

Syndromic Forms of DMS
- Denys-Drash syndrome
  - WT1 mutation
- Pierson syndrome
  - LAMB2 mutation
- Lowe syndrome
  - OCRL1 mutation

Syndromic Forms of FSGS
- Frasier syndrome
  - WT1 mutation
- Nail-patella syndrome
  - LMX1B mutation

DIAGNOSTIC CHECKLIST

Pathologic Interpretation Pearls
- In congenital and infantile nephrotic syndrome, knowledge of syndromic features is essential to diagnosis

SELECTED REFERENCES

1. Pezzella M et al: Galloway-Mowat syndrome: an early-onset progressive encephalopathy with intractable epilepsy associated to renal impairment. Two novel cases and review of literature. Seizure. 19(2):132-5, 2010
2. Akhtar N et al: Galloway-Mowat syndrome. J Coll Physicians Surg Pak. 18(8):520-1, 2008
3. Dietrich A et al: Analysis of genes encoding laminin beta2 and related proteins in patients with Galloway-Mowat syndrome. Pediatr Nephrol. 23(10):1779-86, 2008
4. Sartelet H et al: Collapsing glomerulopathy in Galloway-Mowat syndrome: a case report and review of the literature. Pathol Res Pract. 204(6):401-6, 2008
5. Steiss JO et al: Late-onset nephrotic syndrome and severe cerebellar atrophy in Galloway-Mowat syndrome. Neuropediatrics. 36(5):332-5, 2005
6. Shiihara T et al: Microcephaly, cerebellar atrophy, and focal segmental glomerulosclerosis in two brothers: a possible mild form of Galloway-Mowat syndrome. J Child Neurol. 18(2):147-9, 2003
7. de Vries BB et al: Diagnostic dilemmas in four infants with nephrotic syndrome, microcephaly and severe developmental delay. Clin Dysmorphol. 10(2):115-21, 2001
8. Lin CC et al: Galloway-Mowat syndrome: a glomerular basement membrane disorder? Pediatr Nephrol. 16(8):653-7, 2001
9. Srivastava T et al: Podocyte proteins in Galloway-Mowat syndrome. Pediatr Nephrol. 16(12):1022-9, 2001
10. Hazza I et al: Late-onset nephrotic syndrome in galloway-mowat syndrome: a case report. Saudi J Kidney Dis Transpl. 10(2):171-4, 1999
11. Meyers KE et al: Nephrotic syndrome, microcephaly, and developmental delay: three separate syndromes. Am J Med Genet. 82(3):257-60, 1999
12. Sano H et al: Microcephaly and early-onset nephrotic syndrome--confusion in Galloway-Mowat syndrome. Pediatr Nephrol. 9(6):711-4, 1995
13. Cohen AH et al: Kidney in Galloway-Mowat syndrome: clinical spectrum with description of pathology. Kidney Int. 45(5):1407-15, 1994

GALLOWAY-MOWAT SYNDROME

GMS with Very Early DMS

(Left) These glomeruli from a patient with GMS show early DMS. The glomerulus on the left shows mild mesangial matrix increase with mild mesangial hypercellularity ➡. Overall, these features would be regarded as minimal change disease except that GBM changes on EM (shown below) indicate DMS. *(Right)* This glomerulus shows minimal abnormalities. There is mesangial matrix increase ➡ and a cluster of prominent podocytes ➡. No evidence of capillary loop collapse is present.

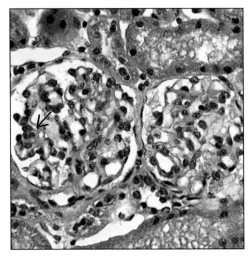
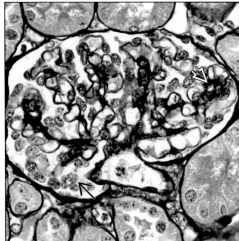

(Left) This glomerulus is nearly normal. It shows mild mesangial hypercellularity ➡ without capillary loop alterations. The podocytes are more prominent than normal but would not in themselves be diagnostic. *(Right)* This electron micrograph shows diffuse effacement of podocyte foot processes ➡. The capillary loop basement membrane shows segmental thickening ➡ with mild lucency and lamellations of the GBM similar to early changes encountered in Alport syndrome.

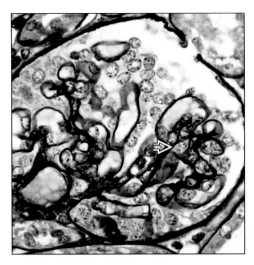
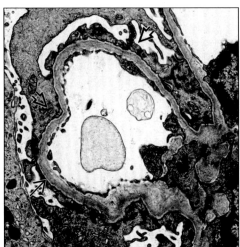

(Left) This capillary loop shows diffuse podocyte foot process effacement ➡. There is a complete sheet of cytoplasm covering the capillary loop. The basement membrane is diffusely thickened and "split" ➡, resulting in a double lamina densa layer. *(Right)* The capillary loop basement membrane is markedly abnormal. There is impressive irregularity and thickening of the lamina rara interna ➡ and lamina rara externa ➡. The lamina densa is irregularly thickened and splayed ➡.

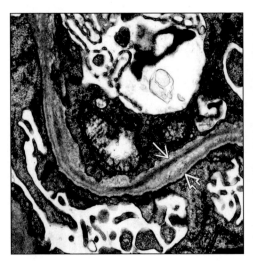
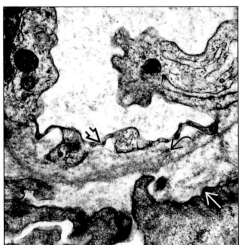

GALLOWAY-MOWAT SYNDROME

3 Year Old with GMS and Severe DMS

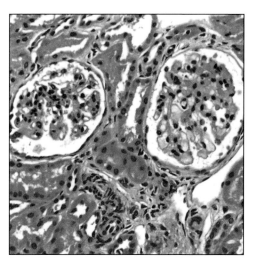

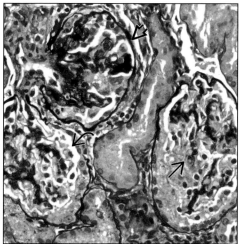

(Left) These 2 glomeruli in a 3 year old with diffuse mesangial sclerosis show variable degrees of mesangial matrix increase. There is also mild mesangial hypercellularity in the glomerulus on the left. *(Right)* This cluster of 3 glomeruli illustrates variable severity of involvement. One glomerulus ⇒ shows pronounced mesangial matrix increase and capillary loop collapse. A 2nd glomerulus shows mild mesangial sclerosis ⇒, and the 3rd appears essentially normal ⇒.

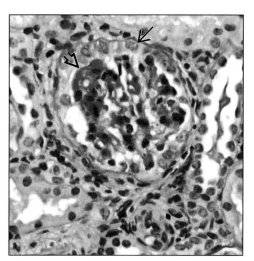

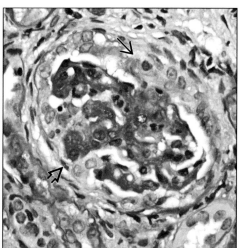

(Left) This glomerulus shows mild mesangial sclerosis and segmental collapse with hyalinosis similar to FSGS ⇒. There is generalized epithelial cell hyperplasia that includes both the parietal ⇒ and visceral epithelial cells. *(Right)* This glomerulus shows advanced mesangial and capillary loop sclerosis with a capsular adhesion ⇒ and disruption of Bowman capsule. There is very prominent epithelial cell hyperplasia involving both parietal ⇒ and visceral epithelial cells.

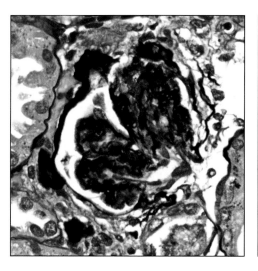

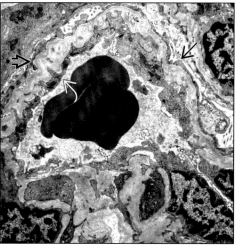

(Left) This glomerulus is completely sclerotic with severe mesangial matrix increase and total capillary loop obliteration. Epithelial hyperplasia is absent, possibly because of the terminal stage of the process. *(Right)* There is diffuse effacement of podocyte foot processes ⇒. The capillary loop basement membrane shows marked thickening ⇒ and irregularity with basement membrane lucencies that contain tiny cell remnants. The endothelial cells lack fenestrations ⇒.

GALLOWAY-MOWAT SYNDROME

5 Year Old with GMS and Advanced DMS

(Left) This 5 year old with GMS shows advanced, approaching end-stage, diffuse mesangial sclerosis. One glomerulus shows severe mesangial matrix increase and diffuse capillary loop collapse ⮡. The other glomerulus shows mesangial sclerosis with residual, but compromised, capillary loops. (Right) This is another glomerulus in a 5 year old with DMS. There is also severe mesangial sclerosis, and most capillary loops are completely obliterated with capsular adhesions.

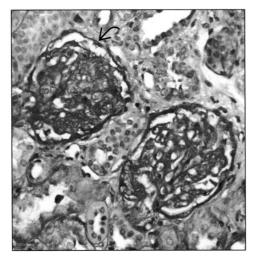
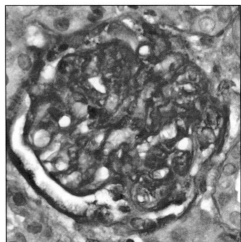

(Left) EM shows complete effacement of podocyte foot processes in this glomerulus. There is also mild variability in the thickness of the capillary loop basement membrane with scalloping along the inner surface. (Right) EM shows the interface with the mesangium that includes portions of 2 mesangial cells. There is podocyte foot process effacement with microvillous transformation ⮡. There is also subepithelial lucency and multilayering of the GBM ⮡.

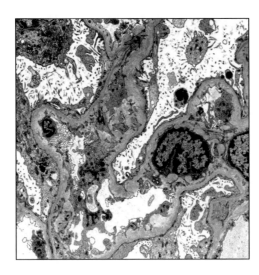
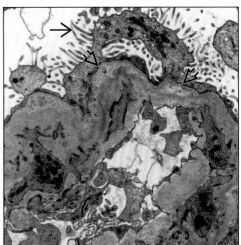

(Left) EM shows diffuse effacement of podocyte foot processes ⮡. The capillary loop basements show irregular thickening with a scalloped contour on both the inner and outer aspects ⮡ and lucencies ⮕ with granularities. (Right) EM shows capillary loop collapse and sclerosis. There is an adhesion composed of strands of matrix material ⮕ that connects the collapsed capillary loop ⮡ to the Bowman capsule. Within the adhesion are epithelial cells.

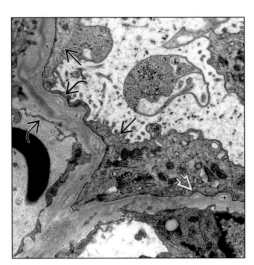
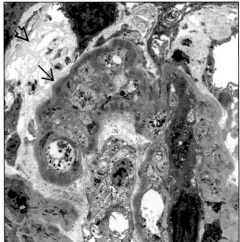

GALLOWAY-MOWAT SYNDROME

2 Year Old with GMS and FSGS

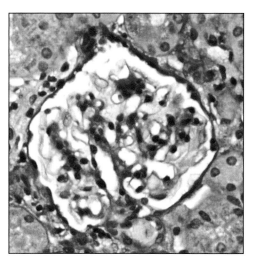

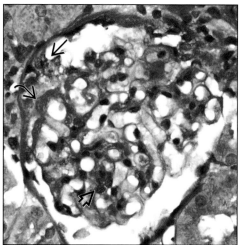

(Left) This 2 year old with GMS and focal segmental glomerulosclerosis shows the usual spectrum of glomerular lesions associated with that diagnostic entity. This glomerulus shows mild segmental mesangial hypercellularity, which occurs in FSGS. The capillary loops remain patent. (Right) This glomerulus shows mild segmental mesangial hypercellularity ➡ and segmental sclerosis ➡. The segmental sclerosing lesion contains hyaline and lipid with overlying epithelial hyperplasia ➡.

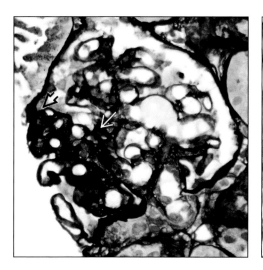

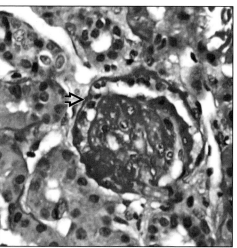

(Left) This is another segmental sclerosing lesion ➡. This lesion is larger than the previous lesion. It contains hyaline, which stains black on silver stain, and a capsular adhesion ➡. The upper left portions of the glomerulus appear normal. (Right) This glomerulus shows the end stage of segmental sclerosis in which the entire glomerulus is sclerotic, known as global glomerulosclerosis. There is residual mild epithelial cell hyperplasia ➡, a feature that will disappear over time.

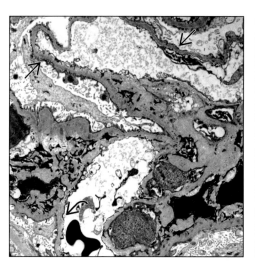

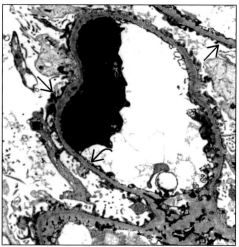

(Left) This glomerulus shows diffuse effacement of podocyte foot processes ➡ by EM. There is mild mesangial matrix increase, far less than in DMS. The capillary loop basement membrane is fairly uniform in thickness, but mild irregularity is present ➡. (Right) This capillary loop shows effacement of podocyte foot processes ➡. The endothelium is normal, and its fenestrations are barely visible. The capillary loop basement membrane ➡ is uniform without irregularity or scalloping.

FABRY DISEASE

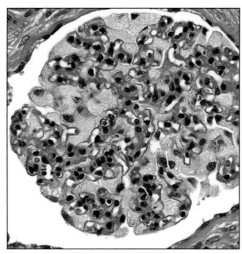

The characteristic podocytes have clear, lacy cytoplasm in Fabry disease. The lipid consists of globotriasolylceremide (GL3), which accumulates in the podocyte more than in other renal structures.

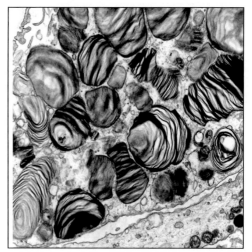

Electron micrograph shows a podocyte with characteristic lipid inclusions that have a striped or "zebra" pattern. The pattern is due to the accumulation of GL3 caused by the deficiency of α-galactosidase A.

TERMINOLOGY

Synonyms
- Anderson-Fabry disease
- Angiokeratoma corporis diffusum

Definitions
- Systemic disease caused by genetic deficiency in α-galactosidase A enzyme (αGal), leading to accumulation of lipid in many cell types, affecting function of kidney, heart, sweat gland, and nerves

ETIOLOGY/PATHOGENESIS

Genetic Disease
- X-linked recessive trait
- Mutation in α-galactosidase A gene (*AGAL*) on long arm of X chromosome (Xq22.1)
  - Over 245 different mutations
  - 5% spontaneous mutations
  - Symptoms and signs vary with mutation and consequent functional level of αGal (more severe with missense than deletion or termination mutations)

Pathophysiology
- α-galactosidase A enzyme (αGal) deficiency in lysosomes
- Globotriaosylceramide (GL3): Major glycosphingolipid that accumulates in endothelial and smooth muscle cells, podocytes, distal tubular cells, collecting ducts, sweat glands, cardiac myocytes, macrophages, dorsal root ganglia, perineurium, cornea stroma, and other cells
  - Other lipids: Galabiosylcerebroside (podocytes) and blood group B substance
- Endothelial involvement leads to microvascular obstruction
  - Proinflammatory and procoagulant effects on endothelium
  - Global and segmental glomerular sclerosis, interstitial fibrosis, tubular atrophy
  - Smooth muscle loss, nodular hyalinosis

CLINICAL ISSUES

Epidemiology
- Incidence
  - Mutation prevalence 1:40,000
    - ~ 0.3% of patients on dialysis, higher in males
  - Often misdiagnosed (mean time to diagnosis is 20 years)

Presentation
- Acroparesthesia: Age 5-25 years
- Renal dysfunction: Age 15-40 years; renal failure at median age of 40 years
- CNS disease (stroke) > 25 years
- Cardiac disease > 35 years
- Hypohidrosis
- Corneal opacities
- Isosthenuria
- Female heterozygote
  - Variable symptoms
    - Asymptomatic to renal failure
- Renal variant
  - Signs and symptoms restricted to kidney
  - 1.2% of male dialysis patients (Japan)
  - Lack classic features: Angiokeratoma, acroparesthesias, hypohidrosis, corneal opacities
- Cardiac variant
  - Occurs in males with partial αGal activity
  - Hypertrophic cardiomyopathy
  - Prominent cardiomyocyte lipid
  - No endothelial GL3
  - No renal failure, neurological disease, or skin lesions

FABRY DISEASE

Key Facts

Terminology
- Caused by mutation in *AGAL* gene, leading to accumulation of lipid globotriaosylceramide (GL3) in blood and many cell types, affecting function of kidney, heart, sweat gland, and nerves

Etiology/Pathogenesis
- X-linked recessive
- Symptoms and signs vary with mutation
- GL3 accumulates in endothelial and smooth muscle cells, podocytes, distal tubules, and many other cells

Clinical Issues
- ~ 0.3% of patients on dialysis
- Renal dysfunction: Age 15-40 years
- Often misdiagnosed clinically

Microscopic Pathology
- Podocyte-expanded cytoplasm appears pale and lacy due to lipid deposits
- EM demonstrates diagnostic feature of laminated, electron-dense lipid deposits in podocytes, endothelial cells, and distal tubular cells
- 1 micron Epon-embedded tissue reveals dense lipid granules by light microscopy
- Female heterozygotes have patchy distribution of podocyte lipid
- FSGS may develop

Top Differential Diagnoses
- Chloroquine toxicity
- Focal segmental glomerulosclerosis (FSGS)
- I-cell disease

Treatment
- Drugs
  - Enzyme replacement therapy (recombinant αGal, Fabrazyme)

Prognosis
- Course is variable depending on severity of enzyme deficiency
- Enzyme replacement benefits pain and quality of life
- Improvement of hypertension and cardiac hypertrophy, as well as reduced rate of loss of renal function reported vs. historical controls
- Long-term effect on renal function and survival remain to be determined

MACROSCOPIC FEATURES

Biopsy Appearance
- Diagnosis may be suspected on renal biopsy
- Glomeruli are paler and whiter compared with red glomeruli in non-Fabry cases

MICROSCOPIC PATHOLOGY

Histologic Features
- Glomeruli
  - Podocytes have expanded cytoplasm that appears pale and lacy due to lipid deposits dissolved in processing
  - Autofluorescent lipid can be appreciated in podocytes in frozen sections with UV illumination
  - Female heterozygotes have patchy distribution of podocyte lipid due to random inactivation of 1 X chromosome
  - Mesangium can be expanded and mildly hypercellular
    - Mesangial cells also contain lipid, but this cannot be easily appreciated in routine sections
  - Glomerular endothelial cells appear normal in routine sections although they also contain lipid
  - Focal segmental glomerulosclerosis (FSGS) can be present, with adhesion to Bowman capsule and segment scars
  - Some glomeruli may show features of collapsing glomerulopathy
- Tubules
  - Distal tubules have abundant lipid deposits, which make them appear pale and vacuolated in routine sections
  - Tubular atrophy is common
- Vessels
  - Endothelium of all vessels accumulate lipid, arteries, arterioles, capillaries, and veins
  - Lipid in arterial endothelium can sometimes be appreciated in routine sections as lacy, vacuolated cytoplasm
  - Lipid in peritubular capillaries is not appreciated in routine sections
  - Lipid in arterial smooth muscle makes them appear pale in routine sections
  - Arteriolar hyalinosis and intimal fibrosis can be prominent
    - Arteriolar hyalinosis may present as peripheral nodular replacement of smooth muscle, indistinguishable from the pattern in calcineurin inhibitor toxicity
- Interstitium
  - Commonly affected by increased fibrosis, with sparse infiltrate
  - Fibroblasts in interstitium also contain lipid
  - Granulomatous interstitial nephritis reported rarely
- 1 micron Epon-embedded tissue
  - Glutaraldehyde/paraformaldehyde fixed tissue as routinely processed for EM is ideal for detecting lipid
  - Lipid granules most conspicuous as dense granules filling podocytes and distal tubular epithelium
  - High power (100x oil) useful for detecting lipid droplets in endothelium
    - Endothelial lipid varies in amounts from rare isolated granules to large aggregates that bulge into lumen

FABRY DISEASE

o Podocyte lipid is decreased in areas of segmental sclerosis and adhesion or collapse
  - Possibly due to increased local podocyte turnover, yielding "young" podocytes with less lipid
- Superimposed diseases have been reported
  o Minimal change disease superimposed on Fabry disease
  o IgA nephropathy (may be incidental)
  o Crescentic glomerulonephritis (± ANCA)

ANCILLARY TESTS

Immunofluorescence
- Generally negative except for IgM and C3 in segmental scars
- Incidental IgA deposition observed in protocol biopsies

Electron Microscopy
- Diagnostic feature is presence of laminated, electron-dense lipid deposits in podocytes, endothelial cells, mesangial cells, smooth muscle cells, distal tubules, and interstitial fibroblasts
- Dense, variegated granules without lamination also present

DIFFERENTIAL DIAGNOSIS

Chloroquine Toxicity
- Lipids that accumulate during therapy with lysosomal inhibitor (chloroquine) are indistinguishable from Fabry disease
- History of chloroquine therapy may not be known to pathologist, but this possibility should be raised
- Diagnosis of Fabry disease generally requires ancillary studies (blood levels of GL3 or genetic testing)

Focal Segmental Glomerulosclerosis (FSGS)
- Fabry patients commonly develop FSGS as consequence of either direct effect of lipid on podocyte or due to decreased nephron mass
- Lipid in podocytes are best clue, but these can be overlooked in light microscopy
- EM is best method to detect lipid, which should be readily detected in podocytes

I-Cell Disease
- Podocyte deposits positive for colloidal iron

Arteriosclerosis
- Vascular disease in Fabry disease is similar to usual arteriosclerosis that arises in hypertension
- If lipid in podocytes (or other sites) is not appreciated, diagnosis may be missed

Subclinical Fabry Disease (in Patients with Other Renal Diseases)
- Lipid deposits may be an "incidental" finding on biopsies taken for other diseases (e.g., crescentic glomerulonephritis, IgA nephropathy, cholesterol emboli)

DIAGNOSTIC CHECKLIST

Pathologic Interpretation Pearls
- 1 micron section (100x oil) useful for detecting and evaluating lipid by light microscopy
- Lipid may be inconspicuous in later stages and may be overlooked
- Diagnosis suggested by pale white bulging glomeruli on macroscopic inspection of biopsy core

SELECTED REFERENCES

1. Fogo AB et al: Scoring system for renal pathology in Fabry disease: report of the International Study Group of Fabry Nephropathy (ISGFN). Nephrol Dial Transplant. 25(7):2168-77, 2010
2. Marchesoni CL et al: Misdiagnosis in Fabry disease. J Pediatr. 156(5):828-31, 2010
3. Ramaswami U et al: Assessment of renal pathology and dysfunction in children with Fabry disease. Clin J Am Soc Nephrol. 5(2):365-70, 2010
4. Rombach SM et al: Vasculopathy in patients with Fabry disease: current controversies and research directions. Mol Genet Metab. 99(2):99-108, 2010
5. Zarate YA et al: A case of minimal change disease in a Fabry patient. Pediatr Nephrol. 25(3):553-6, 2010
6. Abaterusso C et al: Unusual renal presentation of Fabry disease in a female patient. Nat Rev Nephrol. 5(6):349-54, 2009
7. Hirashio S et al: Renal histology before and after effective enzyme replacement therapy in a patient with classical Fabry's disease. Clin Nephrol. 71(5):550-6, 2009
8. Kato T et al: Deceased renal transplantation in patient with Fabry's disease maintained by enzyme replacement therapy. Int J Urol. 16(7):650, 2009
9. Mehta A et al: Enzyme replacement therapy with agalsidase alfa in patients with Fabry's disease: an analysis of registry data. Lancet. 374(9706):1986-96, 2009
10. Mehta A et al: Natural course of Fabry disease: changing pattern of causes of death in FOS - Fabry Outcome Survey. J Med Genet. 46(8):548-52, 2009
11. Bracamonte ER et al: Iatrogenic phospholipidosis mimicking Fabry disease. Am J Kidney Dis. 48(5):844-50, 2006
12. Fischer EG et al: Fabry disease: a morphologic study of 11 cases. Mod Pathol. 19(10):1295-301, 2006
13. Albay D et al: Chloroquine-induced lipidosis mimicking Fabry disease. Mod Pathol. 18(5):733-8, 2005
14. Siamopoulos KC: Fabry disease: kidney involvement and enzyme replacement therapy. Kidney Int. 65(2):744-53, 2004
15. Svarstad E et al: Bedside stereomicroscopy of renal biopsies may lead to a rapid diagnosis of Fabry's disease. Nephrol Dial Transplant. 19(12):3202-3, 2004
16. Nakao S et al: Fabry disease: detection of undiagnosed hemodialysis patients and identification of a "renal variant" phenotype. Kidney Int. 64(3):801-7, 2003
17. Thurberg BL et al: Globotriaosylceramide accumulation in the Fabry kidney is cleared from multiple cell types after enzyme replacement therapy. Kidney Int. 62(6):1933-46, 2002
18. Eng CM et al: Safety and efficacy of recombinant human alpha-galactosidase A--replacement therapy in Fabry's disease. N Engl J Med. 345(1):9-16, 2001

FABRY DISEASE

Microscopic Features

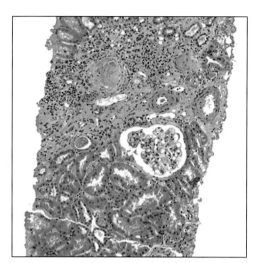

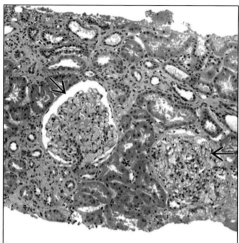

(Left) Low-power view of a renal biopsy from a patient with Fabry disease shows nonspecific findings of interstitial fibrosis and glomerulosclerosis. Demonstration of the lipid accumulation is best shown by electron microscopy or 1 micron sections. *(Right)* Increased size of the podocytes with pale cytoplasm ➡ is suggested in a patient with Fabry disease. Diffuse fine interstitial fibrosis is present and commonly accompanied by patchy tubular atrophy.

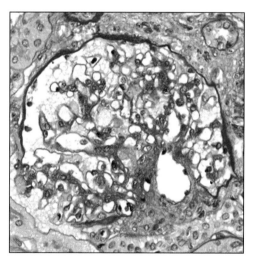

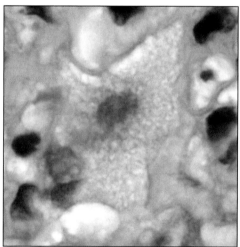

(Left) Periodic acid-Schiff stain of a biopsy from a patient with Fabry disease shows characteristic lacy cytoplasm in the podocytes. The GL3 lipid in the inclusions is dissolved by processing. *(Right)* High power shows a podocyte in a biopsy from a patient with Fabry disease. The podocyte has an enlarged lacy clear cytoplasm, filled with lipid that has been dissolved in processing. This is often the most conspicuous change in routine stains that raises the question of Fabry disease.

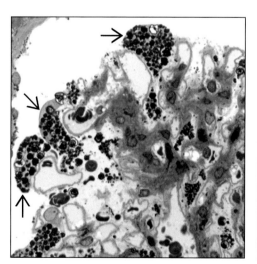

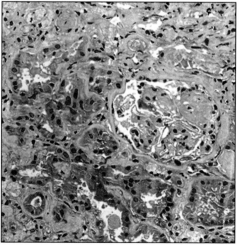

(Left) Toluidine blue stain of 1 micron section shows a prominent accumulation of densely stained lipid (GL3) in podocytes ➡. Podocytes are the most affected cell in Fabry disease. Osmium fixation preserves the lipid. *(Right)* Fabry disease may be deceptively nonspecific on light microscopy, as in this case, which appears to be focal segmental glomerulosclerosis. A careful search for lipid-filled podocytes is generally helpful, and EM is most definitive.

FABRY DISEASE

Electron Microscopy

(Left) Electron micrograph of a podocyte shows characteristic laminated lipid deposits in the cytoplasm ⇨. Other coarser, dense deposits of lipid are also present ➡. These deposits are dissolved in lipid solvents in routine formalin/xylene/paraffin processing. *(Right)* Electron micrograph at high power shows lipid storage deposits with a myelin figure pattern ⇨ in a podocyte in Fabry disease. Some lipid deposits have no substructure ➡.

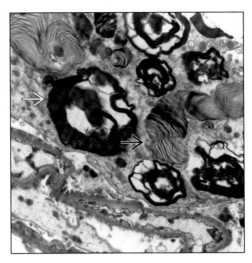
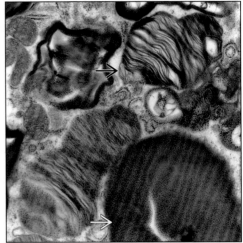

(Left) Electron micrograph of a peritubular capillary shows extensive lipid droplets in the endothelium. This accumulation may affect luminal patency and promote a proinflammatory and procoagulant response and lead to ischemic injury to the affected organ. *(Right)* This electron micrograph shows a peritubular capillary from a patient with Fabry disease. The lipid droplets are typically in a perinuclear location ➡.

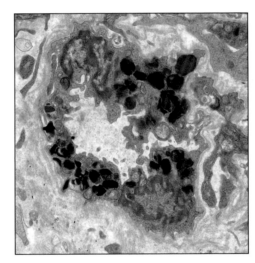
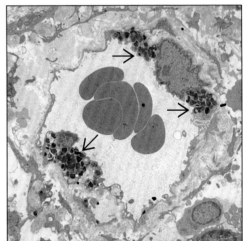

(Left) Electron micrograph of a peritubular capillary from a patient with Fabry disease shows a few lipid droplets near the nucleus ➡. *(Right)* Electron micrograph of a distal tubule from a patient with Fabry disease shows typical laminated lipid deposits in the cytoplasm. The distal tubules and collecting ducts are the most severely affected of the kidney tubules.

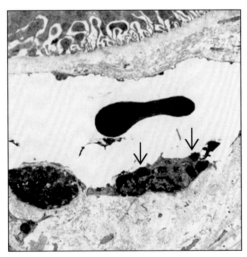
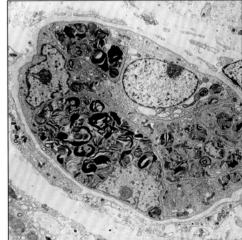

Variant Microscopic Features

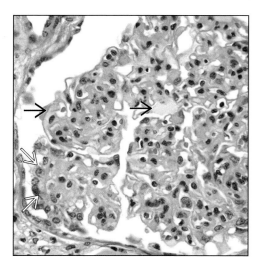
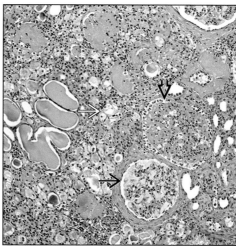

(Left) *Renal biopsy from a heterozygous female with Fabry disease shows variable lipid inclusion in podocytes; some are markedly affected ➡ and some are normal ➡ due to the random inactivation of the X chromosome.* **(Right)** *End-stage renal disease occasionally develops in females with Fabry disease, as in this case. Lipid is evident even at low power in glomeruli ➡ and tubules ➡. Collapsing focal sclerosis is also present ➡.*

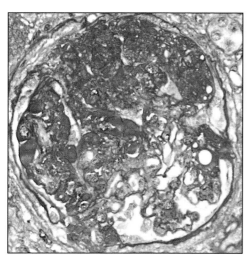
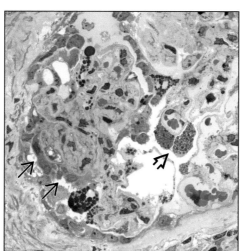

(Left) *Periodic acid-Schiff stain of a glomerulus from a patient with Fabry disease shows focal, segmental glomerulosclerosis.* **(Right)** *Epon-embedded tissue from a patient with Fabry disease shows focal, segmental glomerulosclerosis. Podocytes in the adhesion are relatively free of lipid ➡ compared with podocytes in the normal loops ➡. This suggests that podocytes in the scar are newly divided since the lipids are thought to be present for the life of the cell.*

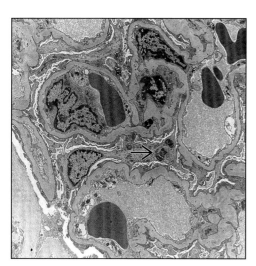
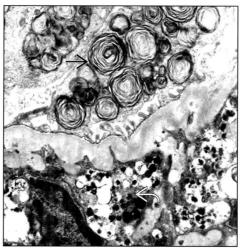

(Left) *Electron micrograph of a transplant kidney from a heterozygous Fabry female shows lipid deposits present in occasional podocytes ➡.* **(Right)** *The principal differential diagnosis with Fabry disease is chloroquine therapy, a drug that inhibits lysosomes. Patients on chloroquine for long periods can show laminated podocyte lipid accumulations ➡, indistinguishable from Fabry disease. Dense lipid granules are present in mesangial cells ➡. (Courtesy A. Cohen, MD.)*

FABRY DISEASE

Arterial Lesions

(Left) The arterial endothelium ⊟ accumulates GL3 lipid in Fabry disease. The endothelial cells show lacy vacuolization on routine paraffin processed material, which can be easily overlooked. Lipid also accumulates in smooth muscle cells, which makes the cytoplasm less dense ⊟. *(Right)* Toluidine blue stain shows a 1 micron section with densely stained granules in arterial endothelial cells ⊟, which bulge into the lumen.

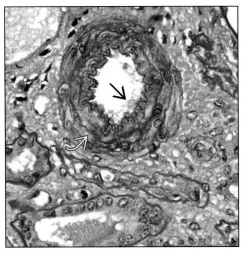
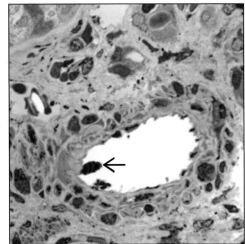

(Left) Toluidine blue stain shows a large artery with lipid in the endothelium ⊟ and media smooth muscle ⊟. One of the postulated mechanisms of tissue injury in Fabry disease is the development of thrombotic occlusion of arteries and capillaries due to lipid in the endothelium. *(Right)* Electron-dense lipid granules ⊟ in arterioles are prominent in untreated Fabry disease, as shown in this electron micrograph. Lipid is also present in the smooth muscle ⊟.

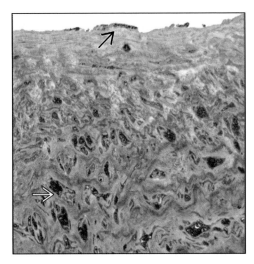
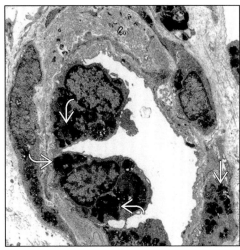

(Left) Toluidine blue stain shows a 1 micron section from a patient with Fabry disease before treatment. Lipid is present in the arterial ⊟ and capillary ⊟ endothelium, as well as in the interstitial fibroblasts ⊟. *(Right)* A 1 micron section from a patient with Fabry disease after 20 weeks of enzyme replacement therapy is shown. Lipid is markedly reduced in arterial ⊟ and capillary ⊟ endothelia as well as in the interstitial fibroblasts ⊟.

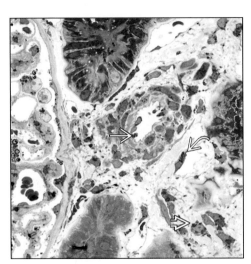
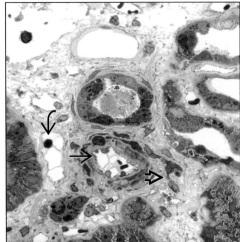

FABRY DISEASE

Effects of Enzyme Therapy

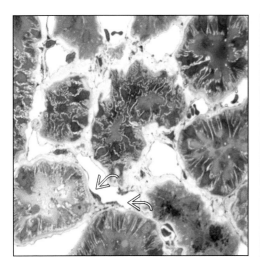

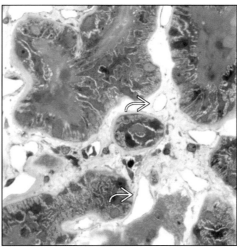

(Left) A 1 micron, Epon-embedded section from a patient with Fabry disease before treatment is shown. Lipid is present in the peritubular capillary ⇗ endothelial cells. *(Right)* A 1 micron section from a patient with Fabry disease after 20 weeks of enzyme replacement therapy (Fabrazyme) is shown. Lipid is markedly reduced in the capillary endothelium ⇗. The endothelial lipid content is the most responsive and most easily assessed to judge response to therapy.

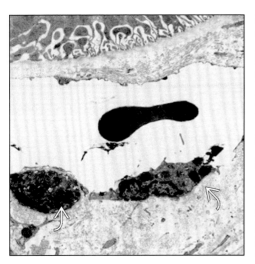

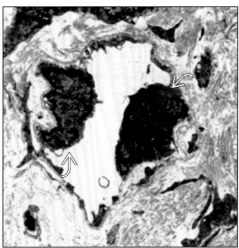

(Left) Electron micrograph from a patient with Fabry disease before treatment is shown. Lipid granules are present in the peritubular capillary endothelial cells ⇗, which are otherwise normal. *(Right)* Electron micrograph of a patient with Fabry disease after 20 weeks of enzyme replacement therapy (Fabrazyme) is shown. Lipid is markedly reduced in capillary endothelium ⇗. The endothelial lipid content is the most responsive and most easily assessed to judge response to therapy.

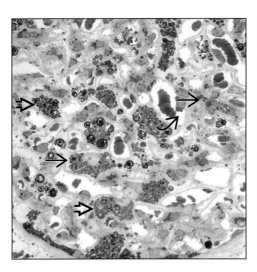

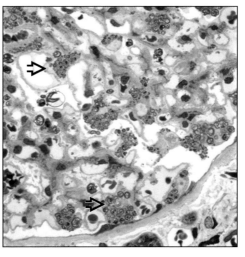

(Left) A 1 micron, Epon-embedded section from a patient with Fabry disease before treatment is shown. Lipid is present in glomerular capillary endothelium ⇗, mesangial cells ⇒, and most conspicuously, podocytes ⇗. *(Right)* A 1 micron, Epon-embedded section from a patient with Fabry disease after 20 weeks of enzyme replacement therapy (Fabrazyme) is shown. Lipid is markedly reduced in glomerular capillary endothelium and mesangial cells but remains in podocytes ⇗.

GAUCHER GLOMERULOPATHY

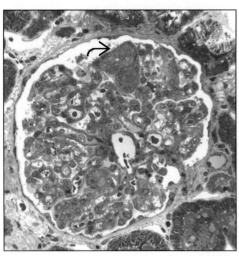

A glomerulus shows a large Gaucher cell in a glomerular capillary loop ⊘ in a 54-year-old woman with Gaucher disease, nephrotic syndrome (7 g/d), and serum creatinine 1.0 mg/dL. (Courtesy A. Cohen, MD.)

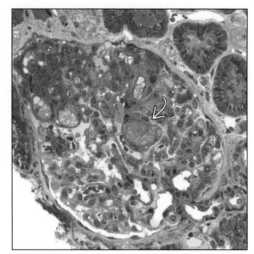

In a 54-year-old woman with Gaucher disease, a glomerular capillary loop contains a large Gaucher cell ⊘, which displays a cytoplasmic "wrinkled paper" appearance. (Courtesy A. Cohen, MD.)

TERMINOLOGY

Definitions
- Accumulation of Gaucher cells in renal parenchyma, particularly in glomerular capillaries

ETIOLOGY/PATHOGENESIS

Developmental Anomaly
- Accumulation of lipid storage material, most notably glucosylceramide
  - Reduced activity of lysosomal enzyme glucosylceramidase
    - Glucosylceramidase typically catalyzes hydrolysis of glucosylceramide into glucose and ceramide
- Renal disease mainly occurs after splenectomy

CLINICAL ISSUES

Epidemiology
- Incidence
  - Most common inherited lipid storage disease
    - Renal involvement rare

Presentation
- Proteinuria
- Hematuria
- Nephrotic syndrome

Natural History
- Type I
  - Classic adult form with hepatic and splenic involvement
  - Central nervous system (CNS) spared
- Type II
  - CNS is involved
- Type III
  - Late form of type I

Treatment
- Drugs
  - Disease may respond to enzyme replacement therapy
    - Proteinuria may essentially disappear

Prognosis
- Gaucher cells 1st accumulate in liver, spleen, and bone marrow
- Gaucher cells accumulate in tissues other than reticuloendothelial system
  - Lungs and heart

MICROSCOPIC PATHOLOGY

Histologic Features
- Glomeruli
  - Gaucher cells present in capillaries and mesangia of glomeruli
    - Gaucher cells are large, having inclusions in a linear configuration, giving appearance of wrinkled paper
    - Gaucher cells belong to monocyte/macrophage lineage
    - Storage material is PAS(+) (2° to glucosyl moiety), Sudan black(+), oil red O(+)
    - Special techniques may demonstrate PAS(+) rod-like inclusions
    - Gaucher cells cannot be distinguished from those present in spleen and liver
- Interstitium
  - Gaucher cells may also accumulate in interstitium

ANCILLARY TESTS

Immunofluorescence
- No specific findings
- ± granular deposits of IgA and IgM

GAUCHER GLOMERULOPATHY

Key Facts

Terminology
- Gaucher cells accumulate in renal parenchyma

Etiology/Pathogenesis
- Glucosylceramide accumulation 2° to ↓ glucosylceramidase activity

Clinical Issues
- Proteinuria, hematuria, nephrotic syndrome

Microscopic Pathology
- Gaucher cells in glomerular capillaries, mesangium, interstitium
  - PAS(+), Sudan black(+), oil red O(+)
  - "Wrinkled paper" inclusions
- EM: Gaucher cells have membrane-bound elongated bodies & tubules with 60-80 nm diameter fibrils
- No specific IF findings

  - Usually only trace if pure Gaucher disease

Electron Microscopy
- Gaucher cells
  - Endothelial cells/monocytes
  - Contain membrane-bound elongated bodies
    - Tubular structures consisting of fibrils 60-80 nm in diameter with twisted arrangement
- Sometimes nonspecific intramembranous dense deposits

DIFFERENTIAL DIAGNOSIS

Fabry Disease
- Deficiency in α-galactosidase A leads to accumulation of glycosphingolipids in many tissues
- Foamy cells in tubules, interstitium, and glomeruli
- Podocytes display osmiophilic inclusions
- Zebra bodies are seen by EM, consisting of whorled cytoplasmic inclusions
- Myelin inclusions/figures are seen in cytoplasm of arterial endothelial cells and myocytes of small arteries

Type III Hyperlipoproteinemia
- Capillary loop foam cells
  - Lamellated, electron-dense material
  - Cholesterol clefts

Other Renal Diseases in Gaucher Patients
- Glomerulopathies such as membranoproliferative GN, focal and segmental glomerulosclerosis, amyloidosis, etc. have been reported
  - Relationship to Gaucher disease is unclear in some reports since glomerular disease may be separate from Gaucher disease
  - Pure Gaucher glomerular disease has characteristic accumulation of Gaucher cells reported here and likely has limited relationship to other glomerulopathies

SELECTED REFERENCES
1. Santoro D et al: Gaucher disease with nephrotic syndrome: response to enzyme replacement therapy. Am J Kidney Dis. 40(1):E4, 2002
2. Faraggiana T et al: Renal lipidoses: a review. Hum Pathol. 18(7):661-79, 1987
3. Siegal A et al: Renal involvement in Gaucher's disease. Postgrad Med J. 57(668):398-401, 1981

IMAGE GALLERY

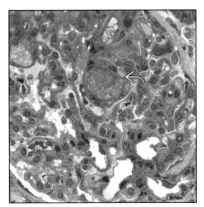 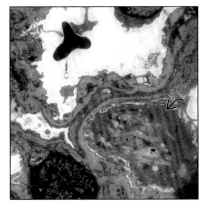 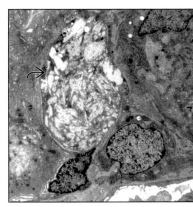

(Left) A 54 year old with Gaucher disease has a large Gaucher cell ➣ with a "wrinkled paper," laminated appearance in the cytoplasm. (Center) A Gaucher cell ➣ with intracytoplasmic inclusions is seen in the glomerulus. (Right) A Gaucher cell ➣ is seen with numerous cytoplasmic inclusions, some of which resemble the microtubular structures classically described in Gaucher cells. (Courtesy A. Cohen, MD.)

I-CELL DISEASE (MUCOLIPIDOSIS II)

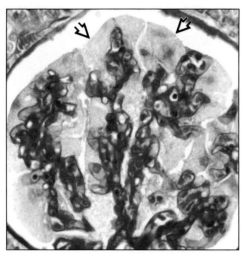

In mucolipidosis II (MLII or I-cell disease), PAS stain highlights the mesangium and capillary loops but does not stain the enlarged, pale vacuolated podocytes ⊵.

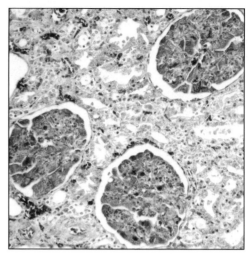

In mucolipidosis II, colloidal iron brilliantly stains the cytoplasm of every podocyte but shows no appreciable staining of other cell types within glomeruli or renal tubules.

TERMINOLOGY

Abbreviations
- Mucolipidosis II (MLII)

Synonyms
- Inclusion cell (I-cell) disease
- Mucolipidosis II α/β

Definitions
- Sialyl oligosaccharide storage disease secondary to N-acetylglucosamine-phosphotransferase deficiency

ETIOLOGY/PATHOGENESIS

Genetic Factors
- Autosomal recessive disorder, chromosome 12q23.3
- Mutation of *GNPTAB* gene
  - Encodes Golgi enzyme, N-acetylglucosamine-phosphotransferase
  - Failure to form mannose-6-phosphate, necessary for trafficking of enzymes to lysosome

CLINICAL ISSUES

Presentation
- Hurler-like syndrome presenting within 1st few years of life
  - Psychomotor retardation
  - Coarse facial features and thickened skin
  - Large joint contractures and deformed long bones
  - Hypertrophic gingiva
- Mitral and aortic valve insufficiency
- Respiratory insufficiency
- Renal abnormalities are usually absent
  - Proximal tubular dysfunction with low-grade proteinuria, hyperphosphaturia, hypercalcuria, aminoaciduria reported

Laboratory Tests
- Increased activity of lysosomal hydrolases (B-D-hexosaminidase, B-D-glucuronidase, B-N-galactosidase and α-l-fucosidase) in plasma and other body fluids
- Increased urinary excretion of oligosaccharides

Treatment
- Symptomatic
- Bone marrow or hematopoietic stem cell transplantation

Prognosis
- Slowly progressive with fatal outcome in early childhood

IMAGE FINDINGS

Radiographic Findings
- Skeletal radiographs show dysostosis multiplex

MICROSCOPIC PATHOLOGY

Histologic Features
- Podocyte cytoplasmic ballooning
  - Clear vacuoles distend cytoplasm
- Podocyte vacuoles do not stain with routine renal biopsy stains
  - PAS negative
  - Trichrome negative
  - Methenamine silver negative
- Vacuolar accumulations of glycolipids and acidic glycosaminoglycans can be stained in routine paraffin-embedded tissues
  - Hale colloidal iron positive
  - Alcian blue-PAS pH 2.5 positive
  - Sudan black positive
  - Oil red O positive in frozen sections
- Rarely, clear vacuoles in proximal tubules and interstitial cells

I-CELL DISEASE (MUCOLIPIDOSIS II)

Key Facts

Terminology
- I-cell disease

Etiology/Pathogenesis
- Autosomal recessive
- Mutation of *GNPTAB* gene, 12q23.3
- N-acetylglucosamine-phosphotransferase forms mannose-6-phosphate necessary for trafficking of enzymes to lysosomes

Clinical Issues
- Usually no renal symptoms
- May rarely have proximal tubular dysfunction
- Increased serum levels of lysosomal enzymes

Microscopic Pathology
- Diffuse podocyte vacuolization
- Vacuole contents can be stained in paraffin sections

  - Hale colloidal iron
  - Alcian blue-PAS pH 2.5
  - Sudan black
- Renal tubule and interstitial cells are rarely affected

Ancillary Tests
- Electron microscopy
  - Podocyte cytoplasm distended by vacuoles
  - Vacuoles largely empty but may contain fibrillogranular or lamellar material
  - Endothelial cells and mesangial cells not affected

Top Differential Diagnoses
- Fabry disease
- GM1 gangliosidosis

ANCILLARY TESTS

Electron Microscopy
- Podocyte cytoplasm is enlarged and vacuolated
  - Most vacuoles appear empty
  - Small amounts of fibrillogranular or lamellar material in some vacuoles
- Endothelial cells and mesangial cells free of vacuoles

DIFFERENTIAL DIAGNOSIS

Storage Diseases Primarily Affecting Podocytes
- Fabry disease
  - Storage material extracted by solvents during preparation cannot be stained
  - Podocyte cytoplasm stains dark blue with toluidine blue in plastic-embedded sections for EM
  - Ultrastructural examination reveals vacuoles filled with whirled lamellar material
- GM1 gangliosidosis
  - Storage material extracted by solvents during preparation cannot be stained
  - EM reveals vacuoles that contain small amount of fibrillogranular or lamellar material

Lysosomal Storage Disorders with Similar Clinical Features
- Hurler disease (mucopolysaccharidosis type 1H)
- Infantile galactosidosis
- Infantile free sialic acid storage disease

DIAGNOSTIC CHECKLIST

Pathologic Interpretation Pearls
- Impressive podocyte vacuolization but no renal disease
- Podocyte lipid not removed by routine processing

SELECTED REFERENCES

1. Cathey SS et al: Phenotype and genotype in mucolipidoses II and III alpha/beta: a study of 61 probands. J Med Genet. 47(1):38-48, 2010
2. Caciotti A et al: Type II sialidosis: review of the clinical spectrum and identification of a new splicing defect with chitotriosidase assessment in two patients. J Neurol. 256(11):1911-5, 2009
3. Leroy JG et al: Mucolipidosis II. GeneReviews [Internet]. Seattle: University of Washington, 2008. Updated July 7, 2009
4. Kudo M et al: Mucolipidosis II (I-cell disease) and mucolipidosis IIIA (classical pseudo-hurler polydystrophy) are caused by mutations in the GlcNAc-phosphotransferase alpha/beta -subunits precursor gene. Am J Hum Genet. 78(3):451-63, 2006
5. Daimon M et al: Surgical treatment of marked mitral valvar deformity combined with I-cell disease 'Mucolipidosis II'. Cardiol Young. 15(5):517-9, 2005
6. Bocca G et al: Defective proximal tubular function in a patient with I-cell disease. Pediatr Nephrol. 18(8):830-2, 2003
7. Renwick N et al: Foamy podocytes. Am J Kidney Dis. 41(4):891-6, 2003
8. Tang X et al: I-cell disease: report of an autopsy case. Tokai J Exp Clin Med. 20(2):109-20, 1995
9. Koga M et al: Histochemical and ultrastructural studies of inclusion bodies found in tissues from three siblings with I-cell disease. Pathol Int. 44(3):223-9, 1994
10. Kitagawa H et al: An autopsy case of I-cell disease. Ultrastructural and biochemical analyses. Am J Clin Pathol. 96(2):262-6, 1991
11. Kashtan CE et al: Proteinuria in a child with sialidosis: case report and histological studies. Pediatr Nephrol. 3(2):166-74, 1989

I-CELL DISEASE (MUCOLIPIDOSIS II)

Ancillary Techniques

(Left) This trichrome-stained glomerulus is from a case of Fabry disease. It is shown for comparison with MLII. In both diseases, the glomeruli show impressive podocyte cytoplasmic expansion by clear vacuoles. **(Right)** In MLII, the trichrome stain highlights mesangial matrix and capillary loop basement membranes, but the podocyte cytoplasmic vacuoles ⊳ remain unstained. This podocyte staining pattern is indistinguishable from the appearance of podocytes in Fabry disease.

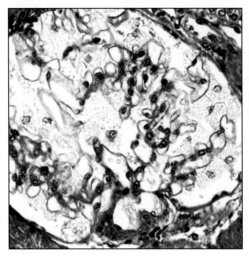
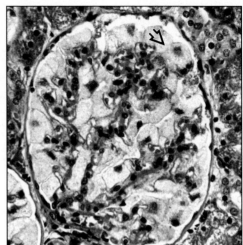

(Left) In MLII, PAS stain highlights the mesangial matrix ➔ and capillary loops ⊳ but not the enlarged vacuolated podocytes. Endothelial cells and mesangial cells do not contain vacuoles and remain inconspicuous and difficult to identify. **(Right)** In MLII, mesangial ➔ and endothelial cells do not stain with Hale colloidal iron stain. The cytoplasm of the podocytes ⊳ is strongly positive with a slightly granular quality that reflects the individually stained vacuoles.

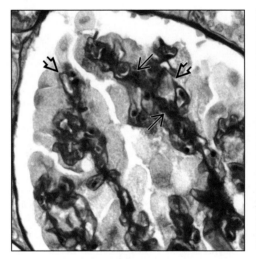
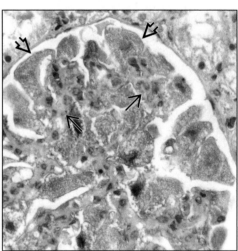

(Left) The podocyte vacuoles ⊳ do not stain with Luxol fast blue stain in MLII. The narrow mesangium and both mesangial ➔ and endothelial ➔ cells are not vacuolated. **(Right)** Sialyl oligosaccharide storage products accumulate in other organs in MLII. This section from a mitral valve shows clusters of macrophages with foamy cytoplasm very similar to podocytes. Although there is no cellular or stromal reaction to this accumulation, valve thickening and insufficiency result.

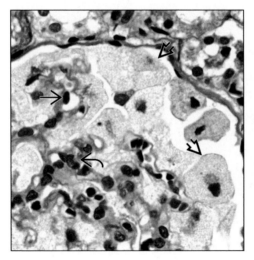
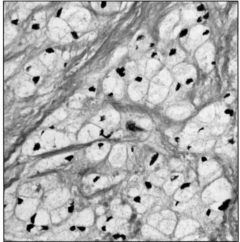

I-CELL DISEASE (MUCOLIPIDOSIS II)

Electron Microscopy

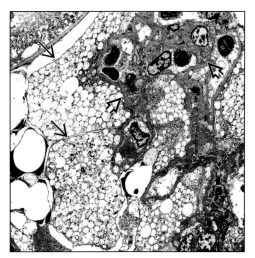
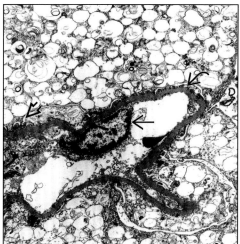

(Left) The cytoplasm of every podocyte is distended by large vacuoles ➡. The vacuoles are largely empty. The mesangium and mesangial cells are negative ⊳. (Right) In MLII, the podocyte cytoplasm is replaced by largely empty vacuoles. There is preservation of some podocyte foot processes ⊳, but others are effaced. The endothelial cells ➡ lining the capillary loop are not affected, and the capillary loop basement membrane ⇗ is normal.

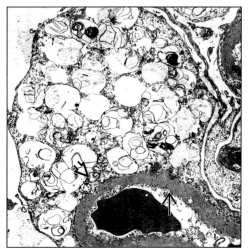
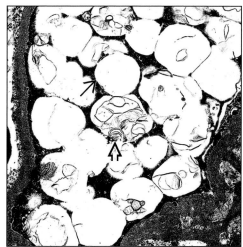

(Left) In MLII, although there is no proteinuria, foot processes are effaced ⊳. Podocyte cytoplasm covers the capillary loop basement membrane ➡. The glomerular basement membrane is normal although the tangential section makes it appear to be mildly thickened. (Right) Some podocyte vacuoles are empty ➡; others contain scant lamellar material ⊳. There is effacement of foot processes with a sheet-like covering of the capillary loop basement membrane.

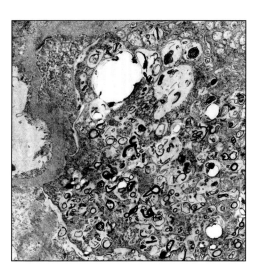
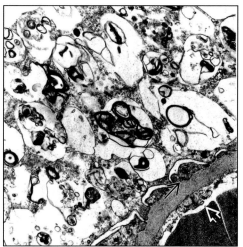

(Left) The podocyte vacuoles in this patient with MLII contain more abundant lamellar and membranous material than typical, reflecting variability in solvent extraction during the dehydration step of tissue processing. (Right) The membranous and lamellar material is more irregular in structure and distribution in MLII than in Fabry disease. There is widening of podocyte foot processes ➡ without complete effacement. The endothelial cell is not affected ⊳.

Vascular Diseases

OVERVIEW AND CLASSIFICATION OF SYSTEMIC VASCULITIDES

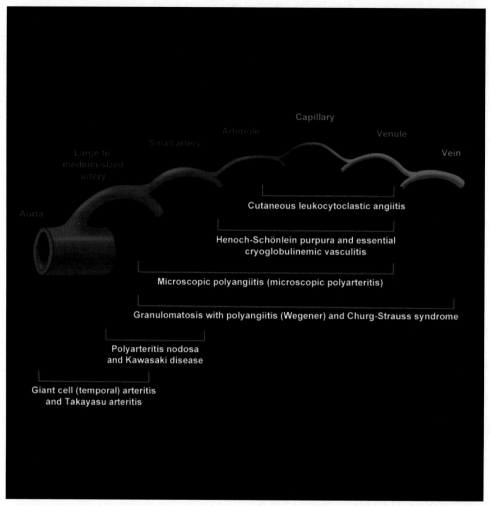

This schematic shows the predominant range of vascular involvement by different vasculitides, as described in the Chapel Hill Consensus Conference on Nomenclature of Systemic Vasculitis. Those that affect capillaries are most likely to cause glomerulonephritis (except for cutaneous leukocytoclastic angiitis). (Courtesy J.C. Jennette, MD.)

TERMINOLOGY

Synonyms
- Primary systemic vasculitides

Definitions
- Pathological
  - Vasculitis is defined as inflammation of blood vessels with demonstrable structural injury such as disruption of elastic lamina ± fibrinoid necrosis
  - Often, occlusive changes due to inflammatory infiltrate or thrombosis are evident
- Clinical
  - Clinical definition is not possible due to organ-specific or multisystemic disease
  - Rapid or prolonged evolution of clinical features over time may impede or delay definitive diagnosis
  - Thorough correlation with pathophysiologic mechanisms, serology, and imaging studies is essential

History
- Vasculitis 1st described by Kussmaul and Maier in 1866; termed "periarteritis nodosa"
- Giant cell arteritis described by Hutchinson in 1890
- Multiple vessel involvement and transmural arterial inflammation led to term "polyarteritis nodosa" by Ferrari in 1903 and later by Dickson in 1908
- Takayasu arteritis described by Takayasu in 1909
- Granulomatosis with polyangiitis (Wegener) described by Klinger and Wegener in 1931 and 1934, respectively
- Allergic granulomatosis and angiitis described by Churg and Strauss in 1951
- Introduction of term "necrotizing angiitis" and attempt to classify vasculitis by Zeek in 1952
- Vasculitis and mucocutaneous lymph node syndrome described by Kawasaki in 1966
- Introduction of the term "microscopic polyangiitis" in 1994 by Jennette et al

Classification Considerations

- No ideal classification
- Vasculitides may be primary or secondary to systemic disease
- Vasculitides can be localized to 1 organ or affect multiple organ systems
- Consensus conferences have developed classifications and criteria based on demographics, clinical characteristics, and pathology

CHAPEL HILL CONSENSUS CONFERENCE NOMENCLATURE OF SYSTEMIC VASCULITIDES (1994)

General

- Most widely used classification system
- Developed definitions and standardized diagnostic terminology
- Classification is based on size of arterial vessel involved and type of inflammatory reaction
- While size-specific vasculitides are identified, significant overlap in size exists between diagnoses, and ANCA testing may be helpful
- Cutaneous leukocytoclastic angiitis is a separate category except for those with immune complex deposits or associated with positive ANCA serology
- Pulmonary renal syndromes of pauci-immune small vessel vasculitides may have similarities and can be distinguished by ANCA serology
- Pathological correlation with clinical and laboratory features may identify specific therapeutic groups

Large Vessel Vasculitis

- Giant cell (temporal) arteritis
  - Granulomatous arteritis of the aorta and its major branches, with predilection for extracranial branches of carotid artery
  - Often involves temporal artery
  - Usually occurs in patients older than 50 and often is associated with polymyalgia rheumatica
- Takayasu arteritis
  - Granulomatous inflammation of aorta and its major branches usually occurring in patients < 50 years

Medium-sized Vessel Vasculitis

- Polyarteritis nodosa (classic polyarteritis nodosa)
  - Necrotizing inflammation of medium-sized, or small arteries without glomerulonephritis or vasculitis in arterioles, capillaries, or venules
- Kawasaki disease
  - Arteritis involving large, medium-sized and small arteries, and associated with mucocutaneous lymph node syndrome
  - Coronary arteries are often involved
  - Aorta and veins may be involved
  - Usually occurs in children

Small Vessel Vasculitis Including Capillaries, Venules, Arterioles, and Arteries

- Granulomatosis with polyangiitis (Wegener)
  - Granulomatous inflammation involving respiratory tract and necrotizing vasculitis affecting small to medium-sized vessels
  - Necrotizing glomerulonephritis is common
- Churg-Strauss syndrome
  - Eosinophil-rich and granulomatous inflammation involving respiratory tract and necrotizing vasculitis affecting small to medium-sized vessels; associated with asthma and eosinophilia
- Microscopic polyangiitis (microscopic polyarteritis)
  - Necrotizing vasculitis with few or no immune deposits, affecting small and medium-sized vessels
  - Necrotizing glomerulonephritis is very common
  - Pulmonary capillaritis often occurs
- Henoch-Schönlein purpura
  - Vasculitis with IgA-dominant immune deposits, affecting small vessels
  - Typically involves skin, gut, and glomeruli, and is associated with arthralgias or arthritis
- Essential cryoglobulinemic vasculitis
  - Small vessel vasculitis with cryoglobulin immune deposits
  - Associated with cryoglobulins in serum
  - Skin and glomeruli are often involved
- Cutaneous leukocytoclastic angiitis
  - Involves cutaneous leukocytoclastic angiitis without systemic vasculitis or glomerulonephritis

OTHER CLASSIFICATION SYSTEMS

American College of Rheumatology (1990)

- Criteria for diagnosis of vasculitides
  - Clinical criteria were developed to standardize cohorts of patients in almost all primary systemic vasculitides
  - Presence of 3 or more criteria were associated with high degree of sensitivity and specificity for diagnosis in appropriate context
  - Application of criteria for individual patients may not be entirely helpful

International Pediatric Consensus Conference (2006)

- Childhood vasculitis
  - Criteria for childhood PAN include histopathological evidence of necrotizing vasculitis or angiographic abnormality along with 1 clinical finding

Birmingham Vasculitis Activity Scores (BVAS)

- BVAS and vascular damage index (VDI) are applied to assess clinical activity and severity in patients with vasculitis

EPIDEMIOLOGY

Incidence

- Depends on specific types of vasculitis and associated primary or secondary systemic diseases

OVERVIEW AND CLASSIFICATION OF SYSTEMIC VASCULITIDES

Ethnicity and Distribution
- Takayasu arteritis and Kawasaki disease most common in Asia and Far East countries
- Granulomatosis with polyangiitis (Wegener) and Churg-Strauss syndrome have predilection for North America and Northern Europe, mainly in Caucasians
- Higher incidence of microscopic polyangiitis in Asia

ETIOLOGY/PATHOGENESIS

Etiology
- Immune complexes
  - Mixed cryoglobulinemia
  - Lupus erythematosus
  - Henoch-Schönlein purpura (presumed)
  - Possibly other vasculitides
- Autoantibodies
  - ANCA
    - Polyangiitis
    - Granulomatosis with polyangiitis (Wegener)
    - Churg-Strauss syndrome
  - Possibly other vasculitides
- Idiopathic
  - Takayasu arteritis
  - Kawasaki disease
  - Giant cell arteritis
- Other factors
  - Infections
    - Bacteria, viruses, fungi, rickettsia, parasites
  - Drug reaction

CLINICAL IMPLICATIONS

Clinical Presentation
- General constitutional symptoms are common with all forms of vasculitis in initial or acute stage
- Specific signs and symptoms depend on several factors
  - Single or multiple organ system involvement
  - Size and type of vessel involved
  - Pathogenetic mechanisms
  - Pathological findings
  - Severity of disease
- Specific presenting symptoms of complications of vasculitis
  - Vascular narrowing
  - Stenosis
  - Occlusion
  - Aneurysm formation with rupture
- Symptoms can be acute, subacute, or chronic
- Clinical features of vasculitis can mimic vasculitis-like diseases, vasculopathies, and, rarely, nonvascular diseases
- Renal findings in vasculitis
  - Hematuria
  - Proteinuria
  - Acute renal insufficiency or failure
  - Rapidly progressive renal failure
  - Slowly progressive renal failure
  - Chronic renal failure
  - Benign or malignant hypertension

Laboratory Findings
- Acute phase response is associated with active vasculitis
  - Rise in C-reactive protein
  - Elevated erythrocyte sedimentation rate
  - Increased plasma viscosity
- Complete blood counts
  - Varied granulocytosis or lymphocytosis
  - Thrombocytosis
  - Anemia
- Specific organ function tests
  - Kidney, lung, heart, liver, pancreas, endocrine
- Serologic tests
  - Various types of infections
  - Autoantibodies
    - Antineutrophil cytoplasmic antibodies
    - Antinuclear antibodies
    - Rheumatoid factor
    - Antiglomerular basement membrane
    - Other less frequent but specific antibodies
  - Complement levels
    - C3, C4, C1q
  - Urinalysis
    - Hematuria
    - Proteinuria
    - Casts
    - Cells

Imaging Findings
- Most useful in large and medium-sized vessel vasculitides
- Specific types of vessel involvement contribute toward definitive diagnosis
- Each diagnostic category may have several vascular patterns by imaging studies
- Variety of imaging modalities may be used to identify specific vascular abnormal patterns
  - Plain x-ray
  - Angiography
    - Computed tomogram
    - Magnetic resonance
  - Doppler studies
  - Tc-99m DMSA scanning

Prognosis
- Vasculitides range from self-limiting to relapsing disease involving different organs
- Significant diagnostic delays occur due to frequent clinical overlap and nonspecific findings leading to worse prognosis
- Varied morbidity and mortality
  - Specific organ involvement
  - Severity of vasculitis
  - Complications
- Sequelae of vasculitis contribute to further organ damage (stenosis, occlusion)
- Infectious complications secondary to immunosuppressive treatment are not uncommon

Treatment
- Ideally, therapeutic approaches should be based on etiology &/or pathophysiology of the vasculitides

OVERVIEW AND CLASSIFICATION OF SYSTEMIC VASCULITIDES

- ○ Corticosteroid therapy alone is useful for giant cell arteritis and Churg-Strauss syndrome without renal involvement
- Clinical heterogeneity and varied immune-mediated pathogenetic mechanisms prompt empirical form of initial therapy
- A number of treatment protocols are in use for primary and secondary vasculitides
  - ○ Cyclophosphamide and steroids in small vessel vasculitides
  - ○ Plasmapheresis and anti-CD20 antibody in severe disease
  - ○ Several immunosuppressive agents including oral steroids, methotrexate, and azathioprine are employed for maintenance of remission

MACROSCOPIC FINDINGS

General Features
- Large and medium-sized vessel vasculitides display distinctive gross characteristics from specimens obtained following excision during surgery or autopsy specimen
- Gross findings of renal vasculitides of all sizes include segmental or total infarction and progressive atrophy in renal artery stenosis
- Cortical petechial hemorrhages in small vessel vasculitides

MICROSCOPIC FINDINGS

General Features
- Several variables have to be considered before histopathological diagnosis is rendered
  - ○ Selection of appropriate tissue for biopsy
  - ○ Sample size
  - ○ Age of disease process
  - ○ Prior immunosuppressive therapy
  - ○ Nonspecific and specific findings
- Types of vascular inflammation in vasculitis
  - ○ Neutrophil rich
  - ○ Eosinophil rich
  - ○ Lymphocytic
  - ○ Granulomatous
  - ○ Necrotizing
  - ○ Focal, segmental
  - ○ Circumferential
- Other findings
  - ○ Endothelial injury and necrosis
  - ○ Disruption of internal &/or external elastic lamina
  - ○ Focal medial laminar lysis of elastic fibers
  - ○ Medial and adventitial inflammation
  - ○ Intravascular thrombosis
  - ○ Tissue infarction
  - ○ Fibromyointimal thickening of healed lesions
- Organ-specific changes
  - ○ Kidneys showing crescentic glomerulonephritis and medullary angiitis
  - ○ Alveolar capillaritis and lung hemorrhage
  - ○ Leukocytoclastic vasculitis in skin
  - ○ Myocardial inflammation and valvulitis

CONDITIONS THAT MIMIC VASCULITIS

Large Arteries
- Fibromuscular dysplasia
- Extensive atherosclerosis
- Other forms of aortitis

Medium-sized Arteries
- Embolic phenomena

Small Vessel Disease
- Atheroemboli
- Bacterial endocarditis
- Thrombotic microangiopathy
  - ○ Antiphospholipid antibody syndrome
- Atrial myxoma
- Amyloid angiopathy

SELECTED REFERENCES

1. Dillon MJ et al: Medium-size-vessel vasculitis. Pediatr Nephrol. 25(9):1641-52, 2010
2. Kobayashi S et al: Anti-neutrophil cytoplasmic antibody-associated vasculitis, large vessel vasculitis and kawasaki disease in Japan. Kidney Blood Press Res. 33(6):442-55, 2010
3. Chan M et al: Pharmacotherapy of vasculitis. Expert Opin Pharmacother. 10(8):1273-89, 2009
4. Mohammad AJ et al: The extent and pattern of organ damage in small vessel vasculitis measured by the Vasculitis Damage Index (VDI). Scand J Rheumatol. 38(4):268-75, 2009
5. Jennette JC et al: Pathologic classification of vasculitis. Pathol Case Rev 12(5): 179-85, 2007
6. Ozen S et al: EULAR/PReS endorsed consensus criteria for the classification of childhood vasculitides. Ann Rheum Dis. 65(7):936-41, 2006
7. Samarkos M et al: The clinical spectrum of primary renal vasculitis. Semin Arthritis Rheum. 35(2):95-111, 2005
8. Ball GV et al: Classification of Vasculitis Syndromes. In Vasculitis, Ball GV, Bridges Jr SL, eds. Oxford University Press, New York, 2002
9. Rao JK et al: Limitations of the 1990 American College of Rheumatology classification criteria in the diagnosis of vasculitis. Ann Intern Med. 129(5):345-52, 1998
10. Lie JT: The Vasculitides. In Biopsy diagnosis in rheumatic diseases, Lie JT eds. Igaku-Shoin, New York, 1997
11. Bajema IM et al: The renal histopathology in systemic vasculitis: an international survey study of inter- and intra-observer agreement. Nephrol Dial Transplant. 11(10):1989-95, 1996
12. Jennette JC et al: Nomenclature of systemic vasculitides. Proposal of an international consensus conference. Arthritis Rheum. 37(2):187-92, 1994
13. Bloch DA et al: The American College of Rheumatology 1990 criteria for the classification of vasculitis. Patients and methods. Arthritis Rheum. 33(8):1068-73, 1990
14. Hunder GG et al: The American College of Rheumatology 1990 criteria for the classification of vasculitis. Introduction. Arthritis Rheum. 33(8):1065-7, 1990

OVERVIEW AND CLASSIFICATION OF SYSTEMIC VASCULITIDES

Differential Diagnosis

Type	Clinical Features	Serology	Pathologic Features	Glomerular Lesion
Large Vessel Vasculitis (Large, Aorta and Major Branches)				
Giant cell arteritis: Usually > 50 years, elderly, M:F = 1:2-6	Polymyalgia rheumatica (50%), mostly head and neck symptoms	ANCA negative	Commonly temporal arteritis, mononuclear cell infiltration with multinucleated giant cells	Ischemic changes; amyloidosis
Takayasu arteritis: Usually 30-50 years, M:F = 1:8	Initial nonspecific symptoms, later ischemic effects of tissues	ANCA negative	Granulomatous panarteritis with multinucleated giant cells	Ischemic changes; mesangial or focal proliferative GN
Medium-sized Vessel Vasculitis (Medium-sized Arteries)				
Polyarteritis nodosa: Peak: 5th-7th decade, M:F = 2:1	Multisystemic, hypertension, symptoms of organ ischemia	Rarely p-ANCA(+); hepatitis B virus (+)	Fibrinoid necrotizing arteritis, transmural, healed lesions, stenosis, aneurysm formation	Ischemic changes; rare pauci-immune crescentic GN
Kawasaki disease: < 3 years in most cases; M:F = 5:1	Mucocutaneous lymph node syndrome; coronary artery vasculitis	Systemic atypical cytoplasmic ANCA(+)	Depending on stage: Acute neutrophilic arteritis, aneurysm formation, chronic inflammation, and scarring	Rare mesangial proliferative GN; patchy interstitial inflammation
Small Vessel Vasculitis (Small Arteries, Arterioles, Venules, Capillaries)				
Granulomatosis with polyangiitis (Wegener): Any age, peak: 30-50 years; M > F	Multisystemic, upper airway, lung and kidneys (90%), rapidly progressive renal failure, no asthma	Antiproteinase-3 ANCA(+) (> 75%), antimyeloperoxidase ANCA(+) (< 25%)	Necrotizing, vascular, or extravascular granulomatous inflammation	Pauci-immune crescentic GN, acute, subacute, and chronic
Microscopic polyangiitis: Any age, peak: 50 years; M = F	Multisystemic, kidney (90-100%), nephritic syndrome, rapidly progressive renal failure, no asthma	Antimyeloperoxidase ANCA(+) (60%), antiproteinase-3 ANCA(+) (15%)	Fibrinoid necrotizing vasculitis	Pauci-immune crescentic GN
Churg-Strauss syndrome: Peak: 40-60 years; M = F	Multisystemic, asthma, eosinophilia, renal manifestations in < 30% of cases	ANCA(+) (40-70%), mostly anti-MPO ANCA	Eosinophil-rich fibrinoid necrotizing vasculitis and granulomatous inflammation	Commonly mesangial, occasional pauci-immune, proliferation, focal GN with crescents
Henoch-Schönlein purpura: 90% before 10 years; M > F; adult/secondary	Multisystemic, kidney, lung, gastrointestinal tract	Sometimes elevated serum IgA level, normal complements, ANCA(-)	Leukocytoclastic vasculitis, dominant IgA and C3 deposits	Mesangial or endocapillary proliferation ± crescents and IgA deposits
Mixed cryoglobulinemic vasculitis: Adults	Multisystemic; skin and kidney frequently involved	Elevated monoclonal IgM κ rheumatoid factor, most HCV(+)	Leukocytoclastic vasculitis with cryoprecipitates, IgM κ, IgG, and C3 deposits	Membranoproliferative GN ± crescents and cryo deposits
Systemic lupus erythematosus: Any age, M:F = 1:9	Multisystemic, skin and kidney (90%)	ANA(+), dsDNA(+), sometimes ANCA(+)	Necrotizing vasculitis	Immune complex GN ± crescents; rarely, pauci-immune crescentic GN

Vascular Diseases Mimicking Vasculitis

Disease	Location	Pathology	Inflammation	Pathogenesis
Antiphospholipid antibody syndrome	All calibers of arteries and veins, capillaries	Fibrin or organizing vascular thrombi, focal recanalization	Rare or none	Antiphospholipid antibodies or lupus anticoagulant
Thrombotic microangiopathy	Small arteries, arterioles, capillaries	Endothelial swelling, intimal mucoid change, fibrin and organizing thrombi; intact elastic lamina	None	Abnormalities of ADAMTS 13; immune complexes; drug induced
Atheroembolism	All calibers of arteries up to capillaries	Luminal occlusion by crystalline cholesterol clefts ± thrombosis	None; foreign body giant cell reaction in older lesions	Embolic phenomenon from atheromas of larger arteries
Amyloid angiopathy	Medium and small arteries, arterioles, and capillaries	Congo red positive, amorphous, acellular, vascular amyloid deposits	None	AL amyloid or monoclonal lambda or kappa chains; rarely other forms of amyloid
Bacterial endocarditis	Small arteries, arterioles, and capillaries	Local ischemic changes, occasional infection-related inflammation, focal glomerulonephritis in kidney	Sometimes	Emboli from cardiac valvular vegetations, which may be bland or septic
Atrial myxoma (intracardiac tumor)	Small arteries, arterioles, and capillaries	Luminal occlusion by fragments of myxoma with ischemic tissue changes	None	Embolic phenomenon from fragments of cardiac tumor

OVERVIEW AND CLASSIFICATION OF SYSTEMIC VASCULITIDES

Large, Medium, and Small Vessel Vasculitis

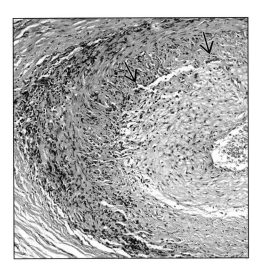 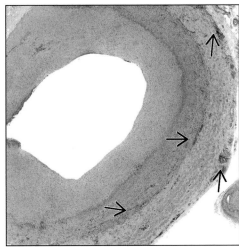

(Left) Segment of temporal artery with giant cell arteritis shows transmural arteritis with inflammatory cell infiltration in the adventitia and the media with marked fibromyointimal thickening. Rare multinucleated giant cells are noted ➡. (Right) Cross section of a thickened large artery from a young female with Takayasu arteritis shows myointimal proliferation with inflammation and focal medial and adventitial inflammation ➡. (Courtesy J.C. Jennette, MD.)

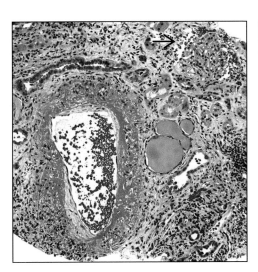 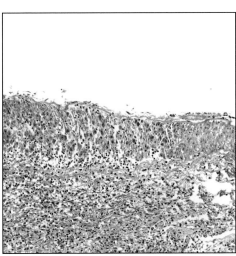

(Left) A renal artery larger than interlobular type with polyarteritis nodosa shows circumferential, transmural fibrinoid necrosis accompanied by primarily neutrophilic infiltrate. An uninvolved glomerulus is seen ➡. (Right) Microscopic section of a coronary artery from a patient with Kawasaki disease shows medial and intimal mixed inflammatory cell infiltrate without significant fibrinoid necrosis. (Courtesy J.C. Jennette, MD.)

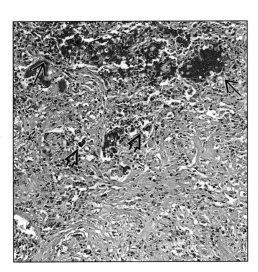 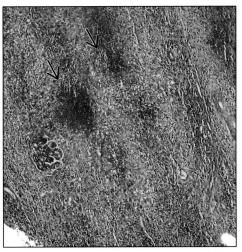

(Left) A section of a lung from a patient with granulomatosis with polyangiitis (Wegener) shows granulomatous inflammation with hemorrhage ➡. Epithelioid and multinucleated giant cells are noted ➡. (Right) PAS-stained kidney section with granulomatosis with polyangiitis (Wegener) shows typical irregular necrotizing granulomatous inflammation with a neutrophilic center ➡. An adjacent glomerulus with ischemic change is noted. (Courtesy W. Travis, MD.)

Small Vessel Vasculitides

(Left) A specimen from a patient with high-titer MPO-ANCA shows full-thickness necrotizing vasculitis of a small intrarenal artery surrounded by active neutrophilic and lymphocytic infiltrate with loss of elastic lamina, consistent with microscopic polyangiitis. There is interstitial inflammation and tubulitis. *(Right)* Glomerulus from a patient with PR3-ANCA(+) shows a large, almost circumferential cellular crescent. Part of the Bowman capsule is disrupted by periglomerular inflammatory infiltrate ➡.

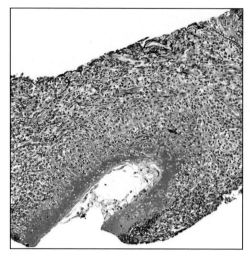
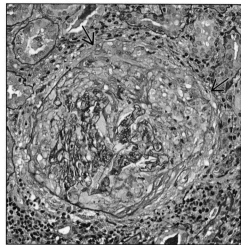

(Left) Subcutaneous medium-sized artery from a patient with Churg-Strauss syndrome shows segmental transmural inflammation with many eosinophils. *(Right)* Intrarenal small artery in a kidney biopsy shows granulomatous vasculitis with fibrinoid necrosis of the intima surrounded by lymphocytes, eosinophils, and epithelioid cells.

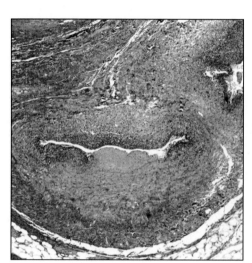
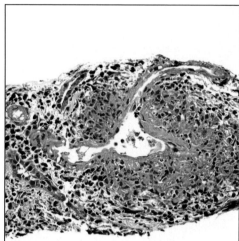

(Left) A section of lung from a patient with pulmonary hemorrhage and positive MPO-ANCA titer shows alveolar hemorrhage and focal capillaritis with neutrophils and lymphocytes ➡. *(Right)* A segment of skin shows extensive leukocytoclastic vasculitis with dominant IgA and C3 deposits (capillaries infiltrated by neutrophils and fragmented neutrophilic nuclei) in a patient with nephritis and palpable Henoch-Schönlein purpuric rash in the legs.

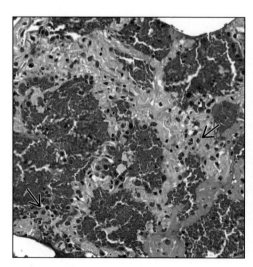
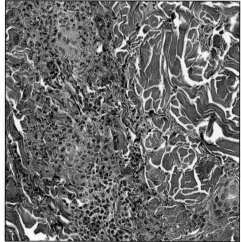

OVERVIEW AND CLASSIFICATION OF SYSTEMIC VASCULITIDES

Differential Diagnosis

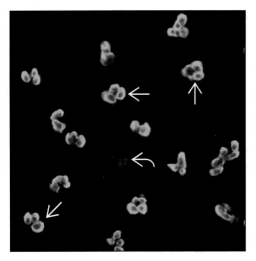 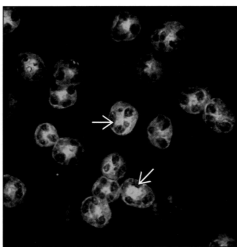

(Left) p-ANCA (perinuclear) pattern ➡ due to MPO IgG antibodies is demonstrated by indirect IF with a patient's serum incubated on alcohol-fixed normal neutrophils. The cytoplasm is not visible. A negative eosinophil is also present ➡. (Courtesy A.B. Collins, BS.) (Right) The c-ANCA (cytoplasmic) pattern ➡ due to PR3 antibodies is demonstrated by indirect IF with a patient's serum incubated on an alcohol-fixed smear of normal neutrophils. (Courtesy A.B. Collins, BS.)

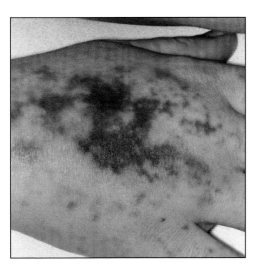 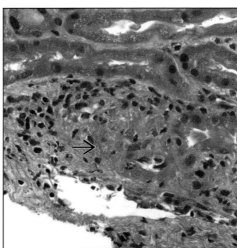

(Left) The rash in a patient with hepatitis C-associated cryoglobulinemia is manifested by focal hemorrhagic palpable purpura. (Courtesy C. Magro, MD.) (Right) The small vessel vasculitis in mixed cryoglobulinemia has eosinophilic material in the vessel wall that somewhat resembles fibrin ➡, but much of it is the precipitated immune complexes of monoclonal IgM rheumatoid factor and IgG. In contrast to fibrin, these deposits are rounded, PAS(+), and stain for IgM and IgG.

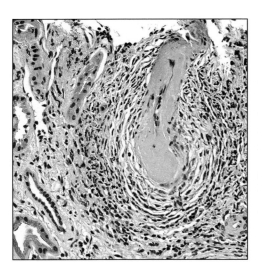 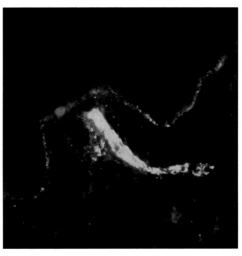

(Left) Cryoglobulin-associated small vessel vasculitis typically has amorphous pale eosinophilic vascular cryoglobulin deposits; here, they narrow the lumen in a kidney biopsy from a patient with HCV and cryoglobulinemic glomerulonephritis. (Right) Immunofluorescence microscopy of skin shows positive cryoglobulin deposits that stain for IgM within the dermal vessels. These deposits also stain for IgG and C3. The IgM is a monoclonal (kappa) rheumatoid factor.

Differential Diagnosis

(Left) Florid arteritis in an SLE patient is manifested by an interlobular artery with transmural fibrinoid necrosis ➡ and inflammatory infiltrate of neutrophils and lymphocytes. (Courtesy B. Fyfe, MD.) *(Right)* Marked destructive arteritis is evident in the kidney of an SLE patient with transmural fibrinoid necrotizing inflammation ➡ of a small artery with obliterative changes. Vasculitis in SLE is due to immune complex deposition. (Courtesy B. Fyfe, MD.)

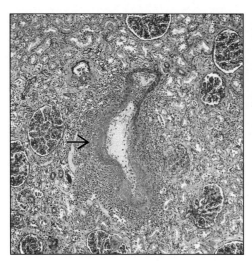
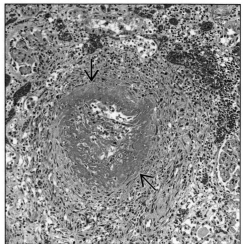

(Left) A renal biopsy from a young female patient shows noninflammatory flocculent PAS-positive intimal arteriolar deposits termed "lupus vasculopathy" ➡. This lesion often accompanies diffuse lupus nephritis and is sometimes mistaken for lupus vasculitis. *(Right)* Skin over the elbow shows a palpable purpuric rash with focal pustular changes in a patient presenting with Henoch-Schönlein purpura. (Courtesy C. Magro, MD.)

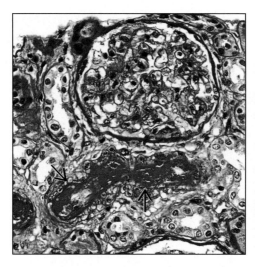
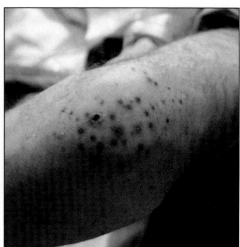

(Left) Skin biopsy shows leukocytoclastic vasculitis and extravasation of red blood cells in a patient with Henoch-Schönlein purpura (HSP). *(Right)* Immunofluorescence of skin biopsy from a patient with Henoch-Schönlein purpura shows dominant granular staining for IgA in the vascular and perivascular areas, enabling the diagnosis of HSP to be made.

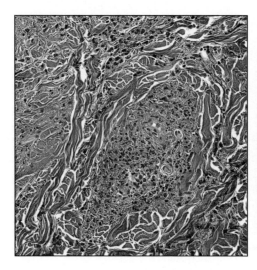
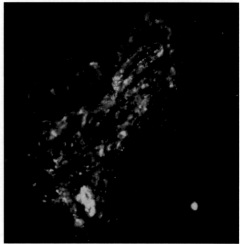

OVERVIEW AND CLASSIFICATION OF SYSTEMIC VASCULITIDES

Lesions that Mimic Vasculitis

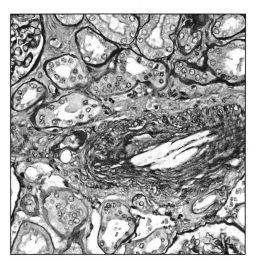

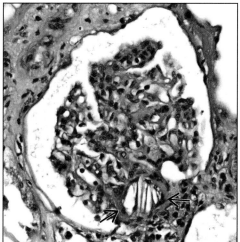

(Left) A biopsy from an elderly patient presenting with acute renal failure, skin rash, and early gangrenous changes of digits in the foot shows atheroemboli within an interlobular artery characterized by needle-shaped spaces signifying cholesterol crystals washed off during processing of the tissue. (Right) A glomerulus shows needle-shaped atheroemboli ⇨ within the hilar arteriole that led to mild to moderate ischemic collapse of the capillary tuft. (Courtesy L. Barisoni, MD.)

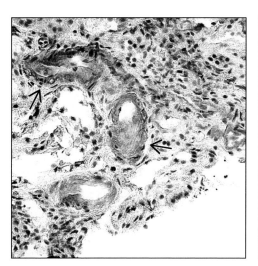

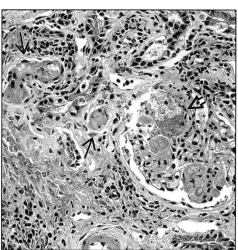

(Left) Amyloid angiopathy. Kidney biopsy from an older patient presenting with heart and liver disease and progressive renal failure with minimal proteinuria shows exclusively vascular and microvascular ⇨ amyloid deposits by Congo red. (Right) A kidney biopsy from a patient with antiphospholipid antibody syndrome having livedo reticularis, stroke, and acute renal failure shows noninflammatory microvascular thrombi within the arterioles ⇨ and glomerulus ⇨.

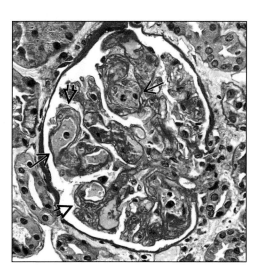

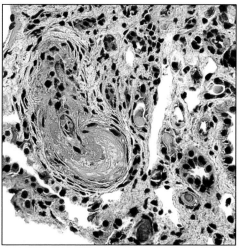

(Left) Glomerulus in a patient with thrombotic thrombocytopenic purpura shows focal intracapillary microthrombi ⇨ and thickening of the peripheral capillary wall with focal double contours ⇨. (Right) Renal biopsy from a patient with thrombotic thrombocytopenic purpura shows noninflammatory endothelial injury of an arteriole with detachment, subendothelial widening, and accumulation of a fibrin thrombus. Focal trapped fragmented RBCs are noted.

ANCA-RELATED GLOMERULONEPHRITIS

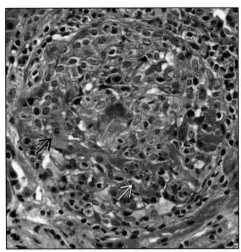

ANCA-related glomerulonephritis (GN) typically has focal necrosis and crescents. Here, the cellular crescent fills most of the Bowman capsule and contains a mitotic figure ➡. Neutrophils ➡ and fibrin are present.

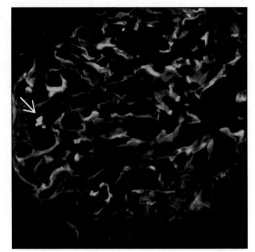

ANCA-related GN classically has little immunoglobulin deposition in glomeruli (pauci-immune) as seen in this IgG stain in a 29 yo woman with hematuria and p-ANCA (MPO). Reabsorption droplets are in podocytes ➡.

TERMINOLOGY

Abbreviations
- Glomerulonephritis related to anti-neutrophil cytoplasmic antibodies (ANCA-GN)

Synonyms
- Pauci-immune glomerulonephritis (PIGN)
- Pauci-immune crescentic glomerulonephritis
- Rapidly progressive glomerulonephritis

Definitions
- Glomerulonephritis related to or caused by ANCA, usually with prominent crescents and little or no immunoglobulin deposition (pauci-immune)
- May occur as an isolated glomerular disease or as part of a systemic ANCA vasculitis syndrome
- History
  - Autoantibody to neutrophil cytoplasmic antigen(s) detected in segmental necrotizing GN (1982)
  - ANCA reported in granulomatosis with polyangiitis (Wegener) (GPA) (1985)
  - Perinuclear antigen (p-ANCA) identified as anti-myeloperoxidase (MPO) in patients with pauci-immune necrotizing GN ± vasculitis (1988)
  - Cytoplasmic antigen (c-ANCA) identified as proteinase 3 (PR3) (1989)

ETIOLOGY/PATHOGENESIS

Autoimmune Disease
- Autoantibodies made to neutrophil lysosomal components (ANCA)
  - T cells, macrophages may also play a role
- Trigger for ANCA production generally unknown
  - Presumed immune dysregulation (Th17/Treg)
  - Evidence for molecular mimicry
  - Can be precipitated by drugs
    - Propothiouracil, hydralazine, penicillamine, minocycline
- Suggested risk factors
  - Leptin receptor gene (LEPR) polymorphism
  - CD226, a leukocyte-endothelial adhesion molecule
  - Epigenetic control of MPO and PR3 expression, which are neutrophil cytoplasmic enzymes

ANCA
- Mechanism of action
  - Autoantibodies react to either PR3 or MPO, constituents of lysosomal proteins in neutrophils and monocytes
    - Patients make either anti-MPO or anti-PR3, but rarely both (~ 6%)
    - Antigens expressed on surface of activated neutrophils
  - Action on neutrophil
    - Presence of ANCA augments neutrophil-mediated cytotoxicity of cultured endothelium
    - ANCA-initiated signal transduction pathways for cell activation, FcR participation
    - Neutrophils activate alternative complement pathway
    - Leukocyte activation → adhesion to primed endothelial cells, resulting in subsequent damage
  - ANCA can be present without overt disease
    - Suggests trigger is needed, such as neutrophil activation from infection
- Measurement of ANCA titers useful in management
- May be other targets, since ~ 20% of PIGN is ANCA(-)
  - Plasminogen antibodies in 25% of ANCA(+) patients
  - Lysosomal-associated membrane protein-2 (LAMP-2)
    - Anti-LAMP-2 reported in most patients with PIGN
    - Not confirmed in a subsequent study

Animal Models
- Adoptive transfer of anti-MPO antibodies precipitates crescentic GN and vasculitis in immunodeficient mice (RAG-1 knockout)

ANCA-RELATED GLOMERULONEPHRITIS

Key Facts

Terminology
- Crescentic GN related to ANCA
- Can be isolated pauci-immune GN or with systemic vasculitis (GPA, MPA, CSS)

Etiology/Pathogenesis
- Autoantibody to neutrophil lysosomal components
  - MPO (p-ANCA) and PR3 (c-ANCA)
- ANCA activates neutrophils
- Neutrophils injure endothelium

Clinical Issues
- Rapidly progressive renal failure
  - Hematuria, proteinuria
- Systemic signs of vasculitis present in majority
- ANCA: 80% sensitive and 96% specific for PIGN

Microscopic Pathology
- Focal, necrotizing glomerulonephritis with prominent crescents
  - Renal vasculitis in 5-35%
  - Variable interstitial inflammation
- IF: Little or no immunoglobulin or complement deposits (pauci-immune)
- EM: Scant or no immune-complex type deposits

Top Differential Diagnoses
- Anti-GBM disease
- Immune complex-mediated crescentic GN
- ANCA superimposed on other diseases

Diagnostic Checklist
- Glomerular lesions correlate with survival
- Glomerular pathology same in PIGN, GPA, MPA, CSS

- Proves that ANCA is not just a marker, but pathogenic
- Requires neutrophils as target
- Enhanced by activation of alternate complement pathway
- No animal models associated with anti-PR3 antibodies yet developed
  - Additional cofactors may be necessary
- Transfer of GN and vasculitis to rats with anti-LAMP-2

CLINICAL ISSUES

Epidemiology
- Incidence
  - 4 per 10^6 patient-years (UK)
  - ~ 60% of patients with crescentic GN (> 50% crescents) are ANCA(+)
  - ~ 60% of pulmonary-renal syndrome are ANCA(+)
- Age
  - Mean age ~ 60 years (increased incidence > 60 years)
  - Occasionally in children (as young as 2 years)
- Gender
  - No gender predilection
- Ethnicity
  - Worldwide

Presentation
- Hematuria, proteinuria
- Rapidly progressive renal failure
- Flu-like syndrome common at onset
  - Fever, arthralgia, myalgia
- Signs of extrarenal vasculitis in ~ 75%
  - Specific features lead to diagnosis of granulomatosis with polyangiitis (Wegener), microscopic polyangiitis, or Churg-Strauss syndrome

Laboratory Tests
- Positive ANCA test by indirect immunofluorescence plus ELISA
  - Sensitivity of 80% and specificity of 96% for PIGN
  - Negative ANCA in ~ 20% of PIGN
- Type of ANCA does not permit specific diagnosis

- MPO ANCA is most common in PIGN, MPA, and CSS (50-60%)
- PR3 ANCA most common in GPA (~ 75%)
- Other ("atypical") ANCA specificities described
  - React with lactoferrin, elastase, and P-cathepsin-G
  - Found in variety of conditions with chronic inflammation or infection
- Negative ANCA associated with absence of disease activity
  - Varied opinions on value of ANCA titers to monitor status
- Normal complement levels

Treatment
- Drugs
  - Cyclophosphamide and prednisolone to induce remission
  - Maintenance therapy with less toxic drugs such as mycophenolate mofitel, azathioprine
  - Plasmapheresis or plasma exchange in refractory cases
  - Rituximab (anti-CD20) in clinical trials
    - May be superior in relapsing disease
  - Novel, less toxic approaches under investigation

Prognosis
- ~ 75% achieve remission
- ~ 30% relapse
- 60-75% 5-year patient and kidney survival
  - Risk factors for early death and ESRD
    - Dialysis dependence at onset
    - Male gender
    - Age > 65 years

MACROSCOPIC FEATURES

Kidney
- Flea-bitten appearance due to blood in tubules and Bowman space

MICROSCOPIC PATHOLOGY

Histopathologic Features

- Glomeruli
  - Focal fibrinoid necrosis with neutrophils
    - GBM is disrupted in areas of necrosis
    - Segmental to global pattern of involvement
  - Crescents prominent, typically > 50% of glomeruli
    - Crescents contain proliferating parietal epithelial cells, neutrophils, and macrophages
    - Crescents of varied age (cellular, fibrocellular, and fibrous)
    - Cellular crescents become fibrotic and can obstruct outlet into proximal tubule
  - GBM of normal thickness on PAS stain
  - No mesangial hypercellularity
  - Normal glomeruli usually present
- Tubules and interstitium
  - Varying degrees of active periglomerular and interstitial inflammation
  - Necrotizing medullary capillaritis
- Vessels
  - Renal vasculitis in 5-35%
    - Involves small arteries, arterioles, capillaries, venules
    - Leukocytoclastic vasculitis pattern (neutrophils, fibrinoid necrosis)
    - Fibrinoid necrotizing arteritis with neutrophils
    - Rarely transmural lymphocytic arteritis
- Later stages
  - Global glomerulosclerosis and progressive interstitial fibrosis and tubular atrophy
  - Arterial vessels heal by sclerosis and narrowing of lumina

ANCILLARY TESTS

Immunofluorescence

- Pauci-immune pattern in glomeruli
  - Typically no more than 1+ granular staining for IgG, IgM, IgA, C3, and C1q (60%)
  - Sclerotic lesions: Nonspecific IgM and C3
- If > 1+ Ig, consider immune complex GN as underlying cause with superimposed ANCA
  - Immune complex GN with granular mesangial/capillary wall immunoglobulin and complement staining (24%)
- If > 1+ linear staining of GBM, probably anti-GBM GN concurrent with ANCA-GN
  - Anti-GBM antibody GN with linear glomerular IgG staining (15%)
- Active crescents and segments with fibrinoid necrosis stain for fibrin/fibrinogen

Electron Microscopy

- Glomerular endothelial swelling, injury, and loss
- Neutrophils, fibrin in capillaries
- Disrupted GBM in necrotic segments associated with crescents
- Scant or no immune-complex deposits
  - May be scattered mesangial and even subepithelial deposits of uncertain significance

DIFFERENTIAL DIAGNOSIS

Anti-GBM Disease

- Accounts for 5-15% of crescentic GN
- Bright, linear staining of GBM for IgG
- Positive serological test for anti-GBM antibodies
- Vasculitis absent
- ~ 30-40% are also positive for ANCA

Immune Complex-mediated Crescentic GN

- Accounts for ~ 30-40% of crescentic GN
- Distinguished by greater deposition of Ig and complement (2+ or greater)
  - Immune complexes also by EM in mesangium and along GBM
- May have mesangial hypercellularity
- Some due to specific diseases such as lupus, cryoglobulinemia, IgA nephropathy, MPGN
  - The rest are heterogeneous, idiopathic, and not well defined

Henoch-Schönlein Purpura/IgA Nephropathy

- Prominent IgA in mesangium
- Mesangial hypercellularity present
- Usually not florid fibrinoid necrosis

Acute Postinfectious GN

- Prominent endocapillary hypercellularity
- Prominent granular IgG and C3 along GBM
- Numerous subepithelial humps by EM

ANCA Superimposed on Other Diseases

- MGN, IgA nephropathy, lupus nephritis may have crescents and necrosis due to superimposed ANCA-GN

DIAGNOSTIC CHECKLIST

Clinically Relevant Pathologic Features

- Pathological classification of ANCA-GN (Berden 2010)
  - Focal
    - > 50% normal glomeruli
    - Glomerular lesions in < 50%
    - Normal = no segmental sclerosis, synechiae, or extensive splitting of Bowman capsule, and > 1 layer of parietal epithelium; may have < 4 leukocytes/glomerulus, segmental GBM wrinkling, slight collapse of tuft
  - Crescentic
    - Cellular or fibrocellular crescents in > 50% of glomeruli
    - Crescents containing > 10% cellularity included
    - Fibrous crescents not counted
  - Mixed
    - Heterogeneous glomerular lesions, none predominating as > 50%
  - Sclerotic
    - Global glomerulosclerosis in > 50% of glomeruli
    - Global glomerulosclerosis defined as > 80% of capillary tuft
- Prognostic significance
  - 5-year renal survival

Frequency of MPO-ANCA & PR3-ANCA by Clinicopathologic Syndromes

	Granulomatosis with Polyangiitis	Microscopic Polyangiitis	Churg-Strauss Syndrome	Renal Limited Crescentic GN
MPO-ANCA (%)	20	50	60	60
PR3-ANCA (%)	75	40	10	20
ANCA(-) (%)	5	10	30	20

Adapted from Jennette JC et al: Pauci-immune and antineutrophil cytoplasmic autoantibody mediated crescentic glomerulonephritis and vasculitis. In Jennette JC et al: Heptinstall's Pathology of the Kidney. 6th ed. Philadelphia: Lippincott Williams & Wilkins. 643-73, 2007.

Comparison Between MPO-ANCA & PR3-ANCA Pauci-immune Crescentic GN

	MPO-ANCA	PR3-ANCA
Extrarenal disease	Lower	Higher
Glomerular lesion	Diffuse	Focal
Chronic renal parenchymal change	Higher	Lower
Intrarenal granulomata	5.5% of cases	2.7% of cases
Kidney survival at 5 years	60%	65%
Patient survival at 5 years	67%	75%

Adapted from Vizjak A et al: Histologic and immunohistologic study and clinical presentation of ANCA-associated glomerulonephritis with correlation to ANCA antigen specificity. Am J Kidney Dis. 41(3):539-49, 2003.

- 93% focal
- 76% crescentic
- 61% mixed
- 50% sclerotic

Pathologic Interpretation Pearls

- Extensive crescents and fibrinoid necrosis with scant immune deposits almost always due to ANCA
- Glomerular pathology does not discriminate the various clinicopathologic conditions caused by ANCA (isolated PIGN, GPA, MPA, CSS)
- % normal glomeruli correlates with outcome at 5 years

SELECTED REFERENCES

1. Berden AE et al: Anti-plasminogen antibodies compromise fibrinolysis and associate with renal histology in ANCA-associated vasculitis. J Am Soc Nephrol. 21(12):2169-79, 2010
2. Berden AE et al: Histopathologic classification of ANCA-associated glomerulonephritis. J Am Soc Nephrol. 21(10):1628-36, 2010
3. Falk RJ et al: ANCA disease: where is this field heading? J Am Soc Nephrol. 21(5):745-52, 2010
4. Stone JH et al: Rituximab versus cyclophosphamide for ANCA-associated vasculitis. N Engl J Med. 363(3):221-32, 2010
5. Pallan L et al: ANCA-associated vasculitis: from bench research to novel treatments. Nat Rev Nephrol. 5(5):278-86, 2009
6. Chen M et al: Antineutrophil cytoplasmic autoantibody-associated vasculitis in older patients. Medicine (Baltimore). 87(4):203-9, 2008
7. Jennette JC et al: New insight into the pathogenesis of vasculitis associated with antineutrophil cytoplasmic autoantibodies. Curr Opin Rheumatol. 20(1):55-60, 2008
8. Kain R et al: Molecular mimicry in pauci-immune focal necrotizing glomerulonephritis. Nat Med. 14(10):1088-96, 2008
9. Jennette JC et al: Pauci-immune and antineutrophil cytoplasmic autoantibody mediated crescentic glomerulonephritis and vasculitis. In Jennette JC et al: Heptinstall's Pathology of the Kidney. 6th ed. Philadelphia: Lippincott Williams & Wilkins. 643-73, 2007
10. Rutgers A et al: Coexistence of anti-glomerular basement membrane antibodies and myeloperoxidase-ANCAs in crescentic glomerulonephritis. Am J Kidney Dis. 46(2):253-62, 2005
11. Jennette JC: Rapidly progressive crescentic glomerulonephritis. Kidney Int. 63(3):1164-77, 2003
12. Slot MC et al: Renal survival and prognostic factors in patients with PR3-ANCA associated vasculitis with renal involvement. Kidney Int. 63(2):670-7, 2003
13. Vizjak A et al: Histologic and immunohistologic study and clinical presentation of ANCA-associated glomerulonephritis with correlation to ANCA antigen specificity. Am J Kidney Dis. 41(3):539-49, 2003
14. Hauer HA et al: Renal histology in ANCA-associated vasculitis: differences between diagnostic and serologic subgroups. Kidney Int. 61(1):80-9, 2002
15. Bajema IM et al: Kidney biopsy as a predictor for renal outcome in ANCA-associated necrotizing glomerulonephritis. Kidney Int. 56(5):1751-8, 1999
16. Franssen CF et al: Determinants of renal outcome in anti-myeloperoxidase-associated necrotizing crescentic glomerulonephritis. J Am Soc Nephrol. 9(10):1915-23, 1998
17. Niles JL et al: Wegener's granulomatosis autoantigen is a novel neutrophil serine proteinase. Blood. 74(6):1888-93, 1989
18. Falk RJ et al: Anti-neutrophil cytoplasmic autoantibodies with specificity for myeloperoxidase in patients with systemic vasculitis and idiopathic necrotizing and crescentic glomerulonephritis. N Engl J Med. 318(25):1651-7, 1988
19. van der Woude FJ et al: Autoantibodies against neutrophils and monocytes: tool for diagnosis and marker of disease activity in Wegener's granulomatosis. Lancet. 1(8426):425-9, 1985
20. Davies DJ et al: Segmental necrotising glomerulonephritis with antineutrophil antibody: possible arbovirus aetiology? Br Med J (Clin Res Ed). 285(6342):606, 1982

Microscopic Features

(Left) ANCA-GN is classically a focal, segmental glomerulonephritis with some glomeruli spared ⇨ and others severely involved ➡. An interstitial inflammation is also commonly encountered. (Right) An early and active lesion in ANCA-GN is fibrinoid necrosis of a segment of the glomerular tuft ⇨, which appears brick in red color and elicits a reaction of the Bowman capsule. Note that the remainder of the glomerulus appears entirely normal. What localizes the inflammation so exquisitely is unknown.

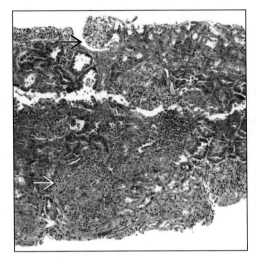
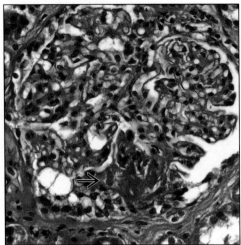

(Left) Segmental destruction ➡ of the glomerulus in ANCA-GN is seen here, with sparing of a portion on the left. Note the marked periglomerular inflammatory response ➡ associated with the segmental necrosis. (Right) This case of ANCA-GN had both active lesions with necrosis and the a segmental glomerular scar ⇨ and adhesion. If only segmental scars were present, this might be mistaken for FSGS. However the GBM is typically disrupted (in contrast to FSGS). This can be seen best on a PAS stain.

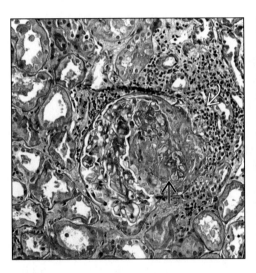
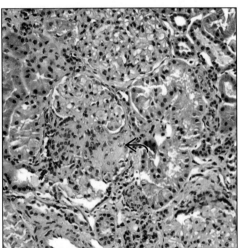

(Left) Anti-MPO-related GN with destruction of the Bowman capsule is accompanied by a marked granulomatous reaction with multinucleated giant cells ➡. Giant cells are also sometimes encountered in anti-GBM nephritis. (Right) A fibrocellular crescent in a patient with ANCA-GN is seen. A Bowman capsule disruption is evident in this PAS stain ⇨. The epithelium has attempted to "recanalize" ➡ the crescent. In animal studies, it takes only a few weeks to reach this stage.

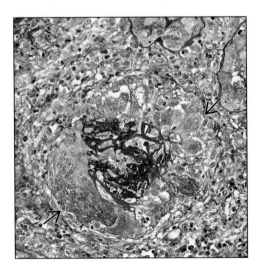
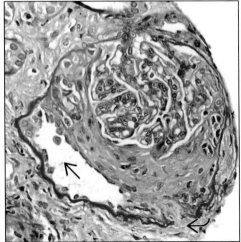

ANCA-RELATED GLOMERULONEPHRITIS

Immunofluorescence and Electron Microscopy

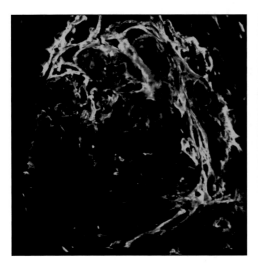 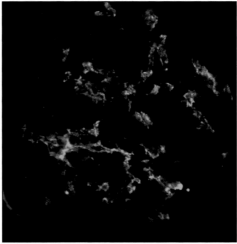

(Left) Fibrin or fibrinogen is a characteristic feature of the active crescents in ANCA-GN, as shown here in a p-ANCA(+) case with isolated GN (no documented vasculitis). *(Right)* Although ANCA-GN usually has little or no immunoglobulin, it is not uncommon to identify scattered immune complex deposits, as seen in this case stained for IgG. In addition, IgM, C3, and even IgA can be seen in small amounts (typically no more than 1+).

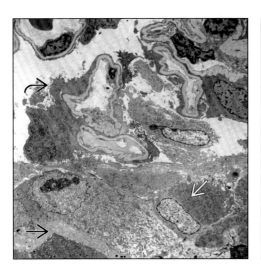 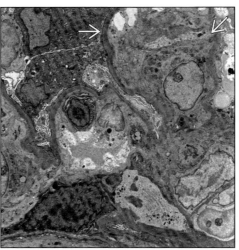

(Left) EM of ANCA-GN shows a crescent ➡ with proliferating cells on the Bowman capsule ➡. The podocytes ➡ are markedly reactive with loss of foot processes. The GBM is normal with no deposits although it is segmentally wrinkled. *(Right)* Electron microscopy of a glomerulus with ANCA-GN shows varying endothelial swelling and segmental separation with a narrow subendothelial lucent zone ➡. No immune deposits are identified.

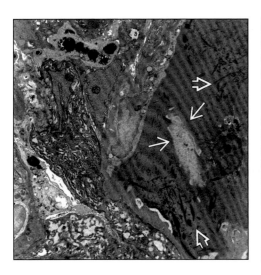 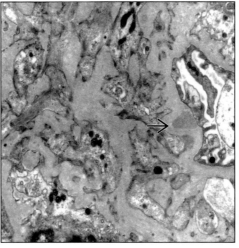

(Left) High magnification of a glomerular capillary in ANCA-GN shows segmental detachment of the endothelial cell with degenerative change ➡. The capillary lumen is filled with proteinaceous material admixed with fibrin tactoids ➡, suggesting the early phase of fibrinoid change. *(Right)* Just as sparse deposits can be seen by IF in ANCA disease, scattered electron-dense deposits can sometimes be seen by EM, as seen here in the subepithelial space ➡. Their significance, if any, is unknown.

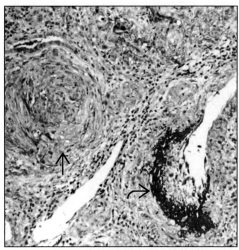

MPO-ANCA-mediated crescentic glomerulonephritis shows segmental transmural necrotizing small vessel vasculitis ➡ adjacent to a glomerulus with circumferential crescent ➡.

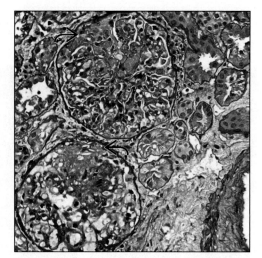

Two glomeruli show segmental pauci-immune type glomerulonephritis with small cellular crescents ➡ in the Bowman space. The remaining portions of the glomeruli are unremarkable.

TERMINOLOGY

Abbreviations
- Microscopic polyangiitis (MPA)

Synonyms
- Microscopic polyarteritis
- p-ANCA mediated small vessel vasculitis
- Systemic or renal limited crescentic glomerulonephritis
- "Pauci-immune" glomerulonephritis

Definitions
- Chapel Hill Consensus Conference
  - Necrotizing vasculitis, with few or no immune deposits, affecting small vessels (i.e., capillaries, venules, or arterioles)
  - Necrotizing arteritis involving small and medium-sized arteries may be present
  - Necrotizing glomerulonephritis is very common
  - Pulmonary capillaritis often occurs

ETIOLOGY/PATHOGENESIS

Environmental Exposure
- Higher rate of onset in winter than summer
  - Similar to granulomatosis with polyangiitis (Wegener)

Pathogenesis
- Anti-neutrophil cytoplasmic antibody (ANCA)-mediated small vessel vasculitis
  - Mainly autoantibodies to antigen myeloperoxidase (p-ANCA)
  - Minority have autoantibodies to antigen proteinase 3 (c-ANCA)
  - Subset of MPO-ANCA small vessel vasculitis is renal-limited necrotizing crescentic glomerulonephritis
  - Subset are ANCA(-) renal-limited necrotizing crescentic glomerulonephritis

- Cell-mediated immune mechanism with T-lymphocytes, neutrophils, and histiocytes are necessary for development of crescentic glomerulonephritis
  - ANCA-activated neutrophils tend to adhere to activated microvascular endothelium to initiate injury
  - Alternate pathway of complement has been shown to initiate and enhance endothelial injury and vasculitis

CLINICAL ISSUES

Epidemiology
- Incidence
  - Varies with geographic locations
    - 1-8/1,000,000 in Europe and United States
    - 10-24/1,000,000 in Asian and Arab countries
- Age
  - All ages affected
  - Average age at onset is 50 years
- Ethnicity
  - Geographic variations may be related to ethnic background

Presentation
- General
  - Pulmonary renal syndrome
  - Constitutional symptoms (up to 75%)
    - Fever, weakness, weight loss
    - Arthralgias, myalgias (25-50%)
    - Hypertension
- Renal (90-100%)
  - Kidney is common organ involved in MPA
  - Hematuria
  - Proteinuria
  - Renal insufficiency
  - Rapidly progressive or oliguric acute renal failure
- Skin

MICROSCOPIC POLYANGIITIS

Key Facts

Terminology
- Necrotizing vasculitis, with few or no immune deposits, affecting small arteries (capillaries, venules, or arterioles)
- Necrotizing glomerulonephritis is common

Etiology/Pathogenesis
- ANCA-mediated small vessel vasculitis
- Cell-mediated immune mechanism

Clinical Issues
- Rapidly progressive or oliguric acute renal failure
- Pulmonary hemorrhage
- p-ANCA/anti-myeloperoxidase positive (60%)
- c-ANCA/anti-PR3 positive (15%)
- Renal (90-100%), lung (25-55%)

Microscopic Pathology
- Crescentic glomerulonephritis with fibrinoid necrosis
- Vasculitis
  - Not always present, even in multiple levels
- Rarely, isolated tubulointerstitial inflammation
- No significant granulomatous inflammation
- IF: Fibrin in crescents but little or no IgG, IgA, or IgM
- Linear IgG in GBM indicates concurrent anti-GBM disease
- EM: Rare deposits, breaks in GBM

Top Differential Diagnoses
- Granulomatosis with polyangiitis (Wegener) and Churg-Strauss syndrome
- Immune complex-mediated glomerulonephritis
- Anti-GBM disease

- Purpuric rash, palpable (45%)
- Lung (25-55%)
  - Hemoptysis
  - Dyspnea
  - Pulmonary hemorrhage
  - Lung infiltrates
- Gastrointestinal (50%)
  - Abdominal pain
    - Severe form with bowel perforation
  - Hepatomegaly
- Neurologic (30%)
  - Peripheral neuropathy less frequent than PAN
  - Central nervous system
- Ear, nose, throat (30-35%)
  - Mouth ulcers
  - Epistaxis
  - Sinusitis

Laboratory Tests
- Anemia (normochromic normocytic)
- Elevation of acute phase proteins
  - Erythrocyte sedimentation rate
  - C-reactive protein
- Leukocytosis and thrombocytosis
- Rheumatoid factor (39-50%)
- Antinuclear antibodies (21-33%)
- p-ANCA/anti-myeloperoxidase positive (60%)
- c-ANCA/anti-PR3 positive (15%)
- Renal
  - Urinalysis shows red cells and RBC casts
  - Varying degrees of proteinuria
  - Elevated serum BUN and creatinine levels

Treatment
- Remission induction, remission maintenance, and relapse treatment are 3 phases of therapy
- Corticosteroids combined with cyclophosphamide is most common induction protocol
- Other forms of immunosuppressive therapy in refractory cases (10%)
- Oral cyclophosphamide, mycophenolate mofetil, or azathioprine used for remission maintenance

Prognosis
- Severe form of glomerular disease with aggressive course
- 1-year mortality rate of untreated cases is 80%
- Early deaths are usually due to fulminant renal disease and lung hemorrhage in MPA
- Frequent relapses occur (25-35%)
  - Different or new organs may be involved during relapses
  - Often associated with rash and arthralgias
  - Generally less severe
- Induction protocol
  - Improvement in > 90% of patients
  - Complete remission in > 75%
- Independent factors that correlate with worse prognosis are older age, higher initial serum creatinine, and pulmonary hemorrhage
- Pathologic parameters representative of recovery of renal function include percent of normal glomeruli at initial biopsy, tubular injury, glomerular crescents, and interstitial inflammation

MACROSCOPIC FEATURES

General Features
- Normal or mildly increased kidney size
- Infarcts when present are small
- Petechial hemorrhages
  - Focal or diffuse
  - Represent glomerular necrosis; hemorrhage in Bowman space or within tubular lumina

MICROSCOPIC PATHOLOGY

Histologic Features
- Glomeruli
  - Pauci-immune crescentic glomerulonephritis
    - Segmental or, rarely, global glomerular necrosis (80-100%)

- Disruption of glomerular basement membranes with accumulation of eosinophilic/fuchsinophilic fibrinoid material
- Majority of glomeruli have crescents (average 45-55%), which frequently accompany necrosis
- Segmental to extensive lysis of Bowman capsule in severe necrotizing glomerular lesions
- Sometimes mild to moderate endocapillary hypercellularity with neutrophils and macrophages
  - ○ Active periglomerular inflammation of varying intensity composed of lymphocytes, neutrophils, eosinophils, and histiocytes
    - Periglomerular granulomatous reaction is unlike that seen in granulomatosis with polyangiitis (Wegener)
  - ○ Subacute or chronic glomerular lesions display fibrocellular or fibrous crescents
    - Segmental and global glomerular necrosis heals by sclerosis
    - Sclerosing glomerular changes are accompanied by tubular atrophy and interstitial fibrosis
- Tubules and interstitium
  - ○ Active disease often associated with acute tubulointerstitial inflammation
  - ○ Rare isolated tubulointerstitial inflammation is noted without glomerular lesions in kidney biopsy
  - ○ No significant granulomatous inflammation is noted
- Renal and extrarenal vessels
  - ○ Interlobular arteries, smaller arteries, arterioles, capillaries, and venules are affected
    - Segmental or circumferential fibrinoid necrosis
    - Palisading mild to intense active inflammatory reaction around necrotic areas
    - Inflammatory cells include neutrophils, activated lymphocytes, and variable eosinophils
    - Focal renal medullary capillaritis with fibrinoid necrosis
  - ○ Healed vascular lesions show intimal thickening, narrowing of lumen, and variable loss of elastic lamina by EVG stain
  - ○ Small vessel vasculitis and capillaritis may be seen in skin, lung, and other organs similar to other small vessel vasculitides
    - Intrarenal small vessel vasculitis often not observed in renal biopsies

ANCILLARY TESTS

Immunofluorescence
- Necrotizing lesions and active crescents stain for fibrinogen
- Pauci-immune glomerular lesions with minimal or no deposits
  - ○ Low-intensity staining of < 1-2+ may be observed for immunoglobulins and complement components
- Intense global, linear IgG staining along GBM indicates concurrent anti-GBM disease

Electron Microscopy
- Earliest change seen in glomeruli is endothelial swelling and widened subendothelial areas

- Later endothelial detachment from basement membranes and microthrombi formation with fibrin tactoids
- On occasion, rare small deposits are noted

DIFFERENTIAL DIAGNOSIS

Granulomatosis with Polyangiitis (Wegener) and Churg-Strauss Syndrome
- Renal histopathological changes are similar to those seen in granulomatosis with polyangiitis (Wegener) (GPA) (i.e., pauci-immune crescentic glomerulonephritis)
- Granulomatous inflammation (GPA), asthma, and eosinophilia (Churg-Strauss) are useful if seen

Immune Complex-mediated Glomerulonephritis with Crescents &/or Small Vessel Vasculitis
- Clinical features, appropriate serology, and immunohistochemistry useful for differentiation

Anti-glomerular Basement Membrane Antibody Disease (Goodpasture)
- Need serology, immunofluorescence for differentiation

DIAGNOSTIC CHECKLIST

Pathologic Interpretation Pearls
- Examination of multiple levels of renal biopsies is helpful to identify focal vasculitis

SELECTED REFERENCES

1. Eriksson P et al: Improved outcome in Wegener's granulomatosis and microscopic polyangiitis? A retrospective analysis of 95 cases in two cohorts. J Intern Med. 265(4):496-506, 2009
2. Jennette JC et al: New insight into the pathogenesis of vasculitis associated with antineutrophil cytoplasmic autoantibodies. Curr Opin Rheumatol. 20(1):55-60, 2008
3. Jennette JC et al: Pauci-immune and antineutrophil cytoplasmic autoantibody-mediated crescentic glomerulonephritis and vasculitis. In Jennette JC et al: Heptinstall's Pathology of the Kidney. 6th ed. Lippincott Williams & Wilkins. 643-674, 2007
4. Rutgers A et al: Coexistence of anti-glomerular basement membrane antibodies and myeloperoxidase-ANCAs in crescentic glomerulonephritis. Am J Kidney Dis. 46(2):253-62, 2005
5. Levy JB et al: Clinical features and outcome of patients with both ANCA and anti-GBM antibodies. Kidney Int. 66(4):1535-40, 2004
6. Hauer HA et al: Determinants of outcome in ANCA-associated glomerulonephritis: a prospective clinico-histopathological analysis of 96 patients. Kidney Int. 62(5):1732-42, 2002
7. Franssen CF et al: Antiproteinase 3- and antimyeloperoxidase-associated vasculitis. Kidney Int. 57(6):2195-206, 2000
8. Bajema IM et al: Kidney biopsy as a predictor for renal outcome in ANCA-associated necrotizing glomerulonephritis. Kidney Int. 56(5):1751-8, 1999

MICROSCOPIC POLYANGIITIS

Small Vessel Vasculitides (Pauci-immune Types)

	MPA	GPA	CSS
Clinical features	Multisystemic	Multisystemic	Multisystemic, associated with asthma or allergy
Serology	ANCA(+) (90%), mainly anti-MPO(+) (50%), PR3(+) (40%)	ANCA(+) (95%), mainly anti-PR3(+) (75%), anti-MPO(+) (20%)	ANCA(+) (50%), mostly anti-MPO(+) (60%)
Organs affected	Thoracic and abdominal viscera, skin, infrequently cerebral vessels	Upper and lower respiratory tract, abdominal viscera, kidney, heart, skin	Upper and lower respiratory tract, kidney, and rarely heart, skin, and brain
Size of vessel involved	Small arteries, arterioles, capillaries	Small arteries and veins, arterioles, capillaries, and venules	Small arteries, veins, arterioles, and rarely capillaries
Pathology of vasculitis	Necrotizing type, polymorphous inflammatory infiltrate and some eosinophils	Necrotizing or granulomatous type, polymorphous inflammatory infiltrate, mild eosinophils	Necrotizing or granulomatous type, eosinophil-rich, inflammatory infiltrate
Other vascular and nonvascular features	Renal limited form seen	Extravascular granulomatous inflammation with "geographic" pattern	Extravascular necrotizing granulomatous inflammation with prominent eosinophils
Glomerular pathology	Acute and chronic forms of crescentic glomerulonephritis and vasculitis, pauci-immune type	Acute and chronic crescentic glomerulonephritis, pauci-immune type	Less frequent crescentic glomerulonephritis, pauci-immune type
Relapse	++	+++	-/+

MPA = microscopic polyangiitis; GPA = granulomatosis with polyangiitis (Wegener); CSS = Church-Strauss syndrome.

Comparison of Anti-GBM and ANCA-associated Diseases

Clinical	ANCA	AGBM + ANCA	AGBM
Age	63 ± 12.7	64 ± 8.7	52 ± 20.6
Gender	M/F	Females	Younger males, older females
Antecedent events	Possible infection	Unknown	Possible smoking, hydrocarbon exposure
Lung hemorrhage	++	+	+
Renal involvement	100%	90%	100%
Multisystemic disease	Yes	20-50%	0
Systemic vasculitis	Yes	10-15%	0
Serology	PR3 or MPO	PR3 or MPO	AGBM
Serum creatinine	+	++	+++
Active urine sediment	+	+	+
Pathology (Crescentic GN)			
Distribution	Focal/diffuse	90-100%	75-100%
Stage of crescents	Acute/subacute/chronic	Mostly acute, some chronic	All acute/one stage
Severity of glomerular necrosis	Segmental	Segmental/global	Segmental/global
Periglomerular granulomatous inflammation	+	+	-
Prognosis			
Relapse	Frequent	+	Rare
1-year survival			
Renal	~ 50%	~ 10%	~ 40%
Patient	~ 85%	~ 55%	~ 75%

9. Guillevin L et al: Microscopic polyangiitis: clinical and laboratory findings in eighty-five patients. Arthritis Rheum. 42(3):421-30, 1999
10. Tervaert JW et al: Silicon exposure and vasculitis. Curr Opin Rheumatol. 10(1):12-7, 1998
11. Bacon PA: Therapy of vasculitis. J Rheumatol. 21(5):788-90, 1994
12. Jennette JC et al: Nomenclature of systemic vasculitides. Proposal of an international consensus conference. Arthritis Rheum. 37(2):187-92, 1994
13. Jennette JC et al: The pathology of vasculitis involving the kidney. Am J Kidney Dis. 24(1):130-41, 1994
14. Gordon M et al: Relapses in patients with a systemic vasculitis. Q J Med. 86(12):779-89, 1993
15. D'Agati V et al: Idiopathic microscopic polyarteritis nodosa: ultrastructural observations on the renal vascular and glomerular lesions. Am J Kidney Dis. 7(1):95-110, 1986
16. Savage CO et al: Microscopic polyarteritis: presentation, pathology and prognosis. Q J Med. 56(220):467-83, 1985

Microscopic Features

(Left) Glomerulus in a p-ANCA positive patient shows early intraglomerular thrombosis or fibrinoid change ➡ prior to a fully developed necrotizing lesion. (Right) Glomerulus shows partial necrosis of the capillary tuft overlaid by a cellular crescent and fuchsinophilic fibrinoid material.

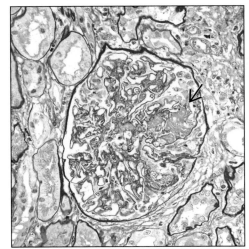 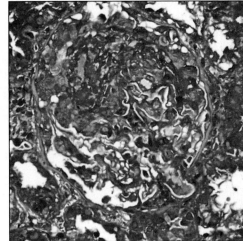

(Left) Glomerulus shows segmental crescentic features with capillary necrosis and disruption of the basement membranes ➡. (Right) Scanning electron microscopy of glomerular capillary basement membrane from a patient with ANCA-mediated crescentic glomerulonephritis shows a frayed and fenestrated appearance, i.e., the GBM is broken, allowing crescent formation.

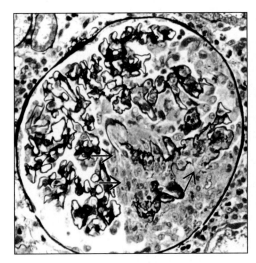 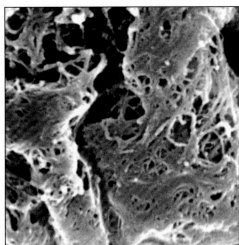

(Left) Crescentic glomerulonephritis with strong staining for fibrinogen is shown within the crescent in the Bowman space. Fibrin is characteristically present in active crescents, regardless of cause. (Right) Pauci-immune crescentic glomerulonephritis typically has little or no immunoglobulin deposits in the glomeruli. Illustrated here is a minor degree of segmental positive IgG staining in the glomerulus, compatible with the diagnosis.

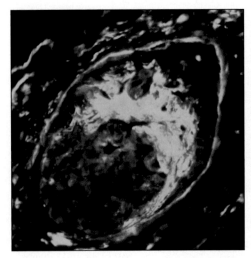 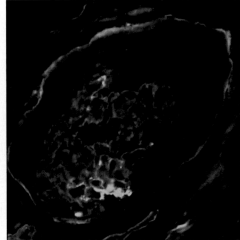

MICROSCOPIC POLYANGIITIS

Microscopic Features

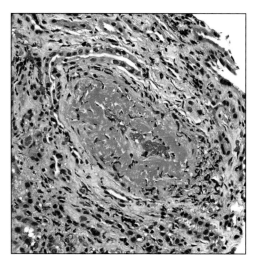
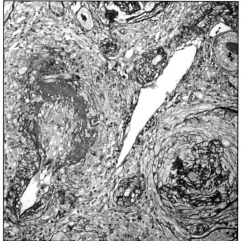

(Left) Intrarenal small vessel necrotizing vasculitis is shown, with transmural and circumferential fibrinoid change accompanied by active inflammation. Intimal and medial layers are not visualized. *(Right)* Crescentic glomerulonephritis accompanied by necrotizing arteritis in a segmental distribution is shown.

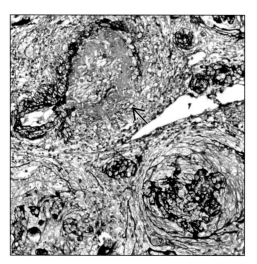
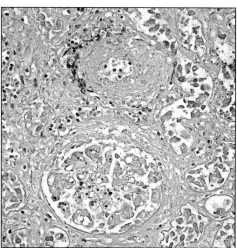

(Left) Crescentic glomerulonephritis with necrotizing arteritis shows disruption of silver positive elastic membranes ➡ in the area of necrosis. *(Right)* Elastic stain from the autopsy kidney of a known case of fulminant polyangiitis shows a healed small artery with fibrointimal thickening, narrowing of the lumen, and almost complete disappearance of internal and external elastic lamina. An adjacent glomerulus is noted.

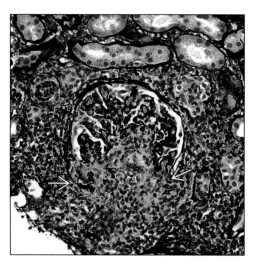
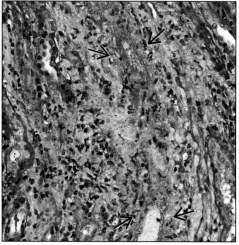

(Left) A case of MPO-ANCA positive with exclusively hilar arteriolar inflammation and necrosis ➡ is shown. No glomerular crescents were identified in this specimen. *(Right)* MPO-ANCA positive case shows predominantly glomerular hilar arteriolitis and medullary capillaritis with fibrinoid change ➡.

Microscopic and Clinical Features

(Left) Medium magnification shows several glomeruli with different stages of healing of crescents. Cellular and fibrocellular crescents ➡ and fibrous crescents ➡ are present. (Right) Glomerulus with segmental fibrinoid necrotizing lesion shows occasional large cells and one multinucleated giant cell ➡. Granulomatous changes in crescentic glomerulonephritis are not unusual.

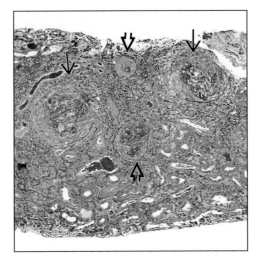

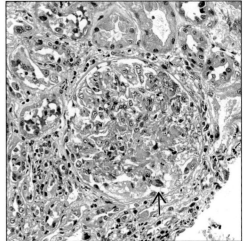

(Left) Glomerulus shows a circumferential fibrocellular crescent along with a pseudotubular space ➡ lined by epithelial cells within the Bowman space. (Right) In polyangiitis associated with ANCA, occasional mesangial ➡ and subepithelial ➡ deposits of uncertain significance can be seen. This does not change the diagnosis. The GBM may also show areas of disruption in glomeruli with crescents.

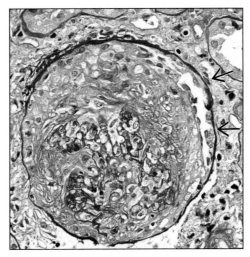

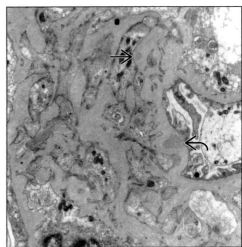

(Left) Clinical photo shows purpuric rash in a patient with microscopic polyangiitis having multisystemic symptoms of lung hemorrhage and acute renal failure. (Right) Dermal capillaries show leukocytoclastic vasculitis ➡.

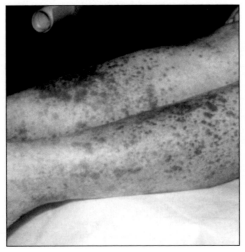

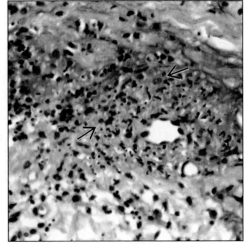

Microscopic Features

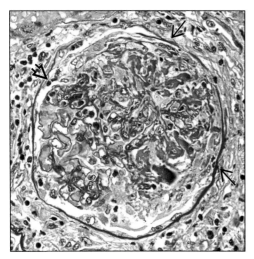 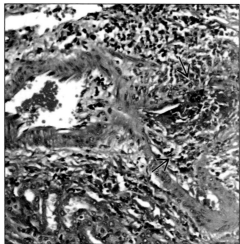

(Left) *Glomerulus shows partial necrosis with fibrinoid change ➡ and focal infiltration of inflammatory cells ➥ within capillary lumina. **(Right)** A section from nephrectomy for renal cell carcinoma with known MPO-ANCA positive serology and hematuria shows segmental necrotizing vasculitis ➡ in an interlobular artery.*

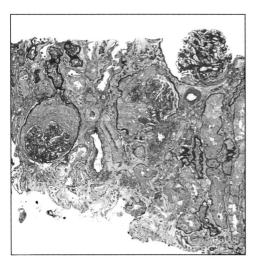 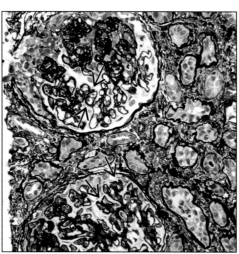

(Left) *Diabetic nephropathy with MPO-ANCA(+) serology superimposed by fibrocellular crescents overlying diabetic glomerular changes shows arteriolar hyalinosis & thickening of the tubular basement membranes. **(Right)** Idiopathic membranous glomerulonephritis stage III superimposed by MPO-ANCA crescentic disease is shown. The uninvolved glomerular capillary walls & portion of the glomerulus below show irregular thickening of the basement membranes ➡.*

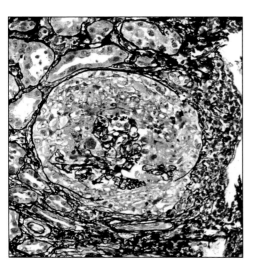 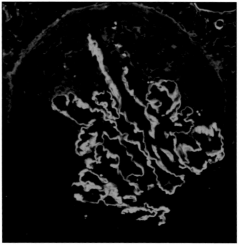

(Left) *Silver-stained glomerulus almost completely compressed by a large cellular crescent in the Bowman space is shown in a case dual positive for anti-GBM antibody and MPO-ANCA. **(Right)** Global, linear glomerular capillary basement membrane fluorescence for IgG is shown, partly compressed by a crescent in a patient with positive serology for ANCA-MPO and anti-GBM antibody.*

GRANULOMATOSIS WITH POLYANGIITIS (WEGENER)

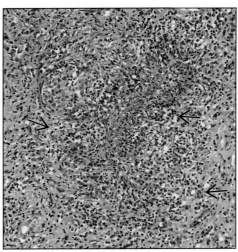

GPA in a kidney shows irregular necrotizing granulomatous inflammation with palisading and giant cells ➔ and a neutrophil-rich infiltrate with lymphocytes and epithelioid cells.

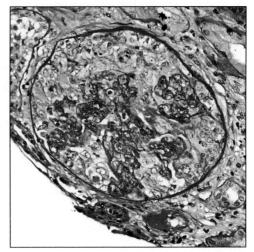

Periodic acid-Schiff shows glomerular tuft mostly compressed by a cellular crescent in the Bowman space mixed with inflammatory cells, typical lesion of GPA, and other ANCA-mediated vasculitides.

TERMINOLOGY

Abbreviations
- Granulomatosis with polyangiitis (GPA)

Synonyms
- Wegener granulomatosis (WG)
- Rhinogenic granulomatosis

Definitions
- Chapel Hill Consensus Conference
  - GPA is granulomatous inflammation of respiratory tract and necrotizing vasculitis of small to medium-sized vessels (capillaries, venules, arterioles, and arteries), commonly with necrotizing glomerulonephritis (GN) with no or very few deposits ("pauci-immune crescentic GN")
- Americal College of Rheumatology (ACR) criteria
  - Nasal or oral inflammation with purulent discharges or oral ulcers
  - Abnormal chest radiograph
    - Cavitating or noncavitating nodules
    - Infiltrates
  - Abnormal urinary finding (e.g., microhematuria)
  - Granulomatous inflammation in vessel wall, perivascular or interstitial locations
  - Any 2 or more of the above have high diagnostic specificity and sensitivity

ETIOLOGY/PATHOGENESIS

Antineutrophil Cytoplasmic Antibody (ANCA)-mediated Small Vessel Vasculitis
- Autoantibodies to proteinase 3 (PR3) in most patients (> 75%)
  - ANCAs react to peptide sequences in complementary PR3-molecule
  - These sequences have significant homology with infectious agents, e.g., *Staphylococcus*

- Minority (< 25%) have antimyeloperoxidase (MPO) ANCA
  - Proteinase-3 (PR3)
    - Serine proteinase related to neutrophil elastase (55% homology)
    - Inactivated by combining with α-1-antitrypsin
  - Neutrophil activation via feedback loop with ANCA
    - Activated neutrophils express PR3 on surface
    - Neutrophils activated via binding of ANCA
    - Release of oxygen radicals, lytic enzymes, and inflammatory cytokines
    - Alternative pathway complement activation and mediation by C5a
  - Increased adhesion of neutrophils to previously activated endothelium and transmigration
    - Mediate endothelial damage and vascular inflammation
  - Disease activity related to inhibition of PR3-α-1-antitrypsin complex formation
- Other antibodies
  - Antiendothelial antibodies identified
    - Lysosomal membrane protein-2, on surface of endothelial cells
- T cells, B cells needed to promote autoimmune response

Genetic Risk Factors
- MHC class II gene *HLA-DRB1*0401*
  - Odds ratio 2-3
  - Retinoid X receptor B (RXRB) polymorphism (nearby on chromosome 6p21.3)
  - *HLA-DRB1*0401* not associated with Churg-Strauss syndrome or microscopic polyangiitis
- *DNAM-1* polymorphism (Gly307Ser)
  - Codes for CD226, DNAX accessory protein
  - Also in type I diabetes, multiple sclerosis, Graves disease
- Limited evidence for other gene polymorphisms

GRANULOMATOSIS WITH POLYANGIITIS (WEGENER)

Key Facts

Etiology/Pathogenesis
- Form of ANCA-mediated small vessel vasculitis
- Usually due to anti-PR3 antibodies (~ 75%), others to MPO

Clinical Issues
- Peak age at onset: 30-50 years
- Kidney, upper airway, and lung involvement in 90% of cases
- Present with acute or rapidly progressive renal failure
- Steroids combined with cyclophosphamide; plasmapheresis beneficial in severe disease
- Poor prognostic factors
  - High initial creatinine, concomitant lung disease
  - Frequency of renal relapses
  - Few preserved glomeruli

Microscopic Pathology
- Fibrinoid necrosis, crescents (cellular, fibrocellular, and fibrous types)
- Occasional interstitial (extravascular) granulomas
- Interlobular and smaller arteries affected by vasculitis
- Granulomatous inflammation in vessel wall, perivascular or interstitial locations
- Isolated or concomitant medullary capillaritis

Ancillary Tests
- Pauci-immune with little or no immunoglobulins or complement components by IF

Top Differential Diagnoses
- ANCA(+) vasculitides (Churg-Strauss syndrome, microscopic polyangiitis), anti-GBM disease, HSP, drug-induced vasculitis

---

- SERPINA1 (α-1-antitrypsin), PTPN22 (protein tyrosine phosphatase), CTLA4, PD-1 gene (also Kawasaki disease), FCGR3B (FcγRIIIb)

Potential Triggers of Autoantibody Response
- Possible triggers of ANCA formation include infections (bacteria, viral)
  - GPA onset more common in winter
- Exposure to allergens
- Exposure to dust, heavy metal, respiratory toxins

Animal Model
- Passive transfer of ANCA (anti-MPO) causes glomerulonephritis with crescents in immunodeficient mice (RAG1 knockout)

CLINICAL ISSUES

Epidemiology
- Incidence
  - 30-60/1,000,000
  - Higher incidence in North America and northern Europe; lower in Asia
  - Increased reporting in last 2 decades due to increased awareness of the disease
- Age
  - GPA can develop at any age
  - Peak age at onset: 30-50 years
  - Mean: 40 years
  - Can also occur in children and the elderly
- Gender
  - Slight male predominance
- Ethnicity
  - No ethnic predilection

Presentation
- Multisystemic involvement, often preceded by constitutional symptoms
  - Kidney, upper airway, and lung involvement in 90% of cases
  - A pulmonary renal syndrome
- 2 phases of disease

- Granulomatous disease of upper respiratory tract
  - Vasculitic phase
- Renal
  - Renal symptoms usually follow but sometimes precede respiratory disease up to several years
  - Macroscopic or microscopic hematuria
  - Red blood cell casts
  - Oliguria
  - Rapidly progressive or acute renal failure
  - Sometimes insidious onset of renal insufficiency with proteinuria &/or hematuria
  - Mass lesion (rare)
  - Occasionally presents with renal mass

Laboratory Tests
- Hematuria, proteinuria, elevated BUN, Cr
- Anemia, elevated ESR
- ~ 95% positive for ANCA
  - ELISA: Anti-PR3 ANCA (~ 75%) or anti-MPO (~ 25%)
  - Indirect IF: c-ANCA (PR3) or p-ANCA (MPO)
- Rheumatoid factor positive (20-30%)

Treatment
- Steroids combined with cyclophosphamide
- Plasmapheresis is beneficial in severe disease
- Maintenance therapies have oral cyclophosphamide, cyclosporine, azathioprine, or mycophenolate mofitel
- Clinical trials to assess benefit of
  - Anti-CD20, targets B cells
  - Blocking tumor necrosis factor-α

Prognosis
- 20% renal morbidity and end-stage renal disease
  - Lack of treatment or late diagnosis leads to ESRD
- Trend toward improved renal and patient survival is observed
- Clinical factors of poor prognosis
  - Older age
  - High creatinine level at initial presentation
  - High serum titer of ANCA (anti-PR3)
  - Severity of initial vascular damage
  - Multisystem involvement
    - Concomitant lung involvement or hemorrhage

3

GRANULOMATOSIS WITH POLYANGIITIS (WEGENER)

- o Increased relapse rate (10-50%)
- Clinical factors of good prognosis
  - o Close to normal baseline renal function

Renal Transplantation

- Patient and graft survival rates are comparable to those observed in non-ANCA patients
- Both renal and extrarenal relapses occur after renal transplantation (though uncommon)
  - o Recurrent disease or relapses are managed effectively by cyclophosphamide therapy

IMAGE FINDINGS

Radiographic Findings

- Chest x-ray shows shifting infiltrates in lungs
- Single or multiple nodular lung lesions
- Diffuse pulmonary infiltrates suggesting hemorrhage

MACROSCOPIC FEATURES

Kidney

- Usually normal in size or slightly enlarged
- In acute phase, small scattered infarcts and petechial hemorrhages in cortex and medulla
- Larger vessels appear grossly normal
- Aneurysms or thrombi are rare
- Focal or diffuse papillary necrosis

MICROSCOPIC PATHOLOGY

Histologic Features

- Glomeruli
  - o Wide range and extent of glomerular lesions with crescents
  - o Segmental to severe capillary tuft thrombosis
    - Fibrinoid necrosis with rupture of basement membranes
    - Accumulation of neutrophils and karyorrhexis of cells in areas of necrosis
  - o Crescents in different stages of healing (such as cellular, fibrocellular, and fibrous types) may be seen in same biopsy
    - Cellular crescent is composed of mainly parietal epithelial cells and exuded inflammatory cells (more than 2-3 layers thick)
    - Segmental/small to large, sometimes circumferential cellular crescents in Bowman space
    - A few crescents acquire granulomatous appearance with epithelioid and giant cells
    - Varying degrees of glomerular tuft compression
  - o Acute and subacute periglomerular inflammation due to disruption of Bowman capsule
  - o No intraglomerular cell proliferation
  - o Later glomerulosclerosis, residual disruption of Bowman capsule
- Tubulointerstitium
  - o Mild to marked active interstitial inflammation may accompany glomerular crescentic lesions

- o Sometimes necrotizing neutrophilic granulomatous interstitial nephritis with palisading histiocytes (geographic pattern) or mass lesion
  - Occasional interstitial (extravascular) granulomas
- o Plasma cells can be prominent
- o Focal microscopic interstitial hemorrhages
- o Tubular red blood cells and RBC casts
- o Active tubulitis and epithelial cell injury
- o Peritubular capillaritis
- o Tubular atrophy and interstitial fibrosis
- Vessels
  - o Interlobular arteries are usual site affected by vasculitis
    - Segmental or circumferential fibrinoid necrosis
    - Cellular reaction composed of neutrophils, histiocytes, and sometimes prominent eosinophils
    - Occasional granulomatous inflammation
  - o Smaller arteries down to pre- and postglomerular arterioles and venules involved
  - o Isolated or concomitant medullary inflammation, capillaritis, and interstitial hemorrhages
  - o Progressive vascular sclerosis with variable loss of elastic lamina by EVG stain
- General comments
  - o Vascular lesions and granulomata are more difficult to find in renal biopsies than in larger samples or autopsy kidneys
  - o Small vessel vasculitis and capillaritis also seen in skin, lung, and other organs similar to other small vessel or ANCA-associated vasculitides

Other Organs

- Lung
  - o Pulmonary (nodular), extravascular granulomatous inflammation is a hallmark lesion
  - o Usually shows irregular necrosis with neutrophilic infiltrate
  - o Progressive, irregular expansion of granuloma affecting bronchial tree and vasculature
  - o Vasculitis can be characterized by fibrinoid necrosis or granulomatous inflammation
  - o Pulmonary capillaritis leads to pulmonary hemorrhage (in 1/3 of cases)
- Skin
  - o Leukocytoclastic vasculitis of dermal capillaries
  - o Granulomatous vasculitis with neutrophilic center
  - o May be accompanied by extravascular palisading granulomatous inflammation
- Sinuses
  - o Necrotizing granulomata and vasculitis

ANCILLARY TESTS

Immunofluorescence

- Strong fibrinogen/fibrin staining is noted in capillary lumina, active necrotizing lesions, or in Bowman space in crescents
- Usually negative glomeruli for immunoglobulins (IgG, IgA, IgM) and complement components (C3, C1q)
  - o Sometimes scant, randomly distributed glomerular immunoglobulin and complement deposits of < 2+ intensity may be localized

GRANULOMATOSIS WITH POLYANGIITIS (WEGENER)

- Presence of unequivocal or significant glomerular deposits leads to overlap of autoimmune or infection-related GN

Electron Microscopy
- Glomerular basement membrane (GBM) contains rare or no deposits (pauci-immune)
- GBM can be disrupted by necrotizing lesions
- Neutrophils in capillaries
- Fibrin in capillaries and crescents
- Podocytes usually have no more than focal foot process effacement
- Endothelial cells may be reactive (loss of fenestrations)

DIFFERENTIAL DIAGNOSIS

Other ANCA(+) Vasculitides (Churg-Strauss Syndrome, Microscopic Polyangiitis)
- Necrotizing granuloma, sinus involvement more common in GPA than in microscopic polyangiitis
- Eosinophilia/asthma in Churg-Strauss syndrome

Anti-GBM Glomerulonephritis
- Linear IgG in GBM distinctive
- Some patients have both ANCA and anti-GBM

Drug-induced Granulomatous Interstitial Nephritis and Vasculitis
- History of drug intake
- Skin rash
- Noncaseating granulomata
- Eosinophilia and tissue infiltration in some cases

Sarcoidosis
- Mediastinal lymphadenopathy and lung involvement
- Nonnecrotizing granuloma
- Rare: Granulomatous angiitis and crescent glomerulonephritis
- Elevated angiotensin converting enzyme levels

Henoch-Schönlein Purpura (HSP)
- IgA prominent in glomeruli

DIAGNOSTIC CHECKLIST

Clinically Relevant Pathologic Features
- Pathology features of poor prognosis
  - Number of fibrous glomerular crescents and fibrinoid necrosis at renal biopsy
  - Extent of tubular atrophy and interstitial fibrosis
- Renal factors of good prognosis
  - High number of preserved glomeruli
  - Low number of cellular crescents
  - Absence of fibrinoid necrosis

Pathologic Interpretation Pearls
- GPA can have just interstitial inflammation/capillaritis without glomerular involvement (possibly due to sampling)
- A negative ANCA does not exclude GPA

- Lack of proliferation in glomerulus helps distinguish ANCA and anti-GBM diseases from other causes of crescentic GN

SELECTED REFERENCES

1. Falk RJ et al: Granulomatosis with Polyangiitis (Wegener's): An alternative name for Wegener's Granulomatosis. Arthritis Rheum. 63(4):863-4, 2011
2. Kamali S et al: Predictors of damage and survival in patients with Wegener's granulomatosis: analysis of 50 patients. J Rheumatol. 37(2):374-8, 2010
3. Mohammad AJ et al: The extent and pattern of organ damage in small vessel vasculitis measured by the Vasculitis Damage Index (VDI). Scand J Rheumatol. 38(4):268-75, 2009
4. Schreiber A et al: C5a receptor mediates neutrophil activation and ANCA-induced glomerulonephritis. J Am Soc Nephrol. 20(2):289-98, 2009
5. Wieczorek S et al: Novel association of the CD226 (DNAM-1) Gly307Ser polymorphism in Wegener's granulomatosis and confirmation for multiple sclerosis in German patients. Genes Immun. 10(6):591-5, 2009
6. Renaudineau Y et al: Renal involvement in Wegener's granulomatosis. Clin Rev Allergy Immunol. 35(1-2):22-9, 2008
7. Geetha D et al: Renal transplantation in the ANCA-associated vasculitides. Am J Transplant. 7(12):2657-62, 2007
8. Gottenberg JE et al: Long-term outcome of 37 patients with Wegener's granulomatosis with renal involvement. Presse Med. 36(5 Pt 1):771-8, 2007
9. Sebastian JK et al: Antiendothelial cell antibodies in patients with Wegener's granulomatosis: prevalence and correlation with disease activity and manifestations. J Rheumatol. 34(5):1027-31, 2007
10. Slot MC et al: Renal survival and prognostic factors in patients with PR3-ANCA associated vasculitis with renal involvement. Kidney Int. 63(2):670-7, 2003
11. Koldingsnes W et al: Predictors of survival and organ damage in Wegener's granulomatosis. Rheumatology (Oxford). 41(5):572-81, 2002
12. Xiao H et al: Antineutrophil cytoplasmic autoantibodies specific for myeloperoxidase cause glomerulonephritis and vasculitis in mice. J Clin Invest. 110(7):955-63, 2002
13. Aasarød K et al: Wegener's granulomatosis: clinical course in 108 patients with renal involvement. Nephrol Dial Transplant. 15(5):611-8, 2000
14. Bajema IM et al: Renal granulomas in systemic vasculitis. EC/BCR Project for ANCA-Assay Standardization. Clin Nephrol. 48(1):16-21, 1997
15. Bonsib SM et al: Necrotizing medullary lesions in patients with ANCA associated renal disease. Mod Pathol. 7(2):181-5, 1994
16. Andrassy K et al: Wegener's granulomatosis with renal involvement: patient survival and correlations between initial renal function, renal histology, therapy and renal outcome. Clin Nephrol. 35(4):139-47, 1991
17. Leavitt RY et al: The American College of Rheumatology 1990 criteria for the classification of Wegener's granulomatosis. Arthritis Rheum. 33(8):1101-7, 1990
18. van der Woude FJ et al: Autoantibodies against neutrophils and monocytes: tool for diagnosis and marker of disease activity in Wegener's granulomatosis. Lancet. 1(8426):425-9, 1985
19. Wegener F: Uber generalisierte, septische Gefaesserkrankungen. Verh Dtsch Ges Pathol. 29:202, 1936

Microscopic Features

(Left) H&E stained glomerulus shows segmental, intracapillary fibrinoid material with early necrosis ➡. The rest of the glomerulus has a normal appearance. *(Right)* A trichrome stained glomerulus shows segmental fibrinoid (fuchsinophilic) necrosis overlaid by a cellular crescent. Mild periglomerular inflammatory infiltrate ➡ adjacent to the area of the necrotizing lesion is noted.

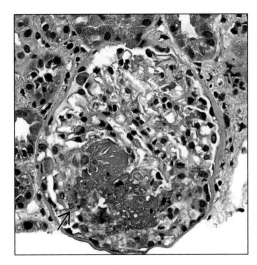 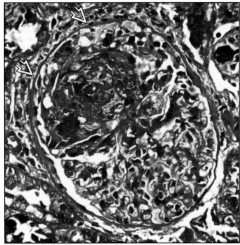

(Left) Glomerulus in GPA with segmental fibrinoid necrotizing lesion and a small cellular crescent are located at the tubular pole of the glomerulus. This can be differentiated from a glomerular tip lesion of focal segmental sclerosis where foam cells and sclerosing changes may predominate. *(Right)* Healed c-ANCA-associated crescentic glomerulonephritis with segmental glomerular sclerosing lesion is covered by a fibrous crescent and capsular adhesion ➡.

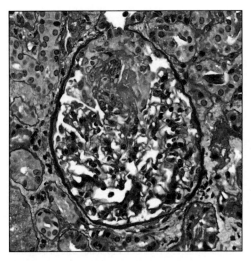 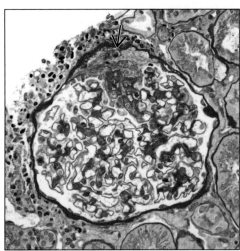

(Left) Glomerulus (PAS stain) shows a larger cellular crescent with an only minimal fibrin deposit in the center ➡. *(Right)* Silver methenamine stained glomerulus showing segmental fibrinoid necrotizing lesion with focal disruption of silver-positive basement membranes ➡ and accumulation of pink fibrinoid material is covered by a cellular crescent.

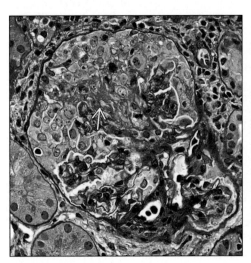 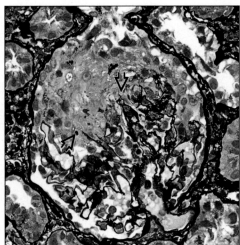

GRANULOMATOSIS WITH POLYANGIITIS (WEGENER)

Microscopic Features

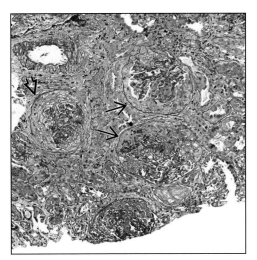 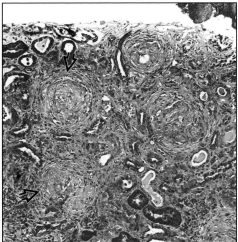

(Left) Low magnification of PAS stained section with 4 glomeruli shows various stages of crescentic glomerulonephritis having fibrinoid necrosis, cellular crescents ➡️, and a fibrocellular crescent ▷.
(Right) Low magnification (trichrome staining) shows glomeruli with varying stages of organizing crescents with fibrosis (blue color) ▷.

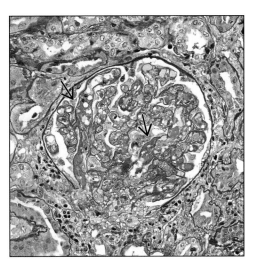 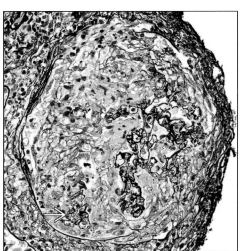

(Left) Glomerulus shows extensive intracapillary fibrinoid thrombosis ➡️ without capillary disruption or inflammation, resembling thrombotic microangiopathy.
(Right) Silver stained section shows extensive glomerular fibrinoid necrosis with residual compressed glomerular capillaries and portion of a cellular crescent. The GBM has been disrupted by the inflammatory process, and fragments ➡️ are disconnected from the tuft.

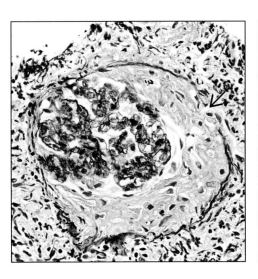 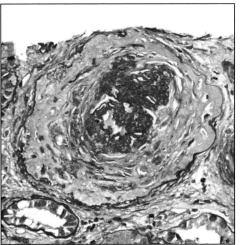

(Left) Silver stained section shows marked collapse of the glomerulus by a fibrocellular/healing crescent. Bowman capsule is disrupted ➡️, a feature that indicates the process was a crescentic glomerulonephritis rather than just ischemic glomerulosclerosis.
(Right) Kidney biopsy shows almost complete collapse and sclerosis of the glomerulus surrounded by a circumferential fibrocellular/fibrous crescent in the Bowman space.

GRANULOMATOSIS WITH POLYANGIITIS (WEGENER)

Microscopic Features

(Left) Immunofluorescence of glomerulus has focal trace positive IgG staining in the mesangial areas and is strongly positive in the hilar arterioles (pauci-immune crescentic glomerulonephritis). The glomerulus itself ➡ does not stain and is not well seen. *(Right)* Positive C3 staining in the mesangial areas in an ANCA-positive crescentic glomerulonephritis without deposits is confirmed by electron microscopy (pauci-immune).

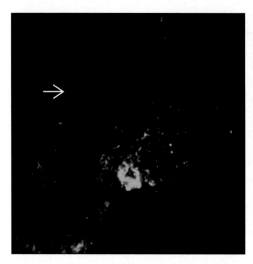

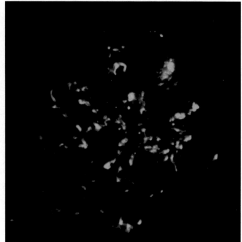

(Left) Glomerulus with necrotizing lesions shows strong immunofluorescence localization of fibrin. *(Right)* H&E stained section shows red cells and RBC casts within tubules ➡, confirming a glomerular origin of the hematuria.

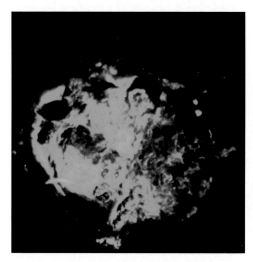

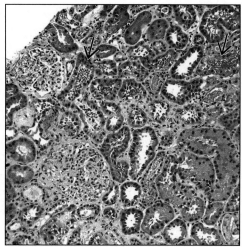

(Left) Electron micrograph shows a glomerular capillary loop with disruption/break ➡ with margination of neutrophils and monocytes in the lumen overlaid by an inflammatory cellular crescent. Breaks in the GBM are a common feature in glomerulonephritis with crescents of any etiology. *(Right)* Electron micrograph shows an uninvolved glomerulus with no significant changes or deposits (pauci-immune).

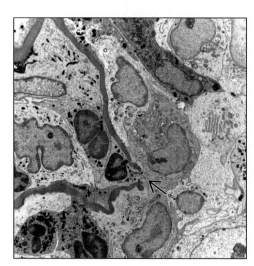

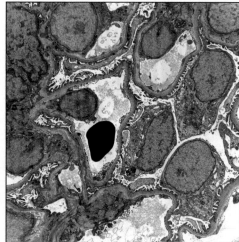

GRANULOMATOSIS WITH POLYANGIITIS (WEGENER)

Microscopic Features: Tubulointerstitial Disease

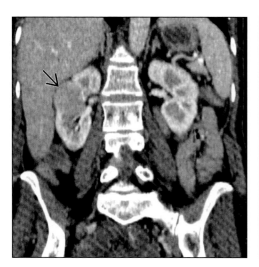

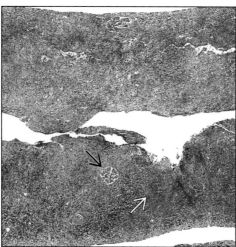

(Left) CT scan shows a renal mass ➡, thought to be neoplastic, an uncommon presentation of GPA. A biopsy showed necrotizing granulomatosis interstitial nephritis. *(Right)* Needle biopsy of a renal mass identified by CT scan in GPA reveals diffuse destruction of tubules and infiltration of the cortex with lymphocytes, plasma cells, and focal necrosis ➡. Glomeruli ➡ were spared. Patient had sinusitis, a saddle nose deformity, and tracheal stenosis. ANCA was negative (~ 10% of GPA).

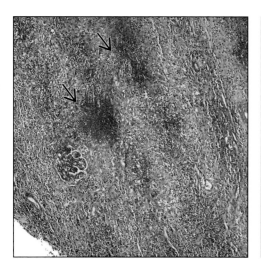

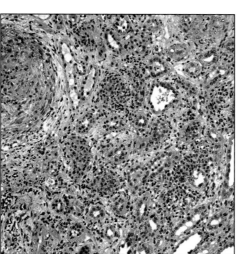

(Left) Low magnification of PAS-stained kidney section shows typical irregular necrotizing granulomatous inflammation with a neutrophilic center ➡. An adjacent glomerulus with ischemic change is noted. (Courtesy W. Travis, MD.) *(Right)* Diffuse, active, nonspecific interstitial inflammation with edema is associated with crescentic GN composed of neutrophils, eosinophils, and lymphocytes.

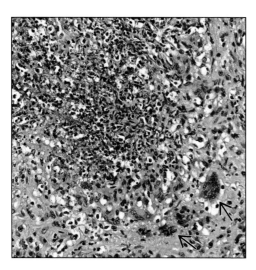

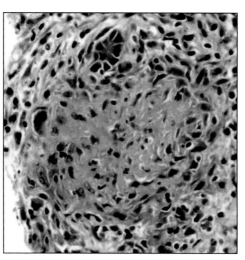

(Left) Interstitial, extravascular granulomatous inflammation with excess neutrophils is surrounded by multinucleated giant cells ➡ resembling a microabscess in the center. (Courtesy W. Travis, MD.) *(Right)* H&E shows a well-developed, small, interstitial, nonnecrotizing granuloma with epithelioid and rare giant cells at the periphery in a patient with GPA.

GRANULOMATOSIS WITH POLYANGIITIS (WEGENER)

Microscopic Features: Spectrum of Renal Vasculitis

(Left) Interlobular artery with marked arteriosclerosis affected by active vasculitis composed of lymphocytes and neutrophils with focal granulomatous features is shown in a patient with GPA. (Right) Trichrome stained interlobular artery shows acute transmural fibrinoid necrotizing vasculitis, where the fibrin is strongly fuchsinophilic ➡.

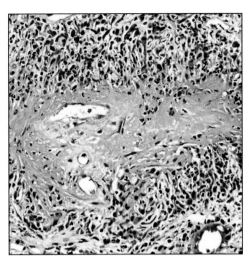
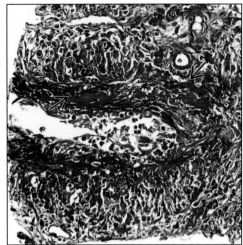

(Left) Intrarenal small artery shows circumferential, transmural fibrinoid necrosis with intense inflammatory reaction. (Right) Elastic (EVG) stain shows partial loss of internal elastic lamina of an interlobular artery ➡ following necrotizing vasculitis in a patient with GPA. An elastic stain is useful to detect old arteritis because the disrupted elastica persists in the fibrous scar.

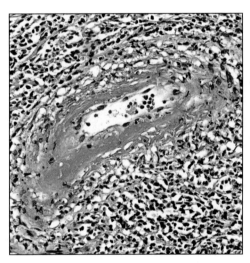
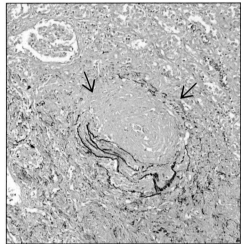

(Left) Fibrinoid necrotizing capillaritis ➡ with interstitial hemorrhages is shown in the renal medulla of a patient with c-ANCA positive GPA. (Right) H&E shows active medullary capillaritis ➡ with extravasation of red cells in the interstitium in a patient with GPA.

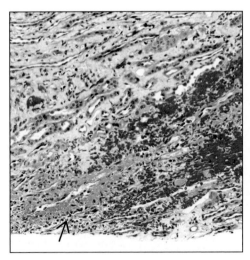
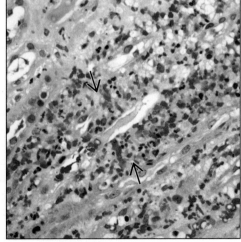

GRANULOMATOSIS WITH POLYANGIITIS (WEGENER)

Microscopic Features: Extrarenal Small Vessel Vasculitis

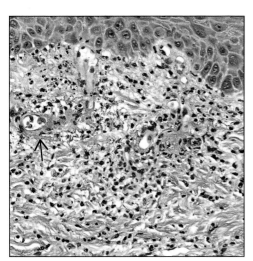

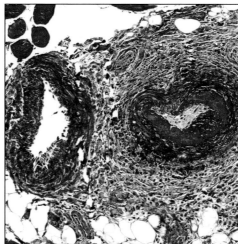

(Left) Skin in GPA shows dermal leukocytoclastic vasculitis of the capillaries, with one showing an early fibrinoid change ➡. *(Right)* A patient with GPA, presenting with a palpable nodule in the leg, shows a segment of a small artery from the subcutaneous tissue with fibrinoid necrotizing vasculitis.

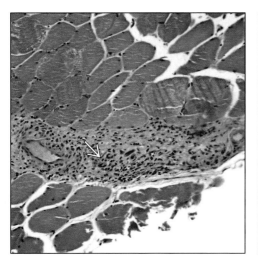

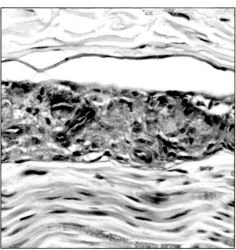

(Left) Skeletal muscle biopsy shows granulomatous inflammation ➡ of an arteriole in the perimysial tissue. *(Right)* Nerve biopsy shows granulomatous arteriolitis associated with acute peripheral neuropathy.

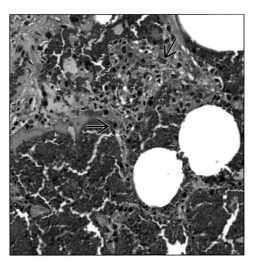

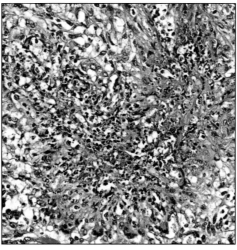

(Left) Section of lung shows extensive alveolar hemorrhage adjacent to capillaritis with neutrophils ➡. This is believed to be an early lesion in GPA. *(Right)* Irregular, necrotizing granulomatous inflammation with palisading of epithelioid and giant cells with a neutrophilic center is shown in the lung of a patient with GPA.

CHURG-STRAUSS SYNDROME

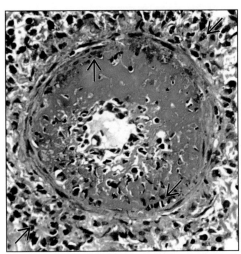

Renal biopsy from a patient with CSS shows circumferential, transmural necrotizing arteritis surrounded by numerous eosinophils and by lymphocytes. Eosinophils invade the media ➡.

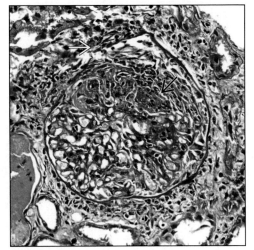

Periodic acid-Schiff stain of a glomerulus in CSS reveals segmental necrosis ➡, a cellular crescent in Bowman space, and rupture of Bowman capsule ➡ with periglomerular inflammation.

TERMINOLOGY

Abbreviations
- Churg-Strauss syndrome (CSS)

Synonyms
- Allergic granulomatosis and angiitis
  - Defined by autopsy study in 1951 by Churg and Strauss

Definitions
- American College of Rheumatology (ACR) criteria differentiate various forms of vasculitides once diagnosis of vasculitis is made
  - CSS diagnosis requires 4 of 6 following features
    - Asthma
    - Eosinophilia > 10%
    - Extravascular eosinophil infiltration
    - Pulmonary infiltrates
    - Paranasal sinus changes
    - Peripheral neuropathy
- Chapel Hill Consensus Conference (pathology)
  - Criteria are diagnostic and generally exclude other forms of systemic vasculitides
  - Eosinophil-rich inflammatory infiltrate and granulomatous inflammation involving respiratory tract
  - Eosinophil-rich necrotizing vasculitis affecting small to medium-sized vessels
  - Associated with asthma and peripheral eosinophilia
- Classified with antineutrophilic cytoplasmic antibody (ANCA) diseases

ETIOLOGY/PATHOGENESIS

Environmental Exposure
- Trigger agents: Allergens, vaccinations, or drugs

Genetic
- Associated with *HLA-DRB4* gene, risk factor

Pathogenesis
- Primarily cell-mediated tissue and vascular injury
  - CD4(+) T cells secrete interferon-gamma (Th-1 cytokine), promoting granulomatous inflammation
  - Eosinophil activation via IL-4, IL-5, and IL-13 secretion and CD95-CD95L pathway
  - Tissue damage by eosinophils due to release of cytotoxic eosinophilic cationic and major basic protein
  - Eotaxin-3 from endothelial cells chemotactic for eosinophils
- ANCA probably contributes to pathogenesis
  - ANCA titers correlate with disease activity

CLINICAL ISSUES

Epidemiology
- Incidence
  - Rare: 3-11/1,000,000 worldwide
  - 16-27% have renal involvement from 3 large series
  - Lesser frequency and milder disease than other small vessel vasculitides involving kidney
- Age
  - Peak age: 40-60 years; mean: ~ 48 years
  - Younger adults may also be affected
- Gender
  - No gender predilection
- Ethnicity
  - No ethnic predisposition

Presentation
- Multisystemic disease
- 4 phases
  - **Allergic**
    - Constitutional symptoms
    - Asthma
    - Rhinitis
  - **Eosinophilic**
    - Peripheral eosinophilia

CHURG-STRAUSS SYNDROME

Key Facts

Terminology
- Synonyms: Allergic granulomatosis and angiitis

Etiology/Pathogenesis
- Triggers: Allergens, vaccines, drugs
- T-helper cell and eosinophil activation

Clinical Issues
- Occurs in any age, mostly 40-60 years
- Asthma, eosinophilia, granulomatous inflammation
- Positive MPO-ANCA (40-70%)
- Typically relapsing disease (35-74%)
- High renal incidence in ANCA(+) cases
- Rapid renal failure, mild renal impairment, hematuria
- Remission after initial treatment (90%)
- Cyclophosphamide in steroid-resistant or relapsing disease

Microscopic Pathology
- Acute, subacute, &/or chronic crescentic GN, pauci-immune
- Occasional isolated eosinophilic interstitial nephritis
- Small vessel vasculitis, fibrinoid necrotizing and granulomatous types

Ancillary Tests
- Negative IF and nonspecific EM
- No immune deposits

Top Differential Diagnoses
- Granulomatosis with polyangiitis (Wegener) with renal involvement
- Drug-induced vasculitis
- Systemic parasitic infestation

- ■ Tissue eosinophil infiltration (e.g., gastrointestinal, sinusitis)
  - ■ Heart
  - o **Vasculitic**
    - ■ Skin purpuric rash
    - ■ Peripheral neuropathy
    - ■ Cerebral vessels
    - ■ Lung
    - ■ Kidney
  - o **Post vasculitic**
    - ■ Sequelae related to major organ damage and hypertension
- Renal disease
  - o Higher incidence in ANCA(+) cases
  - o Progressive renal insufficiency
  - o Acute renal failure (less frequent)
  - o Hematuria (mild to severe)
  - o Subnephrotic proteinuria, usually < 1.0 g/d
  - o Asymptomatic (isolated) urinary abnormalities
  - o Obstructive uropathy caused by ureteral stenosis

Laboratory Tests
- Anemia, leukocytosis
- Peripheral eosinophilia (10-20%)
  - o May be lower or normal in patients previously treated with steroids for asthma
- Elevated erythrocyte sedimentation rate
- ANCA (40-70% positive)
  - o Mainly p-ANCA (antimyeloperoxidase antibodies [MPO]); rarely c-ANCA or atypical
- Rheumatoid factor (25% positive)
- Elevated serum IgE levels and immune complexes containing IgE

Treatment
- Drugs
  - o Immunosuppressive therapy used to treat severe, multisystemic disease manifestations, particularly vasculitis
    - ■ Good response to high-dose corticosteroids
    - ■ Cyclophosphamide in steroid-resistant or relapsing disease
    - ■ Rituximab anti-CD20 antibody in refractory disease
    - ■ Mycophenolate mofetil
  - o Maintenance: Oral cyclophosphamide or azathioprine

Prognosis
- Typically relapsing disease (35-74%)
- Remission after initial treatment (90%)
- Renal flares are rare, and long-term prognosis is favorable
- Factors of poor prognosis
  - o Heart, gastrointestinal, central nervous system involvement
  - o Proteinuria > 1 g/24 hours
  - o Creatinine > 1.5 mg/dL
- Rare: Severe renal vasculitic or crescentic glomerulonephritis and chronic renal failure

MICROSCOPIC PATHOLOGY

Histologic Features
- **Glomeruli** (mild to severe involvement)
  - o Focal glomerulonephritis, pauci-immune
    - ■ Segmental necrotizing lesions
    - ■ Cellular crescents/extracapillary proliferation (5-50% of glomeruli)
    - ■ Crescents in varying stages of healing: Fibrocellular and fibrous types (5-50% of glomeruli)
    - ■ Focal segmental glomerulosclerosis
    - ■ Global glomerulosclerosis, if chronic
  - o Mesangial hypercellularity
    - ■ Mild to moderate
  - o Focal eosinophil or neutrophil infiltration
  - o No endocapillary proliferation or capillary wall abnormalities
- **Tubulointerstitium**
  - o Focal eosinophil-rich interstitial infiltrate
  - o Tissue eosinophils best seen on H&E and trichrome-stained sections
  - o Isolated acute tubulointerstitial nephritis

3

o Focal granuloma formation, rare
o Necrotizing granuloma with eosinophils, necrotic eosinophilic cellular debris, scattered multinucleated giant cells, and epithelioid macrophages in a palisading layer
  ■ Healing of granuloma spontaneous or following treatment
o Free red blood cells, RBC casts, and hemosiderin casts in tubular lumina in acute cases
o Tubular atrophy, interstitial fibrosis, and chronic inflammation
• **Vessels**
o Interlobular (commonly), arcuate, and large branches of renal artery (sometimes) affected
  ■ Necrotizing fibrinoid necrosis involves endothelium and intima 1st and extends to media
  ■ Eosinophils, predominant cell infiltration
  ■ Focal granulomatous change may be seen
o Small vessel vasculitis &/or venulitis
• **Lower urinary tract**
o Renal pelvis, ureter, or prostate
  ■ Eosinophilic and granulomatous inflammation
o Healed lesions lead to
  ■ Obstructive uropathy
  ■ Cause of renal functional impairment
• **Lung and other organs**
o Pulmonary capillaritis with hemorrhage
o Small vessel vasculitis &/or venulitis; other organs and skin with prominent eosinophils

ANCILLARY TESTS

Immunofluorescence
• Generally, no deposits of immunoglobulins (IgG, IgM, IgA) or complement (C3, C1q)
• Strong fibrinogen staining in necrotizing glomerular and vascular lesions

Electron Microscopy
• Glomerular epithelial (parietal and visceral) cell injury in active crescentic lesions
• Variable foot process effacement depending on visceral cell injury
• Normal thickness, contour, and texture of glomerular basement membranes (GBM)
• Variable collapse of capillary tuft due to presence of crescent
• Mild to moderate mesangial hypercellularity and increased matrix
• No immune complex type of electron-dense deposits

DIFFERENTIAL DIAGNOSIS

Granulomatosis with Polyangiitis (Wegener)
• No history of asthma
• Mild or no eosinophilia
• Higher incidence of crescentic GN (90%)
• Almost always c-ANCA positive
• Mild to moderate eosinophil infiltration
• More striking granulomatous inflammation

Drug-induced Vasculitis and Interstitial Nephritis
• History of drug intake
• No history of asthma
• Small proportion associated with MPO-ANCA (hydralazine, antithyroid drugs)
• Less severe eosinophilia (< 10%)
• Rarely, crescentic glomerulonephritis
• Sometimes indistinguishable from CSS

Systemic or Renal Parasitic Infestation
• History of parasitic infection
• Travel to parasite endemic area
• Not associated with positive ANCA serology
• No crescentic glomerulonephritis
o Rare small vessel vasculitis or capillaritis, sometimes varied forms of immune-complex glomerular lesions
• Eosinophil-rich tubulointerstitial nephritis with occasional evidence of parasitic eggs or larvae
• May have episodes of asthma

DIAGNOSTIC CHECKLIST

Pathologic Interpretation Pearls
• Vasculitis with prominent eosinophils and clinical history of asthma should raise possibility of CSS

SELECTED REFERENCES

1. Vaglio A et al: Churg-Strauss syndrome. Kidney Int. 76(9):1006-11, 2009
2. Sinico RA et al: Renal involvement in Churg-Strauss syndrome. Am J Kidney Dis. 47(5):770-9, 2006
3. Sablé-Fourtassou R et al: Antineutrophil cytoplasmic antibodies and the Churg-Strauss syndrome. Ann Intern Med. 143(9):632-8, 2005
4. Sinico RA et al: Prevalence and clinical significance of antineutrophil cytoplasmic antibodies in Churg-Strauss syndrome. Arthritis Rheum. 52(9):2926-35, 2005
5. Keogh KA et al: Churg-Strauss syndrome: clinical presentation, antineutrophil cytoplasmic antibodies, and leukotriene receptor antagonists. Am J Med. 115(4):284-90, 2003
6. Kikuchi Y et al: Glomerular lesions in patients with Churg-Strauss syndrome and the anti-myeloperoxidase antibody. Clin Nephrol. 55(6):429-35, 2001
7. Holloway J et al: Churg-Strauss syndrome associated with zafirlukast. J Am Osteopath Assoc. 98(5):275-8, 1998
8. Jennette JC et al: Nomenclature of systemic vasculitides. Proposal of an international consensus conference. Arthritis Rheum. 37(2):187-92, 1994
9. Vogel PS et al: Churg-Strauss syndrome. J Am Acad Dermatol. 27(5 Pt 2):821-4, 1992
10. Clutterbuck EJ et al: Renal involvement in Churg-Strauss syndrome. Nephrol Dial Transplant. 5(3):161-7, 1990
11. Lanham JG et al: Systemic vasculitis with asthma and eosinophilia: a clinical approach to the Churg-Strauss syndrome. Medicine (Baltimore). 63(2):65-81, 1984
12. Chumbley LC et al: Allergic granulomatosis and angiitis (Churg-Strauss syndrome). Report and analysis of 30 cases. Mayo Clin Proc. 52(8):477-84, 1977
13. Churg J et al: Allergic granulomatosis, allergic angiitis, and periarteritis nodosa. Am J Pathol. 27(2):277-301, 1951

CHURG-STRAUSS SYNDROME

Glomerular Microscopic Features

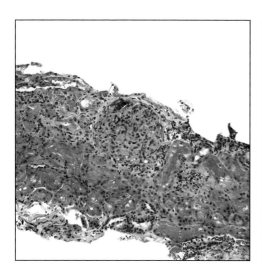
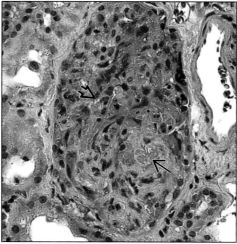

(Left) Low-power view of a renal biopsy from a patient with CSS shows glomerular and periglomerular inflammation with increased eosinophils. (Right) This glomerulus from a patient with CSS is scarcely recognizable due to intraglomerular fibrinoid necrosis ➡, infiltrating eosinophils ➡, and lymphocytes. (Courtesy R. Wieczorek, MD.)

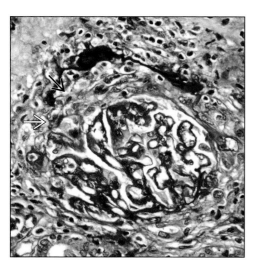
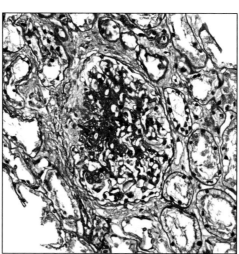

(Left) Periodic acid-Schiff stain of a glomerulus with a fibrocellular crescent ➡ and periglomerular inflammation is partially compressing the glomerulus with rupture of Bowman capsule ➡, typical of crescents of whatever etiology. (Right) PAS-stained glomerulus shows segmental sclerosing lesion with a fibrous crescent and capsular adhesion. Various stages of healing of crescentic GN may be seen in the same renal biopsy as in ANCA disease.

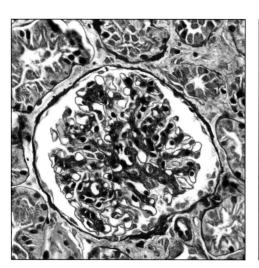
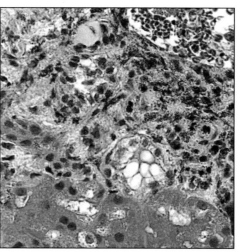

(Left) In CSS, often some degree of mesangial proliferation/hypercellularity may be noted in the glomeruli, in contrast to anti-GBM disease. (Right) This case of CSS shows intense renal interstitial eosinophil infiltration and tubulitis with early necrosis. Eosinophilic infiltration of affected tissue is a hallmark of CSS.

CHURG-STRAUSS SYNDROME

Tubulointerstitial Microscopic Features

(Left) H&E stained renal biopsy shows an isolated eosinophil-rich tubulointerstitial inflammation in a patient with CSS and a recent rise in creatinine. Without the glomerular or arterial lesions, this might be mistaken for a drug reaction. *(Right)* Active interstitial inflammation contains eosinophils sometimes admixed with multinucleated giant cells ⇨ in CSS renal disease, giving it a granulomatous appearance.

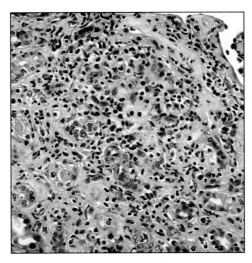
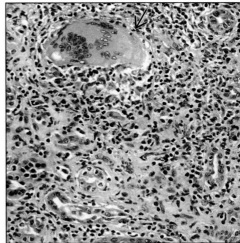

(Left) CSS patient with mild chronic insufficiency and previously treated with steroids shows a focus of sclerosing granulomatous inflammation ⇨ with residual lymphocytic infiltrate and interstitial fibrosis. *(Right)* H&E shows a small interstitial granuloma in a CSS patient with acute renal failure composed of a cuff of lymphocytes, eosinophils, epithelioid macrophages, and a small multinucleated giant cell ⇨ at the edge of the biopsy.

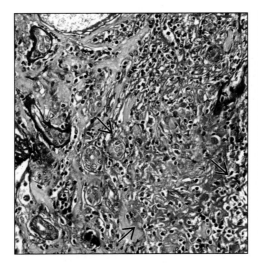
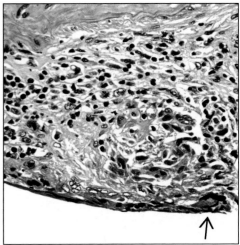

(Left) Kidney biopsy from a CSS patient with progressive renal failure reveals circumscribed interstitial granulomatous inflammation surrounded by a cuff of lymphocytes and eosinophils. *(Right)* A toluidine blue-stained, Epon-embedded section of a kidney biopsy from a CSS patient shows a well-developed nonnecrotizing interstitial granuloma with giant cells. Granulomatous interstitial nephritis can be caused by drugs, sarcoidosis, certain infections, and granulomatosis with polyangiitis (Wegener).

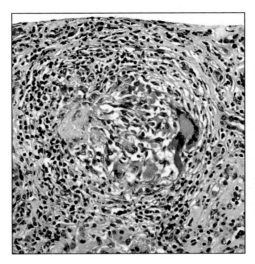
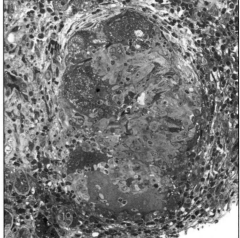

CHURG-STRAUSS SYNDROME

Vascular Microscopic Features

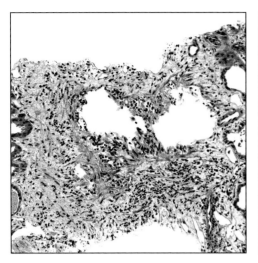

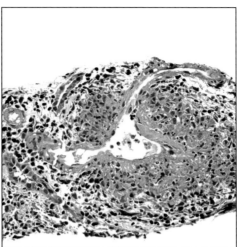

(Left) Corticomedullary junction shows venulitis with prominent adjacent eosinophils. Both small arteries and veins along with capillaries may manifest vascular inflammation in CSS. (Right) Intrarenal small artery in a biopsy shows granulomatous vasculitis with fibrinoid necrosis of the intima, surrounded by lymphocytes, eosinophils, and epithelioid cells. This pattern is typical of ANCA-related diseases.

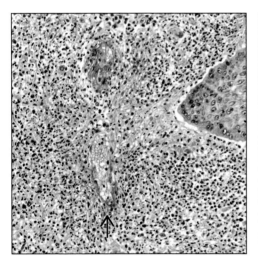

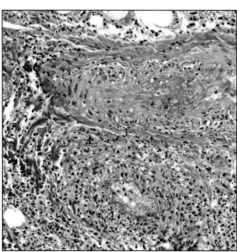

(Left) Skin biopsy from a CSS patient with a severe cutaneous purpuric rash is characterized by eosinophil- and neutrophil-rich dermal inflammation and a fibrinoid necrotizing leukocytoclastic vasculitis of the capillary ➡. (Right) Palpable purpuric rash in the leg from a CSS patient shows subcutaneous transmural arteritis and venulitis. ANCA-related diseases typically involve vasculitis in both arteries and veins.

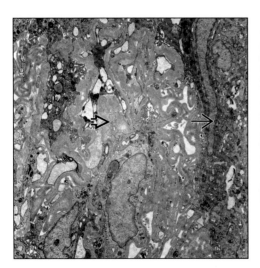

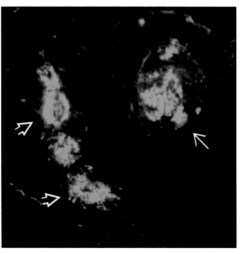

(Left) Electron micrograph of a glomerulus in CSS shows significant compression by a cellular crescent ➡. No conspicuous electron-dense deposits are noted in the glomerular basement membrane ➡, typical of pauci-immune type glomerulonephritis. (Right) Immunofluorescence microscopy demonstrates strong fibrinogen/fibrin deposition in the glomerulus ➡ and small arteries ➡.

POLYARTERITIS NODOSA

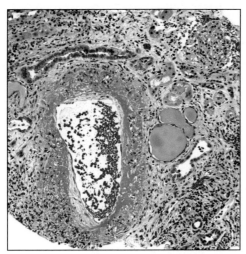

Kidney biopsy in polyarteritis nodosa (PAN) shows circumferential, transmural fibrinoid necrosis and active inflammatory infiltrate composed of neutrophils and lymphocytes.

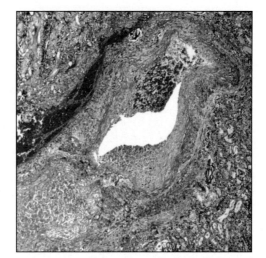

Trichrome-stained kidney section shows a healing PAN of a medium-sized vessel with focal thrombosis and early microaneurysm formation. It is common to have both active and healed lesions in PAN.

TERMINOLOGY

Abbreviations
- Polyarteritis nodosa (PAN)

Synonyms
- Macroscopic polyarteritis
- Classic polyarteritis nodosa
- Kussmaul and Maier periarteritis nodosa

Definitions
- Chapel Hill Consensus Conference criteria
  - Necrotizing inflammation of medium-sized or small arteries without glomerulonephritis or vasculitis in arterioles, capillaries, or venules
- American College of Rheumatology criteria
  - Weight loss ≥ 4 kg, livedo reticularis, testicular pain or tenderness, myalgias, weakness or leg tenderness, mono- or polyneuropathy, diastolic BP > 90 mmHg, elevated BUN or creatinine, hepatitis B virus, biopsy diagnosis of small or medium-sized arteries, arteriography with aneurysms or occlusions in visceral arteries
  - 3 or more of the above criteria have high sensitivity and specificity for diagnosis
- EULAR/PRINTO/PRES criteria for childhood PAN
  - Necrotizing vasculitis, angiographic abnormalities, and either skin involvement, myalgia/muscle tenderness, hypertension, peripheral neuropathy, or renal involvement

ETIOLOGY/PATHOGENESIS

Infectious Agents
- Hepatitis B virus (HBV)
  - Accounts for ~ 36% of PAN cases
- Possibly other bacterial and viral infections
  - Hepatitis C virus (HCV)
  - Rarely HIV, Epstein-Barr virus

Other
- HBV immunization
- Exposure to silica-containing compounds
- In majority, etiology is unknown

Pathogenesis
- Immunologically mediated
  - Believed to be chronic immune-complex mediated disease
    - Resembles chronic serum sickness model
  - Probably a T-cell-mediated immune component
  - Antigen unknown
  - May be microbial or autoantigen in vessel wall
- Participation of neutrophilic and mononuclear inflammatory infiltrate (T cells and macrophages)
  - Weakness in vessel wall leads to thrombosis or fibrosis and microaneurysm formation
- Chronic, cyclic insults support presence of different stages of vasculitis

CLINICAL ISSUES

Epidemiology
- Incidence
  - 2-31/1,000,000 in Europe and USA
    - Some studies have included cases now classified as microscopic polyangiitis
  - Up to 77/1,000,000 in endemic areas for hepatitis B viral infection
- Age
  - Adults: Peak at 5th to 7th decade
  - Children: 7-11 years
    - However, less common in children
- Gender
  - Male predilection (M:F = 2:1)
- Ethnicity
  - 2x higher prevalence in Europeans vs. others
  - Specific HLA haplotypes
  - Involves all ethnic groups

POLYARTERITIS NODOSA

Key Facts

Terminology
- Necrotizing inflammation of medium-sized or small arteries without glomerulonephritis or vasculitis in arterioles, capillaries, or venules

Clinical Issues
- HBV association in ~ 36% of PAN cases
- Up to 77/million in endemic areas for hepatitis B viral infection
- Adult: Peak at 5th to 7th decade
- Multisystemic involvement
- Rarely, ANCA positive
- Kidney frequently involved (70-80%)
- New onset hypertension, sometimes malignant range
- Cyclophosphamide and steroids for severe cases, remission in 90%

Image Findings
- Angiography localizes microaneurysms

Microscopic Pathology
- Intralobar, arcuate, and, rarely, interlobular arteries affected (medium-sized vessels)
- Characteristic features are fibrinoid necrosis and transmural and periarterial inflammation
- Late arterial lesions include aneurysms and stenosis

Top Differential Diagnoses
- Kawasaki disease
- ANCA-related small vessel vasculitides
- Systemic lupus erythematosus
- Fibromuscular dysplasia

Presentation
- Multisystemic involvement
- Clinical symptoms related to ischemia and are dependent on organ involved and disease severity
- Constitutional symptoms: Fever, malaise, weight loss, myalgia, abdominal pain
- Renal
  - Kidney frequently involved (70-80%)
    - Focal renal infarction (~ 30%)
    - Microaneurysms (~ 65%)
    - Hematuria, proteinuria (~ 20%)
    - Loin pain
    - Acute renal failure
  - New onset hypertension, sometimes malignant range
  - Rare: Rupture of kidney with perirenal hematoma
  - Massive retroperitoneal and peritoneal hemorrhage following rupture of arterial aneurysm
- Heart
  - Ischemic heart disease
- Neurologic (10%)
  - Focal defects, hemiplegia, visual loss, mononeuritis multiplex
- Skin
  - Varied lesions: Palpable purpura, necrotic with peripheral gangrene, livedo reticularis, ulcers
  - Subcutaneous nodules
- Skeletal muscle and mesentery (30%)
- Gastrointestinal, peripheral nerves, skin (50%)

Laboratory Tests
- Anemia, leukocytosis, thrombocytosis
- Elevation of ESR and C-reactive protein
- Positive hepatitis B serology in some cases
- No specific serologic tests
- No significant association with ANCA
- Rarely, ANCA positive (usually perinuclear) by indirect IF only, when overlap with microscopic polyangiitis

Treatment
- Steroid therapy is 1st line of therapy; remission in 50% of patients
- Cyclophosphamide and steroids for severe cases; remission in 90%
- Plasma exchange/plasmapheresis in refractory cases
- HBV-associated PAN needs antiviral therapy

Prognosis
- Fulminant disease with < 5-year survival
- 40% of patients have relapse
- 5 factor score (FFS) estimates prognosis
  - Scores renal (Cr > 1.6 mg/dL, proteinuria > 1 gm/24 hr), GI, cardiac, and CNS involvement
  - Lower score correlates with better 5-year survival

IMAGE FINDINGS

Ultrasonographic Findings
- Pulsed and color Doppler ultrasonography
  - Localization of microaneurysm (seen in 50-60%)

Computed Tomography Angiography
- Microaneurysms often seen at artery bifurcations
- Tc-99m DMSA uptake scanning detects patchy renal parenchymal disease

MICROSCOPIC PATHOLOGY

Histologic Features
- Glomeruli
  - Mostly varying degrees of ischemic collapse associated with vessel involvement
  - Global glomerulosclerosis with tubular atrophy in healed cortical scars
  - Normal histology of glomeruli located away from vasculitis
  - Rarely, focal crescentic glomerulonephritis (pauci-immune type)
    - Suggests overlap of PAN and microscopic polyangiitis
    - Rarely, positive ANCA reported
- Tubules and interstitium

o Acute ischemic infarction in distribution of affected artery
o Tubular simplification, atrophy, and mild interstitial fibrosis
o Active &/or chronic interstitial and periarterial inflammation
- Arteries
  o Intralobar, arcuate, and, rarely, interlobular artery affected (medium-sized vessels)
    ▪ Small arterioles and capillaries lacking muscular coat are not affected
  o Obliterative arteritis (acute, subacute, or chronic)
  o Characteristic features are fibrinoid necrosis and transmural and periarterial inflammation
    ▪ Fuchsinophilic/eosinophilic amorphous fibrinoid material in areas of necrosis
    ▪ Destruction of medial smooth muscle
    ▪ Disruption of internal and external elastic laminae
  o Moderate to intense inflammatory infiltrate
    ▪ Neutrophils, eosinophils with karyorrhexis
    ▪ Activated T-lymphocytes and monocytes/ macrophages
  o Varying degrees of luminal narrowing
  o Intravascular thrombosis
  o Acute and chronic/healed lesions can coexist in same vessel
  o Healed lesions show progressive fibrotic and obliterative arteriopathy/endarteritis
    ▪ Late lesions include arterial aneurysms
    ▪ Progressive scarring can lead to stenosis

Other Organs
- Lung, skeletal muscle, liver, pancreas, others
- Obliterative arteritis, fibrinoid necrosis, transmural and periarterial inflammation, thrombosis, and aneurysm as described in kidney
- Spares aorta and its major branches

ANCILLARY TESTS

Immunofluorescence
- Immunoglobulins (IgG, IgM, IgA), complement C3 (nonspecific) staining in areas of fibrinoid necrosis
- Strong staining for fibrinogen in same distribution
- No immune complex deposits in glomeruli

Electron Microscopy
- No glomerular deposits

DIFFERENTIAL DIAGNOSIS

Kawasaki Disease
- Mucocutaneous lymph node syndrome
- Mononuclear infiltrate
- Less fibrinoid necrosis

ANCA-related Small Vessel Vasculitides
- Multisystemic microscopic polyangiitis
- Granulomatosis with polyangiitis (Wegener)
- Churg-Strauss syndrome

Systemic Lupus Erythematosus
- Eosinophils in CSS
- Immune-complex mediated
- PAN-like pauci-immune vasculitis
- Positive serology for SLE

Fibromuscular Dysplasia
- Lesions lack fibrinoid necrosis
- No inflammation
- Disorganized media

DIAGNOSTIC CHECKLIST

Clinically Relevant Pathologic Features
- 3x risk of mortality with renal involvement
- Yield of renal biopsy in polyarteritis nodosa is low
  o Focal and patchy involvement of medium-sized or (rarely) small arteries
  o Increased risk of bleeding in acute cases
  o Rare: Formation of arteriovenous fistulae
  o Biopsy material from affected area (e.g., skin, skeletal muscle) or organ is useful for definitive diagnosis

Pathologic Interpretation Pearls
- Absence of vasculitic lesion (usually a larger vessel) in biopsy does not exclude diagnosis due to sampling problems

SELECTED REFERENCES

1. Dillon MJ et al: Medium-size-vessel vasculitis. Pediatr Nephrol. 25(9):1641-52, 2010
2. Ozen S et al: EULAR/PRINTO/PRES criteria for Henoch-Schönlein purpura, childhood polyarteritis nodosa, childhood Wegener granulomatosis and childhood Takayasu arteritis: Ankara 2008. Part II: Final classification criteria. Ann Rheum Dis. 69(5):798-806, 2010
3. Pagnoux C et al: Clinical features and outcomes in 348 patients with polyarteritis nodosa: a systematic retrospective study of patients diagnosed between 1963 and 2005 and entered into the French Vasculitis Study Group Database. Arthritis Rheum. 62(2):616-26, 2010
4. Dillon MJ et al: A new international classification of childhood vasculitis. Pediatr Nephrol. 21(9):1219-22, 2006
5. Guillevin L et al: Hepatitis B virus-associated polyarteritis nodosa: clinical characteristics, outcome, and impact of treatment in 115 patients. Medicine (Baltimore). 84(5):313-22, 2005
6. Agard C et al: Microscopic polyangiitis and polyarteritis nodosa: how and when do they start? Arthritis Rheum. 49(5):709-15, 2003
7. Stone JH: Polyarteritis nodosa. JAMA. 288(13):1632-9, 2002
8. Fortin PR et al: Prognostic factors in systemic necrotizing vasculitis of the polyarteritis nodosa group--a review of 45 cases. J Rheumatol. 22(1):78-84, 1995
9. Jennette JC et al: Nomenclature of systemic vasculitides. Proposal of an international consensus conference. Arthritis Rheum. 37(2):187-92, 1994
10. Lightfoot RW Jr et al: The American College of Rheumatology 1990 criteria for the classification of polyarteritis nodosa. Arthritis Rheum. 33(8):1088-93, 1990

POLYARTERITIS NODOSA

Gross and Microscopic Features

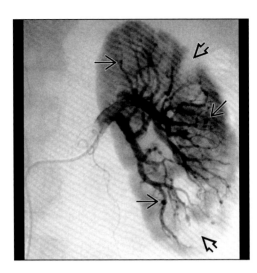
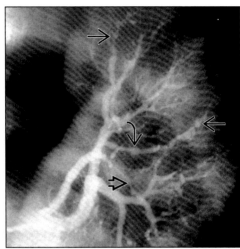

(Left) Digital subtraction angiogram shows characteristic multiple microaneurysms ➡. There are also areas within the kidney parenchyma with decreased perfusion consistent with infarcts ⊡. Infarcts may represent necrosis or thrombosis. Hemorrhage may occur if aneurysms rupture. *(Right)* Catheter angiography shows very severe involvement of renal vessels with multiple microaneurysms ➡, beaded appearance of vessels ⊅, and stenoses ⊡, all characteristic signs of PAN.

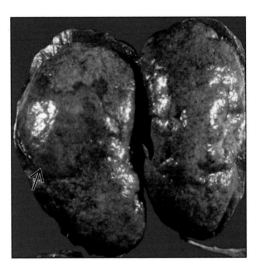
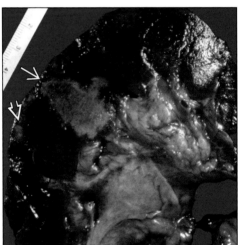

(Left) Gross photograph shows autopsy kidneys from a patient with widespread PAN. Note a large, paler area of the left-sided kidney with a hemorrhagic border representing an infarct ➡. *(Right)* Cut section from the kidney shows large, pale (ischemic) infarct ➡ with a hemorrhagic border. Smaller pale areas ⊡ are also noted in the cortex adjacent to the large infarct, suggesting additional cortical infarcts.

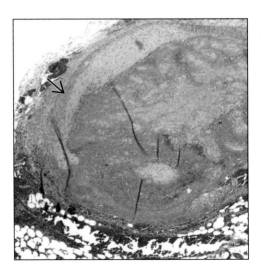
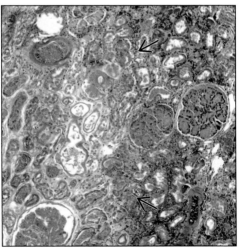

(Left) Section of a large renal artery in the pelvis shows arterial inflammation ➡, fibrinoid necrosis, and thrombosis filling the lumen. This leads to areas of cortical and medullary infarction. *(Right)* Microscopic section from a kidney shows ischemic infarction of the renal cortex with a hemorrhagic border and congestion seen on the right side ➡.

POLYARTERITIS NODOSA

Microscopic Features: Kidney

(Left) Extensive fibrinoid necrosis and thrombosis ⮕ of an arcuate artery are shown surrounded by active inflammatory infiltrate. *(Right)* The artery is stained with EVG, showing lack of elastic lamina ⮕ in the areas of fibrinoid necrosis and thrombosis. A preserved portion of the artery on the right side ⮞ shows multiple layers of elastic lamina consistent with arteriosclerosis.

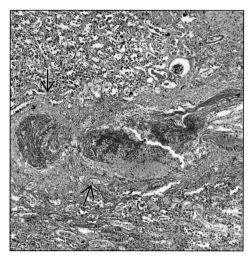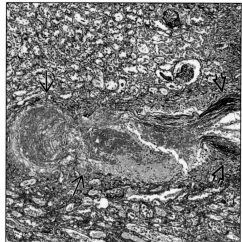

(Left) An interlobular artery in the kidney shows circumferential fibrinoid necrosis (fuchsinophilic) in a trichrome-stained section surrounded by active transmural inflammatory infiltrate. *(Right)* Immunofluorescence of kidney tissue shows strong staining for immunoglobulin IgG within the fibrinoid necrotizing lesion of an interlobular artery. This is nonspecific localization of immunoglobulins, complement C3, as well as fibrinogen.

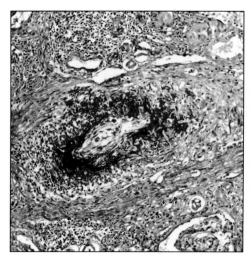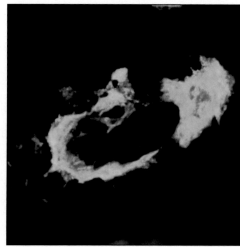

(Left) Low magnification of a kidney biopsy shows mainly mild to moderate ischemic collapse without evidence of crescentic GN ⮕. Ischemic simplification of tubules and mild interstitial inflammation is noted. *(Right)* In addition to a generally unremarkable but ischemic glomerulus, some of the small arteries show evidence of sclerosis and are surrounded by sparse inflammatory infiltrate without significant vasculitis ⮕.

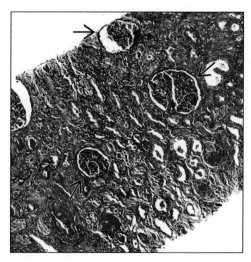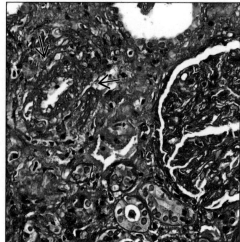

Microscopic Features: Kidney

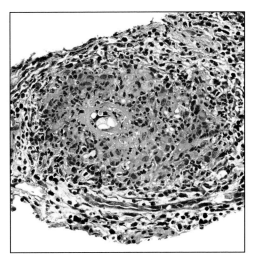

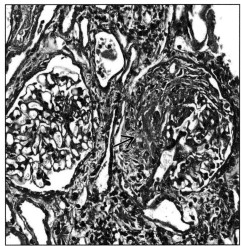

(Left) Renal biopsy shows evidence of a small vessel vasculitis with fibrinoid necrosis in the center surrounded by intense active inflammatory infiltrate composed of lymphocytes, neutrophils, and occasional eosinophils. This is rarely seen in overlapping forms of PAN and microscopic polyangiitis. (Right) In the same case, glomeruli may occasionally show cellular or fibrocellular crescents ➡. An adjacent glomerulus is uninvolved.

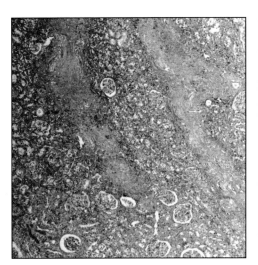

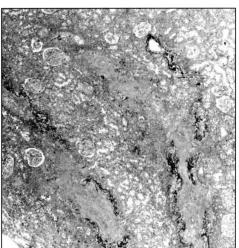

(Left) Trichrome-stained low-magnification kidney section with multiple glomeruli without crescents and 2 medium-sized vessels show obliterative features following acute PAN. (Right) EVG-stained low-magnification kidney section shows interruption and extensive loss of elastic lamina within the obliterated vessel walls.

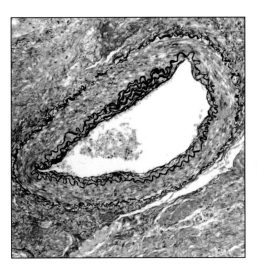

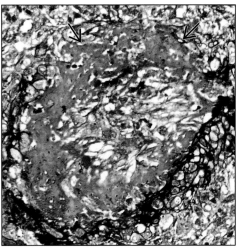

(Left) A medium-sized artery (arcuate type) in the kidney from a patient with PAN shows no evidence of vasculitis with preserved internal and external elastic lamina. (Right) High magnification shows an artery with fibrinoid necrosis and segmental loss of elastic lamina ➡ in a case of PAN (Elastic van Gieson stain).

Microscopic Features: Renal and Nonrenal Vascular

(Left) An interlobular artery from a kidney biopsy shows segmental healing PAN with early microaneurysmal dilatation ➜ while normal preservation is noted in the remaining portions of the artery ⧉. (Right) An interlobular artery in a kidney biopsy shows obliterative arteriopathy with intimal and medial fibrosis, narrowing the lumen.

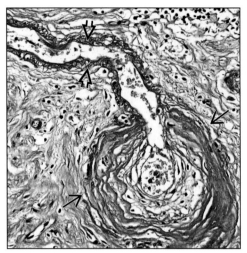 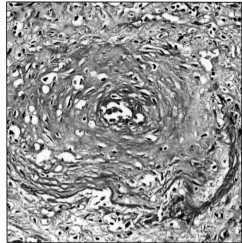

(Left) Kidney biopsy shows an arcuate artery replaced by extensive fibrinoid necrosis and arteritis surrounded by a granulomatous inflammation with scattered giant cells ➜. The granulomatous nature of the inflammatory infiltrate may be seen with PAN. (Right) A medium-sized artery from the subcutaneous tissue (EVG stain) shows residual transmural inflammatory infiltrate along with obliterative arteriopathy and segmental disruption of the elastic lamina.

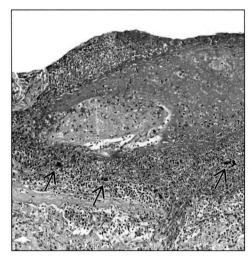 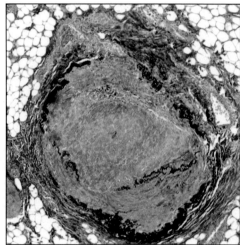

(Left) Low-magnification view of a medium-sized artery in the perimysial area of skeletal muscle shows marked transmural arteritis with central fibrinoid necrosis. (Right) High magnification of an artery shows central fibrinoid necrosis with occlusive features surrounded by active mononuclear infiltrate, composed of lymphocytes and histiocytes, reaching the adventitia.

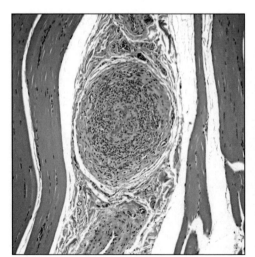 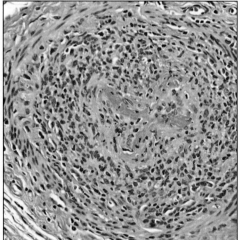

POLYARTERITIS NODOSA

Microscopic Features: Renal and Nonrenal Vascular

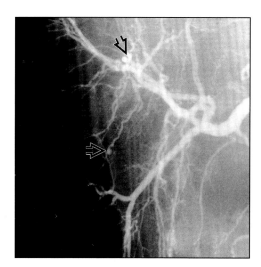

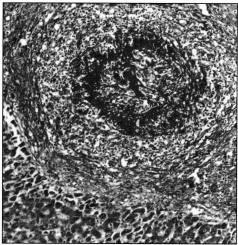

(Left) Angiogram magnification view of the liver shows hepatic artery involvement. Arteries have a very irregular, beaded appearance. Several small aneurysms ⇨ represent a necrotic process involving the arterial wall. These findings would be very difficult to see on CT or MR. *(Right)* A medium-sized artery in the liver parenchyma shows circumferential fibrinoid necrosis along with active inflammatory infiltrate.

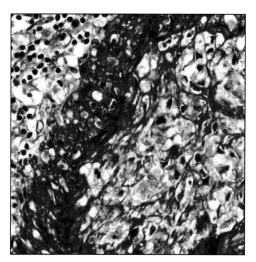

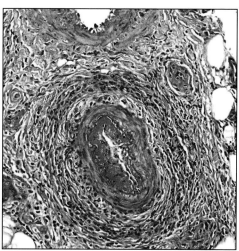

(Left) High magnification of the previous hepatic artery shows adventitial and medial inflammation as well as intimal infiltration of macrophages and lymphocytes from an autopsy case with PAN. *(Right)* A medium-sized artery adjacent to the pancreas from the same autopsy case of PAN shows fibrinoid intimal necrosis and transmural and severe adventitial inflammation and arteritis.

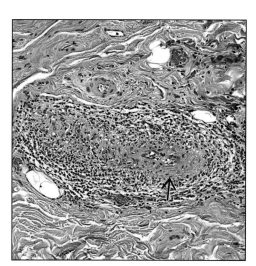

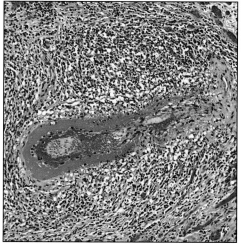

(Left) Adventitial layer of a segment of colon removed for infarction shows circumferential transmural, severe necrotizing arteritis with fibrinoid change in the center ⇨ leading to occlusion of the lumen. *(Right)* The colonic adventitia layer shows circumferential fibrinoid necrosis surrounded by intense active inflammatory infiltrate without evidence of preserved media or adventitia.

KAWASAKI DISEASE

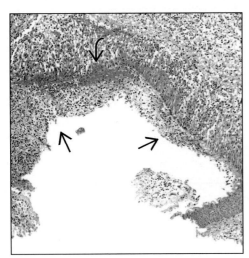

Renal artery branch in Kawasaki disease shows transmural acute inflammation ⇒ with dilatation of the lumen, aneurysm formation, and focal fibrinoid necrosis ⇗. (Courtesy J.C. Jennette, MD.)

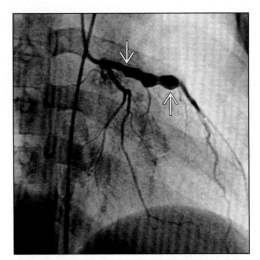

Sagittal oblique angiography shows multiple small aneurysms ⇒ in the left anterior descending coronary artery in a 2-year-old child with Kawasaki disease.

TERMINOLOGY

Abbreviations
- Kawasaki disease (KD)
- Mucocutaneous lymph node syndrome (MCLNS)

Synonyms
- Kawasaki syndrome
- Kawasaki disease arteritis
- Mucocutaneous lymph node syndrome

Definitions
- Chapel Hill Consensus Conference
  - Arteritis involves large, medium, and small arteries and is associated with mucocutaneous lymph node syndrome
  - Coronary arteries are often involved
  - Aorta and veins may be involved
  - Usually occurs in children
- Japan Kawasaki Disease Research Committee Criteria
  - Fever of unknown etiology for 5 days or more (95%)
  - Bilateral congestion of ocular conjunctivae (88%)
  - Reddening of lips and oropharyngeal mucosa and strawberry tongue (at least 1 finding) (90%)
  - Reddening, edema, and desquamation of digits in peripheral extremities (at least 1 finding) (90%)
  - Polymorphous exanthema of body trunk without vesicles or crusts (92%)
  - Acute nonpurulent swelling of cervical lymph nodes of 1.5 cm or more in diameter

ETIOLOGY/PATHOGENESIS

Environmental Exposure
- Exposure to an infectious agent is suggested based on epidemiologic considerations
- Susceptibility in infants with minimal or no immunity with abnormal immune response
- Specific microbe not identified

Genetic
- Interleukin 18 promoter gene polymorphism
- Genome-wide association found with 5 genes with functional relationship to inflammation, apoptosis, and cardiovascular pathology
- *HLA-Bw22* in Japanese, *BW51* or combined *A2*, *B44*, *CW5* in North Americans

Pathogenesis
- Activation of cells of innate and adaptive immunity (e.g., monocytes, lymphocytes)
- Inflammatory cytokines and chemokines activate endothelial cells, leading to vascular inflammation
- Possible role for antiendothelial antibodies
- Vasoactive (endothelin, nitric oxide) and growth factors (VEGF, PDGF) promote vascular permeability and myointimal proliferation

Animal Model
- Candida albicans water-soluble fraction induces severe coronary arteritis with typical histologic features of KD

CLINICAL ISSUES

Epidemiology
- Incidence
  - High prevalence in Japan
    - Epidemic and endemic forms
    - 50/100,000
  - Occurs sporadically or in epidemic form throughout the world
  - Seasonal incidence, spring months
- Age
  - Almost exclusively children
    - 70% of all cases occur < 3 years of age
    - Peaks at age 9-11 months in Japanese
    - Other populations peak at age 1.5-2 years (e.g., North Americans)
- Gender

KAWASAKI DISEASE

Key Facts

Terminology
- Arteritis involves large, medium-sized, and small arteries and is associated with mucocutaneous lymph node syndrome and coronary arteritis

Etiology/Pathogenesis
- Activation of cells of innate and adaptive immunity likely caused by an exogenous trigger
- Role for antiendothelial antibodies

Clinical Issues
- High prevalence in Japan (epidemic and endemic)
- 9-11 months of age in Japanese, 1.5-2 years in North Americans; M:F = 5:1
- Renal, relatively rare
- Leukocytosis (17,000 ± 900 mm³)
- Thrombocytosis, 600,000-1.5 million/mm³

- Combination of aspirin and intravenous gamma-globulin therapy is mainstay

Image Findings
- Angiography (arteritis, dilatation, aneurysm, stenosis)
- DMSA renal SPECT (parenchymal inflammation and scarring)

Microscopic Pathology
- Panarteritis (commonly coronary arteries) involving intima and adventitial layer, with disruption of internal and external elastic lamina
- Arteritis, thrombosis, microaneurysms
- Focal/patchy or diffuse interstitial inflammation or scarring

Top Differential Diagnoses
- Polyarteritis nodosa in childhood

- o Male predominance of 5:1
- Ethnicity
  - o Japanese and Koreans > Chinese > Polynesians > whites and blacks
  - o All racial backgrounds may be affected with lesser frequency (5/100,000 in North Americans)

Presentation
- General constitutional symptoms in the acute phase
- Systemic disease involving skin, mucous membranes, and lymph nodes
- Phases of disease: Acute, subacute, convalescent
- Associated with medium-sized vessel arteritis, frequently affecting coronary arteries (15-25%)
- Exacerbation and recrudescence of symptoms during acute and subacute stages
- Renal
  - o Hypertension related to renal artery disease
  - o Usually mild and clinically silent
  - o Sterile pyuria and proteinuria
  - o Transient microscopic hematuria
  - o Mild renal insufficiency or acute renal failure

Laboratory Tests
- Generally nonspecific and nondiagnostic
- Reflect systemic inflammatory process
  - o Cultures for infective agents are negative
  - o Leukocytosis (17,000 ± 900 mm³)
  - o Increased erythrocyte sedimentation rate
  - o Thrombocytosis/increased platelet counts from 600,000-1.5 million/mm³
  - o Elevated serum acute phase proteins
  - o Diffuse cytoplasmic ANCA pattern, atypical, by direct immunofluorescence

Treatment
- Combination of aspirin and intravenous gamma-globulin therapy is mainstay
  - o For inflammatory symptoms and to reduce coronary artery complications
- Aimed toward symptomatic relief and prevention of serious consequences (e.g., cardiac and coronary involvement)

- Corticosteroids contraindicated due to increased incidence of coronary aneurysms
- Transcatheter coronary intervention thrombolysis

Prognosis
- Factors related to poor prognosis
  - o Involvement of coronary arteries (arteritis, thrombosis, aneurysms)
  - o Involvement of heart (acute interstitial myocarditis and valvulitis)
  - o Recurrence rate of KD (4%) between 5-24 months
  - o Mortality rate with appropriate treatment (0.04%)
  - o Peripheral medium-sized arteritis with infarction (e.g., extremities, central nervous system, small and large intestines)

IMAGE FINDINGS

Radiographic Findings
- Heart and coronary arteries
  - o 2-dimensional echocardiography
    - ▪ Proximal aneurysms of coronary artery
    - ▪ Highly sensitive and specific
  - o Coronary angiography (arteritis, dilatation, or aneurysm)
- Kidney
  - o Ultrasound (increased size, echogenicity)
  - o DMSA renal SPECT (parenchymal inflammation and scarring)
  - o Renal Doppler study (vascular flow pattern and vasculitis)
  - o Renal angiography (arterial stenosis)

MICROSCOPIC PATHOLOGY

Histologic Features
- Arterial changes can be a consequence of acute clinical disease, acute episode followed by subclinical continued activity, recurrent acute attacks, or clinically inapparent disease
- Divided into 4 stages

Medium-sized Vessel Vasculitides

	Polyarteritis Nodosa	Kawasaki Disease
Age of onset	Adults, children	Infants (> 6 months), children (up to 3 years)
Organ system involved	Multisystemic	Mainly heart & coronary arteries; other systems less common
Mucocutaneous lymph node involvement	No	Yes
Level of arterial involvement	Before and after entrance into organ	Before entrance into organ
Size of vessel	Small and medium-sized arteries	Medium-sized arteries
Pathogenesis	Cell-mediated	Cell-mediated
Histopathology	Acute, subacute, and chronic lesions in same organ	All same-stage lesions (acute, subacute, or chronic) in organ affected or may appear in different stages in same artery
Fibrinoid necrosis	Yes	Rare
Vascular infiltrate	Mainly neutrophils and later mononuclear cells	Mainly mononuclear cells (lymphocytes, macrophages)
ANCA serology	Rarely positive ANCA titers	Atypical ANCA or ANCA negative

- o Initiation of arteritis (6-8 days after onset)
- o Aneurysm formation (8-12 days)
- o Persistent arterial inflammation (2-6 weeks)
- o Scarring (> 6 weeks)
- > 1 stage may be observed in different arteries or within different segments of same artery
- Medium-sized arteritis (coronary, renal, intestinal)
  - o Panarteritis involving intima and adventitial layer, with disruption of internal and external elastic lamina
  - o Early neutrophilic infiltration, peak 10 days
  - o Monocytes/macrophages and lymphocytes after 2 weeks
  - o Damage to smooth muscle cells of media
  - o Loss of α-smooth muscle actin and type IV collagen
  - o Rare: Fibrinoid necrosis
- Microaneurysm formation with thrombosis following damage to vascular structure
- Vascular fibrosis and recanalization of thrombi are late features
- Renal parenchyma
  - o Focal/patchy or diffuse interstitial inflammation or scarring
    - Lymphocytes, plasma cells, neutrophils
    - Edema
  - o Normal glomeruli
    - Rare: Mesangial proliferative GN with immune complexes
    - Rare: Interlobular and small arterial vasculitis

DIFFERENTIAL DIAGNOSIS

Polyarteritis Nodosa in Childhood
- Differentiated from Kawasaki disease by absence of mucocutaneous lymph node syndrome
- Pathologic findings of vasculitis frequently show fibrinoid necrotizing features

SELECTED REFERENCES

1. Dillon MJ et al: Medium-size-vessel vasculitis. Pediatr Nephrol. 25(9):1641-52, 2010
2. Takahashi K et al: Administration of human immunoglobulin suppresses development of murine systemic vasculitis induced with Candida albicans water-soluble fraction: an animal model of Kawasaki disease. Mod Rheumatol. 20(2):160-7, 2010
3. Takahashi K et al: Kawasaki disease arteritis and polyarteritis nodosa. Pathol Case Rev. 12:193-99, 2007
4. Wang JN et al: Renal scarring sequelae in childhood Kawasaki disease. Pediatr Nephrol. 22(5):684-9, 2007
5. Falcini F et al: Bilateral renal artery stenosis in Kawasaki disease: a report of two cases. Clin Exp Rheumatol. 24(6):719-21, 2006
6. Sève P et al: Adult Kawasaki disease: report of two cases and literature review. Semin Arthritis Rheum. 34(6):785-92, 2005
7. Grunebaum E et al: The role of anti-endothelial cell antibodies in Kawasaki disease - in vitro and in vivo studies. Clin Exp Immunol. 130(2):233-40, 2002
8. Jennette JC et al: Nomenclature of systemic vasculitides. Proposal of an international consensus conference. Arthritis Rheum. 37(2):187-92, 1994
9. Gribetz D et al: Kawasaki disease: mucocutaneous lymph node syndrome (MCLS). In Churg A et al, eds: Systemic Vasculitides. New York: Igaku-Shoin. 257-72, 1991
10. Salcedo JR et al: Renal histology of mucocutaneous lymph node syndrome (Kawasaki disease). Clin Nephrol. 29(1):47-51, 1988
11. Nardi PM et al: Renal manifestations of Kawasaki's disease. Pediatr Radiol. 15(2):116-8, 1985
12. Ogawa H: Kidney pathology in muco-cutaneous lymphnode syndrome. Nippon Jinzo Gakkai Shi. 27(9):1229-37, 1985
13. Furusho K et al: High-dose intravenous gammaglobulin for Kawasaki disease. Lancet. 2(8411):1055-8, 1984
14. Japan Kawasaki Disease Research Committee: Diagnostic guidelines of Kawasaki disease. Ed 4. Tokyo: Japan Red Cross Medical Center. 1984
15. Kawasaki T et al: A new infantile acute febrile mucocutaneous lymph node syndrome (MLNS) prevailing in Japan. Pediatrics. 54(3):271-6, 1974
16. Kawasaki T: [Acute febrile mucocutaneous syndrome with lymphoid involvement with specific desquamation of the fingers and toes in children.] Arerugi. 16(3):178-222, 1967

KAWASAKI DISEASE

Microscopic and Gross Features

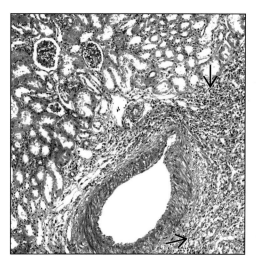
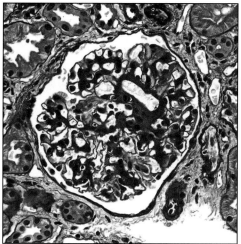

(Left) Low-magnification image of kidney tissue shows an arcuate artery and patchy active interstitial inflammation and edema ➡. The glomeruli are unremarkable. *(Courtesy J.C. Jennette, MD.)* *(Right)* Glomerulus from a 2-year-old girl shows mild, nonspecific mesangial hypercellularity without a significant increase in matrix in an acute case of KD. No immune deposits are localized (PAS).

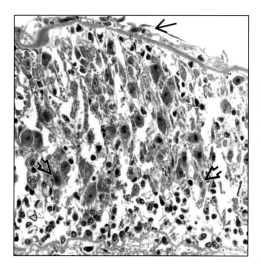
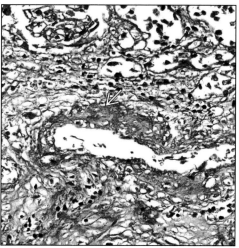

(Left) High magnification of a renal artery in Kawasaki disease shows mild to moderate transmural mononuclear inflammatory infiltrate from tunica intima ➡, media to adventitia ➡, and intercellular edema of the media. *(Courtesy J.C. Jennette, MD.)* *(Right)* On rare occasion, intrarenal healing small vessel vasculitis with obliterative changes ➡ may be seen in Kawasaki disease.

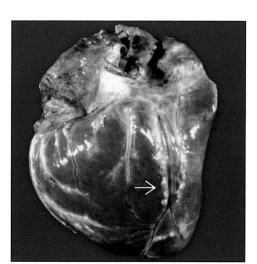
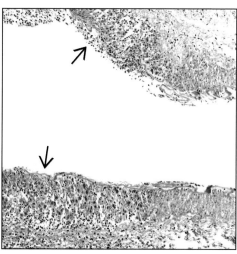

(Left) Gross photograph at autopsy shows the heart of a young patient with Kawasaki disease. Multiple small aneurysms are seen in the left anterior descending coronary artery ➡. *(Courtesy J. Fallon, MD.)* *(Right)* Dilated portion of a renal artery shows segmental transmural inflammation ➡. *(Courtesy J.C. Jennette, MD.)*

GIANT CELL ARTERITIS

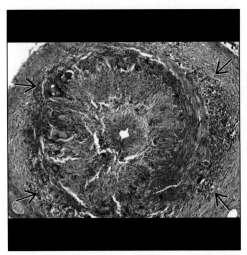

Cross section of a temporal artery shows adventitial, medial, and intimal active arteritis ➡ with occlusive changes. Numerous multinucleated giant cells are noted within the wall.

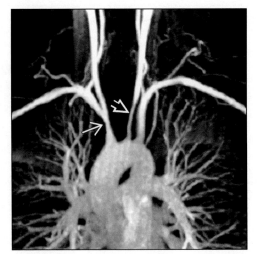

MR angiogram shows an irregular, long-segment stenosis of the left common carotid artery ➡ and brachiocephalic artery stenosis ➡ due to mural thickening. These findings are typical of GCA.

TERMINOLOGY

Abbreviations
- Giant cell arteritis (GCA)

Synonyms
- Temporal arteritis
- Cranial arteritis
- Horton syndrome

Definitions
- Chapel Hill Consensus Conference
  o Granulomatous arteritis of aorta and its major branches, with predilection for extracranial branches of carotid artery
  o Often involves temporal artery
  o Usually occurs in patients > 50 years of age and is often associated with polymyalgia rheumatica
- American College of Rheumatology Criteria
  o Age ≥ 50 years
  o New onset of localized headache
  o Temporal artery tenderness or decreased temporal artery pulse
  o Elevated ESR ≥ 50 mm/hr
  o Biopsy of artery with necrotizing arteritis with mononuclear infiltrates or granulomatous process
  o Presence of any 3 or more of above yields high sensitivity and specificity

ETIOLOGY/PATHOGENESIS

Environmental Exposure
- Etiology unknown
- Possible triggers include exposure to several upper respiratory disease pathogens
  o *Mycoplasma/Chlamydia pneumoniae*
  o Parvovirus B19, human parainfluenza virus type I
  o Herpes simplex virus

Genetic
- Associated with *HLA-DRB1* and *HLA-DR4* gene alleles
- *ICAM-1* gene polymorphism (R241)

Pathogenesis
- Autoimmune cell-mediated mechanism
  o T-cell mediated process
    ▪ CD4(+) T-helper cells in inflammatory site
    ▪ T-cell activation locally in arterial wall following activation of antigen presenting cells (e.g., dendritic cells in adventitia)
  o Activation of monocytes/macrophages responsible for systemic symptom
  o Destructive vascular inflammation may lead to vaso-occlusive intimal proliferation or aneurysm formation depending on type of arterial vessel involved
  o Interferon gamma produced from T cells is crucial in giant cell reaction in GCA
- Role for humoral-mediated immunity is suggested
  o Elevated serum immunoglobulins
  o Detection of circulating immune complexes
  o Rare immune complex deposition

CLINICAL ISSUES

Epidemiology
- Incidence
  o 15-25/100,000 in patients > 50 years of age
  o Low incidence in the Mediterranean and Asian populations
- Age
  o Usually > 50 years
  o Peaks at 75-85 years
- Gender
  o Female predilection (M:F = 1:2-6)
- Ethnicity
  o Highest in patients of northern European descent

GIANT CELL ARTERITIS

Key Facts

Terminology
- Granulomatous arteritis of aorta and its major branches

Etiology/Pathogenesis
- Possible triggers include exposure to several upper respiratory disease pathogens
- Associated with *HLA-DRB1* and *HLA-DR4* gene alleles
- Cell-mediated immune mechanism

Clinical Issues
- Usually > 50 years
- Female predilection (M:F = 1:2-6)
- Symptoms of polymyalgia rheumatica (50-75%)
- Elevation of acute phase reactants in active disease (ESR, CRP)
- Rapid response to steroid treatment

- Microscopic hematuria, particularly with increased disease activity

Image Findings
- MR angiography and high spatial configuration
- Angiography of aorta and great vessels

Microscopic Pathology
- Granulomatous inflammation extending from media to intima and adventitia with disruption of elastic lamina by giant cells

Top Differential Diagnoses
- Takayasu arteritis
- Rheumatoid aortitis
- Atherosclerotic arterial disease
- Other systemic vasculitides
- Fibromuscular dysplasia

Presentation
- Wide variability of clinical symptoms
- Constitutional: Fever, malaise, weight loss
- Symptoms of polymyalgia rheumatica (50-75%)
  - Proximal muscle ache, stiffness, and weakness
  - Bursitis and tenosynovitis
  - Paresthesias
- Vascular
  - Visual disturbance/blindness (optic nerve or retinal ischemia)
  - Jaw claudication, temporal tenderness ± pulsation, headache
  - Peripheral vascular stenotic or occlusive symptoms
    - With decreased pulses in extremities
    - Carotid or subclavian artery bruits
    - Vessels outside head and neck (10-15% of cases)
- Renal
  - Renal manifestations occur infrequently
  - Associated hypertension is uncommon
  - Microscopic hematuria, particularly with increased disease activity
  - Proteinuria or, rarely, nephrotic syndrome
  - Impaired renal function or acute renal insufficiency
  - Glomerular disease, anecdotal

Laboratory Tests
- Elevation of acute phase reactants in active disease (ESR, CRP)
- Anemia, thrombocytosis
- Elevated liver enzymes (50%)
- Serologic studies for autoimmune diseases are negative, including ANCA

Treatment
- Rapid response to steroid treatment
- Immunosuppressive drugs in refractory cases

Prognosis
- Generally self-limiting disease
- Long-term complications
  - Sometimes relapsing-remitting course
  - Thoracic aortic aneurysm (17x risk)

- Abdominal aortic aneurysm (2x risk)
- Aortic dissection
- Myocardial infarction
- Large artery stenosis

IMAGE FINDINGS

General Features
- Findings similar to Takayasu arteritis except in older age groups
- Pre- and post-contrast MR findings
  - T2 identified mural thickening associated with edema and active vasculitis
  - Useful to select mode of therapy
  - MR angiography and high spatial configuration
    - Identifies flow direction and end-organ perfusion
    - Stenosis or occlusion

MICROSCOPIC PATHOLOGY

Renal
- Large vessel vasculitis ± granulomatous features
  - Ischemic renal parenchymal lesions
- Occasionally, small vessel vasculitis with fibrinoid necrosis occurs
  - Concomitant or isolated pauci-immune crescentic glomerulonephritis with fibrinoid necrosis
  - Probably consequence of unrelated or co-incidental small vessel disease or, rarely, GCA
- Glomerular lesions causing nephrotic syndrome
  - Secondary amyloidosis
  - Rare: Membranous glomerulonephritis

Nonrenal
- Temporal arteries commonly affected
- Biopsy diagnosis obligatory to confirm diagnosis of GCA
- Unilateral or bilateral involvement
- Typically focal and segmental in distribution
- Multiple levels of tissue sections suggested to pick up focal lesions

3

- Giant cell arteritis is characterized by
  - Inflammatory infiltrate seen initially in media and extending to intima and adventitia
  - Disruption or fragmentation of internal and external elastic lamina is associated with inflammation
  - Mainly mononuclear cell infiltration composed of mainly T-lymphocytes, macrophages, and dendritic cells is seen
  - Variable number of multinucleated giant cells present (50% of cases), particularly at elastic lamina
  - Occasionally, fibrinoid necrosis of wall is observed
  - Intimal findings include fibroblastic and myointimal cell proliferation, edema, and inflammation
  - Range of healing lesions of intimal and medial fibrosis accompanies active lesions, leading to narrowing or occlusion of lumina

DIFFERENTIAL DIAGNOSIS

Takayasu Arteritis
- Similar vessel size and pathology
- Occurs at younger age (≤ 30-50)
- High incidence in Asian population
- Aortic involvement is frequent

Rheumatoid Aortitis
- Positive rheumatoid serology
- Features suggestive of rheumatoid arthritis
- Typical bone and hand lesions

Atherosclerotic Arterial Disease
- Some (older) age group and radiographic findings
- Clinical symptoms in active disease and polymyalgia rheumatica may help in GCA

Other Systemic Vasculitides
- Primary angiitis of central nervous system
- Polyarteritis nodosa
  - More in small and medium-sized vessels
  - Fibrinoid necrotizing vasculitis by pathology
  - Involvement of kidneys

Fibromuscular Dysplasia
- Younger patients
- No acute constitutional symptoms
- Commonly affects renal and carotid arteries
- Distinct radiographic changes
- Genetic or familial background
- Calcinosis of temporal or larger arteries
  - Age related
  - Calciphylaxis secondary to chronic renal disease
- Drug-induced large vessel vasculitis

SELECTED REFERENCES

1. Awwad ST et al: Calciphylaxis of the temporal artery masquerading as temporal arteritis. Clin Experiment Ophthalmol. 38(5):511-3, 2010
2. Burke AP: Takayasu arteritis and giant cell arteritis. Pathol Case Rev 12(5):186-92, 2007
3. Powers JF et al: High prevalence of herpes simplex virus DNA in temporal arteritis biopsy specimens. Am J Clin Pathol. 123(2):261-4, 2005
4. Müller E et al: Temporal arteritis with pauci-immune glomerulonephritis: a systemic disease. Clin Nephrol. 62(5):384-6, 2004
5. Hamidou MA et al: Temporal arteritis associated with systemic necrotizing vasculitis. J Rheumatol. 30(10):2165-9, 2003
6. Nuenninghoff DM et al: Incidence and predictors of large-artery complication (aortic aneurysm, aortic dissection, and/or large-artery stenosis) in patients with giant cell arteritis: a population-based study over 50 years. Arthritis Rheum. 48(12):3522-31, 2003
7. Weyand CM et al: Medium- and large-vessel vasculitis. N Engl J Med. 349(2):160-9, 2003
8. Nasher G: Giant cell arteritis and polymyalgia rheumatica. In Vasculitis. Ball G et al, eds. Oxford: Oxford University Press. 255-277, 2002
9. Burke A et al: Temporal artery biopsy of giant cell arteritis. Pathol Case Rev 6(6): 265-73, 2001
10. Escribá A et al: Secondary (AA-type) amyloidosis in patients with polymyalgia rheumatica. Am J Kidney Dis. 35(1):137-40, 2000
11. Salvarani C et al: Intercellular adhesion molecule 1 gene polymorphisms in polymyalgia rheumatica/giant cell arteritis: association with disease risk and severity. J Rheumatol. 27(5):1215-21, 2000
12. Strasser F et al: Giant cell arteritis "causing" AA-amyloidosis with rapid renal failure. Schweiz Med Wochenschr. 130(43):1606-9, 2000
13. Lie JT: The vasculitides. In Biopsy Diagnosis of Rheumatoid Diseases. Tokyo: Igaku-Shoin. 61-106, 1997
14. Montoliu J et al: Lessons to be learned from patients with vasculitis. Nephrol Dial Transplant. 12(12):2781-6, 1997
15. Jennette JC et al: Nomenclature of systemic vasculitides. Proposal of an international consensus conference. Arthritis Rheum. 37(2):187-92, 1994
16. Jennette JC et al: The pathology of vasculitis involving the kidney. Am J Kidney Dis. 24(1):130-41, 1994
17. Canton CG et al: Renal failure in temporal arteritis. Am J Nephrol. 12(5):380-3, 1992
18. Hunder GG et al: The American College of Rheumatology 1990 criteria for the classification of giant cell arteritis. Arthritis Rheum. 33(8):1122-8, 1990
19. Shiiki H et al: Temporal arteritis: cell composition and the possible pathogenetic role of cell-mediated immunity. Hum Pathol. 20(11):1057-64, 1989
20. Sonnenblick M et al: Nephrotic syndrome in temporal arteritis. Br J Clin Pract. 43(11):420-1, 1989
21. Sonnenblick M et al: Nonclassical organ involvement in temporal arteritis. Semin Arthritis Rheum. 19(3):183-90, 1989
22. Truong L et al: Temporal arteritis and renal disease. Case report and review of the literature. Am J Med. 78(1):171-5, 1985
23. O'Neill WM Jr et al: Giant cell arteritis with visceral angiitis. Arch Intern Med. 136(10):1157-60, 1976

GIANT CELL ARTERITIS

Microscopic Features

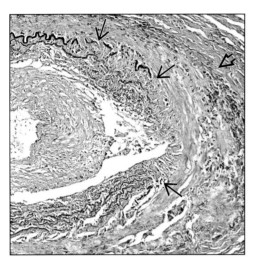

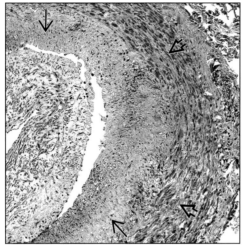

(Left) Section of a temporal artery shows disruption of the elastic lamina and extensive loss of the internal ➡ and external ➡ elastic lamina along with intimal and medial inflammatory infiltrate. Marked fibromyointimal thickening, leading to narrowing of the lumen, is noted. *(Right)* Segment of the temporal artery shows moderate fibrosing changes within the intima ➡ and early fibrocollagenous deposits in the media separating the smooth muscle cells ➡.

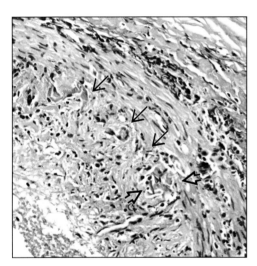

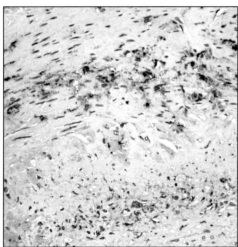

(Left) High magnification shows multinucleated giant cells disrupting and eroding the elastic lamina ➡ and one cell containing fragments of the elastica within the cells ➡. Significant mononuclear cell infiltrate (lymphocytes and macrophages) is also seen in the adventitial layer. *(Right)* Segment of temporal artery shows full thickness arteritis (intimal and medial layer) with increased CD68(+) macrophage infiltration.

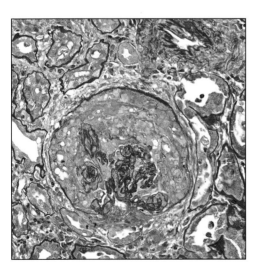

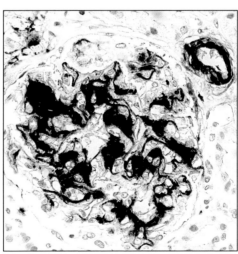

(Left) Biopsy from a 90-year-old Caucasian woman with polymyalgia rheumatica, temporal arteritis, and acute renal failure shows crescentic GN, most probably representing an overlap of concomitant small vessel vasculitis (ANCA negative). *(Right)* Image shows case of giant cell arteritis with nephrotic syndrome. Glomerulus shows mesangial, capillary, and arteriolar staining for amyloid A protein diagnostic of AA amyloidosis. This may be a result of a chronic inflammatory state.

TAKAYASU ARTERITIS

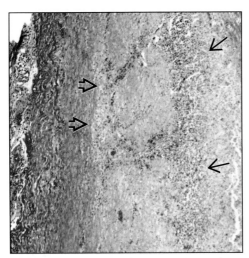

Segment of aortic wall in Takayasu arteritis (TA) shows adventitia ⇨ and a band of medial granulomatous inflammatory infiltrate ⇨.

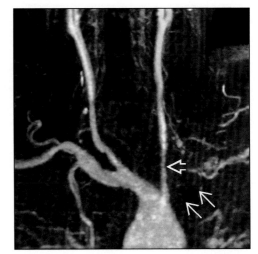

Coronal MR angiogram of the great vessels shows occlusion of the proximal subclavian artery ➡ and irregular diffuse narrowing ⇨ of the left common carotid artery.

TERMINOLOGY

Abbreviations
- Takayasu arteritis (TA)

Synonyms
- Takayasu disease/syndrome
- Pulseless disease
- Obliterative arteritis
- Aortoarteritis
- Idiopathic medial aortopathy and arteriopathy

Definitions
- Chapel Hill Consensus Conference
  - TA is granulomatous inflammation of aorta and its major branches
  - Usually occurs in patients < 50 years of age
- American College of Rheumatology criteria
  - Age ≤ 40 years
  - Claudication of an extremity
  - Decreased brachial artery pulse
  - Systolic blood pressure difference > 10 mmHg (between arms)
  - Bruit over subclavian arteries or aorta
  - Angiographic abnormalities (narrowing or occlusion)
  - Any 3 of the above fulfills requirement for diagnosis of TA with high sensitivity and specificity
- Definitive diagnosis may be problematic and delayed due to slow evolution and low activity of the disease

ETIOLOGY/PATHOGENESIS

Etiology
- Unknown, autoimmune disease

Genetic
- Possible link to various HLA subtypes, particularly *HLA-B22*

- *HLA-BW52* antigen (associated with Crohn disease) is observed in 44% of Japanese patients with TA

Pathogenesis
- Cell-mediated immune mechanism
- Not associated with autoantibodies or immune complexes
- T-lymphocytes, macrophages, antigen presenting dendritic cells, and B-lymphocytes
- Inflammation causes aortic and arterial wall damage
- Crohn disease shows similar mural granulomatous inflammation

CLINICAL ISSUES

Epidemiology
- Incidence
  - Rare: 1-3/10⁶ per year in USA and UK
  - Said to be more common in Asia but may just be more commonly recognized
  - Japan: Higher aortic arch involvement
  - India: Higher thoracic and abdominal aorta
  - USA: Higher great vessel involvement
- Age
  - Patients usually < 30 years (90%)
  - Common in 2nd and 3rd decades of life
- Gender
  - Predominantly female (M:F = 1:8)
- Ethnicity
  - Pattern of disease varies by geographic area

Presentation
- 2 phases of disease
  - Early inflammatory phase
    - Constitutional symptoms of fever, myalgias, arthralgias, weight loss, anemia
    - Pain of involved vessels
    - Hypertension
    - Bruits over great vessels
    - Aortic valve insufficiency

TAKAYASU ARTERITIS

Key Facts

Terminology
- Granulomatous inflammation of aorta and its major branches

Etiology/Pathogenesis
- Cell-mediated immune mechanism

Clinical Issues
- Common in Asia (6/1,000) compared with USA (1-3/1,000)
- Patients usually < 30 years (90%)
- Pain of involved vessels and bruits
- Renovascular hypertension
- Steroid therapy as primary form
- Complications mainly due to hypertension & stroke

Image Findings
- Disease classified by abnormalities of aorta or main branches using angiography ("gold standard")
- Aneurysmal dilatation may alternate with stenosis

Microscopic Pathology
- Granulomatous panarteritis with variable number of multinucleated giant cells
- Multifocal disruption of the medial elastic fibers
- Adventitial and marked intimal thickening

Top Differential Diagnoses
- Isolated granulomatous aortitis
- Giant cell arteritis
- Atherosclerosis
- Fibromuscular dysplasia

- Ischemic effects: Stroke, claudication, mesenteric ischemia
  - Late occlusive or pulseless phase
  - May coexist with other autoimmune diseases (≤ 10%)
    - Rheumatoid arthritis
    - Systemic lupus erythematosus
    - Inflammatory bowel disease (Crohn disease)
  - Initial nonspecific symptomatology may delay definitive diagnosis for months or years
  - Renal
    - Renovascular hypertension (60%) due to obstructive abdominal aortic disease involving renal artery ostia
    - Renal artery stenosis
    - Evidence of glomerular disease (hematuria, proteinuria), anecdotal
    - Progressive renal insufficiency

Treatment
- Steroid therapy as primary form
- Addition of other immunosuppressants or methotrexate in severe/refractory cases or relapse
- Angioplasty or surgical bypass when disease activity is quiescent
- Renal lesions according to the type and frequency of specific lesion

Prognosis
- Complications mainly due to hypertension and stroke
- Mortality mainly due to congestive heart failure
- 15-year survival is 90-95%
- Some have monophasic disease

IMAGE FINDINGS

General Features
- Disease classified by abnormalities of aorta or main branches using angiography ("gold standard")
  - Computerized tomography
  - Magnetic resonance imaging
  - Digital subtraction angiography

- Smooth narrowing of aorta and major vessels
- Patchy distribution of disease
- Aneurysmal dilatation may alternate with stenosis
- Symmetrical great vessel distribution
- 5 patterns of aorta and large vessel involvement seen by angiography
  - Type I: Branches of aortic arch (pulseless disease)
  - Type IIa: Ascending aorta, aortic arch, branches from the aortic arch
  - Type IIb: Ascending aorta, arch, branches, and thoracic descending aorta
  - Type III: Thoracic descending aorta, abdominal aorta, &/or renal arteries (most common, 60%)
  - Type IV: Abdominal aorta &/or renal arteries
  - Type V: Combination of stages IIb and IV

MACROSCOPIC FEATURES

General Features
- On cross section
  - Ridged "tree bark" appearance of intimal surface when very advanced
  - Thickened intimal and medial layers, patchy

MICROSCOPIC PATHOLOGY

Histologic Features
- Glomeruli
  - Nonspecific ischemic glomerular lesions
  - Mesangial proliferative, focal proliferative GN
  - Membranoproliferative and crescentic GN (rare)
  - Amyloidosis (rare)
- Tubules and interstitium
  - Tubulointerstitial scarring
- Renal artery
  - Affected by obliterative inflammatory process
  - Early adventitial inflammation and cuffing of vasa vasorum
  - Granulomatous panarteritis with variable number of multinucleated giant cells

Large Vessel Vasculitis

	Giant Cell Arteritis	Takayasu Arteritis
Age	> 50 years (peak: 75-85 years)	< 50 years (peak: 15-25 years)
Gender	M:F = 1:2	80% women
Ethnicity	Northern European	Asian
Vessels	Carotid arteries/branches, aorta	Aorta, larger branches
Clinical	Polymyalgia rheumatica, localized headache	Nonspecific constitutional symptoms
Pathology	Giant cell arteritis, mainly medial layer	Giant cell arteritis, full thickness, nonnecrotizing
Sequelae	Stenosis, ischemia, CNS symptoms, medial necrosis	Stenosis, dilatation, aneurysm formation, thrombosis
Serology	Negative	Negative
Pathogenesis	CD4, CD8, macrophages, antigen unknown	CD4, CD8, macrophages, genetic basis

- Rare: Lymphoplasmacytic arteritis without giant cells
  - Mainly medial and adventitial inflammation
    - Multifocal disruption of medial elastic fibers
  - Late phase
    - Thickening and occlusive intimal scarring
    - Adventitial and external medial fibrosis

Aorta and Large Vessels
- Generally elastic arteries affected
- Biopsy diagnosis or confirmation of TA can be done with tissues obtained at surgery
- Full-thickness arterial walls or entire endarterectomy specimens essential for histological examination
  - Typically involves subclavian vessels and various parts of aorta giving rise to different radiographic patterns and clinical symptoms
- Autoimmune aortic lymphoplasmacytic valvulitis

DIFFERENTIAL DIAGNOSIS

Isolated Granulomatous Aortitis
- Predilection for ascending aorta
- Medial (cystic) necrosis
- Less adventitial and intimal fibrosis
- Increased risk of aortic dissection
- Occasionally associated with Marfan syndrome

Giant Cell Arteritis
- Age of onset > 50 years
- Associated with polymyalgia rheumatica (50%)
- Pathology is similar
- Temporal artery involvement

Atherosclerosis
- In older individuals
- Mural inflammation may be seen
- Primarily intimal disease with atheromatous deposits, eccentric wall involvement

Fibromuscular Dysplasia
- Young females
- Multiple arteries involved (frequently renal and carotid) with beaded appearance
- Aorta not affected

SELECTED REFERENCES

1. Zhu WH et al: Clinical characteristics, interdisciplinary treatment and follow-up of 14 children with Takayasu arteritis. World J Pediatr. 6(4):342-7, 2010
2. Hijazi R et al: Renal manifestations in toddlers with Takayasu's arteritis and malignant hypertension. Pediatr Nephrol. 24(6):1227-30, 2009
3. Miller DV et al: Surgical pathology of noninfectious ascending aortitis: a study of 45 cases with emphasis on an isolated variant. Am J Surg Pathol. 30(9):1150-8, 2006
4. Tavora F et al: Review of isolated ascending aortitis: differential diagnosis, including syphilitic, Takayasu's and giant cell aortitis. Pathology. 38(4):302-8, 2006
5. Rojo-Leyva F et al: Study of 52 patients with idiopathic aortitis from a cohort of 1,204 surgical cases. Arthritis Rheum. 43(4):901-7, 2000
6. Hata A et al: Angiographic findings of Takayasu arteritis: new classification. Int J Cardiol. 54 Suppl:S155-63, 1996
7. Jennette JC et al: Nomenclature of systemic vasculitides. Proposal of an international consensus conference. Arthritis Rheum. 37(2):187-92, 1994
8. Lie JT: Takayasu's arteritis, Chapter 11. In Churg A et al: Systemic Vasculitides. New York: Igaku-Shoin.159-179, 1991
9. Arend WP et al: The American College of Rheumatology 1990 criteria for the classification of Takayasu arteritis. Arthritis Rheum. 33(8):1129-34, 1990
10. Koumi S et al: A case of Takayasu's arteritis associated with membranoproliferative glomerulonephritis and nephrotic syndrome. Nephron. 54(4):344-6, 1990
11. Long A et al: Takayasu's disease: diagnostic and therapeutic value of subclavian artery biopsy. Ann Vasc Surg. 4(2):151-5, 1990
12. Hellmann DB et al: Takayasu's arteritis associated with crescentic glomerulonephritis. Arthritis Rheum. 30(4):451-4, 1987
13. Lai KN et al: Glomerulonephritis associated with Takayasu's arteritis: report of three cases and review of literature. Am J Kidney Dis. 7(3):197-204, 1986
14. Hall S et al: Takayasu arteritis. A study of 32 North American patients. Medicine (Baltimore). 64(2):89-99, 1985
15. Marquis Y et al: Idiopathic medial aortopathy and arteriopathy. Am J Med. 44(6):939-54, 1968
16. Takayasu M: A case with unusual changes of the central vessels in the retina. Acta Soc Ophthalmol Jap. 112: 554-561, 1908

TAKAYASU ARTERITIS

Microscopic Features: Takayasu Arteritis

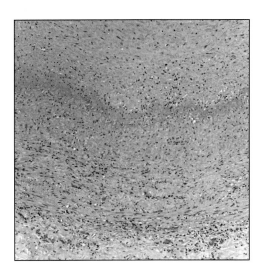
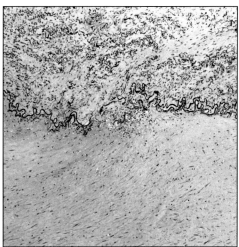

(Left) Segment of a large artery in TA shows the adventitia at the bottom separated by the external elastic lamina. The middle 1/3 shows a sprinkling of inflammatory cells and focal degenerative changes in the media. (Courtesy J.C. Jennette, MD.) (Right) EVG stain shows focal disruption of the external elastic lamina enclosing the media. Note also the fragmentation of the elastic fibers within the media in the upper 1/3 of the picture. (Courtesy J.C. Jennette, MD.)

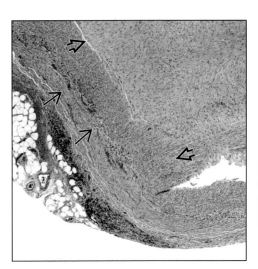
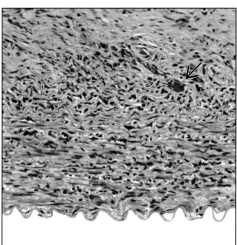

(Left) H&E shows a segment of an internal mammary artery from a 30-year-old Asian woman with chest pain and tenderness. Note adventitial and outer medial inflammatory infiltrate ➡ with marked intimal sclerosis ➡. (Right) Section of internal mammary artery shows active intimal and medial inflammatory infiltrate composed of lymphocytes and macrophages. One giant cell is noted ➡.

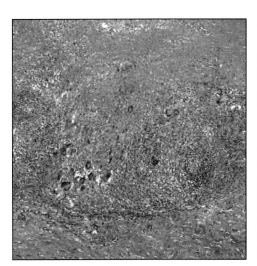
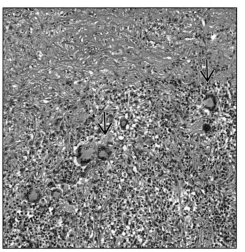

(Left) Segment of an aortic wall shows active medial and adventitial granulomatous inflammation with infiltration of large aggregates of inflammatory cells. (Courtesy A. Shimizu, MD & R. Ohashi, MD.) (Right) High magnification shows frequent multinucleated giant cells ➡ along with other mononuclear cell infiltrates disrupting the medial architecture. (Courtesy A. Shimizu, MD & R. Ohashi, MD.)

Microscopic Features: Takayasu Arteritis & Isolated Aortitis

(Left) Cross section of a renal artery with TA shows focal adventitial and areas of perimedial and medial inflammation along with fibrointimal thickening and sclerosis leading to narrowing of the lumen. (Courtesy L. Salinas, MD.) *(Right)* Axial contrast-enhanced CT shows typical features of abdominal aortic wall thickening ⇒ from Takayasu disease.

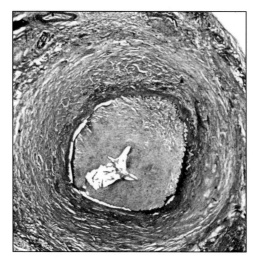
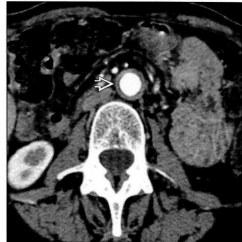

(Left) Giant cell aortitis shows medial and perimedial active inflammatory infiltrate and active granulomatous inflammation with scattered multinucleated giant cells, lymphocytes, and macrophages. *(Right)* Giant cell aortitis shows an area of laminar medial necrosis ⇒ surrounded by mild inflammation and loss of medial cells.

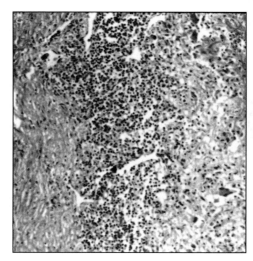
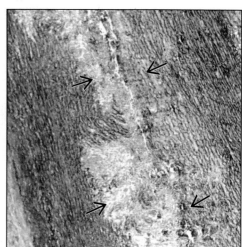

(Left) Inflammatory infiltrate within aortic wall inflammation shows scattered multinucleated giant cells ⇒ mixed with lymphocytes and macrophages. Occasional eosinophils are also noted. *(Right)* Segment of a large artery (aorta) shows focal mild inflammation in the outer portion of the media adjacent to the adventitia with only rare giant cells ⇒ along with lymphocytes.

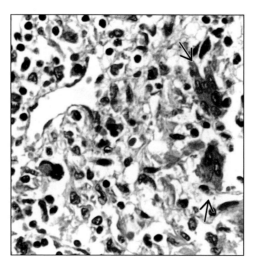
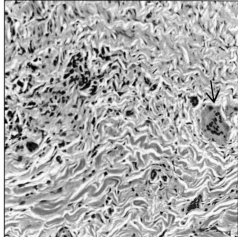

TAKAYASU ARTERITIS

Microscopic Features

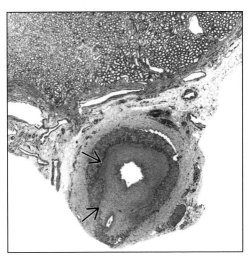

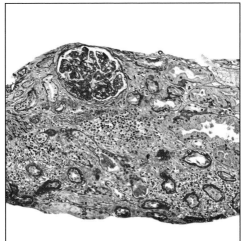

(Left) Large artery in the renal pelvis adjacent to the medulla shows a band of inflammatory infiltrate ➜ in the outer portion of the media adjacent to the adventitial layer almost encircling the entire cross section of the artery. *(Right)* This case of TA, hypertension, and progressive renal insufficiency shows glomerular ischemic collapse with tubular atrophy, interstitial fibrosis, and chronic inflammation.

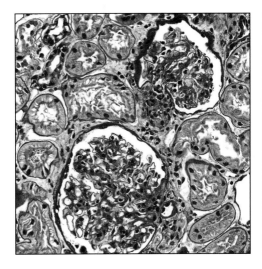

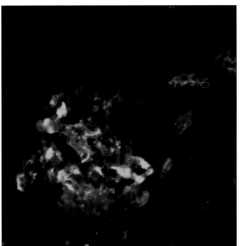

(Left) Renal biopsy following active TA and asymptomatic hematuria shows mild diffuse mesangial proliferation. No chronic tubulointerstitial changes were seen. *(Right)* Immunofluorescence of TA case with mild diffuse mesangial proliferation shows mainly mesangial granular IgM staining confirmed by electron microscopy with small mesangial deposits.

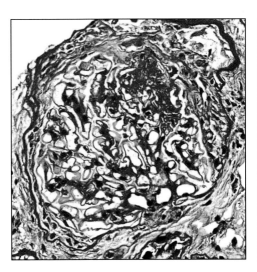

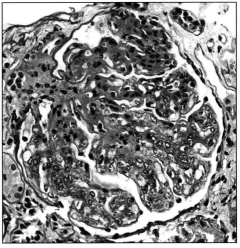

(Left) A case of TA with hematuria and proteinuria shows focal crescentic glomerulonephritis with a fibrocellular crescent in this glomerulus. *(Right)* Glomerulus shows membranoproliferative pattern of injury with a lobulated appearance and hypercellularity. Scant deposits were identified by electron microscopy.

3

INTRODUCTION TO THROMBOTIC MICROANGIOPATHIES

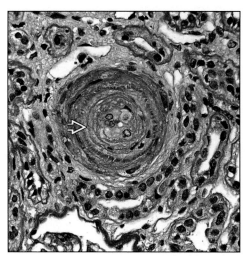

Acute TMA shows classic arteriolar narrowing due to intimal edema and lamination (i.e., "onion skinning") ➡ in this 30-year-old woman with acute renal failure and dilated cardiomyopathy.

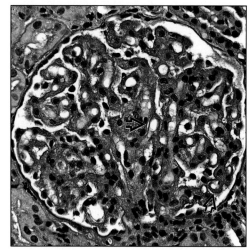

Chronic (or recurrent) TMA is classically manifested by thickened, duplicated GBMs ➡ as seen in this biopsy from a 4 year old with recurrent atypical HUS and a normal serum complement level.

TERMINOLOGY

Abbreviations
- Thrombotic microangiopathy (TMA)

Definitions
- TMA is characterized by microvascular endothelial injury and thrombosis

ETIOLOGY/PATHOGENESIS

Hemolytic Uremic Syndrome (HUS)
- Predominantly due to endothelial injury and activation with secondary prothrombotic state
- Typical HUS
  - Shiga-like and Shiga toxins produced by enteric pathogens
- Atypical HUS
  - Multifactorial

Thrombotic Thrombocytopenic Purpura (TTP)
- Predominantly due to increased thrombosis and secondary endothelial injury
- Deficiency of ADAMTS13 (**A D**istinterin **A**nd **M**etalloprotease with **T**hrombo**S**pondin and type 1 motif, member **13**)
  - ADAMTS13 is a zinc metalloprotease synthesized predominantly in liver
  - ADAMTS13 is required for cleavage of vWF multimers
    - Involved in coagulation pathway, vWF is a glycoprotein synthesized by endothelial cells and megakaryocytes
    - After secretion, vWF is normally proteolyzed to smaller units by ADAMTS13
    - In absence of ADAMTS13, large vWF multimers promote platelet aggregation in microvessels
  - Genetic deficiency of ADAMTS13

- Rare autosomal recessive inheritance results in ADAMTS13 levels < 5% of normal
- Homozygous or compound heterozygous mutations of *ADAMTS13* allele cause clinical disease
- Heterozygous mutations result in ADAMTS13 levels approximately 1/2 of normal and lack clinical disease
  - Autoantibodies against ADAMTS13
    - IgG or IgM antibodies act as inhibitors against ADAMTS13
    - Seen in approximately 30-80% of acquired idiopathic TTP
    - Autoimmunity triggered by environmental or endogenous factors (infections, cytokines, drugs) in susceptible host

CLINICAL IMPLICATIONS

Clinical Presentation
- Varies in HUS and TTP and is also based on etiology
- Atypical HUS etiologically appears to be different from TTP but has significant clinical overlap
  - Hence, clinical syndrome is often referred to as atypical HUS/TTP

Acute Presentation
- Typical HUS
  - Watery diarrhea followed by bloody diarrhea
  - Fever
  - Renal insufficiency
  - Acute renal failure more common in adults
  - Hypertension
  - Other systemic manifestations less common
- Subset of atypical HUS
  - Catastrophic antiphospholipid antibody syndrome and scleroderma renal crisis
    - Abrupt onset of symptoms
    - No prodrome of diarrhea

INTRODUCTION TO THROMBOTIC MICROANGIOPATHIES

Chronic/Insidious Presentation
- TTP and subset of atypical HUS
  - Fever
  - Hypertension
  - Mild proteinuria
  - Microscopic hematuria
  - Chronic renal insufficiency
  - Neurological symptoms predominate in TTP
  - Recurrences and relapses may occur with TTP

LABORATORY INVESTIGATIONS

Microangiopathic Hemolytic Anemia
- Blood flowing through injured or narrowed blood vessels causes erythrocyte fragmentation and platelet consumption
  - Anemia
  - Thrombocytopenia
  - Schistocytes on peripheral smear
  - Elevated serum lactate dehydrogenase
  - Reduced haptoglobin levels
  - Negative Coombs test
  - Normal prothrombin and partial thromboplastin time
- Leukocytosis, especially in typical HUS

Determination of Etiology
- Stool cultures to confirm enteric bacterial infection
- Antiphospholipid antibodies
- Serum complement C3, C4 levels
- ANA, anti-dsDNA for systemic lupus erythematosus (SLE)
- ADAMTS13 antibodies
- Anti-topoisomerase 1 and anti-RNA polymerase (I & III) antibodies if systemic sclerosis is suspected
- Plasma levels of complement factors H, I, and B are recommended in all cases of aHUS, as are CFHR, MCP, and screening for anti-CFH antibodies
- Genotyping of complement genes and *ADAMTS13* gene

MACROSCOPIC FINDINGS

General Features
- Kidneys are enlarged in acute phase
- Petechial hemorrhages are usually seen on external surface
- Patchy cortical necrosis can occur
- In chronic phase, kidneys are small with granular cortical surface

MICROSCOPIC FINDINGS

Acute TMA
- Glomeruli
  - Bloodless appearance
  - Apparent thickening of capillary wall due to subendothelial expansion
  - Mesangiolysis
  - Endothelial swelling
  - Thrombi with fibrinoid necrosis, often at hilum
    - Nuclear debris present but no significant inflammation
    - HUS thrombi are fibrin rich, and TTP thrombi are platelet rich, but difficult to differentiate histologically
  - Rare crescents seen in occasional cases
  - Fragmented RBCs seen entrapped in thrombi, subendothelium, and mesangium
  - In presence of arteriolar changes, downstream glomeruli demonstrate collapse of capillary tufts
    - Segmental sclerosis with collapsing features may be observed
- Tubulointerstitium
  - Acute tubular injury characterized by simplified epithelium, nuclear reactive atypia
  - Interstitial edema
  - Cortical necrosis observed in severe cases
- Blood vessels
  - Arterioles near vascular pole affected frequently
    - Endothelial swelling and luminal occlusion
    - Intimal mucoid edema with entrapped schistocytes
    - Fibrinoid necrosis without evidence of inflammatory infiltrate
  - Interlobular and arcuate arteries show similar changes

Chronic TMA
- Changes may be seen within days of acute onset of TMA
- Glomeruli
  - GBM remodeling results in duplication and double contours
  - Mesangial expansion with features of mesangiolysis
  - Variable focal segmental and global glomerulosclerosis
- Tubulointerstitium
  - Tubular atrophy and interstitial fibrosis
- Arterioles and small arteries
  - Intimal fibrosis with narrowed lumens
  - Concentric lamination of intimal fibrosis causes "onion skin" appearance
  - Recanalized thrombi may be identified

Immunofluorescence Microscopy
- Thrombi in glomeruli and blood vessels stain for fibrinogen
- Nonspecific entrapment of C3 and IgM in glomeruli
- No immune complexes unless associated with connective tissue disorder like SLE

Electron Microscopy
- Acute TMA
  - Endothelial swelling and loss of fenestrations
  - Expansion of subendothelial space by electron-lucent material
    - Entrapped schistocytes and fibrin tactoids in subendothelium
  - Mesangial matrix is also lucent (mesangiolysis)
  - Podocyte foot process effacement is common
  - Thrombi show mixture of platelets, fibrin, and erythrocytes

3

- ○ Myocyte degeneration may be seen in affected arterioles
- Chronic TMA
  - ○ Increased matrix in mesangium and subendothelium
  - ○ Depolymerized fibrin may be identified
  - ○ Mesangial cell interposition
  - ○ Podocyte foot processes are often effaced

DIAGNOSTIC CHECKLIST

Clinically Relevant Pathological Features
- Isolated involvement of glomeruli is associated with better prognosis than when arterioles are affected

Pathologic Interpretation Pearls
- Etiology cannot be distinguished based on biopsy findings
- Anemia, thrombocytopenia, and schistocytes may be absent in mild disease
- Latency period between exposure to radiation and TMA can be very long
- Biopsy with TMA due to malignant hypertension often shows hypertensive arteriopathy
- Significant thrombosis in absence of TMA or arterial remodeling should raise suspicion for antiphospholipid antibody syndrome

SELECTED REFERENCES

1. Batal I et al: Scleroderma renal crisis: a pathology perspective. Int J Rheumatol. 2010:543704, 2010
2. Benz K et al: Thrombotic microangiopathy: new insights. Curr Opin Nephrol Hypertens. 19(3):242-7, 2010
3. Izzedine H et al: VEGF signalling inhibition-induced proteinuria: Mechanisms, significance and management. Eur J Cancer. 46(2):439-48, 2010
4. Ruiz-Irastorza G et al: Antiphospholipid syndrome. Lancet. 376(9751):1498-509, 2010
5. Satoskar AA et al: De novo thrombotic microangiopathy in renal allograft biopsies-role of antibody-mediated rejection. Am J Transplant. 10(8):1804-11, 2010
6. Sánchez-Corral P et al: Advances in understanding the aetiology of atypical Haemolytic Uraemic Syndrome. Br J Haematol. 150(5):529-42, 2010
7. Zipfel PF et al: DEAP-HUS: deficiency of CFHR plasma proteins and autoantibody-positive form of hemolytic uremic syndrome. Pediatr Nephrol. 25(10):2009-19, 2010
8. Zipfel PF et al: Thrombotic microangiopathies: new insights and new challenges. Curr Opin Nephrol Hypertens. 19(4):372-8, 2010
9. Changsirikulchai S et al: Renal thrombotic microangiopathy after hematopoietic cell transplant: role of GVHD in pathogenesis. Clin J Am Soc Nephrol. 4(2):345-53, 2009
10. Gigante A et al: Antiphospholipid antibodies and renal involvement. Am J Nephrol. 30(5):405-12, 2009
11. Moake J: Thrombotic thrombocytopenia purpura (TTP) and other thrombotic microangiopathies. Best Pract Res Clin Haematol. 22(4):567-76, 2009
12. Noris M et al: Atypical hemolytic-uremic syndrome. N Engl J Med. 361(17):1676-87, 2009
13. Copelovitch L et al: The thrombotic microangiopathies. Pediatr Nephrol. 23(10):1761-7, 2008
14. Fine DM et al: Thrombotic microangiopathy and other glomerular disorders in the HIV-infected patient. Semin Nephrol. 28(6):545-55, 2008
15. Stokes MB et al: Glomerular disease related to anti-VEGF therapy. Kidney Int. 74(11):1487-91, 2008
16. Zheng XL et al: Pathogenesis of thrombotic microangiopathies. Annu Rev Pathol. 3:249-77, 2008
17. Chang A et al: Spectrum of renal pathology in hematopoietic cell transplantation: a series of 20 patients and review of the literature. Clin J Am Soc Nephrol. 2(5):1014-23, 2007
18. Desch K et al: Is there a shared pathophysiology for thrombotic thrombocytopenic purpura and hemolytic-uremic syndrome? J Am Soc Nephrol. 18(9):2457-60, 2007
19. Fakhouri F et al: Does hemolytic uremic syndrome differ from thrombotic thrombocytopenic purpura? Nat Clin Pract Nephrol. 3(12):679-87, 2007
20. Fischer MJ et al: The antiphospholipid syndrome. Semin Nephrol. 27(1):35-46, 2007
21. Franchini M et al: Reduced von Willebrand factor-cleaving protease levels in secondary thrombotic microangiopathies and other diseases. Semin Thromb Hemost. 33(8):787-97, 2007
22. Schneider M: Thrombotic microangiopathy (TTP and HUS): advances in differentiation and diagnosis. Clin Lab Sci. 20(4):216-20, 2007
23. Izzedine H et al: Gemcitabine-induced thrombotic microangiopathy: a systematic review. Nephrol Dial Transplant. 21(11):3038-45, 2006
24. Tsai HM: The molecular biology of thrombotic microangiopathy. Kidney Int. 70(1):16-23, 2006
25. Lian EC: Pathogenesis of thrombotic thrombocytopenic purpura: ADAMTS13 deficiency and beyond. Semin Thromb Hemost. 31(6):625-32, 2005
26. Lowe EJ et al: Thrombotic thrombocytopenic purpura and hemolytic uremic syndrome in children and adolescents. Semin Thromb Hemost. 31(6):717-30, 2005
27. Zakarija A et al: Drug-induced thrombotic microangiopathy. Semin Thromb Hemost. 31(6):681-90, 2005
28. Denton CP et al: Scleroderma--clinical and pathological advances. Best Pract Res Clin Rheumatol. 18(3):271-90, 2004
29. Medina PJ et al: Drug-associated thrombotic thrombocytopenic purpura-hemolytic uremic syndrome. Curr Opin Hematol. 8(5):286-93, 2001
30. Ray PE et al: Pathogenesis of Shiga toxin-induced hemolytic uremic syndrome. Pediatr Nephrol. 16(10):823-39, 2001
31. Tsai HM et al: Antibodies to von Willebrand factor-cleaving protease in acute thrombotic thrombocytopenic purpura. N Engl J Med. 339(22):1585-94, 1998
32. Boyce TG et al: Escherichia coli O157:H7 and the hemolytic-uremic syndrome. N Engl J Med. 333(6):364-8, 1995
33. Myers KA et al: Thrombotic microangiopathy associated with Streptococcus pneumoniae bacteremia: case report and review. Clin Infect Dis. 17(6):1037-40, 1993

INTRODUCTION TO THROMBOTIC MICROANGIOPATHIES

Causes of Thrombotic Microangiopathy

Clinical Presentation	Etiology	Mechanism of Action
Typical Hemolytic Uremic Syndrome (HUS)		
	Enteropathogenic infections (*Escherichia coli, Shigella dysenteriae*)	Shiga-like toxin causes endothelial damage by binding to Gb3 receptors
Atypical HUS (Clinical Overlap with TTP)		
	Nonenteric infections (such as *Streptococcus pneumoniae*, HIV, *Mycoplasma pneumoniae*, Coxsackie A and B viruses)	Neuraminidase produced by *Streptococcus pneumoniae* exposes cryptic antigens on erythrocytes, platelets, and glomerular endothelial cells with resultant immunological damage; HIV may infect cells directly or cause immune dysregulation
	Genetic defects in complement activation and regulation	Uncontrolled activation of alternate complement pathway causes endothelial damage and prothrombotic state; environmental triggers may act as "2nd hit" to precipitate HUS
	Drugs (cyclosporine, tacrolimus, anti-VEGF therapy, mitomycin-C, cisplatin, quinine, vaccines)	Direct endothelial injury
	Bone marrow transplantation	Endothelial injury due to chemotherapy, radiation, drugs, or manifestation of graft vs. host disease (GVHD)
	Radiation	Direct endothelial injury, delayed effect
	Pregnancy and postpartum	Increased susceptibility to HUS during postpartum; genetic mutations in complement system appear to have a role
	Systemic sclerosis	Endothelial injury due to antiendothelial antibodies
	Autoimmune (antiphospholipid antibody syndrome, SLE)	Antiphospholipid antibodies cause endothelial damage and hypercoagulability
	Malignant hypertension	Endothelial injury
	Antibody-mediated rejection in transplantation	Endothelial injury
	Neoplasms such as adenocarcinomas (especially mucin producing) and, rarely, leukemia and lymphoma	Possible causes include tumor emboli, tumor procoagulants, impaired fibrinolysis, and possibly low ADAMTS13; may also be triggered by chemotherapeutic agents and radiation
	Idiopathic	Unknown cause
Thrombotic Thrombocytopenic Purpura (TTP)		
	Familial	Mutations in gene encoding ADAMTS13, a vWF cleaving protease; large vWF multimers cause increased platelet aggregation
	Autoimmune	Autoantibodies against ADAMTS13 result in large vWF multimers
	Drugs (Ticlopidine, Clopidogrel)	Deficiency of ADAMTS13 due to autoantibodies in a subset
	Idiopathic	Unknown; may be precipitated by triggering factors

Clinical Parameters of Typical HUS and TTP: Two Ends of a Spectrum

Parameter	Typical HUS	TTP
Age at presentation	Infants and young children	Middle age
Gender predilection	None	More frequent in women
Seasonal variation	Epidemic form usually occurs in summer months	None
Prodrome of diarrhea	Present	Absent
Predisposing factors	Intake of contaminated food or fecal-oral transmission	Nondietary factors
Renal involvement	Present in all cases	Often mild, so patients infrequently undergo renal biopsy
Hemorrhagic colitis	Usually present	Rare
Systemic involvement	Severe cases have systemic manifestations, including neurological	Neurological symptoms predominate with multiorgan involvement
Treatment	Supportive therapy; antibiotics often contraindicated	Plasmapheresis
Morbidity and mortality	Low; most children recover completely	High; can recur in 20-30% of patients
Recurrence in transplanted kidney	Rare	Not uncommon, frequency unknown due to clinical overlap with aHUS

Microscopic Features

(Left) Glomerular fibrin thrombi ➡ are seen with entrapped RBCs, compatible with acute TMA. The biopsy is from a 25-year-old woman with acute renal failure, congestive heart failure, and schistocytes on peripheral smear. Etiology of TMA is undetermined. (Right) Acute TMA is seen with glomerular thrombi ➡ and fragmented RBCs. Patient is 4 months post bone marrow transplantation for follicular lymphoma and has evidence of skin GVHD. Cyclosporine had been discontinued a month prior.

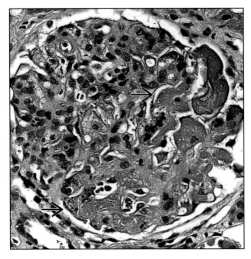
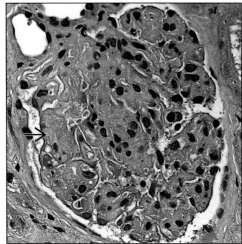

(Left) The interstitium is expanded by edema ➡, and the proximal tubules ➡ are ectatic with simplified epithelium. The patient was clinically diagnosed with TTP, and renal biopsy had characteristic features of TMA. (Right) Several cross sections of interlobular arteries ➡ show intimal edema and narrowed lumens. In this case, TMA changes are due to malignant hypertension. This patient is a 27 year old with a 2-year history of uncontrolled hypertension and noncompliance to medications.

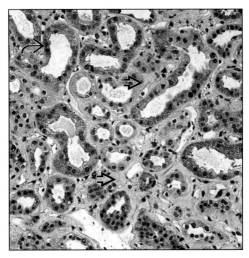
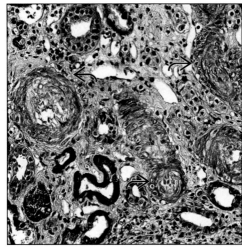

(Left) Chronic TMA is characterized by extensive duplication of GBM due to remodeling and mesangial cell interposition ➡. This patient is a 19 year old with recurrent atypical HUS. A limited work-up at the time of biopsy revealed low C3 and normal factor H levels. (Right) Extensive double contours ➡ and mesangial expansion ➡ are seen in chronic TMA due to recurrent atypical HUS. This patient is a 19-year-old woman with low serum C3 levels, suggestive of a genetic component.

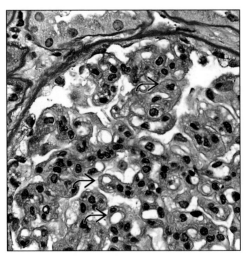
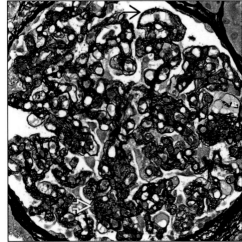

INTRODUCTION TO THROMBOTIC MICROANGIOPATHIES

Microscopic Features

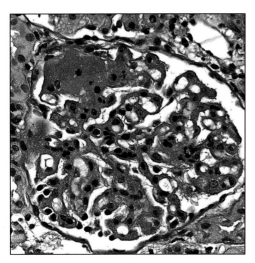

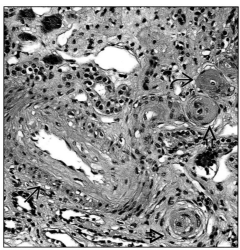

(Left) Segmental glomerulosclerosis is seen along with GBM thickening due to chronic TMA. GBMs appear thickened due to subendothelial expansion and basement membrane remodeling in this 4 year old with recurrent atypical HUS. *(Right)* Malignant hypertension shows hypertensive arteriosclerosis in the background. An interlobular artery ⮕ has mucoid intimal change, and arteriolar hyaline ⮕ is seen. Arterioles ⮕ are edematous with narrowed lumens, consistent with TMA.

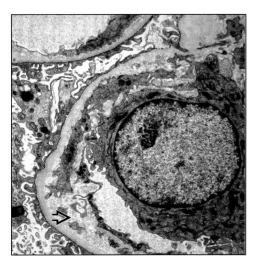

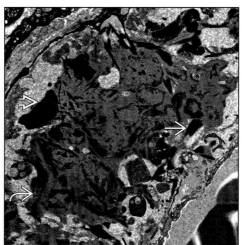

(Left) In TMA, endothelial cells are detached from GBM, and subendothelium is expanded ⮕ by electron-lucent material. Patient presented with fever, microangiopathic hemolytic anemia, and acute renal failure. Clinical diagnosis was TTP. Serological tests included were normal (ANA, C3, anticardiolipin antibody[-], serum C3). *(Right)* Note fibrin thrombus ⮕, fibrin tactoids ⮕, and entrapped fragmented erythrocytes ⮕ in capillary lumen in acute TMA.

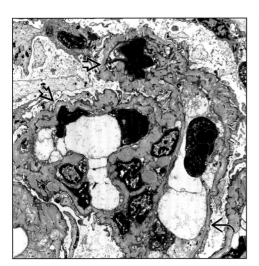

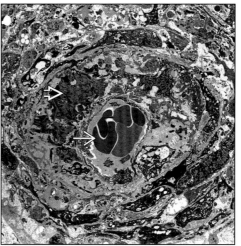

(Left) The GBM shows extensive wrinkling ⮕, and podocyte foot processes are effaced ⮕ in this biopsy of a patient with acute TMA. Arteriolar thrombosis and necrosis result in capillary tuft collapse of downstream glomeruli. *(Right)* Prominent subendothelial edema is seen in this arteriole with luminal narrowing ⮕. Fibrin and cellular debris ⮕ are seen in subendothelial space, compatible with acute arteriolar TMA. No inflammatory infiltrate is present to suggest vasculitis.

HEMOLYTIC UREMIC SYNDROME, INFECTION RELATED

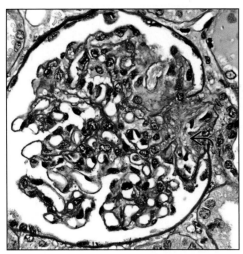

The glomerular capillary lumen near the vascular pole is occluded by an organizing thrombus ➡. This biopsy is from a 37-year-old man with documented E. coli O157:H7-associated HUS.

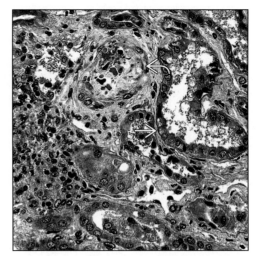

Arteriolar lumen ➡ is occluded by intimal edema with entrapped RBCs and fuchsinophilic fibrin. Acute tubular injury is also seen with simplified epithelium and nuclear atypia ➡.

TERMINOLOGY

Abbreviations
- Diarrhea-associated HUS (D+HUS)

Synonyms
- Epidemic form of HUS
- Classic HUS

Definitions
- HUS caused by enteropathogenic infectious organisms and associated with prodrome of diarrhea

ETIOLOGY/PATHOGENESIS

Infectious Agents
- *Escherichia coli* infection accounts for > 90% of D+HUS in children in United States
  - Route of infection
    - Ingestion of contaminated undercooked hamburgers, raw vegetables, raw milk, or drinking water
    - Animal fecal contact (petting zoos, fairs)
    - Fecal-oral contact, as in child care centers
  - Shiga toxigenic *E. coli* (STEC) or enterohemorrhagic *E. coli* capable of producing Shiga-like toxins (Stx1 and Stx2)
    - Majority of D+HUS in North America and Europe are caused by O157:H7 strain of STEC
    - Genes encoding Stx1 and Stx2 are located on bacteriophages infecting bacteria
    - After colonization of gut epithelium by STEC, locally produced Stx crosses intestinal barrier and enters circulation
  - Shiga toxin (a.k.a. verotoxin) has 1 A and 5 B subunits
    - Stx B subunit binds to glycoprotein receptors, globotriaosylceramide (Gb3)

- Gb3 receptors are expressed in highest concentration in microvascular endothelial cells of kidney, gut, pancreas, and brain and in renal tubular epithelial cells
  - Internalized Stx A subunit in cells has RNA-N-glycosidase activity, inhibits host cell protein synthesis, and causes apoptosis
    - Endothelial damage by Stx causes prothrombotic state, ischemia-induced hemorrhagic enteritis, and thrombotic microangiopathy
    - Microangiopathic anemia caused by shear stress as erythrocytes traverse injured arterioles and glomeruli
- Other STEC virulence factors
  - Subtilase cytotoxin (SubAB)
    - Causes proteolytic cleavage of essential endoplasmic reticulum chaperone molecule and triggers stress response leading to apoptosis
    - Produced by wide range of STEC strains and may be carried on a megaplasmid
    - SubAB receptor is a glycan chain terminating in a sialic acid (Neu5Gc), a glycoprotein not synthesized by humans due to evolutionary loss
    - Neu5Gc is synthesized in nonhuman primates and is present abundantly in red meat and dairy products
    - Neu5Gc from dietary sources can be incorporated metabolically into surfaces of human endothelium and intestinal epithelium
  - Locus of enterocyte effacement (LEE) encodes capacity to adhere to enterocytes and cause effacement of microvilli
  - High pathogenicity island (HPI) contributes to STEC survival
  - Large plasmids encode hemolysin, a pore-forming cytolysin

Other Organisms
- *Shigella dysenteriae* produces Shiga toxin and is most common cause of D+HUS in Asia and Africa

HEMOLYTIC UREMIC SYNDROME, INFECTION RELATED

Key Facts

Terminology
- D+HUS caused by enteropathogenic bacteria and associated with prodrome of diarrhea

Etiology/Pathogenesis
- *Escherichia coli* infection in ~ 90%
- *E. coli* (STEC) producing Shiga-like toxin or Subtilase cytotoxin (SubAB)

Clinical Issues
- 5-10% of patients with *E. coli* O157:H7 infection develop HUS, mainly infants and young children
- Acute renal failure and microangiopathic anemia develop abruptly ~ 1 week after onset of diarrhea
- Most patients (especially children) recover completely with supportive care
  - Antibiotics are contraindicated in STEC infections

Microscopic Pathology
- Fibrinoid necrosis and thrombosis in glomeruli and arterioles
- Mesangiolysis
- Glomerular endothelial swelling and injury
- Cortical necrosis in severe cases

Top Differential Diagnoses
- Thrombotic microangiography due to other causes
- Vasculitis

Diagnostic Checklist
- Isolated glomerular involvement has better prognosis than if blood vessels are affected
- Cause of HUS cannot be distinguished by renal pathology

- *Shigella* directly invade intestinal epithelium and induce apoptosis
- Other enteric infectious agents include *Salmonella*, *Campylobacter*, and *Yersinia*
- Nonenteric pathogens usually result in atypical HUS (without prodrome of diarrhea)
  - Examples include human immunodeficiency virus (HIV), *Streptococcus pneumoniae*, *Mycoplasma pneumoniae*, Coxsackie A and B viruses, *Legionella* infection, histoplasmosis, and brucellosis

Host Risk Factors
- Genetic factors
  - Polymorphisms of genes involved in coagulation, complement activation, and renin angiotensin systems may influence susceptibility or severity
    - Platelet glycoprotein 1bα M allele is associated with increased risk of developing HUS
    - Polymorphism of angiotensin II type I receptor has protective role against long-term sequelae
- Nongenetic factors
  - Gb3 receptors
    - More abundantly expressed in young children
    - Upregulated by cytokines and lipopolysaccharides
    - Upregulated by HIV in renal tubules
  - Consumption of red meat and dairy products causes priming of target cells with SubAB receptors

Animal Model
- Mice given multiple doses of Stx2

CLINICAL ISSUES

Epidemiology
- Incidence
  - ~ 5-10% of patients with *E. coli* O157:H7 infection develop HUS
  - 1-3 cases per 100,000 per year in USA
  - Epidemic *E. coli* outbreaks are often in summer months in North America and Europe
- Age
  - Mainly in infants, young children, and elderly

- Gender
  - Slightly more common in males
- Ethnicity
  - Rare in African Americans

Presentation
- Diarrhea is initially watery and subsequently progresses to bloody diarrhea
- Acute renal failure develops abruptly ~ 1 week after onset of diarrhea
  - Oliguria or anuria
  - Hematuria and proteinuria
  - Elevated BUN and serum creatinine
- Pallor, melena, hematemesis, and petechiae due to anemia and bleeding tendencies
- Hypertension
- Severe disease may have congestive heart failure, acute pancreatitis, headaches, seizures, and visual changes
- *Shigella* infection often has more severe systemic symptoms: Fever, bacteremia, and severe hemolysis
- Incomplete forms of D+HUS are also described

Laboratory Tests
- Microangiopathic hemolytic anemia
  - Schistocytes on peripheral smear
  - Elevated serum lactate dehydrogenase and reduced haptoglobin levels
  - Thrombocytopenia
  - Coombs test negative
  - Normal prothrombin and partial thromboplastin times
- Stool cultures confirm enteric bacterial infection

Treatment
- Supportive care, maintenance of fluid-electrolyte balance, control of hypertension
- Dialysis as needed
- Antibiotics are contraindicated in STEC infections
  - Several antibiotics have been shown to induce Stx-converting bacteriophages and increase Stx production
  - Antibiotics increase risk of HUS in children

Prognosis
- Most patients (especially children) recover completely
- Prognosis of D+HUS is vastly better than D-HUS
- Approximately 3-5% die during acute phase of illness due to cardiovascular or neurological complications
- About 1/3 of D+HUS patients have persistent mild proteinuria &/or renal insufficiency
  - Poor prognostic factors include marked leucocytosis and older age at onset

MICROSCOPIC PATHOLOGY

Histologic Features
- Glomeruli
  - Glomerular endothelial swelling and congestion
    - Mesangiolysis
    - Mesangial hypercellularity
  - Thrombi
    - Ischemic collapse
  - Glomerular necrosis, often contiguous with fibrinoid necrosis in hilar arterioles
    - Apoptotic debris and fragmented erythrocytes in foci of fibrinoid necrosis
    - Glomerular infiltration of neutrophils documented
  - GBM duplication in chronic phase
- Tubules and interstitium
  - Acute tubular injury with simplified epithelium and reactive nuclear atypia
  - Cortical necrosis and infarction seen in severe cases
- Arteries
  - Fibrinoid necrosis and thrombosis of arterioles
    - Little or no inflammation
  - Arteriolar endothelial swelling and mucoid intimal change (can be seen with Alcian Blue stain)
  - Arteriolar fibrin thrombi seen at hilum and in interlobular arteries
- Other organs
  - Similar microvascular endothelial damage also occurs in gastrointestinal tract, brain, pancreas, and liver

ANCILLARY TESTS

Immunofluorescence
- Nonspecific entrapment of C3 and IgM in affected glomeruli and blood vessels
- Fibrin thrombi highlighted on fibrinogen stain
- Fibrinogen in mesangium
- No evidence of immune complex disease

Electron Microscopy
- Endothelial swelling and expansion of subendothelial zone by flocculent material
- Glomerular and arteriolar thrombi show platelets and fibrin tactoids with entrapped fragmented erythrocytes
- Foot process effacement (variable)
- No electron-dense deposits

DIFFERENTIAL DIAGNOSIS

Thrombotic Microangiopathy Due to Other Causes
- Seek evidence for genetic predisposition, autoantibodies, neoplasm, and drug history

Vasculitis
- Fibrinoid necrosis is accompanied by transmural inflammatory infiltrate
- Crescents common

DIAGNOSTIC CHECKLIST

Clinically Relevant Pathologic Features
- Isolated glomerular involvement is associated with better prognosis than if blood vessels are affected

Pathologic Interpretation Pearls
- Cause of HUS cannot be distinguished by pathological features

SELECTED REFERENCES
1. Löfling JC et al: A dietary non-human sialic acid may facilitate hemolytic-uremic syndrome. Kidney Int. 76(2):140-4, 2009
2. Sauter KA et al: Mouse model of hemolytic-uremic syndrome caused by endotoxin-free Shiga toxin 2 (Stx2) and protection from lethal outcome by anti-Stx2 antibody. Infect Immun. 76(10):4469-78, 2008
3. Zheng XL et al: Pathogenesis of thrombotic microangiopathies. Annu Rev Pathol. 3:249-77, 2008
4. Constantinescu AR et al: Non-enteropathic hemolytic uremic syndrome: causes and short-term course. Am J Kidney Dis. 43(6):976-82, 2004
5. Chaisri U et al: Localization of Shiga toxins of enterohaemorrhagic Escherichia coli in kidneys of paediatric and geriatric patients with fatal haemolytic uraemic syndrome. Microb Pathog. 31(2):59-67, 2001
6. Karch H: The role of virulence factors in enterohemorrhagic Escherichia coli (EHEC)--associated hemolytic-uremic syndrome. Semin Thromb Hemost. 27(3):207-13, 2001
7. Ray PE et al: Pathogenesis of Shiga toxin-induced hemolytic uremic syndrome. Pediatr Nephrol. 16(10):823-39, 2001
8. Lingwood CA: Glycolipid receptors for verotoxin and Helicobacter pylori: role in pathology. Biochim Biophys Acta. 1455(2-3):375-86, 1999
9. Inward CD et al: Renal histopathology in fatal cases of diarrhoea-associated haemolytic uraemic syndrome. British Association for Paediatric Nephrology. Pediatr Nephrol. 11(5):556-9, 1997
10. Richardson SE et al: The histopathology of the hemolytic uremic syndrome associated with verocytotoxin-producing Escherichia coli infections. Hum Pathol. 19(9):1102-8, 1988

HEMOLYTIC UREMIC SYNDROME, INFECTION RELATED

Microscopic Features

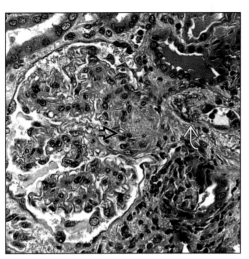

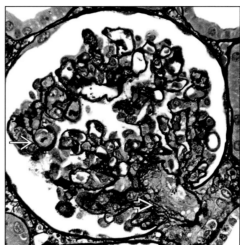

(Left) Typical D+HUS due to E. coli results in glomerular and arteriolar thrombosis. The glomerular organizing thrombus near the vascular pole ⧁ is in continuity with the arteriolar fibrin thrombus ⬈. Fibrin in the arteriole is red on trichrome stain. *(Right)* Diffuse glomerular endothelial swelling ➡ is seen associated with capillary luminal occlusion. Thrombosis is also present near the vascular pole ⧁ in this biopsy with HUS due to a documented E. coli infection.

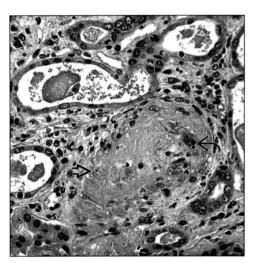

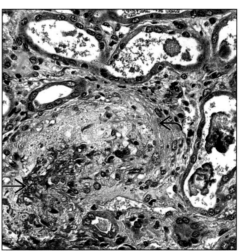

(Left) Fibrinoid necrosis and thrombosis ⧁ of an interlobular artery in a 37-year-old man with E. coli O157:H7 infection is shown. The vessel is expanded and lumen is occluded by fibrin with entrapped erythrocytes. Focal apoptotic debris ⧁ is seen, but inflammatory infiltrate is characteristically absent. *(Right)* Acute thrombotic microangiopathy is seen with thrombosis and intimal edema in an interlobular artery ➡. The fibrin ➡ within the thrombus stains bright red on trichrome.

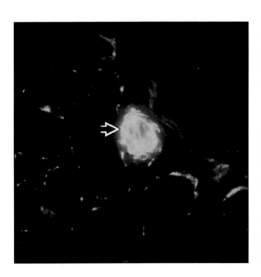

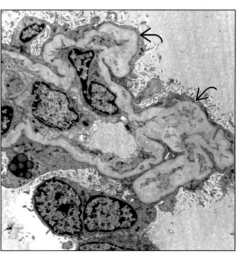

(Left) Fibrin thrombus ⧁ in a renal arteriole detected with antibody to fibrinogen is shown. Characteristic features of acute TMA were present. The pathological features do not typically help distinguish the etiology of thrombotic microangiopathy. *(Right)* Diffuse wrinkling of the GBM is seen with extensive foot process effacement ➡. The characteristic collapse of the capillary tuft is due to E. coli-associated D+HUS in this case.

THROMBOTIC MICROANGIOPATHY, GENETIC

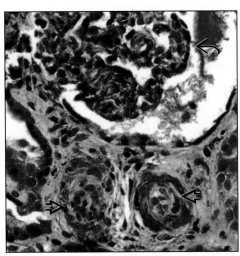

Renal biopsy from a 13-year-old boy with factor H mutation shows arterioles occluded by loose intimal fibrosis ⊵ with trapped red cells. The glomerulus ⊿ demonstrates ischemic collapse.

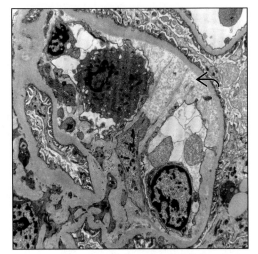

Prominent expansion of the subendothelial space by electron-lucent flocculent material is seen ⊿ in a renal biopsy from an adolescent boy with aHUS due to a missense mutation in the CFH gene.

TERMINOLOGY

Abbreviations
- Atypical hemolytic uremic syndrome (aHUS)

Definitions
- aHUS caused or predisposed by genetic factors

ETIOLOGY/PATHOGENESIS

Genetic Defects in Complement Activation and Regulation
- Mutations in alternate complement pathway account for 50-60% of aHUS cases
  - Excessive generation or defective inactivation of C3b results in uncontrolled complement activation, endothelial damage, prothrombotic state, and, consequently, aHUS
  - Genetic mutations occur in both familial and sporadic aHUS
    - Familial aHUS can have either autosomal dominant or recessive pattern of inheritance
  - These mutations result in defects in either regulators or activators of alternate pathway
    - Regulators: Factor H, MCP, and factor I encoding genes have loss of function mutations
    - Activators: Factor B and C3 encoding genes have gain of function mutations
  - Some aHUS patients present mutations in 2 or more different complement genes
- Complement factor H abnormalities
  - Factor H is a plasma protein that regulates alternative pathway by competing with factor B for C3b, thus resulting in enhanced dissociation of C3 convertase
    - Normally downregulates alternative pathway activation on glomerular basement membranes, which lack complement regulators
  - Vast majority of mutations in CFH, a gene encoding factor H, are heterozygous, but homozygous mutations also occur
  - Point mutations in CFH (chromosome 1q32 locus) account for 40-45% of familial aHUS and 10-20% of sporadic "idiopathic" aHUS
    - Mutant forms have diminished cofactor activity
    - In heterozygous mutations, mutant factor H in serum interacts with normal factor H and impairs its binding to endothelial cells, thus exacerbating defective cofactor activity
    - Homozygous mutations result in quantitative factor H deficiency and low C3 levels
    - Mutant factor H with defective binding to platelets predisposes to platelet activation
    - No correlation between specific CFH mutations and clinical phenotype
  - Mutations in genes encoding complement factor H-related proteins (CFHR1-5) have also been described in 3-5% of patients with aHUS
    - CFHR1 is a complement regulator that inhibits C5 convertase and membrane insertion of terminal complement complex
    - CFHR1 and factor H share an identical surface binding region, and both compete for ligand
    - Deletion of CFHR1 gene also causes abnormalities of terminal complement pathway regulation
    - High degree of sequence homology exists between CFH and CFHR and heterozygous hybrid gene derived from this combination results in gene product with reduced complement regulatory activity
  - Autoantibodies against factor H are detected in 6-10% of patients with aHUS
    - These autoantibodies bind to factor H and reduce its binding to C3b
    - Children with homozygous deletions of CFHR1 and 3 genes develop autoimmune reaction against CFHR1 and 3 in heterozygous mother

THROMBOTIC MICROANGIOPATHY, GENETIC

Key Facts

Etiology/Pathogenesis
- Mutations in alternate complement pathway account for 50-60% of aHUS cases
  - Mutations in *CFH*, *CFHR*, *MCP*, *CFI*, *CFB*, *C3*, and *THBD*
  - Certain high-risk haplotypes
  - Environmental triggers precipitate aHUS

Clinical Issues
- Insidious onset of hypertension and renal manifestations
- Low C3 levels in some patients
  - Genotyping of complement genes recommended even if serum levels are normal
- Plasma levels of complement factors H, I, and B are recommended in all cases of aHUS, as are CFHR, MCP, and screening for anti-CFH antibodies
- Prompt initiation of plasma exchange
- End-stage renal disease in > 50% of patients
- Recurrence rate high after renal transplantation

Microscopic Pathology
- Glomerular fibrinoid necrosis
- Arterial mucoid intimal thickening
- Fibrin thrombi
- Subendothelial zone expansion by EM
  - No electron-dense deposits

Diagnostic Checklist
- Cause of HUS cannot be distinguished by pathologic features
- Low C3 levels in patient with aHUS should raise suspicion for genetic causes

---

- Term DEAP-HUS (**DE**ficiency of CFHR plasma proteins and **A**utoantibody **P**ositive for of **HUS**) has been proposed for this group of patients
- Membrane cofactor protein abnormalities
  - Membrane cofactor protein (MCP) or CD46 is expressed on most cell surfaces, including kidney
  - As a cofactor for factor I, it is essential for prevention of complement activation on glomerular endothelium
  - Mutations in *MCP* gene account for 10-15% of aHUS
  - Mutant forms of MCP result in low expression levels or low C3b binding capability or cofactor activity
- Complement factor I abnormalities
  - Factor I is a serine protease circulating in plasma; regulates all 3 complement pathways by cleaving C3b and C4b
  - Heterozygous mutations in *CFI* (a gene encoding factor I) account for 4-10% of aHUS cases
  - Mutant forms either result in low serum factor I levels or disrupt its cofactor activity
- Complement factor B abnormalities
  - Mutations in *CFB*, a gene encoding complement factor B, occur in only 1-2% of patients with aHUS
  - Mutant forms have more affinity to C3b and form hyperactive C3 convertase resistant to dissociation
  - C3b formation is greater, resulting in chronic activation of alternate complement pathway
- Complement C3 abnormalities
  - Heterozygous mutations in *C3* occur in 4-10% of patients with aHUS
  - Mutant C3 forms result in reduced C3b binding to CFH and MCP and thus impair its degradation
  - Serum C3 levels are often low in these patients
- Thrombomodulin abnormalities
  - Thrombomodulin is a membrane-bound glycoprotein with anticoagulant properties
    - Facilitates complement inactivation by CFI in presence of CFH
  - Heterozygous mutations in *THBD* (gene encoding thrombomodulin) identified in 5% of aHUS

- Mutant variants of thrombomodulin are less efficient in degrading C3b and generating fibrinolysis inhibitors

High-risk Polymorphisms
- Certain haplotypes of *CFH*, *MCP*, *CFI*, *CFB*, *CFHR1*, and *C3* are more frequently seen in aHUS patients than in unaffected population
- These polymorphisms often coexist with other genetic mutations and may account for variability in genetic penetrance among family members

Superimposed Precipitating Factor
- Not all patients with genetic mutations develop aHUS
- Genetic penetrance among carriers of *CFH*, *MCP*, and *CFI* mutations is only 40-50%
- Genetic mutations predispose individuals to environmental triggers that may result in aHUS
- Precipitating factors include infections, pregnancy, oral contraceptive pills, and other drugs

CLINICAL ISSUES

Epidemiology
- Age
  - Genetic aHUS often presents in children and adolescents
  - Environmental triggers can precipitate aHUS in middle age

Presentation
- Mild hematuria and proteinuria
- Hypertension and renal insufficiency
- Diarrhea less common but may precede genetic aHUS precipitated by infections
- Neurological and systemic manifestations less common

Laboratory Tests
- Schistocytes in peripheral smear confirm microangiopathic hemolytic anemia
- Low platelet counts

- Elevated lactate dehydrogenase
- Low C3 and normal C4 levels suggest isolated activation of alternate complement pathway
- Plasma levels of complement factors H, I, and B are recommended in all cases of aHUS, as are CFHR, MCP, and screening for anti-CFH antibodies
- Genotyping of complement genes is recommended even if serum levels are normal

Treatment
- Initiation of plasma exchange within 24 hours after diagnosis
  - Response rates are variable based on specific mutations, but genetic results are not available until long after treatment is instituted
    - Since MCP is a membrane protein, plasma exchange does not provide normal MCP and is thus ineffective
- Monoclonal antibody against complement C5
  - Inhibits terminal component of complement activation
- Renal transplantation
  - Living donor transplantation is contraindicated due to high risk of recurrence
  - Family members may be mutation carriers, and surgical stress may precipitate aHUS
- Liver transplantation
  - To replace deficient protein

Prognosis
- Generally poor prognosis with end-stage renal disease in > 50% of patients
- Renal outcomes vary based on underlying genetic mutation
  - Loss of renal function is more often seen in patients with *CFH, CFI,* and *CFB* mutations (70-80%)
  - *MCP* mutations confer good prognosis with remission rates of 80-90%
- Recurrent aHUS in transplanted kidney is high
  - Rate of recurrent aHUS highest in *CFH* (80-90%) and *CFI* (70-80%) mutations
  - Combined liver-kidney transplantation may be beneficial in patients with *CFH, CFI,* and *CFB* mutations

MICROSCOPIC PATHOLOGY

Histologic Features
- Glomerular fibrinoid necrosis with fragmented RBCs
- Some glomeruli may appear "bloodless" or demonstrate collapse of capillary tuft
- Duplicated glomerular basement membranes seen in subacute or chronic stages
- Acute tubular injury and interstitial edema predominate during acute phase, followed by tubular atrophy and interstitial fibrosis
- Arteriolar fibrin thrombi and intimal mucoid edema

ANCILLARY TESTS

Immunofluorescence
- Granular C3, IgM, and fibrinogen observed in affected glomeruli and arterioles

Electron Microscopy
- Endothelial swelling in glomerular capillaries and arterioles
- Expanded subendothelial zones by flocculent material
  - Fibrin tactoids, fragmented erythrocytes, and platelets are seen in subendothelial zone
- Increased electron lucency of mesangial matrix
- No electron-dense deposits

DIFFERENTIAL DIAGNOSIS

Thrombotic Microangiopathy Due to Other Causes
- Clinical presentation and serological tests help identify cause of thrombotic microangiopathy

Pauci-immune Crescentic Glomerulonephritis
- Glomerular necrosis and crescents associated with basement membrane rupture and leukocyte infiltration
- ANCA serology is positive in most cases

DIAGNOSTIC CHECKLIST

Pathologic Interpretation Pearls
- Low C3 levels in patient with aHUS presentation should raise suspicion for genetic causes

SELECTED REFERENCES
1. Benz K et al: Thrombotic microangiopathy: new insights. Curr Opin Nephrol Hypertens. 19(3):242-7, 2010
2. Noris M et al: Thrombotic microangiopathy after kidney transplantation. Am J Transplant. 10(7):1517-23, 2010
3. Sullivan M et al: Epidemiological approach to identifying genetic predispositions for atypical hemolytic uremic syndrome. Ann Hum Genet. 74(1):17-26, 2010
4. Sánchez-Corral P et al: Advances in understanding the aetiology of atypical Haemolytic Uraemic Syndrome. Br J Haematol. 150(5):529-42, 2010
5. Westra D et al: Genetic disorders in complement (regulating) genes in patients with atypical haemolytic uraemic syndrome (aHUS). Nephrol Dial Transplant. 25(7):2195-202, 2010
6. Zipfel PF et al: Thrombotic microangiopathies: new insights and new challenges. Curr Opin Nephrol Hypertens. 19(4):372-8, 2010
7. Somers MJ et al: Case records of the Massachusetts General Hospital. Case 23-2009. A 13-year-old boy with headache, nausea, seizures, and hypertension. N Engl J Med. 361(4):389-400, 2009
8. Taranta A et al: Genetic risk factors in typical haemolytic uraemic syndrome. Nephrol Dial Transplant. 24(6):1851-7, 2009

Microscopic Features

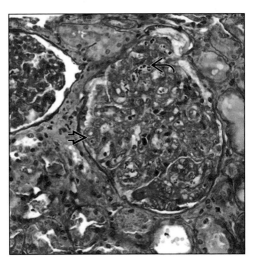 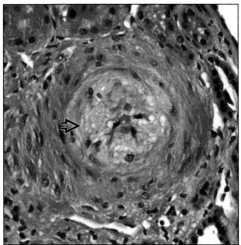

(Left) The glomerulus shows typical features of thrombotic microangiopathy with diffuse endothelial swelling and mesangiolysis ⧉. Focal karyorrhectic debris is seen ⧉, but there is no significant leukocyte infiltration in this patient with genetic form of aHUS. *(Right)* Severe mucoid intimal edema ⧉ is observed in an interlobular artery. These changes of thrombotic microangiopathy in an adolescent boy with seizures and hypertension were determined to be due to genetic aHUS.

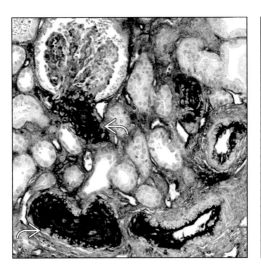 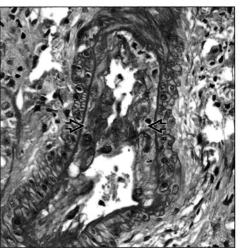

(Left) Numerous fibrin thrombi with factor VIII ⧉ are seen in arterioles and interlobular arteries (compatible with TMA) in an adolescent patient with aHUS due to a complement factor H mutation. *(Right)* Prominent endothelial swelling ⧉ and inflammation are seen in an interlobular artery. Other blood vessels had fibrin thrombi occluding the lumens, compatible with thrombotic microangiopathy due to CFH mutation. This mimics endarteritis in an allograft.

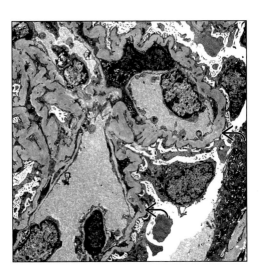 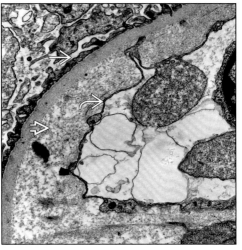

(Left) Extensive glomerular basement membrane wrinkling ⧉ is seen in this glomerulus with ischemic collapse. Characteristic features of thrombotic microangiopathy were seen elsewhere in this biopsy with genetic form of aHUS. *(Right)* Electron micrograph shows expanded subendothelial space ⧉, loss of endothelial cell fenestration ⧉, and podocyte foot process effacement ⧉. The aHUS in this patient was determined to be due to missense mutation in CFH gene.

THROMBOTIC MICROANGIOPATHY, AUTOIMMUNE

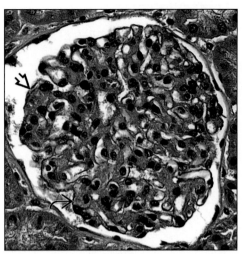

Bloodless glomerulus shows very focal endothelial swelling ⊟ and mesangiolysis ⊟. The patient presented with catastrophic APLS with positive aPLs but negative ANA and normal C3 and C4.

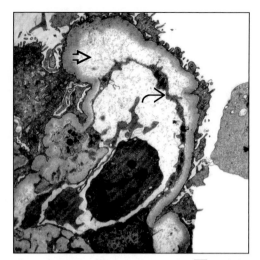

The endothelial cell fenestrations are lost ⊟, and the subendothelium ⊟ is expanded by lucent material. TMA in this 39-year-old woman is due to catastrophic APLS with no evidence of SLE.

TERMINOLOGY

Abbreviations
- Thrombotic microangiopathy (TMA)

Definitions
- TMA due to autoantibodies affecting coagulation system

ETIOLOGY/PATHOGENESIS

Antiphospholipid Autoantibodies (aPLs)
- Heterogeneous group of autoantibodies directed against a broad range of target antigens recognizing phospholipids and phospholipid-binding proteins
  - Subsets of aPLs determined by detection method used; both methods recommended to increase sensitivity of aPL detection
  - Lupus anticoagulant (AL)
    - Functional coagulation assay to detect prolonged clotting times
    - Despite its name, causes prothrombotic state due to preferential inhibition of anticoagulant pathways in vivo
  - Anticardiolipin antibodies (aCL) and anti-β2GPI antibodies
    - Immunoassay to detect binding to anionic phospholipids or phospholipid-binding proteins
- Hypercoagulability in all vascular beds causing antiphospholipid antibody syndrome (APLS)
  - Thrombosis in large caliber vessels and TMA in microvasculature
  - Antibodies interfere with phospholipid-binding proteins involved in coagulation pathways
  - Endothelial cell activation by aPLs causes cytokine secretion and alteration of prostacyclin metabolism
  - Low-density lipoproteins cross react with aPLs, causing oxidant-mediated injury of endothelium

- APLS can be primary (no autoimmune disease) or secondary
  - Infectious organisms trigger aPLs by molecular mimicry
  - Secondary APLS in setting of systemic lupus erythematosus (SLE) or other connective tissue disorders
    - Presence of aPLs can precede clinical onset of disease by 7-8 years in SLE
    - Renal prognosis in SLE patients is worsened by presence of aPLs

ADAMTS13 Autoantibodies
- ADAMTS13 (A Disintegrin And Metalloprotease with ThromboSpondin type 1 repeat)
  - Cleaves von Willebrand factor (vWF) multimers
- Autoantibodies cause severe deficiency of ADAMTS13 in plasma
  - In absence of ADAMTS13, unchecked vWF multimers cause platelet aggregation, thrombi, and consequent end organ damage
  - Known autoantibody triggers include drugs and infections
- Idiopathic thrombotic thrombocytopenic purpura (TTP)
  - IgG or IgM autoantibodies in 30-80% of cases
  - Antibodies against platelet glycoprotein IV (CD36) have been reported in some
- Drug-induced TTP
  - Ticlopidine and clopidogrel

Factor H Autoantibodies
- Affect alternate complement pathway activation
- Identified in children with homozygous deletions of *CFHR1* and *3* genes who develop autoimmune reaction against maternal heterozygous *CFHR1* and *3*
- DEAP-HUS (DEficiency of CFHR plasma proteins and Autoantibody Positive for HUS) proposed for this condition

THROMBOTIC MICROANGIOPATHY, AUTOIMMUNE

Key Facts

Terminology
- TMA due to autoantibodies affecting coagulation system

Etiology/Pathogenesis
- Autoantibodies
  - Lupus anticoagulant (phospholipids)
  - Anticardiolipin antibodies and anti-β2GPI antibodies
  - ADAMTS13 autoantibodies
  - Factor H

Clinical Issues
- Acute or chronic renal failure
- Proteinuria, hematuria, hypertension
- Neurological symptoms predominate in TTP
- Systemic thrombosis in APLS

Microscopic Pathology
- Acute TMA
  - Glomerular and arterial thrombi
  - Endothelial swelling and mesangiolysis
- Chronic TMA
  - GBM duplication and arterial intimal thickening
  - Arterial thrombi of varying ages and recanalized lumens in APLS
- EM: Endothelial swelling, subendothelial flocculent material, duplication of GBM (chronic)
  - No deposits unless associated with lupus nephritis

Top Differential Diagnoses
- TMA due to other causes

TMA Associated with Autoimmune Disease
- Mainly SLE and APLS
  - SLE-TMA without aPLs may be induced by many autoantibodies, including antiendothelial antibodies
  - Subset have ADAMTS13 antibodies
- Reported in scleroderma, mixed connective tissue disorder, rheumatoid arthritis, adult Still disease, Sjögren syndrome, Behçet disease, ulcerative colitis, and myasthenia gravis

CLINICAL ISSUES

Presentation
- Mild renal insufficiency or acute renal failure
- Proteinuria, hematuria, hypertension
- Neurological symptoms may predominate in TTP
- Evidence of systemic thrombosis in APLS

Laboratory Tests
- Assay for autoantibodies
  - Cardiolipin, β2GPI, lupus anticoagulant, ADAMTS13, Factor H
- Schistocytes on peripheral smear
- Thrombocytopenia, elevated LDH

Treatment
- Plasma infusion and exchange in TTP
- Anticoagulation is mainstay of therapy in APLS
- Immunosuppression to inhibit autoantibodies

Prognosis
- Mortality high in untreated TTP or catastrophic APLS
- TTP may be chronic or relapsing

MICROSCOPIC PATHOLOGY

Histologic Features
- Acute TMA
  - Glomerular and arterial thrombi
  - Endothelial swelling, fibrinoid necrosis, and mesangiolysis
  - Acute tubular injury and interstitial edema
- Chronic TMA
  - GBM duplication and arterial intimal thickening
  - Arterial thrombi of varying ages and recanalized lumens in APLS
  - Variable tubular atrophy and interstitial fibrosis

ANCILLARY TESTS

Immunofluorescence
- Glomerular and arterial thrombi stain for fibrinogen
- Immune complexes if associated with lupus nephritis

Electron Microscopy
- Endothelial swelling and subendothelial expansion by flocculent material
- No deposits unless associated with lupus nephritis

DIFFERENTIAL DIAGNOSIS

TMA Due to Other Causes
- Histologically indistinguishable
- Clinical and family history may suggest etiology

SELECTED REFERENCES

1. Zipfel PF et al: Thrombotic microangiopathies: new insights and new challenges. Curr Opin Nephrol Hypertens. 19(4):372-8, 2010
2. Gigante A et al: Antiphospholipid antibodies and renal involvement. Am J Nephrol. 30(5):405-12, 2009
3. Zheng XL et al: Pathogenesis of thrombotic microangiopathies. Annu Rev Pathol. 3:249-77, 2008
4. Fischer MJ et al: The antiphospholipid syndrome. Semin Nephrol. 27(1):35-46, 2007
5. Shelat SG et al: Inhibitory autoantibodies against ADAMTS-13 in patients with thrombotic thrombocytopenic purpura bind ADAMTS-13 protease and may accelerate its clearance in vivo. J Thromb Haemost. 4(8):1707-17, 2006
6. Lian EC: Pathogenesis of thrombotic thrombocytopenic purpura: ADAMTS13 deficiency and beyond. Semin Thromb Hemost. 31(6):625-32, 2005

Microscopic Features

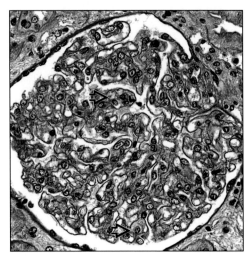
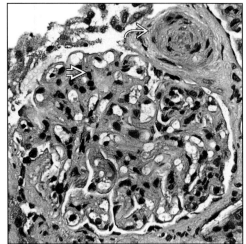

(Left) Mild endothelial swelling ⊟ is observed in this case of TMA. Subsequent to the biopsy, serological tests revealed only IgG and IgM aPLs, compatible with primary APLS. Ultrastructural examination was also consistent with mild TMA. *(Right)* The capillary tuft is mildly retracted, and mesangiolysis ⊟ is seen. An adjacent arteriole ➡ shows TMA features of intimal edema and luminal occlusion. The patient is a 27-year-old man with Still disease and positive aCL.

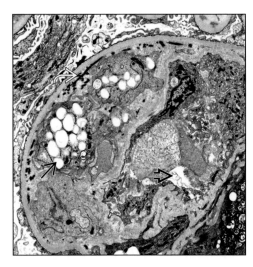
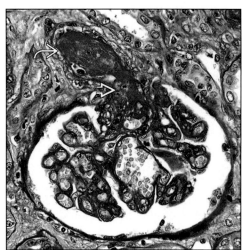

(Left) The capillary lumen ⊟ is severely occluded by a swollen endothelial cell. The subendothelium is expanded by cells ➡, likely macrophages and focal fibrin tactoids ➚, consistent with a diagnosis of acute TMA. *(Right)* An arteriolar luminal thrombus ➚ is seen extending into the vascular pole. Focal apoptotic debris ⊟ is present, but there is no vascular inflammation. The biopsy is from a 20-year-old woman with relapsing TTP.

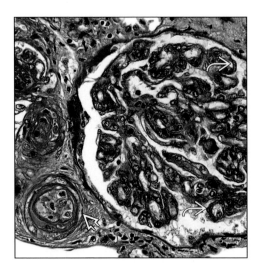
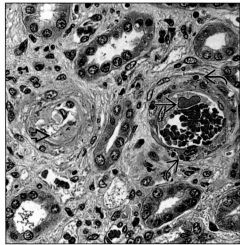

(Left) Endothelial swelling is seen in an arteriole ⊟ with luminal occlusion and mononuclear inflammatory cells. Adjacent glomerulus shows ischemic collapse and also extensive GBM duplication ➚. TMA changes in this patient are attributed to idiopathic TTP. *(Right)* Cross sections of arterioles show intimal edema ⊟ and focal luminal thrombus ➡. Fragmented RBCs ➚ are also seen within the arteriolar wall. These features are characteristic of acute TMA and in this case is due to TTP.

Microscopic Features

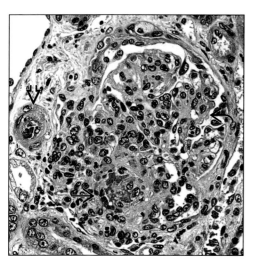

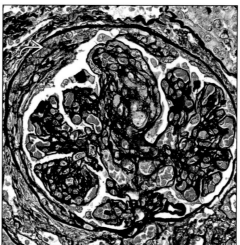

(Left) Glomerulus demonstrates endocapillary proliferation ⇗ and segmental necrosis ⇥. An adjacent arteriole ⇗ has characteristic TMA features of endothelial swelling and luminal fibrin. The patient is 27 years old with proliferative lupus nephritis and detectable aCL. *(Right)* Glomerular endocapillary proliferation and crescent ⇗ are seen in class IV (active and global) lupus nephritis. The patient had positive aCL, and characteristic TMA changes were seen in arterioles.

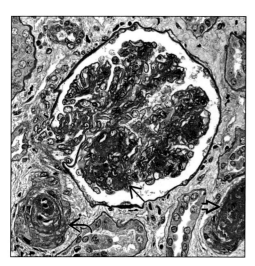

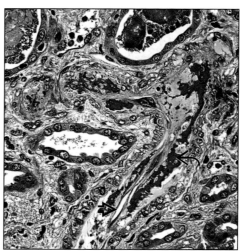

(Left) Diffuse mesangial and segmental endocapillary proliferation ⇗ is seen in this biopsy with proliferative lupus nephritis. Adjacent arterioles show "onion skin" lamination ⇗ as well as luminal thrombosis ⇗. The patient has both lupus nephritis and secondary APLS, confirmed serologically. *(Right)* An interlobular artery shows severe intimal edema with a narrowed lumen ⇗ and fibrin ⇗. These TMA changes are due to APLS occurring in association with lupus nephritis.

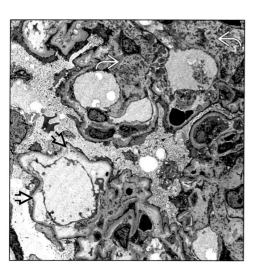

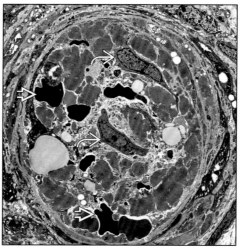

(Left) The endothelial cell is lifted off from the GBM, and the subendothelium is expanded ⇗ by lucent material in TMA. Electron-dense deposits are seen in mesangium ⇗ and capillary walls. The patient is a 22-year-old woman with SLE and positive aCL. *(Right)* The arteriolar lumen is occluded by electron-dense deposits, cellular debris, edema, and fragmented RBCs ⇗. The endothelial nuclei ⇗ are nearly detached. The patient has proliferative lupus nephritis and secondary APLS.

3

THROMBOTIC MICROANGIOPATHY, DRUGS

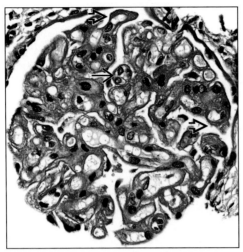

The glomerulus demonstrates extensive duplication of basement membranes ⊵ associated with endothelial swelling ⊷ and mild mesangiolysis. TMA in this 13 year old with renal allografts is attributed to sirolimus.

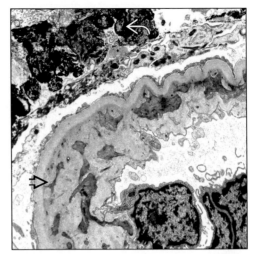

GBM duplication and mesangial cell interposition ⊵ is seen in a 64 year old with TMA. The patient received aflibercept (VEGF trap) for prostate carcinoma. Fibrin ⊷ is also seen in the urinary space.

TERMINOLOGY

Abbreviations
- Thrombotic microangiopathy (TMA)

Definitions
- Atypical hemolytic uremic syndrome (HUS) caused by drugs

ETIOLOGY/PATHOGENESIS

Mechanism of TMA Induction
- Direct endothelial injury due to dose-related toxicity
- Immune-mediated with induction of autoantibodies

Implicated Drugs
- > 60 drugs reportedly associated with TMA, but often difficult to establish causative role
- Chemotherapeutic agents
  - Mitomycin-C
    - Dose-dependent endothelial toxicity
    - Median time from last dose to development of TMA is 75 days
  - Gemcitabine
    - Endothelial damage causes TMA
    - Median time from initiation of therapy to development of TMA is 6-8 months
  - Other agents include bleomycin, cisplatin, daunorubicin, vinblastine, deoxycoformycin
- Anti-vascular endothelial growth factor (VEGF) therapy
  - VEGF receptor blockers (bevacizumab, VEGF trap)
    - VEGF synthesis by podocytes is needed for survival of glomerular endothelial cells that express VEGF receptors
    - TMA due to endothelial damage can occur from 1 week to 9 months after initiation of therapy
    - Symptoms can occur after discontinuation of drug
  - Sunitinib
    - Inhibits receptor tyrosine kinases such as VEGF
    - Endothelial damage causes TMA
- Immunomodulators
  - Calcineurin inhibitors (CNi)
    - Cyclosporine and tacrolimus are associated with TMA
    - Direct endothelial toxicity due to reduced prostacyclin synthesis or reduced formation of activated protein C
    - Toxicity often seen in 1st 6 months after transplantation
  - Sirolimus
    - Mammalian target of rapamycin (mTOR) regulates production of VEGF in addition to its effects on cell cycle
    - Inhibition of VEGF results in endothelial damage
    - Toxicity is exacerbated by concomitant calcineurin inhibitors
- Antiplatelet drugs of thienopyridine family
  - Ticlopidine and clopidogrel
    - TMA occurs within 1st month (or even within 1st week) of exposure
    - Cause direct endothelial toxicity
    - ADAMTS13 levels can be severely deficient (< 5%) in some cases, and inhibitor to ADAMTS13 has been detected
- Miscellaneous drugs
  - Quinine
    - Used for treatment of malaria and nocturnal leg cramps; found in herbal supplements and tonic water
    - Patients develop antibodies to platelet glycoprotein Ib/IX or IIb/IIIa complexes
    - TMA development is not dose related, can occur after years of intake, and recurs after reexposure
  - α-interferon, cocaine, simvastatin, aprotinin, valacyclovir, H2-receptor antagonists, NSAIDs, vaccines, several antibiotics, and hormone supplements

THROMBOTIC MICROANGIOPATHY, DRUGS

Key Facts

Etiology/Pathogenesis
- Direct endothelial injury or immune mediated
- > 60 drugs reportedly associated with TMA, but often difficult to establish causative role
  - Chemotherapeutic agents
  - Anti-vascular endothelial growth factor (VEGF) therapy
  - Immunomodulators (CNi, mTORi)
  - Antiplatelet drugs of thienopyridine family
  - Quinine

Clinical Issues
- Proteinuria ranges from mild to nephrotic
- Mild renal insufficiency or acute renal failure
- Worsening hypertension
- Treatment
  - Withdrawal of offending drug
- Plasma exchange helpful in some settings
- Better prognosis if TMA is limited to kidney
- Diagnosis
  - Thrombocytopenia
  - Schistocytes on peripheral smear
  - Serum lactate dehydrogenase may be elevated
  - ADAMTS13 levels may be low in TMA due to thienopyridines

Microscopic Pathology
- Fibrin thrombi and endothelial swelling in glomeruli and arterioles
- Reduplicated GBM in chronic phase

Top Differential Diagnoses
- TMA due to other causes
- Antibody-mediated rejection in renal allografts

CLINICAL ISSUES

Presentation
- Proteinuria ranges from mild to nephrotic
- Microscopic hematuria
- Mild renal insufficiency or acute renal failure
- Worsening hypertension

Laboratory Tests
- Thrombocytopenia
- Schistocytes may be present on peripheral smear
- Serum lactic acid dehydrogenase may be elevated

Treatment
- Withdrawal of offending drug
- Plasma exchange helpful in some settings

Prognosis
- Variable but usually associated with high morbidity and mortality
- Better prognosis if TMA is limited to the kidney as can occur in renal transplantation

MICROSCOPIC PATHOLOGY

Histologic Features
- Glomeruli
  - Fibrin thrombi and endothelial swelling
  - Ischemic collapse of capillary tuft
  - Mesangiolysis
  - Duplicated GBM in chronic phase
- Tubulointerstitium
  - Acute tubular injury with degenerating epithelium
- Arterioles and interlobular arteries
  - Endothelial swelling and fibrinoid necrosis

ANCILLARY TESTS

Immunofluorescence
- Fibrin in thrombi
- Nonspecific entrapment of C3, IgM in glomeruli and vessels

Electron Microscopy
- Glomeruli
  - Endothelial swelling and subendothelial expansion by lucent material; loss of endothelial fenestrations
  - Platelets and fibrin in capillary lumina
  - No electron-dense deposits

DIFFERENTIAL DIAGNOSIS

TMA Due to Other Causes
- Rule out: Malignant hypertension, postpartum, scleroderma, HUS/TTP
- Clinical history and serological evidence of autoantibodies help determine etiology

Antibody-mediated Rejection
- C4d stain and donor-specific antibodies usually (+)
- Glomerulitis, tubulointerstitial inflammation, and peritubular capillaritis are helpful if present

SELECTED REFERENCES

1. Stokes MB et al: Glomerular disease related to anti-VEGF therapy. Kidney Int. 74(11):1487-91, 2008
2. Roncone D et al: Proteinuria in a patient receiving anti-VEGF therapy for metastatic renal cell carcinoma. Nat Clin Pract Nephrol. 3(5):287-93, 2007
3. Zakarija A et al: Drug-induced thrombotic microangiopathy. Semin Thromb Hemost. 31(6):681-90, 2005
4. Robson M et al: Thrombotic micro-angiopathy with sirolimus-based immunosuppression: potentiation of calcineurin-inhibitor-induced endothelial damage? Am J Transplant. 3(3):324-7, 2003
5. Schwimmer J et al: De novo thrombotic microangiopathy in renal transplant recipients: a comparison of hemolytic uremic syndrome with localized renal thrombotic microangiopathy. Am J Kidney Dis. 41(2):471-9, 2003
6. Medina PJ et al: Drug-associated thrombotic thrombocytopenic purpura-hemolytic uremic syndrome. Curr Opin Hematol. 8(5):286-93, 2001

3

Microscopic Features

(Left) A 39-year-old woman, 3 weeks post renal transplantation, presented with acute renal failure. Fibrin thrombi ⊡ are seen in the capillary lumens, and TMA is attributed to cyclosporine toxicity. *(Right)* The glomerulus shows collapse of the capillary tuft with wrinkling of the GBM ⊡. Characteristic features of TMA with arteriolar and glomerular fibrin thrombi are seen elsewhere in this biopsy from a patient with cyclosporine toxicity.

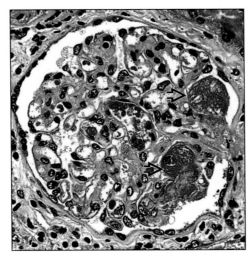
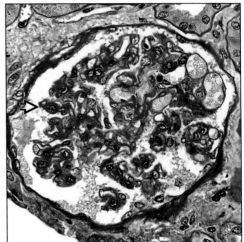

(Left) The patient presented 3 weeks post renal transplantation with acute renal failure, and biopsy revealed TMA. Patchy areas of severe tubular necrosis ⊡ are seen with loss of cellular detail. *(Right)* The glomerulus shows extensive double contours ⊡ with associated endothelial swelling ⊡. TMA in this 13 year old is attributed to sirolimus. The patient is 12 years post renal transplantation and has not been on calcineurin inhibitors for 2 years prior to the biopsy.

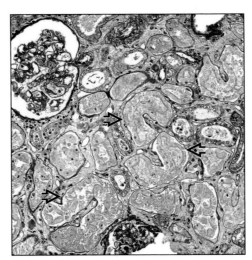
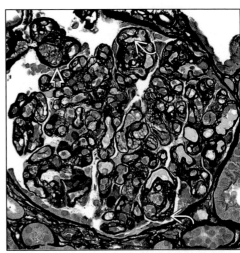

(Left) Glomerular fibrin thrombus ⊡ stains red on trichrome in this biopsy with TMA. Histological features do not help distinguish the etiology of TMA, and in this case, it is clinically attributed to sirolimus toxicity. *(Right)* An interlobular artery shows severe intimal edema ⊡ with luminal occlusion. No inflammatory infiltrate is seen to suggest vasculitis. The arteriolar TMA changes in this post transplantation biopsy are due to sirolimus.

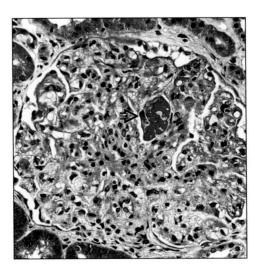
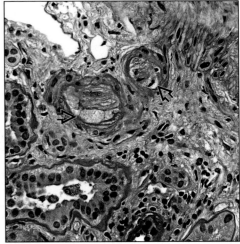

THROMBOTIC MICROANGIOPATHY, DRUGS

Microscopic Features

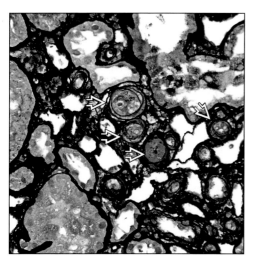

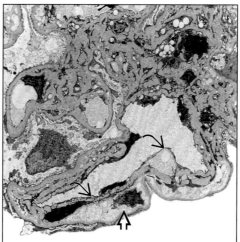

(Left) Cross sections of arterioles show endothelial swelling ➡ with entrapped erythrocytes and apoptotic debris. These TMA changes are due to VEGF trap therapy the patient received for metastatic prostate carcinoma. *(Right)* TMA is characterized by expansion of the subendothelial space as seen in this biopsy. The endothelial membrane ➡ is lifted off the GBM with subendothelial cells and flocculent material ➡. TMA in this case is due to aflibercept, a VEGF trap.

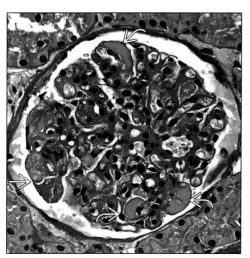

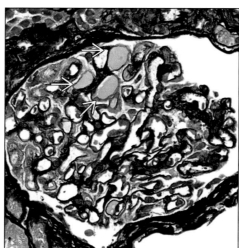

(Left) This glomerulus shows focal mesangiolysis ➡ and amorphous luminal thrombi ➡. The patient is a 51-year-old man with metastatic neuroendocrine carcinoma of an unknown primary site who received bevacizumab (anti-VEGF antibody). *(Right)* The capillary lumens show pale luminal material ➡ confirmed to be fibrin thrombi on ultrastructural examination. Other glomeruli had foci of mesangiolysis and double contours. TMA changes are due to anti-VEGF therapy.

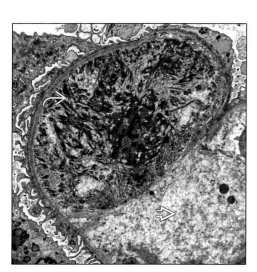

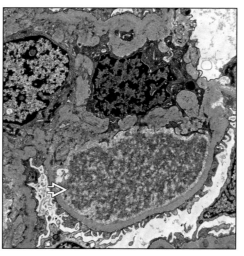

(Left) A fibrin thrombus in the capillary lumen is composed of both fibrin tactoids ➡ and depolymerized fibrin ➡. The patient received bevacizumab for neuroendocrine carcinoma and subsequently presented with proteinuria due to TMA. *(Right)* The capillary lumen in this biopsy with TMA is nearly occluded by depolymerized fibrin ➡. This prothrombotic state is likely caused by anti-VEGF antibody the patient received for a metastatic neuroendocrine carcinoma.

3

POSTPARTUM HEMOLYTIC UREMIC SYNDROME

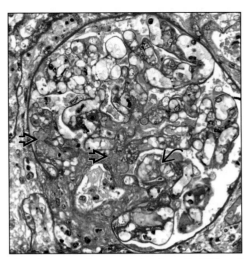

The glomerulus shows endothelial swelling ⇨ and denudation along with capillary lumen fibrin thrombi ⇥ in PHUS. The patient underwent a C-section for HELLP syndrome 6 days prior.

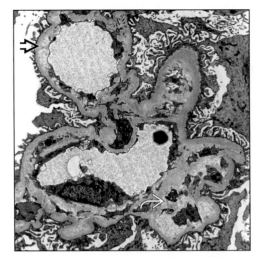

Ultrastructurally, PHUS shows accumulation of electron-lucent material in the subendothelium ⇥ and mesangium ⬊. Glomerular and arteriolar fibrin thrombi were also seen in the biopsy.

TERMINOLOGY

Abbreviations
- Postpartum hemolytic uremic syndrome (PHUS)

Definitions
- HUS occurring in postpartum period, characterized by microangiopathic hemolytic anemia, thrombocytopenia, and acute renal failure
  - Vast majority categorized as atypical HUS although occasional infection-related (verotoxin) classic HUS forms reported

ETIOLOGY/PATHOGENESIS

Genetic Abnormalities in Complement System
- High incidence of mutations in complement genes (86% in one series)
  - Mutations in genes encoding factor H (CFH), factor I, C3, membrane cofactor protein (MCP)
    - These factors regulate alternate complement pathway cascade via their effects on C3 convertase
    - Mutations cause quantitative deficiencies of factors or impaired binding of factors to C3b
    - As a result, C3 convertase causes persistent activation of alternate complement pathway
  - Excessive complement activation causes endothelial injury and, consequently, a prothrombotic state
- Homozygosity for high risk-associated haplotypes of CFH and MCP genes have been detected in > 50% of patients

Increased Susceptibility During Postpartum Period
- Physiological mechanisms protect fetus from maternal complement-mediated immunological attack
  - Complement regulatory factors MCP, decay accelerating factor, and CD59 are expressed on trophoblasts
  - Factor H may be synthesized by trophoblasts
  - All these mechanisms downregulate C3 convertase, preventing complement activation
- Antepartum protective mechanisms may be compromised in immediate postpartum period in susceptible individuals
  - Sudden lack of complement regulatory factors
  - Peripartum inflammation, infections, and hemorrhage potentially activate alternate complement pathway

Other
- Other reported etiological causes include infections and anticardiolipin antibodies

CLINICAL ISSUES

Epidemiology
- Incidence
  - Postpartum subtype accounts for approximately 15% of atypical HUS
    - Risk of PHUS seems highest during 2nd pregnancy

Presentation
- Symptoms manifest postpartum within 24 hours to several weeks
  - Acute renal failure, hematuria, and proteinuria
  - Fever and severe hypertension
- Some patients may have preceding preeclampsia, acute fatty liver of pregnancy, or HELLP syndrome
  - Persistent and severe renal abnormalities postpartum suggest atypical HUS

Laboratory Tests
- Schistocytes in peripheral smear
- Elevated lactate dehydrogenase
- Thrombocytopenia

POSTPARTUM HEMOLYTIC UREMIC SYNDROME

Key Facts

Terminology
- HUS occurring in postpartum period, characterized by microangiopathic hemolytic anemia, thrombocytopenia, and acute renal failure

Etiology/Pathogenesis
- Patients have high incidence of mutations in complement genes
- Antepartum protective mechanisms are compromised in immediate postpartum period in susceptible individuals

Clinical Issues
- Symptoms manifest postpartum within 24 hours to several weeks
- Some patients have preceding preeclampsia, acute fatty liver of pregnancy, or HELLP syndrome

Microscopic Pathology
- Glomerular endothelial swelling, fragmented RBCs, and fibrin thrombi
  ○ Lobulated accentuation and double contours predominate in chronic phase
- Fibrin thrombi and mucoid intimal edema in arterioles
- Cortical necrosis and infarction in severe cases
- Electron microscopy
  ○ Subendothelial expansion by electron-lucent flocculent material and mesangiolysis
  ○ Fibrin tactoids and depolymerized fibrin in capillary lumens or subendothelial areas
  ○ No electron-dense deposits

Treatment
- Plasma exchange and steroids may be beneficial

Prognosis
- Frequent progression to end-stage kidney disease

MICROSCOPIC PATHOLOGY

Histologic Features
- Glomeruli
  ○ Glomerular endothelial swelling, fragmented RBCs, and fibrin thrombi
    ▪ Lobulated accentuation and double contours predominate in chronic phase
- Tubules and interstitium
  ○ Acute tubular injury with loss of brush borders and simplified epithelium
  ○ Cortical necrosis and infarction in severe cases
- Vessels
  ○ Fibrin thrombi and mucoid intimal edema in arterioles

ANCILLARY TESTS

Immunofluorescence
- No evidence of immune complexes
  ○ IgM and C3 along GBM
- Fibrin thrombi in arterioles stain for fibrin

Electron Microscopy
- Glomeruli
  ○ Subendothelial expansion by electron-lucent flocculent material and mesangiolysis
  ○ Fibrin tactoids and depolymerized fibrin in capillary lumens or subendothelial areas
  ○ GBM remodeling with neobasement membrane formation in chronic phase
  ○ No electron-dense deposits

DIFFERENTIAL DIAGNOSIS

Thrombotic Thrombocytopenic Purpura (TTP)
- Due to ADAMTS13 deficiency or autoantibodies directed against it
- Pregnancy may be initial presentation or can exacerbate recurrence in patients with known TTP
  ○ Vulnerability during pregnancy due to progressive physiological decrease in ADAMTS13
- Often presents in late 2nd or 3rd trimesters
- Renal involvement is often mild, and neurological symptoms predominate

Thrombotic Microangiopathy Due to Other Causes
- Clinical and serological tests may identify potential causes such as drugs, infections, neoplasms, or autoimmune diseases

SELECTED REFERENCES

1. Fakhouri F et al: Pregnancy-associated hemolytic uremic syndrome revisited in the era of complement gene mutations. J Am Soc Nephrol. 21(5):859-67, 2010
2. Magee CC et al: Case records of the Massachusetts General Hospital. Case 2-2008. A 38-year-old woman with postpartum visual loss, shortness of breath, and renal failure. N Engl J Med. 358(3):275-89, 2008
3. Martin JN Jr et al: Thrombotic thrombocytopenic purpura in 166 pregnancies: 1955-2006. Am J Obstet Gynecol. 199(2):98-104, 2008
4. Sánchez-Luceros A et al: von Willebrand factor-cleaving protease (ADAMTS13) activity in normal non-pregnant women, pregnant and post-delivery women. Thromb Haemost. 92(6):1320-6, 2004
5. Banatvala N et al: The United States National Prospective Hemolytic Uremic Syndrome Study: microbiologic, serologic, clinical, and epidemiologic findings. J Infect Dis. 183(7):1063-70, 2001

Microscopic Features

(Left) A 27-year-old woman with preeclampsia, 1 week postpartum, underwent a kidney biopsy for acute renal failure. Diffuse endothelial swelling is seen, and focal fibrin thrombi were observed in arterioles, compatible with PHUS. *(Right)* The patient developed acute renal failure 1 week postpartum, and the biopsy had characteristic features of thrombotic microangiopathy. Fibrin thrombus is seen in the arteriole ➡, and the glomerulus had entrapped RBCs ➡ in the mesangium.

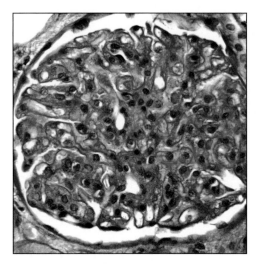

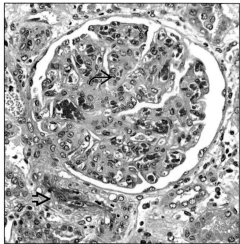

(Left) Nonspecific entrapment of IgM within the glomerulus is seen on immunofluorescence microscopy. Focal segmental staining was also seen with C3. This biopsy is from a young woman who was 1 week postpartum and had persistently elevated levels of serum creatinine. The light microscopy was compatible with thrombotic microangiopathy. *(Right)* Acute tubular injury is evident with loss of brush borders ➡ and sloughed epithelial cells ➡ in this biopsy from a patient with PHUS.

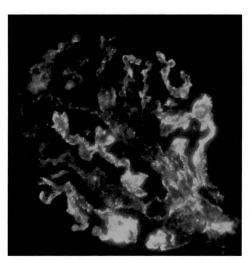

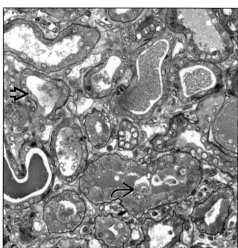

(Left) An aggregate of platelets ➡ is seen in the glomerular capillary lumen. Characteristic features of thrombotic microangiopathy were observed on light microscopy in this 27-year-old woman with acute renal failure and PHUS. *(Right)* The subendothelial zone ➡ is expanded by lucent flocculent material in PHUS. The endothelial cells are reactive and have lost fenestrations ➡. Duplication of the glomerular basement membrane is observed with an entrapped platelet ➡.

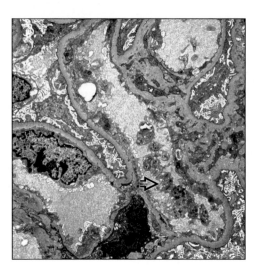

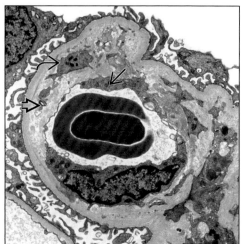

Postpartum HUS and Cortical Necrosis

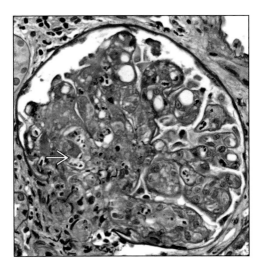

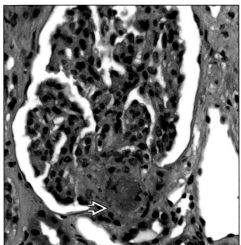

(Left) A 38-year-old woman with postpartum acute renal failure and visual and pulmonary manifestations had characteristic features of TMA on kidney biopsy. Both IgG and IgM anticardiolipin antibodies were positive. The glomerulus shows fibrin deposition and karyorrhexis ➡. (Right) Arteriolar fibrin thrombus is seen at the vascular pole ➡. Serological studies confirmed antiphospholipid antibody syndrome as the cause of PHUS. Approximately 20% of biopsy tissue was infarcted.

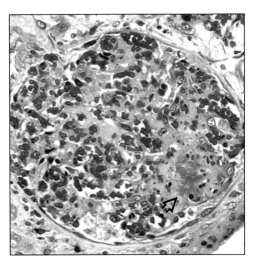

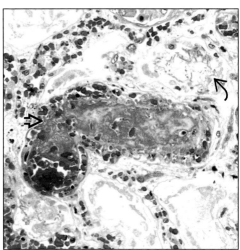

(Left) A 33-year-old woman underwent a C-section at 25 weeks gestation for presumed HELLP syndrome. Within a few days, the patient developed acute renal failure, and renal biopsy showed glomerular fibrin thrombi ➡, compatible with PHUS. Extensive cortical necrosis was also present. (Right) Arteriolar fibrin thrombi ➡ are seen with entrapped RBCs in a biopsy with PHUS. Fibrin strands ➡ are also observed within adjacent tubular lumens.

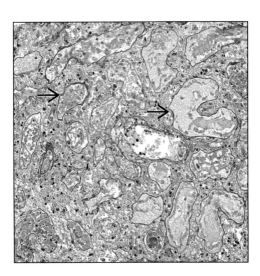

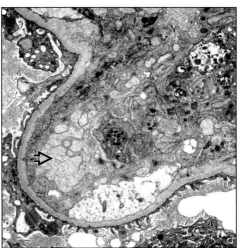

(Left) Extensive cortical necrosis can be observed in severe PHUS. Fibrin thrombi identified in several arterioles likely precipitated cortical necrosis. Only outlines of the tubules ➡ are observed within the infarcted parenchyma. (Right) Severe endothelial cell swelling ➡ and electron-lucent material is seen in the subendothelium. The capillary lumen is occluded. Arteriolar and glomerular fibrin thrombi were identified elsewhere in the biopsy with PHUS.

SCLERODERMA RENAL DISEASE

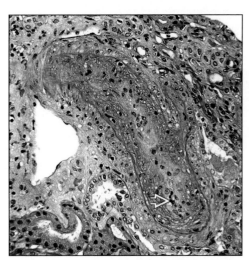

Arterial and arteriolar changes predominate in thrombotic microangiopathy due to scleroderma renal crisis. An interlobular artery is completely occluded by intimal edema ⊳ and proliferation.

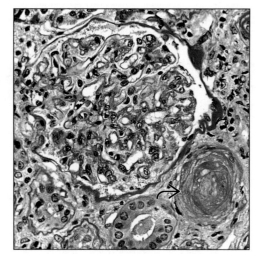

The glomeruli are relatively spared in SRC, as seen in this 37-year-old woman with Raynaud phenomenon and features of scleroderma. An adjacent arteriole with TMA ⊳ has an "onion skin" appearance.

TERMINOLOGY

Synonyms
- Scleroderma

ETIOLOGY/PATHOGENESIS

Endothelial Injury
- Altered vascular permeability, intimal edema, and platelet aggregation
  - Upregulation of growth factors and downregulation of complement regulatory proteins observed
- Cause of endothelial injury unclear
  - Endothelial autoantibodies detected in 25-75% of systemic sclerosis (SS)
    - Uncertain specificities and relevance
  - Pathogenicity of autoantibodies such as anti-RNA polymerase and anti-RNP unknown
- Excessive production of extracellular matrix components by fibroblasts in SS
  - Increased fibroblast expression of TGF-β receptors
  - Other factors include platelet-derived growth factor, connective tissue growth factor, endothelin (ET)-1
    - Certain polymorphisms of ET receptors often seen in patients at risk for scleroma renal crisis (SRC)

Positive Feedback Loop
- Arterial luminal narrowing triggers renin production and exacerbates hypertension

CLINICAL ISSUES

Epidemiology
- Incidence
  - SRC occurs in approximately 10-20% of SS patients
    - Diffuse cutaneous scleroderma is SRC risk factor
    - Corticosteroids are known to precipitate SRC
- Gender
  - Both SS and SRC are more frequent in women

Presentation
- SS disease spectrum includes limited cutaneous, diffuse cutaneous, limited SS, or absent skin sclerosis
  - Nonrenal clinical presentation varies based on extent of involvement
- Scleroderma renal crisis
  - New onset malignant hypertension
  - Elevated serum creatinine and acute renal failure
  - Headaches, fever, and malaise
  - Systemic symptoms of convulsions, visual disturbances, dyspnea, or arrhythmias may be observed due to end organ damage
  - Mild hypertension may precede SS or may represent aborted SRC due to ACE-inhibitor therapy
- Other kidney diseases are uncommon
  - Proteinuria, especially nephrotic range, seen in D-penicillamine-related membranous nephropathy
  - ANCA-related glomerulonephritis (MPO-ANCA) has been reported in SS patients treated with D-penicillamine
  - Mild renal insufficiency due to renal artery stenosis, prerenal, or unrelated causes

Laboratory Tests
- Thrombotic microangiopathy in 50% of SRC cases
  - Peripheral schistocytes, anemia, and low platelets
  - Elevated lactate dehydrogenase, low haptoglobin
- Antinuclear antibodies in > 90% of SS patients
- SS-related autoantibodies
  - Anti-topoisomerase 1 and anti-RNA polymerase (I & III) antibodies often associated with SRC

Treatment
- Adjuvant therapy
  - Many SRC patients require prolonged dialysis
- Drugs
  - Angiotensin converting enzyme (ACE) inhibitor
  - Aggressive control of blood pressure

SCLERODERMA RENAL DISEASE

Key Facts

Etiology/Pathogenesis
- Endothelial injury of uncertain cause
  - Antiendothelial antibodies in ~ 50%
  - Altered vascular permeability and platelet aggregation
  - Increased renin production and positive feedback loop exacerbates hypertension
- Excessive production of extracellular matrix

Clinical Issues
- Scleroderma renal crisis (SRC)
  - New onset malignant hypertension
  - Acute renal failure
  - Angiotensin converting enzyme inhibitor therapy
- Chronic kidney disease is uncommon

Microscopic Pathology
- Arcuate and interlobular arteries more often affected by thrombotic microangiopathy (TMA)
  - Intimal mucoid edema and endothelial swelling result in "onion skin" concentric appearance
  - Luminal occlusion and fragmented RBCs
  - Fibrin thrombi and fibrinoid necrosis
- Predominant arterial involvement results in ischemic collapse of glomerular capillary tufts
- Electron microscopy
  - Endothelial swelling, loss, and reactive changes
  - GBM duplication
  - Expands subendothelial electron-lucent material
  - No immune or electron-dense deposits

Prognosis
- Diffuse cutaneous SS, cardiac involvement, vascular thrombosis, and severe glomerular ischemia on biopsy predict poor renal survival

MICROSCOPIC PATHOLOGY

Histologic Features
- Glomeruli
  - May show fibrin thrombi, endothelial swelling, and fibrinoid necrosis
    - GBM duplication, mesangiolysis in chronic cases
    - Predominant arterial involvement results in ischemic collapse of glomerular capillary tufts
- Tubules
  - Acute tubular injury or variable tubular atrophy and interstitial fibrosis
- Arterial changes predominate in SRC
  - Arcuate and interlobular arteries more often affected by thrombotic microangiopathy (TMA)
    - Luminal occlusion and fragmented RBCs
    - Fibrin thrombi and fibrinoid necrosis
  - Intimal mucoid edema and endothelial swelling result in "onion skin" concentric appearance
    - No associated vessel wall inflammation
    - Duplication of internal elastic lamina and adventitial fibrosis seen in chronic cases
- Non-SRC chronic changes described in autopsy series
  - Increased arterial intimal fibrosis
  - Increased tubular atrophy and interstitial fibrosis
- Superimposed histological changes in SS
  - Penicillamine-induced membranous nephropathy or pauci-immune glomerulonephritis

ANCILLARY TESTS

Immunofluorescence
- Nonspecific entrapment of IgM, C3, and fibrinogen observed in glomeruli &/or arteries
- No evidence of immune complexes

Electron Microscopy
- No electron-dense deposits
- Endothelial swelling and expanded subendothelial space by electron-lucent material
- GBM duplication and mesangial cell interposition in chronic phase

Special Studies
- Endothelin-1 increased in glomeruli and arteries

DIFFERENTIAL DIAGNOSIS

Thrombotic Microangiopathy, Other Causes
- Clinical and serological data help differentiate SRC from other causes of thrombotic microangiopathy
  - Malignant hypertension, drugs, HUS/TTP, pregnancy, rejection, etc.
- Glomerular changes often predominate

Immune Complex-mediated GN
- Variable mesangial or endocapillary proliferation seen
- Immune complexes identified by IF and EM

SELECTED REFERENCES

1. Mouthon L et al: Endothelin-1 expression in scleroderma renal crisis. Hum Pathol. 42(1):95-102, 2011
2. Batal I et al: Scleroderma renal crisis: a pathology perspective. Int J Rheumatol. 2010:543704, 2010
3. Mihai C et al: Anti-endothelial cell antibodies in systemic sclerosis. Ann Rheum Dis. 69(2):319-24, 2010
4. Batal I et al: Renal biopsy findings predicting outcome in scleroderma renal crisis. Hum Pathol. 40(3):332-40, 2009
5. Steen VD et al: Kidney disease other than renal crisis in patients with diffuse scleroderma. J Rheumatol. 32(4):649-55, 2005
6. Denton CP et al: Scleroderma--clinical and pathological advances. Best Pract Res Clin Rheumatol. 18(3):271-90, 2004
7. Steen VD: Scleroderma renal crisis. Rheum Dis Clin North Am. 22(4):861-78, 1996
8. Donohoe JF: Scleroderma and the kidney. Kidney Int. 41(2):462-77, 1992

Microscopic Features

(Left) A 46-year-old woman with dermatomyositis and features suggestive of SS presented with acute renal failure. The interlobular arteries demonstrate intimal edema with luminal fibrin thrombi ➡ while the adjacent glomerulus ➡ shows mild ischemic collapse. *(Right)* Cross sections of interlobular arteries ➡ show fibrin thrombi, karyorrhexis, and entrapped schistocytes. Based on the clinical history of SS, these characteristic features of TMA are attributed to SRC.

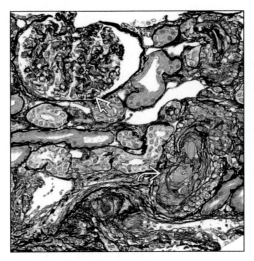
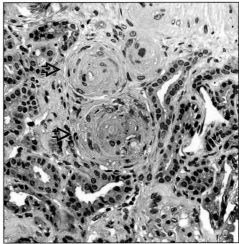

(Left) The interlobular arterial walls show concentric lamination with associated edema and severe narrowing of the lumens ("onion skinning"). Arcuate arteries are also similarly affected in SRC. *(Right)* The glomerulus appears ischemic and "bloodless" in this 63-year-old man with SS and acute renal failure. All interlobular and arcuate arteries sampled in the biopsy had characteristic features of acute thrombotic microangiopathy due to SRC.

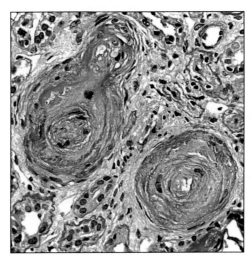
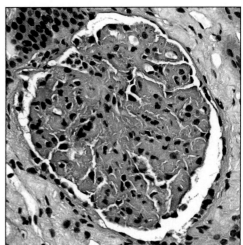

(Left) Severe mucoid intimal edema is seen in this cross section of an arcuate caliber artery. The patient, a 64-year-old man with SS, was biopsied for rapidly progressive renal failure. Almost all arteries sampled in the biopsy were affected. *(Right)* A 36-year-old woman with mixed connective tissue disorder and SS presented with malignant hypertension and nephrotic range proteinuria. Luminal fibrin thrombus ➡ and intimal concentric lamination are seen within an interlobular artery.

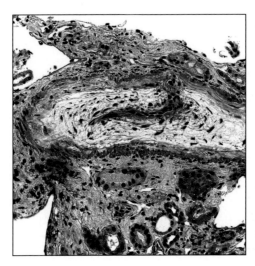
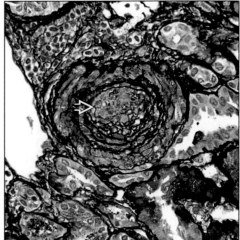

SCLERODERMA RENAL DISEASE

Microscopic Features

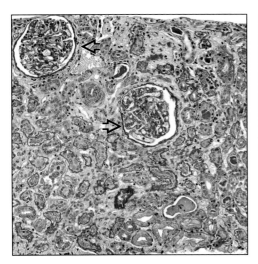

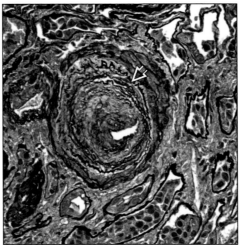

(Left) Extensive glomerular ischemic retraction ⇒ and tubular atrophy are seen in this kidney biopsy. Characteristic arterial wall changes were seen elsewhere in this biopsy from a 36-year-old woman with SRC. *(Right)* Concentric lamination, intimal fibrosis, and internal elastic lamina duplication ⇒ are seen in an interlobular artery. Extensive glomerular ischemia and chronic tubulointerstitial damage in the adjacent parenchyma are compatible with chronic TMA due to SRC.

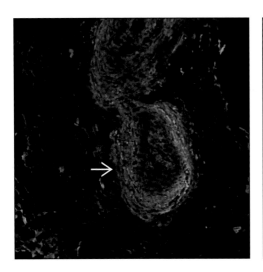

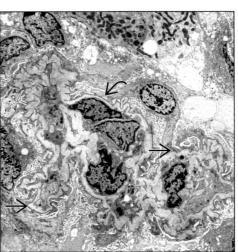

(Left) Antisera to fibrinogen highlights an arcuate caliber artery ⇒ in a biopsy with SRC-related TMA. Fibrin is seen both in the arterial lumen and entrapped within the edematous intima. *(Right)* The glomerular basement membrane shows extensive wrinkling ⇒ with a collapsed capillary tuft. The podocytes demonstrate foot process effacement ⇒, and electron-dense deposits are observed. The arteries in the biopsy had classic features of SRC-related TMA.

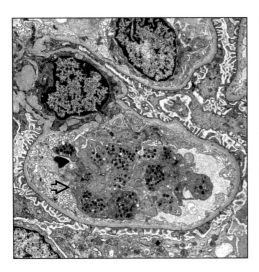

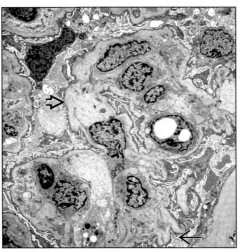

(Left) A platelet thrombus ⇒ is seen within the capillary lumen. The biopsy is from an SS patient with acute renal failure. Endothelial injury in SRC causes altered vascular permeability, intimal edema, and platelet aggregation. *(Right)* Electron-lucent flocculent material ⇒ is seen in the mesangium and subendothelium, compatible with acute TMA. Some capillary loops have lost their endothelium and collapsed ⇒ in this 37-year-old woman with SS and acute renal failure.

PRE-ECLAMPSIA, ECLAMPSIA, HELLP SYNDROME

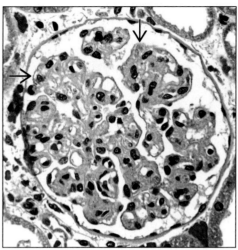

Marked swelling of the endothelial cells ➔ in the glomerular capillaries gives the glomerulus a "bloodless" appearance that is characteristic of pre-eclampsia.

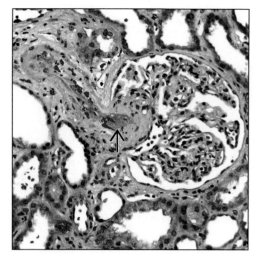

Hematoxylin & eosin reveals an arteriolar thrombus ➔ with entrapped red blood cells and red blood cell fragments from a pregnant woman with HELLP syndrome.

TERMINOLOGY

Abbreviations
- Hemolysis, elevated liver enzymes, low platelets (HELLP) syndrome

Synonyms
- Toxemia of pregnancy
- Pregnancy-induced hypertension

Definitions
- Pre-eclampsia is characterized by hypertension, proteinuria, and edema
- Eclampsia is characterized by of pre-eclampsia with seizures and neurologic symptoms superimposed

ETIOLOGY/PATHOGENESIS

Proposed Mechanism for Pre-eclampsia/ Eclampsia
- Placental factor
  - Upregulation of soluble fms-like tyrosine kinase-1 (sFlt-1)
    - Receptor for vascular endothelial growth factor (VEGF)
  - Endothelial cell injury
  - Symptoms resolve with delivery of placenta
  - Glomerular endothelium is dependent on podocyte for high local levels of VEGF
- Anti-VEGF monoclonal antibody therapy also causes proteinuria

Proposed Mechanism for HELLP Syndrome
- May be related to pregnancy-associated atypical hemolytic uremic syndrome
  - Mutations in complement factors C3, B, H, I, or membrane cofactor protein (MCP)
  - Acquired autoantibodies to factor H

Animal Models
- Homozygous knockout of VEGF in podocytes in mice results in perinatal lethality
  - Heterozygous deletion leads to glomerular endotheliosis mimicking human renal lesions of pre-eclampsia/eclampsia

CLINICAL ISSUES

Epidemiology
- Incidence
  - Pre-eclampsia
    - 5-8% of pregnancies
  - HELLP syndrome
    - 4-12% of pre-eclampsia patients

Presentation
- Hypertension
- Headache
- Proteinuria
  - Often after 20 weeks gestation
- Acute kidney injury
  - Rare

Treatment
- Surgical approaches
  - Delivery of placenta
- Drugs
  - Magnesium sulfate
- Bedrest
- Emergent delivery or termination of pregnancy if life-threatening symptoms present

Prognosis
- Approximately 20% have recurrence with subsequent pregnancies
- If 1st pregnancy is normal, low risk (< 1%) for pre-eclampsia in subsequent pregnancies

PRE-ECLAMPSIA, ECLAMPSIA, HELLP SYNDROME

Key Facts

Terminology
- Toxemia of pregnancy
- Pregnancy-induced hypertension
- Pre-eclampsia is characterized by hypertension, proteinuria, and edema
- Eclampsia is characterized by seizures or convulsions along with signs and symptoms of pre-eclampsia

Etiology/Pathogenesis
- Placental factor
- Upregulation of soluble fms-like tyrosin kinase-1 (sFlt-1)

Clinical Issues
- Pre-eclampsia
  - 5-8% of pregnancies
- HELLP syndrome
  - 4-12% of pre-eclampsia patients
- Hypertension
- Headache

Microscopic Pathology
- "Bloodless" appearance due to occlusion by swollen endothelial cells
- Duplication of glomerular basement membranes
- Mesangiolysis
- Focal segmental glomerulosclerosis
- Glomerular endotheliosis
- Thrombotic microangiopathy

Top Differential Diagnoses
- Other causes of TMA

MACROSCOPIC FEATURES

Size
- Normal to slight enlargement

MICROSCOPIC PATHOLOGY

Histologic Features
- Glomeruli
  - Glomerular endotheliosis
    - "Bloodless" appearance due to occlusion by swollen endothelial cells
    - Normal arterioles
    - Duplication of glomerular basement membranes
    - Focal segmental glomerulosclerosis
    - Collapsing glomerulopathy (rare)
    - Rare crescents
    - Mesangiolysis
- Tubules
  - Ischemic changes
- Interstitium: No specific changes
- Vessels
  - Thrombotic microangiopathy (TMA) may be present
    - May involve glomerular capillaries or arterioles

Predominant Pattern/Injury Type
- Thrombosis

Predominant Cell/Compartment Type
- Endothelial cell

ANCILLARY TESTS

Immunofluorescence
- Fibrin or fibrinogen deposition in some glomerular capillaries
  - IgM may be entrapped in similar distribution as fibrin/fibrinogen
  - Highlights thrombi, if present

Electron Microscopy
- Transmission
  - Reactive endothelium
    - Swelling of endothelial cells
    - Loss of endothelial fenestrations
  - Mesangial cell swelling
  - Podocyte foot processes and slit diaphragms generally well preserved
    - Focal effacement of foot processes may be present
  - Subendothelial space widening by electron-lucent material
    - May not be as prominent as other causes of TMA

DIFFERENTIAL DIAGNOSIS

Other Causes of TMA
- Atypical hemolytic uremic syndrome
  - Mutations in factors C3, B, H, I, or MCP (CD46)
  - TMA with pregnancy in 20% with these mutations
- Anti-phospholipid antibody syndrome
- Thrombotic thrombocytopenic purpura
- Scleroderma
- Malignant hypertension

DIAGNOSTIC CHECKLIST

Pathologic Interpretation Pearls
- Clinical correlation is required to distinguish pre-eclampsia, eclampsia, or HELLP syndrome from each other as well as other etiologies of TMA
- Endotheliosis is highly specific and possibly pathognomonic for pre-eclampsia
  - Poor tissue fixation for electron microscopy may lead to artifactual swelling of endothelial cells

SELECTED REFERENCES

1. Stillman IE et al: The glomerular injury of preeclampsia. J Am Soc Nephrol. 18(8):2281-4, 2007
2. Gaber LW et al: Renal pathology in pre-eclampsia. Baillieres Clin Obstet Gynaecol. 1(4):971-95, 1987

Pre-eclampsia and Eclampsia

(Left) Contrast-enhanced CT in a 30-year-old woman with severe pre-eclampsia and HELLP syndrome shows multiple small areas of renal infarction ➡. The wall of the ascending colon is also thickened ➡ from intramural hemorrhage. *(Right)* Pre-eclampsia manifests glomeruli with a "bloodless" appearance due to prominent swelling of endothelial cells. The glomerular capillary lumina are obscured, which results in a substantial decrease in glomerular filtration.

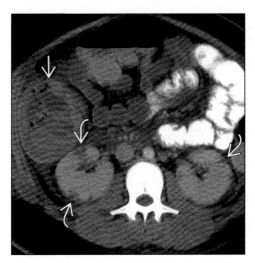

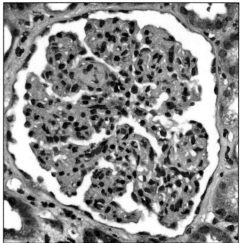

(Left) Periodic acid-Schiff reveals marked swelling of the endothelial cells, which obscures most of the glomerular capillary lumina. *(Right)* Immunofluorescence microscopy highlights some trapping of fibrinogen in subendothelial areas ➡ along a few glomerular capillaries, which supports the diagnosis of pre-eclampsia-associated injury. Evans blue counterstain highlights cell nuclei in red.

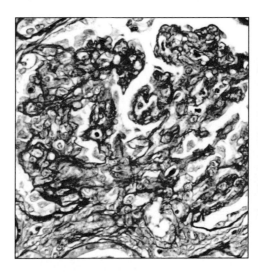

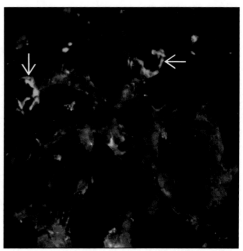

(Left) Diffuse entrapment of fibrinogen is present throughout the glomerular capillaries in subendothelial ➡ and mesangial ➡ areas in this glomerulus from a pre-eclampsia patient. *(Right)* Electron microscopy demonstrates prominent widening of the subendothelial space ➡ and interposition ➡ of foam cells as the overlying endothelial cells show loss of their fenestrations ➡ in this pregnant woman with pre-eclampsia.

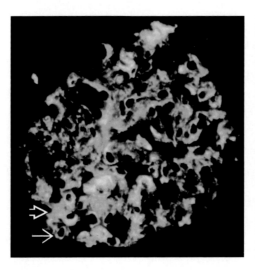

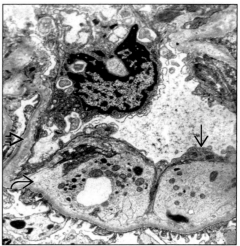

PRE-ECLAMPSIA, ECLAMPSIA, HELLP SYNDROME

HELLP Syndrome

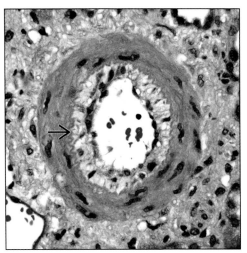 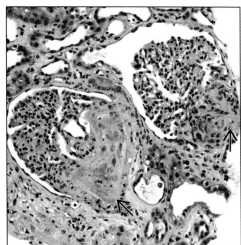

(Left) Hematoxylin & eosin demonstrates marked mucoid intimal change ⮕ in this intralobular artery. This finding is not specific to pre-eclampsia or HELLP syndrome but can also be seen in patients with malignant hypertension or scleroderma. (Right) Hematoxylin & eosin highlights large thrombi with entrapped red blood cells and red cell fragments in the hilar arterioles ⮕ of 2 adjacent glomeruli from a pregnant woman with HELLP syndrome.

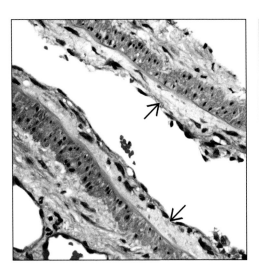 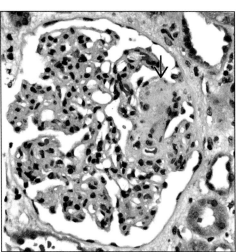

(Left) Hematoxylin & eosin shows marked mucoid intimal change ⮕ in an intrarenal artery of a patient with HFLLP syndrome. This intimal alteration of the artery can also be observed in scleroderma and malignant hypertension. (Right) Hematoxylin & eosin reveals a hilar arteriole with an acute thrombus ⮕ admixed with entrapped red blood cells and red cell fragments. The glomerulus has some ischemic features with mild shrinkage of the glomerular tufts.

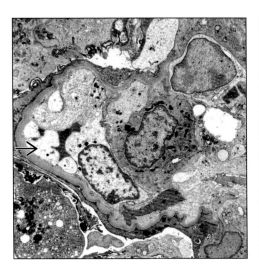 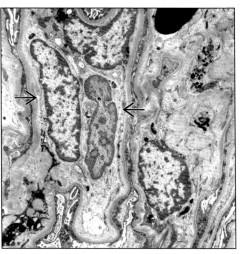

(Left) Electron microscopy reveals prominent swelling ⮕ of the endothelial cells (also termed "endotheliosis"), which decreases the effective glomerular capillary lumen. There is also diffuse effacement of the overlying podocyte foot processes. (Right) These enlarged and swollen endothelial cells ⮕ nearly occupy the entire lumen of this glomerular capillary in a patient with pre-eclampsia. These ultrastructural findings may also be present in HELLP syndrome patients.

RADIATION NEPHROPATHY

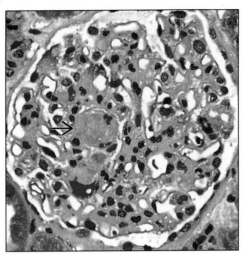

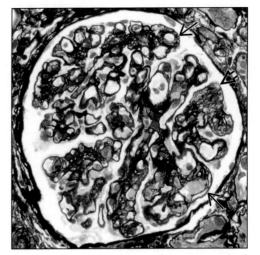

H&E shows a thrombus ➡ *with a few entrapped red blood cells distending a glomerular capillary in a patient with a history of radiation therapy and hematopoietic cell transplantation due to acute myeloid leukemia.*

Jones methenamine silver demonstrates focal mesangiolysis ▷. *There is also frequent duplication of the glomerular basement membranes* ➡, *which is a chronic phase of injury.*

TERMINOLOGY

Synonyms
- Radiation nephritis

Definitions
- Renal injury due to radiation exposure

ETIOLOGY/PATHOGENESIS

Total Body Irradiation Dosage
- 20 to 25 Gy over > 1 month leads to radiation nephropathy

Graft-vs.-Host Disease
- Possible risk factor for developing thrombotic microangiopathy

Additional Risk Factors
- Chemotherapeutic agents may increase risk of developing radiation nephropathy

CLINICAL ISSUES

Epidemiology
- Incidence
  - 20-40% of patients receiving significant radiation
- Age
  - Higher susceptibility in pediatric patients
- Gender
  - No gender predilection
- Ethnicity
  - No ethnic predilection

Presentation
- Renal dysfunction
- Hypertension
- Proteinuria
- Anemia

Prognosis
- Variable
  - Dependent on total radiation dosage

MICROSCOPIC PATHOLOGY

Histologic Features
- Glomeruli
  - Mesangiolysis
  - Capillary thrombi
  - Duplication of GBM
  - Global or segmental glomerular sclerosis
  - Foam cells in glomerular capillaries may be noted
- Interstitium and tubules
  - Interstitial edema
  - Interstitial fibrosis and tubular atrophy
- Arteries and arterioles
  - Mucoid intimal change
  - Thrombi
  - Hyalinosis

Predominant Pattern/Injury Type
- Thrombosis

Predominant Cell/Compartment Type
- Endothelial cell

ANCILLARY TESTS

Histochemistry
- Masson trichrome
  - Reactivity: If present, thrombi stain strongly red

Immunohistochemistry
- CD61 highlights thrombi, if present

Immunofluorescence
- Fibrinogen highlights thrombi, if present

RADIATION NEPHROPATHY

Key Facts

Etiology/Pathogenesis
- 20 to 25 Gy over > 1 month leads to radiation nephropathy
- Possible risk factor for developing thrombotic microangiopathy

Clinical Issues
- Renal dysfunction
- Proteinuria
- Hypertension

Microscopic Pathology
- Thrombi
- GBM duplication if chronic
- Global or segmental glomerulosclerosis
- Interstitial fibrosis and tubular atrophy
- Mucoid intimal change, hyalinosis

Top Differential Diagnoses
- Thrombotic microangiopathy from drugs
- Graft-vs.-host glomerulopathies

- IgM and C3 may demonstrate nonspecific trapping along glomerular basement membranes (GBM) and arterioles

Electron Microscopy
- Transmission
  - Separation of endothelial cells from GBM with widening of subendothelial space by electron-lucent material
  - Duplication of GBM when injury is chronic

DIFFERENTIAL DIAGNOSIS

Thrombotic Microangiopathy Drugs
- Chemotherapeutic agents

Thrombotic Thrombocytopenic Purpura/ Hemolytic Uremic Syndrome
- Correlation with clinical history necessary

Graft-vs.-Host Glomerulopathies
- May occur concurrently with radiation nephropathy

DIAGNOSTIC CHECKLIST

Pathologic Interpretation Pearls
- Clinical history of hematopoietic cell (bone marrow) transplantation

- Chemotherapy often is used in combination with radiation, and both can result in thrombotic microangiopathic injuries

SELECTED REFERENCES

1. Esiashvili N et al: Renal toxicity in children undergoing total body irradiation for bone marrow transplant. Radiother Oncol. 90(2):242-6, 2009
2. Chang A et al: Spectrum of renal pathology in hematopoietic cell transplantation: a series of 20 patients and review of the literature. Clin J Am Soc Nephrol. 2(5):1014-23, 2007
3. Miralbell R et al: Renal insufficiency in patients with hematologic malignancies undergoing total body irradiation and bone marrow transplantation: a prospective assessment. Int J Radiat Oncol Biol Phys. 58(3):809-16, 2004
4. Borg M et al: Renal toxicity after total body irradiation. Int J Radiat Oncol Biol Phys. 54(4):1165-73, 2002
5. Lawton CA et al: Long-term results of selective renal shielding in patients undergoing total body irradiation in preparation for bone marrow transplantation. Bone Marrow Transplant. 20(12):1069-74, 1997
6. Cassady JR: Clinical radiation nephropathy. Int J Radiat Oncol Biol Phys. 31(5):1249-56, 1995
7. Cohen EP et al: Bone marrow transplant nephropathy: radiation nephritis revisited. Nephron. 70(2):217-22, 1995
8. Luxton RW: Radiation nephritis. A long-term study of 54 patients. Lancet. 2(7214):1221-4, 1961

IMAGE GALLERY

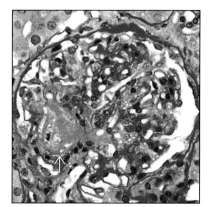 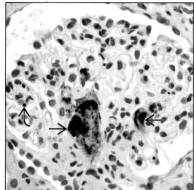 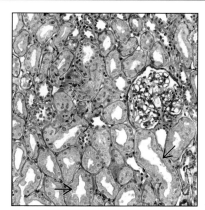

(Left) Periodic acid-Schiff is not the ideal stain for identification of thrombi, but this large hilar thrombus ➡ is easily noted. *(Center)* CD61 highlights the glomerular thrombi ➡. Masson trichrome stain (not shown) can also be useful for identifying thrombi. Normal circulating platelets ➡ are also noted. *(Right)* Features of acute tubular injury with attenuation and loss of the proximal tubular brush borders ➡ correlate with the acute rise in serum creatinine, but other features of thrombotic microangiopathy are not present in this region.

HEREDITARY ENDOTHELIOPATHY, RETINOPATHY, NEPHROPATHY, AND STROKE

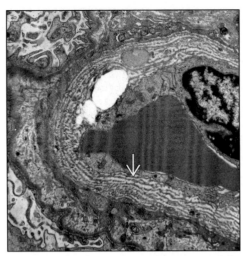

EM reveals the characteristic multilamination of the subendothelial GBM in HERNS ➡. The endothelial cell has an expanded cytoplasm and a deficiency of fenestrations. (Courtesy A. Cohen, MD.)

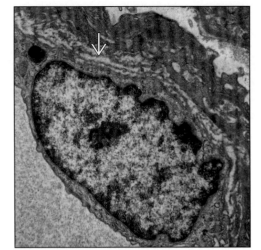

Hereditary endotheliopathy (HERNS) renal biopsy is shown. Electron microscopy of a peritubular capillary shows several layers of new basement membrane ➡. (Courtesy A. Cohen, MD.)

TERMINOLOGY

Abbreviations
- Retinal vasculopathy and cerebral leukodystrophy (RVCL), OMIM 192315
- Hereditary endotheliopathy with retinopathy, nephropathy, and stroke (HERNS)
- 3-prime repair exonuclease (TREX1) mutation, previous termed DNAse III

Synonyms
- RVCL is preferred term for 4 formerly separate syndromes
  - HERNS
  - Cerebroretinal vasculopathy
  - Vascular retinopathy
  - Hereditary systemic angiopathy

Definitions
- Systemic disease causing vascular endothelial injury in brain, retina, kidney, and other sites due to mutation in *TREX1*

ETIOLOGY/PATHOGENESIS

Genetic
- Autosomal dominant trait
- *TREX1* gene on chromosome 3p21
  - Encodes *TREX1*, the most abundant DNA 3'-5' exonuclease
  - Carboxyterminal frameshift mutation
    - *TREX1* becomes diffusely distributed in cytoplasm vs. normal perinuclear space, but exonuclease activity is retained
- 3 generations of Chinese family with 11 affected members
- Other mutations of *TREX1* reported in Aicardi-Goutieres syndrome, familial chilblain lupus, and 3% of systemic lupus erythematosus

Mechanism
- Unknown, probably involving endothelial cell damage/injury
- May involve thrombotic microangiopathy

CLINICAL ISSUES

Presentation
- Chronic renal failure
- Proteinuria, asymptomatic
- Dementia and mood disorders
- Migraine headaches
- Visual field defects due to retinopathy
  - Retinal telangiectasias
  - Macular edema
- Strokes

Natural History
- Onset in middle age
- Progressive dementia, visual loss, and renal dysfunction over 3-4 years

Prognosis
- Uniformly fatal neurological disease over 5-10 years

IMAGE FINDINGS

MR Findings
- Brain MR: Multiple high T2 and gadolinium-enhancing lesions
- Contrast-enhancing lesions in white matter with vasogenic edema

MICROSCOPIC PATHOLOGY

Histologic Features
- Glomeruli
  - Irregularly thickened capillary walls

HEREDITARY ENDOTHELIOPATHY, RETINOPATHY, NEPHROPATHY, AND STROKE

Key Facts

Etiology/Pathogenesis
- Mutation in *TREX1*, encoding a 3'-5' DNA exonuclease

Clinical Issues
- Onset in middle age with neuropsychiatric, retinal, and renal symptoms

Microscopic Pathology
- Glomerular basement membrane thickening

- Arteriolar hyalinosis

Ancillary Tests
- Electron micrograph shows multilaminated basement membranes in capillaries and arteries in kidney and other organs

Top Differential Diagnoses
- Thrombotic microangiopathy (chronic)

---

    o Slightly widened mesangium
- Arteries
    o Subendothelial hyaline and replacement of smooth muscle cells with hyaline
    o Thickened intima with fibrosis
    o Resembles calcineurin inhibitor arteriolopathy
- Endothelial activation described in brain, with enlarged cells, hyperchromatic nuclei, and prominent nucleoli

ANCILLARY TESTS

Electron Microscopy
- Glomeruli
    o Thickened capillary walls
    o Subendothelial multilamination of the glomerular basement membrane (GBM)
        ▪ Original GBM appears normal
    o Mesangial cell interposition
- Peritubular capillaries
    o Multilaminated basement membrane
- Arteries and arterioles
    o Multilaminated basement membrane
- Tubules
    o No distinctive changes in basement membrane
    o Normal mitochondria
- Cerebral vessels
    o Multilamination of capillary basement membrane

DIFFERENTIAL DIAGNOSIS

Thrombotic Microangiopathy (Chronic)
- Thrombi more evident
- Capillaries not affected by multilamination

Chronic Humoral Rejection
- Positive C4d in peritubular capillaries (PTC)
- Limited to kidney

SELECTED REFERENCES

1. Kavanagh D et al: New roles for the major human 3'-5' exonuclease TREX1 in human disease. Cell Cycle. 7(12):1718-25, 2008
2. Winkler DT et al: Hereditary systemic angiopathy (HSA) with cerebral calcifications, retinopathy, progressive nephropathy, and hepatopathy. J Neurol. 255(1):77-88, 2008
3. Richards A et al: C-terminal truncations in human 3'-5' DNA exonuclease TREX1 cause autosomal dominant retinal vasculopathy with cerebral leukodystrophy. Nat Genet. 39(9):1068-70, 2007
4. Seifried C et al: [HERNS. A rare, hereditary, multisystemic disease with cerebral microangiopathy.] Nervenarzt. 76(10):1191-2, 1194-5, 2005
5. Jen J et al: Hereditary endotheliopathy with retinopathy, nephropathy, and stroke (HERNS). Neurology. 49(5):1322-30, 1997

IMAGE GALLERY

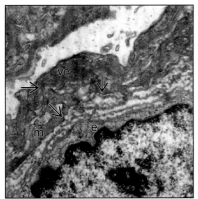 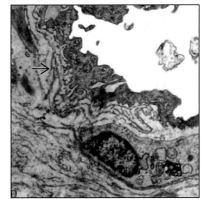 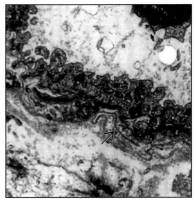

(Left) Glomerular capillary from a patient with RVCL (HERNS) has a multilamination of the GBM ➡ under the endothelial cells (e). Effaced foot processes are present (ve). Mesangial cell (m) interposition is present. (Courtesy A. Cohen, MD.) *(Center)* PTC shows multilamination of the basement membrane ➡. (Courtesy A. Cohen, MD.) *(Right)* Capillaries in other sites, such as the gastric mucosa, also show basement membrane multilamination ➡. (Courtesy A. Cohen, MD.)

SICKLE CELL DISEASE

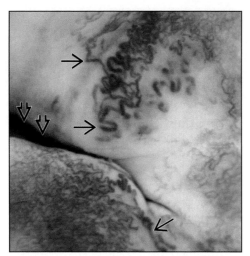

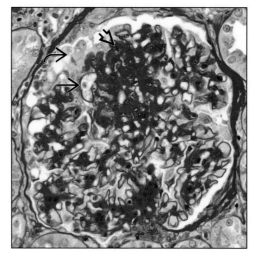

Gross photograph shows marked congestion of the vasa recta ⇨ in the renal pyramid with prominent scarring of the renal papilla ⊃, as shown by the deep horizontal divot. (Courtesy C. Abrahams, MD.)

Periodic acid-Schiff shows segmental sclerosis with accumulation of matrix ⊃ and foam cells ⇨ and focal prominence of adjacent visceral epithelial cells (or podocytes) ⊃.

TERMINOLOGY

Synonyms
- Sickle cell nephropathy

Definitions
- Renal injury due to sickle cell disease

ETIOLOGY/PATHOGENESIS

β-globin Gene Mutation
- Chromosome 11p15.5
- Single nucleotide change leads to a change in amino acid sequence from glutamic acid to valine
- Homozygous mutations
  - Combinations with various thalassemias may cause less severe renal disease

CLINICAL ISSUES

Epidemiology
- Incidence
  - 1 in 500 African American births
- Age
  - 3rd to 5th decade
- Gender
  - No gender predilection
- Ethnicity
  - African American predilection

Site
- Kidney
  - Chronic kidney disease in 4-17%

Presentation
- Proteinuria (25%)
- Nephrotic syndrome (5%)
- Hematuria

- Often unilateral with left > right kidney involvement
- Hyposthenuria

Laboratory Tests
- Hemoglobin electrophoresis

Treatment
- Surgical approaches
  - Renal transplantation
- Drugs
  - Hydroxyurea
  - Angiotensin-converting enzyme inhibitors
  - Nonsteroidal anti-inflammatory agents
    - Should be avoided for pain control
    - May increase risk for papillary necrosis
- Hematopoietic cell transplantation
  - Rare option, possibly curative

Prognosis
- Average life expectancy: 48 years
- Increased risk of medullary renal carcinoma
  - More common with sickle cell trait

MACROSCOPIC FEATURES

General Features
- Papillary necrosis
  - 15-36% incidence
- Vascular congestion of vasa recta in renal medulla
  - Hypoxic milieu enables sickling of red blood cells

Size
- Enlargement in childhood

MICROSCOPIC PATHOLOGY

Histologic Features
- Glomerular hypertrophy
  - More prominent in juxtamedullary glomeruli

SICKLE CELL DISEASE

Key Facts

Terminology
- Sickle cell nephropathy

Etiology/Pathogenesis
- β-globin gene mutation
  - Chromosome 11p15.5

Clinical Issues
- Presentation
  - Chronic kidney disease
  - Proteinuria
- Drugs
  - Angiotensin-converting enzyme inhibitors

Macroscopic Features
- Papillary necrosis
- Vascular congestion of vasa recta in renal medulla

Microscopic Pathology
- Glomerular hypertrophy
- Glomerular sclerosis
  - Global
  - Segmental
- Duplication of glomerular basement membranes
- Hemosiderosis

Ancillary Tests
- Electron microscopy
  - Cytoplasmic rod-like inclusions of polymerized hemoglobin in red blood cells

Top Differential Diagnoses
- Focal segmental glomerulosclerosis
- Chronic thrombotic microangiopathy
- Collapsing glomerulopathy

- Glomerular sclerosis
  - Global
  - Segmental, often perihilar
- Duplication of glomerular basement membranes
  - Resembles chronic TMA
  - No immune complex deposition
- Collapsing glomerulopathy
  - Rare finding in sickle cell nephropathy
  - Possibly related to vascular compromise
- Hemosiderosis
  - Prominent hemosiderin deposition in cytoplasm of tubular epithelial cells
  - Focal hemosiderin deposition in glomerular epithelial cells
  - Confirmed by Prussian blue iron stain
- Thrombosis
- Sickled red blood cells
- Interstitial fibrosis and tubular atrophy

Predominant Pattern/Injury Type
- Glomerulosclerosis, global
- GBM duplication
- Tubules, atrophy

Predominant Cell/Compartment Type
- Glomerulus
- Tubule

ANCILLARY TESTS

Immunofluorescence
- Typical minimal or no immunoglobulin or complement, except IgM and C3 in scarred glomeruli

Electron Microscopy
- Transmission
  - Sickle-shaped red blood cells
    - Cytoplasmic rod-like inclusions represent polymerized hemoglobin
  - Subendothelial space widening
  - Duplication of GBM

DIFFERENTIAL DIAGNOSIS

Focal Segmental Glomerulosclerosis (FSGS)
- No hemosiderin deposition
- Nephrotic range proteinuria

Chronic Thrombotic Microangiopathy
- Clinical differential diagnosis includes
  - Malignant hypertension
  - Hemolytic uremic syndrome
  - Antiphospholipid antibody syndrome

Collapsing Glomerulopathy
- Considered aggressive form of FSGS
- Reported in sickle cell nephropathy

Hemolysis
- Pigmented granular eosinophilic casts in distal nephron segments

End-stage Kidney Disease
- Hemosiderosis

SELECTED REFERENCES

1. Scheinman JI: Sickle cell disease and the kidney. Nat Clin Pract Nephrol. 5(2):78-88, 2009
2. Davenport A et al: Sickle cell kidney. J Nephrol. 21(2):253-5, 2008
3. Marsenic O et al: Proteinuria in children with sickle cell disease. Nephrol Dial Transplant. 23(2):715-20, 2008
4. Nasr SH et al: Sickle cell disease, nephrotic syndrome, and renal failure. Kidney Int. 69(7):1276-80, 2006
5. Falk RJ et al: Prevalence and pathologic features of sickle cell nephropathy and response to inhibition of angiotensin-converting enzyme. N Engl J Med. 326(14):910-5, 1992
6. Bhathena DB et al: The glomerulopathy of homozygous sickle hemoglobin (SS) disease: morphology and pathogenesis. J Am Soc Nephrol. 1(11):1241-52, 1991
7. Bakir AA et al: Prognosis of the nephrotic syndrome in sickle glomerulopathy. A retrospective study. Am J Nephrol. 7(2):110-5, 1987
8. Tejani A et al: Renal lesions in sickle cell nephropathy in children. Nephron. 39(4):352-5, 1985

SICKLE CELL DISEASE

Gross and Microscopic Features

(Left) Gross photograph of a kidney after formalin fixation shows the consequences of papillary necrosis with severe pitting and scarring of the renal papilla ➡ and marked congestion of the vasa recta in the renal medulla ➡. (Courtesy C. Abrahams, MD.) (Right) Gross photograph shows congestion of the vasa recta ➡ in the renal medulla with marked scarring of the renal papilla ➡ in a sickle cell disease patient with papillary necrosis. (Courtesy C. Abrahams, MD.)

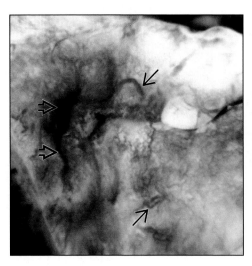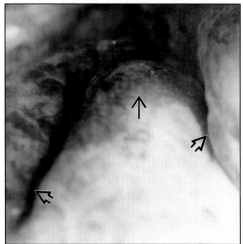

(Left) Periodic acid-Schiff shows an enlarged glomerulus (that fills a 40x field) ➡, which is frequently observed. Features of thrombotic microangiopathy or segmental sclerosis are not present here but may be seen in sickle cell nephropathy. Note hemosiderosis of adjacent tubular epithelial cells ➡. (Right) Periodic acid-Schiff demonstrates segmental sclerosis in 1/2 of this glomerulus ➡. There is substantial interstitial fibrosis ➡ and tubular atrophy ➡ surrounding the scarred glomerulus.

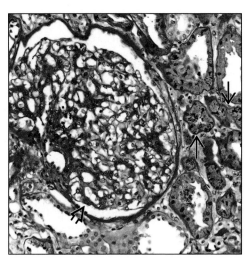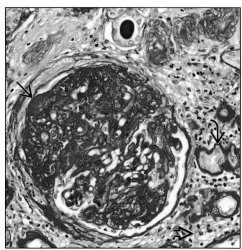

(Left) Hematoxylin & eosin shows marked hemosiderosis of the tubular epithelial cells, which is a diagnostic clue that should raise the consideration of sickle cell nephropathy. (Right) Prussian blue iron stain confirms the presence of severe iron deposition ➡ within the cytoplasm of many proximal tubular epithelial cells. This distinguishes the pigment from melanin, which can be present in the setting of widely metastatic melanoma.

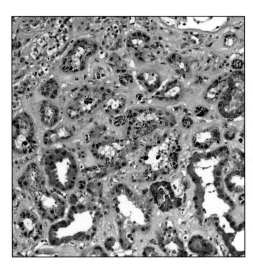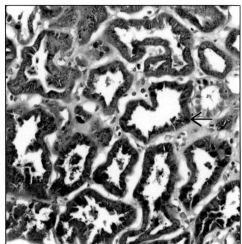

SICKLE CELL DISEASE

Light and Electron Microscopic Features

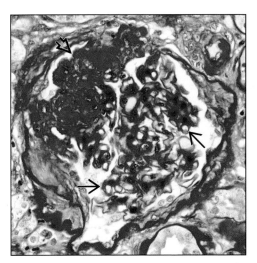

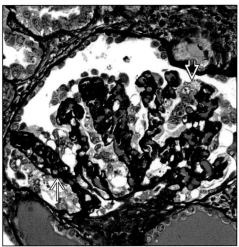

(Left) Periodic acid-Schiff shows segmental sclerosis ⇨ and focal duplication of the GBM →, which are common findings in advanced cases of sickle cell nephropathy. This patient had significant proteinuria and a papillary renal cell carcinoma. *(Right)* Jones methenamine silver shows collapsed glomerular tufts ➡ with prominence of adjacent visceral epithelial cells (podocytes) ⇨ in a patient with nephrotic syndrome due to sickle cell nephropathy. (Courtesy S. Nasr, MD.)

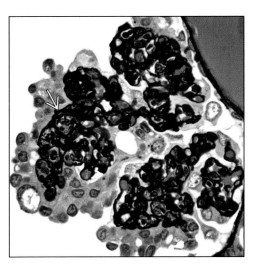

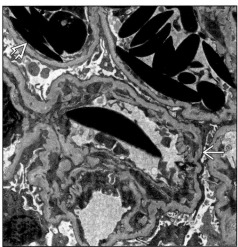

(Left) Jones methenamine silver demonstrates collapsing glomerulopathy, which can rarely occur in sickle cell disease patients. Focal duplication ➡ of the glomerular basement membranes is noted. (Courtesy S. Nasr, MD.) *(Right)* Electron micrograph shows numerous sickled red blood cells ➡ within the glomerular capillaries of a patient with sickle cell disease and nephropathy. Focal duplication of the glomerular basement membranes ➡ is noted in some capillaries.

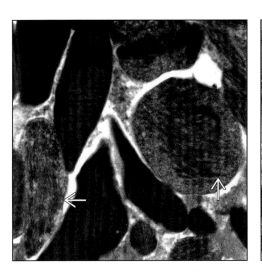

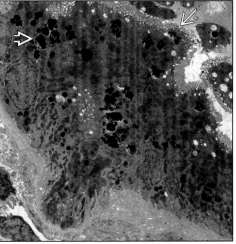

(Left) Electron microscopy at high magnification reveals numerous rod-like inclusions ➡ that represent polymerized hemoglobin within the cytoplasm of several red blood cells in a sickle cell disease patient. *(Right)* Electron microscopy of the proximal tubular epithelial cells, characterized by their brush border ➡ and numerous mitochondria, reveals prominent electron-dense hemosiderin granules ⇨ within the cytoplasm.

HYPERTENSIVE RENOVASCULAR DISEASE

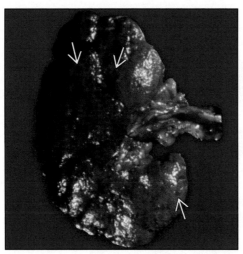

A nephrectomy in a case of hypertensive renovascular disease shows a characteristic coarsely granular, "flea-bitten" surface with scattered petechial hemorrhages ➡.

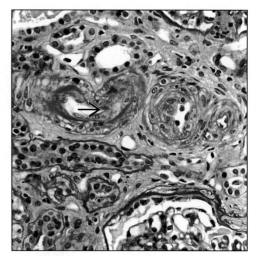

This PAS stain shows arterioles ➡ with plump endothelial cells and muscular hypertrophy in a case of hypertensive renovascular disease.

TERMINOLOGY

Abbreviations
- Hypertension (HTN)
- Arterionephrosclerosis (ANS)

Synonyms
- Arterio-/arteriolonephrosclerosis
- Hypertensive nephrosclerosis
- Benign nephrosclerosis
- Malignant nephrosclerosis

Definitions
- Renal vascular and glomerular disease secondary to hypertension (blood pressure > 120/80 mmHg)
- Accelerated hypertension, mean blood pressure > 140 mmHg, papilledema, retinal hemorrhage

ETIOLOGY/PATHOGENESIS

Essential Hypertension
- 95% of cases
- Evidence for multigenic basis plus environmental factors
- Risk factors include obesity, lack of exercise, salt intake, black race
- Other factors: Low birth weight, decreased nephron number, dysmetabolic syndrome

Secondary Causes of Hypertension
- 5% of cases
- Renal artery stenosis
  - Atherosclerosis, dysplasia, vasculitis, dissection
  - Increased production of renin by ischemic kidney
- Neoplasia
  - Pheochromocytoma
  - Adrenal cortical tumors
  - Renin-producing tumors
- Chronic renal disease
- Cocaine abuse

- Hypercoagulable states

Malignant Hypertension
- May be primary or secondary
- Renin release causes a cycle of vascular injury followed by more renin release
- Features of thrombotic microangiopathy

Effect of Hypertension on Arteries and Arterioles
- Hypertension precedes renal vascular disease
  - Shown in early renal biopsy series of Castleman and Smithwick
  - The more severe the renal vascular disease, the more reduced the glomerular filtration rate and renal blood flow
  - Vascular disease is the result, rather than cause, of hypertension
- Involves direct injury to endothelium
- Plasma (and fibrin) insudates into vascular walls
- Arterial stiffening and increased pulse pressure to afferent arteriolar level leading to hyalinosis
- Severe hypertension causes renal vascular fibrinoid necrosis (Goldblatt)

CLINICAL ISSUES

Epidemiology
- Incidence
  - Approximately 30% of adult Americans have hypertension
  - Hypertension accounts for around 25% of end-stage renal disease (ESRD) cases
  - Malignant nephrosclerosis as result of malignant hypertension occurs at rate of 1-2 cases/100,000 per year
- Age
  - Hypertension appears mostly between mid 40s and mid 50s

HYPERTENSIVE RENOVASCULAR DISEASE

Key Facts

Terminology
- Vascular and glomerular disease 2° to hypertension

Clinical Issues
- ~ 30% of American adults have hypertension
- 95% due to "essential hypertension"
- Causes ~ 25% of ESRD
- Effective drug therapy ameliorates renal sequelae

Macroscopic Features
- Finely granular cortical surface
- Petechiae in malignant hypertension

Microscopic Pathology
- Subcapsular sclerotic scars with sclerotic glomeruli, thickened arterioles, and atrophic tubules
- Global or segmental glomerulosclerosis
- Arterial intimal fibrosis and arteriolar hyalinosis

- "Onion skinning," endothelial swelling, and fibrinoid necrosis of arterioles in accelerated hypertension
- IF may show glomerular and arteriolar IgM, C3, fibrin
- EM: Wrinkled GBMs, and in malignant **hypertension**, may show subendothelial expansion & fibrinoid necrosis

Top Differential Diagnoses
- Diabetic nephropathy
- Renal atheroembolization or severe atherosclerosis from hyperlipidemia
- Primary FSGS
- Renal artery stenosis leading to renal atrophy
- Thrombotic microangiopathy, any cause
- Systemic sclerosis

- Renal damage and dysfunction take years to develop and manifest
- Gender
  - Males have predisposition
- Ethnicity
  - Disproportionately affects black race

Presentation
- Hypertension
- Proteinuria, asymptomatic
  - Related to severity of hypertension
- Renal dysfunction
- Accelerated (malignant) hypertension if mean blood pressure > 160 mmHg
  - Papilledema
  - Retinal hemorrhage
  - Congestive heart failure
  - Stroke
  - Encephalopathy
  - Renal insufficiency
  - Microangiopathic hemolytic anemia (MAHA)

Treatment
- Drugs
  - Antihypertensive agents
    - Diuretics, mineralocorticoid receptor antagonists
    - ACE inhibitors, vasopeptidase inhibitors, renin inhibitors
    - Smooth muscle dilators, endothelin antagonists
    - β-adrenergic blockers, α-adrenoceptor blockers
  - Optimal blood pressure control reduces progression to renal insufficiency and may reverse hypertensive nephrosclerosis

Prognosis
- ESRD develops in mean of 6 years from onset of azotemia
- Factors that predispose to renal failure include
  - Increasing age
  - Poor serum glucose control in diabetic patients
  - Level of systolic blood pressure
  - Male gender
  - Black race

- Elevated uric acid and triglycerides
- High diastolic blood pressure
- **Malignant hypertension**
  - If left untreated, survival is poor (20% 1-year survival)
  - Long-term survival is > 90% if blood pressure is controlled

MACROSCOPIC FEATURES

General Features
- May be normal in size or slightly reduced in size and weight
- Capsular surface is usually finely granular
- Cortical scars may be present
- Simple cysts may be present
- Cortex may be thinned
- **Malignant hypertension**
  - May be normal or increased in weight to 400 g
  - Petechial hemorrhages secondary to arteriolar necrosis gives "flea-bitten" appearance
  - May be mottled yellow and red if infarcts arise

MICROSCOPIC PATHOLOGY

Histologic Features
- Subcapsular scars
  - Composed of sclerotic glomeruli, thickened arterioles, and atrophic tubules
  - Result in granular surface of kidney
  - Bulging areas between depressed scars contain spared and hypertrophied nephrons
- Medium-sized arteries
  - Intimal fibrosis
  - Internal elastic lamina becomes multilayered (fibroelastosis); best seen on elastic stains
  - Smooth muscle hyperplasia
  - Decreased vascular lumen
- Arterioles
  - Hyaline arteriolosclerosis

- Afferent arteriolar media is replaced by homogeneous eosinophilic material positive on PAS or Masson trichrome stains
- Begins under endothelial layer and eventually replaces entire media
- Glomeruli
  o May have swollen endothelial cells and may thus appear "bloodless" and consolidated
  o Glomerular basement membranes may be duplicated
  o Glomerular mesangial matrix may be increased
  o Global glomerulosclerosis
    - Solidified type: Global solidification without collagenous material in Bowman space
    - Obsolescent type: Glomerular tuft sclerosed and Bowman space filled with collagenous material
  o Segmental glomerulosclerosis
    - Secondary focal segmental glomerulosclerosis (FSGS) may occur, typically with GBM corrugation and periglomerular fibrosis and subtotal foot process effacement
  o Glomerular hypertrophy (compensatory) in spared areas
- Interstitium and tubules
  o Interstitial fibrosis and mononuclear inflammation
  o Tubular atrophy
  o Tubular hypertrophy in spared areas
- Histologic features of malignant hypertension
  o Small arteries
    - Mucoid (myxoid) intimal change and endothelial swelling in arterioles, a.k.a. "onion skinning"
    - Fibrinoid necrosis
    - Karyorrhectic debris
    - Occasional neutrophils within endothelium
    - Fibrin thrombi
  o Arterioles
    - Arteriolar occlusion by endothelial swelling/edema-type change
    - Fibrinoid necrosis
    - Fibrin thrombi
  o Glomeruli
    - Segmental necrosis of glomeruli
    - Ischemic retraction of glomeruli with corrugation of GBM
- Treated hypertension
  o As shown by Pickering and Heptinstall
    - Acute lesions of fibrinoid necrosis and mucoid intimal thickening resolve with adequate treatment
    - Intima becomes fibrous with increased cellularity and elastic fibers

Predominant Cell/Compartment Type

- Arterial intima

ANCILLARY TESTS

Immunofluorescence

- IgM and C3 may be present in hyaline layers of arterioles
- C3 may be present in absence of immunoglobulins

- Fibrinogen is most common reactant seen on IF in malignant hypertension (in areas of fibrinoid necrosis and glomerular capillary loops)

Electron Microscopy

- Transmission
  o Glomerular capillary basement membranes may be thickened or wrinkled
  o No electron-dense deposits
  o Thickening and duplication of arteriolar basement membranes
  o Arteriolar hyalinosis
  o Foot process effacement may be present but is usually only segmental
  o In **malignant hypertension**
    - Expanded lamina rara interna (subendothelial expansion) and prominent corrugation of GBM
    - Fibrinoid necrosis

DIFFERENTIAL DIAGNOSIS

Diabetic Nephropathy

- Hyaline arteriosclerosis
  o Afferent and efferent arterioles characteristically involved
- Nodular diabetic glomerulosclerosis
  o Diffuse thickening of GBM

Hyperlipidemia

- May also have hyaline arteriosclerosis
- Relative lack of medium-sized arterial fibroelastosis

Primary FSGS

- Hypertension preceding other manifestations of renal disease are useful in favoring secondary etiology of segmental glomerulosclerosis rather than primary FSGS
- Foot process effacement is more extensive and widespread

Renal Atrophy Due to Ipsilateral Renal Artery Stenosis

- Tubular atrophy can be of "endocrine" type
- Little fibrosis
- May be little intimal fibrosis and arteriolar hyalinosis due to protection from hypertension

Renal Atheroembolization (Cholesterol Crystal Embolization)

- Cholesterol clefts can be identified in vascular lumens upon thorough examination
- Atheromatous debris, thrombosis, leukocytes, or giant cells reacting to atheroemboli may be present
- Interstitial fibrosis can be present

Renal Infarct

- May have similar gross appearance to hypertensive renovascular disease with subcapsular scarring
- Infarcts are usually larger than subcapsular scars of hypertensive renovascular disease
- Are usually single or may be multiple but do not diffusely affect kidney as in hypertensive renovascular disease

HYPERTENSIVE RENOVASCULAR DISEASE

Causes of Hypertensive Renovascular Disease

Category	Associated Etiologies
Primary	
	Benign (essential) hypertension
	Malignant hypertension
Secondary	
	Renal artery stenosis (e.g., from fibromuscular dysplasia, arterio-/atherosclerosis, etc.)
	Glomerulonephritis (similar picture is typically produced by chronic glomerulonephritis)
	Neoplasms (renin-producing tumors, adrenal cortical tumors, pheochromocytoma)
	Endocrine abnormalities (thyrotoxicosis, adrenal cortical hyperplasia, hyperparathyroidism, oral contraceptives)
	Neurogenic disorders
	Thrombotic microangiopathy (TMA) (e.g., hemolytic uremic syndrome [HUS] or thrombotic thrombocytopenic purpura [TTP])
	Antiphospholipid antibody syndrome (APS)
	Preeclampsia
	Systemic sclerosis
	Miscellaneous vascular etiologies (vasculitis or coarctation of aorta)

- PAS stain shows collapsed, condensed glomeruli without collagenous tissue in Bowman space that is seen in benign nephrosclerosis

Primary or Secondary Glomerulonephritis

- Usually has appropriate clinical history of proteinuria &/or hematuria early in course
- Usually, specific features are present that identify glomerular diagnosis
  - Affects glomeruli diffusely throughout cortex rather than in subcapsular areas, which show accentuation in nephrosclerosis from hypertensive renovascular disease
  - May be difficult to identify in late stage

Bartter Syndrome

- Children with hypokalemia, alkalosis, hypercalciuria, hyperreninemia, high angiotensin II, and hyperaldosteronemia
- Have normal blood pressure due to mutation in genes involved with salt resorption in thick ascending limb of Henle
- Hyperplastic juxtaglomerular apparatus (JGA); widespread, macula densa expansion prominent
  - Increased number of cells containing renin granules, particularly in afferent arterioles

Thrombotic Microangiopathy, Any Cause

- Vascular and glomerular lesions similar to malignant hypertension
- Distinguished by clinical correlation
  - Severe hypertension precedes renal failure in hypertensive renovascular disease

Systemic Sclerosis

- Extrarenal and serologic features of systemic sclerosis are usually present
- 5% of systemic sclerosis patients present with renal disease before extrarenal manifestations are present

DIAGNOSTIC CHECKLIST

Pathologic Interpretation Pearls

- Careful clinicopathologic correlation is required in determining etiology of hypertensive renovascular disease since there are many possible causes

SELECTED REFERENCES

1. Hill GS: Hypertensive nephrosclerosis. Curr Opin Nephrol Hypertens. 17(3):266-70, 2008
2. Marcantoni C et al: A perspective on arterionephrosclerosis: from pathology to potential pathogenesis. J Nephrol. 20(5):518-24, 2007
3. Perneger TV et al: Projections of hypertension-related renal disease in middle-aged residents of the United States. JAMA. 269:1272-7, 1993
4. Kasiske BL: Relationship between vascular disease and age-associated changes in the human kidney. Kidney Int. 31(5):1153-9, 1987
5. Kashgarian M: Pathology of small blood vessel disease in hypertension. Am J Kidney Dis. 5(4):A104-10, 1985
6. Ratliff NB: Renal vascular disease: pathology of large blood vessel disease. Am J Kidney Dis. 5(4):A93-103, 1985
7. Pickering GW et al: The reversibility of malignant hypertension. Lancet. 2:952-6, 1952
8. Castleman B et al: The relation of vascular disease to the hypertensive state; the adequacy of the renal biopsy as determined from a study of 500 patients. N Engl J Med. 239(20):729-32, 1948
9. Talbott JH et al: Renal biopsy studies correlated with renal clearance observations in hypertensive patients treated by radical sympathectomy. J Clin Invest. 22(3):387-94, 1943

Microscopic Features

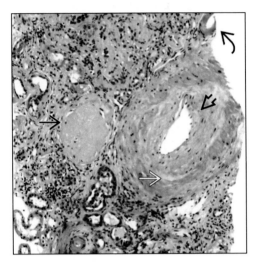
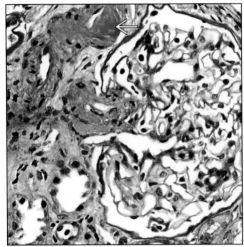

(Left) Typical vascular changes of hypertensive nephrosclerosis include intimal fibrosis of an arcuate-sized artery ⇨ and arteriolar hyalinosis ⇨. The internal elastica, the border between the intima and media, is indicated ⇨. Secondary features are interstitial fibrosis, tubular atrophy, and global glomerulosclerosis ⇨. (Right) Arteriole with hyalinization ⇨ is commonly found in a number of disorders, including hypertension, diabetes, and calcineurin inhibitor toxicity.

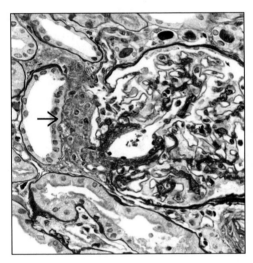
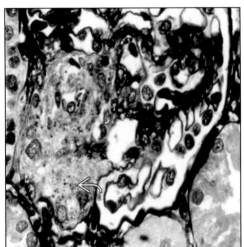

(Left) Periodic acid-Schiff shows a prominent JGA ⇨, a finding that can be seen in hypertensive renovascular disease. (Right) Jones methenamine silver shows hyperplasia of the juxtaglomerular apparatus with renin granules ⇨, a finding that can be seen in hypertensive renovascular disease.

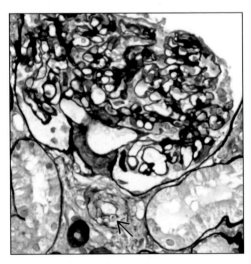
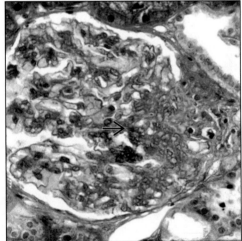

(Left) Jones methenamine silver shows a prominent juxtaglomerular apparatus with a granular consistency, accounted for by renin granules ⇨, a finding that can be seen in hypertensive renovascular disease. (Right) Enlarged juxtaglomerular apparatus (JGA) ⇨ in a case of Bartter syndrome, which is characterized by hypotension or normal blood pressure despite morphologic, biochemical, and hormonal changes suggests that hypertension could be present (Trichrome stain).

HYPERTENSIVE RENOVASCULAR DISEASE

Microscopic Features

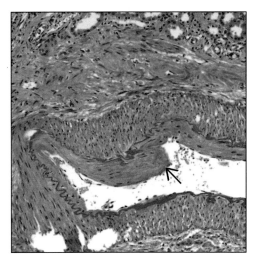

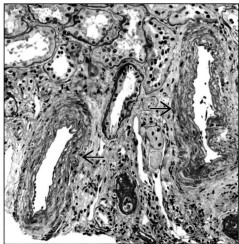

(Left) Intimal fibroplasia ➡ is present in an interlobar-sized artery in a case of hypertensive renovascular disease. *(Right)* A periodic acid-Schiff stain shows thickening and lamellation (reduplication) of the elastic lamellae ➡ of interlobar-sized arteries in a case of hypertensive renovascular disease.

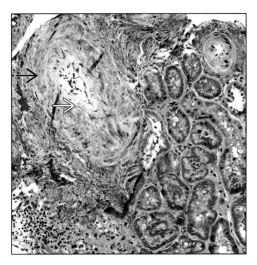

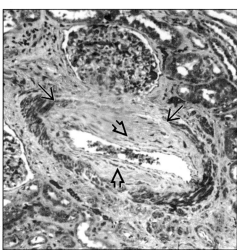

(Left) A trichrome stain shows an interlobar-sized artery with arterial intimal thickening ➡ and medial smooth muscle layer thinning ➡ in hypertensive renovascular disease. *(Right)* In an interlobar-sized artery, a trichrome stain shows arterial medial thinning (between the 2 ➡) with thickening of the arterial intima ➡ in hypertensive renovascular disease. There is a migration of fuchsinophilic medial muscle cells into the intima, a process called intimal fibroplasia.

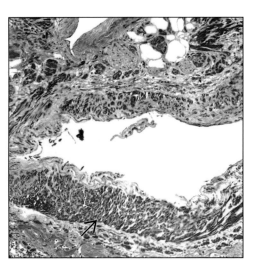

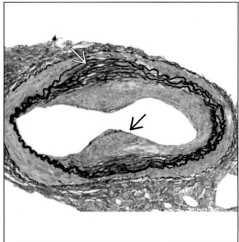

(Left) A trichrome stain shows thickening of the arterial media ➡ in a case of hypertensive renovascular disease. *(Right)* An elastic van Gieson stain shows a reduplication of the internal elastic lamina ➡ and fibrous intimal thickening ➡ in a case of hypertensive renovascular disease.

Glomerular Lesions

(Left) EM from a patient with hypertension and 2 g/d proteinuria shows widespread wrinkling and mild thickening of the GBM and effacement of foot processes, more than is usually seen in hypertension alone. It is difficult to determine the primary disease in this setting. *(Right)* EM shows numerous platelets ➡ in a glomerular capillary loop in a patient with hypertensive renovascular disease. Glomerular capillary loops are wrinkled and variably thickened ➡. Endothelial cells are swollen.

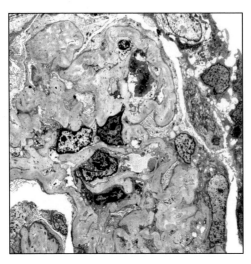
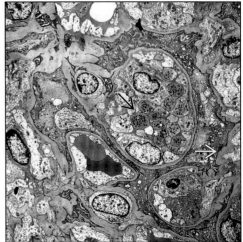

(Left) Electron micrograph shows fibrin tactoids ➡ in a degenerated glomerular capillary loop in a patient with severe hypertensive renovascular disease. *(Right)* An electron micrograph shows swollen endothelial cells ➡, fragmented red blood cells ➡, and platelets ➡ in the glomerular capillary loops in a case of hypertensive renovascular disease. There is focal foot process effacement ➡. There is also widening of the subendothelial zone ➡.

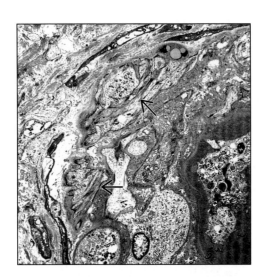
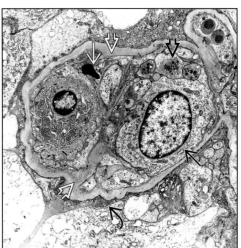

(Left) IF for IgM shows deposition in a glomerulus in a case of hypertensive renovascular disease. *(Right)* IF for C3 shows deposition in a glomerulus in a case of hypertensive renovascular disease.

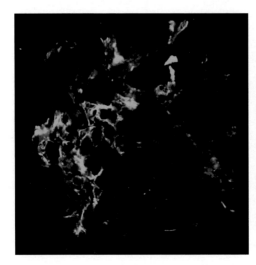
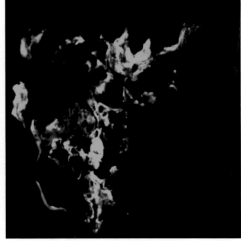

HYPERTENSIVE RENOVASCULAR DISEASE

Malignant Hypertension

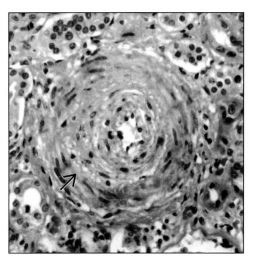

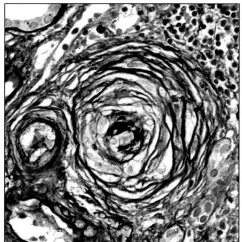

(Left) A higher power image of this renal vessel shows the "onion skin" ➡ change in a vessel wall due to concentric myointimal thickening. (Right) A Jones silver stain shows lamination ("onion skin" changes) of an arteriolar wall with near obliteration of the arteriolar lumen, a process that has been referred to as hyperplastic arteriolosclerosis in malignant hypertension. (Courtesy R. Hennigar, MD.)

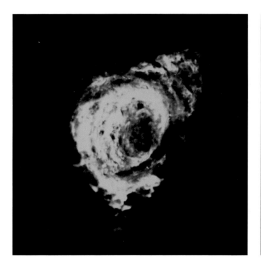

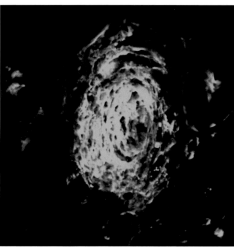

(Left) Immunofluorescence stain for IgM shows accumulation of material in a small artery in a case of severe hypertensive renovascular disease. This should not be confused with vasculitis. (Right) Immunofluorescence for fibrinogen shows accumulation of fibrin in the intima of the small intrarenal artery in severe hypertensive renovascular disease. A similar pattern can be seen in any type of thrombotic microangiopathy.

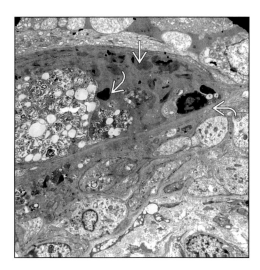

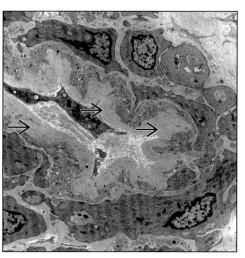

(Left) An electron micrograph shows a capillary with fragmented red blood cells (schistocytes) ➡ in a severe case of hypertensive renovascular disease. The endothelium is severely injured and shows ballooning of the cytoplasm and apoptotic nuclei ➡. (Right) Electron micrograph of a small renal artery shows accumulation of amorphous material between the endothelium and the media ➡, probably the residua of "onion skin" thickening.

RENAL ARTERY STENOSIS

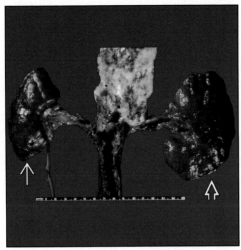

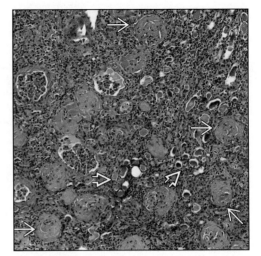

Shown here are a shrunken kidney ➡ affected by renal artery stenosis and a granular kidney ➡ affected by hypertension, likely stimulated by renin production by the shrunken kidney.

There are numerous sclerotic, closely approximated glomeruli ➡ and tubular atrophy in a thyroidization pattern ➡ in this kidney affected by renal artery stenosis.

TERMINOLOGY

Abbreviations
- Renal artery stenosis (RAS)

Synonyms
- Atherosclerotic renovascular disease: Certain cases of RAS
- Fibromuscular dysplasia: Selected cases of RAS
- Renovascular disease

Definitions
- Narrowing of renal artery lumen sufficient to cause ischemic changes in kidney and hypertension

ETIOLOGY/PATHOGENESIS

Causes of RAS
- Atherosclerosis
  o Most common cause of occlusion/stenosis of large renal arteries (70-90% of RAS cases)
  o Autopsy studies show RAS in 5-42% of patients
  o Up to 50% of patients with extensive peripheral vascular disease have RAS
  o RAS is bilateral in 33-39%
    ▪ Bilateral RAS has higher incidence of renal failure
  o Patients often have multifocal occlusive vascular disease, including coronary artery disease or peripheral arterial disease
    ▪ Injury is conceptually semiepisodic, leading to "layers" of injury with vessels that are not able to autoregulate, eventually leading to "critical stenosis"
  o Atheromatous plaques
    ▪ More common with age and in those with risk factors (cigarette smoking, HTN, diabetes, hyperlipidemia)
  o Atheroemboli (cholesterol emboli)

- May occur immediately after or within months of angiographic or surgical procedures involving vessels
  ▪ 0.1-0.8% frequency of symptomatic cholesterol emboli after angiography
  ▪ Incidence of 0.1-3.3% in renal vessels
  ▪ Emboli present in ~ 31% of patients with aortic aneurysms and ~ 77% of patients dying shortly after abdominal aortic surgery
- Thromboembolic
- Fibromuscular dysplasia
- Neurofibromatosis
- Moyamoya disease
- Takayasu arteritis and other arteritides
- Dissecting aneurysms of either aorta or renal artery
- Umbilical artery catheterization in neonates
- Coarctation of the aorta
- Irradiation
- Retroperitoneal fibrosis
- Compression by tumor
- Arteriovenous fistula
- Trauma

Ischemic Renal Disease/Ischemic Nephropathy
- Fundamental mechanism of injury in RAS
- Occurs when renal artery has 70-80% or greater stenosis

Goldblatt Kidney
- Unilateral RAS experimental model developed by Goldblatt has revealed pathophysiology
- Causes hypertension (HTN) by activation of renal-angiotensin-aldosterone system
  o Ischemic kidney produces renin
  o Increased angiotensin II
    ▪ Increased aldosterone production is stimulated
    ▪ Leads to volume retention, hypervolemia, and increased cardiac output
  o Systemic HTN results

RENAL ARTERY STENOSIS

Key Facts

Etiology/Pathogenesis
- Renal artery stenosis from variety of potential causes results in ischemic atrophy
- Atherosclerosis with atheromatous plaques is one of the most important etiologies

Clinical Issues
- Hypertension
- Proteinuria
- Renal dysfunction

Macroscopic Features
- Kidneys small from ischemic atrophy

Microscopic Pathology
- Focal segmental and global glomerulosclerosis (FSGS) can occur
- Glomerular basement membrane (GBM) wrinkling

- Interstitial fibrosis and tubular atrophy (IFTA) and interstitial inflammation
  - Tubular atrophy is of conventional type or may show "endocrine change" or thyroidization
- Atherosclerosis, arteriosclerosis, arteriolar hyalinosis, and sometimes cholesterol emboli
- Electron microscopy may show GBM wrinkling and collapse, foot process effacement, and renin granules in hypertrophic juxtaglomerular apparatus

Top Differential Diagnoses
- Renal artery aneurysms and dissection of aorta or renal artery
- Neurofibromatosis
- Takayasu arteritis and other arteritides
- Fibromuscular dysplasia

- Ischemic kidney is protected from effects of HTN
- Contralateral kidney suffers from effects of HTN (arterial and arteriolar nephrosclerosis)

CLINICAL ISSUES

Epidemiology
- Age
  - Atherosclerotic RAS primarily affects older patients
- Gender
  - 2:1 male to female ratio in atherosclerotic RAS

Presentation
- Renal dysfunction
  - Chronic renal insufficiency
    - Increased serum creatinine and blood urea nitrogen
- Hypertension
- Proteinuria
  - Usually of low or moderate degree
  - Particularly occurs in patients with focal segmental glomerulosclerosis (FSGS)
- Retinopathy
- Abdominal or flank bruits
- Hypokalemia may sometimes be seen
- Family history of HTN may be absent
- Hyperlipidemia, particularly in patients with atherosclerotic RAS
- Diabetes
- Congestive heart failure
- If atheroemboli are associated with RAS
  - Livedo reticularis
  - Acute renal failure
  - HTN
  - Leg pain
  - Gastrointestinal symptoms
  - Vision loss
  - Peripheral eosinophilia
  - Decreased serum complement

Treatment
- Surgical approaches

  - Percutaneous transluminal angioplasty
    - Used more often than stent placement
  - Angioplasty
    - Can be coupled with stent placement
    - Particularly useful when stenosis is at renal artery ostium, where angioplasty has higher failure rate
  - Bypass grafts
- Drugs
  - Antihypertensive agents
    - ACE inhibitors
    - Beta blockers
    - Calcium channel blockers
  - Lipid lowering agents
  - Antidiabetic agents and glucose control

Prognosis
- With 70-80% narrowing of renal artery lumen, ischemic renal disease may occur and may rapidly progress to failure of affected kidney
  - Around 1/2 progress within 2 years

IMAGE FINDINGS

Radiographic Findings
- Intraarterial digital subtraction is "gold standard" to demonstrate RAS
- Other radiographic imaging modalities are useful
  - Magnetic resonance angiography
  - Computed tomographic angiography
  - Color-aided duplex ultrasonography
  - Abdominal aortography
    - If renal artery narrowing, there may be poststenotic dilatation
- Radiography coupled with renal functional measurements are useful in determining contribution of each kidney to overall renal functioning

MACROSCOPIC FEATURES

General Features
- Grossly, narrowing of renal artery may be appreciated

o Origin from aorta involved in approximately 50% of cases
- Aorta may override renal artery ostium
o Bilateral disease in up to 60% of cases
o Can occur from a yellow-white fibroatheromatous plaque (atheroma) in atherosclerotic RAS cases
- Kidneys may be small in ischemic nephropathy from RAS
o Most RAS kidneys are < 50% of normal weight
- Large cortical scars and small cortical cysts may be present
- Granular capsular surface is often evident because of concurrent arteriolosclerosis
- Renal cortex is thinned
- Interlobar and arcuate arteries may appear prominent

MICROSCOPIC PATHOLOGY

Histologic Features
- Glomeruli
o Glomeruli may have basement membrane wrinkling
- Sometimes referred to as an accordion-like wrinkling
- Particularly appreciable on periodic acid-Schiff (PAS) and silver stains
o Glomerular capillary tuft may contract toward vascular pole (a process referred to as glomerulus becoming "simplified"), leading to relative increase in Bowman space
o Intracapsular fibrosis
- Collagen deposition in Bowman space
- Occurs 1st near vascular pole, eventually extending toward urinary pole
o "Atubular glomeruli" may be present
- Typically are present as residual glomeruli in fibrotic scars
- Open capillary loops are not attached to tubules on serial sectioning, and mean glomerular volume tends to be larger than in controls
o FSGS with resultant global sclerosis can occur
- FSGS occurs as secondary form
- Proteinuria may be prominent
o Juxtaglomerular apparatus may be hypertrophic
- Tubulointerstitium
o Interstitial fibrosis and tubular atrophy (IFTA), and interstitial inflammation
- Fibrosis may be diffuse and fine, demonstrable with connective tissue stains (e.g., trichrome)
- Interstitial fibrosis and inflammation may be more severe in hypertensive nephrosclerosis than in RAS
o Dilated tubules ("super tubules")
o "Classic" atrophic proximal tubules
- Thickened tubular basement membranes, possibly due to regeneration from repeated tubular injury
- Numerous mitochondria with decrease in other cellular organelles
o "Endocrine change" form of atrophic tubules
- Decreased tubular diameter with narrowed or inconspicuous lumens
- Cuboidal epithelial cell lining, often with clear cytoplasm

- Often occur in clusters
- Terminology derived from resemblance of these renal tubules to endocrine glands such as parathyroid
o Thyroidization may also be seen, consisting of atrophic tubules filled with proteinaceous cast material
o Tubular atrophy can be potentially reversible
- Reversal of atrophy can be accomplished with reestablishment of blood flow in rat model of RAS
- Atubular glomeruli may be useful prognostic sign (irreversible)
- Vessels
o Atherosclerosis
- Important cause of renal artery stenosis
- Eccentric thickening of intima with fibrosis, amorphous material including matrix proteins, lipid-laden macrophages (foam cells), and myofibroblasts
- Cholesterol clefts may be seen, serving as potential source of cholesterol emboli that may be seen in renal parenchymal vessels
- Medial fibrosis &/or thinning may be present, particularly where there is an overlying plaque
- Endothelial disruption may lead to platelet aggregation and thrombosis
- Saccular or dissecting aneurysms may form
o If vessel narrowing only involves a segmental branch of renal artery, only that portion of that kidney will be affected
o Hyaline arteriolosclerosis and arterial intimal fibrosis may be present
o Cholesterol emboli
- Cholesterol crystals embedded in amorphous debris
- Surrounded by giant cells, sometimes inciting fibrous reaction
- Crystals can be seen as unstained sections under polarized light
- Found in vessels from arcuate arteries to glomerular capillary loops, often at bifurcations
- Seen in biopsies or kidneys removed for renovascular HTN
- Affected parenchyma shows ischemic atrophy and, less frequently, infarcts
- "Protected" (ipsilateral) kidney affected by RAS shows changes mentioned above, and, most classically, shows
o Glomeruli close together because of cortical atrophy, particularly tubular atrophy
o IFTA
o Hypertrophic juxtaglomerular apparatus
- Usually only mild to moderate
- Increased granules are not usually found in setting of prolonged renal artery stenosis, severe atrophy, and scarring
o Arteries and arterioles not usually thickened because they are "protected" from increased blood pressure
- "Unprotected" contralateral kidney (nonstenotic artery)
o Severe arterial and arteriolar sclerosis and nephrosclerosis

○ May show changes of "malignant" HTN

ANCILLARY TESTS

Electron Microscopy
- Transmission
  ○ Glomerular basement membranes are often wrinkled in ischemic pattern, sometimes with collapsing glomerulopathy pattern
  ○ Segmental foot process effacement in secondary FSGS
  ○ Renin granules may be increased in afferent arteriolar granular myoepithelial cells, and these cells may be increased in number
  ○ Atrophic proximal tubular epithelial cells are small with increased number of small mitochondria, reduced number of microvilli, reduced basolateral interdigitations, and reduced number of organelles

DIFFERENTIAL DIAGNOSIS

Fibromuscular Dysplasia (FMD)
- Accounts for 10-30% of cases of RAS in published series
- Renal artery narrowing that particularly affects young women more than men
- Can result in RAS and similar renal parenchymal changes seen in other forms of RAS
- Distinguished by changes to renal arteries
  ○ Narrowing of artery typically concentric as opposed to atheromas, which are typically eccentric
  ○ Alternating constrictions and aneurysmal dilatations may be present
  ○ Intimal fibroplasia of intima composed of loose, hypocellular fibrous tissue
    ▪ Intact internal elastic lamina
    ▪ Adventitia unaffected
  ○ Medial fibroplasia with aneurysm formation may be present
    ▪ Most common variant
    ▪ Often bilateral
    ▪ Has "string of beads" appearance with alternating constriction and dilatation
    ▪ Internal elastic lamina absent in areas of aneurysmal dilatation
  ○ Medial dissection
    ▪ May be present in area of intimal fibroplasia
    ▪ May occur at defect in internal elastic lamina where blood can dissect into media
  ○ Perimedial fibroplasia
    ▪ 10-25% of FMD
    ▪ Medial thickening and replacement of medial smooth muscle cells with mature fibrous tissue (collagen)

Renal Artery Aneurysms and Dissection
- Incidence 0.01-0.1% of all individuals; prevalence 1% in patients screened for renovascular disease
- M:F ratio = 3:2; age range = 20-76 years
- Present with HTN, hematuria, flank pain, sometimes renal failure, and, uncommonly, GI bleeding

- Sometimes associated with polyarteritis nodosa
- 92% in extrarenal portion of renal artery in saccular or fusiform shape, sometimes with dissection
- Usually < 2 cm
- Medial hyperplasia and calcifications can be seen
- Rupture is rare, particularly if < 1 cm
- Repair if > 1 cm, refractory HTN, hematuria, or pain

Aortic Dissection
- May extend into renal artery
- HTN and flank pain may result, sometimes suddenly, eventually followed by renal failure
- May be spontaneous or associated with trauma or renal artery catheterization

Takayasu Arteritis and Other Arteritides
- Takayasu arteritis (also known as Takayasu disease)
  ○ Inflammatory process of aorta and major branches in aortic arch, throughout aorta, or in abdominal aorta
  ○ 3 of 6 criteria: Onset at or < 40 years of age; decreased brachial pulses; > 10 mmHg difference in systolic blood pressure between arms, subclavian artery bruits, extremity claudication, or occlusion or narrowing of aorta &/or its branches
  ○ HTN results from renal artery stenosis or aortic coarctation
    ▪ Stenosis and coarctation can be seen on angiography, along with occlusion, luminal irregularities, ectasia, and aneurysms
    ▪ Renal artery involved in ~ 19% of cases, sometimes bilaterally
  ○ Bruits, absent pulses, claudication, fever, dizziness, HTN, and myalgia
  ○ Most descriptions in Southeast Asia, Japan, India, and Mexico
  ○ Recently also studied in North American Caucasians in which young women were predominantly affected
  ○ RAS, when seen in Asian children, is most commonly caused by Takayasu
  ○ Microscopic acute phase
    ▪ Granulomatous arteritis in media and adventitia composed of lymphocytes, plasma cells, histiocytes, and sometimes giant cells
    ▪ Neovascularization from intima to vasa vasorum
    ▪ Elastic lamellae may be disrupted
    ▪ Thrombosis and aneurysm formation
  ○ Sclerosis eventually results with intimal hyperplasia, adventitial fibrosis, and medial degeneration
- Giant cell aortitis
  ○ Gives similar microscopic appearance to Takayasu disease
  ○ Abdominal aortic and renal artery involvement is more typical of Takayasu than giant cell arteritis

Neurofibromatosis
- Common cause of renal artery stenosis in children and adolescents
- Also known as von Recklinghausen disease
- Associated with HTN in ~ 19% of cases
  ○ HTN 1st appears at mean age of 11 years

Differential Diagnosis of Renal Artery Stenosis (RAS)

Diagnosis	Useful Distinguishing Features in Artery	Useful Distinguishing Features in Kidney
Atherosclerosis	Aortic &/or renal artery atherosclerotic disease with marked narrowing of renal artery or ostium	Cholesterol clefts in vascular lumens and tubular atrophy on affected side; glomerulosclerosis, arterial intimal fibrosis, and arteriolar hyalinosis more severe on contralateral side
Dissecting aneurysm	Plane of dissection in main renal artery	
Fibromuscular dysplasia	Intimal, medial, and perimedial fibroplasia	Larger intrarenal arteries may be affected by dysplastic process; best shown on trichrome and elastin stains
Neurofibromatosis	Occlusion by Schwann cells, fibrosis, smooth muscle cells, and mesodermal dysplasia 1st appearing in adolescent age group	Smaller intrarenal vessels may be affected
Takayasu aortitis	Granulomatous arteritis in the media and adventitia with giant cells	
Giant cell aortitis	Granulomatous arteritis in the media and adventitia, may include giant cells	
Moyamoya disease	Netlike formations with fibrointimal thickening, medial thinning, and sometimes intimal fibroplasia	
Renal artery aneurysm/ dissection	Sometimes due to polyarteritis nodosa	Larger intrarenal arteries may have arteritis; best shown with trichrome and elastin stains
Coarctation of aorta	Aorta itself affected	
Thrombosis	Thrombus in artery, usually organized	May be distal emboli, infarction; can occur in infants with umbilical artery catheterization
Radiation	Intimal fibrosis, periarterial fibrosis	Tubular atrophy and fibrosis increased in field of radiation

- ○ Typically due to renal artery stenosis but can be due to aortic coarctation
  - ▪ Commonly secondary to compression to Schwann cell proliferation and accompanying fibrosis, usually in adventitia but sometimes in intima
  - ▪ Mesodermal dysplasia can be seen in media or intima of smaller vessels, a process whereby cells have nodular proliferation, shown to be smooth muscle cells by electron microscopy and immunohistochemistry
  - ○ Pheochromocytomas can be cause of HTN in these patients also

Moyamoya Disease
- Renovascular HTN in 8.3% of children with moyamoya disease
- Stenosis of vessels through netlike formations, fibrointimal thickening, medial thinning, and sometimes intimal fibroplasia
- 1st described in Japan, typically in carotid artery and branches

DIAGNOSTIC CHECKLIST

Pathologic Interpretation Pearls
- Longitudinal sections of renal artery can be more revealing than cross sections
  - ○ Atherosclerotic disease has multiple atheromas
  - ○ Fibromuscular dysplasia has ridges of hyperplastic tissue

SELECTED REFERENCES

1. Kendrick J et al: Renal artery stenosis and chronic ischemic nephropathy: epidemiology and diagnosis. Adv Chronic Kidney Dis. 15(4):355-62, 2008
2. Textor SC: Atherosclerotic renal artery stenosis: overtreated but underrated? J Am Soc Nephrol. 19(4):656-9, 2008
3. Levin A et al: Controversies in renal artery stenosis: a review by the American Society of Nephrology Advisory Group on Hypertension. Am J Nephrol. 27(2):212-20, 2007
4. Olson JL: Renal disease caused by hypertension. In Jennette JC et al: Heptinstall's Pathology of the Kidney. 6th ed. Philadephia: Lippincott Williams & Wilkins. 965-75, 2007
5. D'Agati VD et al: Atlas of nontumor pathology: Non-neoplastic kidney diseases. Washington DC: American Registry of Pathology. 2005
6. Gröne HJ et al: Characteristics of renal tubular atrophy in experimental renovascular hypertension: a model of kidney hibernation. Nephron. 72(2):243-52, 1996
7. Marcussen N: Atubular glomeruli in renal artery stenosis. Lab Invest. 65(5):558-65, 1991
8. Selye H et al: Pathogenesis of the cardiovascular and renal changes which usually accompany malignant hypertension. J Urol. 56:399-419, 1946
9. Goldblatt H et al: Studies on experimental hypertension : I. The production of persistent elevation of systolic blood pressure by means of renal ischemia. J Exp Med. 59(3):347-79, 1934

RENAL ARTERY STENOSIS

Gross and Low-power Features

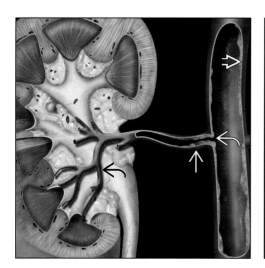

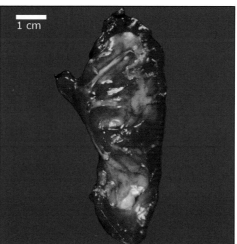

(Left) This image illustrates the common sites of stenosis, which most often occurs in the aorta ⟹, the renal artery ➜, its ostium ⤳, or one of the renal artery branches ↗. *(Right)* An atrophic kidney secondary to renal artery stenosis can be seen.

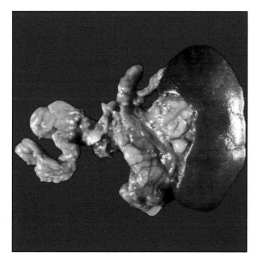

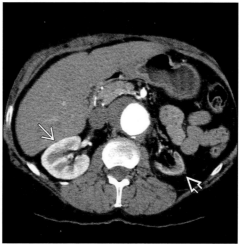

(Left) This is an atrophic kidney with a tortuous, stenotic renal artery. An atrophic kidney purely due to RAS will have a smooth surface since there is no parenchymal scarring. When hypertension damages the kidney before the stenosis, a granular surface due to subcapsular scars is evident. *(Right)* This computed tomography (CT) axial radiologic image shows a shrunken kidney due to renal artery stenosis ⟹, which is in marked contrast with the contralateral kidney ➜.

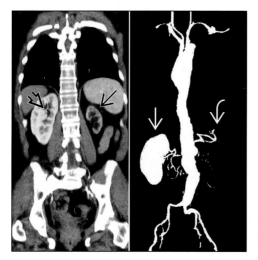

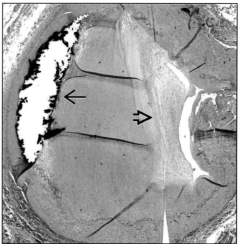

(Left) A coronal CT (left) shows a shrunken kidney ➜ compared with the contralateral kidney ⤳. Angiography (right) shows that the shrunken kidney essentially has no blood supply. The tortuous renal arteries effectively terminate where the kidney is expected to appear ➜, compared with the contralateral kidney ➜. *(Right)* A section of the renal artery shows atherosclerotic disease with intimal thickening by an atheromatous plaque ⤳ and calcification ➜.

Microscopic Features

(Left) At relatively low power, interstitial fibrosis and tubular atrophy (IFTA) can be appreciated with the TA having a thyroidization pattern ➡. *(Right)* This PAS stain of a kidney affected by renal artery stenosis shows global glomerulosclerosis ➡ and prominent tubular atrophy ➡.

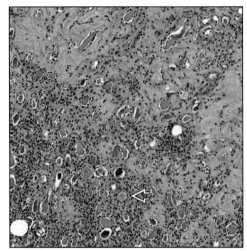 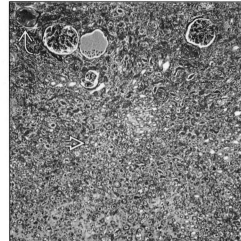

(Left) This higher power image of a PAS stain shows prominent tubular atrophy with a focal "endocrinization"-type pattern ➡, resembling endocrine acinar tissue, proteinaceous casts ➡, and thickened, wrinkled tubular basement membranes ➡. *(Right)* This higher power hematoxylin & eosin stain of a kidney affected by renal artery stenosis shows a globally sclerotic glomerulus ➡ and a glomerulus with segmental sclerosis ➡.

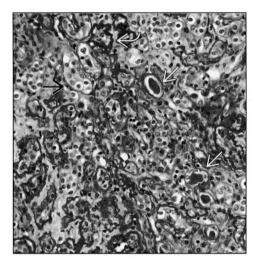 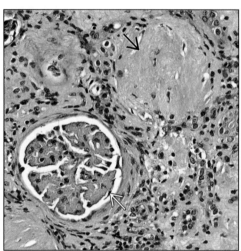

(Left) Dilated tubules with flattened tubular epithelial cells can be seen, denoted here ➡. *(Right)* Proximal tubules have occluded lumens and focally clear cytoplasm ➡, sometimes referred to as endocrine change. Sclerotic glomeruli ➡ and proteinaceous casts ➡ can be seen.

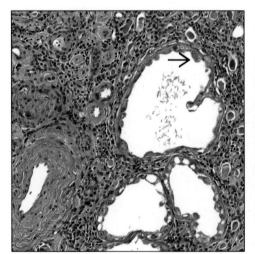 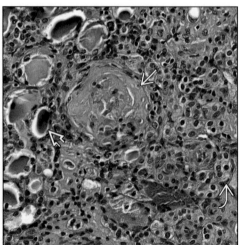

Special Stains and Ancillary Techniques

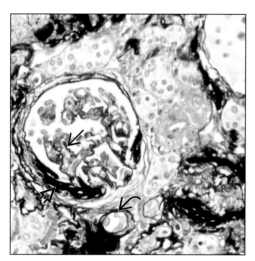

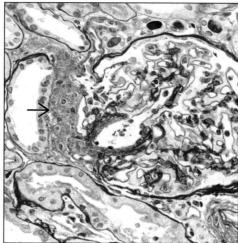

(Left) This Jones methenamine silver (JMS) stain of a kidney affected by renal artery stenosis shows a glomerulus with an ischemic-type, accordion-like wrinkling of the glomerular basement membrane ➡, intracapsular fibrosis ➤, and foci of tubular basement membrane duplication ➡. (Right) This periodic acid-Schiff stain of a kidney affected by renal artery stenosis shows a hypertrophic juxtaglomerular apparatus ➡.

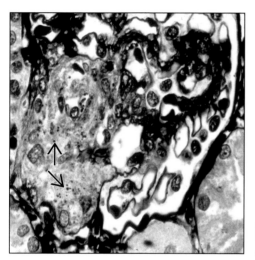

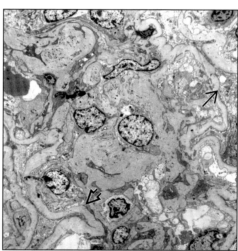

(Left) Renin granules ➡ can be appreciated in the hypertrophic juxtaglomerular apparatus of this kidney affected by renal artery stenosis (JMS stain). (Right) Electron micrograph of a kidney affected by renal artery stenosis shows prominent glomerular basement membrane wrinkling and glomerular capillary loop collapse ➤, essentially occluding glomerular capillary loops. Podocyte foot processes are effaced ➡.

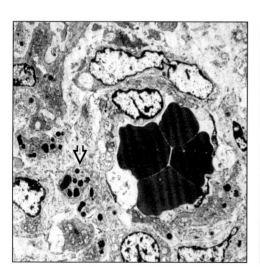

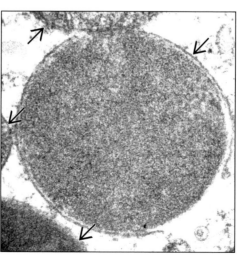

(Left) EM of a juxtaglomerular apparatus in a case of renal artery stenosis shows numerous renin granules in the specialized smooth muscle cells derived from the afferent arteriole ➤, which appear homogeneous and electron dense. (Right) A higher power electron micrograph image of the cells in the juxtaglomerular apparatus shows the ultrastructural characteristics of secretory renin granules ➡, which have no substructure and are bounded by a lipid bilayer membrane.

FIBROMUSCULAR DYSPLASIA

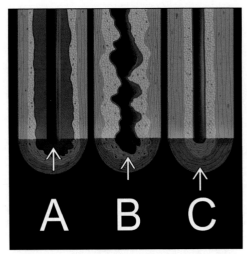

Fibromuscular dysplasia occurs in 3 main varieties: A) intimal fibroplasia, B) medial fibromuscular dysplasia, and C) periarterial (adventitial) fibroplasia.

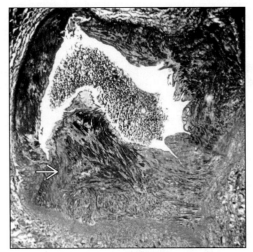

The medial fibroplasia form shows disoriented medial smooth muscle ⇒ that protrudes into the lumen of the renal artery (trichrome stain).

TERMINOLOGY

Abbreviations
- Fibromuscular dysplasia (FMD)

Synonyms
- Arterial fibrodysplasia
- Fibromuscular hyperplasia
- Intimal or periarterial (adventitial) fibroplasia

Definitions
- Idiopathic, segmental, noninflammatory, nonatherosclerotic small and medium-sized artery diseases causing stenosis and aneurysms
- 3 major categories
  - Medial
  - Intimal
  - Periarterial (adventitial)

ETIOLOGY/PATHOGENESIS

Genetic
- Sibling affected in 11% of patients
- Medial fibroplasia form may be congenital since it appears to be malformation
- Occasionally, associated Ehlers-Danlos syndrome type IV or Marfan syndrome
- 1 report of increased prevalence of angiotensin converting enzyme (ACE) I allele

Environment
- Smoking

Female Gender
- No link to estrogens or oral contraceptives proved

CLINICAL ISSUES

Epidemiology
- Incidence
  - Estimated 4/1,000 for symptomatic renal FMD
    - Medial: 60-85%
    - Intimal: 1-5%
    - Periarterial: < 1%
  - 10-20% of patients with renal artery stenosis
- Age
  - Younger (15-50 years) for fibromuscular dysplasia
  - Older (> 50 years) for fibrotic forms
- Gender
  - Female predominance (medial form)
    - 85% affect women under 50 years old
  - Male predominance (intimal form)

Site
- 60-90% involve renal arteries
  - 50% bilateral
  - Distal 2/3 of renal artery
  - Extends into arcuates and interlobular arteries
    - May account for continued hypertension after correction of extrarenal stenosis
  - May have associated aneurysm
- May involve multiple vascular beds
  - Carotid arteries (26%)
  - Mesenteric/intestinal arteries (9%)
  - Iliac arteries (5%)
  - Popliteal, hepatic, coronary, and subclavian arteries (9%)
  - Less commonly, aorta and brachial, superficial femoral, tibial, and peroneal arteries

Presentation
- Hypertension
- Asymptomatic
- Associated with hypertrophic cardiomyopathy

FIBROMUSCULAR DYSPLASIA

Key Facts

Terminology
- Nonatherosclerotic, noninflammatory fibrous, and fibromuscular proliferation of artery, typically leading to stenosis

Clinical Issues
- Mostly young and female
- 60-90% involve renal artery, 50% bilateral
  - Commonly present with hypertension
  - May be asymptomatic
- Percutaneous transluminal renal angioplasty is treatment of choice

Image Findings
- "String of beads" pattern on angiography

Microscopic Pathology
- Intimal

- Intimal hyperplasia resembles atherosclerosis but without lipid deposition
- Medial
  - Medial fibroplasia with abnormally oriented smooth muscle and aneurysms is most common
  - Perimedial fibroplasia with fibrous band in outer media
  - Medial hyperplasia with hyperplastic but otherwise normal media
- Periarterial (adventitial) fibroplasia
  - Circumferential adventitial fibrosis, normal media and intima

Top Differential Diagnoses
- Atherosclerosis
- Vasculitis
- Dissecting aneurysm

Laboratory Tests
- Renin levels elevated

Treatment
- Surgical approaches
  - Surgical correction curative in ~ 70%
  - Percutaneous transluminal renal angioplasty (PTRA) is treatment of choice
  - Complex reconstruction, such as aortorenal bypass, is required in difficult cases
- Drugs
  - Hypertension may respond to ACE inhibitors but not most other antihypertensive agents

Prognosis
- Good, if corrected
- If untreated, progressive narrowing may occur over 10 years, as judged by angiography
  - Obstruction, dissecting aneurysms, and emboli may result
  - Sudden death, particularly in FMD of cardiac arteries (e.g., artery supplying the sinus node) may occur
- Renal failure rare

IMAGE FINDINGS

General Features
- CT and catheter angiography useful in identifying areas of stenosis or classical "string of beads" appearance

MACROSCOPIC FEATURES

General Features
- Beaded pattern of aneurysms and stenosis in renal artery branches

Size
- Kidney may show decreased cortical thickness

MICROSCOPIC PATHOLOGY

Histologic Features
- **Medial fibroplasia**
  - Aneurysms form as a result of loss of smooth muscle and deficient elastic lamina
  - Fibrous and muscular ridges may be formed alternating with areas of marked thinning and even aneurysm formation
  - Renal infarcts are more common with this type of lesion than other types of fibromuscular dysplasia
  - Thrombosis or rupture occurs rarely
  - Medial dissection may also occur in 5-10% of cases
    - Channel forms in outer 1/3 of vessel wall
    - Intimal fibroplasia may occur in area of dissection
- **Perimedial fibroplasia**
  - Dense, pale fibrous tissue in outer media wall is well demarcated from hypertrophied circular muscle of inner media
    - Cellular fibrous tissue may extend transmurally
    - Adventitial fibrosis may extend into adjacent adipose and connective tissue, causing constriction (rare)
  - External elastic lamina outside fibrous zone may be replaced
    - Outer medial border may have circumferential aggregates of elastic tissue, which may appear like dense collagen on light microscopy, but EM shows them to be elastin
  - Thrombosis is more common in this form than in other types of renal artery dysplasia
  - Multifocal stenoses produce irregular beading with beads smaller than vessel diameter on radiographic examination
- **Medial hyperplasia**
  - Medial smooth muscle hyperplasia devoid of fibrosis showing normal orientation
  - Intima, elastica, and adventitia are normal
  - Angiographic appearance similar to intimal fibroplasia
- **Intimal fibroplasia**

FIBROMUSCULAR DYSPLASIA

Fibromuscular Dysplasia Types

Type	General Features	Pathologic Features
Medial		
Medial fibroplasia	Most common variant (60-85% of cases), young women, can have "string of beads" appearance	Fibrous expansion of media, may have fibromuscular ridges, thrombosis, and aneurysms
Perimedial fibroplasia	10-25% of cases, may cause severe or complete stenosis, women and men aged 15-30 years	Hyperplasia of muscle, usually circumferential, particularly in inner media, with fibrous tissue in outer media, thrombosis
Medial hyperplasia	Uncommon (1-15% of cases), may cause severe stenosis, women and men	Smooth muscle hyperplasia devoid of fibrosis
Intimal	Uncommon (1-5% of cases), may cause severe or total stenosis, male and females	Circumferential or eccentric hyperplasia of intima
Periarterial (adventitial)	Rare (< 1% of cases)	Collagenous fibroplasia encircles adventitia and may extend into surrounding tissue

- o Affects major branches of aorta, often bilateral
- o Irregular, long tubular stenosis in the young; smooth, focal stenosis in the elderly
- o Circumferential or eccentric intimal fibrosis
  - ▪ Intimal proliferation of loose, moderately cellular fibrous tissue inside internal elastic lamina without lipid or inflammatory cells
  - ▪ Internal elastic lamina is present
  - ▪ Media and adventitia are normal
- • **Periarterial (adventitial) fibroplasia**
  - o Collagenous fibroplasia encircles adventitia and extends into surrounding periarterial fibroadipose tissue
  - o Few mononuclear cells may be present
  - o Intima, internal elastic lamina, external elastic lamina, and media are usually normal
- • **Parenchymal lesions, affected side**
  - o Atrophy of tubules
    - ▪ Small, back-to-back tubules with simple epithelium and little interstitial fibrosis
  - o Prominent juxtaglomerular apparatus
  - o Small arteries spared changes of hypertension
- • **Parenchymal lesions, contralateral side**
  - o Compensatory hypertrophy of tubules and glomeruli
  - o Vascular lesions related to hypertension
    - ▪ Intimal fibrosis of arcuate-sized arteries
    - ▪ Arteriolar hyalinosis

DIFFERENTIAL DIAGNOSIS

Atherosclerosis
- • Resembles intimal form
- • Lipid-laden cells, foam cells, and often lymphocytes are present

Macroscopic Polyarteritis (Polyarteritis Nodosa)
- • Can resemble perimedial fibroplasia or adventitial form
- • Typically has eccentric scarring, disruption of elastica, and no hyperplasia

Dissecting Aneurysm
- • Healed lesions may resemble perimedial fibroplasia
- • Longer continuous involvement

Normal Artery
- • Occasionally, normal arteries may appear to have disoriented smooth muscle
- • Elastin stains reveal normal layers of elastic lamina

DIAGNOSTIC CHECKLIST

Pathologic Interpretation Pearls
- • Elastin stains valuable for evaluation and classification

SELECTED REFERENCES

1. Olin JW: Recognizing and managing fibromuscular dysplasia. Cleve Clin J Med. 74(4):273-4, 277-82, 2007
2. Plouin PF et al: Fibromuscular dysplasia. Orphanet J Rare Dis. 2:28, 2007
3. Alhadad A et al: Revascularisation of renal artery stenosis caused by fibromuscular dysplasia: effects on blood pressure during 7-year follow-up are influenced by duration of hypertension and branch artery stenosis. J Hum Hypertens. 19(10):761-7, 2005
4. Carmo M et al: Surgical management of renal fibromuscular dysplasia: challenges in the endovascular era. Ann Vasc Surg. 19(2):208-17, 2005
5. Pascual A et al: Renal fibromuscular dysplasia in elderly persons. Am J Kidney Dis. 45(4):e63-6, 2005
6. Slovut DP et al: Fibromuscular dysplasia. N Engl J Med. 350(18):1862-71, 2004
7. Boutouyrie P et al: Evidence for carotid and radial artery wall subclinical lesions in renal fibromuscular dysplasia. J Hypertens. 21(12):2287-95, 2003
8. Bofinger A, Hawley C, Fisher P, Daunt N, Stowasser M, Gordon R Polymorphisms of the renin-angiotensin system in patients with multifocal renal arterial fibromuscular dysplasia. J Hum Hypertens. 15(3):185-90, 2001
9. Pannier-Moreau I et al: Possible familial origin of multifocal renal artery fibromuscular dysplasia. J Hypertens. 15(12 Pt 2):1797-801, 1997
10. Case records of the Massachusetts General Hospital: Weekly clinicopathological exercises. Case 9-1995. A 60-year-old man with hypertrophic cardiomyopathy and ischemic colitis. N Engl J Med. 332(12):804-10, 1995

FIBROMUSCULAR DYSPLASIA

Microscopic Features

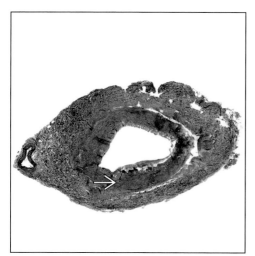 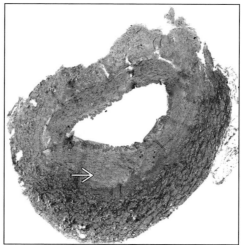

(Left) A low-power view of the renal artery with perimedial fibroplasia shows the outer media is occupied by a layer of blue-staining fibrous tissue ➡, as highlighted on this trichrome stain. (Right) A low-power view shows perimedial fibroplasia of the renal artery in which the outer media is occupied by a layer of fibrous tissue that is paler than the smooth muscle in this H&E stain ➡.

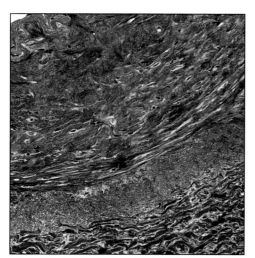 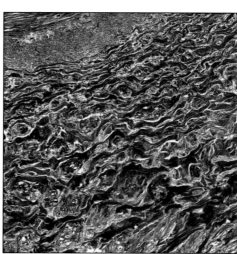

(Left) Higher power trichrome stain of perimedial fibroplasia shows that the majority of the renal artery wall is composed of variably staining fibrous tissue. (Right) Higher power trichrome stain of perimedial fibroplasia of the renal artery shows that the arterial wall smooth muscle is infiltrated by dense fibrous tissue, as shown by this trichrome stain.

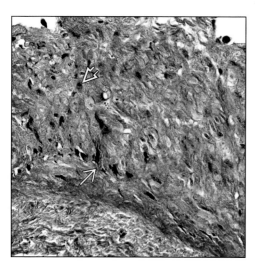 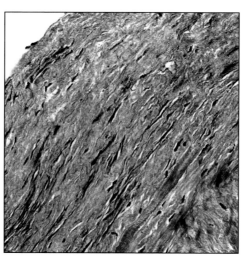

(Left) Higher power trichrome stain of perimedial fibroplasia of the renal artery shows dense fibrous tissue between smooth muscle cells. Smooth muscle cells simulate both a spindled ➡ and epithelioid ➡ morphology. (Right) Higher power trichrome stain of perimedial fibroplasia of the renal artery shows dense fibrous tissue between smooth muscle cells. The smooth muscle cells have acquired a spindled morphology.

Microscopic Features

(Left) Disoriented medial smooth muscle cells protrude into the lumen of a renal artery alternating with abnormally thin regions, typical of the medial fibroplasia variant of fibromuscular dysplasia. This form is probably a congential malformation. *(Right)* Hematoxylin & eosin of the renal artery shows pale-staining loose fibrous tissue in the outer media and darker staining dense fibrous tissue in the inner media in a case of perimedial fibroplasia of the renal artery.

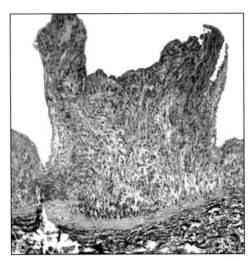
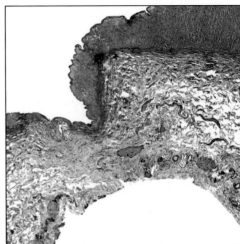

(Left) Periodic acid-Schiff stain of the renal artery shows pale-staining loose fibrous tissue in the outer media ⇨ and denser fibrous tissue admixed with smooth muscle in the inner media ➡ and loose connective tissue in the adventia ⇨ in a case of perimedial fibroplasia of the renal artery. *(Right)* A higher power trichome stain of perimedial fibroplasia of the renal artery shows dense fibrous tissue between smooth muscle cells. Some smooth muscle cells are spindled ⇨, and others simulate an epithelioid morphology ⇨.

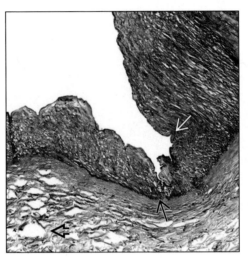
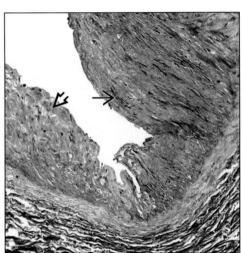

(Left) An elastic stain of the renal artery involved by fibromuscular dysplasia shows pale-staining fibrous tissue filling the outer media with the inner media being filled by a darker layer, which alternates between being thick and thin, focally simulating aneurysm ⇨ formation. *(Right)* Elastic stain of an artery with FMD shows an abnormally thin region of the media, which was probably dilated in vivo, forming an aneurysm ⇨. The outer media has dense bands of elastic fibers.

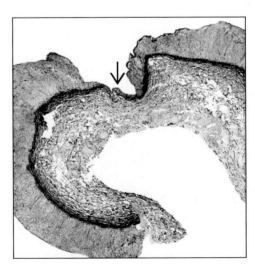
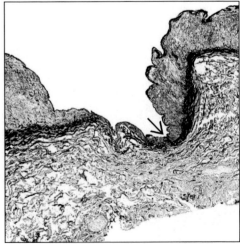

FIBROMUSCULAR DYSPLASIA

Microscopic Features and Patterns

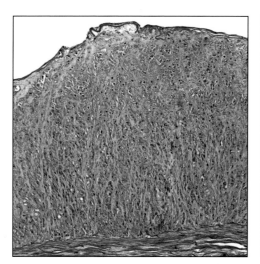

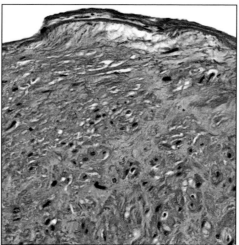

(Left) A medium-power view shows fibromuscular dysplasia due primarily to perimedial fibroplasia in a proliferation in which loose, moderately cellular fibrous tissue leads to narrowing of the renal artery. *(Right)* Hematoxylin & eosin at high power of perimedial fibroplasia with "secondary" intimal fibroplasia shows loose, cellular fibrous tissue expanding the media & extending into the intima, leading to renal artery stenosis. This may simulate "endarteritis" seen in other contexts.

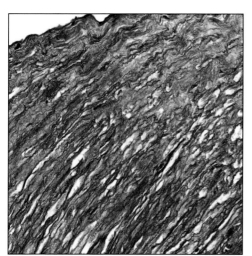

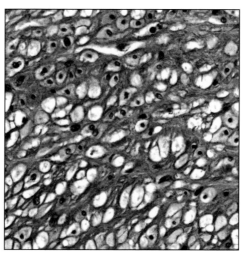

(Left) A higher power view of a PAS stain of the renal artery in FMD shows dense fibrous tissue between smooth muscle cells. *(Right)* A higher power view of perimedial fibroplasia of the renal artery stained with PAS shows dense fibrous tissue between smooth muscle cells. The smooth muscle cells in this case acquire a clear cell appearance that superficially resembles cartilage.

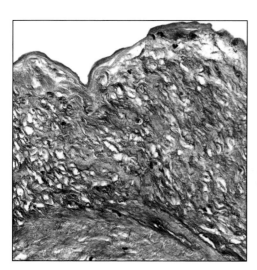

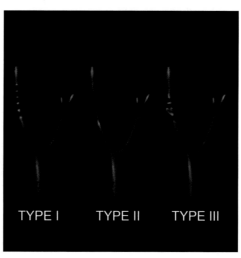

TYPE I   TYPE II   TYPE III

(Left) A higher power image of FMD of the renal artery stained with PAS shows dense fibrous tissue between smooth muscle cells and disoriented smooth muscle cells. *(Right)* A diagram shows the 3 patterns of fibromuscular dysplasia as seen on angiography: Type I) "string of beads" appearance, II) tubular stenosis along a segment of the artery, and III) unifocal abnormality/stenosis.

NEUROFIBROMATOSIS

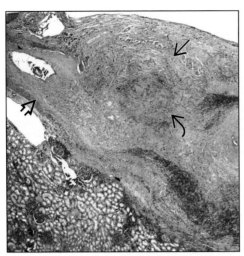

This intralobar artery shows severe occlusion from intimal fibromuscular dysplasia ➡ with secondary formation of an aneurysm ➡. There is also luminal thrombosis ➡ and organization.

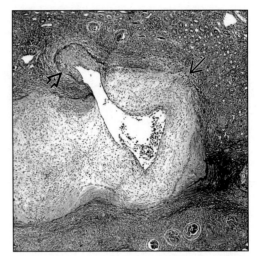

Elastic stain shows an absent media and multifocal disruption of the elastica ➡. This structural alteration leads to aneurysm formation. An arterial branch with intimal thickening ➡ is present.

TERMINOLOGY

Abbreviations
- Neurofibromatosis type 1 (NF1)

Synonyms
- von Recklinghausen disease
- Neurofibromatosis type 1 renal vasculopathy
- Neuroectodermal syndrome

Definitions
- National Institutes of Health consensus statement requires 2 of 7 diagnostic criteria
  - 6 or more café au lait macules
  - 2 or more neurofibromas
  - Axillary freckling
  - 2 or more Lisch nodules (iris hamartomas)
  - Splenoid dysplasia or thinning of long bones
  - 1st-degree relative with NF1
- NF1 vasculopathy is term for arterial or venous aneurysms, stenoses, arteriovenous malformations (AVM), or arterial invasion or compression by neurofibromas

ETIOLOGY/PATHOGENESIS

Genetic Factors
- Autosomal dominant
- 1:3,000 individuals
- Mutation of *NF1*, chromosome 17 (17q11.2)
- *NF1* encodes for neurofibromin, a GTPase activating protein for *RAS*
  - Neurofibromin shares functional and sequence homology with *RAS* oncogene
  - Mutation increases mitogenic signaling and cell proliferation affecting neural, endothelial, and smooth muscle cells

CLINICAL ISSUES

Presentation
- Renovascular hypertension
  - Affects 1% of NF1 patients
  - Most affected patients are pediatric

Treatment
- Surgical repair or bypass if main renal artery affected
- Nephrectomy if intrarenal vessels affected

Prognosis
- Surgical cure of hypertension achieved in most
- Recurrent disease is not uncommon
- Sudden death if rupture of large artery aneurysm or AVM

IMAGE FINDINGS

General Features
- Stenosis of main renal artery or segmental branches in 90%
- Stenosis of intraparenchymal arteries in 12%
- Reduced renal size in 30%
- Bilateral disease in 30%

Radiographic Findings
- Angiography demonstrates intimal stenosis, occasionally with "beading"
  - Short segment stenosis (< 5 mm) in 40%
  - Long segment stenosis (> 10 mm) in 30%
  - Ostia stenosis in 30%
  - Post-stenotic aneurysmal dilatation is common
- Reduced renal size in 30%

MACROSCOPIC FEATURES

General Features
- Arterial stenosis due to fibromuscular dysplasia

NEUROFIBROMATOSIS

Key Facts

Terminology
- Neurofibromatosis type 1 vasculopathies

Etiology/Pathogenesis
- Autosomal dominant
- Mutation of *NF1* gene, 17q11.2

Clinical Issues
- Hypertension is most common presentation
- Life-threatening hemorrhage if rupture occurs

Image Findings
- Angiography demonstrates intimal stenosis, occasionally with "beading"

Macroscopic Features
- Arterial stenosis ± aneurysm
- AVM

- Extra-arterial mass representing a neurofibroma

Microscopic Pathology
- Myxoid intimal fibromuscular dysplasia
- Intimal or medial spindle cell foci
- Attenuation of smooth muscle media
- Disruption of elastica with aneurysm formation
- Thrombosis and organization
- Extravascular hemorrhage

Top Differential Diagnoses
- Fibromuscular dysplasia
- Takayasu arteritis

Diagnostic Checklist
- Consider NF1 vasculopathy when clusters of intimal or medial spindled cells within a myxoid matrix

---

- Arterial or venous aneurysm
- Complex vascular lesion due to AVM
- Periarterial neurofibroma (least common finding)

MICROSCOPIC PATHOLOGY

Histologic Features
- Arterial fibromuscular dysplasia
  - Neointimal proliferation with myxoid stroma
  - Intimal or medial clusters of bland spindle cells
  - Thrombosis, organization, hemorrhage
- Arterial or venous aneurysmal dilatation
  - Medial attenuation or absence
  - Disruption of internal and external elastica
  - Thrombosis and organization
  - Extravascular hemorrhage
- Neurofibroma
  - Disordered proliferation of Schwann cells and fibroblasts
  - S-100 positive
- Intrarenal atherosclerotic changes such as cholesterol clefts, foam cells, and calcification are absent

DIFFERENTIAL DIAGNOSIS

Fibromuscular Dysplasia (FMD)
- Presumed diagnosis in renal artery stenosis of young adults and children
- Angiographic findings indistinguishable from NF1 vasculopathy

Takayasu Arteritis
- Most common cause of renovascular hypertension in Asians

Other Causes of Secondary Hypertension
- Pheochromocytoma
- Coarctation of aorta
- Paraganglioma

DIAGNOSTIC CHECKLIST

Pathologic Interpretation Pearls
- NF1 vasculopathy considered when FMD is associated with clusters of intimal or medial spindled cells within a myxoid matrix

SELECTED REFERENCES

1. Srinivasan A et al: Spectrum of renal findings in pediatric fibromuscular dysplasia and neurofibromatosis type 1. Pediatr Radiol. 41(3):308-16, 2011
2. Malav IC et al: Renal artery stenosis due to neurofibromatosis. Ann Pediatr Cardiol. 2(2):167-9, 2009
3. Chang JB et al: Regarding "Vascular abnormalities in patients with neurofibromatosis syndrome type I: Clinical spectrum, management, and results". J Vasc Surg. 47(6):1378-9; author reply 1379, 2008
4. Oderich GS et al: Vascular abnormalities in patients with neurofibromatosis syndrome type I: clinical spectrum, management, and results. J Vasc Surg. 46(3):475-484, 2007
5. Li F et al: Neurofibromin is a novel regulator of RAS-induced signals in primary vascular smooth muscle cells. Hum Mol Genet. 15(11):1921-30, 2006
6. Han M et al: Renal artery stenosis and aneurysms associated with neurofibromatosis. J Vasc Surg. 41(3):539-43, 2005
7. Porcaro AB et al: Intraparenchymal renal artery aneurysms. Case report with review and update of the literature. Int Urol Nephrol. 36(3):409-16, 2004
8. Fossali E et al: Renovascular disease and hypertension in children with neurofibromatosis. Pediatr Nephrol. 14(8-9):806-10, 2000
9. Devaney K et al: Pediatric renal artery dysplasia: a morphologic study. Pediatr Pathol. 11(4):609-21, 1991
10. DiPrete DA et al: Acute renal insufficiency due to renal infarctions in a patient with neurofibromatosis. Am J Kidney Dis. 15(4):357-60, 1990
11. Finley JL et al: Renal vascular smooth muscle proliferation in neurofibromatosis. Hum Pathol. 19(1):107-10, 1988
12. Zochodne D: Von Recklinghausen's vasculopathy. Am J Med Sci. 287(1):64-5, 1984
13. Greene JF Jr et al: Arterial lesions associated with neurofibromatosis. Am J Clin Pathol. 62(4):481-7, 1974

Arcuate Artery Aneurysms

(Left) Neurofibromatosis characteristically has loose, largely acellular intimal tissue containing small clusters of spindled cells ➡, which in this case occlude an arcuate artery. The media smooth muscle is largely absent with only a couple of short segments remaining ➡. *(Right)* This arcuate artery shows severe dense and fibrotic intimal thickening ➡. In 2 regions, the medial smooth muscle layer is completely absent ➡, and only a single interrupted layer of elastica remains.

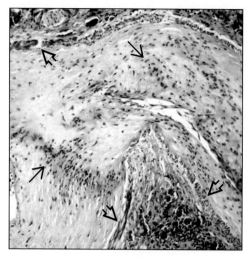
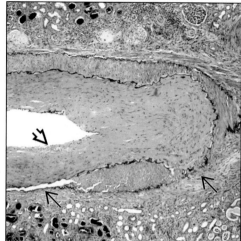

(Left) This is an arcuate artery affected by an aneurysm that has thrombosed and is undergoing organization. There is disruption of the media ➡ with a vigorous proliferation of spindled cells associated with organization. *(Right)* There is thinning ➡ and discontinuity of the media ➡ and exuberant cell proliferation. Some of the cells likely represent the preexisting fibromuscular dysplasia lesion while others represent a cellular reaction to the aneurysmal disruption and hemorrhage.

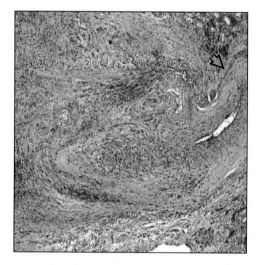
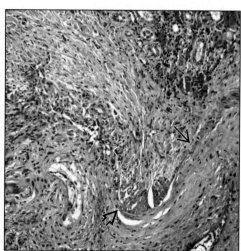

(Left) This arcuate artery shows aneurysm formation. The aneurysm is contained by its external elastic lamina ➡ while the aneurysm lumen is largely filled by loose, edematous paucicellular tissue ➡. *(Right)* This arcuate artery is affected by early aneurysm formation. The media abruptly terminates ➡. The elastica ➡ is focally absent or disrupted. The lumen of the aneurysm and the artery are filled with loose edematous tissue with focal hemorrhage and scattered spindle cells.

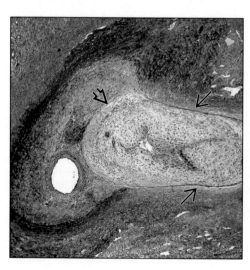
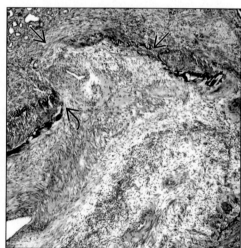

NEUROFIBROMATOSIS

Intralobular Arteries

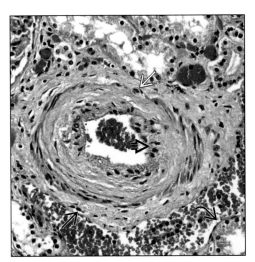

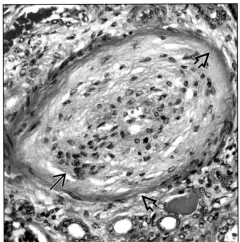

(Left) This intralobular artery has a very thin ⊋ to interrupted media and loose, largely acellular intimal thickening ⊋. There is a similar loose paucicellular alteration of the adventitia ⊋. The adjacent vein ⊋ is normal. Note cortical veins lack a smooth muscle media. *(Right)* This intralobular artery has a very thin media that is focally devoid of all smooth muscle cells ⊋. It also has edematous intimal thickening with focal clusters of bland spindle cells ⊋.

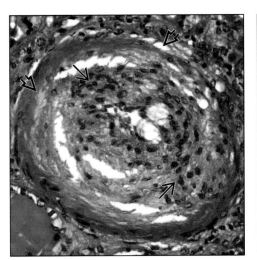

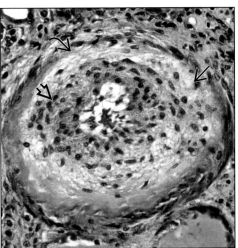

(Left) This intralobular artery has a very thin and focally muscle-deficient media ⊋. There are small clusters of intimal spindle cells ⊋, more numerous than in the preceding images, and acellular areas of intimal thickening. *(Right)* This Movat elastic stain reveals that the internal elastic lamina ⊋ is partially absent and the media smooth muscle ⊋ is greatly attenuated in this intralobular artery. The intima has a myxoid stroma with clusters of oval to spindle cells ⊋.

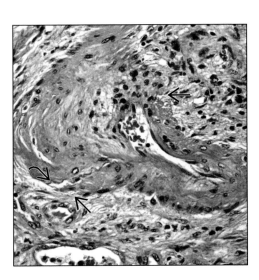

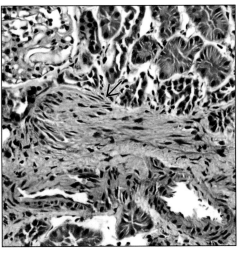

(Left) There is loose intimal thickening that is in continuity with the adventitia and adjacent interstitium. There are 2 areas in which medial smooth muscle cells terminate ⊋ and the internal elastic lamina ends ⊋. *(Right)* This renal biopsy shows a collection of spindled cells ⊋ adjacent to an intralobular artery. The spindle cells are likely related to either an arteriole or a small intralobular artery. Notice that the intralobular artery has a distinct smooth muscle media.

RENAL VEIN THROMBOSIS

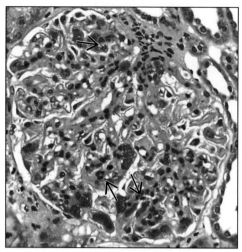

Hematoxylin & eosin demonstrates increased numbers of neutrophils ➡ within the glomerular capillaries of this glomerulus in a patient with renal vein thrombosis.

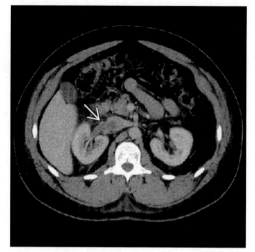

CT scan demonstrates a large opacity leading into the right kidney ➡ that represents a large thrombus in the right renal vein.

TERMINOLOGY

Abbreviations
- Renal vein thrombosis (RVT)

Definitions
- Thrombus involving main renal vein

ETIOLOGY/PATHOGENESIS

Risk Factors
- Nephrotic syndrome
  - RVT is common sequela of severe proteinuria
- Antiphospholipid antibody syndrome
- Neoplasm
  - Renal cell carcinoma
    - Renal vein invasion
  - Urothelial carcinoma
- Infection
- Trauma
- Surgical procedure
- Immobilization
- Dehydration
- Furosemide

CLINICAL ISSUES

Epidemiology
- Incidence
  - 30 to 50% of adults with nephrotic syndrome
  - 2-5% of children with nephrotic syndrome
- Ethnicity
  - No ethnic predilection

Presentation
- Proteinuria, nephrotic range
- Flank pain

Treatment
- Surgical approaches
  - Thrombectomy
    - Rare option
- Drugs
  - Anticoagulation
    - Unfractionated heparin
    - Low molecular weight heparin
  - Fibrinolytic therapy
    - Streptokinase, urokinase

Prognosis
- Poor
  - Due to other thromboembolic events including pulmonary emboli
  - 60% mortality rate in neonates with main renal vein involvement

IMAGE FINDINGS

CT Findings
- Occlusion and distension of main renal vein

MACROSCOPIC FEATURES

General Features
- Enlargement
- Renal vein thrombus
- Vascular congestion

MICROSCOPIC PATHOLOGY

Histologic Features
- Thrombi
  - Renal vein
  - Renal venules
  - Glomerular capillaries
- Glomerular and peritubular capillary dilatation

RENAL VEIN THROMBOSIS

Key Facts

Etiology/Pathogenesis

- Risk factors for RVT
  - Nephrotic syndrome
  - Trauma
  - Infection
  - Antiphospholipid antibody syndrome
  - Neoplasm
  - Dehydration

Clinical Issues

- Treatment
  - Anticoagulation
  - Fibrinolytic therapy

Microscopic Pathology

- Thrombi

Top Differential Diagnoses

- Thrombotic microangiopathy

- Glomerular capillaritis or glomerulitis
  - Leukocyte or neutrophil congestion within glomerular capillaries
- Interstitial edema
- Interstitial foam cells
- Acute tubular injury
- Swelling or prominence of visceral epithelial cells (podocytes)
- Glomerular alterations if concurrent glomerular disease is present
  - Membranous glomerulonephritis, focal segmental glomerulosclerosis

ANCILLARY TESTS

Histochemistry

- Masson trichrome
  - Staining pattern
    - Stains thrombi in red

Immunohistochemistry

- CD61
  - Platelet marker (glycoprotein IIIa)
  - Highlights thrombi

Electron Microscopy

- Subendothelial lucency, endothelial injury

DIFFERENTIAL DIAGNOSIS

Thrombotic Microangiopathy

- Involves capillaries, arterioles, or arteries, **not** veins or venules

Renal Artery Thrombosis

- Hemorrhagic necrosis and infarct

Hydronephrosis

- Dilatation of ureter, renal pelvis, and distal nephron segments

DIAGNOSTIC CHECKLIST

Pathologic Interpretation Pearls

- May have little histologic change on biopsy

SELECTED REFERENCES

1. Arneil GC et al: Renal venous thrombosis. Clin Nephrol. 1(3):119-31, 1973
2. Rosenmann E et al: Renal vein thrombosis in the adult: a clinical and pathologic study based on renal biopsies. Medicine (Baltimore). 47(4):269-335, 1968
3. Eikner WC et al: Renal vein thrombosis. J Urol. 75(5):780-6, 1956

IMAGE GALLERY

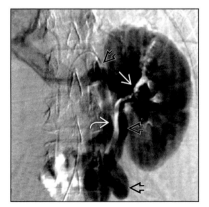 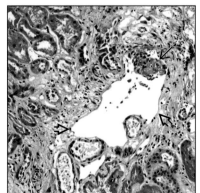 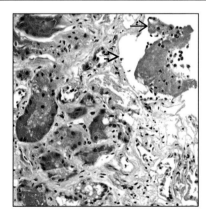

(Left) Venous phase of a right renal arteriogram shows enlarged venous collaterals ⊟ and no main left renal vein. Note the proximity of the collaterals to the renal pelvis ➡ and proximal ureter ➡. *(Center)* Hematoxylin & eosin demonstrates a thrombus ➡ within a portion of the lumen of a renal venule ⊟ in a patient with nephrotic syndrome due to minimal change disease. *(Right)* A thrombus ➡ is slightly detached from this renal venule ⊟ at the edge of this kidney biopsy. This finding may be observed in some patients with nephrotic syndrome.

RENAL ARTERY THROMBOSIS

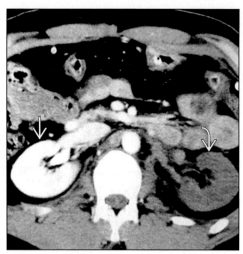

Contrast-enhanced CT shows normal enhancement of the right kidney ➡ with no enhancement of the left kidney ➡, indicating acute thrombosis of the left renal artery. This patient was involved in an MVA.

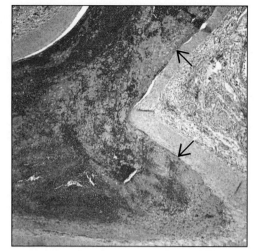

Hematoxylin & eosin reveals a thrombus ➡ at the bifurcation of this large renal artery from a nephrectomy specimen in a female patient with numerous thrombi throughout her vasculature.

TERMINOLOGY

Definitions
- Thrombus of main renal artery

ETIOLOGY/PATHOGENESIS

Risk Factors
- Renal artery stenosis
  - Rupture of atherosclerotic plaques can lead to renal artery thrombosis
- Fibromuscular dysplasia
- Renal artery or abdominal aortic aneurysm
- Trauma
  - Motor vehicle accident (MVA)
  - Complication of surgical procedure or instrumentation
- Hypercoagulable state
  - Antiphospholipid antibody syndrome
  - Factor V Leiden homozygous mutation
  - Protein C deficiency
  - Protein S deficiency
  - Heparin-induced thrombocytopenia
- Inflammation
  - Polyarteritis nodosa
  - Takayasu arteritis
  - Kawasaki disease
- Infection
  - Syphilis
  - Sepsis
- Cocaine use
- Nephrotic syndrome
  - Rare

CLINICAL ISSUES

Epidemiology
- Incidence

  - Dependent on underlying disease or predisposing risk factors

Site
- Kidney

Presentation
- Acute renal failure
- Flank pain
- Hypertension
- Hematuria

Laboratory Tests
- Serologic tests
  - Work-up for hypercoagulable state

Treatment
- Surgical approaches
  - Surgical exploration
  - Thrombectomy
- Drugs
  - Anticoagulation
  - Fibrinolytic therapy

IMAGE FINDINGS

CT Findings
- Occlusion of renal artery with nonenhancement of involved kidney
  - Kidney will infarct and become smaller over time

MACROSCOPIC FEATURES

General Features
- Hemorrhagic necrosis
- Wedge infarct

RENAL ARTERY THROMBOSIS

Key Facts

Etiology/Pathogenesis
- Risk factors
  - Fibromuscular dysplasia
  - Renal artery or abdominal aortic aneurysm
  - Trauma
  - Hypercoagulable state
  - Inflammation
  - Infection

Macroscopic Features
- Hemorrhagic necrosis

Microscopic Pathology
- Arterial thrombus
- Diffuse cortical necrosis

Top Differential Diagnoses
- Thrombotic microangiopathy
- Renal vein thrombosis

MICROSCOPIC PATHOLOGY

Histologic Features
- Arterial thrombus
  - Distension of renal artery
  - Lines of Zahn
    - Indicates thrombus formed gradually in flowing blood
    - Layers of platelets/fibrin alternating with red blood cells
- Diffuse cortical necrosis
- Interstitial hemorrhage
- Acute tubular injury

Predominant Pattern/Injury Type
- Thrombosis

Predominant Cell/Compartment Type
- Artery, intrarenal

DIFFERENTIAL DIAGNOSIS

Thrombotic Microangiopathy
- Thrombi involving arteries, arterioles, or glomerular capillaries

Atheromatous Emboli
- Presence of cholesterol clefts within occluded artery

Renal Vein Thrombosis
- Thrombi in vein, venules, or glomerular capillaries

- Glomerular or peritubular capillary dilatation

Renal Artery Stenosis
- Hypertension
- Marked narrowing of main renal arterial lumen

Acute Tubular Necrosis
- Prominent tubular injury with loss of proximal tubular brush borders or cell sloughing into tubular lumina

SELECTED REFERENCES

1. Tektonidou MG: Renal involvement in the antiphospholipid syndrome (APS)-APS nephropathy. Clin Rev Allergy Immunol. 36(2-3):131-40, 2009
2. Balci YI et al: Nonstroke arterial thrombosis in children: Hacettepe experience. Blood Coagul Fibrinolysis. 19(6):519-24, 2008
3. Tsugawa K et al: Renal artery thrombosis in a pediatric case of systemic lupus erythematosus without antiphospholipid antibodies. Pediatr Nephrol. 20(11):1648-50, 2005
4. Nishimura M et al: Acute arterial thrombosis with antithrombin III deficiency in nephrotic syndrome: report of a case. Surg Today. 30(7):663-6, 2000
5. Klinge J et al: Selective thrombolysis in a newborn with bilateral renal venous and cerebral thrombosis and heterozygous APC resistance. Nephrol Dial Transplant. 13(12):3205-7, 1998
6. Le Moine A et al: Acute renal artery thrombosis associated with factor V Leiden mutation. Nephrol Dial Transplant. 11(10):2067-9, 1996
7. Farkas JC et al: Arterial thrombosis: a rare complication of the nephrotic syndrome. Cardiovasc Surg. 1(3):265-9, 1993

IMAGE GALLERY

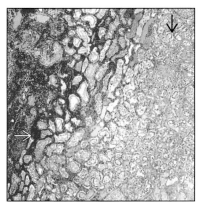 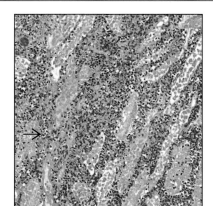 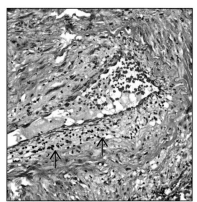

(Left) Hematoxylin & eosin reveals diffuse cortical necrosis ➡ with interstitial hemorrhage ➡ in this young female with a renal artery thrombus. *(Center)* Hematoxylin & eosin shows prominent interstitial neutrophilic infiltration ➡ and hemorrhage between many necrotic tubules. *(Right)* Hematoxylin & eosin demonstrates prominent leukocyte infiltration of the intima ➡ and loose intimal thickening in a segment of a renal artery downstream from a renal artery thrombus.

ATHEROMATOUS EMBOLI

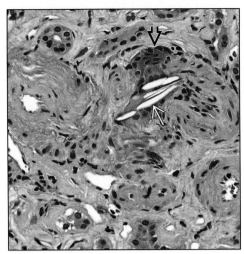

Hematoxylin & eosin shows an atheroembolus with characteristic cholesterol clefts ➡ surrounded by a giant cell reaction ➾ that completely occludes the lumen of an interlobular artery.

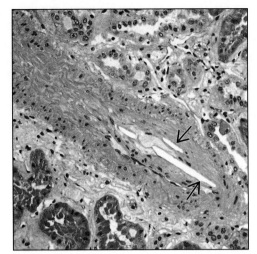

Hematoxylin & eosin reveals several cholesterol clefts ➾ in this interlobular artery. The absence of red cells or fibrin around the clefts is consistent with a remote atheroembolus.

TERMINOLOGY

Synonyms
- Atheroembolic disease
- Atheroemboli
- Cholesterol emboli

ETIOLOGY/PATHOGENESIS

Risk Factors
- Atherosclerosis
  - Risk factors include
    - Hypertension
    - Diabetes mellitus
    - Tobacco use or smoking
    - Hypercholesterolemia
- Invasive vascular procedure
  - Angioplasty or angiography
  - Vascular surgery
    - Coronary artery bypass
    - Aortic aneurysm repair
- Cardiopulmonary resuscitation
- Anticoagulant therapy
- Thrombolytic therapy
- Trauma

CLINICAL ISSUES

Epidemiology
- Incidence
  - 77% of abdominal aortic aneurysm surgical patients
  - Pathology specimens
    - 0.8-4.4% of autopsies
    - 0.5-2% of tumor nephrectomies
- Age
  - > 50 years old
- Gender
  - Male predominance
- Ethnicity
  - Caucasian predilection

Site
- Extremities
- Kidneys

Presentation
- Acute renal failure
- Hypertension
- Hematuria
- Proteinuria
  - May be nephrotic range
- Fever
- Myalgia

Laboratory Tests
- None

Treatment
- Options, risks, complications
  - Primarily symptomatic or preventive measures
- Drugs
  - HMG-CoA reductase inhibitors
    - Stabilize plaques
  - No drug for atheroemboli

Prognosis
- Variable

MACROSCOPIC FEATURES

General Features
- Infarcts
- Scar

MICROSCOPIC PATHOLOGY

Histologic Features
- Atheroembolus

ATHEROMATOUS EMBOLI

Key Facts

Terminology
- Atheroembolic disease
- Cholesterol emboli
- Atheroemboli

Clinical Issues
- Sites of involvement
  - Extremities
  - Kidneys
- Clinical presentation
  - Acute renal failure
  - Hypertension
  - Proteinuria
  - Hematuria

Macroscopic Features
- Infarcts

- Scar

Microscopic Pathology
- Atheroembolus
  - Cholesterol clefts: Crystals dissolved by formalin fixation
  - Acute lesion surrounded by red blood cells, fibrin, or leukocytes
  - Chronic lesion embedded within intimal fibrosis
  - Multinucleated giant cell reaction may be present

Top Differential Diagnoses
- Handling artifact
- Renal artery stenosis
- Arteriosclerosis
- Thrombotic microangiopathy

  - Cholesterol clefts: Crystals dissolved by formalin fixation
  - Acute lesion surrounded by red blood cells, fibrin, or leukocytes
  - Chronic lesion embedded within intimal fibrosis
  - Multinucleated giant cell reaction often present
  - Can involve arteries, arterioles, or glomerular capillaries
  - Recanalization of vessels may occur
- Acute tubular injury
- Vascular disease
  - Intimal fibrosis of arteries
  - Duplication or replication of internal elastic lamina
- Global &/or segmental glomerulosclerosis
- Interstitial fibrosis and tubular atrophy

ANCILLARY TESTS

Electron Microscopy
- Transmission
  - Rare cholesterol clefts in glomerular capillaries
  - Podocyte foot processes may demonstrate substantial effacement

DIFFERENTIAL DIAGNOSIS

Handling Artifact
- Arterioles and small arteries may have slit-like lumen that mimic cholesterol clefts
- Artifact due to compression, handling with forceps, or processing of biopsy specimen

Renal Artery Stenosis
- Hypertension
- Ischemic glomerulopathy, diffuse interstitial fibrosis, and tubular atrophy

Arteriosclerosis
- Severe intimal fibrosis
- No cholesterol clefts within severely narrowed vascular lumen

Thrombotic Microangiopathy
- Thrombi without cholesterol clefts

SELECTED REFERENCES

1. Mittal BV et al: Atheroembolic renal disease: a silent masquerader. Kidney Int. 73(1):126-30, 2008
2. Bijol V et al: Evaluation of the nonneoplastic pathology in tumor nephrectomy specimens: predicting the risk of progressive renal failure. Am J Surg Pathol. 30(5):575-84, 2006
3. Schönermarck U et al: Cholesterol atheroembolic disease in kidney allografts--case report and review of the literature. Clin Nephrol. 66(5):386-90, 2006
4. Scolari F et al: Predictors of renal and patient outcomes in atheroembolic renal disease: a prospective study. J Am Soc Nephrol. 14(6):1584-90, 2003
5. Thériault J et al: Atheroembolic renal failure requiring dialysis: potential for renal recovery? A review of 43 cases. Nephron Clin Pract. 94(1):c11-8, 2003
6. Modi KS et al: Atheroembolic renal disease. J Am Soc Nephrol. 12(8):1781-7, 2001
7. Greenberg A et al: Focal segmental glomerulosclerosis associated with nephrotic syndrome in cholesterol atheroembolism: clinicopathological correlations. Am J Kidney Dis. 29(3):334-44, 1997
8. Liss KA et al: Coexistence of atheroemboli and minimal-change disease. Clin Nephrol. 47(2):125-8, 1997
9. Haqqie SS et al: Nephrotic-range proteinuria in renal atheroembolic disease: report of four cases. Am J Kidney Dis. 28(4):493-501, 1996

ATHEROMATOUS EMBOLI

Microscopic Features

(Left) Hematoxylin & eosin shows an atheroembolus with a large cholesterol cleft ➡ in an arteriole adjacent to a glomerulus ➡. Red blood cells ➡ and leukocytes ⮞ surrounding the clefts indicate an acute lesion. *(Right)* Hematoxylin & eosin shows a large cholesterol cleft ➡ surrounded by many red blood cells ⮞ and foamy macrophages ➡ that is consistent with an acute atheroembolus occluding an artery with severe atherosclerosis.

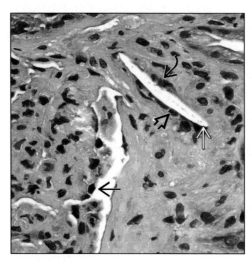
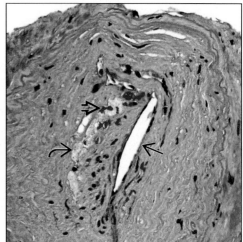

(Left) Periodic acid-Schiff reveals several cholesterol clefts ➡ embedded in this medium-sized renal artery. *(Right)* Periodic acid-Schiff shows an early lesion of segmental sclerosis with obliteration of glomerular capillary lumina ➡. Atheroemboli were present (not shown), which have been observed with focal segmental glomerulosclerosis.

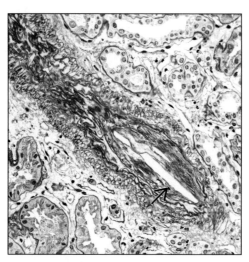
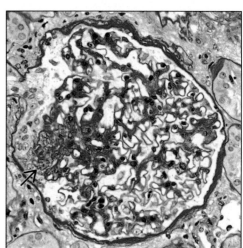

(Left) Periodic acid-Schiff demonstrates segmental sclerosis ➡ with accumulation of hyaline in this patient with tumor nephrectomy for renal cell carcinoma and mild azotemia and proteinuria. A large atheroembolus in an interlobar artery (not shown) was present elsewhere in the biopsy. *(Right)* Hematoxylin & eosin shows a remote atheroembolus completely occluding this interlobar artery with focal giant cell reaction ➡ that extends to the adventitia.

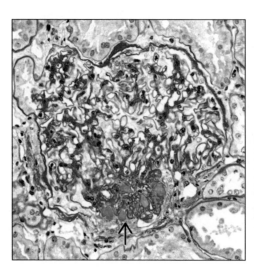
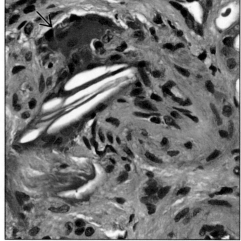

ATHEROMATOUS EMBOLI

Microscopic Features

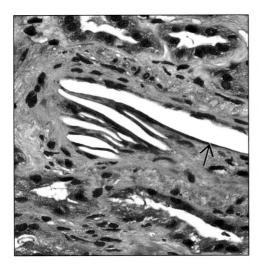 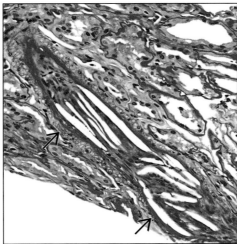

(Left) Hematoxylin & eosin demonstrates the complete occlusion of a renal artery by an atheromatous embolus with giant cell reaction surrounding the cholesterol clefts ➡. Numerous emboli were present in this kidney biopsy. **(Right)** Periodic acid-Schiff reveals numerous cholesterol clefts ➡ of a large atheromatous embolus occluding the entire longitudinal section of this interlobar artery. A giant cell histiocytic reaction surrounds the individual clefts.

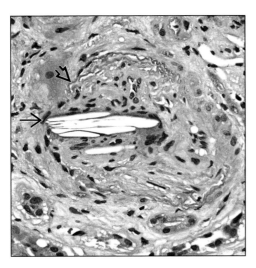 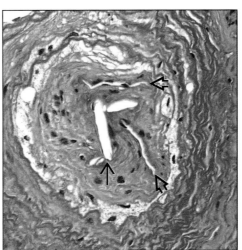

(Left) Hematoxylin & eosin reveals numerous cholesterol clefts ➡, characteristic of an atheroembolus, that are embedded in this occluded artery ➡ with multiple layers of internal elastic lamina and prominent intimal fibrosis. **(Right)** Periodic acid-Schiff shows a remote atheroembolus with cholesterol clefts ➡ embedded within prominent intimal fibrosis. Recanalization of the atheroembolus with slit-like lumens ➡ lined by endothelial cells is also present.

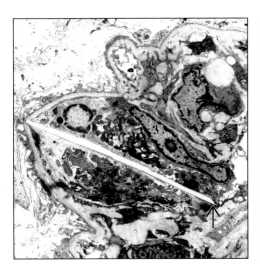 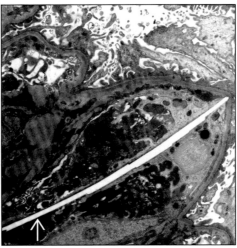

(Left) Electron micrograph reveals a single cholesterol cleft ➡ that distends and occludes the lumen of a glomerular capillary. The clinical significance of this lesion is unclear as no other atheroemboli were identified in this biopsy. **(Right)** Electron micrograph shows a cholesterol cleft ➡, surrounded by a macrophage, occluding the lumen of a glomerular capillary. The irregular distribution of atheroemboli can make this diagnosis difficult to establish.

Tubulointerstitial Diseases

CLASSIFICATION OF TUBULOINTERSTITIAL DISEASES

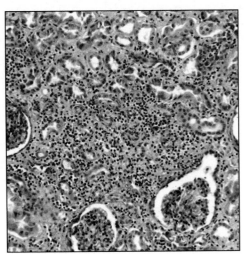

Acute interstitial nephritis was originally described in 1898 by William Councilman as a systemic response to certain extrarenal infections (here an untreated streptococcal infection).

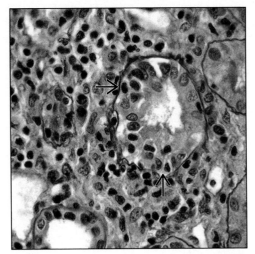

Tubulitis, invasion of tubules by lymphocytes ➔, is a common finding in immunologically mediated tubulointerstitial disease, as illustrated in this example associated with uveitis (TINU syndrome).

TERMINOLOGY

Abbreviations
- Acute interstitial nephritis (AIN)
- Chronic interstitial nephritis (CIN)
- Acute tubular necrosis (ATN)
- Acute tubular injury (ATI)

Synonyms
- Tubulointerstitial nephritis
- Interstitial nephritis

Definitions
- Group of diseases primarily manifested by inflammation &/or injury of renal tubules and interstitium

ETIOLOGY/PATHOGENESIS

Genetic
- Storage diseases, crystal deposition, transport abnormalities, mitochondrionopathies

Infection
- Direct infection of kidney by bacteria, viruses, fungi, protozoa, rickettsia
- Indirect effects of systemic infection
  - *C. diphtheriae*, *Streptococcus*, and many other organisms

Toxic
- Heavy metals, biologic toxins, organic compounds

Metabolic
- Monoclonal protein deposition, milk alkali syndrome, hypokalemia

Immunologic
- Autoimmune, drug allergy, allograft rejection

Ischemia
- Shock
- Hypovolemia

Obstruction
- Stones, reflux, tumor

Radiation
- Late effects of abdominal radiotherapy

Idiopathic
- Sarcoidosis
- Unclassified acute and chronic interstitial nephritis

APPROACH TO DIAGNOSIS OF TUBULOINTERSTITIAL DISEASES

Biopsy
- Appearances often similar despite varied mechanisms
- Search for etiologic agent (organisms) or distinctive pathologic features (granulomata, eosinophils, antibody deposition, crystals, viral inclusions)
- General tools
  - Light microscopy
    - Special stains (PAS, silver methenamine, Giemsa, Brown-Breen, acid fast)
    - Polarized light for crystals, also processing in nonaqueous solutions (urates)
    - Immunohistochemistry or in situ hybridization for organisms (polyoma, EBER, adenovirus, CMV)
  - Immunofluorescence microscopy
    - IgG, IgA, IgM, C3, C1q, fibrinogen, kappa, lambda
    - TBM: Immune complexes, anti-TBM antibodies, monoclonal light chain deposition
  - Electron microscopy
    - Organisms and deposits (viruses, microsporidia) or deposits (light chains)

CLASSIFICATION OF TUBULOINTERSTITIAL DISEASES

Etiologic Classification of Tubulointerstitial Diseases

Genetic	Mitochondrionopathies
	Adenine phosphoribosyl transferase deficiency
Infection	
Direct infection	Polyomavirus nephropathy
	Acute pyelonephritis
	Tuberculosis
Indirect effects	Streptococcal infection
Immunologic	
Allergic	Drug-induced interstitial nephritis
Autoimmune	Sjögren syndrome
Alloimmune	Acute cellular allograft rejection
Unknown antigen	IgG4-associated acute interstitial nephritis
Toxic	Cadmium poisoning
	Analgesic nephropathy
Metabolic	Oxalosis secondary to malabsorption
	Milk alkali syndrome
Ischemia	Acute tubular necrosis in shock
Obstruction	Ureteral-pelvic junction stenosis
Radiation	Radiation interstitial nephritis
Idiopathic	Sarcoidosis
	Balkan nephropathy

Clinical Information

- Careful clinical history may provide clues
  - e.g., drug exposure, work, family history, travel, rash, fever other systemic symptoms

Laboratory Tests

- Blood tests for autoantibodies, functional tests for enzymes, electrolyte and metabolite levels
- Screening for organisms, molecular tests, cultures, antibodies
- Urinalysis for organisms, crystals, leukocytes, eosinophils

Radiologic Studies

- Evidence of obstruction, perfusion, kidney size, stones

SELECTED REFERENCES

1. Michel DM et al: Acute interstitial nephritis. J Am Soc Nephrol. 9(3):506-15, 1998
2. Colvin RB et al: Interstitial nephritis. In Tisher CC et al: Renal Pathology. 2nd ed. Philadelphia: JB Lippincott. 723-68, 1994
3. Cameron JS: Immunologically mediated interstitial nephritis: primary and secondary. Adv Nephrol Necker Hosp. 18:207-48, 1989
4. Papper S: Interstitial nephritis. Contrib Nephrol. 23:204-19, 1980
5. Heptinstall RH: Interstitial nephritis. A brief review. Am J Pathol. 83(1):213-36, 1976
6. Councilman WT: Acute Interstitial Nephritis. J Exp Med. 3(4-5):393-420, 1898

IMAGE GALLERY

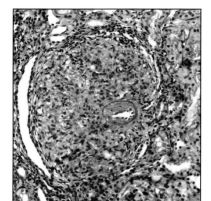 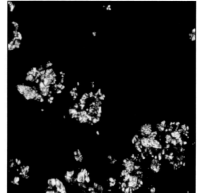 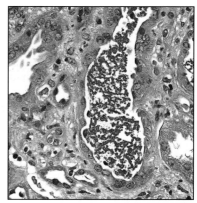

(Left) Granulomas can suggest either an infectious origin, a response to insoluble material, or an immunologic process, as in this case of allergic drug-induced interstitial nephritis. *(Center)* Polarizing light reveals abundant crystals in this fatal case of hereditary oxalosis in a 19-year-old boy. *(Right)* Casts may reveal an etiology, as in this case of rhabdomyolysis due to a statin drug. The granular material stained for myoglobin by immunohistochemistry.

DIFFERENTIAL DIAGNOSIS OF ACUTE INTERSTITIAL NEPHRITIS

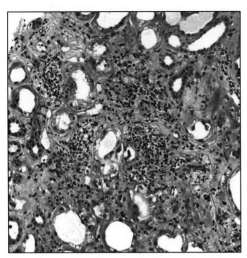

Acute interstitial nephritis is a heterogeneous group of diseases. This case in a 78-year-old man with acute renal failure was due to a recent exposure to antibiotics.

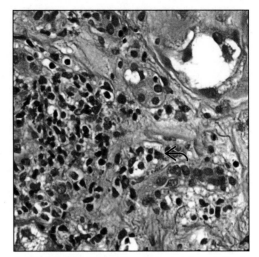

Eosinophilic tubulitis ⇗ is seen in a case of acute allergic interstitial nephritis due to antibiotics, regarded as a useful sign of drug-induced AIN, although the specificity has not been proven.

TERMINOLOGY

Abbreviations
- Acute interstitial nephritis (AIN)

Synonyms
- Acute tubulointerstitial nephritis

ETIOLOGY/PATHOGENESIS

Drugs
- May account for 60-70% of AIN cases
- Allergic (e.g., antibiotics, proton pump inhibitors, nonsteroidal anti-inflammatory drugs [NSAIDs])
- Toxic (e.g., cisplatinum, lithium, NSAIDs)

Autoimmune
- Primary in kidney
  - e.g., anti-tubular basement membrane (TBM) disease, giant cell tubulitis with TBM immune deposits, idiopathic hypocomplementemic tubulointerstitial nephritis (TIN)
- Associated with systemic disease
  - e.g., Sjögren syndrome, tubulointerstitial nephritis with uveitis (TINU) syndrome, IgG4-related systemic autoimmune disease, sarcoid

Infection
- Direct infection
  - Bacteria (e.g., pyelonephritis), mycobacteria
  - Virus (e.g., BK polyomavirus tubulointerstitial nephritis)
  - Other, including parasites
- Reaction to distant infection (e.g., post streptococcal infection)

Hereditary/Toxic/Metabolic
- e.g., hyperoxaluria, gout, heavy metal toxicity
- Typically chronic injury, less inflammation

Idiopathic
- Accounts for ~ 25% of cases

CLINICAL ISSUES

Epidemiology
- Incidence
  - ~ 15-27% of renal biopsies for acute renal failure show AIN

Presentation
- Acute or subacute renal failure
- Proteinuria, subnephrotic
- Microhematuria
- Pyuria
- Eosinophiluria
- In drug-related acute allergic AIN, renal failure may be accompanied by rash, fever, arthralgias, and eosinophilia
- Clinical history important to determine cause of AIN
  - Recent (a week to months) exposure to new drug may suggest allergic AIN
  - Longer period of exposure prior to AIN associated with NSAID use

Treatment
- Drugs
  - Corticosteroids
    - May be of benefit in some cases with more acute onset of AIN
  - Cytotoxic drugs (e.g., cyclophosphamide) and plasmapheresis may be used in anti-TBM disease
- Discontinuation of causative drug in drug-related AIN

DIFFERENTIAL DIAGNOSIS OF ACUTE INTERSTITIAL NEPHRITIS

Key Facts

Etiology/Pathogenesis
- Drugs
  - May account for 60-70% of AIN cases
- Autoimmune
- Infection
- Hereditary/toxic/metabolic

Clinical Issues
- ~ 15-27% of renal biopsies for acute renal failure show AIN
- Treatment: Discontinuation of causative drug in drug-related AIN; corticosteroids (controversial)

Microscopic Pathology
- Interstitial inflammation with lymphocytes, monocytes/macrophages, eosinophils, plasma cells
- High number of eosinophils suggestive of allergic AIN but not specific
- Tubulitis
- Interstitial fibrosis may be present

Top Differential Diagnoses
- Granulomatous AIN
  - Type of AIN; most common causes are drug reaction and sarcoidosis
- Interstitial inflammation associated with glomerular disease
- Neoplasm
- Light chain deposition disease (monoclonal immunoglobulin deposition disease)
- Acute cellular rejection in renal allograft

MICROSCOPIC PATHOLOGY

Histologic Features
- Interstitial inflammation with lymphocytes, monocytes/macrophages, and eosinophils, usually fewer plasma cells than other inflammatory cells
  - High number of eosinophils suggestive of allergic AIN but not specific
  - Increased plasma cells suggestive of autoimmune AIN but not specific
- Interstitial edema
- Tubulitis
  - May be mononuclear cells or eosinophils
- Acute tubular injury
- Granulomatous AIN
  - Nonnecrotizing granulomas in sarcoidosis and drug-related AIN
  - Presence of granulomas or diffuse inflammation in drug-related AIN portends poorer prognosis
- Interstitial fibrosis may be present

Immunofluorescence
- Granular TBM deposits in some cases of autoimmune interstitial nephritis
- Linear TBM deposits in anti-TBM disease

Electron Microscopy
- Amorphous, electron-dense deposits in TBMs in some cases of autoimmune interstitial nephritis

DIFFERENTIAL DIAGNOSIS

Granulomatous AIN
- Type of AIN; most common causes are allergic drug reactions and sarcoidosis
- Rarely direct infection (e.g., tuberculosis)
- May be seen with pauci-immune necrotizing and crescentic glomerulonephritis

Interstitial Inflammation Associated with Glomerular Disease
- Glomerulonephritis
  - Pauci-immune necrotizing and crescentic glomerulonephritis
  - IgA nephropathy
  - Acute postinfectious glomerulonephritis
  - Other
- Focal segmental glomerulosclerosis, collapsing variant

Neoplasm
- Infiltrating lymphoid neoplasm or plasma cell myeloma

Light Chain Deposition Disease (Monoclonal Immunoglobulin Deposition Disease)
- Interstitial inflammation and acute tubular injury by light microscopy
- Linear glomerular and tubular basement membrane staining by monoclonal protein seen by immunofluorescence
- Finely granular, electron-dense deposits in basement membranes seen by electron microscopy

Acute Cellular Rejection in Renal Allograft
- May be impossible to distinguish AIN from acute cellular rejection

SELECTED REFERENCES

1. Perazella MA et al: Drug-induced acute interstitial nephritis. Nat Rev Nephrol. 6(8):461-70, 2010
2. Praga M et al: Acute interstitial nephritis. Kidney Int. 77(11):956-61, 2010
3. Bijol V et al: Granulomatous interstitial nephritis: a clinicopathologic study of 46 cases from a single institution. Int J Surg Pathol. 14(1):57-63, 2006
4. Baker RJ et al: The changing profile of acute tubulointerstitial nephritis. Nephrol Dial Transplant. 19(1):8-11, 2004
5. Baldwin DS et al: Renal failure and interstitial nephritis due to penicillin and methicillin. N Engl J Med. 279(23):1245-52, 1968

Microscopic Features

(Left) H&E shows acute and chronic allergic tubulointerstitial nephritis with diffuse interstitial inflammation. This patient had been taking a number of herbal preparations for many months, after which she was found to have an elevated serum creatinine. Immunofluorescence staining was negative. *(Right)* This case of AIN also showed areas of interstitial fibrosis with inflammation. The fibrosis is indicative of a chronic component of the interstitial nephritis (trichome stain).

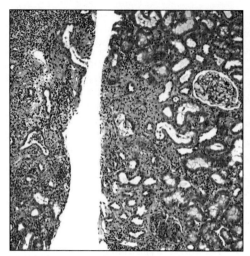
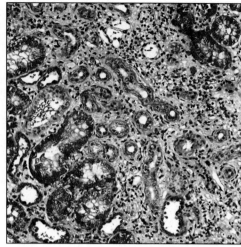

(Left) Acute interstitial inflammation with mononuclear cells and neutrophils is seen in a case of acute pyelonephritis. Neutrophilic casts are present ➥. This biopsy is from a renal transplant patient who had laboratory evidence of a urinary tract infection. *(Right)* A neutrophilic cast ➥ within a tubule is seen in acute pyelonephritis. Neutrophils are also present within the interstitium ➥. Occasional neutrophil casts can be seen for no apparent reason in end-stage kidneys.

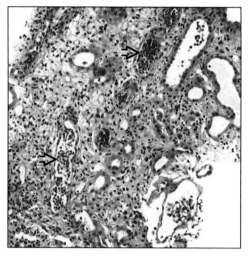
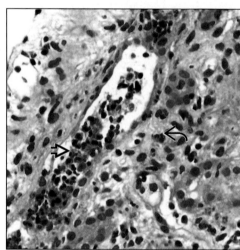

(Left) BK polyomavirus tubulointerstitial nephritis shows interstitial inflammation with increased plasma cells ➥ in an allograft. Some tubular epithelial cells show viral cytopathic effect ➥. *(Right)* In situ hybridization for BK polyomavirus reveals several tubules with positive epithelial cell nuclei ➥. Polyoma can also be readily detected by immunohistochemistry, using an antibody to the large T antigen.

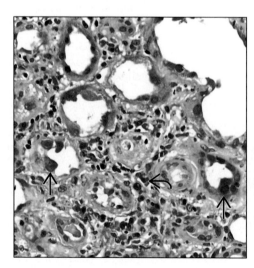
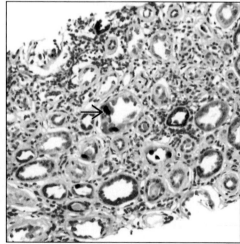

DIFFERENTIAL DIAGNOSIS OF ACUTE INTERSTITIAL NEPHRITIS

Differential Diagnosis

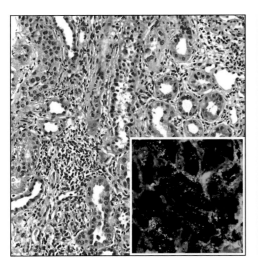

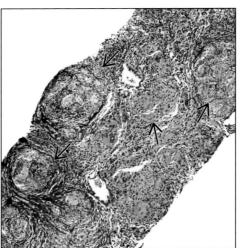

(Left) Tubulointerstitial nephritis with mononuclear cells and plasma cells is seen in Sjögren syndrome. Tubular basement membrane immune complex deposits (inset, immunofluorescence staining for IgG) aid in the diagnosis of an autoimmune interstitial nephritis. (Right) Renal biopsy is shown from a 50-year-old man with a history of sarcoidosis and progressive renal failure over several months. This case shows extensive involvement by nonnecrotizing granulomatous inflammation ➔.

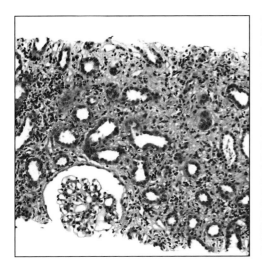

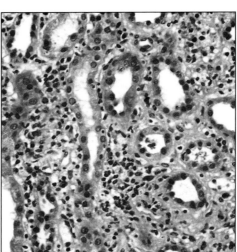

(Left) AIN is seen in a 10-year-old girl who presented with acute renal failure. Several weeks prior, she had cough and fever; no antibiotics were given. 4 months later, the patient developed uveitis and was diagnosed with tubulointerstitial nephritis-uveitis (TINU) syndrome. (Right) The infiltrate in this case of TINU syndrome is composed of mononuclear cells, plasma cells, and eosinophils, mimicking drug-induced AIN, but this patient was on no medications.

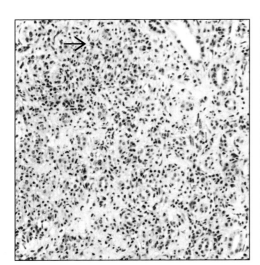

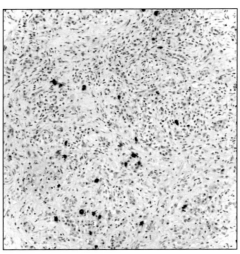

(Left) H&E shows interstitial nephritis associated with IgG4-related systemic disease/autoimmune pancreatitis. This case shows an expansile interstitial fibroinflammatory process with plasma cells and eosinophils ➔. Tubular basement membrane immune complex deposits were present by IF. (Right) Numerous (> 11 cells/40x field) IgG4(+) plasma cells are present in the infiltrate in interstitial nephritis associated with IgG4-related systemic disease.

Other Causes of Interstitial Inflammation

(Left) Hyperoxaluria related to gastric bypass shows interstitial fibrosis and tubular atrophy with interstitial mononuclear cell inflammation ➤. Focal tubules contain calcium oxalate crystals ➚. Usually this condition does not have a florid inflammatory component, in contrast to the usual AIN. *(Right)* A form of hereditary interstitial nephritis is shown with chronic tubulointerstitial nephritis ➤ in a patient with a mutation in the gene for renin.

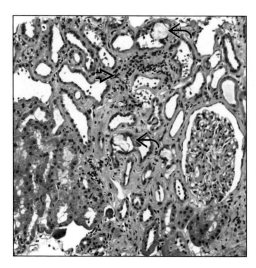
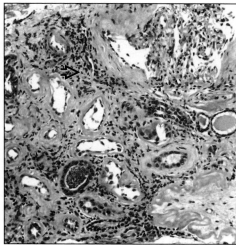

(Left) Urate nephropathy shows interstitial inflammation ➤ surrounding dissolved urate crystals ➚ in a patient with a history of gout and chronic renal failure. *(Right)* Acute postinfectious glomerulonephritis often shows focal interstitial inflammation, including several neutrophils ➤ as shown here. A glomerulus shows an acute exudative glomerulonephritis ➚.

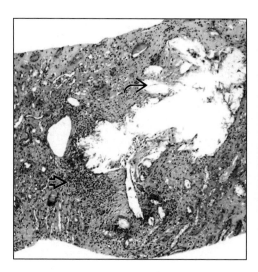
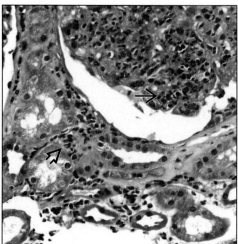

(Left) Interstitial inflammation ➤ is seen in a case of light chain deposition disease (LCDD). A glomerulus shows a nodular glomerulosclerosis ➚. *(Right)* This case showed bright linear glomerular and tubular basement membrane staining for lambda light chain but not kappa light chain by IF, although most cases of LCDD show kappa light chain. Electron microscopy showed finely granular glomerular and tubular basement membrane deposits.

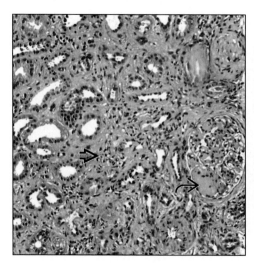
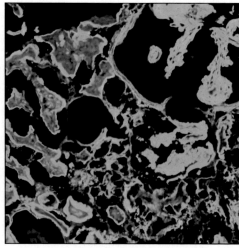

Differential Diagnosis

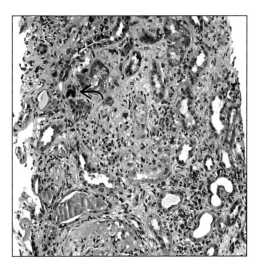

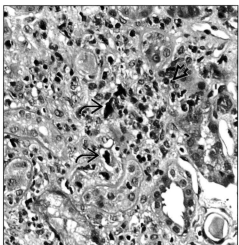

(Left) Extramedullary hematopoiesis shows an interstitial infiltrate at medium magnification. A few cells with large, irregular nuclei stand out ➡. The biopsy is from a 77-year-old man with renal failure and a history of myelofibrosis. *(Right)* Extramedullary hematopoiesis can be confused with AIN. The larger cells can be recognized as megakaryocytes ➡, confirming the diagnosis. Eosinophil and neutrophil precursors are also present ➡.

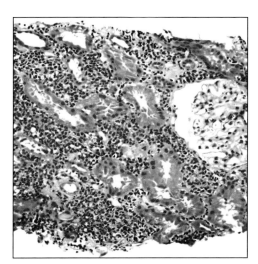

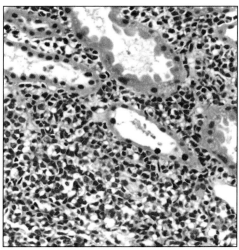

(Left) Acute myeloid leukemia (AML) involving the kidney can resemble AIN. This case has extensive interstitial infiltration by leukocytes. This patient had a history of treated AML and then developed acute renal failure and markedly enlarged kidneys. *(Right)* On higher magnification in this case of AML, atypical cells are seen to be large and monomorphic. Immunohistochemistry revealed blasts positive for CD33 and CD34 and negative for CD3 and CD20.

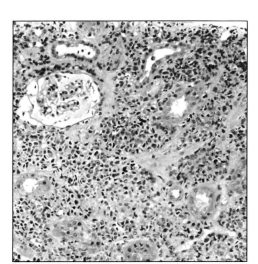

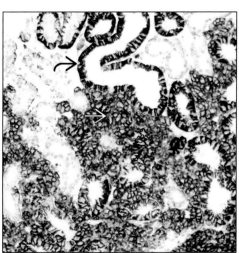

(Left) Plasma cell myeloma in an allograft is shown. Atypical cells are infiltrating the interstitium. No mass lesion was detected; the biopsy was performed for renal dysfunction. *(Right)* Infiltrating cells ➡ are positive for the plasma cell marker CD138, as are some tubular epithelial cells ➡ (a normal finding).

ACUTE TUBULAR NECROSIS

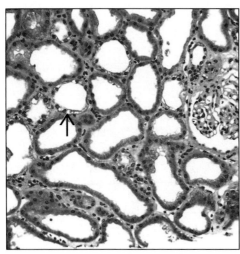

H&E shows epithelial attenuation, loss of apical cytoplasm, prominent dilated tubules, and focal, largely distal, tubular epithelial vacuolization ⊋.

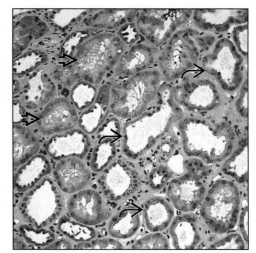

H&E shows patchy tubular epithelial injury with normal appearing segments ⊵, most with attenuated epithelium and open lumens ⊋.

TERMINOLOGY

Abbreviations
- Acute tubular necrosis (ATN)
- Acute tubular injury (ATI)

Synonyms
- Acute tubular injury
- Acute tubular damage

Definitions
- Acute renal failure caused by acute tubular epithelial injury, due to either ischemia or toxins

ETIOLOGY/PATHOGENESIS

Etiology
- Renal ischemia due to reduced renal perfusion (~ 90%)
  - Hypovolemia
    - Blood loss (trauma, surgery, ante- and postpartum hemorrhage)
    - External fluid loss (e.g., burns, sweat, diarrhea)
    - 3rd space fluid loss (e.g., hypoalbuminemia, bowel obstruction, pancreatitis)
  - Decreased perfusion pressure
    - Systemic: Cardiac failure, cardiac tamponade, myocardial infarction, arrhythmia
    - Local: Severe renal artery stenosis, malignant hypertension
  - Reduced effective intravascular volume
    - Sepsis, hepatorenal syndrome, anaphylaxis, vasodilator drugs
- Nephrotoxins (~ 10%)
  - Drugs
    - Antibiotics (e.g., aminoglycosides, vancomycin, amphotericin)
    - Chemotherapeutic agents (e.g., cisplatin, ifosfamide, cytarabine)
    - Nonsteroidal anti-inflammatory agents (NSAIDs)
    - Calcineurin inhibitors (cyclosporine, tacrolimus)
    - Inhibitors of mTOR (rapamycin, sirolimus)
    - Angiotensin-converting enzyme (ACE) inhibitors
    - Anesthetics (halothane)
    - Radiologic contrast agents
  - Organic solvents
    - Ethylene glycol, carbon tetrachloride
  - Heavy metals
    - Mercury, lead, bismuth, uranium, platinum
  - Endogenous substances
    - Hemoglobin (hemolysis, transfusion reactions)
    - Myoglobin (crush injury, statin drugs)
    - Monoclonal immunoglobulin light chains (free or as crystals or casts in myeloma)
    - Intratubular crystals (calcium oxalate, urates)
    - Bile casts (hepatorenal syndrome)

Pathogenesis
- Ischemic or toxic insult to tubular epithelium
- Tubular injury and dysfunction
  - Altered epithelial transport results in reduction of resorption of NaCl
  - Increased delivery of NaCl to macula densa in distal tubule activates tubuloglomerular feedback reducing glomerular filtration rate (GFR)
  - Loss of tubular epithelial adhesion allows leak of glomerular filtrate into interstitium, reducing effective GFR
  - Exfoliated epithelium, increased tubular sodium, and Tamm-Horsfall protein combine to form luminal casts that obstruct flow
- Hemodynamic changes
  - Afferent arteriolar vasoconstriction reduces glomerular hydrostatic pressure
  - Mesangial contraction in tubuloglomerular feedback reduces effective surface area for filtration
  - Endothelial activation increases adhesion molecule expression and procoagulant activity

ACUTE TUBULAR NECROSIS

Key Facts

Etiology/Pathogenesis
- Renal ischemia/reduced renal perfusion (90%)
- Nephrotoxins (10%)

Clinical Issues
- Deterioration of glomerular filtration rate occurs over hours to days
- Urinary microscopy reveals muddy brown casts and sloughed epithelium

Macroscopic Features
- Kidneys are enlarged with increased weight

Microscopic Pathology
- Necrosis of epithelium with bare basement membranes
- Most tubular cells have sublethal injury
- Casts of necrotic cells and debris + lipofuscin pigment

Top Differential Diagnoses
- Causes of ATN
  - Ischemia
  - Drugs
  - Endogenous or exogenous toxins
- Mimics of ATN
  - Acute interstitial nephritis, autolysis

Diagnostic Checklist
- Most epithelial cells have loss of apical cytoplasm, reduced brush border on PAS stain, and open lumens
- Interstitial edema may be prominent, but inflammatory infiltrates are sparse
- Phases of ATN: Initiation, maintenance, and repair
- Ischemia shows little or no overt necrosis in contrast to toxins

CLINICAL ISSUES

Presentation
- Acute renal failure
  - Deterioration of GFR, measured by elevation of serum creatinine or blood urea nitrogen, occurs over hours to days
- Oliguria
  - Nonoliguric ATN uncommon
    - Associated with drug toxicity, especially aminoglycosides and contrast nephropathy
- Hypotension
  - Normotensive patients with prior hypertension, chronic kidney disease, or advanced age may have reduced renal perfusion that is clinically subtle
- Exposure to toxin may be identified in clinical examination
- Urinary microscopy reveals muddy brown casts and sloughed epithelial cells
- Phases
  - Oliguric: Days to weeks; low GFR and urine output < 400 mL/day
  - Early diuretic: Days to weeks; low GFR and increased urinary output
  - Late diuretic: Weeks; normalization of GFR and increased urinary output

Treatment
- Ischemia
  - Restoration of intravascular volume with intravenous fluids
  - Vasodilators may increase renal perfusion but have no effect on recovery of function
- Toxin
  - Cessation of exposure
  - Removal of toxin (dialysis, chelation)
- Restoration of electrolyte balance and pH
  - Hyperkalemia treated using insulin/glucose to increase cellular uptake, sodium polystyrene sulfonate for potassium binding
  - Severe, persistent ATN refractory to medical therapy requires dialysis

- Complications
  - Infection
    - Source of infection: Indwelling vascular or urinary catheters, respiratory tract, urinary tract
    - Most frequent cause of death is sepsis (30-70%)
  - Cardiovascular
    - Congestive heart failure, pulmonary edema, hypertension (25%), cardiac arrhythmia (10-30%)
  - Gastrointestinal
    - Hemorrhage (10-30%)
  - Neurologic
    - Encephalopathy, seizures

Prognosis
- 5-16% of patients with ischemic ATN have irreversible renal failure
- Mortality is ~ 50% and as high as 79% in critically ill patients with ATN requiring dialysis
- Even mild sustained increase of serum Cr is associated with increased mortality in hospitalized patients

MACROSCOPIC FEATURES

General Features
- Kidneys are enlarged with increased weight up to ~ 130% of normal
- Cut surface reveals bulging pale cortex with red medulla

MICROSCOPIC PATHOLOGY

Histologic Features
- Tubular epithelial injury prominent in early phase
  - Necrosis or apoptosis of individual cells
  - Loss of nuclei
  - Denudation of tubular epithelial cells
  - Patchy distribution of changes with variable thickness of tubular epithelium
  - Cell loss most prominent in distal nephron (distal:proximal ~ 4:1)

ACUTE TUBULAR NECROSIS

- Distal tubular casts of necrotic cells and cell debris often with lipofuscin pigment
- Vast majority of tubular cells have nonnecrotizing sublethal injury in ischemic injury
  - Attenuation with reduced apical cytoplasm
  - Reduced or absent brush borders on PAS (= simplification)
  - Open tubular lumen
- Cell necrosis common in toxic injury
  - Most prominent in proximal tubule
- Regeneration prominent in later phases
  - Increased cytoplasmic basophilia
  - Tubular epithelial mitoses
  - Crowding of proximal epithelial nuclei
- Dystrophic calcium phosphate or apatite may be evident
  - Oxalate crystals common but usually sparse
- Interstitial edema common
  - Sparse mononuclear infiltrates; most marked at vasa recta
- Glomeruli generally unremarkable
  - Fibrin thrombi occur in sepsis
  - Parietal epithelium transformed from squamous to cuboidal cell type, called tubularization of Bowman capsule
- Arteries and arterioles generally unremarkable
- Vasa recta may have luminal leukocytes
  - Extramedullary hematopoiesis may occur
- Tubulocapillary anastomosis may form due to ruptured tubules
  - May have red cell casts

Predominant Pattern/Injury Type
- Tubules, acute injury

Predominant Cell/Compartment Type
- Tubule

DIFFERENTIAL DIAGNOSIS

Causes of ATN
- Ischemia
  - Tubular injury without necrosis
- Myoglobinuria/rhabdomyolysis
  - Eosinophilic globular luminal casts that stain for myoglobin by immunohistochemistry
- Lead and bismuth toxicity
  - Tubular nuclear eosinophilic inclusions
- Antiviral agents (e.g., tenofovir, adefovir)
  - Tubular nucleomegaly with pleomorphism
  - Mitochondrial enlargement and loss of cristae on electron microscopy
- Cisplatin and other DNA synthesis inhibitors
  - Tubular nucleomegaly with pleomorphism
- Calcineurin inhibitor toxicity
  - Isometric vacuolization of tubular epithelium
- Ethylene glycol toxicity
  - Oxalate crystals
- Radiocontrast agents
  - Isometric vacuolization of tubular epithelium
- Sulfonamides
  - Drug crystals in tubules
- Acyclovir, indinavir
  - Drug crystals in tubules

Mimics of ATN
- Acute interstitial nephritis
  - Interstitial inflammation and tubulitis more prominent
- Autolysis
  - Kidney weight not increased
  - Loss of cell to cell and cell to tubular basement membrane adhesion
  - No pigment casts
  - No thinned cytoplasm
  - No mitoses

DIAGNOSTIC CHECKLIST

Clinically Relevant Pathologic Features
- Phases of ATN
  - Initiation (hours to days)
    - Cellular injury, loss of polarity and adhesion, exfoliation and obstruction
  - Maintenance (days to weeks)
    - Dedifferentiation, migration, proliferation, microvascular injury (inflammation, coagulopathy)
  - Repair (weeks to months)
    - Differentiation, restoration of polarity

Pathologic Interpretation Pearls
- Necrotic or apoptotic epithelial cells are few
  - Usually seen in casts and associated with bare segments of basement membrane
- Vast majority of epithelial cells have sublethal injury with loss of apical cytoplasm, loss of brush border on PAS stain, and dilated tubules
- Interstitial edema may be prominent, but inflammatory cell infiltrates are sparse
- Hematopoietic precursors are aggregated in vasa recta
- Ischemia has little or no overt necrosis vs. toxins

SELECTED REFERENCES

1. Abuelo JG: Normotensive ischemic acute renal failure. N Engl J Med. 357(8):797-805, 2007
2. Himmelfarb J et al: Acute kidney injury: changing lexicography, definitions, and epidemiology. Kidney Int. 71(10):971-6, 2007
3. Lameire N et al: Acute renal failure. Lancet. 365(9457):417-30, 2005
4. Esson ML et al: Diagnosis and treatment of acute tubular necrosis. Ann Intern Med. 137(9):744-52, 2002
5. Sutton TA et al: Microvascular endothelial injury and dysfunction during ischemic acute renal failure. Kidney Int. 62(5):1539-49, 2002
6. Rosen S et al: Difficulties in understanding human "acute tubular necrosis": limited data and flawed animal models. Kidney Int. 60(4):1220-4, 2001
7. Solez K et al: The morphology of "acute tubular necrosis" in man: analysis of 57 renal biopsies and a comparison with the glycerol model. Medicine (Baltimore). 58(5):362-76, 1979

Microscopic Features

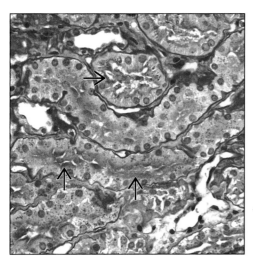
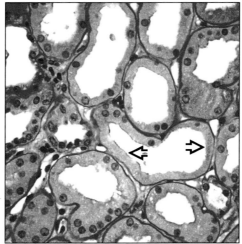

(Left) PAS stain shows a normal proximal tubular brush border ➡ of a normal kidney. Notice that most lumens appears "full" or closed, and the tubules are back-to-back (no edema). *(Right)* Compare the normal appearance with the reduction or absence of brush border (a "crew cut") seen in ATN, which is demonstrated by this PAS stain. The lumens appear dilated but in fact are about the same diameter. Notice the loss of nuclei in some areas, indicating that some cells have sloughed ➡.

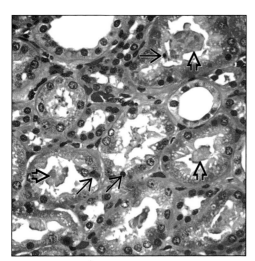
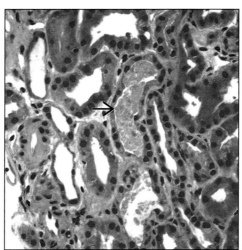

(Left) H&E shows cellular injury in ATN with cytoplasmic debris in tubular lumens ➡ and apoptotic bodies ➡. Frank necrosis is not commonly conspicuous in ischemic ATN, despite its name. Many prefer the term acute tubular injury for that reason. *(Right)* H&E shows ATN with pigmented cast material (lipofuscin) in distal tubules ➡. Lipofuscin is an insoluble metabolic degradation product of lipids, sometimes called a wear and tear pigment.

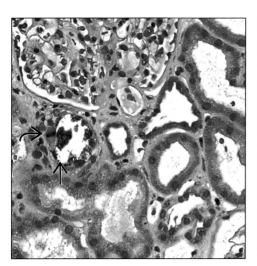
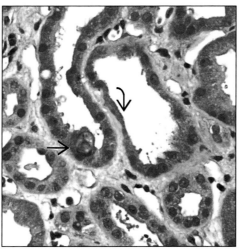

(Left) H&E shows dystrophic calcification ➡ and adjacent epithelial mitosis ➡. The dystrophic calcification was probably formed from the debris of necrotic cells. The glomerulus is unremarkable. *(Right)* H&E reveals an intracellular oxalate crystal ➡. The cytoplasm of the tubular cells is basophilic, indicating increased ribosomal content, a sign of regeneration. Thinning and loss of nuclei are evident ➡, as well as interstitial edema.

Differential Diagnosis

(Left) PAS reveals abundant mitoses in the tubular epithelium ➡ and a loss of brush borders. Interstitial edema is prominent ➡, but the infiltrate is sparse. The tubular basement membranes are intact. *(Right)* PAS shows evidence of tubular regeneration with enlarged nuclei ➡ and mitosis ➡. Note the scattered interstitial inflammation. The tubules have thinned cytoplasm with scattered vacuoles.

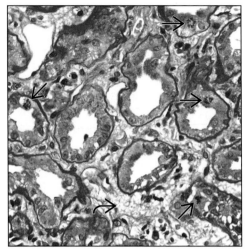
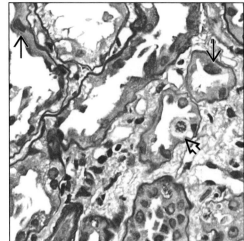

(Left) H&E stain in lead toxicity shows the characteristic eosinophilic nuclear inclusions in proximal tubules ➡. The diagnosis is confirmed by blood or tissue Pb levels. *(Right)* PAS stain of an autolyzed autopsy kidney shows loss of adhesion to the basement membrane in proximal and distal tubular segments. The brush border is attenuated in many segments, and fragments are in the lumen. The brush border fragments are lost from the lumen if the ischemia occurs in vivo.

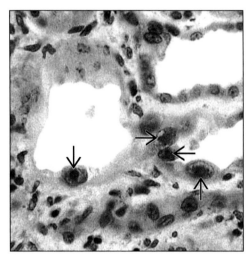
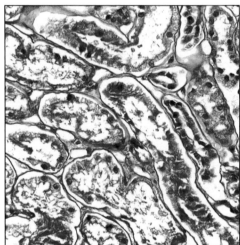

(Left) H&E stain of an autopsy kidney with ATN shows tubular luminal necrotic cellular debris ➡ and autolysis ➡. Congestion of peritubular capillaries is prominent. *(Right)* The same autopsy kidney reveals pigment casts ➡ and autolysis ➡. The presence of pigment casts is a valuable sign that the injury occurred in vivo. Mitoses are usually not frequent in autopsy kidneys with ATN.

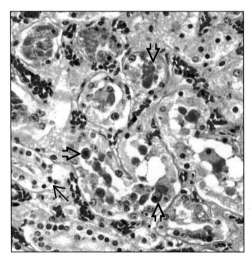
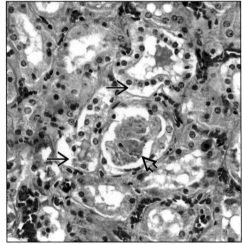

ACUTE TUBULAR NECROSIS

Microscopic Features

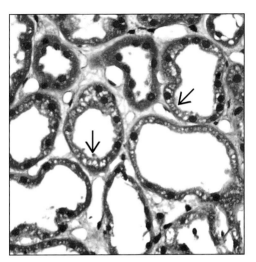

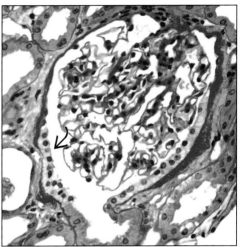

(Left) Light microscopy reveals coarse vacuolization of tubular epithelium ➡. This can be seen in ischemic injury, and therefore is not necessarily due to drugs such as calcineurin inhibitors, contrast agents, or osmotic diuretics. Edema is also prominent. *(Right)* Light microscopy shows ATN with regeneration manifested by "tubularization" of the parietal epithelium ➡. The glomerulus is otherwise unremarkable. Curiously, normal male mice show the same change in Bowman capsule.

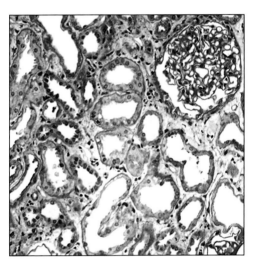

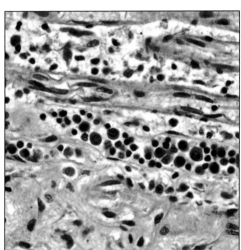

(Left) Low-power microscopy shows ATN with injured flat epithelium, open lumens, interstitial edema, and scattered inflammatory cells. The glomerulus is normal. *(Right)* Venular vasa recta with luminal mononuclear cells with the appearance of granulocytic and erythroid precursors extramedullary hematopoiesis. This is a characteristic feature of ATN and is presumably caused by production of hematopoietic growth factors by the injured kidney.

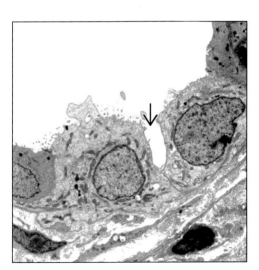

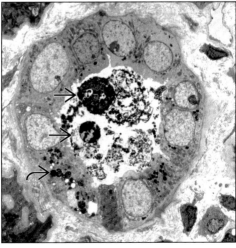

(Left) Electron micrograph shows tubular epithelium in ATN with loss of surface microvilli and separation of the cells due to the loss of intercellular adhesion ➡. Mitochondria are also sparser than normal, and the cell has lost its polarity. *(Right)* Electron micrograph shows a distal tubular segment in ATN with luminal necrotic debris ➡. Phagolysosomes are prominent in some of the cells ➡. The nuclei have an open chromatin pattern, which suggests regeneration.

RENAL CORTICAL NECROSIS

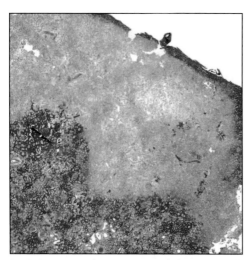

H&E shows coagulation necrosis of the cortex with marked congestion of the subcapsular and deep cortical and juxtamedullary zones in an example of hyperacute antibody-mediated kidney transplant rejection.

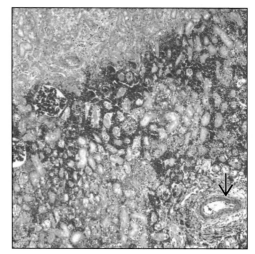

Congestion and hemorrhage at the zone adjacent to necrotic cortical tissue are shown. There is arterial fibrinoid necrosis ➡, consistent with antibody-mediated rejection of a kidney transplant.

TERMINOLOGY

Abbreviations
- Renal cortical necrosis (CN)

Synonyms
- Diffuse renal cortical necrosis
- Bilateral renal cortical necrosis

Definitions
- Bilateral, multifocal or diffuse coagulation necrosis of renal cortex

ETIOLOGY/PATHOGENESIS

Obstetric Complications
- ~ 50-60% of cases
  - Placental abruption with hemorrhage
  - Placenta previa with hemorrhage
  - Puerperal sepsis with placental retention
  - Septic abortion
  - Amniotic fluid embolism
  - Severe eclampsia

Sepsis
- ~ 30-40% of all cases
  - Bacterial infections: *E. coli, Klebsiella*
  - Infantile gastroenteritis

Toxic Causes
- Diethylene glycol
- Snake venom

Miscellaneous Causes
- Shock associated with
  - Acute pancreatitis
  - Diabetic ketoacidosis
  - Blood loss: Postoperative, gastrointestinal hemorrhage
  - Transfusion reactions
  - Burns
- Thrombotic microangiopathy associated with hemolytic uremic syndrome or thrombotic thrombocytopenic purpura
- Atheroembolism
- Antibody-mediated renal allograft rejection

Pathogenesis
- Distribution of renal blood flow: Cortex (80%), medulla (20%)
- High blood flow and metabolic demand increases susceptibility of cortex to ischemic insult
- Outer 1-2 mm of cortex receives blood supply from capsular vessels and is spared in CN
- Widespread thrombosis and vascular spasm of intrarenal vessels results in vascular occlusion, ischemia, and tissue necrosis
  - May also occur secondary to hypertension or shock

CLINICAL ISSUES

Presentation
- Prolonged oliguria or anuria without development of diuresis
- Acute renal failure (ARF) in pregnancy
  - 20% of ARF in pregnancy due to CN

Treatment
- Supportive: Renal replacement therapy
- Correct underlying cause

Prognosis
- ~ 50% develop chronic renal failure
- Duration of oliguria and extent of CN determine renal survival
- Recovery may be complicated by development of hypertension
- In pregnancy, 77% renal recovery rate reported

RENAL CORTICAL NECROSIS

Key Facts

Etiology/Pathogenesis
- Obstetric complications ~ 50-60% of cases
- Sepsis ~ 30-40% of cases
- Thrombotic microangiopathy

Clinical Issues
- Prolonged oliguria or anuria
- 20% of ARF in pregnancy due to CN
- Duration of oliguria and extent of CN determine renal survival

- ~ 50% develop chronic renal failure

Macroscopic Features
- Early: Yellow cortex with subcapsular and juxtamedullary congestion
- Late: Irregular scarring with calcification

Microscopic Pathology
- Multifocal or diffuse coagulation necrosis of cortex
- Thrombi in glomeruli, arterioles, venules, and veins

IMAGE FINDINGS

CT Findings
- Narrow interlobular arteries with prominence of subcapsular vessels
- Dystrophic calcification later in disease

MACROSCOPIC FEATURES

General Features
- Acute phase: Yellow cortex with subcapsular and juxtamedullary congestion
- Late phase: Irregular scarring with thin cortex and calcification

MICROSCOPIC PATHOLOGY

Histologic Features
- Multifocal or diffuse coagulation necrosis of cortex
- Subcapsular cortex (1-2 mm), juxtamedullary cortex, and medulla are spared
- Nonnecrotic tubules have acute tubular injury
- Thrombi in glomeruli, arterioles, venules, and veins

DIFFERENTIAL DIAGNOSIS

Renal Infarction
- Segmental involvement of cortex, with arterial thrombosis or vasculitis

DIAGNOSTIC CHECKLIST

Clinically Relevant Pathologic Features
- Duration of oliguria is proportional to extent of CN
- Extent of necrosis correlates with renal survival

Pathologic Interpretation Pearls
- Coagulation necrosis with microvascular vascular thrombosis (thrombotic microangiopathy)

SELECTED REFERENCES

1. Prakash J et al: Decreasing incidence of renal cortical necrosis in patients with acute renal failure in developing countries: a single-centre experience of 22 years from Eastern India. Nephrol Dial Transplant. 22(4):1213-7, 2007
2. Alfonzo AV et al: Acute renal cortical necrosis in a series of young men with severe acute pancreatitis. Clin Nephrol. 66(4):223-31, 2006
3. Chugh KS et al: Acute renal cortical necrosis--a study of 113 patients. Ren Fail. 16(1):37-47, 1994
4. Kleinknecht D et al: Diagnostic procedures and long-term prognosis in bilateral renal cortical necrosis. Kidney Int. 4(6):390-400, 1973

IMAGE GALLERY

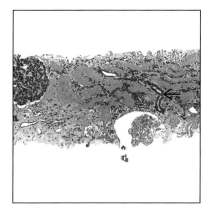 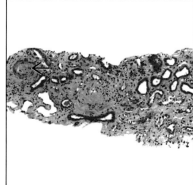 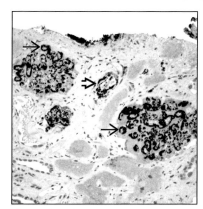

(Left) Needle biopsy specimen demonstrates glomerular and tubular necrosis with congestion and hemorrhage from a patient with severe acute pancreatitis. Necrosis is extensive but spares some tubules ⇒. *(Center)* A scarred medulla without necrosis is seen. Note the obliteration of the arterial lumen ⇒, which indicates an organizing thrombus. *(Right)* Platelet deposits are identified by immunohistochemical staining for CD61 (a platelet integrin) in the glomerular capillaries ⇒ and in the arterioles ⇒.

4

HEPATORENAL SYNDROME/BILE NEPHROSIS

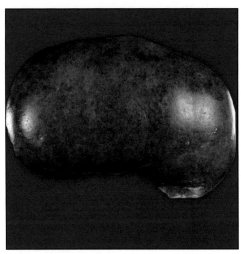

Gross photograph shows the capsular surface of an autopsy kidney from a 32-year-old man with cirrhosis. The green discoloration of the kidney is accentuated after formalin fixation.

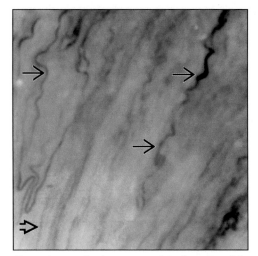

Gross photograph of a cross section of renal medulla shows plugging of nephrons by bile casts ➡ and vasa recta congestion ⊵ in a patient with end-stage liver disease. (Courtesy C. Abrahams, MD.)

TERMINOLOGY

Abbreviations
- Hepatorenal syndrome (HRS)
- Bile nephrosis (BN)

Synonyms
- Cholemic nephrosis
- Jaundice-associated acute kidney injury
- Jaundice-related renal insufficiency

Definitions
- HRS: Renal failure with cirrhosis
  - Type 1: Rapid reduction of renal function
  - Type 2: Slowly progressive loss of renal function
  - Lack of benefit from volume expansion
  - Absence of other causes
- BN: Acute renal failure with bile-containing casts in distal nephron

ETIOLOGY/PATHOGENESIS

Hepatorenal Syndrome
- Circulatory disturbance causing decreased perfusion of kidney
  - Decreased glomerular filtration rate
  - Acute ischemia of tubules
  - Reversible when transplanted into noncirrhotic recipient

Bile Nephrosis
- Distal nephron casts containing bilirubin and bile salts
  - Direct toxicity to tubular epithelium by bile salts
  - Obstruction in distal nephron
    - Propensity of distal nephron due to admixture of Tamm-Horsfall protein with bile components

CLINICAL ISSUES

Presentation
- Hepatic failure
  - Total bilirubin levels often > 20 mg/dL
  - Jaundice
- Acute renal failure
  - Concentrated urine, low Na
- Chronic renal failure

Treatment
- Surgical approaches
  - Liver transplantation if cause of liver failure is irreversible
- Drugs
  - Vasopressors for type 1 HRS
- Supportive therapy
  - Renal replacement therapy

Prognosis
- Poor; dependent on reversibility of liver failure
- Reduction of bilirubin can lead to recovery of renal function

MACROSCOPIC FEATURES

General Features
- Yellow kidneys when fresh or unfixed (bilirubin)
- Green kidneys after formalin fixation (biliverdin)
  - More prominent in pyramids than cortex due to more frequent bile casts in renal medulla

MICROSCOPIC PATHOLOGY

Histologic Features
- BN has intratubular yellow-green pigmented casts
  - Localized predominantly in distal tubules and collecting ducts

HEPATORENAL SYNDROME/BILE NEPHROSIS

Key Facts

Etiology/Pathogenesis

- Elevated blood bilirubin leads to intratubular bile casts
  - Direct toxicity to tubular epithelial cells by bilirubin and bile salts and subsequent ATN
  - Distal nephron obstruction
- Circulatory disturbance causing decreased perfusion of kidney

Clinical Issues

- Presentation
  - Acute renal failure
  - Jaundice

Macroscopic Features

- Yellow when unfixed; green when fixed
- Pigment most prominent in renal pyramids

Microscopic Pathology

- Intratubular yellow-green pigmented casts
  - Hall stain highlights bile casts
- Dark red and some green-yellowish discoloration of sloughed cells
- Acute tubular injury

Top Differential Diagnoses

- Rhabdomyolysis
- Hemolysis
- Acute tubular injury/acute tubular necrosis
- Myeloma cast nephropathy

Diagnostic Checklist

- Identification of pigment in casts by Hall stain diagnostically helpful

---

- Hall stain highlights bile pigment by converting bilirubin to biliverdin and confirms intratubular bile casts
- Sloughed tubular epithelial cells may be admixed with bile casts
- Acute tubular injury
  - Loss or attenuation of proximal tubular brush borders
  - Sloughed cells and cell cytoplasm accumulate within tubular lumina
  - Cellular debris within distal nephron segments admixed with bile and bile salts
- Calcium oxalate crystal deposition
  - Localized to distal nephron segments
  - Refractile with polarized light
  - Green tinged by biliverdin
  - Bile stained crystals **not** to be mistaken for bile casts
- HRS may have little change other than acute tubular injury

DIFFERENTIAL DIAGNOSIS

Acute Tubular Injury/Acute Tubular Necrosis

- Lack of bile-stained casts
- Pigmented granular casts (cell debris)
- Hall stain negative

Rhabdomyolysis

- Pigmented granular eosinophilic casts in distal nephron
  - IHC of casts positive for myoglobin

Hemolysis

- Pigmented granular eosinophilic casts in distal nephron
  - IHC of casts positive for myoglobin

Myeloma Cast Nephropathy

- Intratubular casts with sharp edge or fractured appearance
  - Casts polychromatic on trichome stain
  - Not pigmented

- Multinucleated giant cell reaction around casts
- Monoclonal light chains by immunohistochemistry or immunofluorescence

DIAGNOSTIC CHECKLIST

Pathologic Interpretation Pearls

- Identification of composition of pigmented casts diagnostically helpful
- Hepatorenal syndrome may occur with little bile accumulation

SELECTED REFERENCES

1. Song J et al: Jaundice-associated acute kidney injury. NDT Plus. 2(1):82-83, 2009
2. Moreau R et al: Acute kidney injury: new concepts. Hepatorenal syndrome: the role of vasopressors. Nephron Physiol. 109(4):p73-9, 2008
3. Betjes MG et al: The pathology of jaundice-related renal insufficiency: cholemic nephrosis revisited. J Nephrol. 19(2):229-33, 2006
4. Koppel MH et al: Transplantation of cadaveric kidneys from patients with hepatorenal syndrome. Evidence for the functionalnature of renal failure in advanced liver disease. N Engl J Med. 280(25):1367-71, 1969
5. Sant SM et al: Cholemic nephrosis-an autopsy and experimental study. J Postgrad Med. 11:79-89, 1965
6. Thompson LL et al: The renal lesion in obstructive jaundice. Am J Med Science. 199:305-312, 1940

Gross and Light Microscopic Features

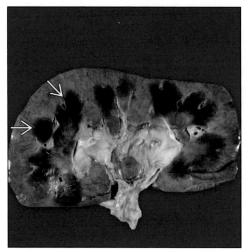

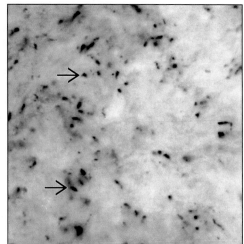

(Left) Gross photograph shows the cut surface of a formalin-fixed kidney with prominent green discoloration, accentuated in the renal pyramids ➡ where bile and bile casts are present in greater numbers and higher concentration compared with the renal cortex. The green color is due to biliverdin. *(Right)* Gross photograph of a cross section of the renal medulla in a jaundiced patient demonstrates numerous bile casts ➡ within the renal tubules. *(Courtesy C. Abrahams, MD.)*

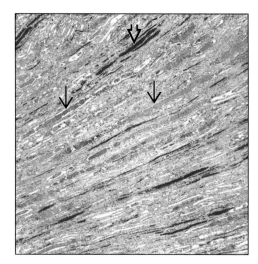

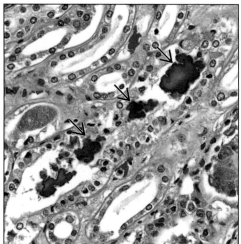

(Left) Hematoxylin & eosin stain of the medulla shows numerous green-yellow ➡ casts within the distal tubules and collecting ducts of the renal medulla with vasa recta ➡ congested by red blood cells in a patient with end-stage liver disease. *(Right)* Hematoxylin & eosin stain of the the the medulla at high power shows green-yellowish red casts with granular and irregular edges within a collecting duct ➡.

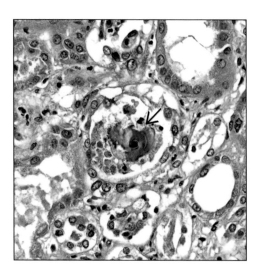

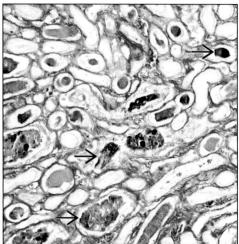

(Left) Hematoxylin & eosin stain shows a calcium oxalate crystal ➡ that is tinged green with bile and should not be confused with a bile cast. Calcium oxalate crystals are uncommon and, when noted, may also be found in distal nephron segments similar to the bile casts. *(Right)* Hall stain shows numerous dark green intratubular casts ➡ in the renal medulla. The Hall stain converts bilirubin to biliverdin, which highlights intratubular bile casts in green to dark green.

HEPATORENAL SYNDROME/BILE NEPHROSIS

Microscopic Features

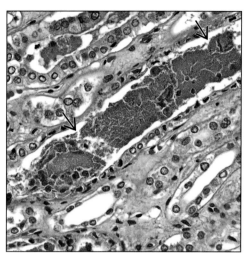 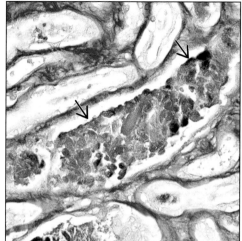

(Left) Hematoxylin & eosin stain shows a dark red cast ➡ within a distal nephron segment that consists of sloughed cells and granular cellular debris. Immunohistochemistry for myoglobin was negative in the tubular casts. *(Right)* Hall stain confirms the presence of bile within the pigmented granular casts ➡ with abundant cellular debris. Bile cast formation in the distal nephron segments may be due in part to the increased concentration of bile and bile salts.

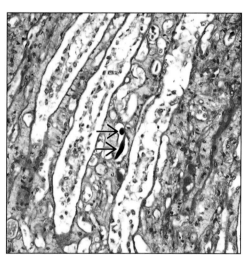 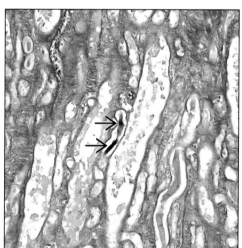

(Left) Periodic acid-Schiff stain reveals a fragmented intratubular bile cast ➡ that has a dark red staining quality and retracted edge. Bile casts do not fill up the entire tubular lumen, which contrasts to intratubular accumulation of Tamm-Horsfall protein. Other proteinaceous casts may show slight retraction from the epithelial cell lining but often not to the extent of bile casts. *(Right)* Hall stain reveals a single intratubular bile cast ➡ in green within the renal medulla.

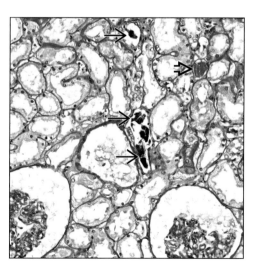 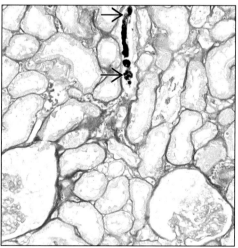

(Left) Periodic acid-Schiff stain reveals intratubular bile casts ➡ that have a dark red staining quality, which contrasts with Tamm-Horsfall protein ⮂ in a nearby tubular lumen that has a much lighter and uneven pink color. *(Right)* Hall stain shows a bile cast ➡ in dark green within a tubule in the renal cortex, which is observed much less frequently in this region compared to the renal medulla.

DRUG-INDUCED ACUTE INTERSTITIAL NEPHRITIS

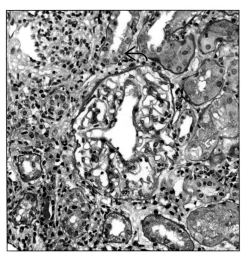

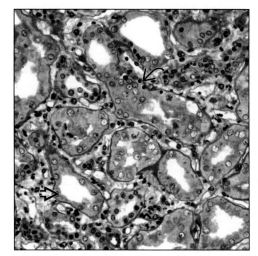

Periodic acid-Schiff shows interstitial infiltrate of mononuclear cells and intraepithelial lymphocytes in tubules ➡. The glomerulus is well preserved with no evidence of proliferation or inflammation.

Infiltrating intraepithelial lymphocytes are seen within nonatrophic tubules (tubulitis) ➡ in a biopsy with AIN. There is evidence of proximal tubular injury with loss of brush borders ➡.

TERMINOLOGY

Abbreviations
- Acute interstitial nephritis (AIN)

Synonyms
- Drug-induced acute tubulointerstitial nephritis

Definitions
- Acute tubulointerstitial inflammation due to allergic reaction to a drug

ETIOLOGY/PATHOGENESIS

Hypersensitivity Reaction
- Usual mechanism believed to be T-cell mediated reaction
- Often associated with systemic hypersensitivity manifestations
- Idiosyncratic reaction, not dose dependent
- Exacerbated response is seen with reexposure
- Cross reactivity with similar class of drugs

Cell-mediated/Delayed Hypersensitivity Reaction
- Positive skin tests to drug "haptens" can be seen in some patients
- Oligoclonal T-cell reactivity to drug in vitro
- Granuloma formation within interstitium
- Drug molecules act as "haptens" and elicit immunological reaction
- Drugs bind covalently to tubular basement membranes (TBM) or tubular epithelial cell components and alter or cross react with endogenous antigens

Antigen/Antibody-mediated Process (Immune Complexes)
- Subset of cases have circulating antibodies to inciting drug (e.g., rifampin)
- Anti-TBM autoantibodies are occasionally identified

IgE Mediated
- IgE antibodies to drugs have been identified in some cases

Drug Classes Implicated
- All drug classes have been implicated in AIN
- Antibiotics
  - Penicillins, cephalosporins, sulfonamides, vancomycin, rifampin, tetracyclines, erythromycin and most others (if not all)
- NSAIDs
  - Both COX-1 and COX-2 inhibitors
  - In some cases, AIN can occur after long-term exposure to NSAIDs
  - Prolonged use can cause analgesic nephropathy
  - Nonallergic mechanism of injury
    - Inhibit renal prostaglandin (vasodilator) synthesis
    - Nephrotoxicity greater with advancing age, dehydration, preexisting renal disease, cirrhosis
  - Can cause minimal change disease (secondary)
- Diuretics
  - Thiazides, furosemide, triamterene
- Miscellaneous drugs
  - Phenytoin, allopurinol, cimetidine, diphenylhydantoin, Chinese herbal medicines, captopril, lithium, valproate, warfarin, interferon-α, lamotrigine
- Antiviral drugs
  - Acyclovir, foscarnet, indinavir

Other Possible Lesions to Accompany Drug-induced AIN
- Granulomatous interstitial nephritis

DRUG-INDUCED ACUTE INTERSTITIAL NEPHRITIS

Key Facts

Terminology
- Acute tubulointerstitial inflammation due to allergic reaction to a drug

Etiology/Pathogenesis
- T-cell-mediated hypersensitivity reaction
- Idiosyncratic reaction, not dose dependent

Clinical Issues
- Triad of fever, rash, eosinophilia in < 50%
- Urine eosinophils
- Subnephrotic proteinuria
- Recovery of renal function in 60-90%

Microscopic Pathology
- Interstitial inflammation with tubulitis, usually with eosinophils
- Other features variably present
  - Granulomata
  - Fibrosis and atrophy with prolonged drug exposure
  - Minimal change disease: NSAIDs and others
  - Papillary necrosis: NSAIDs

Ancillary Tests
- EM may show foot process effacement
- TBM deposits by IF rarely

Top Differential Diagnoses
- Acute tubular injury
- Autoimmune AIN
- Acute pyelonephritis
- Granulomatous AIN due to infection or sarcoidosis

Diagnostic Checklist
- Adverse prognostic features: Fibrosis, granulomata, marked inflammation

---

  - Penicillins, polymyxin, rifampin, spiramycin, sulfonamides, vancomycin, acyclovir, thiazides, triamterene, NSAIDs, allopurinol, captopril, heroin, lamotrigine
- Papillary necrosis
  - NSAIDs (acetaminophen, fenoprofen, ibuprofen, indomethacin)
- Podocytopathy (minimal change disease)
  - Mechanism unknown
  - NSAIDs, penicillins, rifampin, celecoxib, diphenylhydantoin, lithium, interferon-α
- Membranous glomerulonephritis
  - NSAIDs, gold, penicillamine

CLINICAL ISSUES

Presentation
- Maculopapular rash (~ 25% of drug-induced AIN)
  - Onset usually a few days to weeks after drug exposure
  - Predominantly involves trunk and proximal extremities
  - Represents systemic manifestation of hypersensitivity reaction
  - Rash may be absent in NSAID-induced AIN
- Fever (~ 40%)
- Arthralgias
- Oliguria may be seen
- Acute renal failure
  - Often nonoliguric
  - Older patients are more susceptible
- Hypertension and pedal edema occasionally

Laboratory Tests
- Blood
  - Elevated BUN and serum creatinine
  - Eosinophilia (~ 35% > 500/mm³)
  - Serological studies are usually negative or normal (ANA, anti-DNA antibodies, ANCA, complement)
- Urine
  - Sterile pyuria

  - WBC casts
  - Eosinophils in urine
    - Typical, but not specific to AIN
  - Proteinuria
    - Usually subnephrotic, < 1 g/day
    - Nephrotic range proteinuria may be seen with NSAIDs
  - Microscopic hematuria may be seen
  - Fractional excretion of sodium > 1%
  - Urine cultures are negative
  - Evidence of proximal and distal tubular defects
    - Aminoaciduria, glucosuria, phosphaturia, hyperkalemia, urine concentration defects

Natural History
- Acute tubular injury and acute renal failure
- Subset of untreated cases can progress to chronic renal failure

Treatment
- Drugs
  - Removal of offending drug is 1st line of therapy
  - Steroid therapy may improve recovery of renal function, especially if started early
- Supportive measures for acute renal insufficiency and renal failure

Prognosis
- Excellent recovery of renal function in most cases (60-90%) within 1-12 months
- Subset of patients are at risk for chronic renal insufficiency
  - Especially with prolonged intake of offending drug prior to diagnosis, as with over-the-counter NSAIDs
- Minimal change disease resolves on discontinuance of drug but may recur on reexposure to same or similar drug

DRUG-INDUCED ACUTE INTERSTITIAL NEPHRITIS

IMAGE FINDINGS

Ultrasonographic Findings
- Enlarged kidneys may be seen in presence of interstitial edema

MACROSCOPIC FEATURES

General Features
- Gross examination is uncommon as diagnosis is based on kidney biopsy
- Enlarged kidneys due to interstitial edema

MICROSCOPIC PATHOLOGY

Histologic Features
- Interstitial inflammation
  - Predominantly mononuclear cells, plasma cells, and fewer neutrophils
  - Eosinophils are usually present
  - Inflammation may be sparse in NSAID-induced AIN
- Tubulitis with infiltrating mononuclear inflammatory cells
  - Disruption of TBM may be seen on PAS stain
  - Reactive epithelial changes with sloughing, loss of brush border
  - Eosinophils in tubules
- Interstitial edema
- Granulomas in interstitium are not uncommon
  - Noncaseating granulomas with epithelioid histiocytes
  - Occasional multinucleated giant cells may be seen
  - Admixed with interspersed interstitial infiltrate
  - Drug hypersensitivity causes 45% of granulomatous interstitial nephritis in biopsies
- Glomeruli and blood vessels are usually spared
- Prominent tubular protein droplets
  - May be observed in cases of NSAID-induced coexistent minimal change disease
- Chronic changes may be seen with prolonged use of offending drug
  - Mild interstitial fibrosis
  - Thickening of TBMs and tubular atrophy
- Ureteral inflammation has been observed in nephrectomy specimens

ANCILLARY TESTS

Histochemistry
- Acid-fast bacteria and Gomori methenamine silver
  - Reactivity: Negative
  - Staining pattern
    - Organisms may be identified in presence of mycobacterial or fungal infections

Immunohistochemistry
- Usually not needed
- Inflammatory infiltrate is usually mixed and reactive, predominantly T cells

- κ and λ immunohistochemistry or in situ hybridization reveals polyclonal plasma cell infiltrate

Immunofluorescence
- Interstitial fibrin accumulates in edema, as in delayed hypersensitivity reactions in skin
- Linear IgG stain along TBMs can be seen rarely
  - Reported in cases with methicillin and rifampin-induced AIN
- Tubular protein reabsorption droplets may be seen with NSAID-induced minimal change disease on albumin stain

Electron Microscopy
- Tubular epithelial changes such as loss of brush border may be seen
- Glomeruli are normal in most cases
- Diffuse podocyte injury and foot process effacement may be observed
  - Seen in NSAID-induced minimal change disease
- Small, discrete TBM deposits may rarely be seen (probably of no significance)

DIFFERENTIAL DIAGNOSIS

Acute Tubular Injury
- Less interstitial inflammation and tubulitis
- Loss of tubular cell nuclei in areas without inflammation

Glomerulonephritis-associated Interstitial Inflammation
- ANCA-mediated glomerulonephritis can show severe interstitial inflammation including eosinophils
  - If glomerular sampling is inadequate, can be mistaken for AIN
- Presence of RBC casts should raise concern for "missed" crescentic lesions

Acute Pyelonephritis
- Neutrophils may predominate in setting of bacterial infections
- Neutrophil casts may be observed
- Infectious etiology should be ruled out with urine and blood cultures

Toxic Tubular Injury
- More necrosis of tubules, less inflammation

Granulomatous Interstitial Nephritis Due to Infection or Autoimmunity
- Caseating necrosis in granulomas may be present in mycobacterial and fungal infections
- Nonnecrotizing granulomas can be seen in sarcoidosis or granulomatosis with polyangiitis (Wegener)
- Clinical history, presence of glomerular crescents, and special stains (AFB, GMS) are helpful

Lupus Nephritis
- May have predominant tubulointerstitial inflammation
- Immune complex deposits may be seen on immunofluorescence microscopy (granular TBM

deposits and interstitial deposits) and electron microscopy

Idiopathic Hypocomplementemic Tubulointerstitial Nephritis

- Immunofluorescence microscopy and electron microscopy show granular deposits along TBMs and interstitium
- Often seen in elderly males; serum complements are often low

Nephritis Associated with Autoimmune Pancreatitis

- IgG4 in plasma cells seen on IHC and TBM deposits

Sjögren Syndrome

- Clinical renal manifestations may include distal tubular acidosis, impaired urinary concentration ability, Fanconi syndrome
- Serological manifestations include anti-Ro/SSA, anti-La/SSB antibodies, hypergammaglobulinemia, and in some cases ANA
- Tubulointerstitial nephritis is active but may appear more chronic with varying degrees of tubular atrophy and interstitial fibrosis

Interstitial Nephritis with Uveitis (Dobrin Syndrome)

- Rare in adults and has been reported mainly in children
- Clinical manifestations include Fanconi syndrome, renal insufficiency, proteinuria
- Ocular symptoms due to uveitis may precede or follow renal presentation

Primary Antitubular Basement Membrane Antibody Nephritis

- Immunofluorescence microscopy shows linear staining along tubular basement membranes with IgG and often with C3

Lymphoma

- Monomorphic lymphocyte interstitial infiltrates or plasma cell infiltrate
- Evidence of monoclonal population of lymphocytes or plasma cells by immunohistochemistry or in situ hybridization

DIAGNOSTIC CHECKLIST

Clinically Relevant Pathologic Features

- Adverse prognostic features
  o Marked interstitial inflammation
  o Granulomata
  o Tubular atrophy and interstitial fibrosis

Pathologic Interpretation Pearls

- Rule out coincidental pathological changes such as IgA nephropathy or diabetic nephropathy that might explain inflammation

- Diagnosis usually requires detailed clinical history, including all drugs and serologies for autoimmune diseases
- Eosinophils in tubules may be detected and may have diagnostic value

SELECTED REFERENCES

1. González E et al: Early steroid treatment improves the recovery of renal function in patients with drug-induced acute interstitial nephritis. Kidney Int. 73(8):940-6, 2008
2. Cornell LD et al: Pseudotumors due to IgG4 immune-complex tubulointerstitial nephritis associated with autoimmune pancreatocentric disease. Am J Surg Pathol. 31(10):1586-97, 2007
3. Nadasdy T et al: Acute and chronic tubulointerstitial nephritis. In Jennette JC et al: Heptinstall's Pathology of the Kidney. 6th ed. Philadelphia: Lippincott Williams & Wilkins. 1083-1109, 2007
4. Bijol V et al: Granulomatous interstitial nephritis: a clinicopathologic study of 46 cases from a single institution. Int J Surg Pathol. 14(1):57-63, 2006
5. Spanou Z et al: Involvement of drug-specific T cells in acute drug-induced interstitial nephritis. J Am Soc Nephrol. 17(10):2919-27, 2006
6. Rossert J: Drug-induced acute interstitial nephritis. Kidney Int. 60(2):804-17, 2001
7. Whelton A: Nephrotoxicity of nonsteroidal anti-inflammatory drugs: physiologic foundations and clinical implications. Am J Med. 106(5B):13S-24S, 1999
8. De Vriese AS et al: Rifampicin-associated acute renal failure: pathophysiologic, immunologic, and clinical features. Am J Kidney Dis. 31(1):108-15, 1998
9. Michel DM et al: Acute interstitial nephritis. J Am Soc Nephrol. 9(3):506-15, 1998
10. Kleinknecht D: Interstitial nephritis, the nephrotic syndrome, and chronic renal failure secondary to nonsteroidal anti-inflammatory drugs. Semin Nephrol. 15(3):228-35, 1995
11. Ten RM et al: Acute interstitial nephritis: immunologic and clinical aspects. Mayo Clin Proc. 63(9):921-30, 1988
12. Adler SG et al: Hypersensitivity phenomena and the kidney: role of drugs and environmental agents. Am J Kidney Dis. 5(2):75-96, 1985
13. Laberke HG et al: Acute interstitial nephritis: correlations between clinical and morphological findings. Clin Nephrol. 14(6):263-73, 1980
14. Colvin RB et al: Letter: Penicillin-associated interstitial nephritis. Ann Intern Med. 81(3):404-5, 1974
15. Baldwin DS et al: Renal failure and interstitial nephritis due to penicillin and methicillin. N Engl J Med. 279(23):1245-52, 1968

DRUG-INDUCED ACUTE INTERSTITIAL NEPHRITIS

Variant Microscopic Features

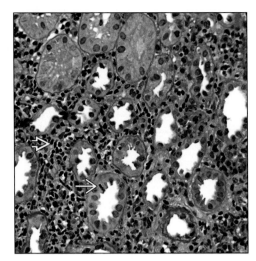 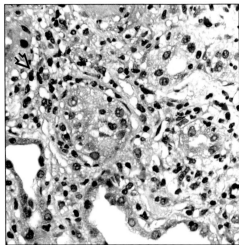

(Left) Periodic acid-Schiff stain of a biopsy with AIN shows predominantly lymphocytic interstitial inflammation ➡️ with a few plasma cells. The history was compatible with a drug-induced process. Acute tubular injury is evident with reactive epithelial changes and mitoses ➡️. (Right) Hematoxylin & eosin shows sparse interstitial infiltrates of lymphocytes and eosinophils ➡️ along with mild interstitial edema. The patient was previously treated with sulphonamide (Bactrim).

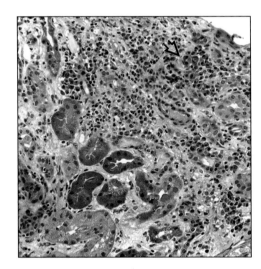 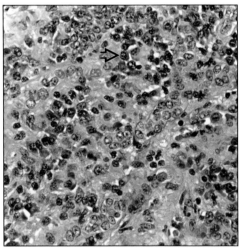

(Left) A biopsy with acute interstitial nephritis shows predominant plasma cell infiltrate ➡️ along with lymphocytes and rare eosinophils. The patient was on multiple potentially nephrotoxic drugs. (Right) A biopsy of suspected drug-induced acute interstitial nephritis demonstrates prominent plasma cell infiltrate ➡️. Lymphocytes and a few eosinophils are also seen. The in situ hybridization studies for κ and λ light chains revealed polyclonal plasma cells.

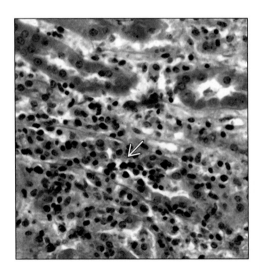 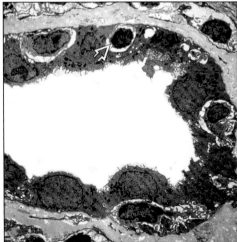

(Left) An eosinophil is seen in a tubule ➡️, accounting for the appearance of these cells in the urine. While no formal test of the diagnostic significance of this finding has been reported, it is regarded as a characteristic feature of drug-induced AIN. Prominent lymphocytic tubulitis is also present. (Right) Electron micrograph of a biopsy with clinical and histological features of drug-induced AIN shows infiltrating intraepithelial lymphocytes ➡️ within a tubule.

DRUG-INDUCED ACUTE INTERSTITIAL NEPHRITIS

Variant Microscopic Features

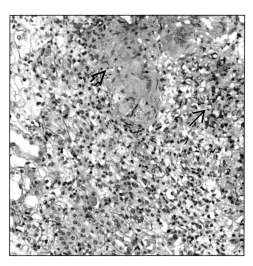
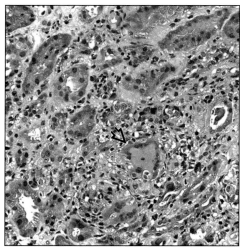

(Left) A case of granulomatous drug-induced AIN due to moxifloxacin has a few noncaseating granulomas ⇰ within the interstitium along with lymphocytes and eosinophils ➔. Multinucleated giant cells are seen in the granuloma. *(Right)* Hematoxylin & eosin shows AIN with interstitial mononuclear infiltrate presumably due to a drug. Although well-formed granulomas were absent, scattered multinucleated giant cells were identified ⇰.

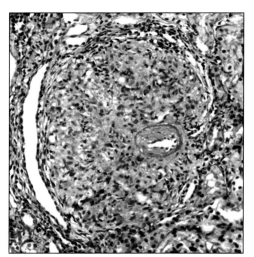
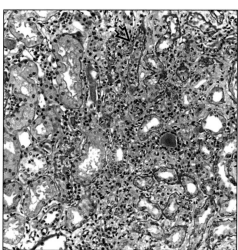

(Left) Perivascular granuloma consisting of epithelioid histiocytes and lymphocytes is seen in a case of drug-induced interstitial nephritis. About 45% of cases of granulomatous interstitial nephritis are caused by drugs. *(Right)* The patient had been on Furosemide for a few months prior to biopsy. Chronic tubulointerstitial damage is evident with TBM thickening in atrophic tubules ⇰. In the absence of other pathology, these changes were attributed to progression of Furosemide-induced AIN.

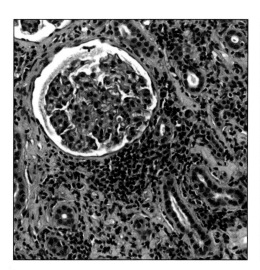
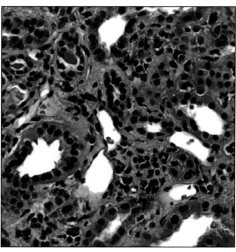

(Left) Chronic drug-induced AIN can be caused by long-term use of over-the-counter NSAIDs (ibuprofen). Diffuse interstitial fibrosis is seen and an intense mononuclear infiltrate separates the tubules, many of which are atrophic. The glomeruli are unremarkable. *(Right)* Renal biopsy shows chronic drug-induced AIN caused by long-term over-the-counter NSAIDs (ibuprofen). Prominent interstitial fibrosis and an intense mononuclear infiltrate with many eosinophils is evident.

4

Variant Microscopic Features

(Left) Periodic acid-Schiff stained section of a biopsy from a patient treated with naproxen shows sparse interstitial infiltrate ⇗ and normal glomerulus. *(Right)* Hematoxylin & eosin of a biopsy from a patient treated with naproxen shows a small collection of eosinophilic infiltrate ⇗ within the medulla. Patients with NSAID-induced acute interstitial nephritis can have only sparse interstitial inflammation.

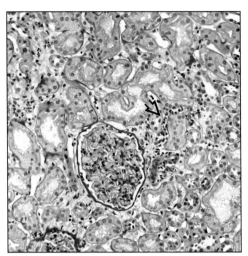
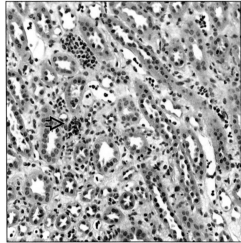

(Left) Periodic acid-Schiff shows mild acute tubular injury characterized by loss of brush borders ⇗ in the proximal tubules and loss of tubular nuclei. The patient presented with acute renal insufficiency subsequent to NSAID treatment. Sparse interstitial infiltrate of AIN was seen elsewhere. *(Right)* Periodic acid-Schiff stain shows prominent protein resorption droplets ⇗ in proximal tubules of a patient with NSAID-induced AIN and minimal change disease.

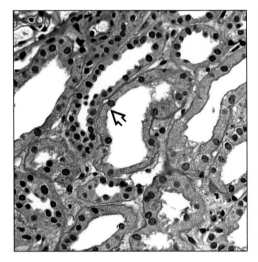
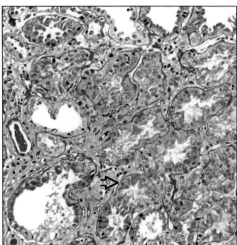

(Left) Immunofluorescence microscopy with antisera to albumin shows prominent protein reabsorption droplets in the tubules. The biopsy is from a patient with NSAID-induced AIN and minimal change disease. Staining for immunoglobulins and complements was negative. *(Right)* Electron micrograph of a glomerulus demonstrates extensive podocyte foot process effacement ⇗. The renal biopsy was compatible with NSAID-induced AIN and minimal change syndrome. No electron-dense deposits were observed.

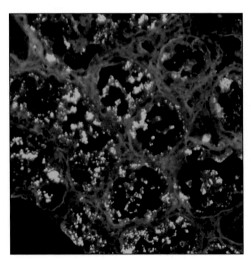
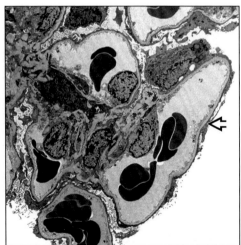

DRUG-INDUCED ACUTE INTERSTITIAL NEPHRITIS

Differential Diagnosis

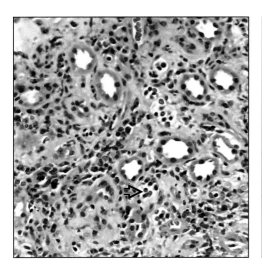

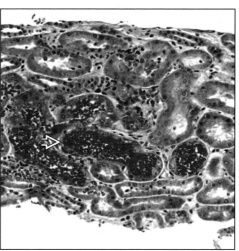

(Left) Pauci-immune glomerulonephritis can have prominent eosinophilic infiltrate ⊵ in interstitium, reminiscent of AIN. Patient presented with acute renal failure & urinalysis revealed RBC casts, which would be unusual in AIN. *(Right)* Presence of RBC casts ⊵ in a suspected case of AIN (clinically and histologically) should raise concern for unsampled crescents in pauci-immune glomerulonephritis. Patient was subsequently found to have positive ANCA serologies.

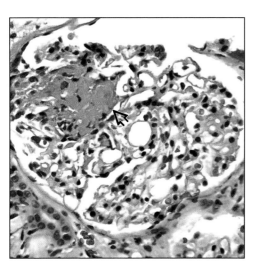

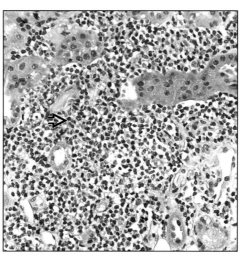

(Left) Focal segmental glomerular necrosis ⊵ was seen in a patient with pauci-immune glomerulonephritis. Tubulointerstitial inflammation in deep cortex & medulla was reminiscent of AIN. *(Right)* Prominent interstitial monomorphic lymphocytic infiltrate ⊵ is seen, atypical for AIN. Immunohistochemical analysis confirmed the presence of a low-grade lymphoma (CD5 & CD10 negative).

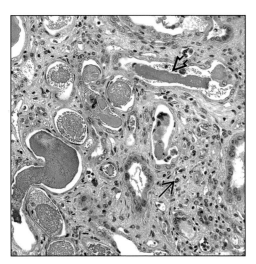

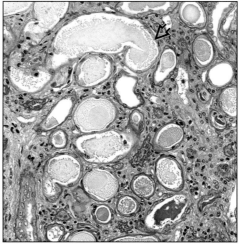

(Left) Hematoxylin & eosin of a kidney biopsy with myeloma cast nephropathy shows several fractured casts ⊵. In addition, mild interstitial inflammation ⊵ is present. The abnormal casts were light chain restricted on immunofluorescence microscopy. *(Right)* Periodic acid-Schiff shows pale fractured casts typical of myeloma cast nephropathy ⊵. The casts showed light chain restriction on immunofluorescence. Mild interstitial inflammation is also observed.

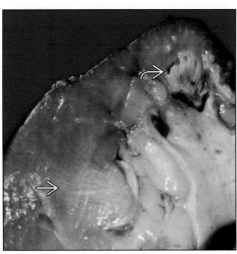

Gross photograph of a kidney shows necrotic papilla ➢ and corresponding atrophic cortex due to analgesic abuse. The line of demarcation of the necrosis is evident. One papilla with its overlying cortex is normal ➢.

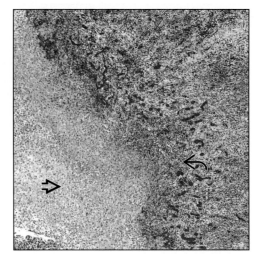

Hematoxylin & eosin of the papillary tip of the renal medulla shows extensive necrosis ➢ with scant inflammation. The periphery of this necrotic area shows intense inflammatory infiltrate ➢.

TERMINOLOGY

Abbreviations
- Renal papillary necrosis (RPN)

Synonyms
- Renal medullary necrosis
- Renal necrotizing papillitis

Definitions
- Coagulative necrosis of papillary tips of medulla

ETIOLOGY/PATHOGENESIS

Medullary Ischemia
- Medulla receives only 8-10% of total renal blood flow
- Rich vascular plexus of vasa recta contribute mainly to countercurrent mechanism
- Nutrient supply for medulla is limited, blood vessels are mostly terminal
- Aggravating factors
  o Luminal occlusion of small arteries and arterioles
    ▪ Diabetic arteriopathy
    ▪ Sickle hemoglobinopathy
    ▪ Transplanted kidney with arteriopathy
    ▪ Age-related arteriolosclerosis
  o Vasoconstrictor effect due to prostaglandin inhibition
    ▪ Nonsteroidal anti-inflammatory drugs (NSAIDs)
  o Volume depletion
    ▪ Dehydration, congestive heart failure

Concentration of Nephrotoxic Agents in Medulla
- Tubular concentration of solute in medulla promotes water reabsorption
- Potentially nephrotoxic agents concentrated in medulla

  o Phenacetin, NSAIDs (ibuprofen, indomethacin, naproxen, tolmetin, benoxaprofen)

CLINICAL ISSUES

Epidemiology
- Incidence
  o Uncommon in absence of predisposing factors
  o Reduced incidence with advent of therapeutic options for aggressive control of predisposing factors, such as diabetes mellitus and acute pyelonephritis
    ▪ Affected patients often have more than 1 causative factor for RPN, such as diabetes mellitus, infection, or analgesic abuse
- Age
  o > 60 years old
  o Can occur at younger age in sickle hemoglobinopathies
- Gender
  o More common in women

Site
- Inner zone of medulla and papillary tip
- Bilateral in 65-70% of cases

Presentation
- Subacute presentation more common
  o Lumbar pain
  o Hematuria
  o Fever
  o Chills
  o Inability to concentrate urine with resultant polyuria and nocturia
  o Renal insufficiency if several papillae are affected
- Acute onset is rare
  o Acute renal failure
  o Sepsis
- Asymptomatic passage of necrotic papillary material

PAPILLARY NECROSIS

Key Facts

Terminology
- Coagulative necrosis of papillary tips of medulla

Etiology/Pathogenesis
- Medullary ischemia
  - Vasoconstriction by NSAIDs
- Concentration of nephrotoxic agents in medulla
- Infection
- Volume depletion exacerbates the risk

Clinical Issues
- > 60 years at presentation
- More common in women, diabetics
- Subacute presentation more common
  - Lumbar pain, hematuria
  - Fever, chills
- Bilateral in 65-70% of cases

- Long history of analgesic use

Microscopic Pathology
- Inner zone of medulla and papillary tip
- Papillae with coagulative necrosis
  - Loss of outlines of tubules and blood vessels
- Necrotic area rimmed by neutrophils in tubules and interstitium
- No inflammatory cells within necrotic area

Top Differential Diagnoses
- Parenchymal infarction
  - Area of involvement not limited to medullary tip

Diagnostic Checklist
- Shed papilla in urine best identified with periodic acid-Schiff stain

Laboratory Tests
- Difficult to diagnose
- Straining of urine for necrotic papillae may be helpful

Treatment
- Options, risks, complications
  - Complications
    - Acute or chronic renal failure
    - Infection and septicemia as necrotic papilla forms nidus for infection
    - Severe hematuria
    - Obstruction of urinary tract by sloughed papillae
- Surgical approaches
  - To relieve urinary tract obstruction, if present
- Adjuvant therapy
  - Removal of offending factor
    - Avoidance of analgesics
    - Treatment of sickle cell crisis
    - Blood sugar control in diabetics
  - Control of aggregating factors for medullary injury
    - Control of hypertension
    - Avoidance of anti-hypertensives that reduce renal blood flow, such as β-blockers
    - Avoidance of volume depletion and dehydration
- Drugs
  - Antimicrobial therapy for acute pyelonephritis, if present
  - Adequate glycemic control in presence of diabetes mellitus

Prognosis
- Variable based on early identification of causative factors and prompt treatment

IMAGE FINDINGS

Radiographic Findings
- Retrograde pyelogram can show calyceal blunting
- Abdominal ultrasonography and CT less sensitive
- Imaging studies may identify evidence of urinary tract obstruction

MACROSCOPIC FEATURES

General Features
- Kidneys may be enlarged in diabetes mellitus
- Edematous kidneys may be seen in acute pyelonephritis
- Yellowish red, sharply defined areas in papillae with congested borders
- Cortical atrophy is restricted to lobes with papillary necrosis
  - Suggests that latter causes former

MICROSCOPIC PATHOLOGY

Histologic Features
- Papillae with coagulative necrosis and loss of outlines of tubules
- No inflammatory cells within necrotic area in early phase
- Necrotic area rimmed by neutrophils in interstitium
- Calcification of rim of necrotic area or tubular basement membranes
- Features of predisposing factors may be seen
  - Diabetic nephropathy with diffuse and nodular mesangial sclerosis, hyalinosis
  - Analgesic nephropathy with
    - Interstitial fibrosis
    - Tubular atrophy
    - Capillary sclerosis
  - Sickle cell disease with evidence of sickled red cells within capillaries
  - Acute pyelonephritis with neutrophil casts

ANCILLARY TESTS

Immunofluorescence
- Usually negative with no evidence of immune complexes

Electron Microscopy
- No electron-dense deposits identified

Clinical Conditions Associated with Renal Papillary Necrosis

Condition	Frequency of Cause	Comments
Diabetes mellitus	50-60%	RPN is 5x more prevalent in diabetic than nondiabetic patients (autopsy series); urinary tract infection is always concurrent complication
Urinary tract obstruction	10-40%	Obstruction of urinary outflow can result in reduced medullary blood flow, mediated by cytokines released from infiltrating monocytes
Analgesic abuse (analgesic nephropathy)	15-20%	More common with phenacetin use and removal of drug from the market > 20 years ago resulted in dramatic decline in diagnosis
Sickle hemoglobinopathy	10-15%	Can occur in both sickle cell disease and sickle cell trait; patients often present with hematuria
Acute pyelonephritis	5%	More often seen in diabetic patients with severe acute pyelonephritis and urinary tract obstruction
Renal transplantation	< 5%	Allograft arteriopathy can predispose to medullary ischemia

- Nonspecific glomerular changes in acute pyelonephritis and analgesic nephropathy
- Diabetic nephropathy features, such as mesangial sclerosis, thickened basement membranes may be seen

DIFFERENTIAL DIAGNOSIS

Parenchymal Infarction

- Nonviable parenchyma with outlines of glomeruli, tubules, and blood vessels seen
- No acute inflammation in area of infarction, but inflammatory infiltrate may be seen at periphery
- Can occur in setting of thromboembolism
  - Fibrin and platelet thrombi may be seen in blood vessels
  - No evidence of transmural inflammatory infiltrate to suggest vasculitis
- Can occur in setting of vasculitis
  - Transmural inflammation of arteries/arterioles with necrosis
  - Glomerular involvement may be present with proliferation &/or crescents
- Can occur in setting of thrombotic microangiopathy
  - Fibrin thrombi and fragmented red blood cells in arterioles &/or glomeruli
  - No evidence of vasculitis
- Clinical history and serological testing is helpful in determining cause of thromboembolism, vasculitis, or thrombotic microangiopathy
- Area of involvement not limited to medullary tip but can include glomeruli and blood vessels
- Usually results in wedge-shaped cortical infarcts

DIAGNOSTIC CHECKLIST

Clinically Relevant Pathologic Features

- Extent of necrosis
- Histological features may suggest causative factor

Pathologic Interpretation Pearls

- Shed necrotic papilla can be identified in urine with periodic acid-Schiff stain

SELECTED REFERENCES

1. Bansal R et al: An unusual cause of renal allograft dysfunction: graft papillary necrosis. J Nephrol. 20(1):111-3, 2007
2. Olson JL et al: Diabetic nephropathy. In Jennette JC et al: Heptinstall's Pathology of the Kidney. 6th ed. Philadelphia: Lippincott Williams & Wilkins. 840-1, 2007
3. Mihatsch MJ et al: Obituary to analgesic nephropathy--an autopsy study. Nephrol Dial Transplant. 21(11):3139-45, 2006
4. Eknoyan G et al: Renal papillary necrosis. In Greenberg A et al: Primer on Kidney Disease. 4th ed. San Diego: National Kidney Foundation. 385-8, 2005
5. Kovacevic L et al: Renal papillary necrosis induced by naproxen. Pediatr Nephrol. 18(8):826-9, 2003
6. Brix AE: Renal papillary necrosis. Toxicol Pathol. 30(6):672-4, 2002
7. Ducloux D et al: Renal papillary necrosis in a marathon runner. Nephrol Dial Transplant. 14(1):247-8, 1999
8. Whelton A: Nephrotoxicity of nonsteroidal anti-inflammatory drugs: physiologic foundations and clinical implications. Am J Med. 106(5B):13S-24S, 1999
9. Fong P et al: Idiopathic acute granulomatous interstitial nephritis leading to renal papillary necrosis. Nephrol Dial Transplant. 12(5):1043-5, 1997
10. Patterson JE et al: Bacterial urinary tract infections in diabetes. Infect Dis Clin North Am. 11(3):735-50, 1997
11. Griffin MD et al: Renal papillary necrosis--a sixteen-year clinical experience. J Am Soc Nephrol. 6(2):248-56, 1995
12. Eknoyan G et al: Renal papillary necrosis: an update. Medicine (Baltimore). 61(2):55-73, 1982

PAPILLARY NECROSIS

Gross and Microscopic Features

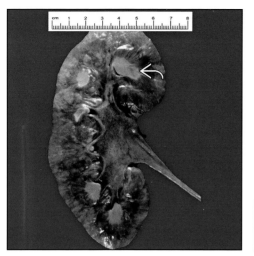
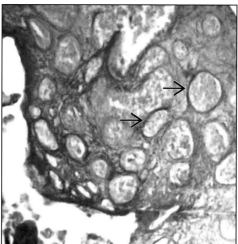

(Left) A kidney is shown with multiple necrotic papillae ⇗ that are pale and distinctly demarcated from the overlying cortex. The etiology of renal papillary necrosis in this instance was acute pyelonephritis. (Courtesy L. Fajardo, MD.) (Right) Periodic acid-Schiff, applied to shed papilla recovered in the urine, highlights the tubular basement membranes ⇨. No cellular elements are preserved.

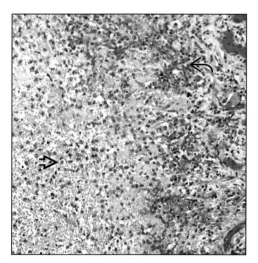
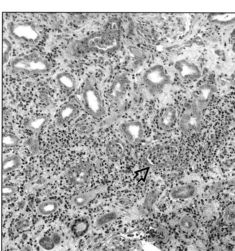

(Left) Hematoxylin & eosin shows an area of necrotic papillae with acellular debris admixed with neutrophils ⇨. Mild chronic inflammation and granulation tissue reaction are seen at the periphery ⇗. (Right) Hematoxylin & eosin shows acute pyelonephritis with interstitial edema and inflammation composed of neutrophils and lymphocytes. Focal neutrophil casts are also seen ⇨. The patient was diabetic, and there was evidence of papillary necrosis elsewhere in the kidney.

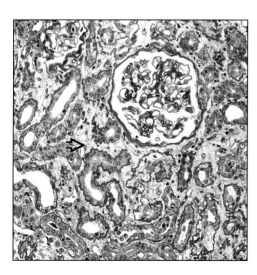
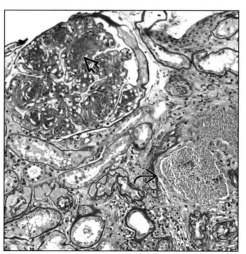

(Left) Diffuse interstitial fibrosis and tubular atrophy are seen ⇨, although the glomeruli are relatively spared in a patient with prolonged use of analgesics and anti-inflammatory drugs. Analgesic abuse may be associated with papillary necrosis. (Right) Biopsy specimen shows nodular sclerosing diabetic nephropathy ⇨ with adjacent tubular debris and neutrophil casts ⇨. Diabetes mellitus is a predisposing factor for acute pyelonephritis and papillary necrosis.

MYOGLOBINURIA/RHABDOMYOLYSIS/HEMOGLOBINURIA

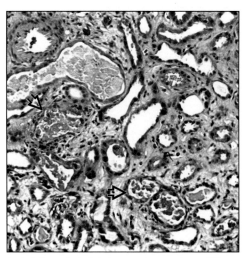

In rhabdomyolysis, light brown pigmented casts ⊵ can be seen within renal tubules. Other tubules show acute injury with simplified epithelium and ectatic lumens separated by interstitial edema.

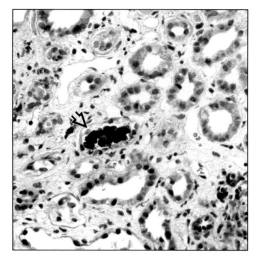

Myoglobin immunohistochemistry stains the myoglobin casts ⊵. Myoglobin, released by rhabdomyolysis, is excreted in the glomerular filtrate and forms tubular casts. (Courtesy M. Troxell, MD, PhD.)

TERMINOLOGY

Synonyms
- Pigment nephropathy

Definitions
- Acute renal failure associated with pigmented tubular casts due to either myoglobinuria or hemoglobinuria

ETIOLOGY/PATHOGENESIS

Myoglobinuria
- Rhabdomyolysis (injury to skeletal muscle)
  - Trauma, such as intense physical exercise, grand mal seizures, pressure injury
  - Drugs, such as cocaine, heroin, amphetamines, HMG-CoA inhibitors (statins)
  - Toxins, such as snake venom, clostridial toxin
  - Inflammation, as in polymyositis
  - Inherited metabolic myopathies
- Precipitating and exacerbating factors for muscle injury
  - Dehydration, fasting, hypo- or hyperthermia, hypoxia, hypokalemia

Hemoglobinuria
- Intravascular hemolysis
  - Mismatched blood transfusions
  - Infections, such as falciparum malaria, *Mycoplasma pneumoniae*
  - Excessive free hemoglobin that exceeds capacity of binding protein haptoglobin is filtered by glomerulus

Mechanisms of Renal Injury by Myoglobin and Hemoglobin
- Myoglobin smaller than hemoglobin (16,700 vs. 64,500 daltons), more easily filtered by glomerulus

- Heme proteins promote vasoconstriction and ischemic tubular injury
- Heme proteins have cytotoxic effects
  - Breakdown product heme and iron are toxic to cell organelles and cause oxidative stress
- Reduced urinary pH, promote formation of myoglobin and hemoglobin casts
- Distal tubular obstruction by pigmented casts and sloughed cells prolongs tubular exposure to denatured heme proteins

CLINICAL ISSUES

Epidemiology
- Gender
  - Men more susceptible to exertional rhabdomyolysis

Presentation
- Acute renal failure
  - Abrupt onset of oliguria
  - Cola-colored urine
- Muscle swelling, bruising, stiffness

Laboratory Tests
- Urinalysis
  - Absence of erythrocytes, but dipstick positive for heme protein
  - Dark pigmented casts on urine microscopy
- Blood tests
  - Elevated serum creatinine (BUN: Creatinine ratio < 5:1)
  - Elevated creatine kinase (CK-MM isoform, often > 100,000 IU/L)
    - Peaks within 48 hours after rhabdomyolysis with half-life of 48 hours
  - Electrolyte imbalances, such as hyperkalemia, hyperphosphatemia, hypocalcemia, hyperuricemia

Treatment
- Supportive

MYOGLOBINURIA/RHABDOMYOLYSIS/HEMOGLOBINURIA

Key Facts

Terminology
- Acute renal failure associated with pigmented tubular casts due to either myoglobinuria or hemoglobinuria

Etiology/Pathogenesis
- Rhabdomyolysis or intravascular hemolysis
- Kidney susceptible to toxicity of heme proteins via vasoconstriction and tubular cytotoxicity

Clinical Issues
- Acute renal failure

Microscopic Pathology
- Acute tubular injury
- Brown pigmented casts in distal tubules

Ancillary Tests
- Myoglobin and hemoglobin stains identify protein in pigmented casts

---

  - Hydration, alkalinization of urine, mannitol, correction of electrolyte imbalances, dialysis
- Elimination of cause if possible (drug, toxin, trauma, infection)

Prognosis
- Recovery with prompt diagnosis and treatment

MICROSCOPIC PATHOLOGY

Histologic Features
- Acute tubular injury
  - Loss of brush borders, sloughed epithelial cells, dilated lumens
  - Hyaline, cellular, and granular casts may be seen
- Brown pigmented casts of hemoglobin or myoglobin, especially in distal tubules
- Interstitial edema is seen, but no significant interstitial inflammation
- Glomeruli are spared
- No evidence of deposits on light microscopy, immunofluorescence, or electron microscopy

ANCILLARY TESTS

Immunohistochemistry
- Myoglobin immunostain positive in myoglobin casts
- Hemoglobin immunostain positive in hemoglobin casts

Electron Microscopy
- Casts contain electron-dense granules

DIFFERENTIAL DIAGNOSIS

Myeloma Cast Nephropathy
- Fractured casts, which are light chain restricted on immunofluorescence microscopy

Acute Ischemic or Toxic Tubular Injury
- Pigmented casts from mitochondrial cytochromes lack myoglobin or hemoglobin

SELECTED REFERENCES

1. Pelletier R et al: Acute renal failure following kidney transplantation associated with myoglobinuria in patients treated with rapamycin. Transplantation. 82(5):645-50, 2006
2. Murali NS et al: Myoglobinuric and hemoglobinuric acute renal failure. In Greenberg A et al: Primer on Kidney Disease. 4th ed. San Diego: National Kidney Foundation. 308-13, 2005
3. Nath KA et al: Intracellular targets in heme protein-induced renal injury. Kidney Int. 53(1):100-11, 1998
4. Zager RA: Rhabdomyolysis and myohemoglobinuric acute renal failure. Kidney Int. 49(2):314-26, 1996
5. Knochel JP: Mechanisms of rhabdomyolysis. Curr Opin Rheumatol. 5(6):725-31, 1993
6. Gabow PA et al: The spectrum of rhabdomyolysis. Medicine (Baltimore). 61(3):141-52, 1982

IMAGE GALLERY

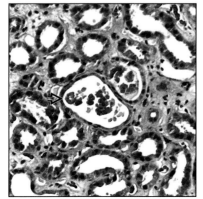 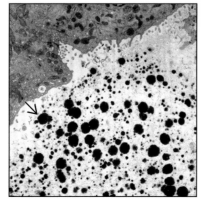 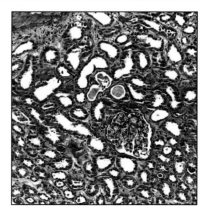

(Left) This renal biopsy is from a patient with acute renal failure after a motor vehicle accident. Pigmented casts due to myoglobin are present ⊇. Features of acute tubular injury are also seen with loss of brush borders, dilated lumens, and basophilic cytoplasm. *(Center)* On electron microscopy, the tubular pigmented cast is composed of electron-dense myoglobin globules ⊇. *(Right)* The renal biopsy shows features of acute tubular injury due to myoglobinuria. The cortex demonstrates interstitial edema, dilated tubules ⊿, and granular casts.

CISPLATIN NEPHROTOXICITY

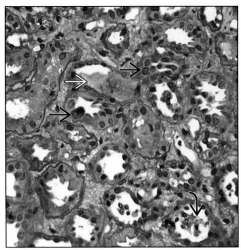

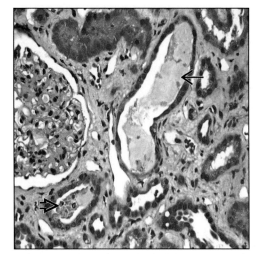

Renal cortex in recent cisplatin nephrotoxicity demonstrates luminal cellular debris ⇒, distal tubular casts ➡, regenerative nuclear atypia ⇒, and interstitial edema.

Kidney cortex shows dilated distal tubular segments with luminal cast material ⇒ and necrotic cellular debris ⇛ from a patient with recent cisplatin exposure. The interstitium is edematous.

TERMINOLOGY

Abbreviations
- Cis-diachlorodiammineplatinum (CDDP)

Synonyms
- Platinum nephrotoxicity, cisplatinum nephrotoxicity, cis-platinum nephrotoxicity, CDDP nephrotoxicity

Definitions
- Nephropathy due to direct toxicity of platinum compounds

ETIOLOGY/PATHOGENESIS

Nephrotoxic Injury
- Cis-diachlorodiammineplatinum II is heavy metal and potent inhibitor of DNA synthesis
  - Concentrated in kidney tissue and excreted in urine
  - Human exposure arises with use of this agent in cancer chemotherapy
- Nephrotoxicity may be detectable after single dose, and severity is dose dependent
- Lesion is initially reversible, but repeated doses increase chance of irreversible injury
- 1/3 of patients develop acute renal failure (acute kidney injury) after dose of 2 mg/kg
- No direct correlation between administered dose, tissue platinum content, severity of histologic injury, and severity of kidney dysfunction
- Preglomerular vasoconstriction with low transcapillary hydrostatic pressure and low single nephron glomerular filtration rate are important determinants of renal failure

CLINICAL ISSUES

Presentation
- Acute renal failure

  - Elevation of serum creatinine develops within days after administration
  - Serum creatinine peaks at about 10 days (8-12)
  - Recovery may take weeks or months
- Proteinuria is subnephrotic
- Hypomagnesemia due to decreased tubular reabsorption
- Impaired urinary concentrating ability with polyuria

Treatment
- Hydration is used as preventive measure
- Cessation of exposure to CDDP

Prognosis
- Majority of patients receiving low dose CDDP have reversible kidney injury
- Small proportion develop chronic renal failure (< 5%)
- Underlying kidney disease may predispose to irreversible injury
- Risk of renal carcinoma is unknown

MACROSCOPIC FEATURES

Gross Examination
- Kidneys are enlarged with pale cortex and red, congested medulla

MICROSCOPIC PATHOLOGY

Histologic Features
- Acute tubular necrosis affects proximal, distal, and collecting tubules
  - Tubular epithelium is flattened, and lumens have granular or hyaline cast material
  - Epithelial cytoplasm may have vacuolar changes, desquamation, and frank coagulative necrosis
  - Tubular epithelial necrosis is patchy and severe
  - Distal tubules may have marked dilation with luminal casts

CISPLATIN NEPHROTOXICITY

Key Facts

Terminology
- Nephropathy due to direct toxicity of platinum compounds

Etiology/Pathogenesis
- Cis-diachlorodiammineplatinum II is heavy metal and potent inhibitor of DNA synthesis

Clinical Issues
- Acute renal failure arises within days of exposure

Microscopic Pathology
- Acute tubular necrosis may be marked and affects proximal, distal, and collecting tubules
- Regeneration is characterized by nuclear atypia and polypoid epithelial proliferations
- Tubular nuclear atypia may persist for months

- o Patchy necrosis may persist for a month or more after therapy
- Interstitial edema with slight mononuclear infiltrate may be evident, but interstitial nephritis is uncommon
- Electron microscopy reveals mitochondrial vacuolar changes in proximal tubules in 2 days with loss of surface microvilli in about 3 days
  - o Platinum particles are not seen and have not been detected by electron probe x-ray analysis
- Glomeruli and vessels have no specific abnormalities
- Regenerative changes are apparent after 10 days
  - o Regeneration is characterized by nuclear enlargement, hyperchromasia, and pleomorphism
  - o Regenerative atypia may be prominent in collecting ducts, and epithelial polypoid lesions may project into tubular lumens
  - o Tubular nuclear atypia may persist for months and be associated with interstitial fibrosis and tubular atrophy

DIFFERENTIAL DIAGNOSIS

Tubular Necrosis with Nuclear Atypia
- Heavy metal toxicity: Mercury, lead, and copper
  - o Eosinophilic nuclear inclusions seen in lead toxicity
- Drugs
  - o Busulphan and foscarnet
- Viral infections
  - o Polyomavirus and adenovirus
- Karyomegalic interstitial nephritis

- o Tubules, endothelium, and interstitial cells have nuclear atypia
- Early neoplasia
  - o Tubular adenoma

DIAGNOSTIC CHECKLIST

Clinically Relevant Pathologic Features
- Tubular necrosis may persist more than a month after cessation of CDDP; regenerative atypia persists for months

Pathologic Interpretation Pearls
- Tubular epithelial necrosis is patchy and severe, and affects all nephron segments
- Regeneration is characterized by nuclear atypia and epithelial polypoid proliferations in collecting ducts

SELECTED REFERENCES

1. Tanaka H et al: Histopathological study of human cisplatin nephropathy. Toxicol Pathol. 14(2):247-57, 1986
2. Madias NE et al: Platinum nephrotoxicity. Am J Med. 65(2):307-14, 1978
3. Gonzales-Vitale JC et al: The renal pathology in clinical trials of cis-platinum (II) diamminedichloride. Cancer. 39(4):1362-71, 1977

IMAGE GALLERY

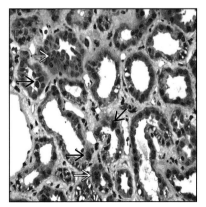 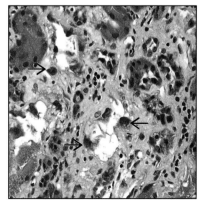 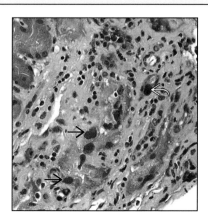

(Left) Acute tubular injury and regeneration in cisplatin toxicity is shown with open lumens, atypical nuclei ➡, and hypercellular collecting ducts ➡. *(Center)* Cisplatin toxicity may have marked atypia of the tubular nuclei ➡ months after exposure. The interstitium has fibrosis with mononuclear inflammation and atrophic tubules. *(Right)* Remote exposure to cisplatin may have interstitial fibrosis and marked nuclear atypia in proximal ➡ and distal ➡ segments.

CHLOROQUINE TOXICITY

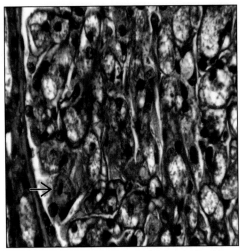

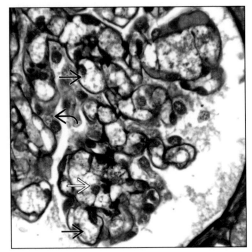

Glomeruli have abundant endocapillary vacuolated foam cells, which appear to partially occlude capillary lumens. Swollen, finely vacuolated podocytes are also evident➡. (Courtesy A. Cohen, MD.)

Endocapillary ➡ and mesangial ➡ cells with finely vacuolated foamy cytoplasm distort the normal architecture of this glomerulus. Some podocytes ➡ are also vacuolated. (Courtesy A. Cohen, MD.)

TERMINOLOGY

Abbreviations
- Chloroquine toxicity (CT)

Synonyms
- Iatrogenic phospholipidosis due to chloroquine; chloroquine-induced (phospho)lipidosis

Definitions
- Type of iatrogenic phospholipidosis characterized by nephropathy due to exposure to chloroquine

ETIOLOGY/PATHOGENESIS

Iatrogenic
- Chloroquine is a weak base and is lysosomotropic
- In lysosomes, chloroquine inhibits activity of numerous enzymes including α-galactosidase A
- ↓ α-galactosidase A enzymatic activity → accumulation of globotriaosylceramide, a sphingolipid
- Mechanism of induction of phospholipidosis is unknown; ceramide accumulates in endothelium, podocytes, smooth muscle, and tubular epithelium

CLINICAL ISSUES

Presentation
- Indications for chloroquine use
  - Treatment of malaria, extraintestinal amebiasis, rheumatoid arthritis, discoid lupus erythematosus, and others
- Toxicity
  - Renal toxicity: Proteinuria, declining renal function
  - Cardiac conduction defects, cardiomyopathy; proximal myopathy, retinopathy, keratopathy, hearing loss

Treatment
- Cessation of exposure to chloroquine

Prognosis
- Proteinuria and reduced glomerular filtration rate are potentially reversible on cessation of exposure to chloroquine

MICROSCOPIC PATHOLOGY

Histologic Features
- Glomerular capillaries and mesangium have cells with vacuolated, foamy cytoplasm
- Some but not all podocytes have swollen foamy cytoplasm
- Proximal and distal tubules may have fine cytoplasmic vacuolization
- Toluidine blue-stained sections have endocapillary vacuolated cells, and cytoplasmic azurophilic granules in podocytes, proximal and distal tubular cells
- Electron microscopy
  - Podocytes have whorled lipid inclusions, called myelin figures or "zebra bodies," in some but not all podocytes and may have curvilinear bodies and variable foot process effacement
  - Glomerular capillaries and mesangium have vacuolated cells with granular, electron-dense inclusions
  - Some myelin figures and vacuoles are evident in endothelium of glomeruli, peritubular capillaries, arterioles, and arteries
  - Smooth muscle cells may have myelin figures also

DIFFERENTIAL DIAGNOSIS

Hereditary Disorders of Lipid Storage
- Fabry disease

CHLOROQUINE TOXICITY

Key Facts

Terminology
- Type of iatrogenic phospholipidosis due to exposure to chloroquine

Microscopic Pathology
- Glomerular capillaries and mesangium have cells with vacuolated, foamy cytoplasm; podocytes have foamy cytoplasm

- Capillary lumens and mesangium have vacuolated cells with granular, electron-dense inclusions; some podocytes have myelin figures

Top Differential Diagnoses
- Fabry disease
- Other lipidoses
- Hydroxychloroquine, amiodarone, and silicon nephropathies

- Hereditary X-linked mutation of α-galactosidase A gene with resultant accumulation of globotriaosylceramide
- Myelin figures or "zebra bodies" seen in podocytes, endothelium, mesangial cells, distal tubules, smooth muscle
- Capillary lumens are not occluded by vacuolated cells, and curvilinear bodies are not seen in podocytes
- Plasma and leukocyte α-galactosidase A activity decreased or absent, but can be normal
- Mutational analysis by DNA sequencing is necessary to exclude this diagnosis
- Gaucher disease
  - Glomeruli have Gaucher ("tissue paper") cells in capillary lumens and in mesangium; podocytes are spared
  - Gaucher cells have PAS and oil red O positive material in cytoplasm
  - By electron microscopy, cytoplasmic elongated lysosomes contain irregular branching fibrils (60-80 nm in diameter)
- Other lipidoses
  - Infantile nephrosialidosis, I-cell disease, ceroid lipofuscinosis, Hurler syndrome, Niemann-Pick disease
    - These disorders have vacuolated podocytes mainly; Niemann-Pick disease may have vacuolated intracapillary cells
    - Differential diagnosis is resolved by DNA mutational analysis

- Lecithin cholesterol acyltransferase deficiency
  - Vacuolated cells in glomerular capillaries and mesangium
  - Extracellular vacuolated structures prominent in glomerular basement membrane and mesangium

Drugs
- Hydroxychloroquine, amiodarone, and silicon nephropathies
  - Pathologic features may be identical to chloroquine toxicity; diagnosis is established by clinical history

DIAGNOSTIC CHECKLIST

Clinically Relevant Pathologic Features
- Pathologic features are not specific and require careful clinical and molecular correlation, especially to exclude Fabry disease

Pathologic Interpretation Pearls
- Segmental podocyte involvement and curvilinear bodies are helpful clues

SELECTED REFERENCES
1. Albay D et al: Chloroquine-induced lipidosis mimicking Fabry disease. Mod Pathol. 18(5):733-8, 2005

IMAGE GALLERY

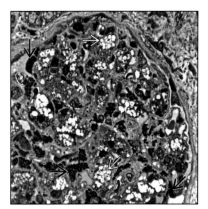 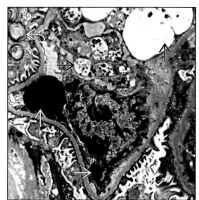 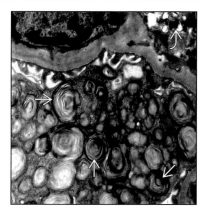

(Left) Plastic-embedded section shows abundant azurophilic granules in podocytes ➡. Endocapillary cells have prominent vacuoles ➡, many that contain granular material. (Courtesy A. Cohen, MD.) *(Center)* EM shows mesangial cytoplasmic vacuoles ➡ with granular debris of variable density. Endothelium has large, electron-dense lysosomes ➡. Myelin figures are in podocytes ➡. (Courtesy A. Cohen, MD.) *(Right)* Podocyte has myelin figures ➡ in abundance. Mesangium has vacuolated cells with electron-dense granules ➡. (Courtesy A. Cohen, MD.)

OSMOTIC TUBULOPATHY

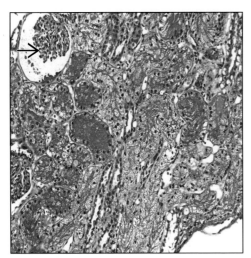

Osmotic tubulopathy in a kidney transplant due to IVIg exposure shows that there is proximal tubular epithelial swelling, luminal obliteration, and vacuolar change. The glomerulus appears shrunken ⊡.

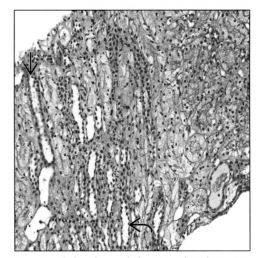

Osmotic tubulopathy in a kidney transplant due to IVIg exposure shows vacuolar changes that are evident in pars recta and pars convoluta, with sparing of collecting ducts ⊡ and loops of Henle ⊡.

TERMINOLOGY

Abbreviations
- Osmotic tubulopathy (OT)

Synonyms
- Osmotic nephrosis, contrast nephropathy, (radio)contrast-induced acute kidney injury, intravenous immunoglobulin-associated tubular toxicity

Definitions
- Tubular epithelial swelling and isometric vacuolization, associated with exposure to parenteral carbohydrate solutions or contrast media, and acute kidney injury

ETIOLOGY/PATHOGENESIS

Causes
- Parenteral infusion of hyperosmolar agents including
  - Parenteral carbohydrate solutions
    - Mannitol: Used as plasma expander and for treatment of cerebral edema
    - Dextran: Used as plasma expander
    - Hydroxyethyl starch (HES): Used as plasma expander and in perfusion preservation of kidney transplants (UW solution)
    - Glucose, sucrose, and maltose: Stabilizing agents
  - Intravenous immunoglobulin (IVIg): Sucrose and maltose used as stabilizing agents
  - Radiologic contrast agents: Iodine-containing agents, ionic or nonionic, high and low osmolality

Pathogenesis
- Hyperosmotic solutions are filtered and then absorbed by proximal tubules by pinocytosis
- Solute is retained in endosomes and not broken down
- Intracellular oncotic gradient is thus created and results in water absorption and hydropic swelling
- Accumulation of pinocytotic vesicles is dose related
- Vacuoles arise by fusion of vesicles with lysosomes
- Experimentally, vacuolar change appears in minutes and disappears in days after exposure
- Direct toxicity from disruption of cellular integrity and possible oxidative injury
- Secondary afferent arteriolar vasoconstriction and efferent vasodilation reduces glomerular filtration rate

Risk Factors
- Age > 65 years
- Preexisting chronic renal failure and diabetic nephropathy
- Concurrent exposure to nephrotoxic agents
- Coexistent ischemic or hypoxic renal injury, especially in kidney transplants
- Dehydration
- Quantity and osmolarity of administered solution, especially for contrast media and mannitol

CLINICAL ISSUES

Epidemiology
- Incidence
  - Incidence varies with agent administered and presence of associated risk factors

Presentation
- Acute deterioration of function of native and transplanted kidneys with exposure to inciting agents
- Renal failure may develop and resolve without clinical symptoms or signs
- Renal failure is typically oliguric
- Renal dysfunction begins within days of infusion and reverses after cessation of infusion
- Persistent impairment is rare
- High osmolal gap (measured osmolality minus calculated osmolality)
- Diagnosis is by kidney biopsy

OSMOTIC TUBULOPATHY

Key Facts

Terminology
- Tubular epithelial swelling and isometric vacuolization, associated with exposure to parenteral carbohydrate solutions or contrast media, and acute kidney injury

Etiology/Pathogenesis
- Parenteral infusion of hyperosmolar agents
  ○ Carbohydrate: Dextrans, mannitol, sucrose
  ○ Contrast agents
- Mechanism includes direct toxic and ischemic tubular injury

Clinical Issues
- Acute oliguric renal failure
- Diagnosis is by kidney biopsy

Microscopic Pathology
- Diffuse or focal clear cell change with luminal narrowing of proximal tubules
- Uniform isometric vacuolization of proximal tubular epithelium

Top Differential Diagnoses
- Tubular calcineurin inhibitor toxicity
- Ischemic tubular injury
- Tubulopathy associated with nephrotic syndrome

Diagnostic Checklist
- Cell swelling with luminal narrowing or obliteration rather than attenuation
- Electron microscopy reveals endosomes and lysosomes, and preserved surface microvilli

Treatment
- Prevention by hydration using iso-osmolar fluids
- Renal replacement therapy necessary in up to 40% of patients
- Plasma exchange for removal of dextran

Prognosis
- Recovery after cessation typically takes days to weeks
- Prolonged renal failure over months may be observed
- End-stage renal failure is rare
- Significant increase in mortality associated with acute renal failure

MACROSCOPIC FEATURES

Gross Examination
- Enlarged and pale kidneys

MICROSCOPIC PATHOLOGY

Histologic Features
- Diffuse or focal clear cell transformation with lumenal narrowing or solidification of proximal tubules
- Uniform isometric vacuolization of proximal tubular epithelium of convoluted and straight segments
- Vacuoles impinge on nuclear membrane imparting scalloped appearance
- Vacuoles are 1-4 microns in diameter and appear empty
- Earliest vacuoles in cell apex
- Vacuoles may persist with protracted renal failure
- Preservation of brush border on PAS staining
- Cellular necrosis and sloughed cells are uncommonly seen
- Immunofluorescence studies are negative
  ○ Immune complex deposits are not seen with IVIg usage
- Electron microscopy
  ○ Abundant cytoplasmic vacuoles and lysosomes
  ○ Surface microvilli are preserved
- Vacuolization of parietal epithelium of Bowman capsule, podocytes, and interstitial cells may be seen
- Mild cortical interstitial edema with scattered inflammatory cells may be evident
- Distal tubules and collecting ducts are unaffected
- Lesions are seen in native and transplanted kidneys
- Lesions may be evident in pre-implantation donor kidneys after perfusion preservation with University of Wisconsin solution (contains HES)

Cytologic Features
- Urinary foamy epithelial cells

DIFFERENTIAL DIAGNOSIS

Proximal Tubular Vacuolization
- Calcineurin inhibitor toxicity
  ○ Isometric vacuolization affects mainly proximal straight segments (medullary rays)
  ○ Focal distribution; rarely, if ever, diffuse
  ○ Ultrastructurally, there is dilation of endoplasmic reticulum
  ○ Evidence of glomerular or arteriolar thrombosis or arteriolar medial nodular hyalinization
- Ischemic acute tubular injury
  ○ Vacuolization typically coarse and irregular
  ○ Accompanied by epithelial flattening rather than swelling
  ○ Loss of brush border on periodic acid-Schiff staining and by electron microscopy
  ○ Focal epithelial necrosis and cellular casts
- Nephrotic syndrome
  ○ Vacuoles typically focal and often basally located in cytoplasm of proximal epithelium
  ○ Interstitial foam cells may be prominent
  ○ Often have abundant PAS-positive granules; protein reabsorption droplets
  ○ Causal glomerular lesions identified
- Alport nephropathy
  ○ Interstitial foam cell clusters
  ○ Characteristic glomerular basement membrane changes

OSMOTIC TUBULOPATHY

Frequency and Natural History

Agent	Frequency	Time to ARF	Duration of ARF	Persistent ARF	ESRD
Contrast media	2-15%	1-5 days	Days-weeks	Uncommon	Uncommon
Intravenous immunoglobulin	1-7%	3 days (range: 1-10 days)	14 days (range: 2-60 days)	Up to 20%	Uncommon
Hydroxyethyl starch	42-80%	10 days (range: 2-30 days)	Weeks-months	Uncommon	Uncommon
Mannitol	Up to 50%	3 days (range: 2-6 days)	Days-weeks	Rare	Not reported
Dextran	Up to 85%	4 days (range: 3-6 days)	Days-weeks	Uncommon	Uncommon

ARF = acute renal failure; ESRD = end-stage renal disease.

Differential Diagnosis of Osmotic Tubulopathy

Diagnosis	Distinguishing Features	Other Helpful Features
Tubular calcineurin inhibitor toxicity	Focal vacuolization, often in medullary rays	Arteriolopathy; dilated endoplasmic reticulum by EM
Ischemic acute tubular injury	Coarse vacuolization, flattened epithelium, necrosis, cellular casts	Loss of brush border on PAS and EM
Nephrotic syndrome	Focal, often basal vacuoles, interstitial foam cells	Glomerular cause of nephrosis
Ethylene glycol toxicity	Coarse large vacuoles, not isometric; calcium oxalate crystals	Mild tubulointerstitial inflammation
Methanol toxicity	No distinguishing features; may see myoglobin casts	
Potassium depletion	Proximal tubules have single well-defined vacuoles	Medullary interstitial cells with PAS(+) granules
Alport nephropathy	Clusters of interstitial foam cells; Alport glomerulopathy	
Armanni-Ebstein tubulopathy	Outer medullary clear cell change; PAS(+) and glycogen	
Intrarenal ectopic adrenal gland	Organoid zonal layers; typically subcapsular	
Xanthogranulomatous pyelonephritis	Interstitial foamy macrophages, mixed inflammatory infiltrate	
Renal cell carcinoma	Abrupt change in architecture, nuclear atypia or prominent nucleoli	

- Ethylene glycol toxicity
  - Coarse large vacuoles in proximal tubules
  - Calcium oxalate crystals
- Methanol toxicity
  - No morphologic distinguishing features
  - May see myoglobin casts
- Hypokalemia/potassium depletion
  - Proximal tubules have single coarse cytoplasmic vacuoles
- Hyperglycemia with glycosuria; Armanni-Ebstein tubulopathy
  - Clear cell change mainly in outer medulla
  - Clear cells are PAS positive and diastase digestible indicating glycogen
- Intrarenal adrenal gland
  - Typically subcapsular with recognizable zona glomerulosa, fasciculata, reticularis
- Xanthogranulomatous pyelonephritis
  - Interstitial clusters of foamy macrophages
  - Mixed neutrophilic and mononuclear inflammation
  - Gram-negative bacilli in exudates and neutrophils
- Clear cell renal cell carcinoma
  - Abrupt change in tubular architecture
  - Nuclear atypia

DIAGNOSTIC CHECKLIST

Clinically Relevant Pathologic Features
- Diffuse proximal tubular cytoplasmic swelling and vacuolization in setting of acute renal failure

Pathologic Interpretation Pearls
- Cell swelling with luminal narrowing or obliteration rather than attenuation with scant evidence of cellular necrosis
- Electron microscopy reveals endosomes and lysosomes, and preserved surface microvilli

SELECTED REFERENCES

1. Dickenmann M et al: Osmotic nephrosis: acute kidney injury with accumulation of proximal tubular lysosomes due to administration of exogenous solutes. Am J Kidney Dis. 51(3):491-503, 2008
2. Haas M et al: Isometric tubular epithelial vacuolization in renal allograft biopsy specimens of patients receiving low-dose intravenous immunoglobulin for a positive crossmatch. Transplantation. 78(4):549-56, 2004
3. Verhelst D et al: Acute renal injury following methanol poisoning: analysis of a case series. Int J Toxicol. 23(4):267-73, 2004
4. Cantú TG et al: Acute renal failure associated with immunoglobulin therapy. Am J Kidney Dis. 25(2):228-34, 1995

OSMOTIC TUBULOPATHY

Microscopic Features

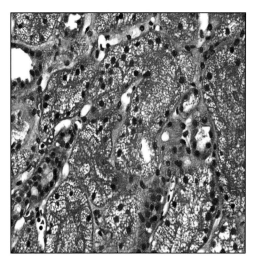

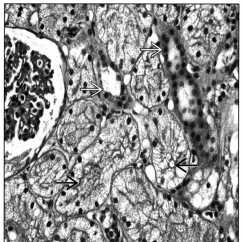

(Left) This kidney transplant has proximal tubular cytoplasmic swelling, luminal obliteration, and abundant small isometric vesicles. The changes are due to IVIg exposure. *(Right)* A kidney transplant has proximal tubules with extensive lumenal obliteration, cytoplasmic swelling, vacuolization, and preservation of the brush borders ➡. Distal tubular segments are spared ➡.

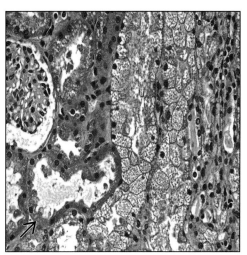

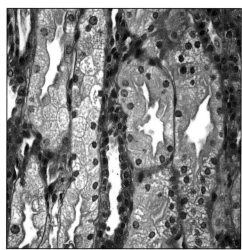

(Left) Tubular isometric vacuolization may persist for weeks after removal of the inciting injury, associated with use of IVIg in this instance. Clinically, there was persistent renal transplant dysfunction for 3 weeks. Note acute tubular injury ➡ in addition. *(Right)* Persistent epithelial vacuolization and diminished PAS-positive brush borders are seen in a transplant kidney with persistent dysfunction for 3 weeks after diagnosis of IVIg toxicity and cessation of exposure.

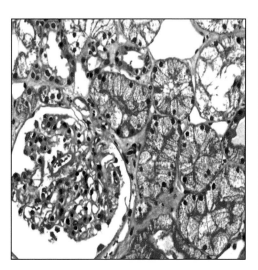

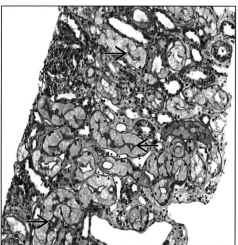

(Left) Diffuse vacuolization is seen in the proximal tubules in this case of osmotic tubulopathy from exposure to radiologic contrast. The glomerulus and interstitium are unremarkable. *(Right)* Osmotic tubulopathy associated with use of radiologic contrast shows tubular profiles that have cytoplasmic swelling, vacuolization, and preservation of the brush borders ➡.

4

Microscopic Features and Differential Diagnosis

(Left) Tubular injury with epithelial flattening and abundant coarse cytoplasmic vacuoles is shown in the pre-implantation biopsy from a perfusion preserved kidney transplant. The findings are probably a combination of ischemic and osmotic tubulopathy from HES in the University of Wisconsin perfusion solution. *(Right)* Clear cell change and isometric vacuolization are shown in a pre-implantation biopsy specimen exposed to HES in UW perfusion solution.

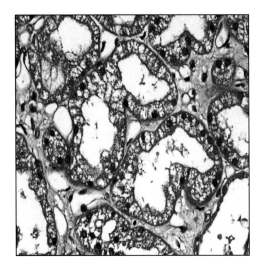
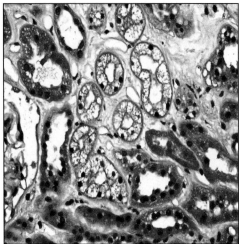

(Left) Focal isometric vacuolization in a straight segment of proximal tubule from a kidney transplant with tubular calcineurin inhibitor toxicity. Other tubular segments, including a loop of Henle ➡ and a collecting duct ➡, are spared. *(Right)* Acute ischemic tubular injury in the native nontransplant kidney with coarse irregular vacuolization of the proximal tubular cytoplasm ➡ shows that the interstitium has mild edema with scattered inflammatory cells (lower middle).

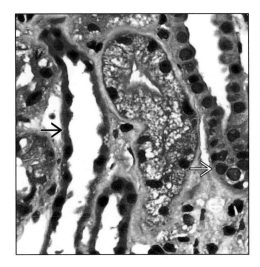
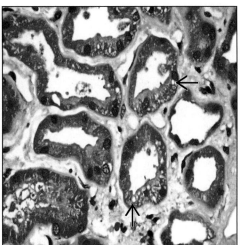

(Left) Coarse irregular cytoplasmic vacuolization of proximal tubules is seen in a native nontransplant kidney with ischemic acute tubular injury. *(Right)* Tubular cytoplasmic vacuolization without hydropic change associated with lipiduria in nephrotic syndrome is shown. Small, even-sized vacuoles are mainly basal in distribution, but they fill the cytoplasm in some instances ➡.

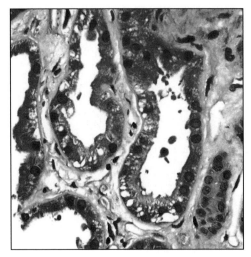
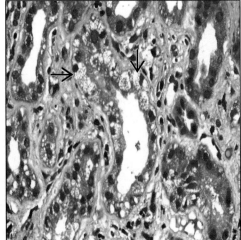

OSMOTIC TUBULOPATHY

Differential Diagnosis

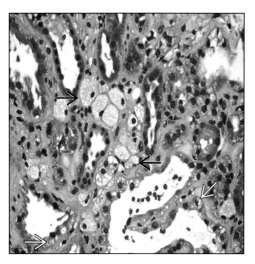
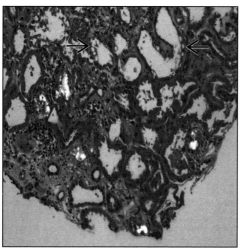

(Left) In this case of interstitial foam cells associated with the nephrotic syndrome, collections of interstitial foam cells ⮕ are seen in a patient with IgA nephropathy and nephrotic range proteinuria. Subtle tubular vacuoles are also evident ⮕. *(Right)* Partially polarized light microscopic view of a kidney from a patient with ethylene glycol toxicity demonstrates calcium oxalate crystals and large proximal tubular vacuoles ⮕.

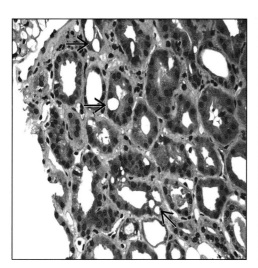
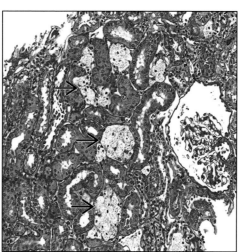

(Left) H&E shows single "punched out" coarse vacuoles in proximal tubules ⮕ of a kidney transplant patient with acute tubular injury and severe hypokalemia. *(Right)* Clear cell clusters with cytoplasmic vacuolization ⮕ in the interstitium are shown in this biopsy specimen from a patient with Alport nephropathy and nephrotic range proteinuria.

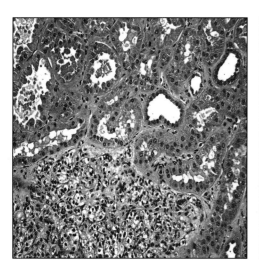
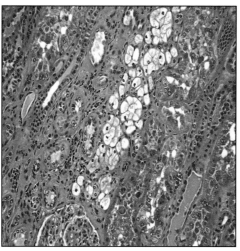

(Left) An abrupt change from normal renal tubules to a discrete nodule composed of clear cell clusters is seen. The clear cells have small regular nuclei and interstitial vessels are prominent. The patient's kidney had multiple satellite nodules of renal cell carcinoma, clear cell type. *(Right)* A tiny satellite cluster of clear cells in the interstitium is shown. The clear cells have small regular nuclei and abundant foamy cytoplasm. This satellite was distant from a primary renal cell carcinoma, clear cell type.

ANTIVIRAL DRUG NEPHROTOXICITY

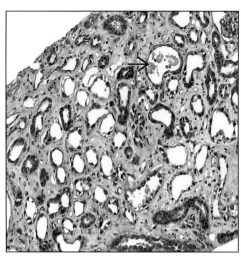

H&E shows acute tubular injury with severe attenuation of the epithelium, luminal widening, and necrotic debris ⇒ in an HIV-positive patient exposed to tenofovir. There is also diffuse interstitial fibrosis.

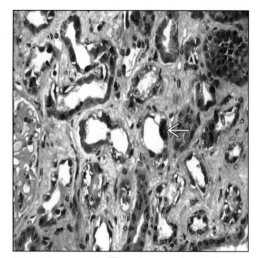

Tubular karyomegaly ⇒ and acute tubular injury are evident in this biopsy specimen from a patient with tenofovir toxicity. The interstitium has extensive fibrosis.

TERMINOLOGY

Synonyms
- Antiviral nephrotoxicity

Definitions
- Kidney dysfunction due to exposure to antiviral agents

ETIOLOGY/PATHOGENESIS

Environmental Exposure
- Antiviral agents with known nephrotoxicity
  - Nucleoside analogs (reverse transcriptase inhibitors): Acyclovir, valacyclovir, ganciclovir, abacavir, lamivudine, didanosine
  - Nucleotide analogs (reverse transcriptase inhibitors): Tenofovir, adefovir, cidofovir
  - Peptide analogs (protease inhibitors): Indinavir, ritonavir, atazanavir
  - Pyrophosphate analogs: Foscarnet (trisodium phosphonoformate)
  - Fusion or entry inhibitors: Enfurtivide
  - Other agents: Intravenous immunoglobulin, interferon-α
- Risk factors for nephrotoxicity
  - Kidney
    - Drugs are concentrated in specific nephron segments; proximal tubules are at greatest risk of injury
    - Organic anion transporter system concentrates tenofovir and cidofovir in proximal tubules
  - Patient
    - Infection, e.g., HIV
    - Underlying chronic kidney disease and dehydration
    - Pharmacogenetics and immune response genes
  - Drug
    - Dose dependent: High dose increases risk of renal injury
    - Solubility: Concentration and pH dependent
    - Immune stimulatory potential
- Pathogenesis
  - Direct tubular toxicity: Tenofovir, adefovir, acyclovir, cidofovir
    - Mitochondrial toxicity: Antiviral nucleoside and nucleotide analogs (ANA) act as competitive alternative substrate for mitochondrial thymidine kinase
    - ANA triphosphate inhibits mitochondrial DNA polymerase-γ, resulting in altered mitochondrial DNA
    - Mitochondrial depletion and mitochondrial DNA depletion are associated with tenofovir, adefovir, and cidofovir
  - Tubulointerstitial nephritis (TIN): Indinavir, atazanavir, abacavir, efavirenz, foscarnet
    - Dysfunction associated with inflammatory injury
    - Injury may be precipitated by tubular injury or idiosyncratic immunologic reactions ± effects of HIV infection
  - Crystal nephropathy: Acyclovir, indinavir
    - Crystals may be toxic to epithelium and may obstruct tubules
    - Crystal precipitation often associated with tubulointerstitial nephritis
  - Glomerulopathy: Foscarnet, valacyclovir, acyclovir, enfuvirtide
    - Glomerular crystal deposition

CLINICAL ISSUES

Presentation
- Proximal tubulopathy and Fanconi syndrome: Cidofovir, tenofovir, adefovir, foscarnet, stavudine, lamivudine
  - Frequency: Tenofovir (0.3-2%), adefovir (up to 50% at high dose)
- Distal tubular acidosis: Foscarnet

ANTIVIRAL DRUG NEPHROTOXICITY

Key Facts

Terminology
- Kidney dysfunction due to exposure to antiviral agents

Etiology/Pathogenesis
- Direct tubular toxicity: Tenofovir, adefovir, acyclovir, cidofovir
- Tubulointerstitial nephritis (TIN): Indinavir, atazanavir, abacavir, efavirenz, foscarnet
- Crystal nephropathy: Acyclovir, indinavir
- Glomerulopathy: Foscarnet, valacyclovir, acyclovir, enfuvirtide

Microscopic Pathology
- Acute tubular injury or necrosis ± TIN
  - Karyomegaly + megamitochondria
  - Proximal tubules are most severely affected

- Interstitial fibrosis may be prominent
- Crystal nephropathy: Intrarenal precipitation of crystallized salts of antiviral agent (indinavir and foscarnet)
- TIN: Acute and chronic
- Glomerular crystals (foscarnet), thrombotic microangiopathy (acyclovir)

Ancillary Tests
- Mitochondrial enlargement, dysmorphism, distortion of cristae; mitochondrial depletion on electron microscopy
- Infrared spectroscopy allows definitive identification of crystal composition

- Nephrogenic diabetes insipidus: Foscarnet, didanosine, abacavir
- Acute renal failure/kidney injury: Acyclovir, ganciclovir, cidofovir, indinavir, tenofovir, adefovir, foscarnet
  - Frequency: Tenofovir (0.5-1.5%), acyclovir (10%)
- Crystalluria, lithiasis: Acyclovir, indinavir
  - Frequency: Indinavir (10-20%), acyclovir (12-48% with intravenous infusions), atazanavir (0.01%)
  - Crystalluria may be associated with acute kidney injury
- Proteinuria: Cidofovir, foscarnet, interferon-α
- Chronic renal failure: Cidofovir, indinavir, tenofovir

Treatment
- Drug withdrawal or substitution
- Hydration and restoration of high urinary output

Prognosis
- Most acute dysfunction due to antiviral agents is reversible
  - Most acute kidney injuries and acute crystal nephropathies are reversible
  - TIN ± crystal deposits are reversible if interstitial fibrosis is limited
  - Lesions have limited reversibility if there is extensive scarring on biopsy
- Anecdotal reports of end-stage renal failure due to cidofovir and foscarnet toxicity

MICROSCOPIC PATHOLOGY

Histologic Features
- Acute tubular injury or necrosis
  - Tubular injury can be associated with most antiviral agents
    - Proximal tubules are most severely affected with loss of apical cytoplasm, brush border, irregular tubular luminal boundary
    - Karyomegaly with nuclear enlargement, irregular nuclear membrane, hyperchromatism, coarse nucleoli
    - Proximal tubular megamitochondria are rounded eosinophilic cytoplasmic inclusions; fuchsinophilic on trichrome stain; PAS negative
    - Megamitochondria are characteristic of tenofovir, but also described in cidofovir, adefovir, lamivudine, and stavudine toxicity
    - Distal tubular segments and collecting ducts also have evidence of injury with regeneration
    - Interstitial fibrosis may be prominent
  - Myoglobinuric acute tubular necrosis has been described with use of didanosine and zidovudine in patients with HIV infection
  - Intravenous immunoglobulin may be associated with osmotic tubulopathy
- Crystal nephropathy: Intrarenal precipitation of crystallized salts of antiviral agent
  - Acyclovir
    - Distal tubular crystal deposits and mild tubulointerstitial inflammation without crystal deposits are both described
  - Foscarnet
    - Crystal deposits detectable in air-dried or alcohol-fixed frozen sections
    - Rhomboid and clustered polyhedral yellow crystals; washed out by aqueous fixatives
    - Birefringent on polarization microscopy
    - Sites of proximal tubular crystal deposition have luminal macrophages, giant cells, and tubular injury, all with cytoplasmic crystal clefts
    - Similar-appearing crystal clefts are seen in glomerular capillaries, associated with fibrin deposition and, rarely, crescent formation
    - Crystals are von Kossa positive
    - Infrared spectroscopy reveals trisodium foscarnet, as well as sodium and calcium phosphate salts containing foscarnet
  - Indinavir
    - Crystals are detectable in frozen sections as polyhedric, rectangular, or needle-shaped structures; birefringent on polarization

- Tubular luminal cellular casts are composed of macrophages containing sharp-ended clefts in cytoplasm
- Focal distal tubular and collecting ductal crystal deposits are associated with widespread tubular injury and tubulointerstitial nephritis with fibrosis
  - Infrared spectroscopy reveals indinavir monohydrate
  - Crystal nephropathy is accompanied by TIN
  - Nephrolithiasis is associated with acyclovir and indinavir
- TIN
  - Described in foscarnet, atazanavir, abacavir, efavirenz, and indinavir toxicity
  - Patchy or diffuse interstitial inflammation, edema, and focal tubulitis
  - Infiltrates composed of predominantly mononuclear cells and fewer polymorphonuclear neutrophils
  - Tubular nuclear atypia is common
  - Interstitial fibrosis and tubular atrophy are of variable severity
- Glomerular disorders
  - Glomerular crystal deposits in foscarnet toxicity; may be associated with crescent formation
  - Thrombotic microangiopathy: Acyclovir, valacyclovir
  - Membranoproliferative glomerulonephritis: Enfurtivide
  - Focal segmental glomerulosclerosis rarely associated with interferon-α therapy for hepatitis C infection

ANCILLARY TESTS

Electron Microscopy
- Acute tubular injury in tenofovir and cidofovir toxicity
  - Mitochondrial enlargement, dysmorphism, distortion of cristae; mitochondrial depletion
- Crystal clefts in glomerular capillaries and mesangium, in tubules in foscarnet toxicity
- Crystal clefts in intratubular macrophages in indinavir toxicity

Infrared Spectroscopy
- Allows definitive identification of crystal composition

Immunofluorescence
- Nonspecific

DIFFERENTIAL DIAGNOSIS

Acute Tubular Injury
- Tubular injury can be caused by many therapeutic agents
- Megamitochondria are uncommon but may be seen in calcineurin inhibitor toxicity and mitochondrial cytopathies
- HIV infection can have renal tubular injury and mitochondrial dysmorphism in absence of exposure to antiretroviral agents

Tubulointerstitial Nephritis (TIN)
- TIN can be caused by many different agents
  - Specific cause difficult to determine in most instances
- Reactive tubular nuclear karyomegaly and atypia is uncommon in TIN
  - Viral infections (adenovirus, polyomavirus, HIV), cisplatinum/busulfan toxicity, and karyomegalic interstitial nephropathy must be excluded

Crystal Nephropathy
- Oxalate nephropathy: Birefringent sheaf-like arrays of yellow crystals in tubular epithelium, lumens, and interstitium
- Uric acid nephropathy: Intratubular needle-like clefts in tubular epithelium or in interstitial granulomas (tophi)
- Other drugs: Sulfadiazine, triamterene, ampicillin, methotrexate, vitamin C, ciprofloxacin, orlistat may also cause crystal nephropathy
- Intratubular precipitates of cholesterol crystals in nephrotic states can resemble indinavir crystals

DIAGNOSTIC CHECKLIST

Clinically Relevant Pathologic Features
- Acute tubular necrosis and TIN, ± intratubular crystal deposition, are most common lesions associated with acute kidney injury

Pathologic Interpretation Pearls
- Megamitochondria are characteristic of tenofovir and cidofovir toxicity
- Intratubular crystals in indinavir toxicity and glomerular crystals in foscarnet toxicity

SELECTED REFERENCES

1. Herlitz LC et al: Tenofovir nephrotoxicity: acute tubular necrosis with distinctive clinical, pathological, and mitochondrial abnormalities. Kidney Int. 78(11):1171-7, 2010
2. Justrabo E et al: Irreversible glomerular lesions induced by crystal precipitation in a renal transplant after foscarnet therapy for cytomegalovirus infection. Histopathology. 34(4):365-9, 1999
3. Martinez F et al: Indinavir crystal deposits associated with tubulointerstitial nephropathy. Nephrol Dial Transplant. 13(3):750-3, 1998

ANTIVIRAL DRUG NEPHROTOXICITY

Acute Tubulopathy and Megamitochondria

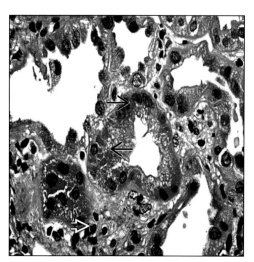

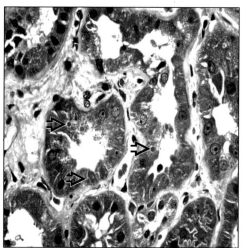

(Left) Megamitochondria may be seen singly and in clusters → in tubular epithelium in tenofovir toxicity. There is acute tubular injury and interstitial mononuclear inflammation ⇒. (Courtesy L. Herlitz, MD.) (Right) Acute tubular injury with prominent brightly fuchsinophilic megamitochondria ⇒ are seen in this trichrome stain of a biopsy specimen from a patient with hepatitis B infection treated with tenofovir. (Courtesy L. Herlitz, MD.)

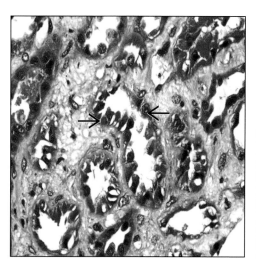

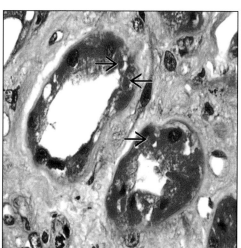

(Left) Markers of antiviral toxicity include megamitochondria → often in tubules with other features of acute injury. Coarse cytoplasmic vacuolization and karyomegaly are also apparent. The interstitium is edematous with early fibrosis. (Right) Megamitochondria may be quite subtle and require careful search for their identification →. These were identified in an HIV-positive patient treated with tenofovir. These proximal segments are shrunken, and there is background fibrosis.

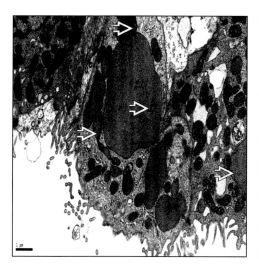

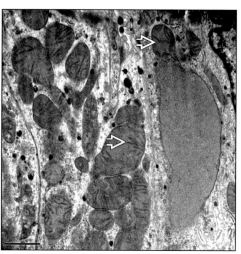

(Left) EM shows enlarged dysmorphic mitochondria with shrunken and misshapen cristae ⇒ are seen in this injured proximal tubular epithelial cell from a patient treated with tenofovir for hepatitis B infection. (Courtesy L. Herlitz, MD.) (Right) A cluster of dysmorphic mitochondria with varied sizes and shapes, and distorted cristae ⇒, are evident in the proximal tubular epithelium of a patient with HIV infection and tenofovir toxicity (EM).

Tubular Injury and Interstitial Nephritis

(Left) Distal tubular segments with acute epithelial injury ➡ are shown in an example of tenofovir toxicity. The macula densa ➡ appears intact, but the remaining epithelium is attenuated. (Right) Periodic acid-Schiff shows tubulointerstitial nephritis in a biopsy specimen from a patient with HIV infection and exposure to atazanavir, ritonavir, abacavir, and lamivudine. Tubulitis ➡, mitoses ➡, and tubular atrophy ➡ indicate active and chronic tubulointerstitial nephritis.

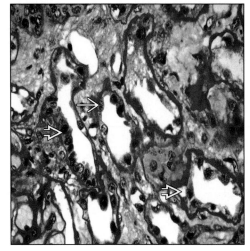
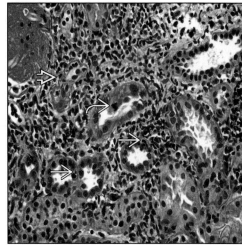

(Left) H&E shows tubular epithelial injury with attenuation of epithelium, karyomegaly ➡, and luminal basophilic crystalline material in the tubule ➡. This material may contain foscarnet salts. There is interstitial fibrosis and mononuclear infiltrate. (Right) Periodic acid-Schiff shows large atypical tubular epithelial nuclei and a luminal sawtooth pattern in tubular injury associated with the use of foscarnet.

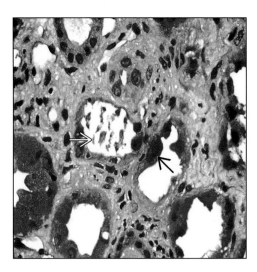
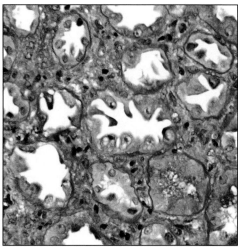

(Left) H&E shows granulomatous interstitial nephritis ➡ associated with foscarnet exposure in a renal transplant biopsy from a patient with systemic Cytomegalovirus infection. The inflammatory infiltrate is composed of mononuclear and granulocytic cells. There is acute tubular injury ➡. (Right) Chronic tubulointerstitial nephritis associated with foscarnet exposure is shown. Tubules have nuclear atypia ➡.

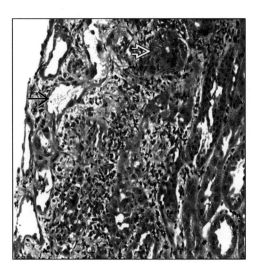
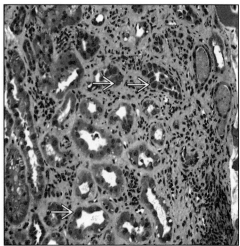

Crystal Nephropathy

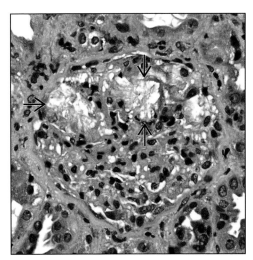
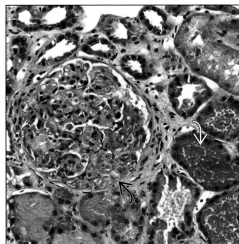

(Left) H&E shows glomerular crystalline clefts ➡ in a biopsy specimen from a patient with CMV infection treated with foscarnet. *(Right)* Crescentic glomerulonephritis is shown in this example of foscarnet toxicity. Crescents ➡ and red cell casts ➡ were prominent in this biopsy, mimicking glomerulonephritis, but they were caused by crystals lodging in glomerular capillaries. Crystals appear as clear spaces in capillaries and are difficult to identify at medium power.

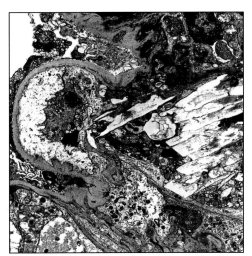
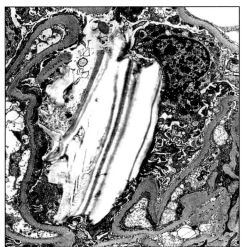

(Left) EM shows angulated cytoplasmic crystal clefts in a mesangial phagocyte associated with foscarnet toxicity. Foscarnet salts are uncommon but characteristic of toxicity from this agent. *(Right)* EM shows crystal clefts compressing the podocyte in Bowman space in a case of foscarnet toxicity. Similar clefts can be seen in capillaries, in mesangium, and in proximal tubules.

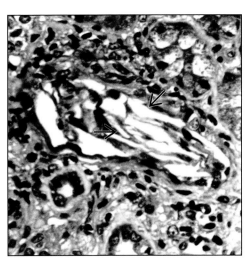
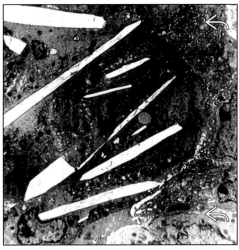

(Left) This intratubular cellular cast composed of macrophages contains needle-like clefts ➡. Crystals of indinavir salts were washed out in tissue preparation. There is mononuclear inflammation and fibrosis in the interstitium. *(Courtesy S. Rosen, MD.)* *(Right)* This example of indinavir toxicity demonstrates needle and rhomboid crystal clefts in the cytoplasm of intratubular macrophages. Note the tubular epithelium at the right ➡. *(Courtesy S. Rosen, MD.)*

ACUTE PHOSPHATE NEPHROPATHY

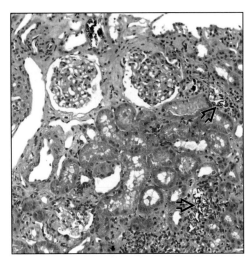

Calcium phosphate precipitates ⊳ are seen within tubular lumens in a case of acute phosphate nephropathy related to ingestion of oral sodium phosphate solution for bowel preparation.

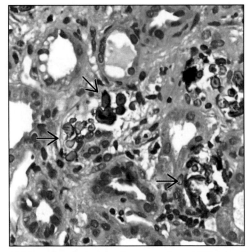

Calcium phosphate deposits are purple on H&E stained sections ➜ and are characteristically prominent in acute phosphate nephropathy.

TERMINOLOGY

Synonyms
- Phosphate-induced nephrocalcinosis

Definitions
- Tubular injury or atrophy with abundant intratubular calcium phosphate precipitates

ETIOLOGY/PATHOGENESIS

Calcium Phosphate Precipitation in Tubules
- Related to elevated calcium phosphate product (CPP) within distal tubules and collecting ducts
  - CPP elevation exacerbated by volume depletion

Clinical Causes of Phosphate Nephropathy
- Oral sodium phosphate (OSP) ingestion as part of bowel preparation for colonoscopy
  - Phospho-soda solution or Visicol (sodium phosphate) tablets
    - Decreased phosphate content in more recent formulations
  - Risk factors for phosphate nephropathy with OSP use
    - Inadequate hydration while receiving OSP
    - History of hypertension
    - Use of angiotensin converting enzyme inhibitor or angiotensin receptor blocker or diuretics
    - Older patients
    - Female gender
  - Increased risk of acute renal failure with OSP than with polyethylene glycol bowel preparation for colonoscopy
    - Incidence of acute renal failure estimated between 1 in 1,000 to 1 in 5,000 patients receiving OSP bowel preparation
- Phosphate supplementation in renal transplant patients
  - Post-transplant hyperparathyroidism and hypophosphatemia in early post-transplant period
  - Allograft biopsies may show calcium phosphate precipitates within tubular lumens
- Nephrocalcinosis in children with hypophosphatemic rickets
  - Calcium phosphate deposition in kidney associated with oral vitamin D and phosphate administration

CLINICAL ISSUES

Presentation
- Acute renal failure
  - Renal function may improve after initial insult, but most patients develop some degree of chronic renal failure
- Chronic renal failure
  - May be discovered months to > 1 year following recognized exposure to OSP

Prognosis
- High risk for chronic renal failure

MICROSCOPIC PATHOLOGY

Histologic Features
- Calcium phosphate crystals within tubular lumens
  - Deposits present within distal tubules and collecting ducts
    - Appear purple on H&E stained sections
    - Nonpolarizable crystals
    - Calcium phosphate deposits positive (black) on von Kossa stain
  - Interstitial calcium phosphate deposits as residua of atrophic tubule
- Acute tubular injury
- Tubular atrophy and interstitial fibrosis
- Focal mild interstitial inflammation

ACUTE PHOSPHATE NEPHROPATHY

Key Facts

Etiology/Pathogenesis
- Oral sodium phosphate (OSP) ingestion as part of bowel preparation for colonoscopy
- Risk factors for phosphate nephropathy with OSP use
  - Inadequate hydration while receiving OSP
  - Use of angiotensin converting enzyme inhibitor or angiotensin receptor blocker or diuretics

Clinical Issues
- Acute or chronic renal failure

Microscopic Pathology
- Calcium phosphate crystals within tubular lumens, positive (black) on von Kossa stain
- Tubular atrophy and interstitial fibrosis

Top Differential Diagnoses
- Nephrocalcinosis
  - Clinical in setting of chronic hypercalcemia

- No specific glomerular or vascular involvement, except as related to underlying hypertensive disease

Electron Microscopy
- Electron-dense, radially oriented crystals around a central nidus

ANCILLARY TESTS

Laboratory Testing
- Serum calcium and phosphorus levels usually normal
  - Serum phosphorus levels may be transiently elevated at time of OSP administration; if elevated, serum levels decrease to normal within days after administration

DIFFERENTIAL DIAGNOSIS

Nephrocalcinosis
- Occurs in setting of chronic hypercalcemia
  - e.g., hyperparathyroidism, malignancy, granulomatous disorders, milk alkali syndrome, vitamin D intoxication, and some medications
- No history of oral sodium phosphate ingestion
- May have tubular basement membrane calcium phosphate deposits along with tubular lumen and interstitial deposits

Oxalate Nephropathy
- Calcium oxalate crystals within tubular lumens

- Calcium oxalate crystals are clear and polarizable on H&E stained sections

Other Crystalline Nephropathies
- e.g., drug crystals

SELECTED REFERENCES

1. Heher EC et al: Nephrocalcinosis, oral sodium phosphate solution, and phosphate nephropathy. Nephrol Rounds. 5(2):1-6, 2007
2. Hurst FP et al: Association of oral sodium phosphate purgative use with acute kidney injury. J Am Soc Nephrol. 18(12):3192-8, 2007
3. Bhan I et al: Post-transplant hypophosphatemia: Tertiary 'Hyper-Phosphatoninism'? Kidney Int. 70(8):1486-94, 2006
4. Markowitz GS et al: Acute phosphate nephropathy following oral sodium phosphate bowel purgative: an underrecognized cause of chronic renal failure. J Am Soc Nephrol. 16(11):3389-96, 2005
5. Markowitz GS et al: Renal failure due to acute nephrocalcinosis following oral sodium phosphate bowel cleansing. Hum Pathol. 35(6):675-84, 2004
6. Desmeules S et al: Acute phosphate nephropathy and renal failure. N Engl J Med. 349(10):1006-7, 2003
7. Alon U et al: Metabolic and histologic investigation of the nature of nephrocalcinosis in children with hypophosphatemic rickets and in the Hyp mouse. J Pediatr. 120(6):899-905, 1992

IMAGE GALLERY

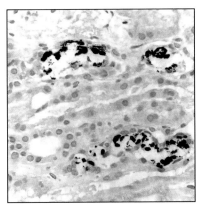 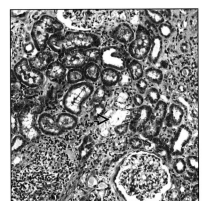 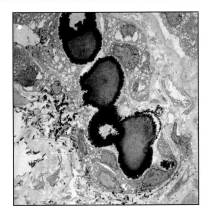

(Left) Calcium phosphate crystals stain positively (black) on a von Kossa stain (detects phosphate). *(Center)* Calcium phosphate deposits ➡ are less conspicuous on a trichrome stain. *(Right)* Electron microscopy shows calcium phosphate precipitates present within the tubular lumens. The crystals are electron-dense and appear radially oriented around a central nidus.

LITHIUM-INDUCED RENAL DISEASE

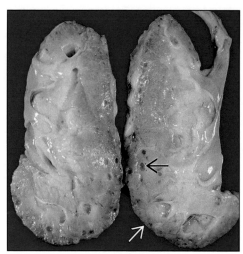

Numerous cysts ⇨ are present throughout the kidney of a 43-year-old man with renal failure on long-term lithium therapy. The renal cortex is thinned ⇨.

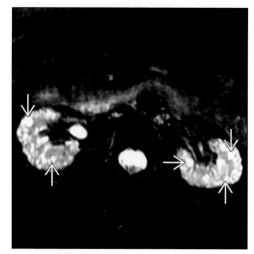

Axial T2-weighted MR shows innumerable tiny bright lesions ⇨ throughout both kidneys, which represent fluid in microcysts (a typical feature of lithium-induced nephropathy). The patient had long-term lithium use.

TERMINOLOGY

Synonyms
- Lithium-induced nephropathy, lithium nephrotoxicity

Definitions
- Renal disease affecting tubules, glomeruli, and interstitium related to chronic lithium treatment

ETIOLOGY/PATHOGENESIS

Lithium Exposure
- Principal cells of collecting ducts are primary target of lithium toxicity
  - Decreased ratio of principal cells to intercalated cells of collecting ducts after lithium therapy
  - Epithelial sodium channel (ENaC) expressed on apical surface
    - Permeable to only sodium and lithium
    - Nearly 2x higher permeability for lithium compared to sodium
    - Important mechanism in development of nephrogenic diabetes insipidus
  - Glycogen synthase kinase type 3β (GSK-3β)
    - Inhibited by lithium
  - Cyclooxygenase-1 and -2 expression in renal medulla reduced by lithium
- Tubular dysfunction
  - Marked downregulation of aquaporin-2 expression
- Increased rate of proliferation
  - May increase sensitivity to other tubular injury

Lithium Pathophysiology
- Freely filtered by glomeruli
  - 80% reabsorbed, primarily by proximal tubules

Idiosyncratic Factors
- Possible contribution of other drugs/toxins or genetic factors

CLINICAL ISSUES

Epidemiology
- Incidence
  - Chronic kidney disease (Cr > 150 μM/L) in 1.2% of lithium-treated patients (Sweden)
    - 0.53% develop end-stage renal disease
    - 6x risk compared with general population
  - Nephrogenic diabetes insipidus
    - 40% of all patients treated with lithium
    - 80% of patients with lithium nephrotoxicity

Presentation
- Nephrogenic diabetes insipidus
  - Polydipsia, polyuria
- Chronic renal failure
- Proteinuria
  - Nephrotic-range (> 3.5 g/24 hours) in 25%

Natural History
- Chronic kidney disease
  - Occurs after 10-20 years of lithium use
  - Can develop up to 10 years after lithium use is stopped
- Hypercalcemia
  - Long-term sequelae

Treatment
- Drugs
  - Amiloride
    - Targets and inhibits ENaC, which may reduce lithium nephrotoxic effects
- Reduction or discontinuation of lithium therapy
  - Not effective when cystic change and marked glomerular and tubulointerstitial scarring present

Prognosis
- Less than 1% of patients treated with lithium progress to end-stage renal disease
  - Average of 20 years of lithium therapy

LITHIUM-INDUCED RENAL DISEASE

Key Facts

Etiology/Pathogenesis
- Principal cells of collecting ducts are primary target of lithium toxicity
- Exposure for more than 10 years

Clinical Issues
- Nephrogenic diabetes insipidus
- Occurs in up to 40% of patients treated with lithium
- Proteinuria
- Amiloride targets and inhibits ENaC, which may reduce lithium nephrotoxic effects
- Reduction or discontinuation of lithium therapy
- Less than 1% of patients treated with lithium progress to end-stage renal disease
- Sequelae
  - Chronic kidney disease
  - Hypercalcemia

Image Findings
- Multiple (several to innumerable) tiny cysts

Microscopic Pathology
- Renal cysts
  - Hobnail appearance of the tubular epithelial cells may be present
- Segmental glomerulosclerosis
- Tubular dilation
- Glomerulosclerosis, focal, segmental
- Foot process effacement

Top Differential Diagnoses
- Other forms of FSGS or minimal change disease
- Other forms of cystic and tubulointerstitial disease

IMAGE FINDINGS

General Features
- Kidneys are small to normal size
- Multiple (several to innumerable) tiny cysts
  - Usually 2-5 mm
  - Best seen on T2-weighted MR where they appear as small bright dots

MICROSCOPIC PATHOLOGY

Histologic Features
- Renal cysts
  - Cortex
  - Medulla
- Cystic dilation of distal tubules and collecting ducts
  - Accumulation of Tamm-Horsfall protein and cellular debris
  - Hobnail appearance of tubular epithelial cells may be present
- Glomerular alterations
  - Segmental glomerulosclerosis
    - Present in 50% of cases
    - Secondary to hyperfiltration
    - Usually correlates with presence of proteinuria
  - Global glomerulosclerosis
  - Glomerular hypertrophy
    - Secondary to hyperfiltration
  - Mesangial hypercellularity
  - Mesangial sclerosis
  - Crescents, rarely
- Interstitial fibrosis and tubular atrophy
- Interstitial inflammation
  - May be sufficient for additional diagnosis of acute interstitial nephritis

ANCILLARY TESTS

Immunohistochemistry
- *Arachis hypogaea* lectin (peanut) may help identify collecting ducts
- Epithelial membrane antigen identifies both distal tubules and collecting ducts

Electron Microscopy
- Transmission
  - Podocyte foot process effacement is common
  - Mitochondrial abnormalities reported
    - Small, elongated, very dense
    - Large, less dense

DIFFERENTIAL DIAGNOSIS

Other Forms of FSGS or Minimal Change Disease
- No history of lithium use
- Lack ectatic collecting ducts, hobnail cells

Other Forms of Cystic or Tubulointerstitial Disease
- No history of lithium use
- Lack ectatic collecting ducts, hobnail cells

SELECTED REFERENCES

1. Bendz H et al: Renal failure occurs in chronic lithium treatment but is uncommon. Kidney Int. 77(3):219-24, 2010
2. Grünfeld JP et al: Lithium nephrotoxicity revisited. Nat Rev Nephrol. 5(5):270-6, 2009
3. Markowitz GS et al: Lithium nephrotoxicity: a progressive combined glomerular and tubulointerstitial nephropathy. J Am Soc Nephrol. 11(8):1439-48, 2000
4. Walker RG: Lithium nephrotoxicity. Kidney Int Suppl. 42:S93-8, 1993
5. Aurell M et al: Renal function and biopsy findings in patients on long-term lithium treatment. Kidney Int. 20(5):663-70, 1981

LITHIUM-INDUCED RENAL DISEASE

Microscopic Features

(Left) H&E shows cross section of the cortex from a 50 year old who developed renal failure after long-term lithium therapy for bipolar disorder. Many cortical cysts are present ⮕ as well as one elongated space that is probably an ectatic collecting duct ⮕. *(Right)* Complete cysts may not be present in needle core biopsies, but careful examination may reveal a significant length of tubular epithelial cells lining basement membranes such as these 2 partial cysts ⮕.

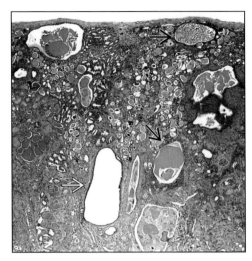
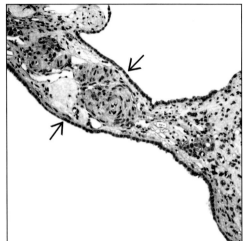

(Left) Periodic acid-Schiff shows typical, nonspecific pattern of lithium-associated chronic tubulointerstitial nephritis, with foci of mononuclear cells ⮕, atrophic tubules ⮕, and diffuse, fine, interstitial fibrosis. Glomeruli are normal in this field, except for periglomerular fibrosis ⮕. *(Right)* H&E shows focal segmental glomerulosclerosis in a patient on long-term lithium. Glomerular hypertrophy, hyaline ⮕, and adhesions ⮕ are also present.

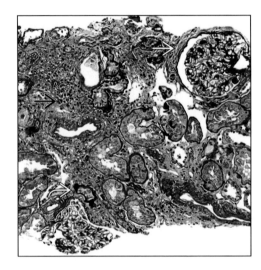
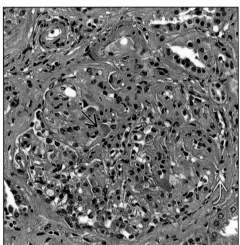

(Left) Diffuse mesangial hypercellularity and mesangial sclerosis are noted in this glomerulus that is hypertrophied. Podocytes ⮕ are prominent, correlating with proteinuria and FSGS. *(Right)* H&E shows a large tubular cyst filled with Tamm-Horsfall protein admixed with cellular debris and lined by collecting duct type epithelium. Microcysts 1-2 mm in diameter are common in late stages of lithium nephrotoxicity and appear to be derived from the distal nephron, especially the collecting ducts.

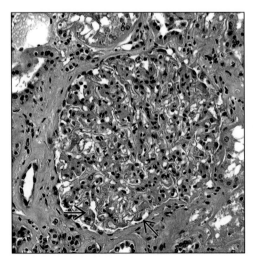
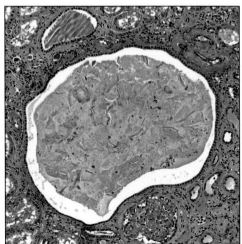

LITHIUM-INDUCED RENAL DISEASE

Light and Electron Microscopic Features

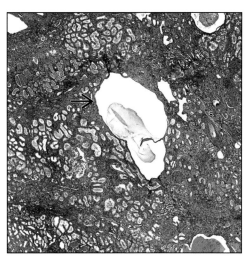
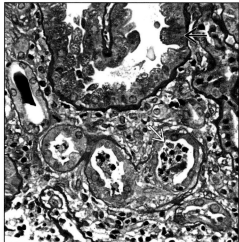

(Left) This ectatic collecting duct ➡ is a characteristic feature of chronic lithium nephrotoxicity. This patient required a renal transplant. *(Right)* Periodic acid-Schiff shows acute tubular injury in lithium toxicity. Tubular epithelial cells have a hobnailed appearance ➡ and PAS-positive reabsorption droplets. Other tubules have cell debris in their lumen ➡ and thinned cytoplasm. A mononuclear interstitial infiltrate is present.

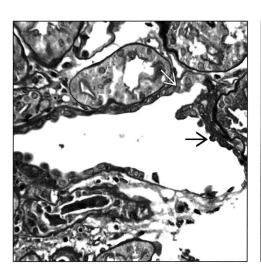
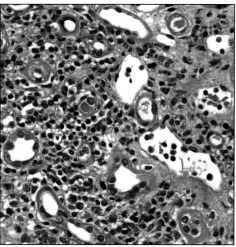

(Left) Cortical collecting duct in a patient with lithium toxicity shows rounded hobnailed cells ➡ typical of acute lithium toxicity in a rat. These hobnailed cells have a high proliferative index. The collecting duct is the only tubule in the cortex that branches ➡. *(Right)* Periodic acid-Schiff demonstrates prominent interstitial inflammation with a mixture of lymphocytes, eosinophils, and plasma cells among many atrophic tubules.

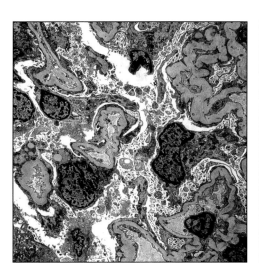
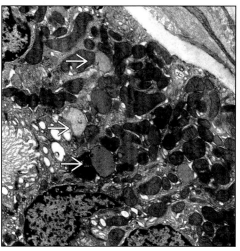

(Left) EM shows widespread effacement of foot processes and villous hypertrophy of podocytes are seen in this patient on lithium with nephrotic syndrome and focal segmental glomerulosclerosis. Minimal change disease is also associated with lithium therapy. *(Right)* Abnormal mitochondria have been described in chronic lithium nephrotoxicity in the form of abnormally large, less-dense mitochondria ➡. The reproducibility and relevance to the pathophysiology is unknown (EM).

CALCINEURIN INHIBITOR TOXICITY

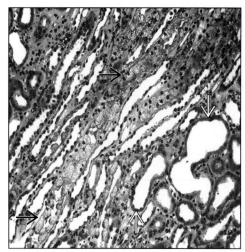

Isometric vacuolization of straight segments of the proximal tubules ➡ with acute tubular injury ➡ is shown in a kidney transplant with CI toxicity.

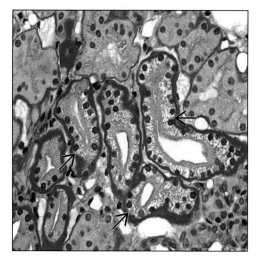

Focal tubular isometric vacuolization ➡ is evident in a renal transplant biopsy with tacrolimus toxicity. The affected tubules have thickened basement membranes, a nonspecific finding.

TERMINOLOGY

Abbreviations
- Calcineurin inhibitor (CI)
- Calcineurin inhibitor toxicity (CIT)

Synonyms
- Cyclosporine toxicity, cyclosporine A (CsA) toxicity, tacrolimus toxicity, FK506 toxicity

Definitions
- Acute or chronic kidney dysfunction attributable to direct injury from calcineurin inhibitor drugs

ETIOLOGY/PATHOGENESIS

Types of CI Toxicity
- Functional CIT: Reversible acute renal dysfunction associated with afferent arteriolar vasoconstriction
- Structural CIT: Characterized by cellular injury and matrix remodeling
  - Tubular CIT: Acute tubular injury with vacuolization of epithelium
  - Vascular CIT: Direct toxic injury to endothelium of arterioles and glomeruli, as well as to smooth muscle of arterioles
    - May manifest as thrombotic microangiopathy or chronic hyaline arteriolopathy
- Tubular and vascular toxicity typically coexist
- Native and transplanted kidneys are affected by CIT; histologic manifestations are similar

Mechanisms
- Histologic lesions are dose related
  - Acute CIT with markedly elevated blood levels of CI
  - Chronic CIT with long-term exposure to CI
- May also be dose-independent susceptibility factors
- CsA and tacrolimus bind intracellular receptors called immunophilins
  - Immunophilin/CI complexes bind and inhibit calcineurin
  - Calcineurin is T-cell activator via nuclear factors of activated T cells (NFAT)
  - NFAT activate transcription of inflammatory mediators like interleukin-2, interferon γ, and tumor necrosis factor α
- Immunosuppressive potency and renal toxicity of CI are pharmacologically inseparable
- Renal toxic effects of CsA and tacrolimus are identical
- CIT affects endothelium, vascular smooth muscle, and tubular epithelium
  - Endothelium: Increased thromboxane A2, endothelin-1, superoxide and peroxynitrite, decreased prostaglandin and prostacyclin, apoptosis, necrosis
  - Smooth muscle: Vacuolization, necrosis, apoptosis, hyalinization
  - Tubular epithelium: Vacuolization, megamitochondria, calcification, necrosis

CLINICAL ISSUES

Epidemiology
- Incidence
  - In kidney transplants
    - Thrombotic microangiopathy (TMA) in 2-5%; chronic CIT in 60-70% at 2 years and > 90% at 10 years

Presentation
- Acute or chronic elevation of serum creatinine; CIT may arise at any time after initiation of therapy
- Elevated trough blood levels of CI may confirm diagnosis, but correlation of structural tissue injury and blood level is not strong
- TMA may be localized to kidney (40%) or may be systemic

CALCINEURIN INHIBITOR TOXICITY

Key Facts

Terminology

- Kidney dysfunction attributable to injury from calcineurin inhibitor immunosuppressive therapy

Etiology/Pathogenesis

- Transplanted and native kidneys affected by CIT
- CIT is dose related
- Functional CIT: Reversible acute renal dysfunction associated with afferent arteriolar vasoconstriction
- Structural CIT: Tubular and vascular CIT

Clinical Issues

- Acute or chronic elevation of serum creatinine
- Elevated blood or serum levels of CI
- Correlation of structural tissue injury and blood levels is not strong

Microscopic Pathology

- Tubular toxicity: Acute tubular injury with focal isometric vacuolization of proximal tubular segments
- Acute arteriolopathy: Smooth muscle loss and expansion of intima and media by loose matrix
- Thrombotic microangiopathy (TMA)
- Chronic arteriolopathy: Nodular medial hyalinization

Diagnostic Checklist

- Exposure to CI is a sine qua non for diagnosis
- Absence of pathologic lesions in kidney biopsy does not exclude CIT
- Observation of combined tubulopathy and vasculopathy increases diagnostic certainty

Treatment

- Dose reduction or cessation of CI therapy

Prognosis

- Acute CIT is typically reversible and associated with resolution of histologic changes
- Chronic CIT is less likely to be reversible; however, resolution of arteriolopathy has been observed with cessation of CI

MICROSCOPIC PATHOLOGY

Histologic Features

- Functional CIT
  - No morphologic tissue injury by definition
- Tubular CIT
  - Acute
    - Focal proximal tubular epithelial isometric vacuolization affecting straight more than convoluted segments
    - Vacuolar changes may be accompanied by acute tubular injury
    - Proximal tubules may have large eosinophilic cytoplasmic granules corresponding to megamitochondria (CsA toxicity) or lysosomes (tacrolimus toxicity)
    - Tubular calcium phosphate deposition
  - Chronic
    - Cortical tubular atrophy and interstitial fibrosis in striped pattern
    - Striped fibrosis is characterized by radial fibrosis affecting cortex with intervening nonscarred parenchyma
    - Striped fibrosis may arise as result of chronic ischemia from arteriolopathy in addition to direct tubular toxicity
  - Tubular CIT is typically accompanied by vascular CIT, which may be very focal
- Vascular CIT
  - Vasculopathies of CIT tend to be focal and mainly affect arterioles
  - Acute CIT has spectrum of severity from acute arteriolopathy to TMA
  - Chronic CIT is characterized by hyalinization of arterioles
  - Acute and chronic vasculopathy may be evident in same biopsy
  - Acute arteriolopathy
    - Loss of definition of smooth muscle cells
    - Myocyte cytoplasmic vacuolization and dropout from necrosis or apoptosis
    - Medial swelling and thickening with separation of myocytes
    - Clear or basophilic medial or intimal loose matrix accumulation
    - Intimal or medial platelet insudates may be identifiable by immunohistochemistry for CD61
  - Thrombotic microangiopathy (TMA)
    - Arteriolar thrombi
    - Arteriolar intimal and medial fibrinoid exudate with erythrocytolysis
    - Obliterative arteriolopathy has stenosis, intimal and medial interstitial swelling, and hypercellularity ("onion skinning")
    - Arteries may have intimal myxoid thickening in TMA
  - Chronic arteriolopathy
    - Early lesions have hyaline replacement of individual medial smooth muscle cells
    - Nodular hyalinization is seen in outer media; imparting an eosinophilic, PAS-positive "beaded necklace" appearance
    - Over months to years, entire vessel wall is hyalinized
    - Arteriolopathy mainly affects afferent arterioles but can involve vasa recta and small arteries
    - Striped interstitial fibrosis, tubular atrophy, calcification, and glomerular sclerosis may be present
- Glomerulopathy and CIT
  - TMA
    - Capillary thrombi; glomerular hilar thrombi (so-called "pouch lesions")

CALCINEURIN INHIBITOR TOXICITY

- Capillary double contours; mesangiolysis
  - o Chronic lesions
    - Ischemic capillary collapse with pericapsular fibrosis (ischemic glomerulopathy)
    - Focal segmental and global glomerular sclerosis
- Immunohistology
  - o Acute arteriolopathy and TMA
    - Direct immunofluorescence (DIF) may reveal arteriolar mural IgM, C3, and fibrinogen
    - Glomeruli may have IgM, C3, and fibrinogen deposits in TMA
    - Immunoperoxidase staining for CD61 or CD62 reveals luminal and mural platelet deposits in arterioles and in glomeruli
  - o Chronic arteriolopathy
    - DIF may reveal IgM, C3, and C1q in hyaline deposits
    - Platelets are rare in hyaline arteriolopathy
- Electron microscopy
  - o Tubular CIT
    - Isometric vacuoles appear as dilated endoplasmic reticulum; multiple large lysosomes, megamitochondria, endocytotic vesicles may also be seen
  - o Vascular CIT
    - Endothelial swelling, cytoplasmic vacuolization, detachment from basal lamina and apoptosis or necrosis
    - Myocyte vacuoles, disruption of myofibrils, detachment from basal lamina, apoptosis
    - Electron-dense hyaline material accumulates within basal lamina of medial smooth muscle
    - Glomerular endothelial swelling, subendothelial widening with double contours, mesangial lysis
    - Glomerular capillary basement membrane wrinkling, focal segmental and global sclerosis

DIFFERENTIAL DIAGNOSIS

Tubulopathy

- Osmotic tubulopathy associated with exposure to parenteral carbohydrates, intravenous immunoglobulin, or radiocontrast agents
  - o Vacuolar changes tend to be diffuse rather than focal
  - o Epithelium is swollen with preserved proximal tubular brush border
  - o Vacuoles are endosomes and phagolysosomes
- Ischemic acute tubular injury
  - o Vacuoles tend to be coarse and irregular, with focal epithelial necrosis and apoptosis
- Tubulopathy associated with lipiduria in nephrotic syndrome
  - o Vacuoles are isometric, focal, and contain lipid
  - o Associated with interstitial foam cells
  - o Periodic acid-Schiff positive protein droplets in tubules; stain for Ig and albumin by DIF
  - o Causal glomerulopathy is typically identified

Vasculopathy

- Lesions outlined below affect native and transplant kidneys, with exception of humoral rejection

- TMA
  - o Humoral rejection
    - Transplant glomerulopathy
    - Peritubular capillaritis and capillary basement membrane multilayering
    - Peritubular capillary mural C4d deposits
    - Donor-specific antibodies detected serologically
  - o Malignant hypertension
    - Clinical history of severe hypertension
  - o Hemolytic uremic syndrome/thrombotic thrombocytopenic purpura
    - Clinical history
    - Lesions in kidney tend to be diffuse in contrast to focal distribution in CI toxicity
  - o Antiphospholipid nephropathy
    - Detectable antiphospholipid antibodies or anticardiolipin antibodies
- Acute arteriolopathy
  - o Indistinguishable changes seen in severe hypertensive arteriolosclerosis
- Hyaline arteriolosclerosis of diabetic nephropathy and hypertension
  - o Initial lesions classically intimal rather than medial
  - o Peripheral nodular medial hyalinization may be seen rarely in other conditions such as severe hypertension
  - o Transmural hyalinization in advanced disease, making determination of etiology difficult
  - o Hyaline deposits in afferent and efferent vessels in diabetic arteriolopathy
- Amyloid vasculopathy deposits are not typically nodular and are Congo red positive

DIAGNOSTIC CHECKLIST

Clinically Relevant Pathologic Features

- Absence of pathologic lesions in kidney biopsy does not exclude CIT
- Exposure to CI inhibitors is a sine qua non for diagnosis of CIT
- Observation of combined tubulopathy and vasculopathy increases diagnostic certainty

Pathologic Interpretation Pearls

- Acute CIT: Tubulopathy with isometric vacuolization, acute tubular injury, acute arteriolopathy, and TMA
- Chronic CIT: Nodular arteriolar hyalinization, striped fibrosis, calcifications, global and segmental glomerular sclerosis

SELECTED REFERENCES

1. Nankivell BJ et al: Calcineurin inhibitor nephrotoxicity: longitudinal assessment by protocol histology. Transplantation. 78(4):557-65, 2004
2. Mihatsch MJ et al: The side-effects of ciclosporine-A and tacrolimus. Clin Nephrol. 49(6):356-63, 1998

Microscopic Features

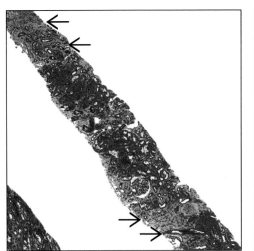

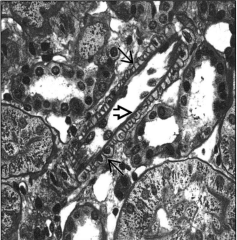

(Left) Kidney transplant biopsy core demonstrates band-like fibrosis ⇒ with atrophic tubules in a striped pattern. Relatively nonscarred cortex is seen between the fibrotic bands. *(Right)* The profile of a normal-appearing arteriole is seen, with PAS highlighting the basal laminae of the medial smooth muscle cells ⇒. The endothelial basal lamina is also evident ⇒.

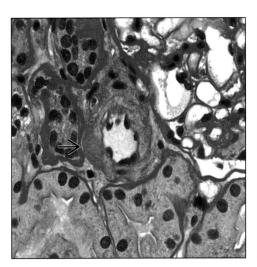

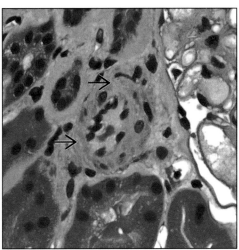

(Left) One of the earliest detectable features of CI-associated vascular toxicity is loss of myocyte definition and medial thickening, as seen in this PAS-stained section. There is also focal hyaline in the outer media ⇒. *(Right)* Medial thickening, loss of definition of medial smooth muscle, and accumulation of medial myxoid blue matrix ⇒ are early features of acute arteriolopathy of CIT.

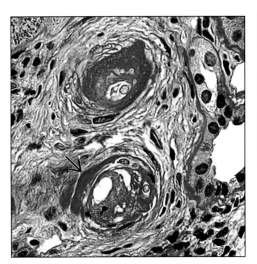

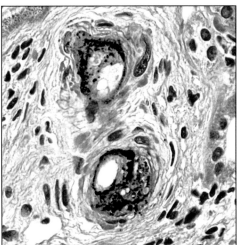

(Left) Arterioles have luminal narrowing and intimal PAS-positive "fibrinoid" matrix material in a biopsy obtained from a kidney transplant with CIT-associated TMA. Medial hyaline deposition is also apparent ⇒. *(Right)* A kidney transplant biopsy demonstrating arteriolar intimal matrix material contains platelet deposits with CD61 expression in TMA from CIT.

Microscopic Features

(Left) A kidney transplant biopsy with severe obliterative arteriolopathy from CIT is shown. These arteriolar profiles have luminal obliteration, loss of smooth muscle, and matrix accumulation ➔, and were observed in the context of greatly elevated blood levels of tacrolimus. *(Right)* Obliterative arteriolopathy attributable to CIT may have unrecognized mural deposits of platelets. Immunohistochemical staining for CD61 reveals granular platelets and platelet microparticles in the intima and media.

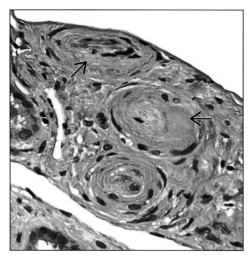
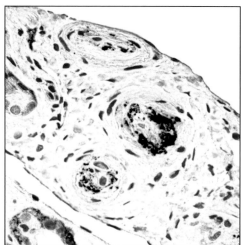

(Left) H&E shows occlusive luminal fibrin-platelet thrombus in an arteriole with extensive loss of smooth muscle nuclei ➔, obtained from a kidney transplant with acute CIT associated TMA. The adjacent glomerulus has marked congestion without apparent thrombi. *(Right)* TMA in CI toxicity demonstrates mural fibrin deposition ➔ with medial erythrocytolysis ➔ and luminal stenosis. The lower arteriolar profile has prominent endothelium with preserved medial smooth muscle.

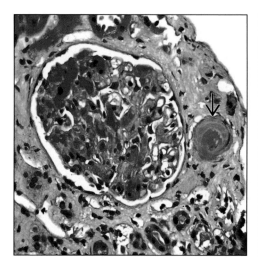
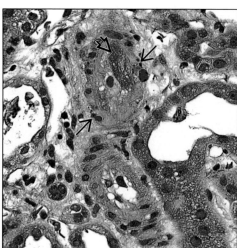

(Left) H&E shows segmental glomerular capillary fibrin-platelet thrombi in a glomerulus from a kidney transplant with CI toxicity and TMA. Pericapsulitis is nonspecific. *(Right)* Nonthrombotic lesions of TMA in CIT have segmental or global double contours of the glomerular capillary basement membrane ➔. These lesions represent repair of endothelial injury from CIT and must be distinguished from transplant glomerulopathy. Thrombi may be absent from glomeruli with these lesions.

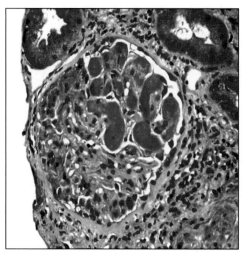
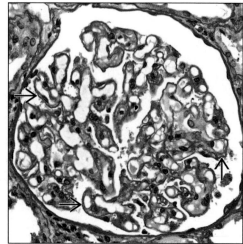

CALCINEURIN INHIBITOR TOXICITY

Microscopic Features

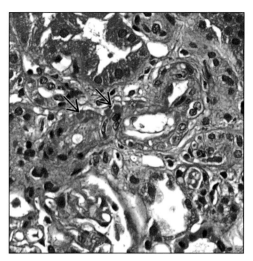

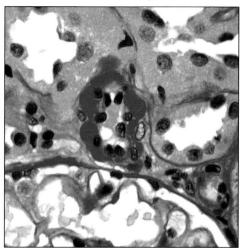

(Left) Eosinophilic nodular hyaline material ➡ is evident in the outer media in arteriolopathy due to CIT. The hyaline material often replaces dead or dying myocytes. The intima appears thickened. (Right) Periodic acid-Schiff shows PAS-positive medial nodular hyalinization identified in the media of an arteriole from a renal allograft with CI toxicity. Hyaline material surrounds and displaces myocyte nuclei and imparts a characteristic "beaded necklace" appearance.

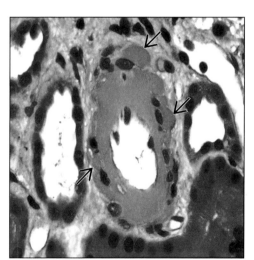

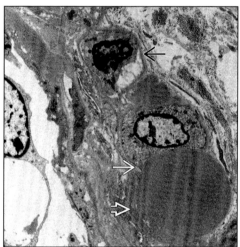

(Left) Transmural hyalinization is shown in chronic arteriolopathy of CIT in a renal allograft. Hyaline material fills the intima and media. Hyalinization retains a nodular pattern in outer media ➡. (Right) EM shows nodular hyaline arteriolosclerosis in a kidney transplant with CIT. Upper myocyte shows shrinkage & detachment from basal lamina ➡. Rounded amorphous hyaline material ⏩ fills the basal lamina, replacing the myocyte and compressing adjacent cell ➡.

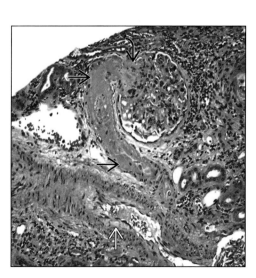

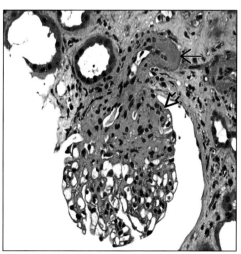

(Left) An afferent arteriole has luminal occlusion from extensive accumulation of hyaline material ➡. The glomerular hilus is sclerotic ➡. The interlobular artery has segmental myxoid thickening of the intima ➡. The patient had renal transplant dysfunction, hypertension, and elevated blood levels of tacrolimus. (Right) H&E shows perihilar segmental glomerular sclerosis ⏩ associated with arteriolar hyalinization ➡ in a renal allograft with exposure to CI for 7 years.

mTOR INHIBITOR TOXICITY

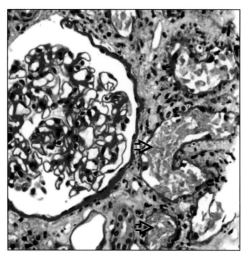

PAS shows acute rapamycin toxicity with PAS-negative casts ⊡ and severe acute tubular injury. The material consists of cytoplasmic debris from damaged tubular epithelial cells.

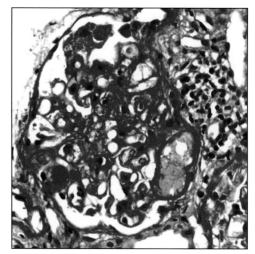

Patients develop proteinuria as part of chronic mTOR inhibitor toxicity; biopsies of these patients sometimes show focal segmental glomerulosclerosis.

TERMINOLOGY

Abbreviations
- Mammalian target of rapamycin (mTOR)

Definitions
- mTOR inhibitors used in renal transplantation
  - Rapamycin (sirolimus)
  - Everolimus
    - Structurally similar to sirolimus; shorter half-life

ETIOLOGY/PATHOGENESIS

mTOR Inhibitor (Rapamycin/Sirolimus): Drug Effects
- Sirolimus binds FK binding protein 12 to form a complex, sirolimus effector protein (SEP)
- SEP complex inhibits the mTOR pathway
  - Sirolimus blocks cytokine-mediated signal transduction pathways, affecting T-cell cycle progression
  - Decreases lymphocyte proliferation
- mTOR expressed in kidney, including in tubular epithelial cells
  - Repair response to acute tubular injury requires tubular epithelial cell turnover and proliferation
  - Sirolimus inhibits tubular epithelial cell proliferation and apoptosis in setting of acute injury
- Sirolimus decreases VEGF synthesis
  - Thought to be mechanism of thrombotic microangiopathy

mTOR Inhibitor Effect on Podocyte
- Focal segmental glomerulosclerosis (FSGS) lesions in mTOR inhibitor toxicity show abnormal podocyte phenotype, suggestive of podocyte dedifferentiation
  - PAX2 and cytokeratin expression in proliferating podocytes
  - Loss of synaptopodin and VEGF expression
  - Downregulated nephrin expression in podocytes, both in vitro and in vivo
  - Staining pattern does not distinguish between sirolimus-related FSGS and other types of FSGS
  - Abnormal podocyte phenotype provides evidence for glomerular, rather than tubular, origin of proteinuria
- In vitro podocyte culture model showed decreased VEGF synthesis and Akt phosphorylation by podocytes in presence of sirolimus and decreased synthesis of WT1, a protein required for podocyte integrity

CLINICAL ISSUES

Presentation
- Delayed graft function (DGF)
  - More common in patients treated with mTOR inhibitor (25%) than without (9%); DGF correlates with mTOR inhibitor dose
- Acute renal failure
  - Acute mTOR inhibitor toxicity
- Proteinuria
  - Chronic mTOR inhibitor toxicity

Treatment
- Drugs
  - Discontinuation or reduced dose of mTOR inhibitor
  - Initiation of alternative immunosuppressive therapy

MICROSCOPIC PATHOLOGY

Histologic Features
- Acute mTOR inhibitor toxicity
  - Severe acute tubular injury
    - Dilatation of tubules, epithelial flattening, loss of tubular brush border
    - Epithelial cell necrosis
    - Atypical, eosinophilic PAS-negative casts reminiscent of myeloma cast nephropathy

mTOR INHIBITOR TOXICITY

Key Facts

Etiology/Pathogenesis

- mTOR drugs
  - Inhibit tubular epithelial cell proliferation and apoptosis in setting of acute injury
  - Decreases VEGF synthesis, related to development of FSGS

Clinical Issues

- Acute renal failure, delayed graft function (acute toxicity)
- Proteinuria (chronic toxicity)

Microscopic Pathology

- Acute mTOR inhibitor toxicity
  - Severe acute tubular injury
  - Epithelial cell necrosis
  - Atypical, eosinophilic PAS-negative casts reminiscent of myeloma cast nephropathy
  - Thrombotic microangiopathy (TMA)
- Chronic mTOR inhibitor toxicity
  - Focal segmental glomerulosclerosis
  - Abnormal podocyte phenotype, suggestive of podocyte dedifferentiation

Top Differential Diagnoses

- Acute mTOR inhibitor toxicity
  - Severe acute tubular necrosis
  - Acute humoral rejection
  - Light chain (myeloma) cast nephropathy
- Chronic mTOR inhibitor toxicity
  - Focal segmental glomerulosclerosis due to other factors

- Irregular, sharply demarcated cast edges
- Casts may appear "fractured"
- Casts may have surrounding cellular reaction
- Atypical casts stain for cytokeratin by immunohistochemistry
- Myoglobin-appearing casts; stain for myoglobin by immunohistochemistry
- Resolution of histologic features upon removal of sirolimus
  - Thrombotic microangiopathy (TMA)
    - Associated with decreased VEGF expression in glomeruli
    - Some cases may be associated with laboratory evidence of acute TMA: Thrombocytopenia, anemia, low haptoglobin levels
    - Increased risk of TMA in patients on both sirolimus and cyclosporine
- Chronic mTOR inhibitor toxicity
  - Focal segmental glomerulosclerosis
    - May have pattern of collapsing FSGS
    - Some patients on mTOR inhibitor have proteinuria without histologic lesion of FSGS

DIFFERENTIAL DIAGNOSIS

Severe Acute Tubular Necrosis

- Due to causes other than an mTOR inhibitor

Rhabdomyolysis

- Myoglobin casts present in both rhabdomyolysis and mTOR inhibitor toxicity

Acute Humoral Rejection

- C4d-positive peritubular capillaries
- May show acute tubular necrosis &/or TMA

Light Chain (Myeloma) Cast Nephropathy

- Monotypic light chain staining by immunofluorescence
- Serum or urine paraprotein usually detectable
- Unusual in renal allograft

Focal Segmental Glomerulosclerosis

- Recurrent or de novo in allograft
- FSGS pattern may be result of chronic calcineurin inhibitor (CNI) toxicity
  - Arteriolar hyalinosis also present in chronic CNI toxicity

SELECTED REFERENCES

1. Biancone L et al: Loss of nephrin expression in glomeruli of kidney-transplanted patients under m-TOR inhibitor therapy. Am J Transplant. 10(10):2270-8, 2010
2. Letavernier E et al: Sirolimus interacts with pathways essential for podocyte integrity. Nephrol Dial Transplant. 24(2):630-8, 2009
3. Vollenbröker B et al: mTOR regulates expression of slit diaphragm proteins and cytoskeleton structure in podocytes. Am J Physiol Renal Physiol. 296(2):F418-26, 2009
4. Letavernier E et al: High sirolimus levels may induce focal segmental glomerulosclerosis de novo. Clin J Am Soc Nephrol. 2(2):326-33, 2007
5. Pelletier R et al: Acute renal failure following kidney transplantation associated with myoglobinuria in patients treated with rapamycin. Transplantation. 82(5):645-50, 2006
6. Straathof-Galema L et al: Sirolimus-associated heavy proteinuria in a renal transplant recipient: evidence for a tubular mechanism. Am J Transplant. 6(2):429-33, 2006
7. Izzedine H et al: Post-transplantation proteinuria and sirolimus. N Engl J Med. 353(19):2088-9, 2005
8. Sartelet H et al: Sirolimus-induced thrombotic microangiopathy is associated with decreased expression of vascular endothelial growth factor in kidneys. Am J Transplant. 5(10):2441-7, 2005
9. Smith KD et al: Delayed graft function and cast nephropathy associated with tacrolimus plus rapamycin use. J Am Soc Nephrol. 14(4):1037-45, 2003

mTOR INHIBITOR TOXICITY

Microscopic Features

(Left) Acute mTOR inhibitor toxicity here shows a thrombus ⊅ within a glomerulus in a renal transplant patient on sirolimus and tacrolimus. Either sirolimus or tacrolimus by itself may cause TMA; there is greater risk of TMA in combined sirolimus and tacrolimus therapy than in sirolimus without a calcineurin inhibitor. *(Right)* A CD61 stain for platelets highlights a thrombus near the glomerular vascular pole in a patient on mTOR inhibitors.

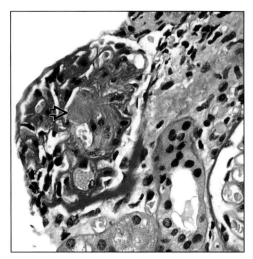
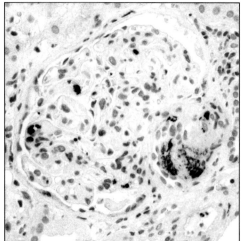

(Left) PAS-negative cast material within a tubular lumen is seen in a patient on mTOR inhibitors. Casts become more compact with time and bear more resemblance to those in light chain cast nephropathy. *(Right)* Immunohistochemical stain for keratin reveals positive staining of the intratubular material ➡, indicative of cellular debris. This contrasts with the casts of myeloma cast nephropathy, which contain immunoglobulin light/heavy chains.

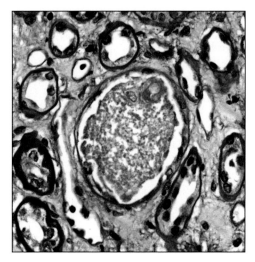
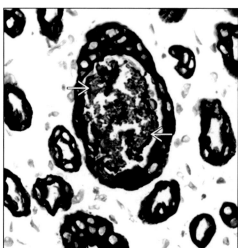

(Left) PAS-negative casts ➡ are seen in acute mTOR inhibitor toxicity. Tamm-Horsfall proteins, produced by the distal tubule, comprise the usual proteinaceous casts and are strongly PAS positive. *(Right)* Casts stain for myoglobin by immunohistochemistry in mTOR inhibitor toxicity, similar to those in rhabdomyolysis. This is presumptive evidence of muscle injury.

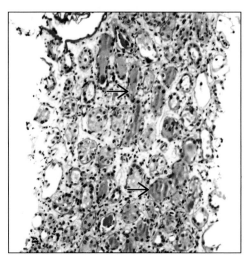
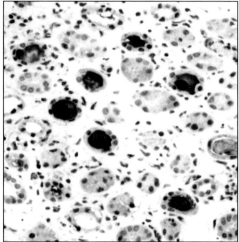

mTOR INHIBITOR TOXICITY

Microscopic Features

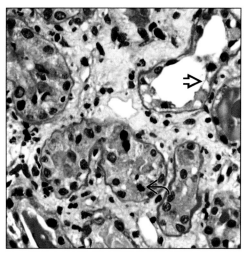
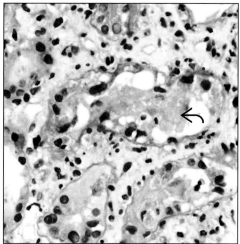

(Left) Acute tubular injury is seen in acute mTOR inhibitor toxicity, with tubular epithelial cell flattening, vacuolization, and loss of the brush border ⮞, and a tubular epithelial cell mitotic figure ➚. *(Right)* Acute tubular injury is seen with reactive tubular epithelial cells and early formation of an atypical-appearing cast ➙. This case also showed tubulitis and interstitial inflammation and qualified for an additional diagnosis of acute cellular rejection type I.

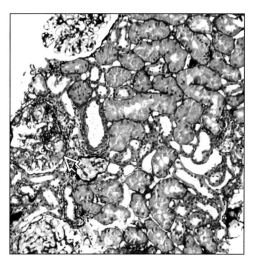
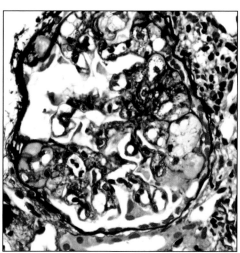

(Left) De novo FSGS ⮞ is due to chronic mTOR inhibitor toxicity in a 58-year-old man with 425 mg/d proteinuria 2.5 years post transplant. The patient was on rapamycin, prednisone, and mycophenolate mofetil, and had never been on a calcineurin inhibitor. The tubules, interstitium, and vessels appear normal. *(Right)* Focal segmental glomerulosclerosis due to chronic mTOR inhibitor toxicity is seen 2.5 years post transplant. There was no evidence of thrombotic microangiopathy.

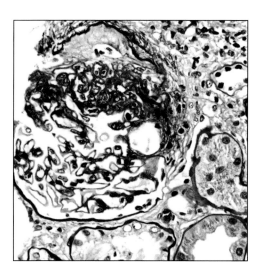
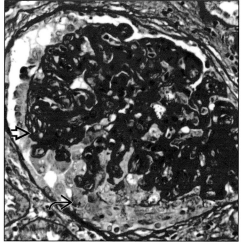

(Left) Focal segmental glomerulosclerosis is seen in a renal allograft patient on rapamycin with proteinuria. There was no evidence of calcineurin inhibitor toxicity. *(Right)* Focal segmental glomerulosclerosis, collapsing type, is seen in a patient with nephrotic syndrome 8 years post renal transplant. Note the proliferating podocytes ➚ overlying the collapse of the glomerular capillary loops ⮞. This patient had been on sirolimus and had never been on a calcineurin inhibitor.

LEAD AND OTHER HEAVY METAL TOXINS

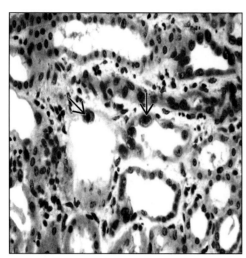

Acute tubular injury with prominent eosinophilic nuclear inclusions ⬅ is evident in this example of acute lead nephropathy. There is mild interstitial edema and inflammatory exudates.

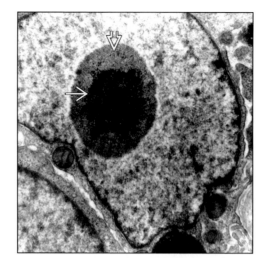

Acute lead nephropathy has nuclear inclusions composed of central, electron-dense spicules ➡ and a halo of less electron-dense material ⬅ by electron microscopy. (Courtesy A. Cohen, MD.)

TERMINOLOGY

Definitions
- Group of disorders characterized by renal dysfunction due to toxic effects of lead and other metals

ETIOLOGY/PATHOGENESIS

Toxic Renal Injury
- Principal toxic metals encountered include lead (Pb), mercury (Hg), gold (Au), cadmium (Cd), copper (Cu), chromium (Cr), bismuth (Bi), antimony (Sb), arsenic (As), uranium (U), platinum (Pt), iron (Fe), and lithium (Li)
- Exposure to toxic metals may be environmental, occupational, iatrogenic, or secondary to metabolic and hematologic disease states
- Routes of entry include ingestion, inhalation, and absorption through skin
  - Environmental exposure
    - Ingestion: Contamination of water supplies in lead pipes or lead soldered joints, moonshine stills, lead paint, contaminated foods
    - Inhalation: Lead, mercury, and cadmium vapors, fumes, or dust
    - Application of mercury-containing skin lightening products
    - Mercuric chloride and colloidal bismuth ingestion in suicide
  - Occupational exposure
    - Paint manufacture and spraying, plumbing, welding, smelting, mining, pesticides, thermometer manufacturing, and others
  - Iatrogenic exposure
    - Gold therapy in rheumatoid arthritis
    - Colloidal bismuth in treatment of peptic ulcer and syphilis
    - Copper intrauterine contraceptive devices
    - Lithium in bipolar disorders

- Platinum in cancer chemotherapy
- Iron for deficiency states
  - Metabolic and hematologic diseases
    - Hemochromatosis
    - Wilson disease
    - Hemolysis
- Metals may be absorbed through gastrointestinal tract, lungs, or skin, entering bloodstream
- Circulating metals are filtered by glomeruli, often secreted by tubules and excreted in urine
- Renal injury is by 2 principal mechanisms
  - Direct tubular toxicity causes tubular injury
    - High-dose exposure leads to acute nephropathy
    - Low-dose prolonged exposure leads to chronic nephropathy
  - Glomerular immune complex deposition results in membranous glomerulopathy
    - Associated with gold and mercury toxicity
    - Neither metal is detected in immune deposits

CLINICAL ISSUES

Presentation
- Acute nephropathy
  - Toxic metal exposures to Pb, Hg, Au, Cd, Cu, Cr, Bi, Sb, U, Pt, Fe can be associated with acute kidney injury
  - Proximal tubulopathy is often an early manifestation
    - Characterized by aminoaciduria, glycosuria, phosphaturia (Fanconi syndrome) and increased urinary β2-microglobulin excretion
  - Blood and urinary levels of toxic metals are elevated
- Chronic nephropathy
  - Lead
    - Gouty arthropathy and hyperuricemia in 50%, chronic renal failure, hypertension, positive calcium-EDTA mobilization test
  - Mercury and gold

LEAD AND OTHER HEAVY METAL TOXINS

Key Facts

Terminology
- Renal disease due to toxic effects of lead and other metals

Etiology/Pathogenesis
- Principal toxic metals encountered include lead (Pb), mercury (Hg), gold (Au), and cadmium (Cd)
- Direct tubular toxicity may be acute (high-dose toxicity) or chronic (low-dose prolonged toxicity)
- Membranous glomerulopathy in Hg and Au toxicity due to immune complex deposition

Clinical Issues
- History of recent or past exposure to toxic metals is critical for diagnosis
- Blood and urinary levels of toxic metals are elevated in acute nephropathy

Microscopic Pathology
- Acute nephropathy: Acute tubular injury
  - Eosinophilic nuclear inclusions (lead, bismuth) or pigment (iron, copper)
  - Hg and Au particles in proximal tubules by EM
- Nonspecific chronic tubulointerstitial nephritis
- Membranous glomerulonephritis in Hg and Au toxicity
- Radiographic fluorescence or spectroscopy may be used to quantify metal content in tissues

Top Differential Diagnoses
- Acute tubular injury/necrosis from drugs and infection
- Chronic tubulointerstitial diseases (lithium, Balkan nephropathy, aristolochic acid)

- Proteinuria and chronic renal dysfunction
  - Cadmium
    - Chronic renal failure
    - Hypercalciuria and nephrolithiasis
    - Osteomalacia
  - Lithium
    - Chronic renal failure and proteinuria
- History of recent or past exposure to toxic metals is critical for diagnosis

Treatment
- Cessation of toxic exposure
- Chelation therapy
- Dialysis

Prognosis
- Acute tubular necrosis is generally reversible with appropriate therapy
- Reversibility of chronic nephropathy depends on extent of renal scarring
- Membranous nephropathy may persist for months or years after cessation of toxic exposure; however, recovery of function occurs in most patients

MACROSCOPIC FEATURES

Gross Findings
- Acute nephropathy: Diffuse enlargement with cortical swelling in acute kidney injury
- Chronic nephropathy: Bilateral shrunken kidneys with granular outer surface
- Cadmium toxicity: Calcium phosphate stones

MICROSCOPIC PATHOLOGY

Histologic Features
- Lead
  - Acute nephropathy
  - Glomeruli normal
  - Tubules

- Acute tubular injury with characteristic eosinophilic nuclear inclusions in proximal tubules and loops of Henle
- Inclusions are of variable size and shape and composed of lead-protein complexes and are periodic acid-Schiff, acid fast, and Giemsa positive
- Inclusions may persist for years after cessation of exposure to lead
  - Chronic nephropathy
    - Glomeruli normal
    - Tubules: No inclusions, only patchy interstitial fibrosis and tubular atrophy with mild mononuclear infiltrates (chronic tubulointerstitial nephritis)
    - Gouty tophi in renal medulla
    - Hypertensive vascular sclerosis
- Mercury
  - Acute nephropathy
    - Glomeruli normal
    - Acute tubular necrosis with primary and most severe involvement of straight proximal tubule
    - Hg particles are detectable by electron microscopy in cytoplasm of injured tubules
  - Chronic nephropathy
    - Glomeruli have membranous glomerulopathy, typically Ehrenreich and Churg stage I-II, with subepithelial immune complex deposits
    - Tubules have epithelial flattening and interstitium has fibrosis and tubular atrophy
- Gold
  - Acute nephropathy
    - Glomeruli may have membranous glomerulopathy
    - Acute tubular necrosis with gold inclusions in proximal tubules
  - Chronic nephropathy
    - Membranous glomerulopathy
    - Minimal change disease
    - Mesangial proliferative glomerulonephritis
    - Chronic tubulointerstitial nephritis
- Cadmium
  - Glomeruli: Normal

- Chronic tubulointerstitial nephritis
- Bland outer cortical interstitial fibrosis and tubular atrophy
- Calcium phosphate stones
- Arsenic
  - Glomeruli: Normal
  - Acute tubular necrosis with hemoglobin casts secondary to hemolysis
  - Cortical necrosis
  - Chronic tubulointerstitial nephritis
- Iron
  - Glomeruli: Normal
  - Acute tubular injury with iron detectable in tubular epithelium by Prussian blue stain
- Copper
  - Glomeruli: Normal
  - Acute tubular injury with copper detectable in tubular epithelium using Rubeanic acid stain

ANCILLARY TESTS

Immunofluorescence
- Glomerular capillary wall IgG and C3 in membranous nephropathy associated with mercury and gold

Electron Microscopy
- Lead
  - Tubular nuclei have discrete inclusions composed of electron-dense spicules in less electron-dense matrix
  - Tubular cytoplasm may contain abundant lysosomes with electron-dense material containing lead
- Mercury
  - Tubules have cytoplasmic clusters of electron-dense, amorphous, particulate matter containing mercury
  - Subepithelial electron-dense deposits ± spikes (usually Ehrenreich-Churg stage I-II)
- Gold
  - Tubules have clustered spicular material in cytoplasm associated with lysosomes
  - Subepithelial electron-dense deposits ± spikes
- Cadmium
  - Increased proximal tubular cytoplasmic lysosomes with electron-dense material containing cadmium
- Bismuth
  - Tubular nuclear inclusions are rounded and uniformly electron dense
  - Tubular mitochondria have small, rounded, smooth electron densities containing bismuth

Imaging
- Radiographic fluorescence or spectroscopy may be useful to quantify metal content in tissues

DIFFERENTIAL DIAGNOSIS

Acute Tubular Necrosis with Inclusions
- Lead and bismuth nuclear inclusions are characteristically rounded and eosinophilic ± halos
- Nuclear inclusions need to be distinguished from Cytomegalovirus tubulopathy, a rare cause of acute tubular injury

- Mercury containing electron-dense bodies are in tubular cytoplasm but absent from the nucleus

Acute Tubular Necrosis with Nuclear Atypia
- Tubular nuclear atypia may be associated with platinum toxicity
- Nuclear atypia also seen in karyomegalic interstitial nephritis, an idiopathic systemic disorder
- Drug toxicity due to busulphan, foscarnet, tenofovir, and other agents can have atypical reactive nuclear changes
- Viral infections, especially Cytomegalovirus, polyomavirus, and adenovirus

Acute Tubular Necrosis with Pigmentation
- Iron toxicity with hemosiderosis
  - Prussian blue positive cytoplasmic granules
- Copper toxicity
  - Rubeanic acid positive cytoplasmic granules
- Acute tubular necrosis with lipofuscinosis

Chronic Tubulointerstitial Nephropathy
- Histologic features of chronic tubulointerstitial nephropathies are generally nonspecific
  - Important considerations include lithium, aristolochic acid, and Balkan nephropathy
- Membranous glomerulopathy and chronic TIN may suggest gold or mercury toxicity
  - This combination of glomerular and tubulointerstitial lesions may be seen in nephropathy associated with nonsteroidal anti-inflammatory agents or lupus

DIAGNOSTIC CHECKLIST

Clinically Relevant Pathologic Features
- Acute tubular necrosis with nuclear inclusions suggests lead or bismuth toxicity and with cytoplasmic pigment suggests copper or iron toxicity

Pathologic Interpretation Pearls
- Acute tubular injury with nuclear inclusions in acute lead and bismuth nephropathy
- Gold and mercury particles are detectable in tubular cytoplasm by EM in acute nephropathy from these agents
- Membranous nephropathy ± chronic tubulointerstitial nephritis suggests gold or mercury toxicity

SELECTED REFERENCES

1. Li SJ et al: Mercury-induced membranous nephropathy: clinical and pathological features. Clin J Am Soc Nephrol. 5(3):439-44, 2010
2. Brewster UC et al: A review of chronic lead intoxication: an unrecognized cause of chronic kidney disease. Am J Med Sci. 327(6):341-7, 2004
3. Goyer RA: Mechanisms of lead and cadmium nephrotoxicity. Toxicol Lett. 46(1-3):153-62, 1989
4. Bennett WM: Lead nephropathy. Kidney Int. 28(2):212-20, 1985

LEAD AND OTHER HEAVY METAL TOXINS

Microscopic Features

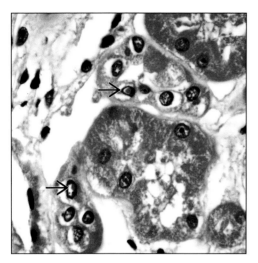 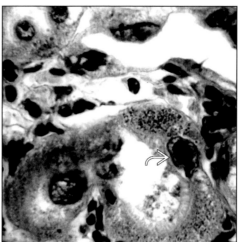

(Left) Lead nephropathy has characteristic bright eosinophilic nuclear inclusions ➡ in the proximal tubular nuclei. (Courtesy A. Cohen, MD.) (Right) H&E shows proximal tubule nuclear inclusion ➡ in a case of chronic lead toxicity. The inclusion is typically slightly eosinophilic and nearly fills the nucleus, somewhat resembling Cytomegalovirus. These inclusions are infrequent in chronic lead nephropathy (black and white photo). (Courtesy M. Mihatsch, MD.)

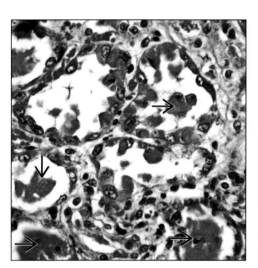 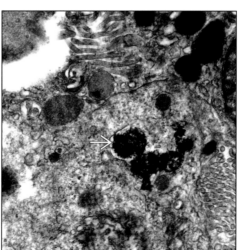

(Left) Mercury ingestion leads to acute tubular necrosis affecting proximal straight segments most severely. All segments may be affected, however. Tubules have flat epithelium & luminal cell debris ➡. Mild interstitial inflammation is also apparent. (Courtesy A. Cohen, MD.) (Right) Cytoplasmic spicular gold particles ➡ may be seen in acute gold nephrotoxicity. Glomeruli in such cases may have membranous glomerulopathy (EM). (Courtesy A. Cohen, MD.)

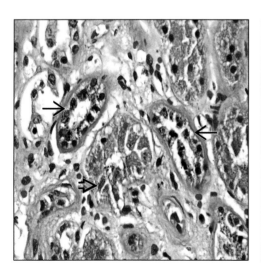 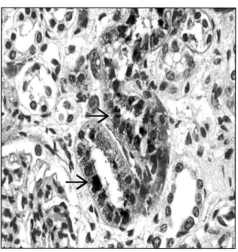

(Left) Tubular hemosiderosis in a patient with hemochromatosis has granular brown hemosiderin deposits in the epithelium of the proximal ➡ and distal ➡ tubules. Heavy deposits of iron may cause acute tubular necrosis. (Right) A Prussian blue stain for iron highlights granular deposits in the tubular epithelial cytoplasm ➡ in hemosiderosis. This patient had symptomatic primary hemochromatosis.

ARISTOLOCHIC ACID NEPHROPATHY

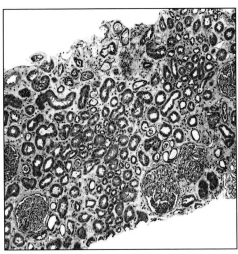

Early features of aristolochic acid nephropathy include acute tubular injury, early tubular atrophy, and diffuse fine interstitial fibrosis with little inflammation. Glomeruli are spared.

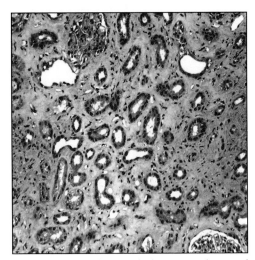

Tubules are shrunken, and there is widening of the interstitial compartment with myxoid matrix accumulation and characteristically minimal infiltrate of mononuclear cells.

TERMINOLOGY

Abbreviations
- Aristolochic acid nephropathy (AAN)

Synonyms
- Chinese herb nephropathy

Definitions
- Tubulointerstitial nephropathy and urothelial carcinoma associated with exposure to aristolochic acid in herbal remedies

ETIOLOGY/PATHOGENESIS

Plant-derived Toxin from Genus Aristolochia
- Used in traditional Chinese, Indian, and European medical preparations
- Aristolactams derived from reduction of aristolochic acid (AA) bind adenine and guanine residues on DNA, forming DNA-adducts
  - Proximal tubule is most affected in animal models of disease
  - AA-related DNA adducts cause activation of H-ras and p53, and may be important in carcinogenesis
    - A:T → T:A transversions are signature mutations of p53 from exposure to AA
- Severity of renal injury is dose dependent
  - Cumulative intake of > 100 grams is associated with chronic renal failure
  - Cumulative intake of > 200 grams is associated with development of end-stage kidney disease and increased risk of urothelial carcinoma
  - Injury appears to be progressive even after discontinuation of exposure to toxin
- AA toxicity is confounded by simultaneous exposure to appetite suppressants fenfluramine and diethylpropion
  - These compounds have vasoconstrictive properties

- Thought to be etiologic agent in Balkan nephropathy

CLINICAL ISSUES

Presentation
- Acute renal failure
  - Progression to end-stage renal disease in months
- Chronic renal failure
  - May be asymptomatic
- Proteinuria, asymptomatic
  - Tubular proteinuria, < 1.5 g per day
- Fanconi syndrome uncommon
- Many patients give history of intake of herbal preparations for weight loss

Prognosis
- Risk of progression to end-stage disease is proportional to duration of exposure
- Stable chronic renal failure may be seen in patients with serum creatinine less than 2 mg/dL
- Renal failure tends to be progressive
- Increased risk of urothelial carcinoma

MACROSCOPIC FEATURES

- Asymmetrically shrunken kidneys
- Papillary or papular lesions in urothelium of pelvis, ureter, or bladder

MICROSCOPIC PATHOLOGY

Histologic Features
- Glomeruli
  - Typically unremarkable
- Tubules and interstitium
  - Early lesions have acute tubular injury with interstitial myxoid change and scattered mononuclear cell infiltrates

ARISTOLOCHIC ACID NEPHROPATHY

Key Facts

Terminology
- Progressive tubulointerstitial nephropathy and urothelial carcinoma related to aristolochic acid in herbal remedies

Etiology/Pathogenesis
- Patients give history of intake of herbal preparations containing aristolochic acid for weight loss
- Severity of renal injury is dose dependent

Microscopic Pathology
- Early lesions have acute tubular injury with interstitial myxoid change and scattered mononuclear cell infiltrates
- Late interstitial fibrosis tends to be paucicellular and most pronounced in outer cortex
- Papillary urothelial carcinoma may arise in pelvis, ureter, or bladder

○ Later lesions have marked interstitial fibrosis and tubular atrophy; mast cells may be prominent
○ Late interstitial fibrosis tends to be paucicellular and most pronounced in outer cortex
○ Tubular injury and atrophy affects mainly proximal tubular segments
- Arteries and arterioles
  ○ Intimal fibrosis of small arteries
- Urothelium
  ○ Urothelial hyperplasia, dysplasia, in situ or invasive carcinoma in medullary collecting ducts, pelvicaliceal system, ureter, or bladder
    ▪ Dysplastic nuclei are p53 positive by immunohistochemistry
  ○ Highest frequency of urothelial carcinoma is in upper urinary tract
- Aristolochic acid-DNA adducts can be detected in tissue
- Electron microscopy and immunofluorescence findings are nonspecific

DIFFERENTIAL DIAGNOSIS

Cortical Interstitial Fibrosis and Tubular Atrophy
- Chronic renal ischemia
  ○ Ischemic nephropathies usually have ischemic glomerulopathy or global glomerular sclerosis
    ▪ In AA nephropathy, glomeruli are relatively spared

- Advanced chronic tubulointerstitial nephritis associated with infection or drugs

Cortical Interstitial Fibrosis, Tubular Atrophy, and Urothelial Carcinoma
- Other types of toxic injury
  ○ Balkan endemic nephropathy (probably same toxin)
  ○ Analgesic nephropathy, associated with papillary necrosis

DIAGNOSTIC CHECKLIST

Pathologic Interpretation Pearls
- Paucicellular interstitial fibrosis, most pronounced in outer cortex, is an initial clue to diagnosis

SELECTED REFERENCES
1. Debelle FD et al: Aristolochic acid nephropathy: a worldwide problem. Kidney Int. 74(2):158-69, 2008
2. Grollman AP et al: Aristolochic acid and the etiology of endemic (Balkan) nephropathy. Proc Natl Acad Sci U S A. 104(29):12129-34, 2007
3. Chang CH et al: Rapidly progressive interstitial renal fibrosis associated with Chinese herbal medications. Am J Nephrol. 21(6):441-8, 2001
4. Depierreux M et al: Pathologic aspects of a newly described nephropathy related to the prolonged use of Chinese herbs. Am J Kidney Dis. 24(2):172-80, 1994

IMAGE GALLERY

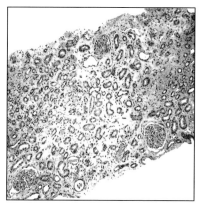 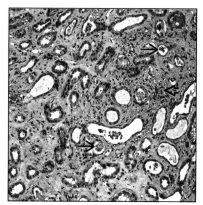 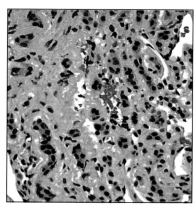

(Left) There is typically rapid progression of interstitial fibrosis with diffuse severe tubular atrophy. *(Center)* The predominant lesion is interstitial fibrosis, but tubular injury with necrotic casts ➡ and scattered mononuclear infiltrates ➡ are also described. *(Right)* Rapid progression to severe tubular atrophy and bland collagenous interstitial fibrosis is typical in aristolochic acid nephropathy.

BALKAN ENDEMIC NEPHROPATHY

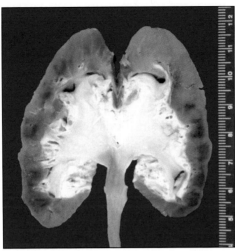

This atrophic kidney (7 cm in length) shows the typical features of Balkan endemic nephropathy (BEN) with marked thinning of the cortex and a smooth capsular surface. (Courtesy D. Ferluga, MD.)

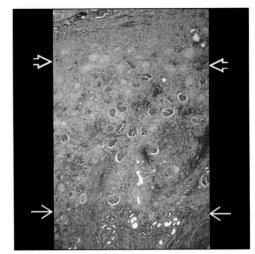

BEN characteristically has a zonal distribution, with progressively more severe interstitial fibrosis and glomerular sclerosis from the juxtamedullary ➡ to the subcapsular cortex ➡. (Courtesy D. Ferluga, MD.)

TERMINOLOGY

Abbreviations
- Balkan endemic nephropathy (BEN)

Synonyms
- Balkan nephropathy, Yugoslavian chronic endemic nephropathy, southeastern Europe endemic nephropathy, Danubian endemic familial nephropathy

Definitions
- Chronic tubulointerstitial nephropathy with high risk of urothelial carcinoma, endemic in specific regions of Balkan countries, Romania, and Bulgaria

ETIOLOGY/PATHOGENESIS

Unknown
- Tubulopathy is earliest lesion, and proximal tubules are probably major site of renal injury
- Environmental toxin(s) are strongly suspected
  - Aristolochic acid (AA)
    - Metabolites of AA form DNA adducts; may induce mutations of p53 with A:T → T:A transversions
    - Specific p53 mutations are found with high frequency in upper urinary tract malignancies associated with BEN
    - DNA adducts detected in kidney tissue
  - Ochratoxin A
    - Nephrotoxic mycotoxin that causes porcine nephropathy with pathologic similarity to BEN
    - No clear examples of ochratoxin A-associated kidney disease in humans
- Chromosomal breakage in several bands, most frequently 3q25, containing oncogenes *src* and *raf-1*
  - Possibly reflect environmentally induced DNA injury

CLINICAL ISSUES

Epidemiology
- Incidence
  - Up to 10% in endemic areas
  - Discrete geographic distribution
    - Farming populations most affected
    - Familial clustering but not hereditary
  - Immigrants to endemic areas at risk after 15-20 years

Presentation
- Tubular dysfunction early in course
  - Impaired concentrating ability and salt wasting
  - Tubular proteinuria
    - Increased urinary β2-microglobulin
- Slowly progressive renal failure beginning at 30-50 years
- Late features
  - Copper-toned skin, orange palms and soles, weight loss, anemia, Fanconi syndrome

Prognosis
- Survival varies from months to more than 10 years
  - 33% progression of BEN to end-stage kidney disease in 15 years (1 study)
  - Mortality of 43% in Bulgaria from 1961-1970
  - A few studies indicate mortality rate of 50% within 2 years of diagnosis
  - Recent studies from Serbia suggest no change in mortality from unaffected individuals
- Urothelial carcinoma develops in 30-50% of individuals with BEN

MACROSCOPIC FEATURES

Bilateral Shrunken Kidneys
- Finely granular surface and smooth contour
- Down to 20 grams in advanced disease
- Obstructive hydronephrosis with urothelial carcinoma

BALKAN ENDEMIC NEPHROPATHY

Key Facts

Etiology/Pathogenesis
- Environmental toxin(s)
  - Aristolochic acid (AA) suspected

Clinical Issues
- Slowly progressive renal failure in 30-50 year olds
  - Impaired concentrating ability and salt wasting, Fanconi syndrome later
  - Copper-toned skin, orange palms and soles, weight loss, anemia

- Urothelial carcinoma develops in 30-50% of individuals with BEN

Microscopic Pathology
- Interstitial fibrosis and tubular atrophy
  - Begins in outer cortex and expands to involve inner cortex
  - Scanty inflammatory infiltrate
- Upper tract urothelial malignancy

MICROSCOPIC PATHOLOGY

Histologic Features
- Tubules and interstitium
  - Interstitial fibrosis and tubular atrophy
    - Begins focally in outer cortex and expands centripetally to involve inner cortex over years
    - Inflammatory infiltrates are scanty
  - Early cases with tubular dysfunction may have normal histology
- Glomeruli
  - Spared early
  - Global glomerular sclerosis in advanced disease
    - FSGS and focal GBM duplication described
- Blood vessels
  - Hyalin arteriolosclerosis and arteriosclerosis
- Urothelium
  - Urothelial dysplasia and papillomas; malignancy develops in up to 50%
  - Urothelial carcinomas affect mainly pelvis and ureter
  - Squamous carcinomas are also described
- IF and EM are nonspecific

DIFFERENTIAL DIAGNOSIS

Aristolochic Acid Nephropathy
- Similar distribution with sparing of glomeruli but more rapid course
- May be causal agent of BEN

Chronic Tubulointerstitial Nephritis, Any Cause
- Especially chronic pyelonephritis, obstructive uropathy, and radiation nephropathy

Chronic Renal Ischemia
- Ischemic glomerulopathy, with intrarenal or extrarenal vascular stenosis

DIAGNOSTIC CHECKLIST

Pathologic Interpretation Pearls
- Outer cortical paucicellular interstitial fibrosis and upper urinary tract urothelial carcinoma are characteristic

SELECTED REFERENCES

1. Bukvic D et al: Today Balkan endemic nephropathy is a disease of the elderly with a good prognosis. Clin Nephrol. 72(2):105-13, 2009
2. Grollman AP et al: Role of environmental toxins in endemic (Balkan) nephropathy. October 2006, Zagreb, Croatia. J Am Soc Nephrol. 18(11):2817-23, 2007
3. Ferluga D et al: Renal function, protein excretion, and pathology of Balkan endemic nephropathy. III. Light and electron microscopic studies. Kidney Int Suppl. 34:S57-67, 1991

IMAGE GALLERY

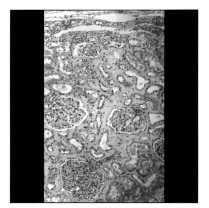 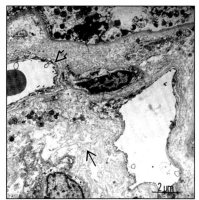 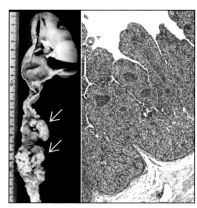

(Left) Balkan endemic nephropathy (BEN) characteristically has hypocellular interstitial fibrosis and tubular atrophy, with sparing of glomeruli. *(Courtesy D. Ferluga, MD.)* *(Center)* The interstitial fibrosis in BEN consists of loose collagen fibrils ➡, with mild duplication of the basement membrane of peritubular capillaries ➡. *(Courtesy D. Ferluga, MD.)* *(Right)* Multifocal exophytic ureteral tumors ➡ and hydronephrosis are shown in BEN with a papillary pattern on histology. *(Courtesy D. Ferluga, MD.)*

ETHYLENE GLYCOL

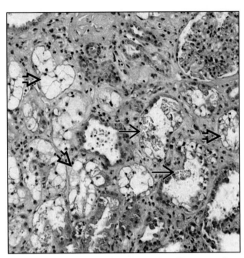

Cortex with intratubular, refractile, pale yellow, crystalline calcium oxalate ➡, epithelial injury with macrovesicular (ballooning) vacuolization ⪧, and interstitial edema with scattered inflammation. (Courtesy T. Nadasdy, MD.)

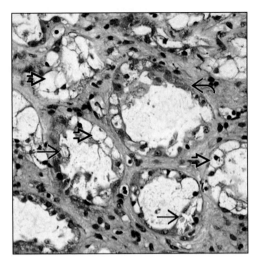

Refractile, pale yellow crystals of calcium oxalate within the cytoplasm of proximal tubular cells ➡. Crystals are associated with severe tubular injury ⤳ & epithelial cytoplasmic vacuoles ⪧. (Courtesy T. Nadasdy, MD.)

TERMINOLOGY

Abbreviations
- Ethylene glycol-oxalosis (EGO)

Synonyms
- Ethylene glycol toxicity

Definitions
- Oxalosis due to ethylene glycol ingestion

ETIOLOGY/PATHOGENESIS

Toxic Exposure
- Colorless, odorless fluid with bitter-sweet flavor; given by HO-CH2-CH2-OH
  - Commonly component of anti-freeze radiator fluid
  - Also in hydraulic brake fluid, de-icing solutions, lacquers, and polishes
- Acute toxicity arises by oral ingestion
  - Deliberate in suicides and homicides
  - Inadvertent in cases of contamination
- Ethylene glycol (EG) is rapidly absorbed with peak serum concentration in 1-4 hours
- Minimum lethal dose for adults is 1-1.5 mL/kg
- EG metabolized in liver to glycoaldehyde by alcohol dehydrogenase
  - Glycoaldehyde → glycolic acid → glyoxylic acid → oxalic acid + calcium → calcium oxalate
  - Glycolic acid and glyoxylic acid contribute to metabolic acidosis
- Calcium oxalate is deposited in kidneys, myocardium, vasculature, brain, liver, and spleen
- Renal injury is attributed to calcium oxalate deposition
- Severe tubular injury with balloon vacuoles may be due to other toxins like glycolic acid

CLINICAL ISSUES

Presentation
- Pattern of presentation depends on dose of EG ingested
  - Phase 1: Neurologic (0.5-12 hours after ingestion)
    - Inebriation, altered mental status, seizures, coma
  - Phase 2: Cardiopulmonary (12-24 hours)
    - Tachycardia, congestive heart failure, respiratory distress syndrome
  - Phase 3: Renal (24-72 hours)
    - Oliguric acute renal failure, flank pain, hematuria, crystalluria
- Diagnosis
  - Inebriation or altered mental state with high anion gap metabolic acidosis
  - Urinary calcium oxalate crystals on microscopy
    - Octahedral- or tent-shaped crystals typical of calcium oxalate dihydrate more specific for EGO
    - Prism- or dumbbell-shaped crystals of calcium oxalate monohydrate not specific
  - Urinary fluorescence in Wood light indicates excretion of sodium fluorescein (component of anti-freeze)

Treatment
- Supportive using intravenous fluids to control shock and sodium bicarbonate for acidosis
- Hemodialysis for acute renal failure and removal of EG
- Antidotes include ethanol and fomepizole (4-methylpyrazole)
  - Competitive inhibitors of alcohol dehydrogenase reduce formation of toxic metabolites of EG

Prognosis
- Permanent renal insufficiency is uncommon in nonfatal cases

ETHYLENE GLYCOL

Key Facts

Terminology
- Oxalosis due to ethylene glycol ingestion

Etiology/Pathogenesis
- Renal injury due to calcium oxalate deposition and other toxins like glycolic acid

Clinical Issues
- Phase 1: Neurologic (0.5-12 hours after ingestion)
- Phase 2: Cardiopulmonary (12-24 hours)
- Phase 3: Renal (24-72 hours)

Microscopic Pathology
- Acute tubular injury and necrosis
- Proximal tubular cytoplasmic ballooning vacuolization
- Tubular calcium oxalate crystals

Top Differential Diagnoses
- Primary and secondary oxalosis

MACROSCOPIC FEATURES

Gross Examination
- Enlarged swollen kidneys with bulging cut surface and gritty texture
- Imprint or "scrimp" specimens reveal calcium oxalate crystals on polarization microscopy

MICROSCOPIC PATHOLOGY

Histologic Features
- Acute tubular injury and necrosis
- Cytoplasmic vacuolization (macrovesicular or ballooning or hydropic) in proximal tubules
- Intraepithelial and intraluminal refractile calcium oxalate in proximal tubules; birefringent in polarized light
- Interstitial edema with mild inflammation
- Glomeruli are unremarkable
- Rare findings include crystals with multinucleated giant cells and cortical necrosis

Predominant Pattern/Injury Type
- Crystals, calcium oxalate

Predominant Cell/Compartment Type
- Proximal tubular epithelium

DIFFERENTIAL DIAGNOSIS

Primary and Secondary Oxalosis
- Intratubular and interstitial calcium oxalate with foreign body giant cell reaction and inflammation
- Severe acute tubular injury with macrovesicles not a feature of this group of disorders

DIAGNOSTIC CHECKLIST

Clinically Relevant Pathologic Features
- Acute renal failure due to acute tubular injury
- Calcium oxalate and ballooning vacuoles are typical

Pathologic Interpretation Pearls
- Severe acute tubular injury, large vacuoles, intraepithelial and intraluminal calcium oxalate

SELECTED REFERENCES

1. Friedman EA et al: Consequences of ethylene glycol poisoning. Report of four cases and review of the literature. Am J Med. 32:891-902, 1962
2. Smith DE: Morphologic lesions due to acute and subacute poisoning with antifreeze (ethylene glycol). AMA Arch Pathol. 51(4):423-33, 1951
3. Pons CA et al: Acute ethylene glycol poisoning; a clinico-pathologic report of eighteen fatal cases. Am J Med Sci. 211:544-52, 1946

IMAGE GALLERY

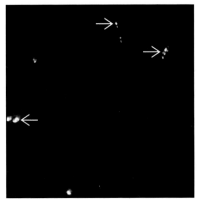 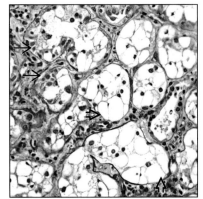 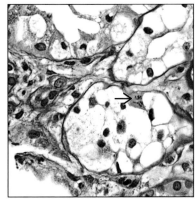

(Left) Birefringent intratubular calcium oxalate crystals ➡, some of which are highlighted, are seen using partially polarized light. *(Courtesy T. Nadasdy, MD.)* *(Center)* An extensive tubular epithelial injury with cellular dyshesion ➡ is seen, with large, ballooning, cytoplasmic vacuoles ➡ and scattered interstitial inflammation. *(Courtesy T. Nadasdy, MD.)* *(Right)* Also visible are severely injured, vacuolated, tubular epithelium with regeneration indicated by mitosis ➡. *(Courtesy T. Nadasdy, MD.)*

KARYOMEGALIC INTERSTITIAL NEPHRITIS

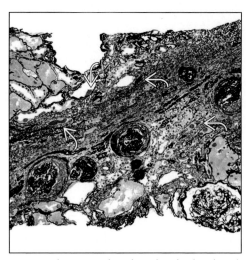

Karyomegalic interstitial nephritis has focal, enlarged, abnormal tubular epithelial nuclei ➚ *accompanied by tubular atrophy, glomerulosclerosis, interstitial inflammation and fibrosis. (Courtesy A. Friedl, MD.)*

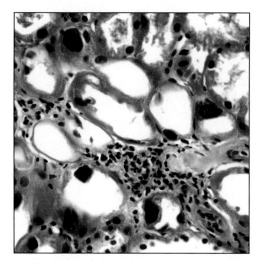

In KIN, enlarged, hyperchromatic nuclei are most prominent in tubular cells. Similar nuclear changes occur in most other organs, including liver, lung, brain, and endocrine glands. (Courtesy G. Monga, MD.)

TERMINOLOGY

Abbreviations
- Karyomegalic interstitial nephritis (KIN)

Synonyms
- Systemic karyomegaly

Definitions
- Chronic tubulointerstitial nephritis with prominent karyomegaly in tubular epithelium
- Initially reported by Mihatsch and colleagues in 1979

ETIOLOGY/PATHOGENESIS

Sporadic and Familial Cases
- Genetic risk factor suspected, but unproved
- Possible association with HLA (B27/35)

Environmental Toxins
- Suspected in some cases
- Ochratoxin has been implicated in cases in Tunisia

Animal Models
- Various toxins in rats
  - Ochratoxin
  - Cisplatin
  - Glutathione depletion (1-cyano-3,4-epithiobutane)

CLINICAL ISSUES

Epidemiology
- Incidence
  - Rare; < 30 cases reported
  - Presents at 9-51 years of age (median: 33 years)
  - No gender preference

Presentation
- Proteinuria, asymptomatic
  - Low molecular weight (tubular)
- Microhematuria
- Chronic renal failure
- Recurrent respiratory infection
- Elevated liver enzymes

Treatment
- None identified

Prognosis
- Usually leads to chronic renal failure at 30-40 years of age

MICROSCOPIC PATHOLOGY

Histologic Features
- Glomeruli
  - Global and segmental sclerosis
  - Occasional karyomegaly in glomerular cells
- Tubules
  - Karyomegaly in scattered tubules throughout the nephron
    - Nuclei 2-5x larger than normal
    - Hyperchromatic
    - Increased DNA ploidy
    - No mitotic figures
  - Tubular atrophy in affected areas
- Interstitium
  - Nonspecific mononuclear infiltrate
  - Not well characterized
  - Fibrosis in areas of tubular atrophy
- Vessels
  - Karyomegaly of occasional smooth muscle cells

Other Organs
- Karyomegaly in most organs studied
  - Smooth muscle cells of vessels and bowel, Schwann cells and astrocytes, pulmonary and bronchial epithelium, liver
- No associated inflammation or fibrosis except in kidney

KARYOMEGALIC INTERSTITIAL NEPHRITIS

Key Facts

Etiology/Pathogenesis

- Idiopathic
  - Genetic risk factor suspected, but unproved
  - DNA toxins suspected in some cases (ochratoxin)

Clinical Issues

- Rare; < 30 cases reported
- Proteinuria, asymptomatic
- Chronic renal failure

Microscopic Pathology

- Karyomegaly in tubules throughout the nephron
- Interstitial nephritis, fibrosis and tubular atrophy
- Karyomegaly in most organs
- Probably overlooked diagnosis

Top Differential Diagnoses

- Viral infection due to adenovirus, Polyomavirus, Cytomegalovirus

ANCILLARY TESTS

Cytology

- Karyomegalic cells are shed in urine

Immunohistochemistry

- Ki-67 and PCNA do not stain enlarged nuclei (they are not in cell cycle)

Immunofluorescence

- No specific findings
  - IgM and C3 in scarred glomeruli

Electron Microscopy

- Little or no foot process effacement in glomeruli
- Abnormal nuclei have expanded loose matrix and convoluted nuclear membranes

DIFFERENTIAL DIAGNOSIS

Nonspecific Nuclear Atypia Found with Cytotoxic Drugs

- Azathioprine in transplant recipients

Viral Infection Due to Adenovirus, Polyomavirus, Cytomegalovirus

- No viral antigens by IHC

DIAGNOSTIC CHECKLIST

Pathologic Interpretation Pearls

- Potential to be misinterpreted as carcinoma in urine cytology
- Probably underdiagnosed

SELECTED REFERENCES

1. Palmer D et al: Karyomegalic interstitial nephritis: a pitfall in urine cytology. Diagn Cytopathol. 35(3):179-82, 2007
2. Baba F et al: Karyomegalic tubulointerstitial nephritis--a case report. Pathol Res Pract. 202(7):555-9, 2006
3. Monga G et al: Karyomegalic interstitial nephritis: report of 3 new cases and review of the literature. Clin Nephrol. 65(5):349-55, 2006
4. Hassen W et al: Karyomegaly of tubular kidney cells in human chronic interstitial nephropathy in Tunisia: respective role of Ochratoxin A and possible genetic predisposition. Hum Exp Toxicol. 23(7):339-46, 2004
5. Bhandari S et al: Karyomegalic nephropathy: an uncommon cause of progressive renal failure. Nephrol Dial Transplant. 17(11):1914-20, 2002
6. Spoendlin M et al: Karyomegalic interstitial nephritis: further support for a distinct entity and evidence for a genetic defect. Am J Kidney Dis. 25(2):242-52, 1995
7. Mihatsch MJ et al: Systemic karyomegaly associated with chronic interstitial nephritis. A new disease entity? Clin Nephrol. 12(2):54-62, 1979

IMAGE GALLERY

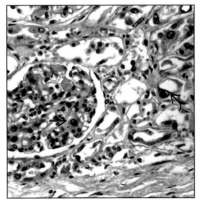 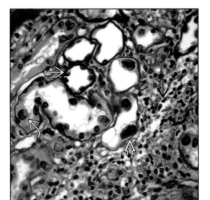 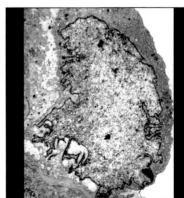

(Left) Tubular cells appear to be the main target in KIN ➡ although glomerular cells ➡ also show focal enlargement. (Courtesy G. Monga, MD.) *(Center)* KIN nuclei range from normal ➡ to moderately enlarged ➡ to immense ➡. Lymphocytes, which are conspicuous in the accompanying interstitial infiltrate, are 6-8 microns in diameter ➡. *(Right)* Enlarged nuclei in KIN have convoluted nuclear membranes and expanded loose chromatin without prominent nucleoli (EM). (Courtesy A. Friedl, MD.)

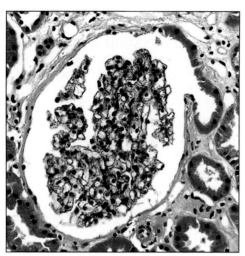

Argyria is caused by chronic intake of silver. The silver precipitates in the glomerular basement membrane and appears as black grains in unstained or stained sections. (Courtesy M. Mihatsch, MD.)

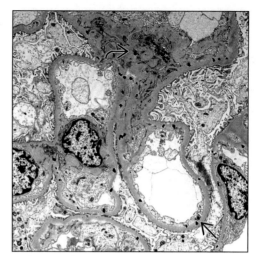

In this case of argyria, electron microscopy reveals the characteristic electron-opaque silver deposits along the endothelial side of the GBM ➡ and in the mesangium ➥. (Courtesy M. Mihatsch, MD.)

TERMINOLOGY

Synonyms

- Argyrosis (pigmentation of conjunctiva)

Definitions

- Systemic disease caused by accumulation of silver (Ag) or silver salts in skin and other tissues due to chronic exposure to silver colloid or salts
  - Localized form due to topical silver exposure

ETIOLOGY/PATHOGENESIS

Environmental Exposure

- Silver salts or colloid ingestion
  - Silver salts used as antibacterial agent
    - Ag+ is bacteriocidal (not metallic Ag)
    - Declining use of silver salts and colloids as antibiotic
    - Silver colloid available as over-the-counter drug promoted in alternative medicine
    - Nanoparticles of Ag used as coating of materials
- Exposure measured in years

Silver Precipitates in Tissues

- Deposits are elemental silver, Ag_2S or Ag-protein complexes
  - Ag+ binds to sulfhydryl (e.g., glutathione), amino, carboxyl, phosphate and imidazole groups
  - Light catalyzes reduction of Ag+ to silver metal (as in photographic film)
  - Ag oxidized in tissue to Ag_2S
- Debatable evidence that renal disease is caused by silver deposition alone
  - Some cases with chronic renal dysfunction had exposure to heavy metals, solvents, or other nephrotoxins

Animal Models

- Heavy oral exposure to silver nitrate (mice, rats) or 56 nm nanoparticles of silver shows GBM deposition, but no renal disease
- Used to show turnover of GBM in vivo

CLINICAL ISSUES

Presentation

- Slate gray discoloration of light exposed skin and conjunctiva
- Usually no other systemic manifestations
  - Questionable link to silver deposition
    - Variable loss of renal function
    - Nephrotic syndrome
    - Hypertension

Treatment

- Laser treatment of skin
- No effective treatment to remove systemic deposits
  - No chelating agents active

MACROSCOPIC FEATURES

General Features

- Renal biopsy cores have prominent black glomeruli easily visible to naked eye

MICROSCOPIC PATHOLOGY

Histologic Features

- Glomeruli
  - Granular black deposits along GBM
  - Marked accumulation in sclerotic glomeruli
  - Membranous glomerulonephritis described
- Tubules and interstitium
  - No silver deposition in TBM
  - Peritubular capillary BM deposits of silver

ARGYRIA

Key Facts

Terminology
- Accumulation of silver salts in skin and other tissues

Etiology/Pathogenesis
- Deposits are elemental silver, Ag₂S, or Ag-protein complexes

Clinical Issues
- Slate gray discoloration of light-exposed skin and conjunctiva

- Uncertain link to renal disease

Microscopic Pathology
- Granular black deposits along GBM
- Also described in peritubular capillary BM and arteries
- Dense black grains in GBM and mesangium by EM

Diagnostic Checklist
- Black glomeruli in renal biopsy core

- Vessels
  - Deposits along internal elastica of arteries described at autopsy
  - Some cases with arteriosclerosis
    - Not clearly related to silver deposition

ANCILLARY TESTS

Electron Microscopy
- Dense black grains about 100-200 nm in GBM and mesangium
  - Deposited primarily along subendothelial side of GBM
- No deposits in cells, including lysosomes
- No obvious effect on podocytes, endothelial cells

Energy-filtered Transmission Electron Microscopy
- Able to identify elements in tissue deposits
  - Higher resolution than energy dispersive x-ray scanning electron microscopy
- Deposits have energy spectrum of silver

Skin Biopsy
- Black silver deposits in dermis, macrophages

DIAGNOSTIC CHECKLIST

Pathologic Interpretation Pearls
- Black glomeruli in renal biopsy core

SELECTED REFERENCES

1. Mayr M et al: Argyria and decreased kidney function: are silver compounds toxic to the kidney? Am J Kidney Dis. 53(5):890-4, 2009
2. Schroeder JA et al: Ultrastructural evidence of dermal gadolinium deposits in a patient with nephrogenic systemic fibrosis and end-stage renal disease. Clin J Am Soc Nephrol. 3(4):968-75, 2008
3. Drake PL et al: Exposure-related health effects of silver and silver compounds: a review. Ann Occup Hyg. 49(7):575-85, 2005
4. Watanabe Y et al: [Case of membranous nephropathy associated with argyria.] Nippon Jinzo Gakkai Shi. 47(5):547-51, 2005
5. Day WA et al: Silver deposition in mouse glomeruli. Pathology. 8(3):201-4, 1976
6. Owens CJ et al: Nephrotic syndrome following topically applied sulfadiazine silver therapy. Arch Intern Med. 134(2):332-5, 1974
7. Zech P et al: [Nephrotic syndrome with silver deposits in the glomerular basement membranes during argyria.] Nouv Presse Med. 2(3):161-4, 1973
8. Walker F: Basement-membrane turnover in man. J Pathol. 107(2):123-5, 1972
9. Walker F: Experimental argyria: a model for basement membrane studies. Br J Exp Pathol. 52(6):589-93, 1971
10. Zollinger HU: Niere und Ableitende Harnwege. Heidelberg: Springer Verlag. 282, 1966

IMAGE GALLERY

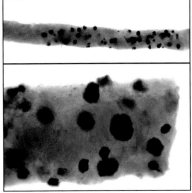 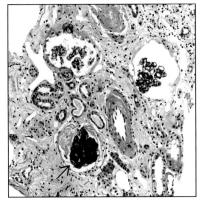 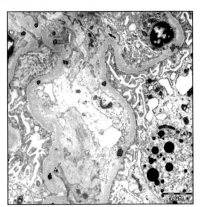

(Left) The diagnosis of argyria can be made by visual inspection of the renal biopsy cores. The glomeruli stand out as black balls. *(Courtesy M. Mihatsch, MD.)* *(Center)* Black silver grains can be appreciated in H&E sections predominantly in the GBM, shown here in functional and globally sclerotic glomeruli ➡. *(Courtesy M. Mihatsch, MD.)* *(Right)* Energy-filtered electron microscopy identifies the grains as silver (colored red here). *(Courtesy M. Mihatsch, MD and J.A. Schroeder, MD.)*

TUBULOINTERSTITIAL NEPHRITIS WITH UVEITIS

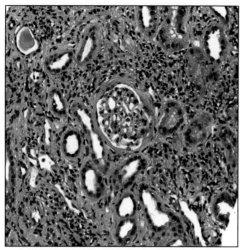

Hematoxylin & eosin shows a diffuse interstitial infiltrate with interstitial fibrosis and tubular atrophy in a case of tubulointerstitial nephritis with uveitis (TINU).

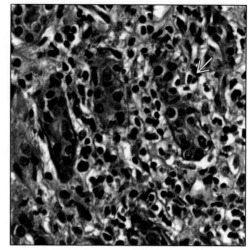

Periodic acid-Schiff stain shows a tubulointerstitial nephritis with a focus of tubulitis ➡ in a case of TINU.

TERMINOLOGY

Abbreviations
- Tubulointerstitial nephritis with uveitis (TINU)

Synonyms
- Dobrin syndrome

Definitions
- Tubulointerstitial nephritis associated with uveitis and, in some cases, identifiable bone marrow granulomas

ETIOLOGY/PATHOGENESIS

Environmental Exposure
- Environmental exposures such as insect bites have been proposed in selected cases

Infectious Agents
- A few of the multiple suggested associated pathogens include: *Klebsiella*, *Chlamydia*, *Mycoplasma*, herpes zoster, Epstein-Barr virus (EBV), and *Toxoplasma*

Autoimmune
- Most likely cause in most cases
- Lymphocyte reactions and circulating antibodies to renal tubular epithelia
- Antibodies may also be directed against uveal cells

Genetic
- Reports of identical twins and siblings with identical haplotypes suggest genetic predisposition

CLINICAL ISSUES

Epidemiology
- Incidence
  - ~ 5% of lymphocytic interstitial nephritis cases
- Age
  - Mostly adolescents
    - Median age of onset 15 years; range: 9-74 years
    - First 2 patients were Caucasian females, 14 and 17 years old, respectively (Dobrin, 1975)
- Gender
  - F > M

Presentation
- Eye abnormalities: Anterior uveitis (by definition in all and usually bilateral) and eye pain or redness (32%)
- Renal dysfunction: Proteinuria and sometimes a form of Fanconi syndrome (proximal tubule dysfunction)
- Fever (53%)
- Weight loss (47%) and anorexia (28%)
- Fatigue, malaise (44%) &/or weakness, asthenia (28%)
- Abdominal or flank pain (28%)
- Arthralgias/myalgias (17%)
- Uncommonly: Rash (1%) and lymphadenopathy (1%)
- Concurrent chronic sialadenitis has been described

Laboratory Tests
- Anemia (96%)
- Increased creatinine (90%)
- Increased erythrocyte sedimentation rate (ESR) (89%)
- Increased IgG (83%)
- Urine: Protein (86%), leukocytes (55%), normoglycemic glucosuria (47%), microscopic hematuria (42%), urinary eosinophils (3%), aminoaciduria (3%)
- Usually seronegative for typical autoimmune diseases

Treatment
- Drugs
  - Steroids (corticosteroids) are often used to facilitate recovery

Prognosis
- Spontaneous remission can occur
- Permanent renal dysfunction may persist

TUBULOINTERSTITIAL NEPHRITIS WITH UVEITIS

Key Facts

Terminology
- Tubulointerstitial nephritis with uveitis (TINU)

Etiology/Pathogenesis
- Autoimmune, infectious, environmental, and genetic
  - Most likely cause in most cases is autoimmune

Clinical Issues
- Mostly children
- Females affected more than males
- Uveitis and other eye abnormalities
- Renal dysfunction: Proteinuria & Fanconi syndrome
- Multitude of signs/symptoms (e.g., fever, weight loss, anorexia)
- Laboratory abnormalities such as anemia, increased creatinine, increased ESR, proteinuria, urinary leukocytes, normoglycemic glucosuria, hematuria

- Spontaneous remission can occur but recovery is usually facilitated with steroids
- Permanent renal dysfunction may persist

Microscopic Pathology
- Tubulointerstitial nephritis with mononuclear cells (lymphocytes and macrophages), plasma cells, eosinophils, and neutrophils
- Acute tubular injury
- Noncaseating granulomata in kidneys, bone marrow, and lymph nodes

Top Differential Diagnoses
- Drug-induced acute interstitial nephritis
- Sarcoidosis
- Sjögren syndrome

MICROSCOPIC PATHOLOGY

Histologic Features
- Tubulointerstitial nephritis sometimes accompanied by interstitial fibrosis and tubular atrophy
  - Mononuclear cells
    - Frequent lymphocytes with fewer plasma cells and macrophages
    - Mononuclear inflammation centered on proximal tubules, sometimes arranged in circular arrays
  - Eosinophils (34%) and neutrophils (25%)
- Acute tubular injury
  - Flattened tubular epithelium
- Noncaseating granulomata in kidneys (reportedly in 13%), bone marrow, and lymph nodes

ANCILLARY TESTS

Immunohistochemistry
- Inflammatory cells mostly CD4(+) and CD8(+) T cells

Immunofluorescence
- Immunoreactants usually not in glomeruli or tubules (only in ~ 14%)

DIFFERENTIAL DIAGNOSIS

Drug-induced Acute Interstitial Nephritis
- Clinical history and features helpful
  - History of drug exposure, rash, lack of uveitis
- Pathology similar or indistinguishable
  - Eosinophils typically more numerous, particularly when allergic/hypersensitivity reaction is suspected
  - Some drugs have characteristic patterns of injury
    - Lithium, for example, may lead to prominent interstitial fibrosis and tubular cystic change with only mild inflammation

Sarcoidosis
- Granulomas are usually quite prominent, which is less common in TINU

Sjögren Syndrome
- Usually characterized by xerostomia and xerophthalmia
- Antinuclear antibody (ANA) usually positive vs. TINU (usually ANA negative)

DIAGNOSTIC CHECKLIST

Pathologic Interpretation Pearls
- Often more chronic injury/atrophy of tubules with TBM thickening than in typical drug-related interstitial nephritis

SELECTED REFERENCES

1. Neilson EG et al: Case records of the Massachusetts General Hospital. Case 21-2009. A 61-year-old woman with abdominal pain, weight loss, and renal failure. N Engl J Med. 361(2):179-87, 2009
2. Abed L et al: Presence of autoantibodies against tubular and uveal cells in a patient with tubulointerstitial nephritis and uveitis (TINU) syndrome. Nephrol Dial Transplant. 23(4):1452-5, 2008
3. Izzedine H: Tubulointerstitial nephritis and uveitis syndrome (TINU): a step forward to understanding an elusive oculorenal syndrome. Nephrol Dial Transplant. 23(4):1095-7, 2008
4. Herlitz LC et al: Uveitis and acute renal failure. Kidney Int. 72(12):1554-7, 2007
5. Litwin M et al: Tubulointerstitial nephritis with uveitis: clinico-pathological and immunological study. Pediatr Nephrol. 17(8):683-8, 2002
6. Mandeville JT et al: The tubulointerstitial nephritis and uveitis syndrome. Surv Ophthalmol. 46(3):195-208, 2001
7. Grefer J et al: Tubulointerstitial nephritis and uveitis in association with Epstein-Barr virus infection. Pediatr Nephrol. 13(4):336-9, 1999
8. Dobrin RS et al: Acute eosinophilic interstitial nephritis and renal failure with bone marrow-lymph node granulomas and anterior uveitis. A new syndrome. Am J Med. 59(3):325-33, 1975

TUBULOINTERSTITIAL NEPHRITIS WITH UVEITIS

Microscopic Features

(Left) There is severe interstitial nephritis in this case of TINU with an inflammatory infiltrate composed of mononuclear cells, many of which appear to be macrophage-type cells. Tubules contain proteinaceous cast material. (Right) Trichrome stain shows severe fibrosis and tubular atrophy with a predominantly mononuclear lymphoid infiltrate in a case of TINU. Tubules contain proteinaceous cast material.

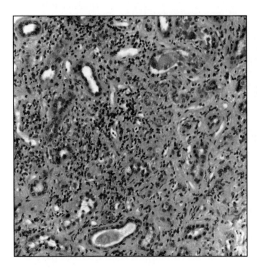
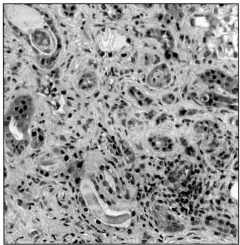

(Left) Periodic acid-Schiff shows markedly disrupted tubules in a case of tubulointerstitial nephritis with uveitis (TINU). Ring-like duplication of the TBM is evident ➡, indicative of chronic or repeated tubular damage and repair. (Right) A prominent tubulointerstitial nephritis with frequent eosinophils is seen in this case of TINU. Eosinophils can be quite prominent, also a feature of drug-induced acute interstitial nephritis.

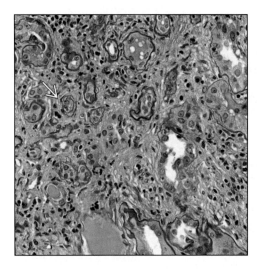
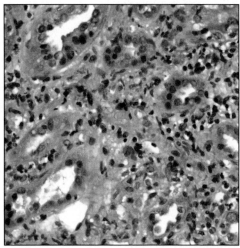

(Left) A prominent tubulointerstitial nephritis is present in this case of TINU with a predominantly mononuclear infiltrate composed primarily of lymphocytes and macrophage-type cells. Tubules appear injured and contain proteinaceous cast material. (Right) Hematoxylin & eosin stain shows fibrosis, tubular atrophy, and edema with a predominantly mononuclear infiltrate with occasional eosinophils ➡ in a case of TINU.

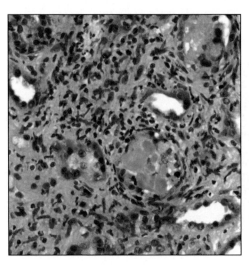
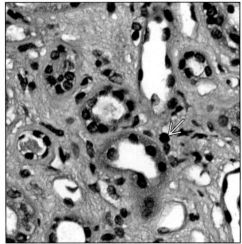

Ancillary Techniques

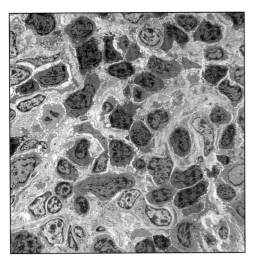

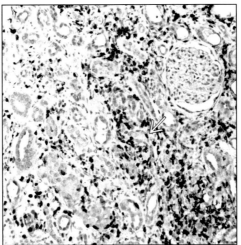

(Left) Electron micrograph shows a dense infiltrate of mononuclear cells in a case of TINU, which includes mostly small, activated lymphocytes. *(Right)* CD3 immunohistochemical stain shows numerous CD3(+) lymphocytes in a case of TINU and highlights areas of tubulitis ➡. These cells are believed to be autoreactive T cells (primarily CD4) but the putative autoantigen in the tubules is unknown.

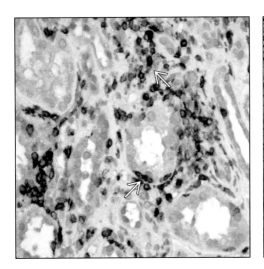

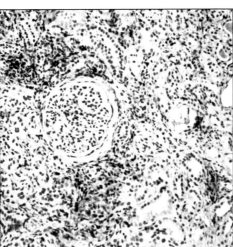

(Left) CD3 immunohistochemical stain shows numerous CD3(+) lymphocytes with foci of tubulitis ➡ in TINU. Tubulitis with intratubular T cells is seen in other forms of acute interstitial nephritis, such as that due to drugs and allograft rejection. *(Right)* On this CD4 immunohistochemical stain, numerous lymphocytes are CD4(+) in this case of TINU.

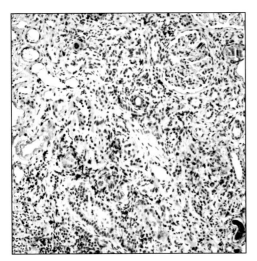

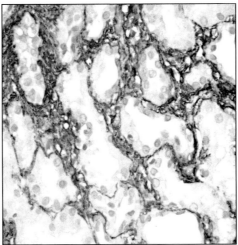

(Left) Many of the lymphocytes in this case of TINU are CD8(+) (as demonstrated in this CD8 immunohistochemical stain) as well as CD4(+). *(Right)* In this TINU case, α-smooth muscle actin immunohistochemical stain is positive in the expanded, fibrotic interstitium. Expression of α-smooth muscle actin is indicative of active fibrosis, and the myofibroblasts may be derived in part from epithelial to mesenchymal transition, as shown in experimental models.

SJÖGREN SYNDROME

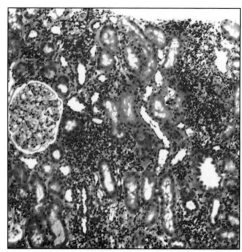

Renal biopsy in Sjögren syndrome typically shows a patchy but heavy interstitial infiltrate. The glomeruli are usually normal. The infiltrate forms broad sheets of cells that separate the tubules.

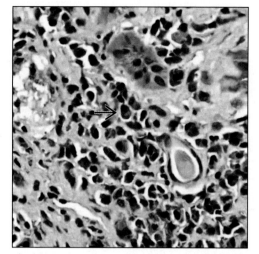

This biopsy in Sjögren syndrome shows the plasma cell-rich ⇒ nature of the infiltrate. The interstitium is greatly expanded and tubular atrophy and interstitial fibrosis has developed.

TERMINOLOGY

Abbreviations
- Sjögren syndrome (SS)

Synonyms
- Sicca syndrome

Definitions
- Autoimmune disorder involving exocrine glands, particularly salivary and lacrimal glands
  - May be primary or a component of other autoimmune disorders
    - Rheumatoid arthritis in 50%
    - Systemic sclerosis in 5%
    - Systemic lupus erythematosus in 5%

ETIOLOGY/PATHOGENESIS

Etiology Not Clear
- May be multifactorial
- Initiation by an exogenous factor, possibly viral
  - Epstein-Barr virus implicated
  - Genetic predisposition
- Lymphoplasmacytic inflammation with atrophy of eccrine, salivary, and lacrimal glands
  - T-lymphocyte response
  - B-lymphocyte hyper-reactivity
    - Autoantibodies: Rheumatoid factor (RF), SS-A (Ro) and SS-B (La)
  - Injury to salivary gland epithelium

CLINICAL ISSUES

Epidemiology
- Age
  - 45-55 years
- Gender
  - Female predominance (F: M = 9:1)

Presentation
- Renal disease ~ 5%
  - Tubulointerstitial disease
    - Distal renal tubular acidosis 70-80%
    - Renal failure 25-30%
    - Tubular proteinuria 20%
    - Hypercalcuria, occasionally hypokalemia
    - Fanconi syndrome (rare)
  - Glomerulonephritis 5-15%
    - Proteinuria &/or hematuria &/or renal failure
- Keratoconjunctivitis (dry eyes) > 95%
- Xerostomia (dry mouth) > 95%
- Cutaneous vasculitis 10-30%
  - Associated with cryoglobulins in 30%
  - Small to medium-sized vessels
- Peripheral neuropathy ~ 10%
- Interstitial lung disease ~ 10%
- Lymphoma 40x increased risk
  - B-cell lymphoma or Waldenström macroglobulinemia

Laboratory Tests
- 50-90% have SS-A antibodies
  - ANA, anti-SS-B, and RF often positive
- Hypergammaglobulinemia
- Organ-specific antibodies
  - Thyroid microsome
  - Thyroglobulin
  - Salivary duct epithelium
  - Gastric parietal cells
- Low C4, C3 (9%)

Treatment
- Immunosuppression: Corticosteroids, Rituximab

Prognosis
- Tubulointerstitial disease an early manifestation
- Glomerulonephritis develops later
- Renal function improves with treatment in most

SJÖGREN SYNDROME

Key Facts

Terminology
- Progressive autoimmune disorder involving exocrine glands, particularly salivary and lacrimal glands
- May be primary or a component of other autoimmune disorders

Clinical Issues
- Female predominance; age range 45-55
- Keratoconjunctivitis and xerostomia most common
- Renal disease
  - Renal failure
  - Renal tubular acidosis
  - Proteinuria and hematuria
- Risk of non-Hodgkin lymphomas
  - B-cell lymphoma or Waldenström macroglobulinemia
- Cutaneous vasculitis
  - Cryoglobulins in 30%
  - Small- to medium-sized vessels

Microscopic Pathology
- Chronic tubulointerstitial nephritis
  - Plasma cell-rich infiltrate
  - Tubular atrophy and interstitial fibrosis
- Acute tubulointerstitial nephritis
  - Tubulitis and edema
- Glomerulonephritis
  - Many forms described

Top Differential Diagnoses
- Primary SS vs. association with other autoimmune disorder
- Allergic or other interstitial nephritis such as sarcoid
- IgG4-related systemic disease

MICROSCOPIC PATHOLOGY

Histologic Features
- Glomeruli
  - Involved in minority (25-30%)
    - Membranoproliferative glomerulonephritis
    - Membranous glomerulonephritis
    - Mesangial proliferative glomerulonephritis
    - Crescentic glomerulonephritis &/or arteritis
    - IgA nephropathy
- Tubules and interstitium
  - Chronic tubulointerstitial nephritis 40-50%
    - Dense, patchy, plasma cell and lymphocytic infiltrate
    - Eosinophils usually absent
    - Tubular atrophy and interstitial fibrosis
    - Nephrocalcinosis in 30%
  - Acute tubulointerstitial nephritis 25%
    - Tubulitis and interstitial edema

ANCILLARY TESTS

Immunofluorescence
- Usually negative unless glomerulonephritis is present
- Occasionally TBM or interstitial deposits of IgG and C3
  - Resembles cryoglobulinemia or lupus, either may be associated with Sjögren syndrome

Electron Microscopy
- Interstitium rich in plasma cells
- Usually no detectable deposits in interstitium or TBM
- Variable glomerular pathology

DIFFERENTIAL DIAGNOSIS

Primary Sjögren Syndrome
- Clinical and serologic data required to discriminate

Sjögren Syndrome Secondary to Other Autoimmune Diseases
- Clinical and serologic data required to discriminate

Allergic or Other Causes of Tubulointerstitial Nephritis
- Lack of eosinophils argues against allergic etiology
- Absence of granulomas argues against sarcoidosis
- Lack of IgG4 deposits in TBM and few IgG4(+) plasma cells argue against IgG4-related systemic disease

DIAGNOSTIC CHECKLIST

Pathologic Interpretation Pearls
- If plasma cell-rich interstitial nephritis, think SS

SELECTED REFERENCES

1. Maripuri S et al: Renal involvement in primary Sjögren's syndrome: a clinicopathologic study. Clin J Am Soc Nephrol. 4(9):1423-31, 2009
2. Kaufman I et al: Sjögren's syndrome - not just Sicca: renal involvement in Sjögren's syndrome. Scand J Rheumatol. 37(3):213-8, 2008
3. Kim YK et al: Acquired Gitelman syndrome in a patient with primary Sjögren syndrome. Am J Kidney Dis. 52(6):1163-7, 2008
4. Ramos-Casals M et al: Primary Sjögren syndrome in Spain: clinical and immunologic expression in 1010 patients. Medicine (Baltimore). 87(4):210-9, 2008
5. Ren H et al: Renal involvement and followup of 130 patients with primary Sjögren's syndrome. J Rheumatol. 35(2):278-84, 2008
6. Aasarød K et al: Renal involvement in primary Sjögren's syndrome. QJM. 93(5):297-304, 2000
7. Winer RL et al: Sjögren's syndrome with immune-complex tubulointerstitial renal disease. Clin Immunol Immunopathol. 8(3):494-503, 1977

SJÖGREN SYNDROME

Microscopic Features

(Left) The interstitial infiltrate in Sjögren syndrome is broad, widely separating the renal tubules. This pattern of infiltration simulates a malignant lymphoma involving the kidney. The cytologic features of the infiltrate are usually sufficient to resolve any diagnostic concern. **(Right)** This infiltrate consists predominately of mature-appearing plasma cells ⊳. The tubules appear intact, but early interstitial fibrosis is present. One tubule ⊿ shows lymphocytic tubulitis.

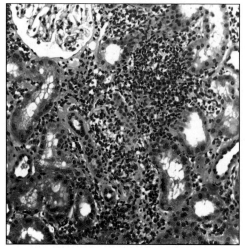
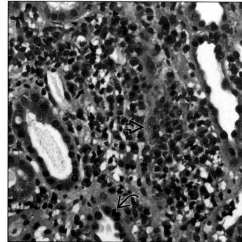

(Left) This is a renal biopsy in a patient with Sjögren syndrome. It shows a broad expanse of interstitial inflammation. The tubules are atrophic and contain protein casts. The infiltrating cells are primarily plasma cells. **(Right)** This renal biopsy in Sjögren syndrome contains tight clusters of interstitial plasma cells ⊿ with a few lymphocytes. There is mild interstitial fibrosis. Although most tubules are not atrophic, there are several small atrophic tubules present ⊿.

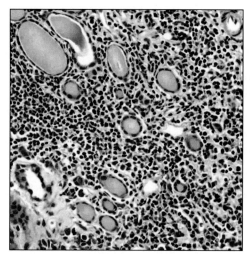
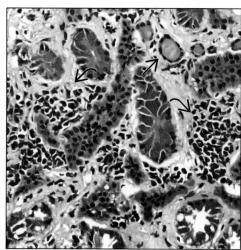

(Left) Tubulitis ⊿ is prominent in this biopsy from a 58-year-old woman with Sjögren syndrome. She also had finely granular interstitial deposits of IgG and positive Ro and La antibodies and ANA, but negative dsDNA. **(Right)** Tubulitis is present in this case. Although the interstitial infiltrate is primarily composed of plasma cells ⊳, the cells within the tubules are lymphocytes ⊿, likely T cells. There is interstitial expansion due to edema.

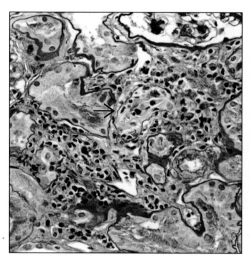
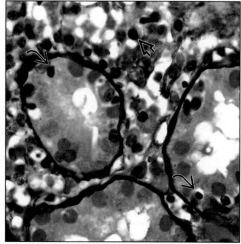

SJÖGREN SYNDROME

Immunofluorescence and Electron Microscopy

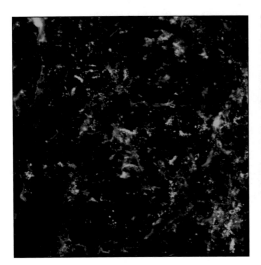
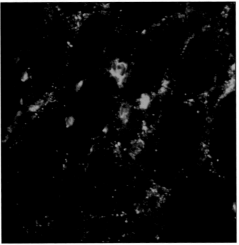

(Left) Immunofluorescence shows fine granular interstitial deposits of IgG in a patient with Sjögren syndrome without definitive evidence of lupus. This 58-year-old woman had a low complement and positive Ro and La antibodies and ANA, but negative dsDNA and no glomerular deposits. A minority of patients with Sjögren syndrome have such deposits. *(Right)* There are IgM granular interstitial deposits in this patient with Sjögren syndrome, mixed cryoglobulinemia and rheumatoid arthritis.

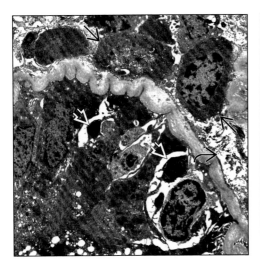
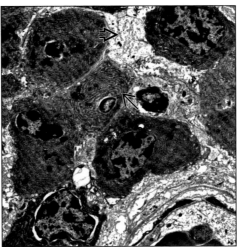

(Left) This tubule shows lymphocytic tubulitis. Notice that there are lymphocytes ⇒ on the inside of the tubular basement membrane and between tubular epithelial cells. The interstitium shows edema ⇒, and all of the interstitial cells are plasma cells ⇒. *(Right)* This electron micrograph shows interstitial edema ⇒ and a cluster of plasma cells. Plasma cells are distinctive because their cytoplasm is filled with rough endoplasmic reticulum ⇒.

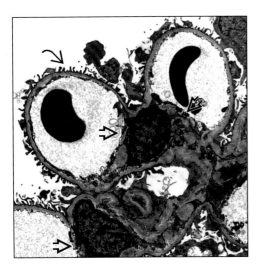
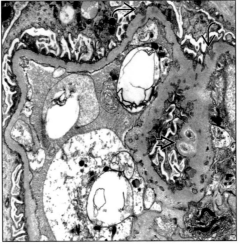

(Left) In most cases of Sjögren syndrome the glomerulus is normal, as shown in this case. There is preservation of the podocyte foot processes ⇒, no deposits, and the mesangium ⇒ is not expanded. *(Right)* Notice the scattered subepithelial deposits ⇒ in this slide from a patient with Sjögren syndrome. Some are undergoing reabsorption ⇒. This is an immune complex disease, perhaps a forme fruste of membranous glomerulonephritis occasionally seen in Sjögren syndrome.

4

IgG4-RELATED SYSTEMIC DISEASE

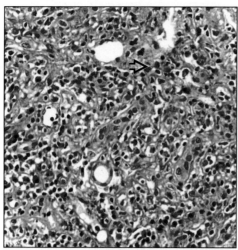

H&E shows IgG4-related systemic autoimmune disease (IgG4-RSD). A plasma cell-rich, expansile interstitial nephritis is characteristic with fibrosis and destruction of the tubules and scattered eosinophils ⊡.

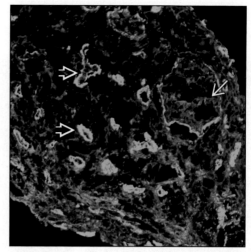

Immunofluorescence for IgG reveals granular tubular basement membrane and Bowman capsule deposits ⊡. Similar staining was seen for C3, kappa, and lambda. A glomerular tuft is negative ⊡.

TERMINOLOGY

Abbreviations
- IgG4-related tubulointerstitial nephritis (IgG4-TIN)

Synonyms
- IgG4-related systemic disease (IgG4-RSD)
- Autoimmune pancreatitis (AIP)-associated tubulointerstitial nephritis (TIN)

Definitions
- Autoimmune TIN with increased IgG4(+) plasma cells and often tubulointerstitial immune complex deposits; usually associated with systemic autoimmune inflammatory disease

ETIOLOGY/PATHOGENESIS

Systemic Autoimmune Disease
- Renal involvement by multiorgan IgG4-associated autoimmune immune complex disease

Proposed Autoantigens
- Plasminogen-binding protein (PBP) peptide
  - Homologue of PBP of *Helicobacter pylori* and of ubiquitin-protein ligase E3 component n-recognin 2, an enzyme expressed in pancreatic acinar cells
  - PBP peptide antibodies in 95% of patients with AIP
- Carbonic anhydrase-II and -IV
- Lactoferrin
- Pancreatic secretory trypsin inhibitor
- α-fodrin

IgG4 Distinctive Subclass
- Thought to serve as "anti-inflammatory" antibodies
- Weaker interchain disulfide bridges
  - IgG4 immunoglobulin half-molecules dissociate from each other, reassociate with other IgG4 half-molecules, including those with different antigen specificities

- Does not fix complement
  - May block antigen binding site for more pathogenic IgG1

Propensity to Form Pseudotumors
- May be due to production of anti-inflammatory cytokines, including IL-10, tumor necrosis factor-α, and fibrogenic IL-13, and resultant expansion of IgG4-secreting plasma cells

CLINICAL ISSUES

Presentation
- Renal mass(es), enlarged kidneys, or heterogeneous appearance on CT scan
- Acute or chronic renal failure
- Other organ involvement may be present concurrently, previously, or may present in future
  - Autoimmune pancreatitis (AIP)
  - Sclerosing cholangitis
  - Lymphoplasmacytic sclerosing cholecystitis
  - Inflammatory bowel disease
  - Sialadenitis/Mikulicz disease
  - Inflammatory aortic aneurysm
  - Retroperitoneal fibrosis
  - Lymph nodes
  - Inflammatory masses in liver, lung, breast, heart, prostate, pituitary, other organs
  - Skin rash
- Not all renal cases have evidence of other organ involvement

Laboratory Tests
- Eosinophilia in some patients (~ 30%)
- Hypergammaglobulinemia
  - Typically no monoclonal protein
- Elevated serum IgG4 or total IgG in ~ 80%
  - Elevated serum IgG4 present in 70-75% of AIP patients
- Hypocomplementemia (50%)

IgG4-RELATED SYSTEMIC DISEASE

Key Facts

Terminology

- Autoimmune TIN with increased IgG4(+) plasma cells and often tubulointerstitial immune complex deposits; usually associated with systemic autoimmune inflammatory disease

Etiology/Pathogenesis

- Autoimmune, autoantigen unknown
- IgG4 is an "anti-inflammatory" IgG subclass

Clinical Issues

- Renal mass(es)
- Acute or chronic renal failure
- Steroid-responsive
- Steroid therapy usually effective

Microscopic Pathology

- Plasma cell-rich interstitial inflammation

- Many plasma cells produce IgG4
  - Polyclonal
- Granular TBM immune complex deposits by IF
  - Contain IgG4, C3, kappa and lambda light chains
- Glomeruli negative by IF unless concurrent MGN
- Amorphous, electron-dense deposits within tubular basement membranes and in interstitium by EM

Top Differential Diagnoses

- Idiopathic hypocomplementemic interstitial nephritis with extensive tubulointerstitial deposits
- Sjögren syndrome
- Tubulointerstitial lupus nephritis
- Lymphoma or leukemia
- Inflammation may be misinterpreted as nondiagnostic in biopsy taken for "mass"

Treatment

- Drugs
  - Steroids
    - Most cases very sensitive to steroid therapy
    - Steroid responsiveness is one diagnostic criterion for AIP
    - Despite steroid responsiveness, high rate of relapse in AIP patients
  - Rituximab
    - Anti-CD20 drug has been used with success in some cases of AIP
  - Mycophenolate mofetil
    - Has been used with steroids in some TIN cases

IMAGE FINDINGS

CT Findings

- Single or multiple low-attenuation lesions, usually bilateral, in renal cortex
- Findings suggestive of vasculitis or lymphoma
- Inflammatory lesions may extend beyond kidney
- Masses in other organs (e.g., pancreas, liver, lung) may give clue to renal diagnosis

MICROSCOPIC PATHOLOGY

Histologic Features

- Plasma cell-rich interstitial inflammation
  - Eosinophils often present and may be prominent
- Interstitial fibroinflammatory process, expansile interstitial fibrosis
- Tubular atrophy and destruction of tubules by interstitial fibrosis
- Thickened tubular basement membranes
- Membranous glomerulonephritis (MGN) present in a subset of cases
  - ~ 8% of cases in one series showed MGN
  - MGN deposits are also IgG4-dominant
- Range of appearances

  - Some cases show more interstitial inflammation and less fibrosis
  - Other cases show more sclerosis and less inflammation
    - Cases with less inflammation often show fewer IgG4(+) plasma cells, but still > 10/HPF in the most concentrated areas
- Fibroinflammatory process may extend outside of kidney and involve surrounding organs

ANCILLARY TESTS

Immunohistochemistry

- Increased IgG4(+) plasma cells
  - At least moderate increase: > 10 IgG4(+) cells/40x field in most concentrated area
  - Some cases show marked increase, > 30 IgG4(+) cells/40x field
  - IgG4 staining ~ 100% sensitive and ~ 92% specific for detecting TIN related to IgG4(+) TIN vs. other types of plasma cell-rich interstitial nephritis
    - False-positives in interstitial infiltrate associated with pauci-immune necrotizing and crescentic glomerulonephritis

Immunofluorescence

- Granular tubular basement membrane (TBM) immune complex deposits in > 80% of cases
  - IgG, C3, kappa and lambda light chains; rarely dim accompanying IgM &/or C1q
  - IgG4(+) deposits; other IgG subclasses also present in varying degrees
  - Deposits may be focal; present in most but not all cases
- Granular interstitial deposits may be present
- Glomeruli usually negative by IF unless concurrent MGN
  - Rare cases of concurrent IgA nephropathy or membranoproliferative glomerulonephritis with IgG4-RSD

IgG4-RELATED SYSTEMIC DISEASE

Electron Microscopy
- Amorphous electron-dense deposits within tubular basement membranes and in interstitium
- Thickened and laminated TBM
- Normal glomeruli unless concurrent MGN

DIFFERENTIAL DIAGNOSIS

Idiopathic Hypocomplementemic Interstitial Nephritis with Extensive Tubulointerstitial Deposits
- Some cases may represent disease in spectrum of IgG4-RSD and show increased IgG4(+) plasma cells
- Not part of systemic autoimmune disease

Sjögren Syndrome-associated Tubulointerstitial Nephritis
- May be related to IgG4-associated autoimmune disease
- Usually no increase in IgG4(+) plasma cells
- Tubulointerstitial immune complex deposits

Giant Cell Tubulitis with Tubular Basement Membrane Immune Deposits
- May represent allergic drug reaction
- Giant cells in tubules
- TBM deposits

Tubulointerstitial Lupus Nephritis
- Usually glomerular disease with immune deposits along with TBM or interstitial immune deposits
- Lupus serologies positive, nonrenal lupus involvement

Chronic Pyelonephritis
- May have appearance of mass on imaging studies
- Neutrophils in infiltrate
- Evidence of urinary tract bacterial infection

Pauci-immune Necrotizing and Crescentic Glomerulonephritis
- Granulomatosis with polyangiitis (Wegener) may be mass-forming
- 25% of cases show at least moderate increase in IgG4(+) plasma cells in interstitial infiltrate
- Areas of necrosis in interstitial infiltrate may be present in granulomatosis with polyangiitis (Wegener)
  ○ Necrosis not present in IgG4-associated TIN
- Most cases ANCA(+)
- Absence of tubulointerstitial immune complex deposits

Lymphoma or Leukemia
- May be mass-forming on radiographic studies
- Atypical and monotypic cellular infiltrate
- Rare cases show TBM immune complex deposits by IF
- Immunohistochemical studies can confirm monoclonal infiltrate

Interstitial Inflammation with TBM Deposits Associated with Glomerular Disease
- Minority of cases of MGN or other immune complex GN show TBM immune complex deposits

Monoclonal Immunoglobulin Deposition Disease
- Linear vs. granular TBM deposits
- Monoclonal immune deposits by IF

Renal Neoplasm
- Imaging studies often suggest neoplasm
- Inflammation may be misinterpreted

DIAGNOSTIC CHECKLIST

Pathologic Interpretation Pearls
- Needle biopsy sometimes performed for renal mass
- Inflammatory process may be mistaken for reaction around tumor, and specimen considered inadequate for diagnosis

SELECTED REFERENCES

1. Raissian Y et al: Diagnosis of IgG4-related tubulointerstitial nephritis. J Am Soc Nephrol. In press, 2011
2. Saeki T et al: Clinicopathological characteristics of patients with IgG4-related tubulointerstitial nephritis. Kidney Int. 78(10):1016-23, 2010
3. Aalberse RC et al: Immunoglobulin G4: an odd antibody. Clin Exp Allergy. 39(4):469-77, 2009
4. Frulloni L et al: Identification of a novel antibody associated with autoimmune pancreatitis. N Engl J Med. 361(22):2135-42, 2009
5. Cornell LD et al: Pseudotumors due to IgG4 immune-complex tubulointerstitial nephritis associated with autoimmune pancreatocentric disease. Am J Surg Pathol. 31(10):1586-97, 2007
6. Deshpande V et al: Autoimmune pancreatitis: a systemic immune complex mediated disease. Am J Surg Pathol. 2006 Dec;30(12):1537-45. Erratum in: Am J Surg Pathol. 31(2):328, 2007
7. Ghazale A et al: Value of serum IgG4 in the diagnosis of autoimmune pancreatitis and in distinguishing it from pancreatic cancer. Am J Gastroenterol. 102(8):1646-53, 2007
8. Zhang L et al: IgG4-positive plasma cell infiltration in the diagnosis of autoimmune pancreatitis. Mod Pathol. 20(1):23-8, 2007
9. Chari ST et al: Diagnosis of autoimmune pancreatitis: the Mayo Clinic experience. Clin Gastroenterol Hepatol. 4(8):1010-6; quiz 934, 2006
10. Deshpande V et al: Autoimmune pancreatitis: more than just a pancreatic disease? A contemporary review of its pathology. Arch Pathol Lab Med. 129(9):1148-54, 2005
11. Aalberse RC et al: IgG4 breaking the rules. Immunology. 105(1):9-19, 2002
12. Kambham N et al: Idiopathic hypocomplementemic interstitial nephritis with extensive tubulointerstitial deposits. Am J Kidney Dis. 37(2):388-99, 2001

IgG4-RELATED SYSTEMIC DISEASE

Light Microscopy

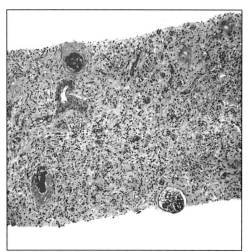

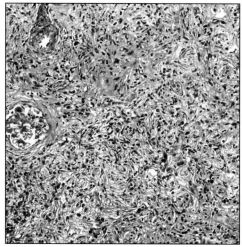

(Left) This biopsy came from a 72-year-old man with chronic renal failure and heterogeneous renal masses; he had elevated serum IgG levels and a history of primary biliary cirrhosis. The biopsy reveals a diffuse, expansile interstitial nephritis within the cortex. In this case, the inflammation accounts for the renal masses. *(Right)* A trichrome stain reveals extensive interstitial fibrosis, which was present diffusely throughout the cortex, and profound loss of tubules.

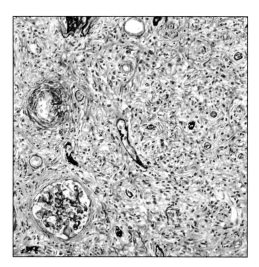

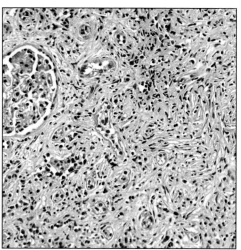

(Left) A silver stain nicely highlights the residual basement membranes of destroyed tubules. Glomeruli show only secondary changes of periglomerular fibrosis and global glomerulosclerosis. *(Right)* This case of IgG4-RSD has a more sclerotic, less cellular fibroinflammatory pattern, probably representing a late stage in the disease.

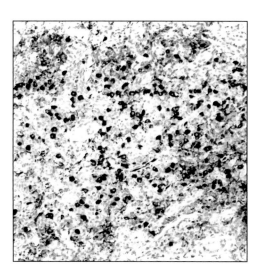

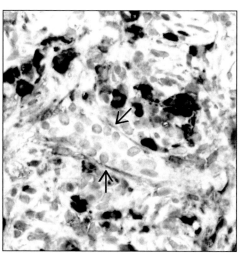

(Left) An immunohistochemical stain for IgG4 reveals numerous (> 30/HPF) IgG4-positive plasma cells, a feature that distinguishes IgG4-RSD from other types of TIN. *(Right)* Tubular basement membrane granular deposits ⇨ can be seen in this IgG4 immunohistochemical stain. The densely stained cells are plasma cells.

IgG4-RELATED SYSTEMIC DISEASE

Immunofluorescence

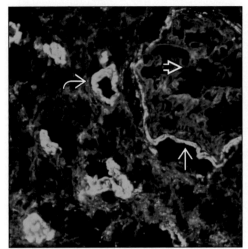 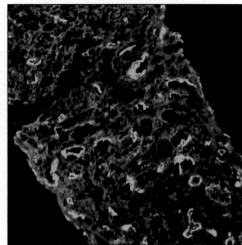

(Left) Immunofluorescence for IgG reveals granular TBM staining ⮕ in a case of IgG4-TIN. A glomerular tuft is negative for IgG ⮞ but shows granular staining of Bowman capsule ⮕. *(Right)* Tubular basement membrane granular staining for C3 is also present, but it was less bright than for IgG in this case of IgG4-RSD.

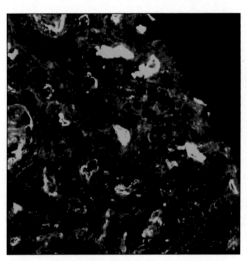 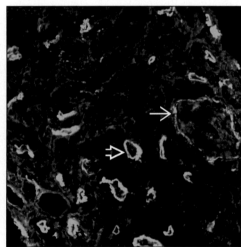

(Left) Immunofluorescence for kappa light chain shows the same staining pattern as IgG, with granular tubular basement membrane staining, and was equal to lambda staining. *(Right)* Immunofluorescence for lambda light chain shows the same staining pattern as IgG and kappa light chain ⮞. Note the glomerulus that shows Bowman capsule staining but no glomerular tuft staining ⮕.

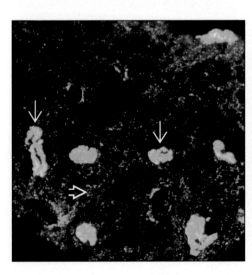 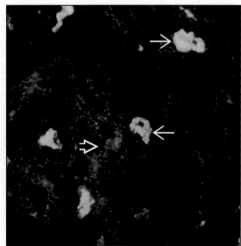

(Left) Immunofluorescence staining for IgG subclasses revealed granular TBM ⮕ and interstitial ⮞ staining for all 4 subclasses, with brightest staining for IgG4. IgG4 is usually the least common subclass of IgG, typically < 5% of circulating IgG. *(Right)* Immunofluorescence for IgG1 reveals positive granular staining of TBMs ⮕ and granular interstitial ⮞ staining, to a lesser degree than IgG4.

IgG4-RELATED SYSTEMIC DISEASE

Electron Microscopy

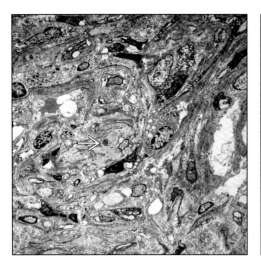

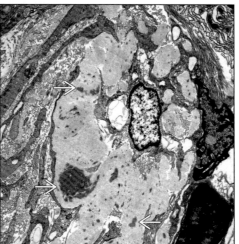

(Left) Electron microscopy reveals interstitial leukocytes, increased collagen deposition in the interstitium, and a few residual tubular basement membranes containing immune deposits ➡. *(Right)* On higher magnification, a ruptured tubular basement membrane of a destroyed tubule can be seen. Immune deposits are present within this tubular basement membrane ➡.

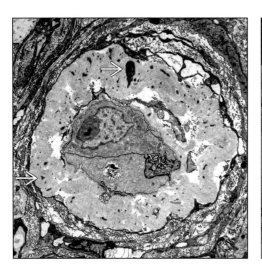

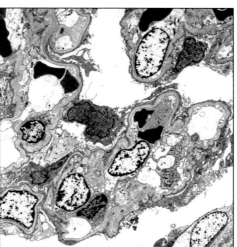

(Left) This residual destroyed tubule shows a markedly thickened basement membrane that contains electron-dense immune deposits ➡. *(Right)* IgG4-RSD is shown. Glomeruli usually do not show immune deposits. Rare cases of IgG4-associated tubulointerstitial nephritis have been associated with membranous glomerulonephritis.

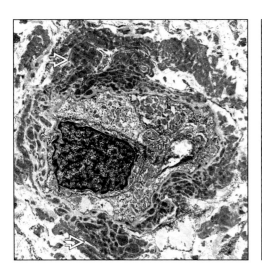

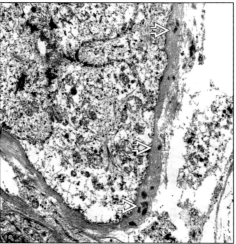

(Left) Massive immune deposits ➡ within and surrounding a tubular basement membrane are evident in this case and were seen in trichrome stains by light microscopy. *(Right)* EM performed on a pancreas specimen in a patient with autoimmune pancreatitis/systemic IgG4-associated autoimmune disease is shown. Electron-dense, immune-type deposits are seen within a basement membrane ➡, analogous to what is seen in tubular basement membranes of the kidney.

IDIOPATHIC HYPOCOMPLEMENTEMIC TUBULOINTERSTITIAL NEPHRITIS

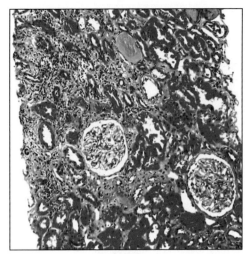

Idiopathic hypocomplementemic interstitial nephritis with extensive tubulointerstitial deposits (HTIN) shows prominent interstitial inflammation with fibrosis. The glomeruli are normal.

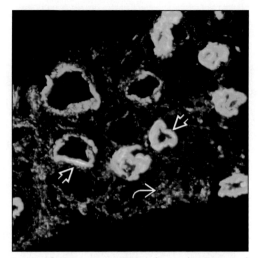

Immunofluorescence in HTIN shows distinctive and prominent granular tubular basement membrane ➡ and finely granular interstitial ➤ deposits that stain for IgG and usually C3 and C1q.

TERMINOLOGY

Abbreviations
- Hypocomplementemic tubulointerstitial nephritis (HTIN)

Synonyms
- Idiopathic hypocomplementemic tubulointerstitial nephritis with extensive tubulointerstitial deposits
- Kambham disease

Definitions
- Tubulointerstitial nephritis with polyclonal tubular basement membrane (TBM) deposits and hypocomplementemia

ETIOLOGY/PATHOGENESIS

Antibody Deposition in TBM
- Immune complexes formed, probably locally
  o Antigen unknown
- Local complement fixation
  o Promotion of inflammation, tubular injury

Animal Model: Heymann Nephritis
- Immunization with tubular cell components (Fx1a)
- Immune complex deposition in TBM and GBM

CLINICAL ISSUES

Epidemiology
- Age
  o Average ~ 65 years
- Gender
  o Male predominance (M:F = 7:1 in 1 series)

Presentation
- Renal dysfunction
- No significant proteinuria or hematuria

- No history of Sjögren syndrome or SLE
- Hypocomplementemia

Laboratory Tests
- Low serum complement levels
- Negative ANA or low-titer positive ANA

Treatment
- Drugs
  o May respond to prednisone
  o Reported case of subacute renal failure reversed with mycophenolate mofetil and corticosteroids

Prognosis
- Usual improvement of serum creatinine with immunosuppressive therapy

IMAGE FINDINGS

Radiographic Findings
- No cases reported to be mass forming, in contrast to IgG4-associated TIN

MICROSCOPIC PATHOLOGY

Histologic Features
- Glomeruli
  o No specific findings
  o May have secondary glomerulosclerosis in advanced cases
- Tubules
  o Tubulitis, mononuclear
  o Thickened TBM
  o Destruction and atrophy of tubules in advanced cases
- Interstitium
  o Marked mononuclear inflammation
    ▪ Polytypic infiltrate
    ▪ T cells, B cells, plasma cells

IDIOPATHIC HYPOCOMPLEMENTEMIC TUBULOINTERSTITIAL NEPHRITIS

Key Facts

Clinical Issues
- Renal dysfunction with little proteinuria
- No history of Sjögren syndrome or SLE
- Low serum complement levels
- Negative or low-titer positive ANA

Microscopic Pathology
- Prominent tubulointerstitial nephritis
  - Lymphocytes, plasma cells, and sometimes eosinophils
- Destruction of tubules and interstitial fibrosis
- Glomeruli relatively spared

Ancillary Tests
- Granular TBM and interstitial deposits of IgG and C3
  - IgG in all cases; often C3 deposits
  - IgE(+) TBM deposits may be present
- Kappa and lambda equal
- Glomeruli usually negative
- TBM and interstitial deposits by EM
  - Usually amorphous; few cases with fingerprint substructure
  - No glomerular deposits

Top Differential Diagnoses
- IgG4-related tubulointerstitial nephritis
- Sjögren syndrome
- Lupus nephritis
- Monoclonal immunoglobulin deposition disease
- Giant cell tubulitis with TBM immune deposits
- Anti-TBM nephritis
- TIN associated with glomerular disease

- Lymphocytes may appear atypical, suggesting extranodal marginal zone B-cell lymphoma
- Eosinophils sometimes present

ANCILLARY TESTS

Immunofluorescence
- Granular TBM and interstitial deposits of immunoglobulin and complement components
  - IgG and complement in all cases; usually C3 and C1q
  - Variable staining for IgM; rare staining for IgA
  - IgE(+) TBM deposits may be present
  - Kappa and lambda equal
- Glomeruli sometimes have mesangial deposits with same reactants

Molecular Genetics
- B cells and T cells usually polyclonal
- 1 case with clonal B cells

Electron Microscopy
- TBM and interstitial immune complex deposits
  - Usually amorphous; few cases with fingerprint substructure
- Endothelial tuboreticular inclusions rare (1 case)
- No glomerular deposits

DIFFERENTIAL DIAGNOSIS

IgG4-related Tubulointerstitial Nephritis
- Systemic disease: Autoimmune pancreatitis, sclerosing cholangitis, inflammatory mass lesions in other organs
  - May be mass forming on radiographic studies
- Increased IgG4(+) plasma cells in infiltrate
- Elevated serum IgG4
- May also have hypocomplementemia
  - May be related to HTIN

Sjögren Syndrome
- Patients may also show hypocomplementemia and tubulointerstitial immune complex deposits

Giant Cell Tubulitis with Tubular Basement Membrane Immune Deposits
- Multinucleated giant cells surrounding tubules

Lupus Nephritis
- Very rare cases of lupus TIN have no glomerular immune complex deposits

Monoclonal Immunoglobulin Deposition Disease
- Linear TBM staining by IF of single light chain type
- Distinctive finely granular deposits by electron microscopy

Anti-TBM Nephritis
- Linear polyclonal TBM immunoglobulin deposits

TIN Associated with Glomerular Disease
- Rare cases of membranoproliferative glomerulonephritis, membranous glomerulonephritis, and other glomerular diseases may show TBM deposits

SELECTED REFERENCES

1. Cornell LD et al: Pseudotumors due to IgG4 immune-complex tubulointerstitial nephritis associated with autoimmune pancreatocentric disease. Am J Surg Pathol. 31(10):1586-97, 2007
2. Vaseemuddin M et al: Idiopathic hypocomplementemic immune-complex-mediated tubulointerstitial nephritis. Nat Clin Pract Nephrol. 3(1):50-8, 2007
3. Mihindukulasuriya JC et al: Idiopathic hypocomplementemic interstitial nephritis with extensive tubulointerstitial deposits: Reversal of subacute renal failure with mycophenolate mofetil and corticosteroids [Abstract]. J Am Soc Nephrol 14: 800A, 2003
4. Kambham N et al: Idiopathic hypocomplementemic interstitial nephritis with extensive tubulointerstitial deposits. Am J Kidney Dis. 37(2):388-99, 2001
5. Tokumoto M et al: Acute interstitial nephritis with immune complex deposition and MHC class II antigen presentation along the tubular basement membrane. Nephrol Dial Transplant. 14(9):2210-5, 1999

4

IDIOPATHIC HYPOCOMPLEMENTEMIC TUBULOINTERSTITIAL NEPHRITIS

Light Microscopy

(Left) Advanced cases of HTIN show extensive interstitial fibrosis, tubular destruction and atrophy, and global glomerulosclerosis, along with interstitial inflammation. *(Right)* The predominant lesion in HTIN is focal interstitial inflammation ⊳ with tubular damage and fibrosis; glomeruli are relatively spared. This specimen is from a 69-year-old man who had progressive chronic renal failure, a low-titer ANA, and no clinical evidence of liver disease, pancreatitis, or systemic lupus.

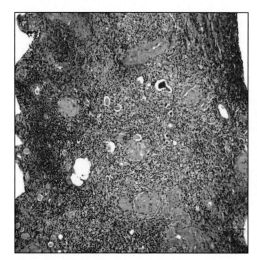
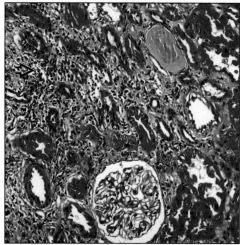

(Left) In HTIN, a trichrome stain highlights the interstitial fibrosis, areas of which show inflammation and tubular destruction. Remnants of tubules are evident ⊡. *(Right)* In HTIN, the infiltrate is composed of mononuclear cells, a few eosinophils, and plasma cells. Tubulitis is present ⊡, and there is extensive destruction of tubules, leaving residual structures ⊡.

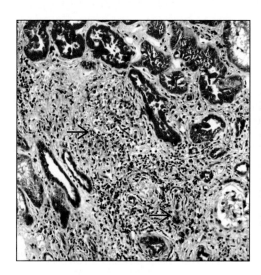
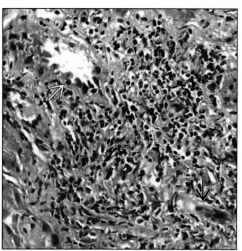

(Left) The infiltrate is composed mostly of CD3(+) T cells, here seen at low power. The glomerulus stands out as a negative area ⊡. *(Right)* Many CD20(+) B cells are also present in HTIN. Stains for kappa and lambda light chains revealed polytypic plasma cells.

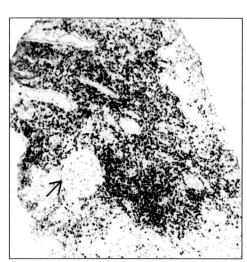
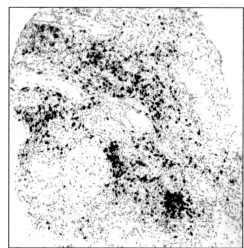

IDIOPATHIC HYPOCOMPLEMENTEMIC TUBULOINTERSTITIAL NEPHRITIS

Immunofluorescence and Electron Microscopy

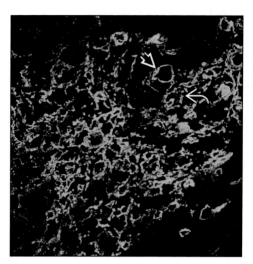

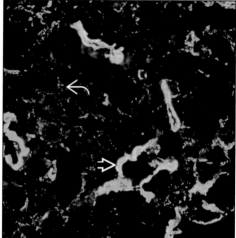

(Left) Immunofluorescence staining for IgG in HTIN reveals prominent granular tubular basement membrane ⇨ and interstitial deposits ➘. *(Right)* Granular tubular basement membrane ⇨ and interstitial ➚ deposits for IgG are seen in HTIN. Similar staining was seen for C1q, C3, and kappa and lambda light chains. The glomeruli were negative by immunofluorescence. The TBM deposits appear coarse and confluent.

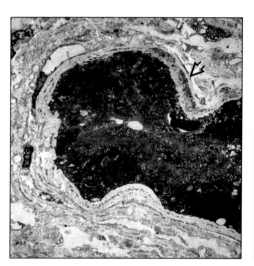

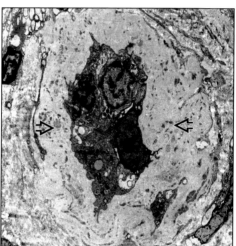

(Left) By electron microscopy, the tubular basement membranes are thickened and duplicated. Electron-dense, immune-type deposits are widespread in the TBM ⇨. *(Right)* A thickened tubular basement membrane contains immune deposits ⇨. The tubule is markedly damaged and likely nonfunctional. The process probably evolves over time with recurrent episodes of deposits and repair.

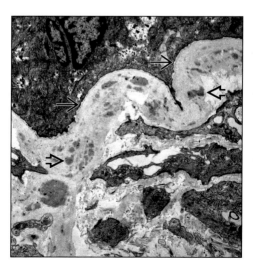

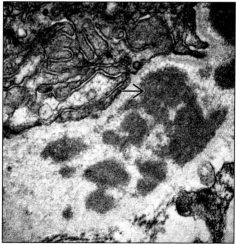

(Left) At high power by electron microscopy, immune complex deposits ⇨ are present within a thickened tubular basement membrane. A thin layer of newly formed TBM ⇨ is present under the tubular epithelial cells, probably in response to the injury mediated by the deposits. *(Right)* On high magnification, the deposits ⇨ are amorphous and lack substructure, typical of immune complex deposits. Occasional cases with a "fingerprint" pattern have been described.

ANTI-TUBULAR BASEMENT MEMBRANE DISEASE

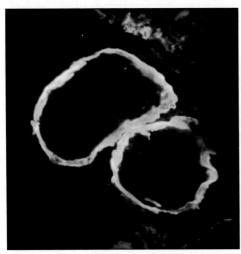

Linear staining of the proximal tubular basement membrane (TBM) is the 1st clue that anti-TBM antibodies are present. This case was associated with methicillin interstitial nephritis.

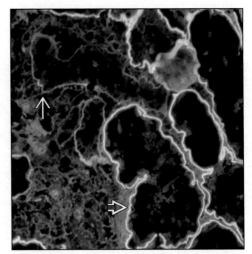

Anti-TBM disease de novo in a renal transplant. Note linear staining of IgG in the proximal TBMs ⮞. Distal TBMs ➡ are negative, presumably due to lack of the TBM antigen in the recipient. (Courtesy V. Pardo, MD.)

TERMINOLOGY

Abbreviations
- Anti-TBM (aTBM) disease

Definitions
- Renal disease caused by autoantibodies to the tubular basement membrane (TBM); antibodies arise as primary or secondary event

ETIOLOGY/PATHOGENESIS

Antibody-mediated Disease
- TBM antigen (TIN antigen)
  - Expressed only in kidneys (adult and fetal)
    - Chromosome 6p11.2-12
    - Homologies to follistatin, agrin, osteonectin/ SPARC; laminin-α1, vitronectin; cathepsin family of cysteine proteases
  - Noncollagenous 54-58 Kd protein in proximal tubular basement membranes
  - Regulates tubulogenesis
    - Interacts with type IV collagen, laminin, and integrins
    - Reduced or absent expression in some cases of juvenile nephronophthisis

Conditions in Which Anti-TBM Antibodies Arise
- Primary diseases
  - Idiopathic tubulointerstitial nephritis
  - Membranous glomerulonephritis (MGN) in children, familial
- Secondary to other renal diseases
  - Drug-induced tubulointerstitial nephritis
    - Antibiotics
  - Aristolochic acid (Chinese herb nephropathy)
  - Kimura disease
  - Oxalosis post-jejunal-ileal bypass

- Renal allografts
  - Alloantibodies to TBM may arise in transplant setting
    - Presumably due to lack of TBM alloantigen in recipient

Cell-mediated Component
- Mononuclear cells likely contribute to damage

Animal Models
- Strain 13 guinea pigs immunized with autologous TBM
  - Develop interstitial nephritis over several weeks
    - Anti-TBM antibodies
    - Prominent giant cell reaction (macrophages) around tubules
- Transplantation aTBM disease
  - Fisher 344 kidney to Lewis rat
    - Lewis rats lack TBM antigen, develop aTBM disease in graft

CLINICAL ISSUES

Presentation
- Polyuria
- Polydipsia
- Chronic renal failure
- Microhematuria
- Proteinuria
  - Nephrotic in some
    - Associated with MGN

Treatment
- Steroids often used
- Stop drug use if disease is drug associated

Prognosis
- Outcome uncertain; cases rare
- Can lead to renal failure

ANTI-TUBULAR BASEMENT MEMBRANE DISEASE

Key Facts

Etiology/Pathogenesis
- Primary idiopathic disease (rare)
  - Familial MGN anti-TBM syndrome
- Associated with other diseases
  - Drug-induced tubulointerstitial nephritis
  - Renal allograft rejection

Clinical Issues
- Chronic renal failure
- Polyuria, polydipsia, proteinuria

Microscopic Pathology
- Mononuclear infiltrate, rarely giant cells
- Tubulitis
- Tubular atrophy and fibrosis

Ancillary Tests
- Linear staining of proximal TBM for IgG and C3

Diagnostic Checklist
- Requires demonstrating serum anti-TBM antibodies

MICROSCOPIC PATHOLOGY

Histologic Features
- Glomeruli normal, unless other disease
- Tubules
  - Tubulitis
  - Atrophy
  - Destruction of TBM on PAS stains
- Interstitium
  - Mononuclear infiltrate
    - T cells, macrophages
    - Eosinophils usual in setting of drug-induced interstitial nephritis
    - Fibrosis
    - Rarely giant cells
- Vessels have no specific changes

ANCILLARY TESTS

Immunofluorescence
- Linear staining of proximal tubules for IgG and C3
  - Occasionally other reactants, IgA, C4, IgM
- No glomerular staining unless superimposed on glomerular disease (such as MGN)
- Test serum for anti-TBM activity by indirect immunofluorescence (IF)
  - Reacts with normal proximal TBM, not GBM or distal tubules
  - Anti-type IV collagen antibodies in Goodpasture syndrome that react with GBM and distal TBM

DIAGNOSTIC CHECKLIST

Pathologic Interpretation Pearls
- Requires linear IgG along TBM: C3 alone is present commonly in TBM as nonspecific finding
- Must demonstrate anti-TBM activity in serum (indirect IF with normal kidney)

SELECTED REFERENCES

1. Dixit MP et al: Kimura disease with advanced renal damage with anti-tubular basement membrane antibody. Pediatr Nephrol. 19(12):1404-7, 2004
2. Iványi B et al: Childhood membranous nephropathy, circulating antibodies to the 58-kD TIN antigen, and anti-tubular basement membrane nephritis: an 11-year follow-up. Am J Kidney Dis. 32(6):1068-74, 1998
3. Clayman MD et al: Isolation and characterization of the nephritogenic antigen producing anti-tubular basement membrane disease. J Exp Med. 161(2):290-305, 1985
4. Hyman LR et al: Immunopathogenesis of autoimmune tubulointerstitial nephritis. II. Role of an immune response gene linked to the major histocompatibility complex. J Immunol. 117(5 Pt, 1976
5. Bergstein J et al: Interstitial nephritis with anti-tubular-basement-membrane antibody. N Engl J Med. 292(17):875-8, 1975

IMAGE GALLERY

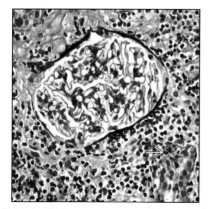 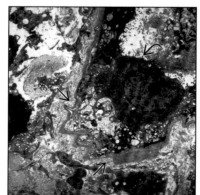 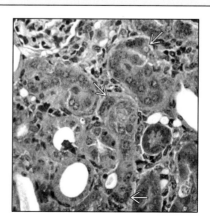

(Left) Methicillin hypersensitivity with aTBM antibodies is shown. An extensive infiltrate is present, which focally invades the tubules ➡. *(Center)* The TBM ➡ is disrupted, frayed, and laminated in this anti-TBM disease associated with methicillin hypersensitivity. An injured, reactive tubular epithelial cell is detached from the TBM ➡ (EM). *(Right)* Image shows mononuclear giant cells ➡ surrounding tubules in aTBM disease in a guinea pig (this is rarely seen in humans).

SARCOIDOSIS

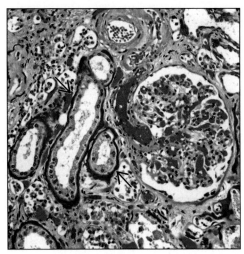

Sarcoidosis is often associated with hypercalcemia, which may cause azotemia, tubular dysfunction with polyuria, or rarely, nephrocalcinosis with calcification of nephron basement membranes ➡.

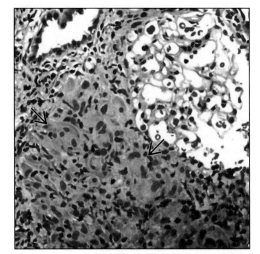

Renal involvement in sarcoidosis is often characterized by well-defined noncaseating granulomas. This granuloma is composed of epithelioid histiocytes, lymphocytes, and multinucleated giant cells ➡.

TERMINOLOGY

Definitions
- Systemic granulomatous disease

ETIOLOGY/PATHOGENESIS

Etiology Unclear
- Possibly multifactorial
  - Disordered immune regulation affecting T cells and histiocytes leading to tissue injury
  - Inflammatory cytokines stimulate synthesis of 1,25 OH vitamin-D3 leading to hypercalcemia
  - Genetic susceptibility &/or environmental factors

CLINICAL ISSUES

Epidemiology
- Incidence
  - 1-40 per 100,000 population
- Age
  - Most common in 2nd-4th decades
- Gender
  - More common in males than females
- Ethnicity
  - 3.5-10x higher in African-Americans than whites

Presentation
- Nonspecific systemic symptoms
  - Lymphadenopathy
  - Cough, dyspnea, fever
- Renal involvement in 15-45% of patients
  - Tubular dysfunction due to hypercalcemia
    - Urine concentration defect with polyuria
  - Acute or chronic renal failure
  - Hydronephrosis from retroperitoneal lymphadenopathy

Laboratory Tests
- Hypercalcemia (50-60%)
- Elevated angiotensin-converting enzyme (ACE) level
- Azotemia
- Hematuria &/or proteinuria, low grade to nephrotic

Treatment
- Drugs
  - Steroids

Prognosis
- Usually good, most patients respond to steroids
  - Worse outcome in African-Americans and elderly
- Recurrent or resistant disease
  - Acute or chronic renal failure
  - Death

IMAGE FINDINGS

Radiographic Findings
- Mediastinal lymphadenopathy

MACROSCOPIC FEATURES

General Features
- Renal enlargement
  - Severe tubulointerstitial nephritis with edema
  - Hydronephrosis from retroperitoneal lymphadenopathy

MICROSCOPIC PATHOLOGY

Histologic Features
- Noncaseating granulomatous tubulointerstitial nephritis
  - Well-formed, sharply defined granulomas
    - Epithelioid histiocytes and giant cells
    - Schaumann bodies (intracellular calcific bodies)

SARCOIDOSIS

Key Facts

Etiology/Pathogenesis
- Unclear etiology; disordered immune regulation
- Renal dysfunction related to nature and extent of involvement

Clinical Issues
- More common in African-Americans than whites
- Involves multiple organs
- Isolated renal sarcoidosis rarely occurs
- Elevated calcium and ACE levels help diagnosis

Image Findings
- Hilar lymphadenopathy

Macroscopic Features
- Usually unremarkable

Microscopic Pathology
- Well-formed noncaseating granulomas
- Interstitial fibrosis in chronic recurrent renal sarcoidosis
- Glomerulonephritis rarely occurs

Top Differential Diagnoses
- Allergic (drug-induced) tubulointerstitial nephritis
  - Most common
  - Granulomas less distinct, often with eosinophils
- Granulomatous infections
  - Caseation may be present
  - Special stains for organisms required
- Granulomatous vasculitis
  - Granulomatosis with polyangiitis (Wegener)
  - Giant cell arteritis

- Active interstitial inflammation
  - Lymphoplasmacytic infiltrate
  - Tubular injury and interstitial edema
  - Eosinophils rare
- Tubular atrophy and interstitial fibrosis, if recurrent or resistant to therapy
- Nephrocalcinosis
  - Tubular basement membrane calcification
  - Tubular epithelial cell calcification
- A variety of glomerulonephritides reported
  - Membranous glomerulonephritis is most common
  - Focal segmental glomerulosclerosis
  - IgA nephropathy

ANCILLARY TESTS

Immunofluorescence
- Negative or nonspecific reactions
  - IgM, C3 in mesangium due to nonspecific trapping

Electron Microscopy
- Normal glomeruli without immune complex deposits

DIFFERENTIAL DIAGNOSIS

Granulomatous Allergic Reaction (Most Common)
- Granulomas less distinct
- Eosinophils more numerous

Granulomatous Infections
- Acid-fast infection
- Fungal infection

Granulomatous Angiitis
- Granulomatosis with polyangiitis (Wegener)
- Giant cell arteritis

DIAGNOSTIC CHECKLIST

Pathologic Interpretation Pearls
- Noncaseating granulomas: Think drugs and sarcoidosis
  - Rule out infection and systemic vasculitis

SELECTED REFERENCES

1. Mahévas M et al: Renal sarcoidosis: clinical, laboratory, and histologic presentation and outcome in 47 patients. Medicine (Baltimore). 88(2):98-106, 2009
2. Monge M et al: Sarcoidosis and the kidney: not only the granulomatous interstitial nephritis. Clin Nephrol. 71(2):192-5, 2009
3. Saeed A et al: Sarcoidosis presenting with severe hypocalcaemia. Ir J Med Sci. Epub ahead of print, 2009
4. Hawrot-Kawecka A et al: Acute renal failure as the first extrapulmonary presentation of sarcoidosis. Intern Med. 47(24):2201; author reply 2203, 2008
5. Mayer C et al: Isolated renal relapse of sarcoidosis under low-dose glucocorticoid therapy. J Gen Intern Med. 23(6):879-82, 2008
6. Shetty AK et al: Childhood sarcoidosis: A rare but fascinating disorder. Pediatr Rheumatol Online J. 6:16, 2008
7. Javaud N et al: Renal granulomatoses: a retrospective study of 40 cases and review of the literature. Medicine (Baltimore). 86(3):170-80, 2007
8. Joss N et al: Granulomatous interstitial nephritis. Clin J Am Soc Nephrol. 2(2):222-30, 2007
9. Rybicki BA et al: Genetic linkage analysis of sarcoidosis phenotypes: the sarcoidosis genetic analysis (SAGA) study. Genes Immun. 8(5):379-86, 2007
10. Darabi K et al: Nephrolithiasis as primary symptom in sarcoidosis. Scand J Urol Nephrol. 39(2):173-5, 2005
11. Thumfart J et al: Isolated sarcoid granulomatous interstitial nephritis responding to infliximab therapy. Am J Kidney Dis. 45(2):411-4, 2005
12. Bergner R et al: Frequency of kidney disease in chronic sarcoidosis. Sarcoidosis Vasc Diffuse Lung Dis. 20(2):126-32, 2003
13. Asakura K: Renal involvement in sarcoidosis. Intern Med. 41(12):1088-9, 2002

4

Microscopic Features in Renal Sarcoidosis

(Left) Renal sarcoidosis often shows granulomatous interstitial nephritis with multinucleated giant cells ⇥. Note the Schaumann body ⇥. The granulomatous inflammation is destructive and replaces a large portion of the interstitial compartment. (Right) This granuloma is composed of histiocytes without multinucleated giant cells. Numerous lymphocytes are present but no eosinophils are identified. The discrete granuloma and lack of eosinophils make an allergic reaction unlikely.

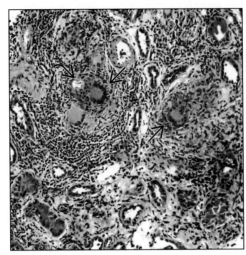
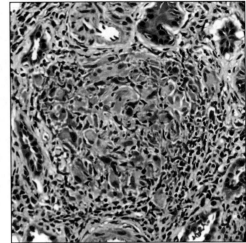

(Left) This granuloma, composed of histiocytes and lymphocytes, was present in a nephrectomy performed for a renal neoplasm. The cells ⇥ above the granuloma are tumor cells and the tumor is a benign oncocytoma. (Right) Noncaseating granulomatous inflammation is not pathognomonic of sarcoidosis. However, the presence of a Schaumann body (intracytoplasmic laminated &/or centrally calcified body) ⇥ within a giant cell greatly increases the likelihood of sarcoidosis.

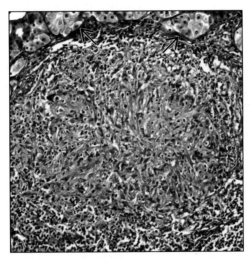
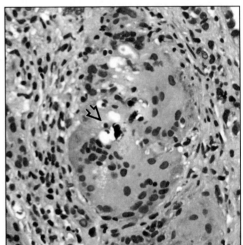

(Left) Granulomatous inflammation rarely directly involves glomeruli, which are usually completely normal. This micrograph shows a multinucleated giant cell ⇥ in the vicinity of a normal glomerulus. (Right) Some patients with sarcoidosis have recurrent episodes of renal involvement or steroid-resistant disease. This can result in interstitial fibrosis and tubular atrophy, as shown here, where there is marked dropout of tubules with replacement fibrosis and persistent inflammation.

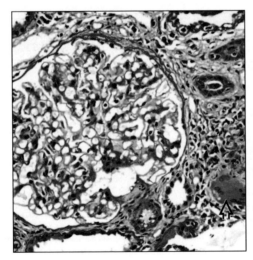
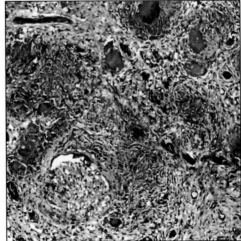

SARCOIDOSIS

Nonsarcoid Granulomatous Diseases

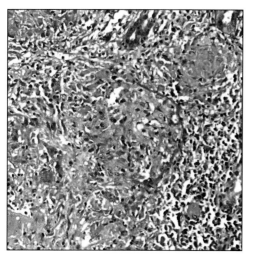

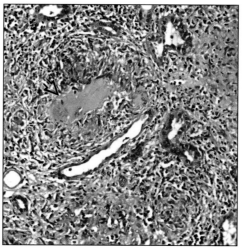

(Left) Renal sarcoidosis needs to be distinguished from other forms of granulomatous tubulointerstitial nephritis, such as infection, allergic reaction, and granulomatous angiitis. This micrograph from a case of renal TB shows active granulomatous inflammation. Although caseous necrosis is not present, special stains for organisms must be performed. (Right) This is a case of renal TB. The granuloma shows central caseous necrosis ⊵, making an infectious etiology likely.

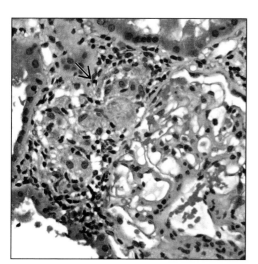

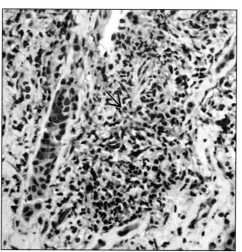

(Left) Allergic reactions are the most common cause of a granulomatous interstitial nephritis. In this situation, the granulomas are often less distinct. This micrograph shows a drug-induced interstitial nephritis with a small granuloma ⇒. Other areas contained frequent eosinophils. (Right) This antibiotic-induced tubulointerstitial nephritis shows a cluster of histiocytes ⇒ without a well-defined granuloma. Numerous lymphocytes, plasma cells, and eosinophils are also present.

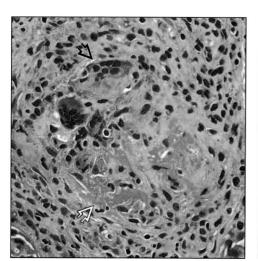

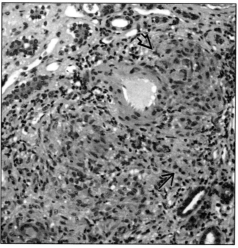

(Left) ANCA-associated necrotizing and granulomatous arteritis may involve renal arteries. This is a case of granulomatosis with polyangiitis (Wegener) with necrotizing arteritis that includes multinucleated giant cells ⊵ associated with fibrinoid necrosis ◼ of the arterial wall. (Right) This is a case of organ-isolated giant cell arteritis. There are numerous granulomas ⊵ centered on small arteries and arterioles. There is also acute interstitial nephritis associated with eosinophils ⇒.

NEPHROCALCINOSIS

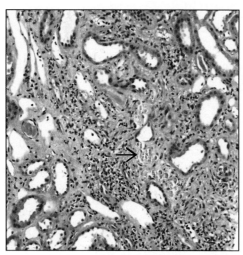

Nephrocalcinosis, with purple-staining calcium phosphate ⊟ deposits in the interstitium, is associated with interstitial inflammation in this case.

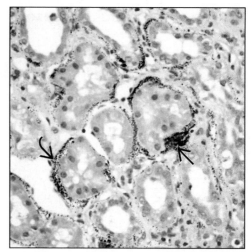

A von Kossa stain reveals tubular basement membrane ⊟ and interstitial calcification ⊟.

TERMINOLOGY

Definitions
- Deposition of abundant calcium phosphate precipitates within renal tubules, tubular basement membrane, and interstitium
- "Nephrocalcinosis" usually refers to calcium phosphate deposits in setting of hypercalcemia
  - Calcium oxalate deposits in other conditions (e.g., primary hyperoxaluria, usually termed "oxalosis")

ETIOLOGY/PATHOGENESIS

Calcium Precipitation Within Kidney
- Increased urinary concentration of calcium and phosphate that allows for precipitation
- Almost all calcium (98%) filtered by glomerulus is reabsorbed by tubule
- Randall plaques (calcium deposits at or near papillary tip) may be initial site of calcification, at least in some types of nephrocalcinosis
  - Randall plaques show deposits in interstitium, tubular basement membranes, and tubular lumens

Hypercalcemia Due to Various Conditions
- Nephrocalcinosis usually in setting of chronic hypercalcemia
- Sarcoidosis
- Hypercalcemia of malignancy
- Milk-alkali syndrome
- Hypervitaminosis A or D
- Hyperparathyroidism (primary)

Inherited Tubulopathies
- Dent disease, cystinosis, and others

CLINICAL ISSUES

Epidemiology
- Age
  - Childhood through older adulthood
  - Neonates, especially those receiving loop diuretics

Presentation
- Chronic renal failure
- Nephrolithiasis
  - Not always present
- No or little proteinuria
- Benign urine sediment
- Hypercalcemia
- Hypercalciuria
- Nephrocalcinosis may be found in presence of other renal disease

Treatment
- Directed at underlying cause

Prognosis
- Depends on cause

IMAGE FINDINGS

Radiographic Findings
- Diffuse, fine renal parenchymal calcifications

MICROSCOPIC PATHOLOGY

Histologic Features
- Calcium phosphate deposits within tubular lumens, interstitium, and tubular basement membranes
  - Deposits are purple on H&E stained sections
  - Deposits are positive (black) on von Kossa stain, which stains phosphate
  - Alizarin Red used to stain calcium specifically
  - Crystals not polarizable

NEPHROCALCINOSIS

Key Facts

Terminology

- Deposition of abundant calcium phosphate precipitates within renal tubules and interstitium
- "Nephrocalcinosis" usually refers to calcium phosphate deposits in setting of hypercalcemia

Etiology/Pathogenesis

- Hypercalcemia due to various conditions
  - Nephrocalcinosis usually in setting of chronic hypercalcemia
- Inherited tubulopathies

Clinical Issues

- Chronic renal failure
- Hypercalcemia
- Hypercalciuria

Image Findings

- Diffuse, fine renal parenchymal calcifications

Microscopic Pathology

- Calcium phosphate deposits within tubular lumens, interstitium, and tubular basement membranes
  - Deposits are purple on H&E stained sections
  - Deposits are positive (black) on von Kossa stain, which stains phosphate
  - Interstitial fibrosis and tubular atrophy and interstitial inflammation

Top Differential Diagnoses

- Phosphate nephropathy
  - Usually related to ingestion of oral sodium phosphate

- Interstitial fibrosis and tubular atrophy
- Focal mild interstitial inflammation with mononuclear cells
- No specific glomerular or vascular changes, except as relates to chronic tubulointerstitial disease

ANCILLARY TESTS

Metabolic Workup

- Hyperparathyroidism
- Hypercalcemia
- Hyperphosphatemia
- Hypercalciuria, hyperphosphaturia, or hyperoxaluria

DIFFERENTIAL DIAGNOSIS

Phosphate Nephropathy

- Calcium phosphate deposits in tubular lumens
- Usually related to ingestion of oral sodium phosphate
- Absence of chronic hypercalcemia

Dent Disease

- Deposition of calcium phosphate or calcium oxalate crystals in kidney
- X-linked, affects children
- Renal stone disease, hypercalciuria, proximal tubular dysfunction, low molecular weight proteinuria

Other Tubulopathies Causing Nephrocalcinosis

- Lowe syndrome, Bartter syndrome, cystic fibrosis, distal renal tubular acidosis, cystic fibrosis, autosomal dominant hypocalcemia, hypomagnesemic hypercalciuric nephrocalcinosis, X-linked hypophosphatemia, Williams syndrome, Wilson disease, Liddle syndrome

Nephrogenic Systemic Fibrosis (NSF)

- Extensive TBM calcium phosphate deposition present in all cases in an autopsy series
- Calcific deposits in other organs as well

Medullary Sponge Kidney

- Medullary nephrocalcinosis
  - Calcium phosphate precipitates within renal cysts

Calcium Oxalate Deposition in Kidney

- Clear, polarizable crystals on H&E stained sections

Gout/Urate Nephropathy

- Needle-like crystals within interstitium dissolved by routine processing
- Surrounding inflammatory reaction that may be granulomatous

Adenine Phosphoribosyltransferase Deficiency/2,8-Dihydroxyadenine Crystalluria

- Reddish-brown, polarizable crystals within tubular lumens, tubular epithelial cell cytoplasm, and interstitium

SELECTED REFERENCES

1. Herlitz LC et al: A case of nephrocalcinosis. Kidney Int. 75(8):856-9, 2009
2. Koreishi AF et al: Nephrogenic systemic fibrosis: a pathologic study of autopsy cases. Arch Pathol Lab Med. 133(12):1943-8, 2009
3. Troxell ML et al: Glomerular and tubular basement membrane calcinosis: case report and literature review. Am J Kidney Dis. 47(2):e23-6, 2006
4. Markowitz GS et al: Renal failure due to acute nephrocalcinosis following oral sodium phosphate bowel cleansing. Hum Pathol. 35(6):675-84, 2004
5. Sayer JA et al: Nephrocalcinosis: molecular insights into calcium precipitation within the kidney. Clin Sci (Lond). 106(6):549-61, 2004
6. Randall A: The origin and growth of renal calculi. Ann Surg. 105(6):1009-27, 1937

Microscopic Features

(Left) This biopsy specimen came from a 75-year-old woman with hypercalcemia and chronic renal failure with a creatinine of 2.3 mg/dL. Calcium phosphate is seen within the interstitium ⊳ surrounding a tubule. The biopsy also shows interstitial fibrosis and tubular atrophy. *(Right)* Calcium phosphate is deposited in large clumps ⇒ and in finer granules ⊳ in tubular lumens and the interstitium.

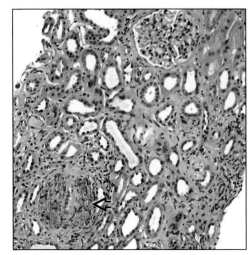
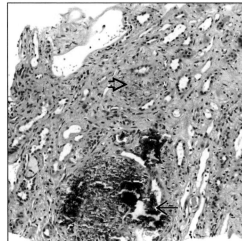

(Left) Calcium phosphate is deposited in the interstitium in this case (von Kossa). The patient was found to have an enlarged spleen and a splenic marginal zone lymphoma. After splenectomy and rituximab treatment, the patient's hypercalcemia resolved. The creatinine remained stable, although elevated. *(Right)* Calcium phosphate surrounds a tubule stained with von Kossa stain, which detects phosphate.

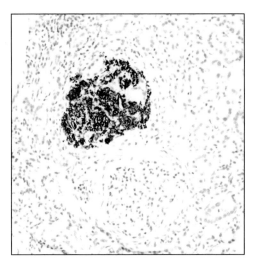
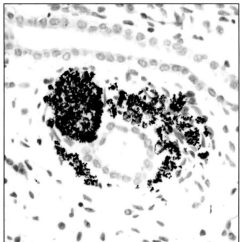

(Left) Shown here is a biopsy of a Randall plaque in a patient with renal stone disease. Randall plaques may represent the earliest manifestations of stone formation and serve as a nidus for precipitation of minerals. Interstitial calcium phosphate deposits are present ⇒. *(Right)* Randall plaque biopsy shows tubular basement membrane ⇒ calcium phosphate deposits.

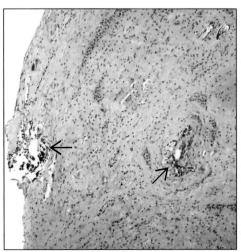
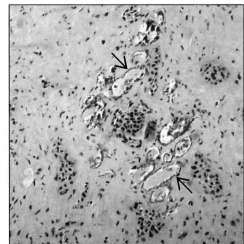

NEPHROCALCINOSIS

Microscopic Features

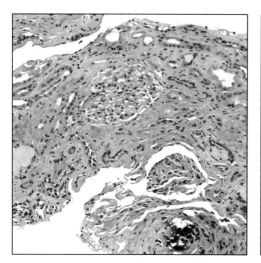

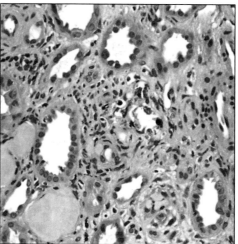

(Left) H&E shows recurrent nephrocalcinosis in an allograft 2 years post transplant from a patient with Pearson Kearns-Sayre syndrome (a mitochondrial genetic disease). The original renal disease was nephrocalcinosis. *(Right)* H&E shows recurrent nephrocalcinosis, along with interstitial fibrosis.

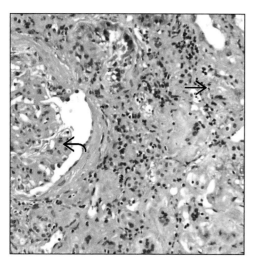

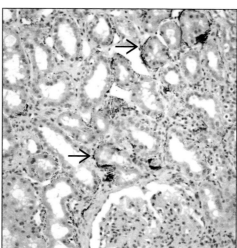

(Left) H&E shows a case of nodular diabetic glomerulosclerosis ➔ with the additional subtle finding of diffuse fine interstitial and tubular basement membrane calcification ➔. *(Right)* A von Kossa stain on a case of diabetic glomerulosclerosis reveals diffuse tubular basement membrane and interstitial calcification ➔. The patient had a normal serum calcium level at the time of biopsy. The cause of nephrocalcinosis is unknown.

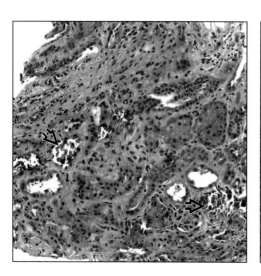

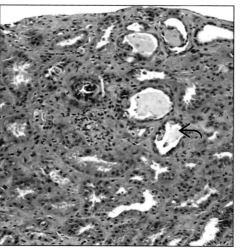

(Left) H&E shows acute nephrocalcinosis in a patient with acute renal failure, hypercalcemia, and multiple myeloma. Several calcium phosphate ➔ deposits are within the tubular lumens. There was no evidence of light chain deposition disease or of light chain cast nephropathy. *(Right)* H&E shows acute nephrocalcinosis. Focal acute tubular injury is also present, with dilated tubules with flattened epithelium ➔.

URIC ACID NEPHROPATHY/GOUT

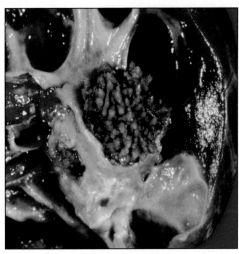

Gross photograph reveals a brown calculus with a rough surface in the renal pelvis. There is marked calyceal dilation, pyramidal effacement, and parenchymal thinning. (Courtesy V. Nickeleit, MD.)

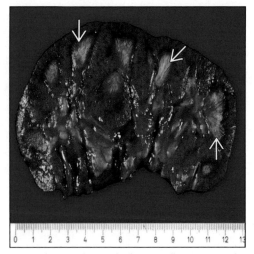

Gross photograph reveals distinct yellow striae in the medulla ➡, with congestion at the corticomedullary junction, of a kidney with acute uric acid nephropathy. (Courtesy V. Nickeleit, MD.)

TERMINOLOGY

Abbreviations
- Uric acid nephropathy (UAN)

Synonyms
- Urate nephropathy, gouty nephropathy with tophi, gout nephropathy

Definitions
- Intrarenal precipitation of uric acid associated with hyperuricemia or hyperuricosuria

ETIOLOGY/PATHOGENESIS

Normal Metabolism
- Uric acid is final degradation product of purine metabolism
- Sources are endogenous from adenine or guanine nucleotides or exogenous from diet
- Uric acid can be generated in all cells but most markedly by hepatocytes
- Urate is filtered freely, reabsorbed, secreted, and undergoes post-secretory reabsorption, all in proximal tubules
- 10% of filtered load is excreted in urine

Hyperuricemia
- Defined as plasma uric acid > 7 mg/dL
  - Due to
    - Decreased excretion (75-90%)
    - Overproduction (10-25%)
- Decreased tubular secretion/increased reabsorption
  - Idiopathic
  - Drugs: Thiazide diuretics, cyclosporine A, low dose salicylates
  - Chronic heavy metal toxicity: Lead (saturnine gout), beryllium
  - Metabolic: Ketoacidosis, lactic acidosis, dehydration, Bartter syndrome, chronic renal failure

- Endocrine: Hypothyroidism, hyperparathyroidism
  - Genetic: Familial juvenile hyperuricemic nephropathy (uromodulin storage disease)
  - Miscellaneous: Sickle cell anemia, Down syndrome, sarcoidosis, eclampsia
- Overproduction/excessive release
  - Idiopathic (60%)
  - Massive tissue destruction
    - Hematologic diseases: Leukemia, lymphoma, myeloma, polycythemia
    - Tumor lysis syndrome: Treatment of leukemia, lymphoma, multiple myeloma, and solid tumors with cytotoxic agents or radiation
    - Crush injury, rhabdomyolysis, seizures (prolonged, severe)
  - Hereditary enzyme deficiencies
    - X-linked: Hypoxanthine guanine phosphoribosyl transferase deficiency; complete (Lesch-Nyhan syndrome) or partial
    - Autosomal recessive: Glucose-6-phosphatase deficiency in glycogen storage disease type 1

Hyperuricemia and Kidney Disease
- Deposits of uric acid in tissue are in form of monosodium urate monohydrate or rarely ammonium urate
  - Deposits are doubly refractile on polarization microscopy
- Kidney is involved in 3 ways
  - Intratubular uric acid deposits: Acute UAN
  - Interstitial deposits: Chronic UAN
  - Lithiasis: Uric acid or mixed uric acid and calcium oxalate stones
- Severe hyperuricemia (plasma levels 20-50 mg/dL)
  - Associated with tissue destruction, hematologic disease, enzyme deficiency
  - Marked hyperuricosuria exceeds urinary solubility with resultant precipitation
  - May be compounded by acidic urine, high urinary calcium phosphate in cases with tissue destruction

URIC ACID NEPHROPATHY/GOUT

Key Facts

Terminology
- Intrarenal precipitation of uric acid associated with hyperuricemia

Etiology/Pathogenesis
- Decreased uric acid excretion (75-90%)
- Overproduction of uric acid (10-25%)

Clinical Issues
- Acute UAN: Acute oliguric or anuric renal failure
- Chronic UAN: Chronic renal failure and hypertension

Macroscopic Features
- Acute UAN: Medullary and papillary yellow radial striations
- Chronic UAN: Medullary yellow flecks corresponding to tophi or microtophi

- Uric acid stones

Microscopic Pathology
- Acute UAN: Birefringent urate crystals in collecting ducts forming linear streaks, acute tubular injury
- Chronic UAN: Medullary foreign body-type granulomas containing needle-like urate crystals or crystal clefts (= microtophus)

Top Differential Diagnoses
- Acute tubular injury with crystal deposits: Indinavir, acyclovir, sulfadiazine, light chain proximal tubulopathy
- Chronic nephropathy with granulomas: Cholesterol granulomas, oxalate nephropathy, indinavir or acyclovir nephropathy, sarcoidosis

---

- o Usually associated with acute UAN
- Kidney injury in acute UAN has at least 4 potential contributing mechanisms
  - o Intrarenal tubular obstruction: Precipitated uric crystals in lumens of collecting ducts
  - o Direct toxicity to tubular epithelium: Release of lysosomal contents resulting in epithelial injury
  - o Indirect tubular epithelial injury: Release of chemokines with secondary inflammation
  - o Vasoconstriction, impaired autoregulation, and renal ischemia

CLINICAL ISSUES

Presentation
- Acute UAN
  - o Acute oliguric or anuric renal failure
  - o Severe hyperuricemia (> 15 mg/dL)
  - o Urinalysis reveals birefringent uric acid crystals
  - o Typically arises in tissue destruction associated with tumor lysis syndrome or crush injury
  - o Flank pain if nephrolithiasis
- Chronic UAN (classical gouty nephropathy)
  - o Arises in patients with gout, chronic hyperuricemia, and hypertension
  - o Chronic renal failure is uncommonly caused by pure chronic UAN (1.5% in 1 series)
  - o Significantly increased odds of developing chronic renal failure with chronic UAN (odds ratio 4.6)
- Uric acid calculi
  - o May arise in acute UAN
  - o Are identified in 15-20% of patients with gout
    - ▪ Associated with hyperuricemia, low urinary pH, and low fractional excretion of uric acid
    - ▪ Chronic obstructive pyelonephritis may be significant cause of chronic renal failure

Treatment
- Acute UAN: Prevention is mainstay of treatment in acute disease
  - o Volume expansion, loop diuretics

- o Allopurinol blocks xanthine oxidase activity and hence uric acid formation
- o Recombinant urate oxidase converts urate to more water soluble allantoin
- o Hemodialysis to remove uric acid load
- Chronic UAN
  - o Hydration
  - o Uricosuric agents: Probenecid, sulfinpyrazone

Prognosis
- Acute UAN
  - o High rates of reversal of acute renal failure with full recovery if treated early
- Chronic UAN
  - o No therapy: 40% develop chronic renal failure and 10% develop uremia
  - o Gouty nephropathy is rare with uricosuric therapy
  - o < 1% of end-stage renal failure is attributable to chronic UAN

MACROSCOPIC FEATURES

Gross Examination
- Acute UAN: Medullary yellow striations converging on papilla
- Chronic UAN: Medullary yellow flecks corresponding to tophi or microtophi
- Chronic renal disease with reduced renal mass, cortical thinning, and surface granularity
- Uric acid stones
  - o Yellow-brown, hard, rough or smooth, multiple, small (2 cm or less)
  - o Dilated pelvis or ureter
  - o 6-25% with chronic UAN have features of pyelonephritis

MICROSCOPIC PATHOLOGY

Histologic Features
- Acute UAN

o Intraluminal clusters of birefringent urate crystals in collecting ducts forming linear streaks
o Acute tubular injury
o Tubulointerstitial inflammation is mild
o Tubular ectasia associated with obstruction
o Tubular rupture with interstitial extrusion of T-H protein is uncommonly seen
o Glomeruli usually are unremarkable and rarely have a lobular form of glomerulopathy
o Needle-like birefringent crystals of monosodium urate best seen in alcohol-fixed or frozen tissue
o De Galantha and Schultz stains identify uric acid in tissue
o Electron microscopy reveals injured epithelial cells with cytoplasmic angulated crystals in collecting ducts

• Chronic UAN
o Microtophi are granulomas containing birefringent, needle-like sodium urate crystals or crystal clefts, or occasionally basophilic crystalline deposits
o Cellular components include syncytial giant cells, epithelioid macrophages, lymphocytes, and eosinophils
o Microtophi may be intratubular or interstitial
o Microtophi are mainly medullary; cortical microtophi are uncommon
o Interstitial fibrosis and tubular atrophy, arterial and arteriolar sclerosis, glomerular sclerosis are variable
o Glomerular changes include mesangial sclerosis and capillary double contours
o Features of pyelonephritis may also be evident, especially if there are calculi

DIFFERENTIAL DIAGNOSIS

Acute Tubular Injury with Crystal Deposits

• Distinction from other crystal deposits based on clinical drug exposure and spectroscopic analysis
• Drugs: Antivirals and antibiotics
o Indinavir and acyclovir
▪ Acute tubular injury, interstitial inflammation, and granulomas
▪ Cortical and medullary collecting duct crystals
o Sulfadiazine
▪ Collecting duct crystals mixed with secreted protein and cell debris
▪ Acute tubular injury
▪ Acute tubulointerstitial nephritis, eosinophils, granulomas
• Light chain proximal tubulopathy (Fanconi syndrome)
o Proximal tubular needle-like crystals or crystal clefts in epithelial cytoplasm
o Monotypic light chains by immunofluorescence (kappa more frequently than lambda)

Chronic Nephropathy with Granulomas

• Cholesterol granulomas: Associated with nephrotic syndrome
• Oxalate nephropathy: Characteristic birefringent crystals on polarization microscopy
• Indinavir or acyclovir nephropathy

o Needle-like birefringent crystals with granulomas and fibrosis
o Indinavir sulfate lithiasis
o Distinction from other crystals based on clinical drug exposure and spectroscopic analysis

• Sarcoidosis
o Noncaseating "tight" granulomas ± Schaumann bodies (psammomatous calcium phosphate) or asteroid bodies (eosinophilic stellate inclusions) in cytoplasm of giant cells
o Rim of lymphocytes around granulomas

DIAGNOSTIC CHECKLIST

Clinically Relevant Pathologic Features

• Acute UAN
o Linear intratubular precipitates of uric acid crystals in medullary collecting ducts: Apparent on gross exam
o Acute tubular injury with interstitial inflammation on light microscopy
o Acute renal failure associated with
▪ Toxic tubular injury
▪ Tubular obstruction
▪ Tubulointerstitial inflammation
▪ Secondary ischemia associated with hyperuricemia
• Chronic UAN
o Medullary tubulointerstitial microtophi
o Interstitial fibrosis, tubular atrophy, and glomerular sclerosis
o Glomerular mesangial sclerosis and double contours

Pathologic Interpretation Pearls

• Acute UAN: Massive intratubular deposits of uric acid with acute tubular injury, ectasia, and inflammation
• Chronic UAN: Noncaseating granulomas with radial clefts or needle-like crystals, localized to medulla
o Often accompanied by interstitial fibrosis, tubular atrophy, and vascular sclerosis
• De Galantha or Schultz stains identify uric acid deposits in alcohol fixed or frozen sections

SELECTED REFERENCES

1. Shimada M et al: A novel role for uric acid in acute kidney injury associated with tumour lysis syndrome. Nephrol Dial Transplant. 24(10):2960-4, 2009
2. Nickeleit V et al: Uric acid nephropathy and end-stage renal disease--review of a non-disease. Nephrol Dial Transplant. 12(9):1832-8, 1997
3. Robinson RR et al: Acute uric acid nephropathy. Arch Intern Med. 137(7):839-40, 1977
4. Kanwar YS et al: Leukemic urate nephropathy. Arch Pathol. 99(9):467-72, 1975

Microscopic Features

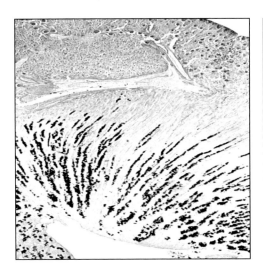

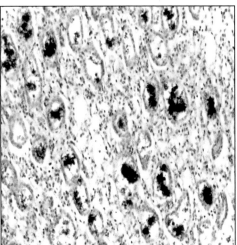

(Left) Acute uric acid nephropathy has radial striations composed of intratubular uric acid crystal precipitates, mainly in the collecting ducts; highlighted by the Schultz stain performed on frozen or alcohol-fixed tissue. *(Courtesy V. Nickeleit, MD)*. *(Right)* Uric acid stain reveals extensive intratubular angulated crystalline deposits associated with tubular injury and tubulointerstitial inflammation in acute urate nephropathy. *(Courtesy V. Nickeleit, MD.)*

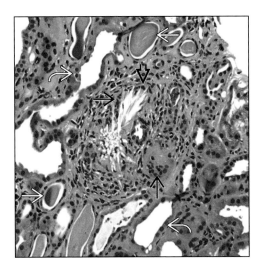

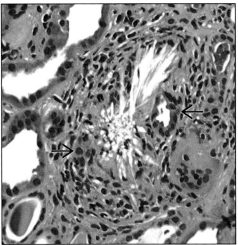

(Left) A discrete medullary interstitial microtophus is composed of a collection of macrophages and foreign body giant cells ➡, some of which contain needle-like clefts ➡, with lymphocytes, plasma cells, and eosinophils. Surrounding tubules have epithelial flattening ➡ and casts ➡. *(Right)* A high-power view reveals radial needle-like clefts, mononuclear and eosinophilic infiltrates, and shrunken tubular profiles ➡ within the granuloma.

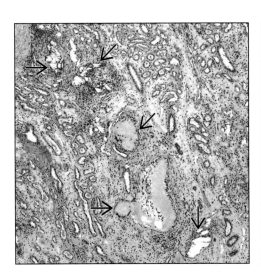

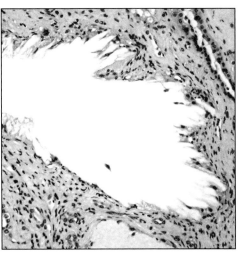

(Left) Multiple medullary tophi are evident, with and without crystal clefts ➡. There is interstitial fibrosis, mononuclear inflammation, and tubular loss in the surrounding medulla. *(Right)* A medullary interstitial microtophus is shown with cleft-like spaces remaining after dissolution of urate crystals during formalin fixation. There is fibrosis and mild mononuclear inflammation in the surrounding medulla.

FAMILIAL JUVENILE HYPERURICEMIC NEPHROPATHY

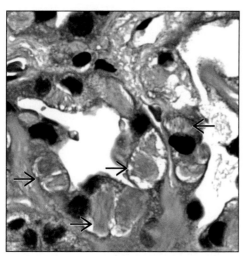

Hematoxylin & eosin shows characteristic intracytoplasmic fibrillar inclusions ⇒ in thick ascending limb of Henle (TALH). (Courtesy S. Nasr, MD and V. D'Agati, MD.)

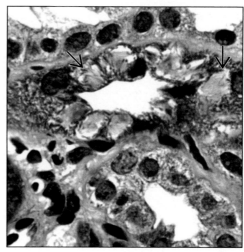

Masson trichrome stain shows fibrillar inclusions ⇒ in epithelial cytoplasm of TALH. (Courtesy S. Nasr, MD and V. D'Agati, MD.)

TERMINOLOGY

Abbreviations
- Familial juvenile hyperuricemic nephropathy (FJHN)

Synonyms
- Uromodulin (Tamm-Horsfall protein) storage disease
- Uromodulin-associated nephropathy
- Medullary cystic disease type 2
- Familial glomerulocystic disease variant

Definitions
- Autosomal dominant tubulointerstitial disorder with chronic renal failure, hyposthenuria, hyperuricemia, and frequently uromodulin gene mutations

ETIOLOGY/PATHOGENESIS

Genetic Disorder
- Autosomal dominant inheritance with genetic heterogeneity
- Phenotype associated with mutations of uromodulin (UMOD) gene (on chromosome 16p12) in ~ 30%
- Other potential mutations in genes located on chromosome 1, probably associated with UMOD secretion
- Up to 40% of families with this phenotype have no identifiable UMOD mutation
- Different mutations associated with spectrum of disorders including
  - FJHN
  - Medullary cystic kidney disease type 2
  - Familial glomerulocystic disease variant

Pathogenesis
- UMOD mutation gives rise to protein folding disorder
- Impaired protein trafficking and secretion
- Retention in cells of thick ascending limb of loop of Henle (TALH)

- Retained protein may incite tubulointerstitial inflammation
- Hyperuricemia related to reduced excretion of uric acid

CLINICAL ISSUES

Presentation
- Males > females
- Hyperuricemia in childhood or adolescence
- Gout in teenage years (precocious gout) in ~ 50%
- Hyposthenuria, polyuria, and enuresis
- Progressive chronic renal failure by age 20
- Minimal or no proteinuria
- Fractional excretion of uric acid < 5% even with normal glomerular filtration rate (hypouricosuria)
- Bland urinalysis with no urate crystals
- Decreased urinary UMOD excretion

Treatment
- No specific therapy; allopurinol for gout
- Supportive for end-stage renal failure

Prognosis
- End-stage renal failure by age 30-60

IMAGE FINDINGS

General Features
- Bilateral small kidneys
- Medullary cysts uncommon despite name

MACROSCOPIC FEATURES

General Features
- Bilateral shrunken scarred kidneys with rare medullary cysts

FAMILIAL JUVENILE HYPERURICEMIC NEPHROPATHY

Key Facts

Terminology
- Autosomal dominant tubulointerstitial disorder with chronic renal failure and hyperuricemia

Etiology/Pathogenesis
- Mutations of uromodulin (UMOD) gene (on chromosome 16p12) in ~ 30%

Clinical Issues
- Early hyperuricemia with precocious gout

- Reduced urinary uric acid and UMOD
- Chronic renal failure by 20 years
- End-stage renal failure by age 30-60

Microscopic Pathology
- Tubular atrophy and interstitial fibrosis with inclusions in TALH
- Lamellated bundles of ER and dilated ER by EM
- UMOD cytoplasmic aggregates in TALH by IHC

MICROSCOPIC PATHOLOGY

Histologic Features
- Tubular atrophy and interstitial fibrosis
- Tubular basement membrane lamellation and thickening
- Eosinophilic fibrillar inclusions in TALH (trichrome positive, PAS positive)
- Electron microscopy reveals lamellated bundles of endoplasmic reticulum (ER) and dilated ER containing granular storage material
- Immunohistochemistry (IHC) for UMOD shows cytoplasmic aggregates (inclusions) in TALH
- No tophi or uric acid crystal deposits

Predominant Pattern/Injury Type
- Tubules, atrophy

Predominant Cell/Compartment Type
- Epithelial, tubular

DIFFERENTIAL DIAGNOSIS

Light Chain Fanconi Syndrome
- Crystalline inclusions in proximal tubules
- Positive for kappa or lambda light chains by immunofluorescence
- Cytoplasmic crystals with herringbone substructure by EM

Refsum Disease
- Vacuolar changes in podocytes and tubular epithelium (proximal and distal)
- Vacuoles stain for fat using oil red O (on frozen tissue only)
- EM reveals cytoplasmic inclusions of clustered tubular structures with quadrangular profiles

DIAGNOSTIC CHECKLIST

Pathologic Interpretation Pearls
- Eosinophilic PAS(+) inclusions in TALH
- Atrophic tubules have thickened, split, basement membranes
- Interstitial fibrosis and tubular atrophy
- EM reveals lamellated ER and granular material in dilated ER in TALH
- IHC confirms UMOD aggregates in TALH
- DNA sequencing identifies UMOD gene mutation

SELECTED REFERENCES

1. Nasr SH et al: Uromodulin storage disease. Kidney Int. 73(8):971-6, 2008
2. Kumar S: Mechanism of injury in uromodulin-associated kidney disease. J Am Soc Nephrol. 18(1):10-2, 2007
3. Vylet'al P et al: Alterations of uromodulin biology: a common denominator of the genetically heterogeneous FJHN/MCKD syndrome. Kidney Int. 70(6):1155-69, 2006
4. Scolari F et al: Uromodulin storage diseases: clinical aspects and mechanisms. Am J Kidney Dis. 44(6):987-99, 2004

IMAGE GALLERY

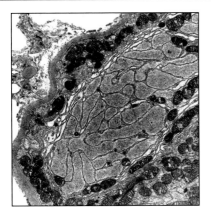 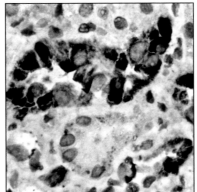 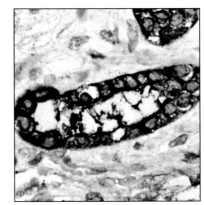

(Left) Electron micrograph shows dilated endoplasmic reticulum with UMOD accumulations seen as granular amorphous material. (Courtesy S. Nasr, MD and V. D'Agati, MD.) *(Center)* TALH with cytoplasmic aggregates of UMOD are identified using anti-UMOD IHC. (Courtesy S. Nasr, MD and V. D'Agati, MD.) *(Right)* Normal TALH stained for UMOD by immunohistochemistry shows the absence of cytoplasmic aggregates of UMOD as seen in the previous image. (Courtesy S. Nasr, MD and V. D'Agati, MD.)

PRIMARY OXALOSIS

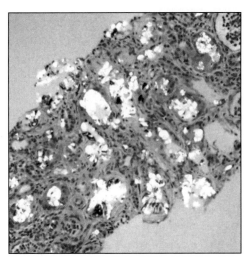

Hematoxylin & eosin using partially polarized light shows abundant anisotropic calcium oxalate in the cortex of a 4-month-old male with primary oxalosis type 1.

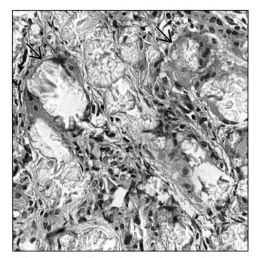

Refractile, pale yellow, calcium oxalate crystals are seen, some of which are in giant cells ➡ in the renal cortex.

TERMINOLOGY

Abbreviations
- Primary oxalosis (PO)
  - Type 1 (PO1), type 2 (PO2)

Synonyms
- Primary hyperoxaluria (PH), primary hyperoxalemia

Definitions
- Oxalate overproduction due to gene mutations affecting enzymes that catalyze glyoxylate breakdown, with systemic calcium oxalate deposition

ETIOLOGY/PATHOGENESIS

Hereditary Disorder
- Autosomal recessive mutations of alanine glyoxylate aminotransferase gene (PO1) or glyoxalate reductase gene (PO2)
- Alanine glyoxylate aminotransferase (AGT) gene on chromosome 2q36-37
  - AGT converts glyoxylate to glycine in hepatic peroxisomes
- Glyoxylate reductase (GR) gene on chromosome 9c
  - GR converts glyoxylate to glycolate in hepatocyte cytoplasm
- Mutations are multiple (50 identified for AGT and 14 for GR), have varying effects
  - e.g., loss of catalytic function, accelerated degradation, and mistargeting
- Loss of function of these enzymes results in excess glyoxylate, which is converted to oxalate by lactate dehydrogenase
- Hyperoxalemia leads to widespread calcium oxalate deposition in tissues (oxalosis)
- Oxalate is excreted in urine
  - Excess excretion predisposes to renal calcium oxalate deposition and lithiasis

- Stones are composed of > 95% calcium oxalate monohydrate (whewellite)

CLINICAL ISSUES

Presentation
- PO1
  - Renal colic, hematuria, and renal failure beginning in childhood
  - Marked hyperoxaluria (> 100 mg/d, normal 20-55 mg/d), ↑ urinary glycolate
  - Heterogeneous mutations associated with clinical variation; 10% have infantile onset
- PO2
  - Marked hyperoxaluria, ↑ urinary L-glyceric acid, mild renal impairment
- Renal oxalate deposition causes renal failure and compounds systemic oxalosis
  - Systemic oxalosis: Retinopathy, neuropathy, osteoarthropathy, cardiomyopathy, and bone marrow deposits with pancytopenia
- Diagnosis is made by assay of enzyme activity in liver tissue

Treatment
- Hydration, pyridoxine (vitamin B6), pyridoxamine
- Combined liver and kidney transplantation

Prognosis
- End-stage renal failure frequent in PO1
- PO2 is milder and rarely causes end-stage renal failure

MACROSCOPIC FEATURES

Stones
- Rounded, white or pale yellow with smooth surface
  - Ultrastructure: 50 μm plates that aggregate to form rounded structures resembling balls of wool

PRIMARY OXALOSIS

Key Facts

Etiology/Pathogenesis
- Autosomal recessive mutations of *AGT* (PO1) or *GR* (PO2) genes

Clinical Issues
- PO1: Hyperoxaluria (> 100 mg/d), increased urinary glycolate, renal failure
- PO2: Hyperoxaluria, increased urinary L-glyceric acid, mild renal failure
- Diagnosis by assay of enzyme activity in liver tissue

- End-stage renal failure frequent in PO1

Macroscopic Features
- Stones are composed of > 95% calcium oxalate monohydrate (whewellite)

Microscopic Pathology
- Extensive birefringent crystal deposits, in rosettes and sheaves, in tubules and interstitium with giant cell reaction and fibrosis

Kidney
- Shrunken, scarred kidney with gritty texture on cut surface
- Dilated pelvicalyceal system with crystalline stone material

MICROSCOPIC PATHOLOGY

Histologic Features
- Early disease: Intratubular yellow, birefringent calcium oxalate crystal deposits in rosettes and sheaves
- Later disease: Extensive crystal deposit in cortical and medullary tubules
- Proximal and distal tubular epithelium is injured and necrotic
- Tubules rupture with extrusion of crystals to interstitium
- Crystals are contained in giant cells
- Tubulointerstitial inflammation and fibrosis
- Calcium oxalate may be observed in walls of muscular blood vessels
- Glomeruli are devoid of crystal deposits but may have segmental or global sclerosis in advanced disease

DIFFERENTIAL DIAGNOSIS

Extensive Secondary Renal Calcium Oxalate Deposition
- Excess ingestion: Ethylene glycol toxicity

  o Shows large vacuoles in proximal tubular epithelium
- Excess enteric absorption: Inflammatory bowel disease, ileal resection or bypass

Hyperoxaluria
- No parenchymal deposits
- Defect in reabsorption

DIAGNOSTIC CHECKLIST

Clinically Relevant Pathologic Features
- Extensive calcium oxalate deposition and tubulointerstitial inflammation associated with chronic renal failure

Pathologic Interpretation Pearls
- Intratubular, interstitial, and vascular calcium oxalate deposits; giant cell reaction and fibrosis

SELECTED REFERENCES

1. Danpure CJ: Molecular aetiology of primary hyperoxaluria type 1. Nephron Exp Nephrol. 98(2):e39-44, 2004
2. Asplin JR: Hyperoxaluric calcium nephrolithiasis. Endocrinol Metab Clin North Am. 31(4):927-49, 2002
3. Milliner DS et al: Phenotypic expression of primary hyperoxaluria: comparative features of types I and II. Kidney Int. 59(1):31-6, 2001

IMAGE GALLERY

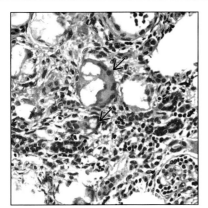 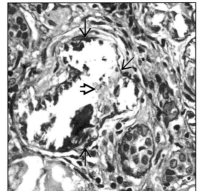 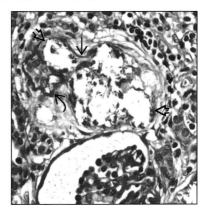

(Left) Interstitial calcium oxalate deposits in giant cells ⇨ are associated with mononuclear inflammation, interstitial fibrosis, and tubular atrophy. *(Center)* PAS stain shows crystal material that is partially surrounded by the tubular basement membrane ⇨ and associated with tubular epithelial cell injury ⇨. *(Right)* Interstitial crystalline material ⇨ is seen adjacent to a ruptured ⇨ and fragmented ⇨ PAS-positive tubular basement membrane, with inflammation of the surrounding interstitium.

SECONDARY OXALOSIS

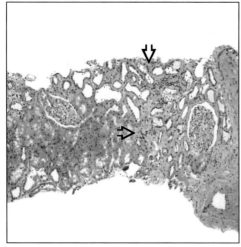

Oxalosis and chronic renal failure developed 1 year after gastric bypass surgery in a 69-year-old woman (Cr 2.7 mg/dL). Focal interstitial fibrosis and tubular atrophy ⊵, along with calcium oxalate crystals, are evident.

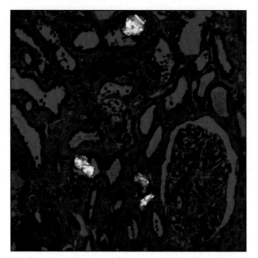

Oxalate crystals are easily appreciated with polarized light, as shown here in a biopsy performed for chronic renal failure after gastric bypass.

TERMINOLOGY

Synonyms
- Oxalate nephropathy
- Oxalosis

Definitions
- Deposition of excessive calcium oxalate within kidney parenchyma due to excessive intake or decreased excretion

ETIOLOGY/PATHOGENESIS

Increased Blood Oxalate Levels
- Caused by increased intake, increased absorption, decreased excretion, or vitamin deficiency
- Enteric hyperoxaluria (malabsorptive states)
  - Increased oxalate absorption by gut; causes include
    - Gastric/intestinal bypass surgery
    - Prolonged use of antibiotics
    - Crohn disease/celiac sprue
    - Pancreatic insufficiency
- Ingestion of ethylene glycol
  - Oxalate is metabolite of ethylene glycol
- Increased ingestion of oxalate-containing foods
  - Rhubarb, parsley, spinach, beet greens, starfruit, peanuts
- Excessive vitamin C intake (rare)
  - Vitamin C is precursor to oxalic acid
- Exposure to methoxyflurane anesthetic
  - Used in 1960s-1970s

CLINICAL ISSUES

Presentation
- Acute renal failure
  - Especially with high ingestion (dietary) of ethylene glycol

- Chronic renal failure
  - Slowly progressive rise in serum Cr, one to several years after gastric bypass
- Nephrolithiasis
  - Calcium oxalate stones
- Progressive nephrocalcinosis

Treatment
- Remove source of excess oxalates
- Remove gastric bypass
- Hemodialysis
  - Removes excess oxalate
- Some respond to pyridoxine therapy

Prognosis
- Leads to irreversible renal failure if not treated

MICROSCOPIC PATHOLOGY

Histologic Features
- Calcium oxalate crystals within tubular lumens, tubular epithelial cytoplasm, and interstitium
  - Crystals are translucent on H&E stain and have fan-like or irregular shapes
  - Crystals strongly birefringent upon examination under polarized light
  - May have massive deposits in advanced cases
  - In a study of oxalate nephropathy secondary to gastric bypass, biopsies showed on average 3.5 calcium oxalate crystals per glomerulus (range: 1.5-7.9)
- Tubular injury
- Interstitial fibrosis and tubular atrophy (nonspecific)
- Focal mononuclear cell inflammation in areas of interstitial fibrosis
- Granulomatous reaction to calcium oxalate crystals

SECONDARY OXALOSIS

Key Facts

Etiology/Pathogenesis
- Oxalate accumulation in kidney
  - Enteric malabsorption (gastric bypass)
  - Ingestion of oxalate-containing foods
  - Pyridoxine deficiency
  - Ingestion of ethylene glycol

Clinical Issues
- Acute or chronic renal failure
- Nephrolithiasis/progressive nephrocalcinosis

Microscopic Pathology
- Calcium oxalate crystals within tubular lumens, tubular epithelial cytoplasm, and interstitium
- Crystals translucent and strongly birefringent

Top Differential Diagnoses
- Primary oxalosis
- Other crystals, such as 2,8-dihydroxyadenine, urate, drugs
- Acute tubular injury

DIFFERENTIAL DIAGNOSIS

Primary Oxalosis
- Young age
- More extensive deposition (e.g., arterial media, bone marrow)

2,8-Dihydroxyadeninuria (DHA)
- Polarizable crystals within renal parenchyma
- Reddish-brown crystals, vs. clear crystals of calcium oxalate

Tubulointerstitial Nephritis, Granulomatous Interstitial Nephritis
- Usual interstitial nephritis cases do not show calcium oxalate crystals

Urate Crystals
- Large, amorphous deposits; nonpolarizing crystals
- Surrounding granulomatous reaction

Leucine Crystals
- Seen in patients with liver failure
- Polarizable

Drug Crystals
- e.g., antibiotics and antiviral drugs
- Some may be polarizable

Crystals Due to Monoclonal Immunoglobulin
- Light chain cast nephropathy

- Light chain proximal tubulopathy (light chain Fanconi syndrome)
- Crystal-storing histiocytosis

Acute Tubular Injury
- May have very focal calcium oxalate crystals within tubular lumens

---

SELECTED REFERENCES

1. Bergstralh EJ et al: Transplantation outcomes in primary hyperoxaluria. Am J Transplant. 10(11):2493-501, 2010
2. Hoppe B et al: The primary hyperoxalurias. Kidney Int. 75(12):1264-71, 2009
3. Nasr SH et al: Oxalate nephropathy complicating Roux-en-Y Gastric Bypass: an underrecognized cause of irreversible renal failure. Clin J Am Soc Nephrol. 3(6):1676-83, 2008
4. Nasr SH et al: Secondary oxalosis due to excess vitamin C intake. Kidney Int. 70(10):1672, 2006
5. Alkhunaizi AM et al: Secondary oxalosis: a cause of delayed recovery of renal function in the setting of acute renal failure. J Am Soc Nephrol. 7(11):2320-6, 1996

IMAGE GALLERY

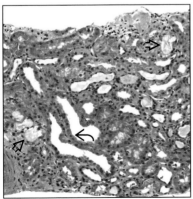 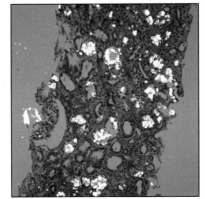 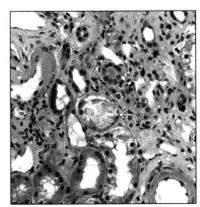

(Left) Dietary oxalosis: For 6-8 weeks prior to this biopsy, the patient was on a high oxalate diet (fruits and vegetables). The biopsy shows acute tubular injury ➡ and oxalate crystals ⊳. *(Center)* Suspected ethylene glycol intoxication has numerous calcium oxalate crystals, highlighted by polarized light. *(Right)* Bile-stained oxalate crystals ➡ in a patient with renal failure and jaundice appear similar to 2,8-dihydroxyadenine crystals. (Courtesy S. Nasr, MD.)

2,8-DIHYDROXYADENINURIA

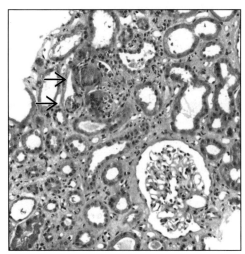

2,8-DHA crystals have a brown-tinged appearance on H&E stain ➡ and are birefringent under polarized light, which may lead the pathologist to misinterpret them as calcium oxalate crystals.

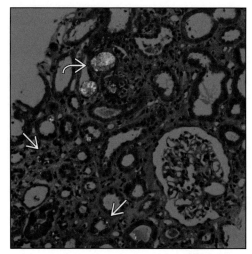

Strongly birefringent 2,8-DHA crystals ➡ are seen under partially polarized light. Numerous additional small crystals are appreciable under polarized light ➡ that are not initially apparent.

TERMINOLOGY

Abbreviations
- 2,8-dihydroxyadeninuria (2,8-DHA)

Synonyms
- Adenine phosphoribosyltransferase (APRT) deficiency

Definitions
- Autosomal recessive trait caused by genetic deficiency in APRT, which leads to increased production and renal excretion of 2,8-DHA as stones or intratubular crystals

ETIOLOGY/PATHOGENESIS

Genetic Basis
- Autosomal recessive, *APRT* gene located on 16q24
- 2 forms with complete in vivo deficiency of APRT
  - Type I complete in vitro deficiency of APRT (APRT*QO)
    - Commonest form in Caucasians
    - Heterogeneous mutations: Missense, nonsense, insertion or deletion
    - Most common (40%) in France: Mutation in intron 4 splice donor site resulting in truncated protein (IVS4+2insT)
    - Most common (100%) in Iceland: D65V
  - Type II: Some in vitro activity of APRT (APRT*J)
    - Commonest in Japanese
    - Single missense mutation in *APRT* (M136T)

Metabolic Pathway
- APRT is a purine salvage enzyme
- Converts adenine to 5'-AMP from 5-phosphoribosyl-1-pyrophosphate
- Adenine otherwise metabolized to 2,8-DHA by xanthine oxidase
- 2,8-DHA poorly soluble and crystalizes in water over wide range of pH

CLINICAL ISSUES

Epidemiology
- Incidence
  - Frequency of heterozygosity at the *APRT* locus has been estimated to be 0.4-1.1% in whites, suggesting homozygosity of 1 in 50,000 to 1 in 100,000
    - Fewer cases, however, are diagnosed; may be due to patients being asymptomatic, unrecognized, or misdiagnosed

Site
- Kidney; no known extrarenal manifestations of APRT deficiency

Presentation
- Clinical presentation is variable, typically diagnosed late (> 30 years old)
- Nephrolithiasis, recurrent (90%)
  - Patients do not always have history of nephrolithiasis
  - 2,8-DHA stones are radiolucent; may be misdiagnosed as uric acid stones
- Chronic renal failure (31%)
- Acute renal failure (18%)
- Renal transplant recipient with idiopathic graft dysfunction (15%)
- Infection, urinary tract
- Crystalluria
  - 2,8-DHA is insoluble in urine at physiologic pH

Laboratory Tests
- 2,8-DHA crystals can be detected by urine microscopy
- APRT enzyme activity in erythrocytes
- Elevated oxalate levels in blood, but to lesser degree than in primary hyperoxaluria

Treatment
- Drugs
  - Allopurinol

2,8-DIHYDROXYADENINURIA

Key Facts

Terminology
- Autosomal recessive trait caused by genetic deficiency in APRT, which leads to increased production and renal excretion of 2,8-DHA as stones or intratubular crystals

Clinical Issues
- Underdiagnosed
  - 2,8-DHA stones are radiolucent; may be confused with uric acid stones
- Nephrolithiasis, recurrent
- Chronic renal failure
- Renal transplantation: In patients with undiagnosed 2,8-DHA, original diagnosis may be made when disease recurs in allograft

Microscopic Pathology
- Birefringent intratubular crystals under polarized light; reddish brown-tinged crystals on H&E stained sections
- Numerous 2,8-DHA crystals in tubular lumens, tubular epithelial cell cytoplasm, and interstitium
- Crystals may show foreign body giant cell reaction

Top Differential Diagnoses
- Oxalate crystals/oxalate nephropathy

Diagnostic Checklist
- Red-brown color distinguishes 2,8-DHA crystals from oxalates

---

- Low purine diet
- Renal transplantation
  - If not treated, disease will recur in transplant
    - Diagnosis may be first made with recurrence

Prognosis
- Excellent if started on allopurinol before renal failure develops

MICROSCOPIC PATHOLOGY

Histologic Features
- Numerous 2,8-DHA crystals in tubular lumens, tubular epithelial cell cytoplasm, and interstitium
  - Very fine deposits within tubular epithelial cells
  - Most crystals are in renal cortex
  - Range from single crystals to small aggregates to large aggregates; needle, rod, or rhomboid-shaped crystals
  - Reddish brown-tinged crystals on H&E and PAS, light blue crystals on trichrome, black crystals on silver stains, birefringent under polarized light
- Acute tubular injury in nonatrophic tubules
- Interstitial fibrosis and tubular atrophy
- Mild to moderate interstitial inflammation
  - Crystals may show foreign body giant cell reaction
  - Lymphocytes and monocytes; no significant eosinophilic infiltrate

DIFFERENTIAL DIAGNOSIS

Oxalate Crystals/Oxalate Nephropathy
- Calcium oxalate crystals are colorless and 2,8-DHA crystals are red-brown

Phosphate Nephropathy
- Intratubular calcium phosphate deposits appear purple/blue on H&E stained sections, rather than brown 2,8-DHA crystals, and do not polarize

Urate Nephropathy/Gout
- Urates dissolve in routine processing (need alcohol-fixed tissue)
  - Needle-like, colorless crystals

Cystinosis
- Crystals dissolve in routine processing (need alcohol-fixed tissue)
  - Hexagonal, colorless crystals, often in cells
- Multinucleated podocytes

DIAGNOSTIC CHECKLIST

Pathologic Interpretation Pearls
- Red-brown color distinguishes 2,8-DHA crystals from oxalates

SELECTED REFERENCES

1. Bollée G et al: Phenotype and genotype characterization of adenine phosphoribosyltransferase deficiency. J Am Soc Nephrol. 21(4):679-88, 2010
2. Nasr SH et al: Crystalline nephropathy due to 2,8-dihydroxyadeninuria: an under-recognized cause of irreversible renal failure. Nephrol Dial Transplant. 25(6):1909-15, 2010
3. Edvardsson V et al: Clinical features and genotype of adenine phosphoribosyltransferase deficiency in iceland. Am J Kidney Dis. 38(3):473-80, 2001
4. Brown HA: Recurrence of 2,8-dihydroxyadenine tubulointerstitial lesions in a kidney transplant recipient with a primary presentation of chronic renal failure. Nephrol Dial Transplant. 13(4):998-1000, 1998
5. Ceballos-Picot I et al: 2,8-Dihydroxyadenine urolithiasis, an underdiagnosed disease. Lancet. 339(8800):1050-1, 1992
6. Simmonds H et al: 2,8-Dihydroxyadenine urolithiasis. Lancet. 339(8804):1295-6, 1992

Microscopic Features

(Left) Clear to brown-tinged small crystals are seen within the tubular epithelial cell cytoplasm ➡. The interstitium has a fine fibrosis with minimal inflammation. *(Right)* A few small crystals ➡ are visualized on this PAS-stained section. Proximal tubules appear generally normal and there is no fibrosis. The diagnosis could easily be missed on this sample.

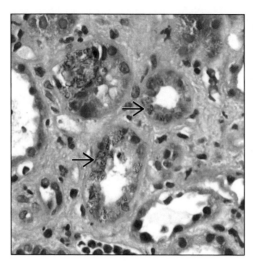
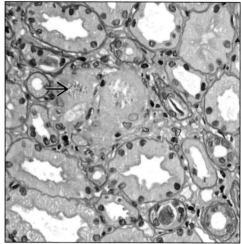

(Left) Recurrent 2,8-DHA deposition is seen in a renal transplant recipient. The disease was first diagnosed in this patient at the time of recurrence, 8 months after transplant. The interstitium has marked fibrosis and the tubules are atrophic. A few foci of brown crystals are present ➡. *(Right)* Fine brown crystals of 2,8-DHA are seen in the interstitium of the cortex, probably in macrophages.

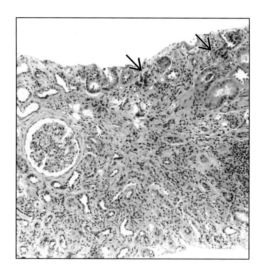
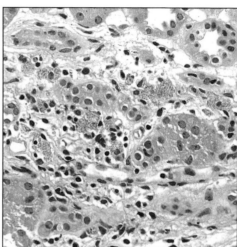

(Left) By light microscopy 2,8-DHA crystals resemble calcium oxalate, except for the brown color. Here the crystals are primarily in tubules, with an accompanying interstitial inflammation and fibrosis. *(Right)* By polarizing light microscopy more extensive 2,8-DHA crystals can be appreciated, including some in the interstitium ➡ and within tubular cells ➡.

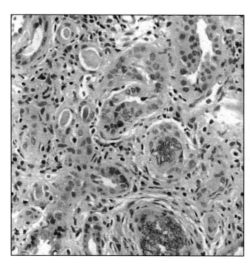
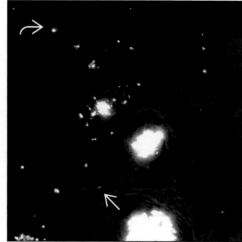

2,8-DIHYDROXYADENINURIA

Microscopic Features

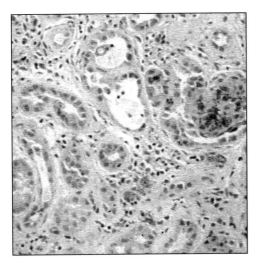

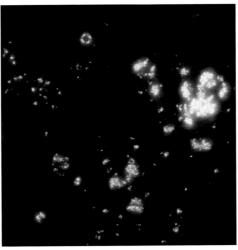

(Left) Brown crystals of 2,8-DHA are seen largely within tubules with accompanying cellular reaction. *(Right)* Polarized light reveals extensive crystal accumulation in the interstitium as well as in the tubules.

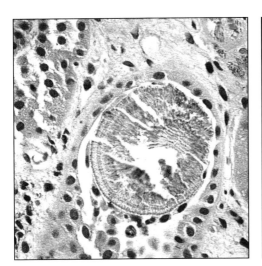

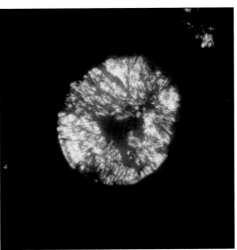

(Left) High-power view shows an intratubular cast of brown 2,8-DHA crystals with a vague radial and ring pattern. *(Right)* Polarized light microscopy at high power shows an intratubular cast of brown 2,8-DHA crystals with the characteristic birefringence.

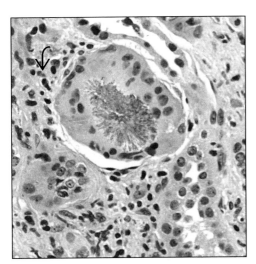

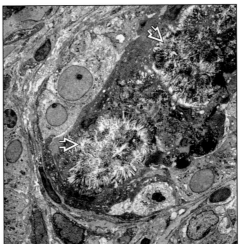

(Left) Intratubular 2,8-DHA crystals in a patient with APRT deficiency sometimes provoke a giant cell response and inflammation, as shown in this field. An eosinophil is also present ➚. *(Right)* Crystals are seen within tubules by electron microscopy, appearing as radiating spicules within cells and free in the lumen ➥.

CYSTINOSIS

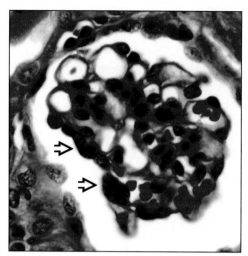

Multinucleated podocytes ⊵ are characteristic of cystinosis even in the absence of Fanconi syndrome. Pathogenesis may involve aberrant podocyte division without cytokinesis.

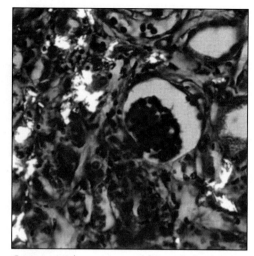

Cystine crystals are water soluble and dissolve with formalin fixation; rhomboid or polymorphous crystals are best seen on frozen sections under polarized light. (Courtesy J. Bernstein, MD.)

TERMINOLOGY

Definitions
- Autosomal recessive lysosomal storage disease secondary to mutations in *CTNS* gene resulting in intralysosomal accumulation of cystine and multiorgan damage

ETIOLOGY/PATHOGENESIS

Genetics
- *CTNS*
  - Encodes cystinosin
    - Lysosomal membrane cystine transporter
  - Maps to chromosome 17p13
  - Autosomal recessive inheritance
  - More than 90 mutations reported
  - Infantile form
    - 75% of European patients are homozygous for 57 kb deletion
    - Eliminates protein expression
  - Juvenile and adult forms
    - Point mutations or missense mutations affecting transmembrane loops or N-terminus

Pathophysiology
- Cystinosin mutations cause defective cystine transport and accumulation in lysosomes
- Renal failure may be due to atubular glomeruli

CLINICAL ISSUES

Epidemiology
- Incidence
  - Infantile form
    - 1 in 100,000 to 200,000 live births
  - Juvenile and adult forms
    - Rare; 5% of all cystinosis cases

- Age
  - Infantile form
    - Typically presents at 6-12 months
  - Juvenile and adult forms
    - Onset of symptoms at 3-50 years

Presentation
- Fanconi syndrome (infantile)
  - Polyuria, polydipsia, electrolyte abnormalities, dehydration, rickets, growth retardation
  - Not always present in juvenile and adult forms
- Hypothyroidism: 5-10 years
- Retinopathy
- Pulmonary dysfunction: 21-40 years
- Male hypogonadism
- Swallowing abnormalities
- Myopathy
- Corneal deposits (only adults)

Laboratory Tests
- Cystine levels in blood polymorphonuclear leukocytes
  - Tandem mass spectrometry most sensitive
    - Homozygotes: > 1 nmol cystine/mg protein
    - Heterozygotes: 0.14-0.57 nmol cystine/mg protein
    - Normal range: 0.04-0.16 nmol cystine/mg protein

Treatment
- Drugs
  - Cysteamine
    - Aminothiol
    - Binds intralysosomal cystine, allowing excretion from lysosome and cytoplasmic degradation
    - Slows disease progression

Prognosis
- Infantile form
  - If untreated, ESRD develops at mean of 9.2 years
- Juvenile form
  - May progress to ESRD, but at later age (12-28 years)

CYSTINOSIS

Key Facts

Etiology/Pathogenesis
- *CTNS* gene mutations
- 75% of European patients homozygous for 57 kb deletion

Clinical Issues
- Presents with Fanconi syndrome
- > 1 nmol cystine/mg protein in peripheral blood neutrophils
- Treat with cysteamine

Microscopic Pathology
- Podocyte and tubular epithelial multinucleation
- Proximal tubule "swan neck" deformity, atubular glomeruli
- Polarizable cystine crystals on frozen section

Top Differential Diagnoses
- Renal oxalosis, Fabry disease, cystinuria

MICROSCOPIC PATHOLOGY

Histologic Features
- Glomerular findings
  - Podocyte multinucleation
  - FSGS, typically seen in juvenile form
  - Endothelial and podocyte cystine crystals
- Tubular findings
  - Cystine crystal deposition
    - Polarizable, hexagonal, rhomboid, or polymorphous
    - Water soluble, best seen in frozen sections under polarized light
  - Proximal tubule "swan neck" deformity
    - Shortened, atrophic early proximal tubule after 6 months of age
  - Epithelial multinucleation
- Interstitium
  - In allografts, infiltrating macrophages contain hexagonal crystals

ANCILLARY TESTS

Immunofluorescence
- No specific findings reported

Electron Microscopy
- Intracellular spaces (plate, hexagon) where crystals located

DIFFERENTIAL DIAGNOSIS

Renal Oxalosis
- Fan-shaped, needle-like polarizable crystals
  - Preserved after formalin fixation

Fabry Disease
- Lacey podocytes
- Laminated deposits by EM

Cystinuria
- Recurrent nephrolithiasis without intracellular accumulation

DIAGNOSTIC CHECKLIST

Pathologic Interpretation Pearls
- Multinucleated podocytes pathognomic

SELECTED REFERENCES

1. Larsen CP et al: The incidence of atubular glomeruli in nephropathic cystinosis renal biopsies. Mol Genet Metab. 101(4):417-20, 2010
2. Wilmer MJ et al: Cystinosis: practical tools for diagnosis and treatment. Pediatr Nephrol. Epub ahead of print, 2010
3. Servais A et al: Late-onset nephropathic cystinosis: clinical presentation, outcome, and genotyping. Clin J Am Soc Nephrol. 3(1):27-35, 2008
4. Spear GS: Pathology of the kidney in cystinosis. Pathol Annu. 9(0):81-92, 1974

IMAGE GALLERY

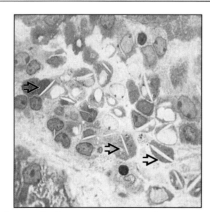
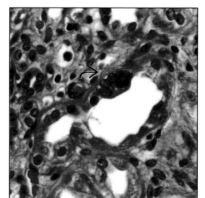
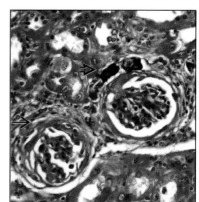

(Left) Needle-shaped colorless crystals in interstitial macrophages ➔ are characteristic of cystinosis, as shown on toluidine blue stained sections. *(Courtesy G. Spear, MD.)* *(Center)* Tubular epithelial cells may also show giant cell transformation ➔, in spite of absent cystine crystals. *(Right)* Chronic cystinosis features include periglomerular fibrosis ➔, tubular atrophy, interstitial inflammation, and calcium-containing deposits ➔.

BARTTER SYNDROME

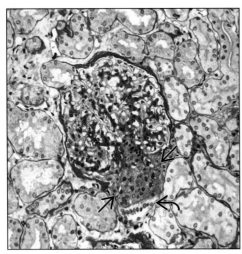

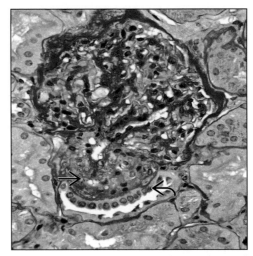

Bartter syndrome shows a hyperplastic and hypertrophic juxtaglomerular apparatus ⇒ with prominent macula densa ⇒. This reaction to Na loss is the primary histologic feature in Bartter syndrome.

Hyperplastic JGA with increased cytoplasmic volume and granularity ⇒, and prominence of the macula densa ⇒, is shown in an example of Bartter syndrome.

TERMINOLOGY

Definitions
- Normotensive hyper-reninemic hyperaldosteronism with hypokalemic alkalosis and hyperplasia of juxtaglomerular apparatus

ETIOLOGY/PATHOGENESIS

Autosomal Recessive Inheritance
- 5 types of loss-of-function mutations are described in Bartter syndrome
  - Type I: *NKCC2* gene on chromosome 15 for NKCC2 (a Na-K-Cl cotransporter)
  - Type II: *KCNJ1* gene on chromosome 11 for ROMK (renal outer medullary K channel)
  - Type III: *CLCNKB* gene on chromosome 1 for ClCKB (a Cl transporter)
  - Type IV: *BSND* gene, which encodes protein barttin and is involved in Cl transport
  - Type V: *CASR* gene which encodes CaSR (a calcium sensing receptor)

Dysfunction of Ion Channels
- Location mainly in ascending loop of Henle and distal nephron
- Failure of transport mechanisms results in delivery of excess NaCl to distal tubule and collecting duct
  - Promotes NaCl loss, volume depletion, K and acid secretion
- Electrolyte and water depletion with hypovolemia activates renin-angiotensin-aldosterone (RAA) system
  - Aldosterone promotes further K loss
  - Angiotensin II (AT II) promotes prostaglandin synthesis (especially PGE2) and may influence interstitial cell hyperplasia
  - Prolonged RAA activation leads to hyperplasia of juxtaglomerular apparatus (JGA)

CLINICAL ISSUES

Presentation
- Growth retardation, polyuria, dehydration
  - Hyper-reninemia, high AT II, hyperaldosteronism
  - Hypokalemia, alkalosis, hypochloremia
- Classic form
  - Presents in 1st few months to years of life
  - Failure to thrive, growth retardation, dehydration
  - Associated with type III mutations
- Neonatal form
  - Polyhydramnios, severe growth retardation, hypercalciuria, nephrocalcinosis
  - Neonatal Bartter syndrome is associated with type I and II mutations

Treatment
- Drugs
  - Nonsteroidal anti-inflammatory agents and potassium-sparing diuretics
  - Potassium and sodium replacement

Prognosis
- Limited data suggests chronic renal functional impairment occurs in ~ 20% of patients

MICROSCOPIC PATHOLOGY

Histologic Features
- Glomeruli and blood vessels
  - Diffuse JGA enlargement is due to hypertrophy of individual cells and hyperplasia
  - JGA cells and modified epithelioid smooth muscle of afferent and efferent arterioles have increased cytoplasmic granularity
    - Granules stain positively with periodic acid-Schiff and silver stains
    - Renin localized to granules by IHC

BARTTER SYNDROME

Key Facts

Terminology
- Normotensive hyper-reninemic hyperaldosteronism with hypokalemic alkalosis and hyperplasia of juxtaglomerular apparatus

Etiology/Pathogenesis
- 5 types of loss-of-function mutations of genes affecting ion channels are described in Bartter syndrome

Clinical Issues
- Growth retardation, polyuria, dehydration

Microscopic Pathology
- Diffuse enlargement of the JGA with renin and AT II expression
- Hypertrophy and hyperplasia of medullary interstitial cells

---

- Clusters of sclerotic and immature glomeruli are typically seen in cortex; most glomeruli are normal
  - Rarely focal segmental glomerulosclerosis, C1q nephropathy and medullary sponge kidney have been described
- Afferent arterioles have intimal and medial hyalinization
- Tubules and interstitium
  - Hypertrophy and hyperplasia of medullary interstitial cells
    - Cytoplasm of interstitial cells has vacuoles and PAS-positive granules
    - May arise from chronic hypokalemia and AT II
  - Proximal tubules may have prominent coarse vacuoles (secondary to hypokalemia)
  - Neonatal Bartter syndrome is associated with nephrocalcinosis
- Immunofluorescence findings are nonspecific
- Electron microscopy
  - JGA and epithelioid smooth muscle cells of arterioles have prominent endoplasmic reticulum and Golgi complexes and cytoplasmic, electron-dense secretory granules, some of which have a rhomboid appearance
  - Hyperplastic interstitial medullary cells have cytoplasmic, membrane-bound granules and myelin figures

DIFFERENTIAL DIAGNOSIS

Juxtaglomerular Apparatus Hyperplasia
- Chronic renal ischemia
  - Renal artery stenosis
  - Cardiac failure
  - Intrarenal vascular sclerosis
    - Hypertension, scleroderma, chronic thrombotic microangiopathies
- Drugs
  - AT II receptor antagonists, cyclosporine, diuretics
- Addison disease

DIAGNOSTIC CHECKLIST

Pathologic Interpretation Pearls
- Enlarged JGA is characteristic but not diagnostic

SELECTED REFERENCES

1. France R et al: Intracellular granules of the renal medulla in a case of potassium depletion due to renal potassium wasting. Electron microscopic comparison with renal medullary granules in the potassium-depleted rat. Am J Pathol. 91(2):299-312, 1978
2. Bartter FC et al: Hyperplasia of the juxtaglomerular complex with hyperaldosteronism and hypokalemic alkalosis. A new syndrome. Am J Med. 33:811-28, 1962

IMAGE GALLERY

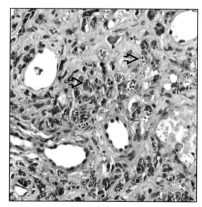 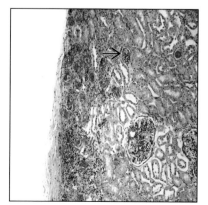 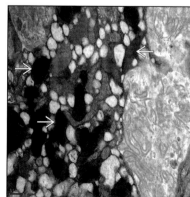

(Left) Hyperplasia of the medullary interstitial cells is shown with prominent PAS-positive granules ⊳. These have been described in association with chronic hypokalemia. (Courtesy S. Nasr, MD and L. Cornell, MD.) *(Center)* Clustering of atrophic and immature glomeruli ➡ in the outer cortex is described in Bartter syndrome in children. *(Right)* Ultrastructural (EM) features of a juxtaglomerular cell demonstrate membrane-bound granules of varying density ➡ and numerous vesicles.

DENT DISEASE

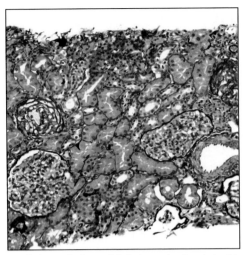

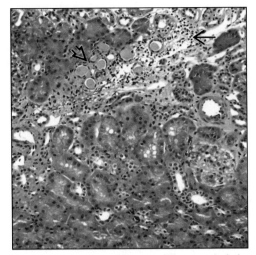

Focal glomeruli show global glomerulosclerosis in this biopsy from a 9-year-old boy with a family history of Dent disease. The serum creatinine was normal and he had 2+ proteinuria on urinalysis.

This case showed very mild interstitial fibrosis and tubular atrophy ⊟, with focal sparse interstitial inflammation ⊟.

TERMINOLOGY

Synonyms
- X-linked recessive nephrolithiasis
- X-linked recessive hypophosphatemic rickets
- Idiopathic low molecular weight proteinuria

ETIOLOGY/PATHOGENESIS

Gene Mutations
- Both identified genes located on X chromosome
- *CLCN5* gene, "Dent disease 1"
  - Mutation in 2/3 of Dent disease patients
  - Encodes electrogenic chloride/proton exchanger ClC-5
  - Deficiency in ClC-5 protein alters membrane trafficking via receptor-mediated endocytic pathway in proximal tubular epithelial cells
- *OCRL1* gene, "Dent disease 2"
  - Encodes a protein (OCRL1) with phosphatidylinositol-4,5-bisphosphate 5-phosphatase activity
  - OCRL1 protein is present on clathrin-coated intermediates, early endosomes, and Golgi apparatus and may facilitate trafficking between these compartments in tubular epithelial cells
  - Lowe syndrome, a related disease, also has mutation in *OCRL1* gene
    - Lowe syndrome (oculocerebrorenal) has more severe renal and systemic phenotype than Dent disease 2
- Some patients with Dent disease phenotype have neither mutation

CLINICAL ISSUES

Presentation
- Usually presents in childhood

- Nephrocalcinosis
- Nephrolithiasis
- Hypercalciuria
  - Normal serum calcium level
- Proteinuria, asymptomatic
  - Usually < 2 g/day total proteinuria
  - Low molecular weight proteinuria (100%)
- Proximal tubular dysfunction, partial Fanconi syndrome
  - Glycosuria, aminoaciduria, concentrating defect
  - Rickets (uncommon)
- Hematuria
- Chronic renal failure
  - Age 25-50 years
- Dent disease is likely underdiagnosed
  - Should be suspected in young male patient with nephrolithiasis and any degree of proteinuria
- No known clinical disease in female carriers
  - May have low molecular weight proteinuria

Treatment
- Surgical approaches
  - Kidney transplantation for end-stage renal disease
    - Disease not known to recur in allograft
- Drugs
  - Thiazide diuretics to stimulate reabsorption of calcium in distal tubules
- Other
  - Restrict dietary sodium intake
    - Sodium excretion promotes calcium excretion
  - Dietary calcium restriction reduces calciuria but increases risk of bone disease

MICROSCOPIC PATHOLOGY

Histologic Features
- Nonspecific features
- Interstitial fibrosis and tubular atrophy

DENT DISEASE

Key Facts

Etiology/Pathogenesis
- *CLCN5* or *OCRL1* gene, both located on X chromosome

Clinical Issues
- Nephrolithiasis
- Hypercalciuria
- Low molecular weight proteinuria
- Chronic renal failure
- Dent disease is likely underdiagnosed

- ○ Should be suspected in young male patient with nephrolithiasis and any degree of proteinuria

Microscopic Pathology
- Interstitial fibrosis and tubular atrophy
- Focal global or segmental glomerulosclerosis

Ancillary Tests
- Urinary retinol binding protein

- ○ Focal deposition of calcium phosphate or calcium oxalate may be present
- ○ Focal mild interstitial inflammation
- Focal global glomerulosclerosis
- Focal segmental glomerulosclerosis

Electron Microscopy
- Glomeruli may show mild segmental podocyte foot process effacement
- No specific features in tubules

ANCILLARY TESTS

Molecular Genetics
- Dent disease-specific mutations in *CLCN5* or *OCRL1*

Urine Testing
- Retinol binding protein
- β2-microglobulin
- α1-microglobulin

DIFFERENTIAL DIAGNOSIS

Other Causes of Partial Fanconi Syndrome
- Heavy metal toxicity
- Interstitial nephritis/nephropathy
- Cystinosis
- Mitochondriopathy
- Lowe syndrome

Focal Global Glomerulosclerosis Due to Other Causes
- Nonspecific light microscopy pattern

Focal Segmental Glomerulosclerosis
- Some cases may be familial

Nephrolithiasis
- Calcium phosphate and/or calcium oxalate stones
- If low molecular weight proteinuria is present, Dent disease should be suspected

DIAGNOSTIC CHECKLIST

Pathologic Interpretation Pearls
- May be overlooked as cause of FSGS in males

SELECTED REFERENCES

1. Claverie-Martín F et al: Dent's disease: clinical features and molecular basis. Pediatr Nephrol. Epub ahead of print, 2010
2. Frishberg Y et al: Dent's disease manifesting as focal glomerulosclerosis: Is it the tip of the iceberg? Pediatr Nephrol. 24(12):2369-73, 2009
3. Hodgin JB et al: Dent disease presenting as partial Fanconi syndrome and hypercalciuria. Kidney Int. 73(11):1320-3, 2008
4. Copelovitch L et al: Hypothesis: Dent disease is an underrecognized cause of focal glomerulosclerosis. Clin J Am Soc Nephrol. 2(5):914-8, 2007

IMAGE GALLERY

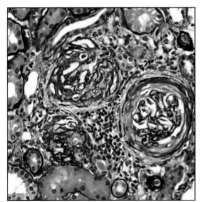 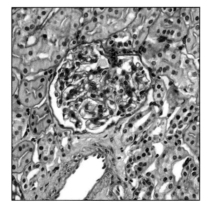 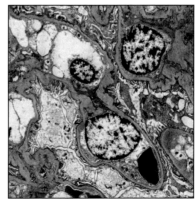

(Left) Focal glomeruli show global glomerulosclerosis. No segmental scars were identified in this case, although focal segmental glomerulosclerosis may be seen in Dent disease. *(Center)* A nonglobally sclerotic glomerulus appears normal by light microscopy. *(Right)* With electron microscopy the glomeruli show largely preserved podocyte foot processes, with very mild segmental foot process effacement. No glomerular basement membrane features of Alport syndrome are present.

OCULOCEREBRORENAL SYNDROME OF LOWE

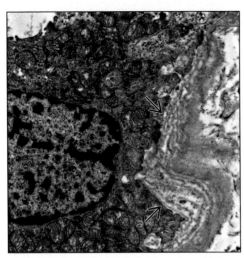

This proximal convoluted tubule in a patient with Lowe syndrome shows marked thickening of the tubular basement membrane. There is also prominent tubular basement membrane lamellar ➔ alteration.

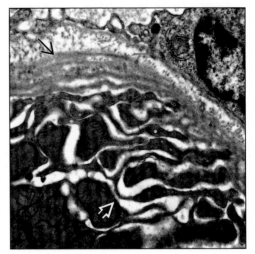

This proximal convoluted tubule in a patient with Lowe syndrome shows prominent dilatation of the tubular infolding ⬃ and marked tubular basement membrane lamellar ➔ alteration.

TERMINOLOGY

Abbreviations
- Oculocerebrorenal syndrome of Lowe (OCRL)

Synonyms
- Oculocerebrorenal dystrophy

Definitions
- Disease triad of renal tubular dysfunction, congenital cataracts, and mental retardation due to mutations in *OCRL* (OMIM #309000)

ETIOLOGY/PATHOGENESIS

X-linked Genetic Disease
- Mutations in *OCRL* gene (Xq26.1)
  - Heterogeneous: Premature stop codons, insertion/deletion, splice site, and missense mutations
- *OCRL* encodes OCRL1 protein
  - Phosphatidylinositol 4,5-biphosphate 5-phosphatase
  - Binds to clathrin
    - Regulates clathrin-mediated protein trafficking
  - Affects vesicle-dependent proximal tubule reabsorption and trafficking of transporter proteins
    - Small molecular weight proteins, albumin, aminoacids, bicarbonate, calcium
    - Lysosomal enzymuria due to altered trafficking
    - Glucose transport not affected

CLINICAL ISSUES

Epidemiology
- Incidence
  - 1:200,000-1:500,000 births
  - Pan-ethnic disorder
- Gender
  - Almost all males
  - Females with X-autosomal translocations reported

Presentation
- Hypotonia and cataracts at birth
  - Glaucoma (~ 50%)
- Severe mental retardation (~ 33%)
  - Seizures (~ 50%)
- Metabolic acidosis
  - Bicarbonate wasting, moderate
  - Not Fanconi syndrome, no glycosuria, mild phosphaturia
- Low-grade proteinuria
- Chronic renal disease by 2nd decade
- Cryptorchidism

Laboratory Tests
- Hypokalemia, hypocalcemia, low bicarbonate
- Assessment of proximal tubular function
  - Low molecular weight proteinuria (e.g., retinol binding protein) (100%)
  - Lysosomal enzymuria (N-acetyl-β-d-glucosaminidase) (100%)
  - Generalized aminoaciduria (~ 90%)
  - Hypercalcuria (~ 95%)
- Increased alkaline phosphatase
- Genetic tests for *OCRL* mutations

Treatment
- Renal tubular acidosis
  - Monitor acid-base status and electrolyte levels
    - Potassium and calcium supplementation
    - ~ 50% require bicarbonate supplementation

Prognosis
- Renal failure occurs in 2nd to 4th decade
- Dialysis and transplantation plays limited role

IMAGE FINDINGS

Radiographic Findings
- Metaphyseal flaring, osteopenia of wrists and long bones

OCULOCEREBRORENAL SYNDROME OF LOWE

Key Facts

Terminology
- Oculocerebrorenal syndrome (OCRL)

Etiology/Pathogenesis
- Inherited mutation caused by *OCRL1* gene mutation
- Affects protein trafficking and cellular metabolism

Clinical Issues
- X-linked disorder; 1:200,000-1:500,000 births
- Proximal tubular dysfunction, congenital cataracts, and cognitive impairment

Microscopic Pathology
- Tubular and interstitial abnormalities most frequent
  - Dilated tubules with protein casts
  - Tubular atrophy and interstitial fibrosis
  - Medullary nephrocalcinosis
- Glomerular disease is rare
  - Diffuse mesangial sclerosis

Ancillary Tests
- Electron microscopy
  - Dilated proximal tubular infolding
  - Proximal tubular basement membrane lamellar thickening
  - Tubular mitochondrial swelling and irregularity
  - Irregular glomerular basement membrane thickening

Top Differential Diagnoses
- Dent disease
- Cystinosis
- Fanconi syndrome
- Hypophosphatemic rickets

Ultrasonographic Findings
- Medullary nephrocalcinosis (~ 50%) and nephrolithiasis

MR Findings
- Periventricular white matter abnormalities in brain

MICROSCOPIC PATHOLOGY

Histologic Features
- Glomeruli
  - Rarely, diffuse mesangial sclerosis
    - Glomerular hypercellularity and matrix increase
    - Capillary loop collapse with podocyte hyperplasia
  - Nonspecific glomerulosclerosis
- Tubules and interstitium
  - Dilated tubules with protein casts
  - Tubular atrophy and interstitial fibrosis
  - Medullary nephrocalcinosis described radiologically

ANCILLARY TESTS

Immunofluorescence
- Negative for immune reactants and complement

Electron Microscopy
- Glomerulus: Diffuse mesangial sclerosis
  - Capillary loop GBM irregular thickening
  - Mesangial matrix increase ± hypercellularity
- Proximal tubule
  - Proximal tubule dilatation
  - Mitochondrial swelling
  - Basement membrane lamellar thickening
  - Small vesicles adjacent to TBM changes
  - Dilation of proximal tubular infolding

DIFFERENTIAL DIAGNOSIS

Dent Disease
- Lacks systemic features (cataracts, mental retardation)
- Nephrolithiasis and nephrocalcinosis prominent
- Mutation in *CLCN5* (Dent1) or *OCRL1* (Dent2)
  - Genotype does not distinguish Dent2 from OCRL

Cystinosis
- Multinucleated podocytes
- Thin 1st part of proximal tubule: Swan-neck deformity
- Typical Fanconi syndrome with glucosuria

Fanconi Syndrome
- Various causes
- Glycosuria present by definition

Hypophosphatemic Rickets
- Inability to establish normal ossification
- Phosphate wasting more severe

SELECTED REFERENCES

1. Cui S et al: OCRL1 function in renal epithelial membrane traffic. Am J Physiol Renal Physiol. 298(2):F335-45, 2010
2. Bockenhauer D et al: Renal phenotype in Lowe Syndrome: a selective proximal tubular dysfunction. Clin J Am Soc Nephrol. 3(5):1430-6, 2008
3. Cho HY et al: Renal manifestations of Dent disease and Lowe syndrome. Pediatr Nephrol. 23(2):243-9, 2008
4. Monnens L et al: Evaluation of the proximal tubular function in hereditary renal Fanconi syndrome. Nephrol Dial Transplant. 23(9):2719-22, 2008
5. Erdmann KS et al: A role of the Lowe syndrome protein OCRL in early steps of the endocytic pathway. Dev Cell. 13(3):377-90, 2007
6. Laube GF et al: Early proximal tubular dysfunction in Lowe's syndrome. Arch Dis Child. 89(5):479-80, 2004
7. Charnas LR et al: Clinical and laboratory findings in the oculocerebrorenal syndrome of Lowe, with special reference to growth and renal function. N Engl J Med. 324(19):1318-25, 1991

OCULOCEREBRORENAL SYNDROME OF LOWE

Microscopic Features

(Left) Light microscopy from a patient with oculocerebrorenal syndrome shows a glomerulus that appears essentially normal. There is no obvious capillary wall thickening or mesangial matrix expansion or increased cellularity.
(Right) In patients with Lowe syndrome, glomerular lesions by light microscopy are usually not observed until chronic tubulointerstitial disease develops. This silver stain shows no significant abnormalities of the GBM or mesangium regions.

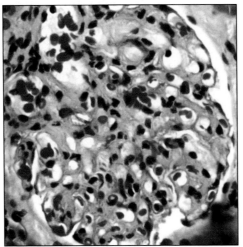
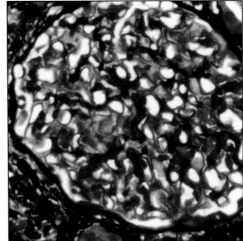

(Left) This patient with Lowe syndrome has developed progressive renal injury. The glomerulus shows a moderate mesangial expansion and compromise of the capillary loops. There is prominent periglomerular fibrosis ➡ associated with tubular atrophy and interstitial fibrosis.
(Right) This patient with Lowe syndrome has developed chronic tubulointerstitial disease. This glomerulus shows early alterations consisting of mild increase in mesangial matrix with mild hypercellularity ➡.

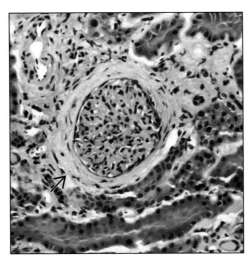
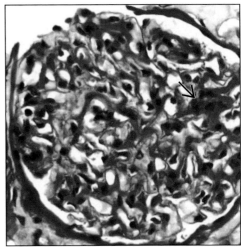

(Left) The tubules in Lowe syndrome show nonspecific changes. Here is an atrophic tubule containing a protein cast ➡. The background tubules show early epithelial atrophy and interstitial fibrosis ➡. *(Right)* Diffuse mesangial sclerosis is rarely encountered in Lowe syndrome. It is characterized by mesangial hypercellularity and increased mesangial matrix ➡.
There is distinctive marked epithelial cell hyperplasia and enlargement ➡ with collapse of the capillary loops.

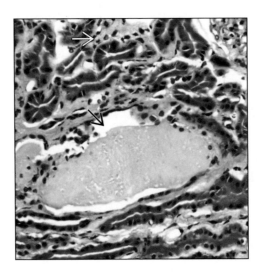
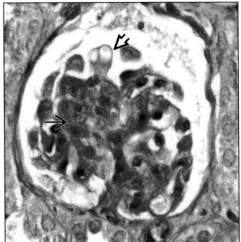

OCULOCEREBRORENAL SYNDROME OF LOWE

Electron Microscopy

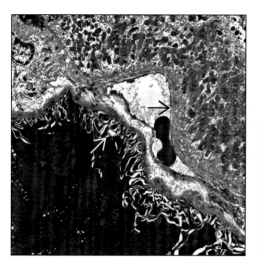

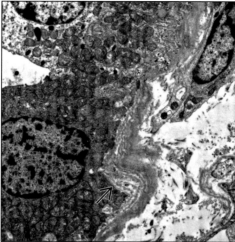

(Left) In patients with Lowe syndrome, electron microscopy shows distinctive tubular changes. There is often dilatation of the plasma membrane infoldings ➡ and lamellar thickening of the basement membrane ➡ *(Right)* In this patient with Lowe syndrome, there is marked thickening and lamellation of the tubular basement membrane ➡, somewhat similar to glomerular changes in Alport syndrome. The brush border disappears and the cytoplasm may protrude into the tubular lumen.

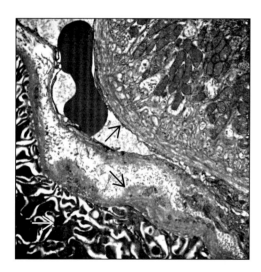

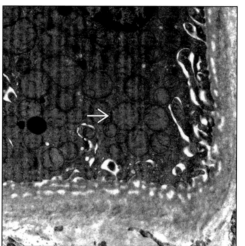

(Left) The plasma membrane infoldings ➡ of the proximal tubules frequently appear quite dilated in patients with Lowe syndrome. Both tubules in this image also show the characteristic tubular basement membrane thickening and lamellation ➡ of Lowe syndrome. *(Right)* Mitochondrial changes in the proximal tubules include swelling and irregularity with a pronounced circular profile ➡. The cristae also appear less numerous, and may be disrupted and shorter or completely absent.

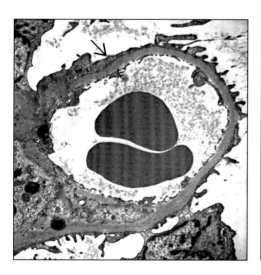

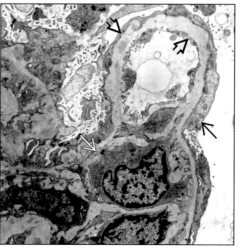

(Left) The glomerular capillary loops in Lowe syndrome with tubulopathy may be normal or demonstrate mild irregular thickening of the glomerular basement membrane (GBM). Endothelial cell swelling and segmental effacement of podocyte foot processes ➡ are often observed. *(Right)* In diffuse mesangial sclerosis there is mesangial hypercellularity ➡, matrix expansion, and marked irregularity of the GBM ➡ with diffuse effacement of the podocyte foot processes ➡.

METHYLMALONIC ACIDEMIA

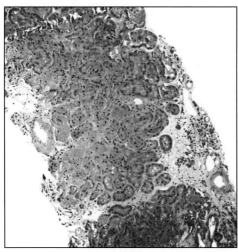

H&E shows focal interstitial fibrosis and tubular atrophy in a biopsy from a 26-year-old man with vitamin B12-responsive methylmalonic acidemia. He had chronic renal failure with a serum creatinine of 2.7 mg/dL.

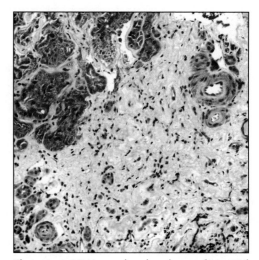

The cortex in MMA may show broad areas of interstitial fibrosis and tubular atrophy with little inflammation. The disease may be either genetic or caused by vitamin B12 deficiency.

TERMINOLOGY

Abbreviations
- Methylmalonic acidemia (MMA)

Synonyms
- Methylmalonic aciduria

ETIOLOGY/PATHOGENESIS

Impaired Metabolism of Methylmalonic Acid
- Methylmalonic acid is generated during metabolism of amino acids isoleucine, methionine, threonine, and valine, and odd-chain fatty acids

Genetic
- Metabolic defect caused by complete or partial deficiency of adenosylcobalamin-dependent enzyme methylmalonyl-CoA mutase
  - Several different genetic defects identified
- May be detected by newborn screening exams
- Inherited in autosomal recessive fashion
- Incidence ~ 1:48,000

Severe Vitamin B12 (Cobalamin) Deficiency
- Vitamin B12 is cofactor of methylmalonyl-CoA mutase

CLINICAL ISSUES

Epidemiology
- Incidence
  - Estimated incidence in Europe is 1:115,000 to 1:277,000
- Age
  - Genetic forms have usually early onset
    - Neonatal period through early childhood

Presentation
- Chronic renal failure

- Renal disease develops in patients with longer survival
- Proximal renal tubular acidosis
- Nonrenal manifestations (inherited MMA)
  - Developmental delay, failure to thrive, lethargy, vomiting, seizures, muscular hypotonia
  - Metabolic acidosis, hyperammonemia
- Variable patterns and severity of presentation
- Hypertension in some patients

Laboratory Tests
- Diagnosis of MMA
  - Plasma and urine concentrations of methylmalonic acid

Treatment
- Surgical approaches
  - Renal transplantation
    - Treats end-stage renal disease
    - Some methylmalonyl-CoA mutase is produced by allograft kidney; renal transplantation treats, in part, the original metabolic defect
  - Liver transplantation
    - Most methylmalonyl-CoA mutase is produced in liver
- Drugs
  - Hydroxy-cobalamin therapy if B12-responsive disease
    - Patients with mutations in methylmalonyl-CoA mutase do not respond
  - Antibiotics
    - Reduce levels of gut bacteria that produce particular amino acids
  - Angiotensin II inhibition in patients with renal disease
- Low-protein diet to reduce precursors of methylmalonic acid
  - Amino acids
    - Reduced intake of isoleucine, methionine, threonine, valine

METHYLMALONIC ACIDEMIA

Key Facts

Etiology/Pathogenesis
- Impaired metabolism of methylmalonic acid
- Genetic
  - Metabolic defect caused by complete or partial deficiency of adenosylcobalamin-dependent enzyme methylmalonyl-CoA mutase
- Severe vitamin B12 (cobalamin) deficiency
  - Vitamin B12 is a cofactor of methylmalonyl-CoA mutase

Clinical Issues
- Chronic renal failure
- Variable patterns and severity of presentation
- Hydroxy-cobalamin therapy if B12-responsive disease
- Low-protein diet to reduce precursors of methylmalonic acid

Microscopic Pathology
- Interstitial fibrosis and tubular atrophy
- Chronic interstitial nephritis

  - Reduced intake of odd-chain fatty acids and polyunsaturated fat

MICROSCOPIC PATHOLOGY

Histologic Features
- Interstitial fibrosis and tubular atrophy
- Chronic interstitial nephritis
  - Sparse inflammation
- Nonspecific histologic findings
  - Biopsy needed to exclude other causes of renal failure

DIFFERENTIAL DIAGNOSIS

Chronic Tubulointerstitial Nephropathy
- Other causes of chronic tubulointerstitial nephropathy/nephritis may have similar histologic appearance
- Other potential causes include urinary tract obstruction or infection, vascular diseases, toxins or drugs, renal structural defects, and other inherited disorders

SELECTED REFERENCES

1. Manoli I et al: Methylmalonic acidemia. GeneReviews [Internet]. Seattle: University of Washington. Posted August 16, 2006; updated September 28, 2010
2. Ha TS et al: Delay of renal progression in methylmalonic acidemia using angiotensin II inhibition: a case report. J Nephrol. 21(5):793-6, 2008
3. Lubrano R et al: Renal transplant in methylmalonic acidemia: could it be the best option? Report on a case at 10 years and review of the literature. Pediatr Nephrol. 22(8):1209-14, 2007
4. Deodato F et al: Methylmalonic and propionic aciduria. Am J Med Genet C Semin Med Genet. 142C(2):104-12, 2006
5. Lubrano R et al: Kidney transplantation in a girl with methylmalonic acidemia and end stage renal failure. Pediatr Nephrol. 16(11):848-51, 2001
6. Rutledge SL et al: Tubulointerstitial nephritis in methylmalonic acidemia. Pediatr Nephrol. 7(1):81-2, 1993
7. Molteni KH et al: Progressive renal insufficiency in methylmalonic acidemia. Pediatr Nephrol. 5(3):323-6, 1991
8. Thompson GN et al: The use of metronidazole in management of methylmalonic and propionic acidaemias. Eur J Pediatr. 149(11):792-6, 1990
9. Coulombe JT et al: Massachusetts Metabolic Disorders Screening Program. II. Methylmalonic aciduria. Pediatrics. 67(1):26-31, 1981
10. Rosenberg LE et al: Methylmalonic aciduria. An inborn error leading to metabolic acidosis, long-chain ketonuria and intermittent hyperglycinemia. N Engl J Med. 278(24):1319-22, 1968

IMAGE GALLERY

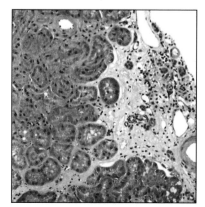 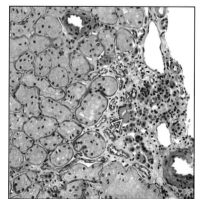 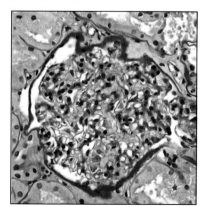

(Left) Minimal focal interstitial fibrosis with sparse mononuclear cell inflammation is evident in this case of MMA. *(Center)* Periodic acid-Schiff shows focal interstitial fibrosis and tubular atrophy. Focal arterioles show intimal hyalinosis ➡ in this case. *(Right)* A nonglobally sclerotic glomerulus appears normal. This case showed focal glomeruli with global sclerosis.

4

MITOCHONDRIOPATHIES

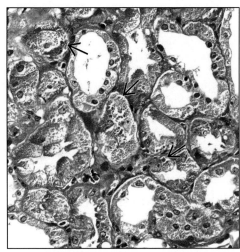

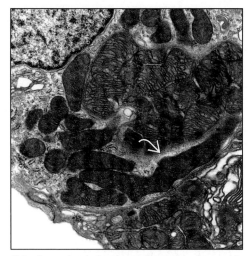

Renal tubules show prominent eosinophilic tubular inclusions indicating giant mitochondria ⮞ in 9-year-old girl with Fanconi syndrome, opaque cornea, and deafness (traits suggestive of inherited mitochondrial defect).

EM of renal tubule shows increased dysmorphic mitochondria with crowding, irregular size and shape ⮞, and varied loss of cristae in a patient treated with Viramune, a reverse transcriptase inhibitor.

TERMINOLOGY

Abbreviations
- Mitochondriopathies (MCP)

Definitions
- Genetic defect of oxidative phosphorylation due to deficiency of one of the mitochondrial respiratory chain complexes; also acquired form due to drug toxicity (e.g., Viramune)

ETIOLOGY/PATHOGENESIS

Genetic
- Abnormal mitochondrial components from mutated mitochondrial (mtDNA) or nuclear DNA (nDNA)
- Mitochondria have own DNA, a circular strand (mtDNA)
  - Genes that encode for enzymes, structural signaling, carrier/shuttle, channel receptor, tRNAs, rRNAs, or heat shock or assembling proteins are affected
  - DNA polymerase and tRNA different from nucleus
  - Maternal inheritance pattern for mtDNA

Drugs
- Acquired MCP is secondary to drugs that interfere with mtDNA replication
  - Reverse transcriptase inhibitors given for HIV infection (HAART) and rifampin affect mitochondrial DNA polymerase

Etiology
- Biochemical classification is based on different types of defects or deficiency in metabolic cell cycle in the mitochondria
  - Lack of cytochrome oxidase isotypes and succinate dehydrogenase are common defects

Mechanism
- Interference with oxidative metabolism

- Organs/cells most dependent on oxidative phosphorylation are affected
  - Brain, heart, eye, kidney

CLINICAL ISSUES

Epidemiology
- Incidence
  - Genetic forms
    - 4-5/100,000 live births
    - 1/50,000 prevalence of mtDNA mutations (adults)
    - 50% of children with MCPs have renal disease
- Age
  - Birth to 6 years at onset of symptoms

Presentation
- MCPs are clinically, biochemically, and genetically heterogeneous with single or multiorgan involvement
- Varied effects on organs: Ophthalmoplegia, seizures, lactic acidosis, ataxia, deafness, short stature, cardiomyopathy, hypopituitarism
- DeToni-Debré-Fanconi syndrome
  - Tubular dysfunction including aminoaciduria, glucosuria, phosphaturia, hyperuricemia
    - Occurs in Kearns-Sayre syndrome (KSS); Pearson syndrome; myoclonic epilepsy and ragged red fibers (MERRF); and mitochondrial encephalopathy, lactic acidosis, and stroke-like episodes (MELAS)
- Chronic renal failure
- Nephrotic syndrome (rare)

Laboratory Tests
- Blood lactic acid, ketones
- Urine: Amino acids, glucose, ketones, carnitines
- Genetic studies for mtDNA or nDNA mutations and COQ2

Treatment
- No specific treatment for inherited form

MITOCHONDRIOPATHIES

Key Facts

Etiology/Pathogenesis
- Rare genetic disorder of mtDNA
- Drug induced with reverse transcriptase inhibitors

Clinical Issues
- Clinically, biochemically and genetically heterogeneous
- 50% have renal involvement
- Renal disease occurs in KSS, Pearson syndrome, MERRF, and MELAS
- DeToni-Debré-Fanconi syndrome
  - Urine amino acids, glucose, ketones, carnitines

Microscopic Pathology
- Most common lesion is proximal tubulopathy with dysmorphic mitochondria
- Definitive diagnosis is based on integration of clinical, electrophysiological, neuroimaging, histopathological, biochemical, and genetic investigations

---

- Discontinuation of drugs implicated in acquired MCP usually reverses renal failure

Prognosis
- High mortality rate for inherited forms

MICROSCOPIC PATHOLOGY

Histologic Features
- Glomeruli
  - Focal segmental sclerosis progressing to parenchymal scarring
  - Collapsing glomerulopathy in *COQ2* defect
- Tubules
  - Eosinophilic coarsely granular cytoplasm indicating large mitochondria in proximal tubulopathy
  - Tubular cystic changes and obstruction by casts
  - Acute proximal tubular injury is seen in acquired form of toxicity during tenofovir therapy
- Interstitium
  - Interstitial fibrosis and tubular atrophy
  - Minimal inflammation
- Vessels
  - No specific changes
- Extrarenal
  - Depending on the type of mitochondriopathy, other organs affected include skeletal muscle, heart, liver, central nervous system, and endocrine organs
    - Muscle biopsy with specific features

- Definitive diagnosis is based on integration of clinical, electrophysiological, neuroimaging, histopathological, biochemical, and genetic investigations

ANCILLARY TESTS

Electron Microscopy
- Renal tubular dysmorphic mitochondrial changes
  - Increased number
  - Irregularly shaped, large-sized mitochondria
  - Fragmented, disoriented or variable loss of cristae

DIFFERENTIAL DIAGNOSIS

Nonspecific Tubulointerstitial Nephritis
- Mitochondrial EM abnormalities point to MCP

SELECTED REFERENCES

1. Herlitz LC et al: Tenofovir nephrotoxicity: acute tubular necrosis with distinctive clinical, pathological, and mitochondrial abnormalities. Kidney Int. 78(11):1171-7, 2010
2. Diomedi-Camassei F et al: COQ2 nephropathy: a newly described inherited mitochondriopathy with primary renal involvement. J Am Soc Nephrol. 18(10):2773-80, 2007
3. Finsterer J: Overview on visceral manifestations of mitochondrial disorders. Neth J Med. 64(3):61-71, 2006
4. Martín-Hernández E et al: Renal pathology in children with mitochondrial diseases. Pediatr Nephrol. 20(9):1299-305, 2005

IMAGE GALLERY

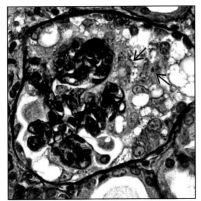 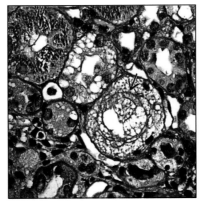 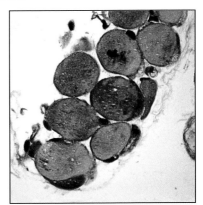

(Left) Collapsing glomerulopathy with hyperplastic, vacuolated epithelial cells having giant dysmorphic mitochondria seen as coarsely granular inclusion bodies ⇒ in an 18 month old with COQ2 deficiency. (Courtesy L. Barisoni, MD.) (Center) Proximal tubular cells show vacuolization ⇒ with focal protein resorption droplets in COQ2 defect. (Courtesy L. Barisoni, MD.) (Right) Myopathy with COQ2 mutation shows ragged red fibers in which PAS(+) granules aggregate & accumulate at periphery of the myocyte below the sarcolemma. (Courtesy L. Barisoni, MD.)

Infections of the Kidney

ACUTE PYELONEPHRITIS

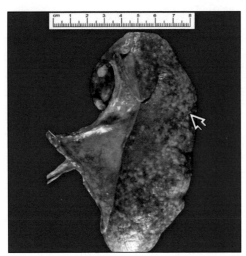

An autopsy kidney with gross features of acute bacterial pyelonephritis is shown. The renal capsule has been peeled, and the cortical surface shows multiple small abscesses ➡. (Courtesy L. Fajardo, MD.)

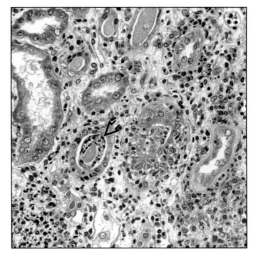

H&E stain of a renal biopsy shows neutrophils within the tubular lumens ➡ and interstitium, along with mononuclear cells, eosinophils, and plasma cells. Mild interstitial edema is also seen.

TERMINOLOGY

Abbreviations
- Acute pyelonephritis (APN)

Synonyms
- Upper urinary tract infection (UTI)
- Acute bacterial nephritis (used when no pyelitis)

Definitions
- Acute inflammation of kidney parenchyma due to bacterial infection

ETIOLOGY/PATHOGENESIS

Ascending Infection
- Retrograde infection via urethra, urinary bladder, and ureters
- Most common route of infection (95%)
- Usually associated with predisposing factor
  - Obstruction
  - Reflux
  - Instrumentation
  - Urolithiasis
  - Diabetes
  - Pregnancy
- Gram-negative bacteria from gastrointestinal tract (fecal flora) most common
  - *Escherichia coli* most common organism
    - Uropathogenic and virulence factors include fimbriae/pili and serotypes O, K, and H
    - Can colonize urinary bladder efficiently
  - P fimbriae (mannose resistant)
    - Attach to digalactoside residue on urothelial cells and facilitate persistent infection
    - Enhance host innate inflammatory response by interaction with Toll-like receptor 4 (TLR4), resulting in IL-6 and IL-8 production
    - Most important for renal involvement

- Type 1 fimbriae (mannose sensitive)
  - Binds to Tamm-Horsfall protein
- *Proteus, Klebsiella, Enterobacter, Pseudomonas, Streptococcus faecalis*
- Fungal organisms can produce similar pathology

Hematogenous Infection
- In septicemia or bacterial endocarditis
  - *Staphylococcus aureus* common pathogen
  - Fungal organisms in immunocompromised hosts
- No obstruction or reflux required for pathogenesis

Asymptomatic Bacteriuria
- Bacterial counts of > 100,000 colony forming units/mL of urine in relatively asymptomatic patient
- Frequently encountered in pregnant women
  - Antimicrobial therapy recommended as it can progress to overt bacteriuria and pyelonephritis

CLINICAL ISSUES

Epidemiology
- Age
  - Infants
    - Associated with anatomic abnormalities of urinary tract
  - Elderly males
    - Prostatic hypertrophy is risk factor
- Gender
  - Women more susceptible, especially during pregnancy

Site
- Pelvic urothelium (pyelitis)
- Renal tubules and interstitium (pyelonephritis)
- Renal cortical abscesses (bacterial nephritis)

Presentation
- Fever
- Chills

ACUTE PYELONEPHRITIS

Key Facts

Terminology
- Acute inflammation of kidney parenchyma due to bacterial infection

Etiology/Pathogenesis
- Retrograde infection via urethra, urinary bladder, and ureters
  - *E. coli* common organism
- Hematogenous infection in septicemia
  - *S. aureus* common organism

Clinical Issues
- Associated with lower tract problems, obstruction, reflux, pregnancy, diabetes
- Fever
- Costovertebral angle tenderness
- Leukocyte casts

- Acute uncomplicated pyelonephritis responds to antimicrobial therapy in > 90% of cases

Microscopic Pathology
- Neutrophilic infiltrate and casts in tubules
- Abscesses and papillary necrosis may arise
- Glomeruli and blood vessels relatively spared
- Early infection in medulla and collecting ducts
- Pelvic inflammation in ascending infection

Top Differential Diagnoses
- Drug-induced interstitial nephritis
- Glomerulonephritis associated severe tubulointerstitial inflammation
- Myeloma cast nephropathy
- Ischemic or toxic tubular injury
- Acute humoral rejection in transplants

- Flank pain
- Nausea and vomiting
- Costovertebral angle tenderness
- May be subclinical
- If lower UTI is present
  - Dysuria
  - Frequency of micturition
  - Suprapubic tenderness may be present
- Acute renal failure
  - Severe and bilateral cases
  - Emphysematous pyelonephritis
  - Single kidney
  - Transplant kidney

Laboratory Tests
- Urine microscopy
  - Pyuria (white blood cells in urine)
  - Leukocyte casts
  - Gram stain may be positive
- Urine cultures
  - Midstream urine needed to minimize contamination
- Blood examination
  - Leukocytosis with shift to left
  - Blood cultures positive in septicemia

Treatment
- Surgical approaches
  - Correction of anatomical defect or source of obstruction
  - Nephrectomy uncommon as most patients respond to antibiotic therapy
- Drugs
  - Antimicrobials
  - Empiric antimicrobial therapy with Gram-negative coverage until culture results are obtained

Prognosis
- Severe complications more common in patients with diabetes mellitus and urinary obstruction
  - Papillary necrosis: Coagulative necrosis of papillary tips
  - Pyonephrosis: Accumulation of pus in renal pyelocalyceal system

  - Perinephric abscess: Suppurative inflammation extends beyond kidney into perinephric fat
  - Emphysematous pyelonephritis: Presence of gas within renal parenchyma
  - Septicemia
- Scarring ensues in 30% of children with APN
- Acute uncomplicated pyelonephritis responds to antimicrobial therapy in > 90% of cases
  - Lack of response in
    - Drug-resistant bacterial strains
    - Presence of anatomic abnormality (reflux, etc.)
    - Urinary tract obstruction
- Recurrent episodes of pyelonephritis can lead to chronic pyelonephritis and chronic renal failure

IMAGE FINDINGS

General Features
- Imaging is indicated in select cases
  - Patients with recurrent UTI, especially adult males and children < 5 years of age
  - Patients with diabetes mellitus
- Tests include
  - Cystoscopy
  - Retrograde pyelogram
  - Voiding cystourethrogram
  - Abdominal CT scan and plain radiograph
  - Technetium-99m dimercaptosuccinic acid (DMSA) renal scintigraphy

MACROSCOPIC FEATURES

General Features
- Enlarged and edematous kidney
- Ascending pyelonephritis
  - Characteristic straight yellow streaks may be seen in medulla
    - Correspond to collecting ducts filled with pus
    - Typical of ascending APN
  - Pyelitis usual

5

3

ACUTE PYELONEPHRITIS

o Pyelocalyceal system may be dilated in setting of obstruction or reflux
o Scarred areas may be present as residua of prior episodes
  ▪ Cortical scars in ascending APN often overlie pelvic calyces
o Inflammation may extend into perirenal fat with perinephric abscess
o Calculi or strictures may be seen in pelvis or ureters
• Hematogenous bacterial nephritis
  o Small subcapsular yellow abscesses measuring a few millimeters in diameter
    ▪ Typical of hematogenous APN
• Emphysematous pyelonephritis
  o Empty (gas-filled) rounded spaces in cortex and perirenal fat and dissection planes under capsule associated with abscesses

MICROSCOPIC PATHOLOGY

Histologic Features
• Patchy neutrophilic infiltrate in tubules and interstitium, typically with spared areas
  o Neutrophil casts in tubular lumens, sometimes with associated bacteria
  o Abscesses with tubular destruction in severe cases
• Lymphocytes, plasma cells, eosinophils, and macrophages are seen within a few days
• Acute tubular injury
  o Loss of proximal tubule brush border
  o Simplified tubular epithelium
  o Sloughed epithelial cells in tubular lumens
• Tubular basement membranes disrupted
• Severe cases may have papillary necrosis
  o Usually tip of papilla vs. papillary necrosis from analgesic abuse
• Glomeruli and blood vessels relatively spared
• Bacterial and fungal stains often useful

Variants
• Ascending infection
  o Acute inflammation of pelvis usual
  o Early infection in medulla and collecting ducts
  o Organisms invade via fornix of calyx and intrarenal reflux through collecting ducts
• Hematogenous infection
  o Randomly scattered abscesses in cortex
  o Occasionally, septic emboli in glomeruli containing organisms in endocarditis
  o Little or no inflammation of pelvis
• Emphysematous pyelonephritis
  o Round empty spaces and planes of dissection in tissue due to gas-forming organisms
• Acute lobar nephronia
  o Variant that suggests mass lesions in imaging studies
  o Focal areas of intense inflammation and edema in cortex

ANCILLARY TESTS

Histochemistry
• Gram
  o Reactivity: Detects Gram-positive or Gram-negative organisms
  o Staining pattern
    ▪ Bacteria typically not conspicuous in tubules but can be detected in abscesses
• Grocott methenamine silver
  o Reactivity: Positive in tubules and abscesses if fungal organisms present
  o Staining pattern
    ▪ Infection

Immunofluorescence
• Glomeruli and tubular basement membranes negative for immunoglobulins and complement
• C4d binds to bacterial surfaces in APN via activation of lectin pathway in ring pattern

Electron Microscopy
• Glomerular and tubular basement membranes negative for electron-dense deposits
• Bacteria rarely encountered

DIFFERENTIAL DIAGNOSIS

Drug-induced Interstitial Nephritis
• Clinical history of drug exposure
  o Neutrophilic infiltrate less prominent
  o Urine and blood cultures are negative unless it is superimposed on UTI

Myeloma Cast Nephropathy
• Neutrophilic infiltrate can be associated with myeloma casts
• Tubular casts are typically fractured and weakly PAS(+)
• Should be carefully excluded in elderly patients with acute renal failure
• Tubular casts are light chain restricted on immunofluorescence microscopy

Glomerulonephritis-associated Severe Tubulointerstitial Inflammation
• Glomerular hypercellularity and crescents indicate primary glomerular process
• Neutrophilic infiltrate less prominent
• No abscesses
• Immunofluorescence and electron microscopy may indicate presence of immune complexes

Ischemic or Toxic Tubular Injury
• Less neutrophilic infiltrate
• No abscesses
• Tubular injury in area without inflammation

Acute Humoral Rejection in Transplants
• Neutrophils in tubules sometimes mimic APN
• C4d in peritubular capillaries
• Abscesses not seen

Predisposing Factors for Ascending Bacterial Pyelonephritis

Mechanisms	Protective Factors	Predisposing Factors
Bacterial properties	Normal vaginal and urethral flora, such as lactobacilli	P-fimbriated *E. coli*
Entry into bladder	Long urethra (male)	Short urethra (females), trauma (sexual intercourse, catheterization)
Urine properties	Low pH, low glucose, high osmolality, high urea	Diabetes mellitus raises glucose concentration
Flushing mechanism of micturition	Residual volume of urine in bladder only a few mL	Large residual volume (in obstruction, neurogenic bladder, nephrolithiasis)
Ureteral vesicle junction	Competent vesicoureteral valve mechanism	Congenital vesicoureteral reflux, secondary reflux due to obstruction
Intrarenal reflux	Prevented by convex papillae that close with increased pelvic pressures	Compound papillae with flattened tips fail to close, common in the upper and lower poles
Secretion of blood group substances	Secretion of blood group substances (ABO) inhibits bacterial adherence to urothelial cells	Nonsecretor status of host has higher risk of recurrent UTI and scarring
Secreted molecules in urine	Tamm-Horsfall protein binds type 1 fimbriae of *E. coli*	
Bladder epithelium	Anti-adherence mechanisms of bladder mucosa (lining glycosaminoglycans, oligosaccharides)	Denudation and inflammation
Immune system	Cervicovaginal antibody in women; secreted (IgA) or systemic (IgG) antibody to bacterial antigens in urine	Deficiency of antibody, new bacterial strain

DIAGNOSTIC CHECKLIST

Clinically Relevant Pathologic Features

- Abscess formation
- Papillary necrosis
- Histological evidence of chronic pyelonephritis
  - Numerous hyaline casts in atrophic tubules reminiscent of thyroidization
  - Can indicate prior episodes of APN or presence of urinary outflow obstruction

Pathologic Interpretation Pearls

- Neutrophils occasionally found in end-stage kidneys without other evidence of APN, presumably due to sterile tubular injury
- Always check for fungi, which can be easily missed (PAS and silver stain)
- Persistent infection may have abundant eosinophils

SELECTED REFERENCES

1. Pontin AR et al: Current management of emphysematous pyelonephritis. Nat Rev Urol. 6:272-9, 2009
2. Schmidt S et al: Emphysematous pyelonephritis in a kidney allograft. Am J Kidney Dis. 53:895-7, 2009
3. Chung SD et al: Emphysematous pyelonephritis with acute renal failure. Urology. 72:521-2, 2008
4. Hewitt IK et al: Early treatment of acute pyelonephritis in children fails to reduce renal scarring: data from the Italian Renal Infection Study Trials. Pediatrics. 122:486-90, 2008
5. Cheng CH et al: Comparison of urovirulence factors and genotypes for bacteria causing acute lobar nephronia and acute pyelonephritis. Pediatr Infect Dis J. 26:228-32, 2007
6. Lane MC et al: Role of P-fimbrial-mediated adherence in pyelonephritis and persistence of uropathogenic Escherichia coli (UPEC) in the mammalian kidney. Kidney Int. 72(1):19-25, 2007
7. Smaill F: Asymptomatic bacteriuria in pregnancy. Best Pract Res Clin Obstet Gynaecol. 21(3):439-50, 2007
8. Weiss M et al: Pyelonephritis and other infections, reflux nephropathy, hydronephrosis and nephrolithiasis. In Jennette JC et al: Hepinstall's Pathology of the Kidney. 6th ed. Philadelphia: Lippincott Williams & Wilkins. 991-1004, 2007
9. D'Agati VD et al: Infectious tubulointerstitial nephritis. In Jennette JC et al: Non-neoplastic kidney diseases. AFIP: American Registry of Pathology. 547-53, 2005
10. Joss N et al: Lobar nephronia in a transplanted kidney. Clin Nephrol. 64:311-4, 2005
11. Webb NJ et al: Cytokines and cell adhesion molecules in the inflammatory response during acute pyelonephritis. Nephron Exp Nephrol. 96(1):e1-6, 2004
12. Ahmed E et al: Acute graft dysfunction due to pyelonephritis: value and safety of graft biopsy. Ren Fail. 25:509-12, 2003
13. Weiser AC et al: The role of gadolinium enhanced magnetic resonance imaging for children with suspected acute pyelonephritis. J Urol. 169:2308-11, 2003
14. Hooton TM et al: A prospective study of asymptomatic bacteriuria in sexually active young women. N Engl J Med. 343(14):992-7, 2000
15. Kumar PD et al: Focal bacterial nephritis (lobar nephronia) presenting as renal mass. Am J Med Sci. 320:209-11, 2000
16. Patterson JE et al: Bacterial urinary tract infections in diabetes. Infect Dis Clin North Am. 11(3):735-50, 1997
17. Rosenfield AT et al: Acute focal bacterial nephritis (acute lobar nephronia). Radiology. 132:553-61, 1979

ACUTE PYELONEPHRITIS

Gross and Microscopic Features

(Left) A bivalved kidney with acute bacterial pyelonephritis due to an ascending infection is shown. The pelvic calyceal system is mildly dilated with necrosis of the medullary pyramids ➡. Focal pale abscesses are also seen ➡. *(Courtesy L. Fajardo, MD.)* *(Right)* A cross section of the autopsy kidney shows multiple small, yellow abscesses within the renal cortex ➡. The patient had septicemia due to bacterial endocarditis, which resulted in acute pyelonephritis due to bacterial seeding.

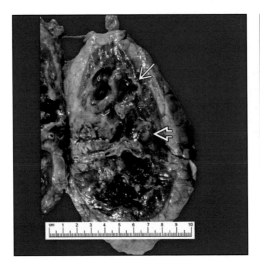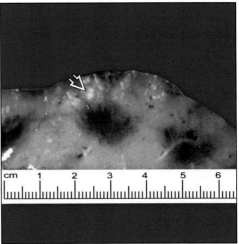

(Left) Hematoxylin & eosin shows pelvic urothelium infiltrated by neutrophils and lymphocytes ➡, compatible with acute pyelonephritis. Neutrophil exudate is seen in the lumen along with bacteria ➡. *(Right)* Periodic acid-Schiff shows neutrophil casts ➡ within the collecting ducts of the medulla. Mild interstitial edema is seen. Early acute pyelonephritis due to ascending infection can be localized to the medulla only.

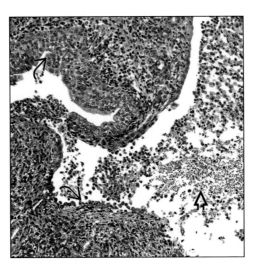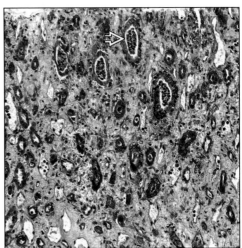

(Left) Periodic acid-Schiff of a kidney biopsy shows neutrophil casts within the cortical tubules ➡, compatible with acute bacterial pyelonephritis. Interstitial neutrophils were seen elsewhere. *(Right)* Periodic acid-Schiff stain of the kidney biopsy with acute pyelonephritis is shown. Areas of normal cortex with well-preserved glomeruli are seen. Neutrophilic infiltrates in the tubulointerstium were visible elsewhere in the biopsy.

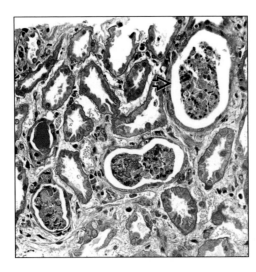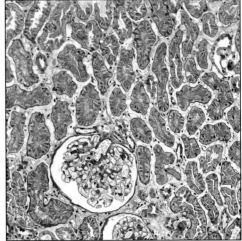

ACUTE PYELONEPHRITIS

Gross and Microscopic Features

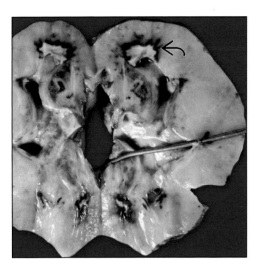
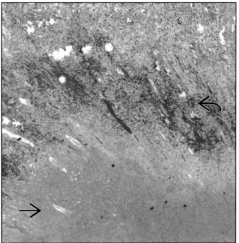

(Left) Bivalved transplant kidney nephrectomy with severe acute pyelonephritis with papillary necrosis is shown. The necrotic papillae are sharply demarcated by a hemorrhagic zone ➡. *(Right)* Transplant kidney nephrectomy with severe acute pyelonephritis with papillary necrosis is shown. The necrotic papillae are sharply demarcated by a hemorrhagic zone ➡. The necrotic area shows no residual viable cells ➡.

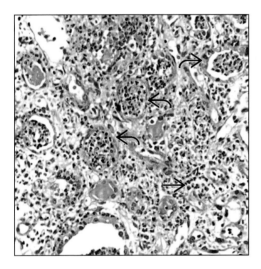
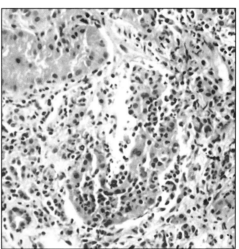

(Left) Light microscopy shows a case of acute pyelonephritis in a renal transplant. Abundant neutrophils are present in the edematous interstitium ➡, prominently as casts ➡. *(Right)* Light microscopy of a renal transplant biopsy shows intense neutrophilic infiltrate forming a cast. The patient had a positive urine culture. This pattern strongly favors APN over rejection, although in acute humoral rejection, neutrophils in tubules are not uncommonly observed.

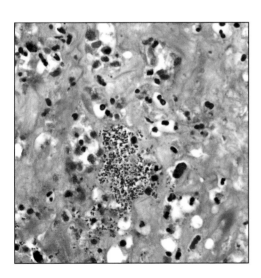
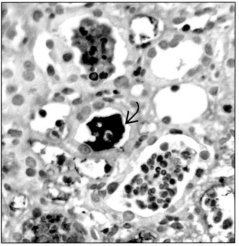

(Left) Hematoxylin & eosin at high power reveals a cluster of bacteria in the medulla of a transplant with severe pyelonephritis. In contrast to calcium deposits, bacteria are more uniform and are typically smaller. *(Right)* C4d stain of a biopsy with acute pyelonephritis shows a cluster of positive-staining cocci in the tubular lumen ➡. C4d is activated by bacterial surface carbohydrates via the lectin pathway (mannose-binding lectin, ficolin).

ACUTE PYELONEPHRITIS

Emphysematous Pyelonephritis

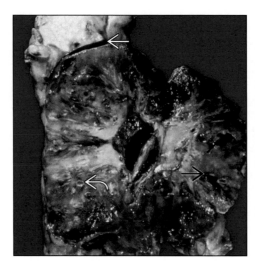 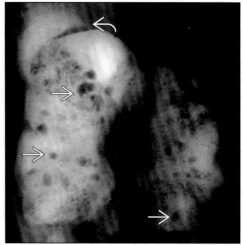

(Left) Nephrectomy with emphysematous pyelonephritis. Dissection is evident between the kidney and the perinephric fat ➡. Many abscesses are seen with empty centers ➡ that contained gas. A streak of pus in a dilated collecting duct can be seen ➡. *(Right)* Specimen radiograph of bivalved kidney with emphysematous pyelonephritis. Gas has dissected between the kidney and the perinephric fat ➡. The rounded spaces are due to gas-forming *E. coli* ➡.

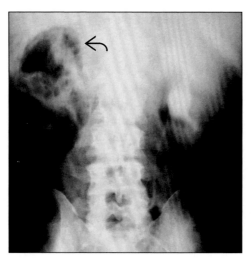 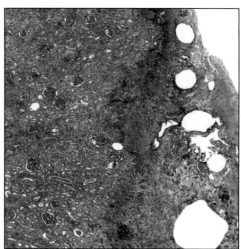

(Left) Intravenous pyelogram reveals a nonfunctioning kidney ➡ with many lucent areas caused by gas-producing *E. coli*. A nephrectomy was performed. The contralateral kidney is unremarkable. *(Right)* Light microscopy of the outer cortex at low power reveals rounded empty spaces, which were originally filled with gas, due to a gas-producing *E. coli* infection in a diabetic patient. This condition is termed emphysematous pyelonephritis.

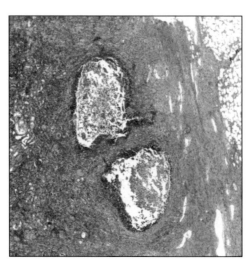 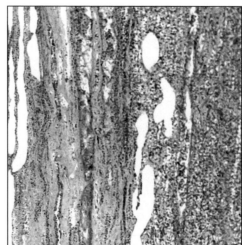

(Left) Light microscopy of the outer cortex at medium power reveals rounded abscesses filled with debris and air spaces surrounded by an intense neutrophilic inflammatory infiltrate. This is a case of emphysematous pyelonephritis due to a gas-producing *E. coli* infection in a diabetic patient. *(Right)* The medulla shows streaks of neutrophilic infiltrates in collecting ducts in a diabetic patient with emphysematous pyelonephritis. This pattern is typical of ascending APN.

Acute Lobar Nephronia

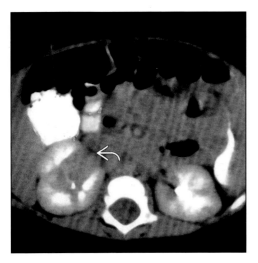
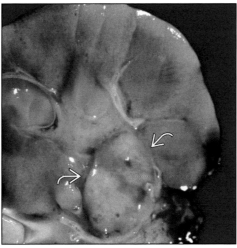

(Left) Abdomen CT of a 4-year-old girl shows nodular masses in the kidney ➔. These were interpreted as possibly neoplastic, and the kidney was removed. The masses were due to localized bacterial infection (acute lobar nephronia). *(Right)* Gross photograph of kidney from a 4-year-old girl with acute pyelonephritis presenting as a localized mass on a CT scan. The focus of inflammation is evident as a bulging yellow mass ➔. This form of APN is sometimes termed acute lobar nephronia.

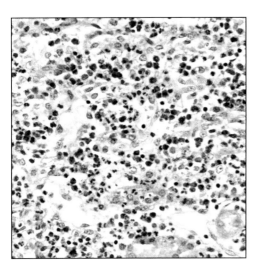
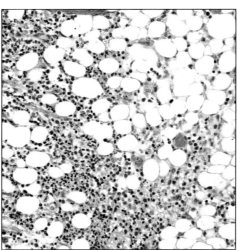

(Left) Light microscopy of the cortex from a patient with acute lobar nephronia shows intense infiltration by granulocytes, including both eosinophils and neutrophils. Destruction of the tubular architecture is evident. *(Right)* Light microscopy shows extension of the inflammation into the perinephric fat in this patient with acute lobar nephronia (focal acute pyelonephritis).

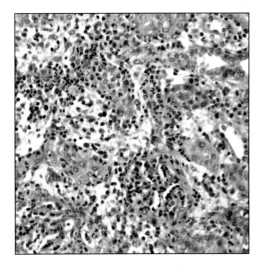
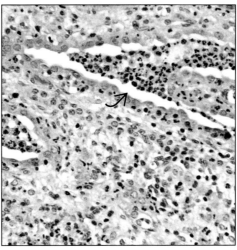

(Left) Light microscopy shows separation of the tubules by edema and an intense infiltrate of mostly neutrophils in this nephrectomy specimen with acute lobar nephronia. *(Right)* Light microscopy of a cortical collecting duct shows a neutrophil cast ➔ filling the lumen. The tubular epithelium is attenuated and basophilic, indicting injury and reactive changes, respectively. The only tubules with branches in the kidney are the collecting ducts.

CHRONIC PYELONEPHRITIS

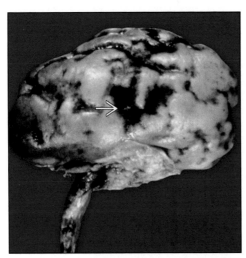

Gross photograph of a kidney with chronic pyelonephritis demonstrates large irregular cortical scars ➜ that often overlie the pelvic calyces.

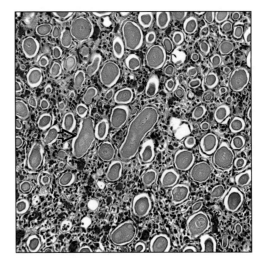

Hematoxylin & eosin of nephrectomy performed for chronic pyelonephritis is shown. Although not specific, characteristic hyaline casts ⊵ are seen in atrophic tubules (thyroidization).

TERMINOLOGY

Abbreviations
- Chronic pyelonephritis (CPN)

Definitions
- Renal damage due to repeated bacterial infection and scarring

ETIOLOGY/PATHOGENESIS

Urinary Outflow Tract Obstruction or Urinary Reflux
- Prostatic disease
- Nephrolithiasis
- Neurogenic bladder
- Ureteral stenosis or dysfunction
- Vesicoureteral reflux, congenital or acquired
  - Role of infection debated

CLINICAL ISSUES

Epidemiology
- Gender
  - More common in females

Presentation
- Chronic renal failure if bilateral
  - Loss of urinary concentration ability
  - Proteinuria
  - Hypertension
- Silent clinical course if unilateral
  - Hypertension
- Repeated episodes of acute pyelonephritis
  - Fever, chills, flank pain

Laboratory Tests
- Elevated BUN, serum creatinine
- Urinalysis: Proteinuria, pyuria

Treatment
- Surgical approaches
  - Correct anatomic defect
  - Nephrectomy in unilateral disease to control hypertension
- Drugs
  - Antimicrobial therapy if bacterial infection
  - Antihypertensives

Prognosis
- Progression slowed only if detected early

IMAGE FINDINGS

General Features
- Plain radiographs, CT scan of abdomen for obstruction
- Voiding cystourethrogram for reflux nephropathy

MACROSCOPIC FEATURES

General Features
- Large irregular scars on cortical surface
  - Adjacent cortical surface can be smooth or granular if associated with arterionephrosclerosis
  - Cortical scars more common in upper and lower poles of kidney
  - Thickness of cortex can be reduced to 2-3 mm
  - Cortical scars overlie deformed calyces
    - Indicative of ascending infection
- Dilated pelvis and calyces
- Calyces are blunted or deformed
- Calculi may be seen in pelvis

MICROSCOPIC PATHOLOGY

Histologic Features
- Patchy chronic tubulointerstitial inflammation

CHRONIC PYELONEPHRITIS

Key Facts

Terminology
- Renal damage due to repeated bacterial infection and scarring

Etiology/Pathogenesis
- Urinary tract obstruction
- Reflux nephropathy

Clinical Issues
- Insidious onset of renal insufficiency if bilateral
- Progression to end-stage kidney disease
- Hypertension
- Proteinuria due to secondary FSGS

Macroscopic Features
- Large irregular scars on cortical surface
- Dilated pelvis
- Calyces are blunted or deformed
- Cortical scars overlie deformed calyces

Microscopic Pathology
- Patchy chronic tubulointerstitial inflammation with spared areas
- Thyroidization of tubules
- Inflammation and scarring involves pelvis and calyces
- Glomeruli are relatively spared but often show periglomerular fibrosis
- Secondary FSGS may be present

Top Differential Diagnoses
- Chronic tubulointerstitial nephritis
- Glomerulonephritis with severe interstitial inflammation

- Lymphocytes, plasma cells, and monocytes predominate
- Tubular atrophy and interstitial fibrosis
- Thyroidization of tubules
  - Atrophic tubules with attenuated epithelium and luminal colloid-like hyaline casts
  - Not specific for chronic pyelonephritis
- Inflammation and scarring of pelvis and calyces
- Sharp demarcation between areas of inflammation and preserved parenchyma
- Neutrophil casts in setting of acute pyelonephritis
- Extravasated Tamm-Horsfall protein may be abundant
- Glomeruli are relatively spared
  - Periglomerular fibrosis common
  - With progression, focal segmental glomerulosclerosis (FSGS) may develop due to loss of renal mass
- Arteriosclerosis if hypertension

ANCILLARY TESTS

Immunofluorescence
- Segmental glomerular IgM and C3 if FSGS present

Electron Microscopy
- Mild foot process effacement if secondary FSGS

DIFFERENTIAL DIAGNOSIS

Chronic Tubulointerstitial Nephritis
- Pelvicalyceal inflammation and thyroidization of tubules more prominent in chronic pyelonephritis
- No selective destruction of medulla or evidence of obstruction
- Uniform involvement; no spared lobes

Primary FSGS
- Lacks pelvicalyceal inflammation and destruction of medulla

Hypertensive Renal Disease
- Lacks pelvicalyceal inflammation and destruction of medulla

DIAGNOSTIC CHECKLIST

Pathologic Interpretation Pearls
- Diagnosis almost impossible on biopsy alone; clinical and radiographic correlations needed
- Sterile reflux produces similar pathology; difficult to be certain infection played a role

SELECTED REFERENCES

1. Craig WD et al: Pyelonephritis: radiologic-pathologic review. Radiographics. 28(1):255-77; quiz 327-8, 2008
2. Tolkoff-Rubin NE et al: Urinary tract infection, pyelonephritis, and reflux nephropathy. In Brenner BM et al: Brenner & Rector's The Kidney. 8th ed. Philadelphia: WB Saunders. 1203-30, 2007
3. Roberts JA: Mechanisms of renal damage in chronic pyelonephritis (reflux nephropathy). Curr Top Pathol. 88:265-87, 1995
4. Morita M et al: The glomerular changes in children with reflux nephropathy. J Pathol. 162(3):245-53, 1990
5. Woodard JR et al: Reflux uropathy. Pediatr Clin North Am. 34(5):1349-64, 1987
6. Brenner BM: Nephron adaptation to renal injury or ablation. Am J Physiol. 249(3 Pt 2):F324-37, 1985
7. Ransley PG et al: The pathogenesis of reflux nephropathy. Contrib Nephrol. 16:90-7, 1979
8. Cotran RS: The renal lesion in chronic pyelonephritis: immunofluorescent and ultrastructural studies. J Infect Dis. 120(1):109-18, 1969
9. Heptinstall RH: The enigma of chronic pyelonephritis. J Infect Dis. 120(1):104-8, 1969
10. Angell ME et al: "Active" chronic pyelonephritis without evidence of bacterial infection. N Engl J Med. 278(24):1303-8, 1968

CHRONIC PYELONEPHRITIS

Microscopic Features

(Left) Hematoxylin & eosin shows an abrupt transition from the normal cortex ⇒ to an area of scarring ⇨, characterized by tubular atrophy, interstitial fibrosis, and inflammation. Note the sparing of the glomeruli ⇒ by sclerosis. (Right) Hematoxylin & eosin shows dense chronic inflammation involving the pelvis. Lymphocytic infiltrates are seen within the urothelium ⇒. Pelvicalyceal involvement is always seen in chronic pyelonephritis.

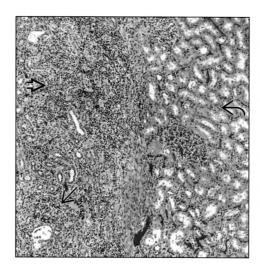
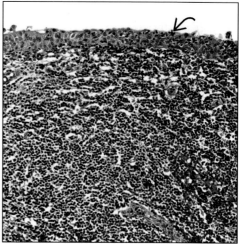

(Left) Hematoxylin & eosin of nephrectomy with chronic pyelonephritis shows columns of chronic inflammation extending into the cortex in a patchy distribution ⇒. Note the concavity of the blunted papillary tip ⇨, which predisposes to intrarenal reflux. (Right) Periodic acid-Schiff of the kidney with CPN shows intense inflammation with a germinal center formation ⇨ adjacent to extravasated Tamm-Horsfall protein ⇒. These changes may be due to urinary obstruction.

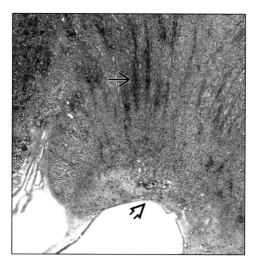
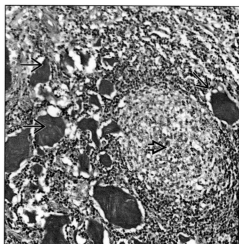

(Left) Hematoxylin & eosin shows the patchy nature of the tubulointerstitial inflammation in chronic pyelonephritis. Residual proximal tubules show compensatory hypertrophy ⇨. A few globally sclerosed glomeruli are seen ⇒. (Right) Periodic acid-Schiff shows segmental sclerosis ⇨ in a glomerulus with Bowman capsular adhesion. Focal segmental glomerulosclerosis is due to the loss of renal mass in chronic pyelonephritis and hyperfiltration in remnant nephrons.

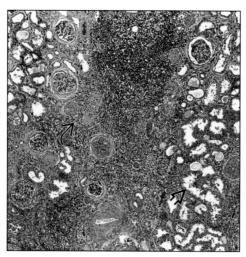
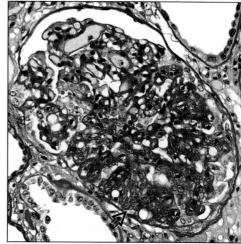

CHRONIC PYELONEPHRITIS

Gross and Microscopic Features

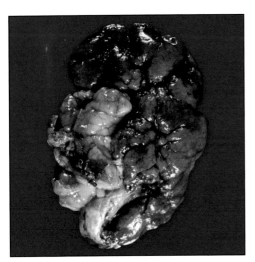
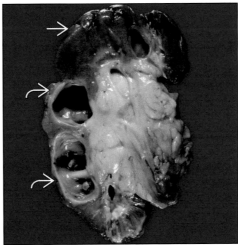

(Left) External surface of a nephrectomy specimen from a 41-year-old woman with unilateral CPN due to repeated episodes of Enterococcus infections shows a coarsely nodular pattern caused by focal scars with intervening hypertrophy. (Right) Cross section of a nephrectomy specimen with CPN due to Enterococcus shows a few calyceal stones. The cortex and medulla are markedly thinned in some areas ➡, but other areas are spared ➡.

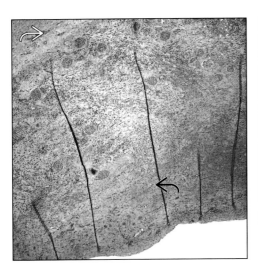
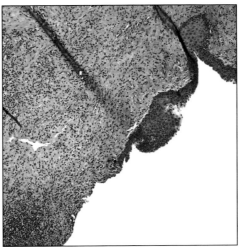

(Left) Full-thickness section through the cortex and medulla of a lobe involved with CPN is shown. The capsule is fibrotic ➡, and the medulla is markedly atrophic ➡. (Right) Squamous metaplasia of the urothelium is evident in a portion of the pelvis from a nephrectomy specimen with CPN and calyceal stones. Stone disease can lead to squamous metaplasia and increased risk of squamous carcinoma.

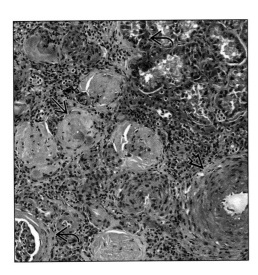
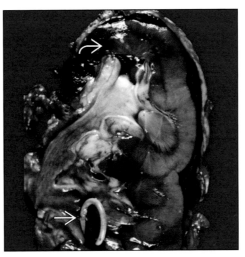

(Left) Widespread global glomerulosclerosis ➡ is evident in an area of scarring in CPN. The patient had severe hypertension, and prominent intimal fibrosis is seen in a small artery ➡. One glomerulus has periglomerular fibrosis ➡. (Right) Nephrectomy specimen from a patient with CPN due to inadvertent ureteral injury during ovarian surgery 1 year prior is shown. The poles are most severely affected ➡. A nephrostomy tube is in place in the lower pole ➡.

XANTHOGRANULOMATOUS PYELONEPHRITIS

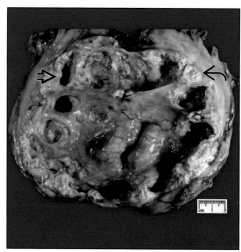

Gross photograph shows a kidney with xanthogranulomatous pyelonephritis. Note the dilated pelvicalyceal system with deformed papillae ➡ and also tan-yellow mass lesions ➡.

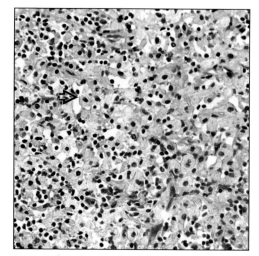

Hematoxylin & eosin of renal "mass" shows foamy histiocytes ➡ admixed with lymphocytes. The pelvis is scarred with acute and chronic inflammation in this kidney with xanthogranulomatous pyelonephritis.

TERMINOLOGY

Abbreviations
- Xanthogranulomatous pyelonephritis (XPN)

Definitions
- Variant of chronic pyelonephritis characterized by mass lesion with abundant foamy macrophages

ETIOLOGY/PATHOGENESIS

Infectious Agents
- *Proteus mirabilis*, *E. coli*, *Pseudomonas* sp, *Klebsiella* sp
  - *Proteus mirabilis* most common (> 50%)

Predisposing Factors
- Urinary tract obstruction
- Nephrolithiasis
  - Staghorn calculi most common
- Diabetes mellitus

CLINICAL ISSUES

Epidemiology
- Age
  - 5th and 6th decades
  - Can occur in children
- Gender
  - Common in females (M:F = 1:4)

Site
- Predominantly in pelvicalyceal areas
- Often unilateral

Presentation
- Fever, malaise, flank pain, weight loss, loin tenderness; palpable mass in some patients

Laboratory Tests
- Leukocytosis

- Elevated ESR
- Mild proteinuria, pyuria
- Urine cultures negative in > 30% of patients

Treatment
- Surgical approaches
  - Unilateral nephrectomy is treatment of choice
  - Partial nephrectomy for focal disease
- Drugs
  - Intense antimicrobial therapy may be helpful

Prognosis
- Renal function maintained after unilateral nephrectomy

IMAGE FINDINGS

General Features
- Ultrasonography, CT scan, and plain radiographs
  - Evidence of urinary tract obstruction, stones
  - Extent of renal and perirenal involvement can be assessed

MACROSCOPIC FEATURES

General Features
- Enlarged kidneys with perirenal adhesions
- Dilated pelvicalyceal system
- Deformed papillae and yellow necrotic material in calyces
- Renal cortical abscesses may be present
- Large yellow nodules mimic renal cell carcinoma
- Large calculi may be present
- Extrarenal extension in ~ 30% (pitfall for malignant gross appearance)

XANTHOGRANULOMATOUS PYELONEPHRITIS

Key Facts

Terminology
- Variant of chronic pyelonephritis characterized by abundant foamy lipid-laden macrophages

Etiology/Pathogenesis
- *E. coli*, *Proteus* sp, *Pseudomonas* sp, *Klebsiella* sp
- Urinary tract obstruction
- Nephrolithiasis
- Diabetes mellitus

Clinical Issues
- 5th and 6th decades
- Common in females (M:F = 4:1)
- Predominantly in pelvicalyceal areas
- Often unilateral
- Unilateral nephrectomy is treatment of choice
- Fever, malaise
- Flank pain

Macroscopic Features
- Dilated pelvicalyceal system
- Deformed papillae and yellow necrotic material in calyces

Microscopic Pathology
- Calyceal areas show sheets of foamy lipid-laden macrophages
- Other admixed cells include mononuclear cells, lymphocytes, and plasma cells

Top Differential Diagnoses
- Clear cell renal cell carcinoma
- Renal medullary tuberculosis

MICROSCOPIC PATHOLOGY

Histologic Features
- Involved calyces show sheets of foamy, lipid-laden macrophages
- Admixture of mononuclear cells, lymphocytes, and plasma cells
- Neutrophils within necrotic areas
- Zonal distribution of inflammation may be seen
  - Neutrophils and necrosis adjacent to collecting system
  - Macrophages with fibrosis and chronic inflammation at periphery
- Occasional multinucleated giant cells may be present
- Tubular atrophy and interstitial fibrosis in adjacent areas
- Glomeruli are relatively spared

DIFFERENTIAL DIAGNOSIS

Renal Cell Carcinoma
- Clinical, gross, and microscopic resemblance to xanthogranulomatous pyelonephritis
- Clear cells of renal cell carcinoma may mimic foamy macrophages
- Immunohistochemical stains are helpful
  - Macrophage markers CD163, CD68 are negative in lesion cells
  - Epithelial markers such as CKAE1/CAM5.2 and EMA are positive in renal cell carcinoma

Renal Medullary Tuberculosis
- Necrotizing granulomas with epithelioid histiocytes and multinucleated giant cells
- AFB or Fite stain demonstrates acid-fast mycobacteria

DIAGNOSTIC CHECKLIST

Pathologic Interpretation Pearls
- Immunohistochemistry and bacterial stains helpful in differential

- Inflammation occurs around calyces
- Macrophages often have indistinct cell borders compared with epithelial cells
- Renal cell carcinoma may coexist with xanthogranulomatous pyelonephritis

SELECTED REFERENCES

1. Afgan F, Mumtaz S, and Ather MH, Preoperative diagnosis of xanthogranulomatous pyelonephritis. Urol J. 4 (3):169-73, 2007
2. Weiss M et al: Pyelonephritis and other infections, reflux nephropathy, hydronephrosis, and nephrolithiasis. In Jennette JC et al: Hepinstall's Pathology of the Kidney. 6th ed. Philadelphia: Lippincott Williams & Wilkins. 1006-7, 2007
3. Zugor V et al: Xanthogranulomatous pyelonephritis in childhood: a critical analysis of 10 cases and of the literature. Urology. 70(1):157-60, 2007
4. D'Agati VD et al: Infectious tubulointerstitial nephritis. In D'Agati VD et al: Nonneoplastic Kidney Diseases. AFIP: American Registry of Pathology. 559-61, 2005
5. Clapton WK et al: Clinicopathological features of xanthogranulomatous pyelonephritis in infancy. Pathology. 25(2):110-3, 1993
6. Antonakopoulos GN et al: Xanthogranulomatous pyelonephritis. A reappraisal and immunohistochemical study. Arch Pathol Lab Med. 112(3):275-81, 1988
7. Parsons MA et al: Xanthogranulomatous pyelonephritis: a pathological, clinical and aetiological analysis of 87 cases. Diagn Histopathol. 6(3-4):203-19, 1983
8. Goodman M et al: Xanthogranulomatous pyelonephritis (XGP): a local disease with systemic manifestations. Report of 23 patients and review of the literature. Medicine (Baltimore). 58(2):171-81, 1979

XANTHOGRANULOMATOUS PYELONEPHRITIS

Gross and Microscopic Features

(Left) Gross photograph shows a nephrectomy specimen with xanthogranulomatous pyelonephritis associated with a "staghorn" calculus (not shown). Calyces are dilated and lined with yellow nodular plaques ➡. *(Right)* Hematoxylin & eosin of a kidney with xanthogranulomatous pyelonephritis shows sheets of lipid-laden foamy histiocytes admixed with lymphocytes. The histiocytes have indistinct cell borders with apparent clearing of cytoplasm.

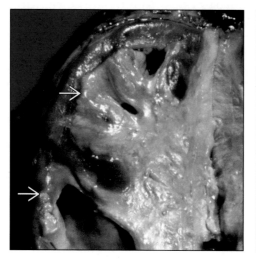
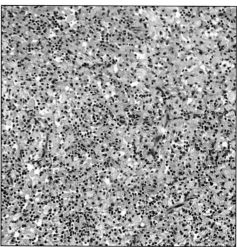

(Left) The renal pelvis in XPN shows a neutrophilic infiltrate ➤ and necrosis. Xanthogranulomatous inflammation can show a zonal distribution with acute inflammation near the collecting system surrounded by lymphohistiocytic infiltrate at the periphery. *(Right)* XPN appeared as a tan mass lesion composed of spindled cells, mimicking a sarcomatoid renal cell carcinoma. These cells, however, stain positive for CD163, indicative of macrophages.

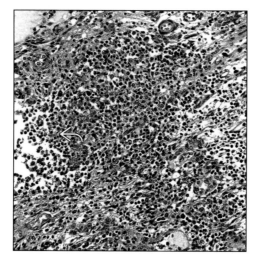
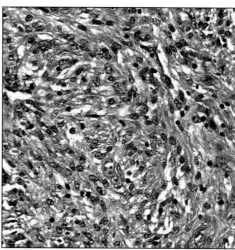

(Left) CK8/18/CAM5.2 keratin stain shows a renal mass with sheets of spindle cells. Although the histology is suggestive of sarcomatoid renal cell carcinoma, the keratin stain is negative, strongly favoring XPN. *(Right)* A renal mass shows sheets of CD163(+) cells identified as macrophages. The lesional cells were foamy and negative for cytokeratin stain, confirming the diagnosis of XPN.

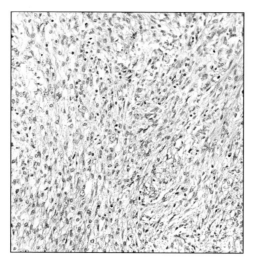
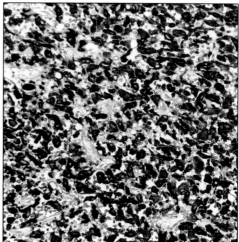

XANTHOGRANULOMATOUS PYELONEPHRITIS

Differential Diagnosis

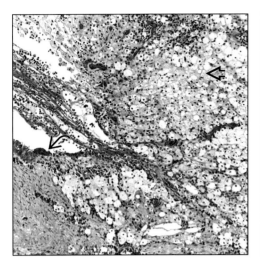

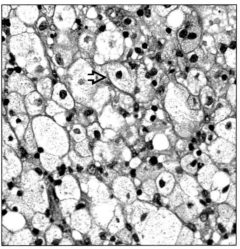

(Left) Hematoxylin & eosin shows the pelvis ➔ with adjacent mass lesion composed of clear foamy cells ⇨ of XPN. Renal calculi with acute and chronic pyelonephritis were seen elsewhere in the kidney. *(Right)* Light microscopy findings of XPN show typical sheets of foamy histiocytes ⇨. The clinical, gross, and microscopic findings may resemble a low-grade renal cell carcinoma, clear cell type.

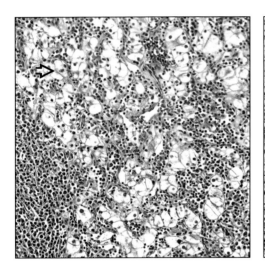

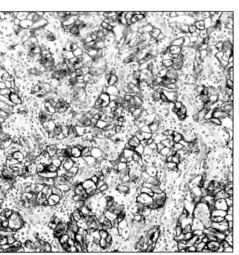

(Left) Cells in this clear cell renal cell carcinoma have a clear cytoplasm and distinct cell borders ⇨. Other areas in the kidney have typical features of XPN, possibly due to obstruction by the renal cell carcinoma. *(Right)* Clear cell renal cell carcinoma is positive for CK8/18/CAM5.2 keratins. The neoplastic cells with clear cytoplasm and low-grade nuclei mimic the histiocytes of XPN.

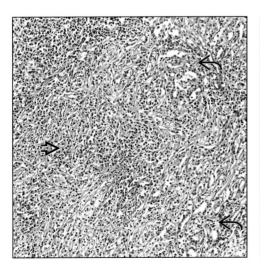

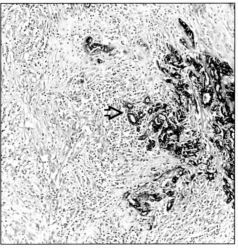

(Left) This renal cell carcinoma, collecting duct type, has a histiocytic infiltrate ⇨ mimicking XPN. Indistinct glands of low-grade collecting duct carcinoma are admixed ➔. *(Right)* Glandular structures ⇨ of a low-grade collecting duct carcinoma of kidney are positive for AE1/AE3 keratin. The mass was initially misdiagnosed as XPN due to a prominent histiocytic infiltrate. HMW cytokeratin is also positive.

MALAKOPLAKIA

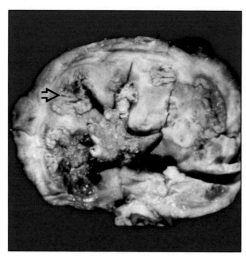

Gross photograph of a kidney with malakoplakia shows multiple tan-yellow masses ⧫ mimicking a neoplasm. (Courtesy R. Rouse, MD.)

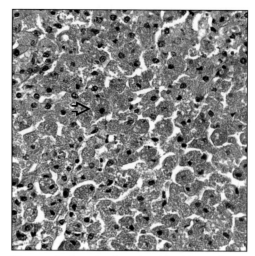

Hematoxylin & eosin of renal malakoplakia is shown. The mass identified in the nephrectomy specimen is composed of sheets of macrophages with granular eosinophilic cytoplasm ⧫.

TERMINOLOGY

Synonyms
- Malakoplakia

Definitions
- Chronic bacterial infection with abundant macrophages containing granular eosinophilic cytoplasm and Michaelis-Gutmann bodies often forming plaque or mass lesion

ETIOLOGY/PATHOGENESIS

Infectious Agents
- *E. coli* most common

Defective Intracytoplasmic Macrophage Bactericidal Function
- Decreased lysosomal degradation of bacteria
- Inability of cells to release lysosomal enzymes
- Partially digested bacterial products form a nidus for calcium and iron deposition

Altered Immune Status
- Predisposing factor for malakoplakia
- AIDS
- Immunosuppressive therapy
  - Renal transplants
  - Rheumatoid arthritis, systemic lupus erythematosus
- Malignancies

CLINICAL ISSUES

Epidemiology
- Age
  - Infancy to 9th decade
    - 5th decade most common
- Gender
  - M:F = 1:4

Site
- Most common site is urinary bladder
- Renal pelvicalyceal system and parenchyma
  - Bilateral involvement common (30-50% of cases)
- Other reported sites include skin, prostate, gastrointestinal tract, testis

Presentation
- Fever
- Chills
- Flank pain
- Loin tenderness
- Palpable mass may be present
  - Frequently mistaken for neoplasm
- Acute renal failure in bilateral involvement or in renal transplants

Laboratory Tests
- Urinalysis shows pyuria and proteinuria
- Urine cultures may be positive for *E. coli*

Treatment
- Surgical approaches
  - Nephrectomy if suspected malignancy
  - Surgical therapy now less common with antibiotics and better imaging techniques
- Drugs
  - Fluoroquinolone

Prognosis
- High mortality rate (70%) in early reports
- Significant improvement in mortality rate with early diagnosis and antibiotic therapy with fluoroquinolone

IMAGE FINDINGS

General Features
- Mass lesion detected on ultrasound and CT scan

MALAKOPLAKIA

Key Facts

Terminology
- Chronic bacterial infection with abundant macrophages containing Michaelis-Gutmann bodies

Etiology/Pathogenesis
- *E. coli* most common
- Defective intracytoplasmic macrophage bactericidal function
- Altered immune status

Clinical Issues
- M:F = 1:4
- Bilateral involvement common (30-50% of cases)
- Frequently mistaken for neoplasm
- Surgical therapy now less common with antibiotics and better imaging techniques

Macroscopic Features
- Yellow-tan nodules in calyces and renal parenchyma

Microscopic Pathology
- Sheets of macrophages with foamy eosinophilic cytoplasm in mass lesion
- Characteristic cytoplasmic inclusions (Michaelis-Gutmann bodies)
- Calcium positive (von Kossa stain)
- Iron positive (Prussian blue stain)

Top Differential Diagnoses
- Renal cell carcinoma
- Xanthogranulomatous pyelonephritis
- Megalocytic interstitial nephritis

MACROSCOPIC FEATURES

General Features
- Enlarged kidneys
- Yellow tan nodules in calyces and parenchyma
- Dilated pelvicaliceal system if urinary obstruction
- Renal calculi rare

MICROSCOPIC PATHOLOGY

Histologic Features
- Sheets of macrophages with foamy eosinophilic cytoplasm in mass lesion
- Characteristic cytoplasmic inclusions (Michaelis-Gutmann bodies)
  - 4-10 microns in diameter, basophilic
  - Periodic acid-Schiff positive
  - Calcium positive (von Kossa stain positive)
  - Iron positive (Prussian blue stain)
- Admixed lymphocytes and plasma cells
- Tubular atrophy and interstitial fibrosis in adjacent parenchyma

ANCILLARY TESTS

Electron Microscopy
- Michaelis-Gutmann bodies have central crystalline core, intermediate lucent area, and peripheral lamellar rings of deposited mineral

DIFFERENTIAL DIAGNOSIS

Renal Cell Carcinoma
- Immunohistochemistry with CKAE1/CAM5.2 (epithelial cells), CD163, and CD68 (macrophages) is helpful
- Special stains for Michaelis-Gutmann bodies negative

Xanthogranulomatous Pyelonephritis
- Macrophages foamy and lipid laden
- Absence of Michaelis-Gutmann bodies
- Usually associated with "staghorn" calculus

Megalocytic Interstitial Nephritis
- Macrophages have strongly PAS-positive granular eosinophilic cytoplasm
- Absence of Michaelis-Gutmann bodies

DIAGNOSTIC CHECKLIST

Pathologic Interpretation Pearls
- High level of suspicion needed for biopsy diagnosis
- von Kossa stains and immunohistochemical stains are useful

SELECTED REFERENCES

1. Kobayashi A et al: Malakoplakia of the kidney. Am J Kidney Dis. 51(2):326-30, 2008
2. Weiss M et al: Pyelonephritis and other infections, reflux nephropathy, hydronephrosis and nephrolithiasis. In Jennette JC et al: Hepinstall's Pathology of the Kidney. 6th ed. Philadelphia: Lippincott Williams & Wilkins. 1007-9, 2007
3. Tam VK et al: Renal parenchymal malacoplakia: a rare cause of ARF with a review of recent literature. Am J Kidney Dis. 41(6):E13-7, 2003
4. van der Voort HJ et al: Malacoplakia. Two case reports and a comparison of treatment modalities based on a literature review. Arch Intern Med. 156(5):577-83, 1996
5. August C et al: Renal parenchymal malakoplakia: ultrastructural findings in different stages of morphogenesis. Ultrastruct Pathol. 18(5):483-91, 1994
6. al-Sulaiman MH et al: Renal parenchymal malacoplakia and megalocytic interstitial nephritis: clinical and histological features. Report of two cases and review of the literature. Am J Nephrol. 13(6):483-8, 1993
7. Dobyan DC et al: Renal malacoplakia reappraised. Am J Kidney Dis. 22(2):243-52, 1993
8. Esparza AR et al: Renal parenchymal malakoplakia. Histologic spectrum and its relationship to megalocytic interstitial nephritis and xanthogranulomatous pyelonephritis. Am J Surg Pathol. 13(3):225-36, 1989
9. McClure J: Malakoplakia. J Pathol. 140(4):275-330, 1983

Microscopic Features

(Left) Hematoxylin & eosin of a renal malakoplakia mass shows sheets of macrophages with eosinophilic cytoplasm. The clinical, gross, and microscopic features mimic renal cell carcinoma. *(Right)* Hematoxylin & eosin of renal malakoplakia shows sheets of histiocytes extending into the pelvic adipose tissue ⮞. Similar changes in the capsular surface cause perinephric adhesions. The macroscopic findings of a nephrectomy closely resemble renal cell carcinoma.

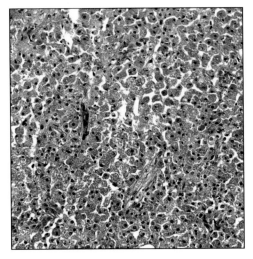
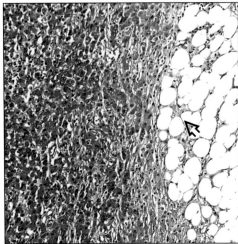

(Left) Renal malakoplakia can show areas of necrosis and acute inflammation ⮞ along with the characteristic macrophages with eosinophilic cytoplasm ⮞. *(Right)* Scattered foci of necrosis and acute inflammation ⮞ can be seen in renal malakoplakia along with macrophages with granular cytoplasm. Renal tuberculosis, on the other hand, has caseating granulomas with central acellular necrosis surrounded by epithelioid histiocytes.

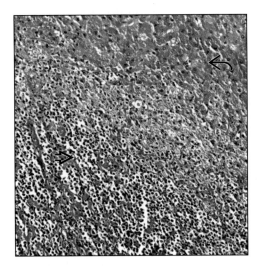
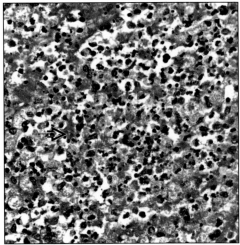

(Left) Hematoxylin & eosin of renal malakoplakia at high magnification shows the typical basophilic Michaelis-Gutmann bodies ⮞ within the cytoplasm of the macrophages. *(Right)* End-stage native kidney with multiple cysts ⮞ was removed for a suspected renal neoplasm. The microscopic examination of the mass was compatible with renal malakoplakia. The patient had undergone renal transplantation 2 years earlier.

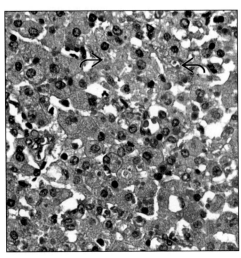
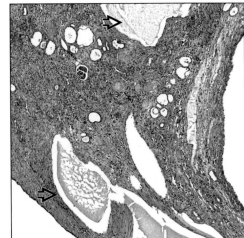

MALAKOPLAKIA

Ancillary Techniques

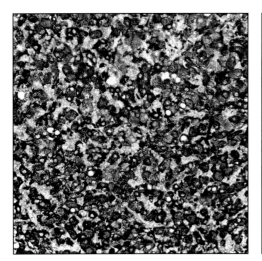

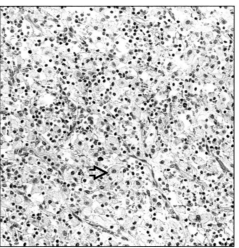

(Left) CD163 (macrophage marker) of the renal mass lesion diagnosed as malakoplakia is shown. The macrophages are positive for CD163. The cytokeratin stain is negative, ruling out the possibility of renal cell carcinoma. *(Right)* CKAE1/AE3 of the native kidney mass diagnosed as renal malakoplakia in a renal transplant recipient is shown. The lesional cells have granular cytoplasm and lack staining for cytokeratin ⇨ but are positive for CD163 (macrophage marker).

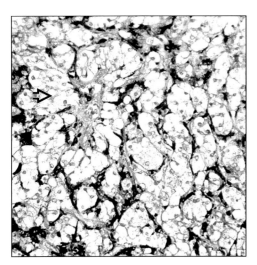

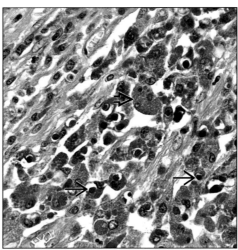

(Left) CD163 stain of a renal cell carcinoma demonstrates the lack of staining in the lesional neoplastic cells ⇨ while the admixed histiocytes are positive. Renal malakoplakia is composed of sheets of macrophages, and the histological findings can be mistaken for renal cell carcinoma. *(Right)* Periodic acid-Schiff of renal malakoplakia highlights the granular cytoplasm of the macrophages ⇨ and also stains the characteristic Michaelis-Gutmann bodies ⇨.

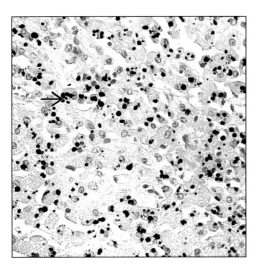

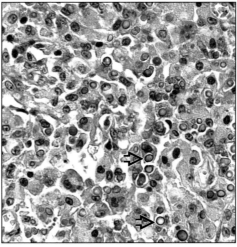

(Left) von Kossa highlights the Michaelis-Gutmann bodies ⇨ in malakoplakia. Partially digested bacterial products form the nidus for the calcium (von Kossa[+]) and iron deposition in these bodies. *(Right)* Giemsa of renal malakoplakia fails to reveal organisms, but the Michaelis-Gutmann bodies ⇨ are highlighted by their refractile appearance. Other stains for microorganisms such as AFB, Gram, Gomori methenamine-silver were also negative.

MEGALOCYTIC INTERSTITIAL NEPHRITIS

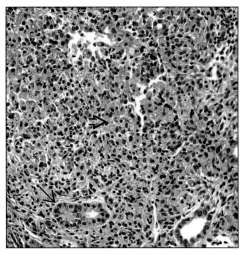

Hematoxylin & eosin of a kidney biopsy with megalocytic interstitial nephritis shows diffuse interstitial macrophage infiltrate ⊟, but the tubules are spared ⇥. (Courtesy C. Nast, MD.)

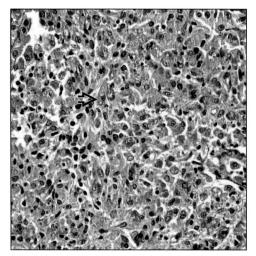

Periodic acid-Schiff of a kidney biopsy with megalocytic interstitial nephritis shows diffuse interstitial infiltrate of histiocytes with granular cytoplasm ⊟. (Courtesy C. Nast, MD.)

TERMINOLOGY

Abbreviations
- Megalocytic interstitial nephritis (MIN)

Definitions
- MIN is closely related to malakoplakia and is characterized by infiltration of histiocytes with eosinophilic granular cytoplasm

ETIOLOGY/PATHOGENESIS

Chronic Bacterial Infection
- *E. coli* and other Gram-negative bacteria

Host Immune Factors
- Leukocyte bactericidal defects
- Immunodeficiency state
  - Transplantation
  - Immunosuppressive therapy
  - Systemic lupus erythematosus, Behçet disease

CLINICAL ISSUES

Epidemiology
- Incidence
  - Rare condition
- Age
  - Middle-aged adults

Site
- Renal cortex
- Can be bilateral

Presentation
- Fever, chills
- Dysuria, urgency
- Flank pain
- Acute renal failure may be present

Laboratory Tests
- Urinalysis shows white blood cells
- Urine and blood cultures may be positive for *E. coli*

Treatment
- Surgical approaches
  - Nephrectomy may be needed if unresponsive to antibiotic therapy
- Drugs
  - Antibiotic therapy directed against Gram-negative bacteria

Prognosis
- Good with early diagnosis on biopsy and aggressive antibiotic therapy

IMAGE FINDINGS

Ultrasonographic Findings
- Enlarged kidneys
- Mass lesions may be present

MACROSCOPIC FEATURES

General Features
- Diffuse involvement of cortex by multiple yellow-gray lesions or discrete nodules

MICROSCOPIC PATHOLOGY

Histologic Features
- Extensive interstitial histiocytic infiltrate with abundant granular and eosinophilic cytoplasm
- Fewer lymphocytes may be seen admixed with histiocytes
- Glomeruli are uninvolved

MEGALOCYTIC INTERSTITIAL NEPHRITIS

Key Facts

Terminology
- MIN is closely related to malakoplakia

Etiology/Pathogenesis
- *E. coli* and other Gram-negative bacteria
- Leukocyte bactericidal defects, immunodeficiency

Microscopic Pathology
- Interstitial histiocytic infiltrate with abundant granular eosinophilic cytoplasm

Ancillary Tests
- Periodic acid-Schiff positive cytoplasmic granules

Top Differential Diagnoses
- Malakoplakia
- Xanthogranulomatous pyelonephritis
- Atypical mycobacterial infection
- Renal cell carcinoma

ANCILLARY TESTS

Histochemistry
- Periodic acid-Schiff
  - Reactivity: Positive
  - Staining pattern
    - Cytoplasmic granules in histiocytes

Immunofluorescence
- Negative for immunoglobulins and complement components

Electron Microscopy
- Macrophages have large intracytoplasmic phagolysosomes filled with granular material and electron-lucent crystalloids

DIFFERENTIAL DIAGNOSIS

Malakoplakia
- Michaelis-Gutmann bodies identified
- Calcium/von Kossa(+), PAS(+)

Xanthogranulomatous Pyelonephritis
- Often associated with urinary outflow tract obstruction
- Involvement of pelvicalyceal system
- Often admixed with more lymphocytes & neutrophils

Atypical Mycobacterial Infection
- Acid-fast bacillus stain positive for mycobacteria

Renal Cell Carcinoma
- Clear cell carcinoma may have PAS(+) granular cytoplasm
- Immunohistochemistry for cytokeratin is helpful

SELECTED REFERENCES

1. Jo SK et al: Anuric acute renal failure secondary to megalocytic interstitial nephritis in a patient with Behcet's disease. Clin Nephrol. 54(6):498-500, 2000
2. Krupp G et al: Tumefactive megalocytic interstitial nephritis in a patient with Escherichia coli bacteremia. Am J Kidney Dis. 25(6):928-33, 1995
3. al-Sulaiman MH et al: Renal parenchymal malacoplakia and megalocytic interstitial nephritis: clinical and histological features. Report of two cases and review of the literature. Am J Nephrol. 13(6):483-8, 1993
4. Esparza AR et al: Renal parenchymal malakoplakia. Histologic spectrum and its relationship to megalocytic interstitial nephritis and xanthogranulomatous pyelonephritis. Am J Surg Pathol. 13(3):225-36, 1989
5. Cledes J et al: Diminished bactericidal activity in megalocytic interstitial nephritis. Clin Nephrol. 23(2):101-4, 1985
6. Garrett IR et al: Renal malakoplakia. Experimental production and evidence of a link with interstitial megalocytic nephritis. J Pathol. 136(2):111-22, 1982
7. Kelly DR et al: Megalocytic interstitial nephritis, xanthogranulomatous pyelonephritis, and malakoplakia. An ultrastructural comparison. Am J Clin Pathol. 75(3):333-44, 1981

IMAGE GALLERY

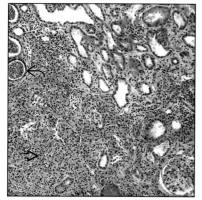 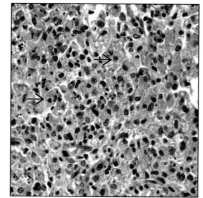 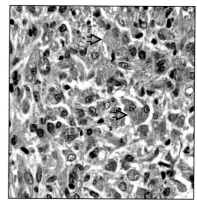

(Left) Megalocytic interstitial nephritis demonstrates interstitial macrophage infiltrate ➡. A few neutrophil casts are seen within the tubular lumens ➡. *(Courtesy C. Nast, MD.)* *(Center)* The macrophages ➡ in megalocytic interstitial nephritis are admixed with fewer lymphocytes and have granular cytoplasm. Michaelis-Gutmann bodies are not identified. *(Courtesy C. Nast, MD.)* *(Right)* Periodic acid-Schiff of a kidney biopsy with megalocytic interstitial nephritis shows sheets of macrophages with characteristic granular cytoplasm ➡. *(Courtesy C. Nast, MD.)*

TUBERCULOSIS

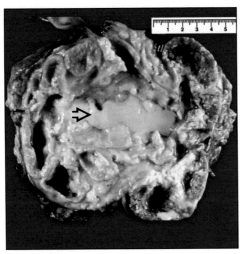

Gross photograph of a nephrectomy specimen with renal tuberculosis shows a dilated pelvicalyceal system with ulcerated papillae and caseous necrotic material ➡. (Courtesy L. Fajardo, MD.)

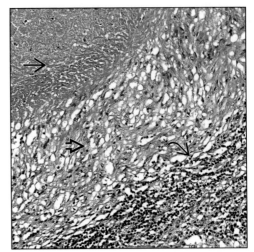

Mycobacterium tuberculosis infection in the kidney is characterized by large caseating granulomas with central caseous necrosis ➡ rimmed by histiocytes ➡ and lymphocytes ➡.

TERMINOLOGY

Abbreviations
- Tuberculosis (TB)

Definitions
- Infection of kidney by *Mycobacterium tuberculosis*

ETIOLOGY/PATHOGENESIS

Infectious Agents
- *M. tuberculosis*: Most common organism
- *M. bovis*: Bovine bacillus can rarely cause disease
- *M. avium-intracellulare* in immunosuppressed state

Pathogenesis
- Acute infection
- Hematogenous dissemination of active pulmonary infection
  o Immune status of host determines susceptibility
- Reactivated latent infection

CLINICAL ISSUES

Epidemiology
- Incidence
  o Genitourinary TB accounts for 30% of extrapulmonary TB in developed countries
    ▪ Higher frequency in immunosuppressed individuals (HIV, transplantation, dialysis), endemic areas, and drug-resistant TB infection
- Gender
  o More common in men with genital tuberculosis
    ▪ Role of antegrade infection of kidney

Site
- Pelvic calyces and renal medulla

Presentation
- Lower urinary tract infection symptoms
  o Dysuria, frequency, and sometimes blood in urine
- Constitutional symptoms of fever, weight loss unusual

Laboratory Tests
- Urine
  o White blood cells on microscopy
  o Urine bacterial cultures negative (sterile pyuria)
  o Mycobacterial cultures positive in 6-8 weeks
- Mantoux skin test
- PCR detection of mycobacterial nucleic acid
- Interferon-γ release assay (ELISA blood test)
  o *M. tuberculosis* antigens in latent and active infection stimulate production of host interferon-γ
  o Negative in other mycobacterial infections and Bacillus Calmette-Guérin vaccine

Treatment
- Options, risks, complications
  o Hypertension, chronic renal failure
- Surgical approaches
  o Nephrectomy for cavitary lesions
  o Relief of obstruction for ureteral strictures
- Drugs
  o Multidrug therapy with isoniazid, rifampicin, pyrazinamide, and ethambutol (or streptomycin) for several months based on regimen
  o 2nd-line drugs for multidrug-resistant TB

Prognosis
- Treatment failure due to nonadherence to regimen or drug-resistant organisms

IMAGE FINDINGS

Radiographic Findings
- Calyceal distortion, ureteric strictures on intravenous pyelography (IVP)
- Calcification of necrotic papillae

TUBERCULOSIS

Key Facts

Terminology
- Infection by *M. tuberculosis*

Etiology/Pathogenesis
- Reactivated latent infection or hematogenous dissemination of active pulmonary infection

Clinical Issues
- Sterile pyuria

Macroscopic Features
- Destruction of the pelvic calyces and papillae with caseous cheesy material

Microscopic Pathology
- Caseating granulomatous inflammation with acid-fast bacilli

Top Differential Diagnoses
- *M. avium-intracellulare* infection, sarcoidosis

MACROSCOPIC FEATURES

General Features
- Ulceration and destruction of pelvic calyces and papillae with caseous cheesy material
- Hydronephrosis if associated with ureteral strictures
- Large tumor-like nodules of chalky material may replace the renal parenchyma

MICROSCOPIC PATHOLOGY

Histologic Features
- Caseating granulomatous inflammation
  - Early infection in renal medulla but can affect entire kidney
  - Central necrosis rimmed by histiocytes, plasma cells, and lymphocytes and few multinucleated giant cells
- Extensive tubular atrophy, interstitial fibrosis, and variable glomerulosclerosis
- Severe interstitial inflammation may be present
- Amyloid deposition due to longstanding infection may be seen
- *M. avium-intracellulare* infection lacks caseation but is characterized by sheets of histiocytes

ANCILLARY TESTS

Histochemistry
- Acid-fast bacteria stain (Ziehl-Neelsen)

  - Reactivity: Positive
  - Staining pattern
    - Rare organisms at the periphery of necrosis

DIFFERENTIAL DIAGNOSIS

M. avium-intracellulare Infection
- Lacks caseation
- Sheets of macrophages

Sarcoidosis
- Granulomas lack caseating necrosis

BCG Granulomatous Interstitial Nephritis
- Temporal association to BCG therapy

Drug-induced Interstitial Nephritis
- Granulomas lack caseating necrosis

SELECTED REFERENCES

1. Pai M et al: Systematic review: T-cell-based assays for the diagnosis of latent tuberculosis infection: an update. Ann Intern Med. 149(3):177-84, 2008
2. Guerra RL et al: Use of the amplified mycobacterium tuberculosis direct test in a public health laboratory: test performance and impact on clinical care. Chest. 132(3):946-51, 2007
3. Wise GJ et al: Genitourinary manifestations of tuberculosis. Urol Clin North Am. 30(1):111-21, 2003
4. Eastwood JB et al: Tuberculosis and the kidney. J Am Soc Nephrol. 12(6):1307-14, 2001

IMAGE GALLERY

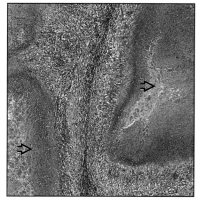 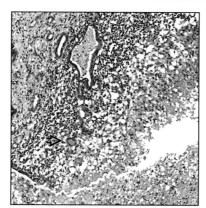 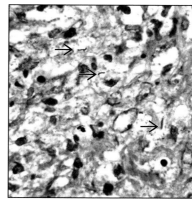

(Left) Caseating granulomatous inflammation is seen in a kidney resected for renal tuberculosis. Extensive necrosis ⊵ is present in the granulomas with associated lymphohistiocytic infiltrate. *(Center)* Necrotizing granulomas are seen in the pelvic wall, extending into the medulla of a kidney with tuberculous infection. In addition to the histiocytes, occasional multinucleated giant cells ⊵ are seen rimming the necrosis. *(Right)* Acid-fast bacteria stain of the kidney shows scattered acid-fast bacilli ⊳ in the granulomas. (Courtesy G. Berry, MD.)

BCG GRANULOMATOUS INTERSTITIAL NEPHRITIS

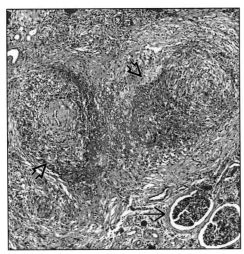

Granulomatous inflammation ⊳ of the kidney is seen in a patient treated with intracavitary BCG therapy for in situ urothelial carcinoma of the pelvis. The glomeruli are relatively spared ⊳.

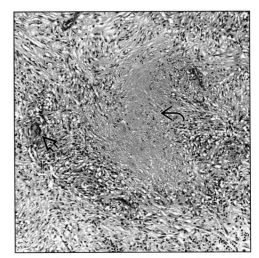

BCG nephritis in a patient with prior in situ urothelial carcinoma of the pelvis is seen. The granulomas show extensive necrosis ⊳ with surrounding histiocytes and a rare multinucleated giant cell ⊳.

TERMINOLOGY

Abbreviations
- Bacillus Calmette-Guérin (BCG)

Synonyms
- BCG nephritis

Definitions
- Granulomatous inflammation of kidney due to intracavitary BCG for treatment of in situ urothelial carcinoma

ETIOLOGY/PATHOGENESIS

Mechanisms of Granulomatous Reaction
- Hypersensitivity reaction to BCG
  - Urine and blood cultures are often negative
  - Corticosteroid therapy helpful if anti-tuberculous therapy fails
- Direct infection of tissues by live attenuated organism in BCG vaccine
- Vesico-ureteral and intrarenal reflux is predisposing factor

Local Immune Mechanisms
- Triggered by macrophage phagocytosis of BCG antigen and presentation to helper T cells
- Upregulation of chemokines and cytokines by T cells, macrophages, and neutrophils contributes to antitumor properties of BCG
- Exaggerated immune response combined with host factors may lead to BCG nephritis

CLINICAL ISSUES

Epidemiology
- Incidence
  - Symptomatic BCG nephritis is uncommon

- BCG nephritis less frequent than granulomatous cystitis secondary to intravesical BCG therapy
- Asymptomatic granulomatous inflammation of renal pelvis occurs in 25% of patients treated with BCG for noninvasive renal urothelial carcinoma
- BCG nephritis can occur in 2% of patients who receive intravesical BCG therapy for urothelial carcinoma of bladder

Site
- Renal cortex and medulla

Presentation
- Urinary frequency, dysuria
- Low-grade fever, malaise
- Flank pain, tenderness
- Temporal association to BCG therapy

Laboratory Tests
- Urine
  - White blood cells
  - Negative cultures (sterile pyuria)
- Blood cultures for mycobacteria are usually negative

Treatment
- Surgical approaches
  - Nephrectomy if aggressive medical therapy fails
- Drugs
  - Anti-tuberculosis drug regimens
  - Trial of steroid therapy if cultures are negative

Prognosis
- Most patients respond to combination anti-tuberculosis therapy and corticosteroids

BCG GRANULOMATOUS INTERSTITIAL NEPHRITIS

Key Facts

Terminology
- Granulomatous inflammation of kidney due to intracavitary BCG therapy for in situ urothelial carcinoma

Etiology/Pathogenesis
- Hypersensitivity reaction to BCG
- Direct infection of tissues by live attenuated organism in BCG vaccine

- Exaggerated immune response combined with host factors may lead to BCG nephritis

Microscopic Pathology
- Granulomas ± caseating necrosis are seen

Top Differential Diagnoses
- Drug-induced interstitial nephritis
- Sarcoidosis
- Fungal infection

MACROSCOPIC FEATURES

Multiple Renal Masses in Cortex and Medulla
- Nephrectomy performed only in therapeutically unresponsive cases

MICROSCOPIC PATHOLOGY

Histologic Features
- Tubulointerstitial inflammation with lymphocytes, histiocytes, plasma cells, and few eosinophils
- Granulomas ± caseating necrosis are seen
- Multinucleated giant cells may be seen
- Glomeruli are relatively spared
- Residual in situ urothelial carcinoma may be identified

ANCILLARY TESTS

Histochemistry
- Ziehl-Neelsen (acid-fast bacteria) stain
  - Reactivity: Negative

Immunofluorescence
- Faint mesangial IgM and C3 staining reported in a few cases (mesangial glomerulonephritis)

Electron Microscopy
- Normal with no electron-dense deposits

DIFFERENTIAL DIAGNOSIS

Drug-induced Interstitial Nephritis
- Noncaseating granulomas ± eosinophils
- Recent history of drug exposure

Sarcoidosis
- Noncaseating "tight" granulomas with rim of lymphocytes
- Extrarenal manifestations of sarcoidosis may be present

Fungal Infection
- Immunocompromised individuals are susceptible
- GMS (Gomori methenamine-silver) stain positive

SELECTED REFERENCES

1. Bijol V et al: Granulomatous interstitial nephritis: a clinicopathologic study of 46 cases from a single institution. Int J Surg Pathol. 14(1):57-63, 2006
2. Kennedy SE et al: Acute granulomatous tubulointerstitial nephritis caused by intravesical BCG. Nephrol Dial Transplant. 21(5):1427-9, 2006
3. Tavolini IM et al: Unmanageable fever and granulomatous renal mass after intracavitary upper urinary tract bacillus Calmette-Guerin therapy. J Urol. 167(1):244-5, 2002
4. Prescott S et al: Mechanisms of action of intravesical bacille Calmette-Guérin: local immune mechanisms. Clin Infect Dis. 31 Suppl 3:S91-3, 2000
5. Soda T et al: Granulomatous nephritis as a complication of intrarenal bacille Calmette-Guérin therapy. Urology. 53(6):1228, 1999

IMAGE GALLERY

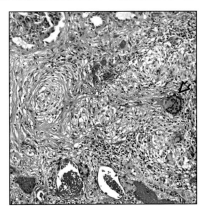
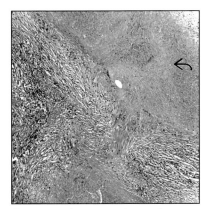
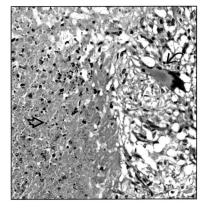

(Left) Hematoxylin & eosin shows granulomatous inflammation due to BCG therapy for in situ urothelial carcinoma of the kidney. The granulomas have scant necrosis but demonstrate lymphohistiocytic infiltrate and multinucleated giant cells ⮡. *(Center)* BCG granulomatous interstitial nephritis is characterized by large areas of caseating necrosis ⮡. *(Right)* Renal granulomatous inflammation due to BCG therapy with areas of necrosis ⮡ rimmed by histiocytes and a multinucleated giant cell ⮡ is seen. The acid-fast bacteria stain was negative.

LEPROSY

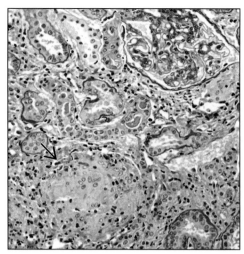

PAS stain shows granulomatous interstitial nephritis in a patient with leprosy. A granuloma is present ➡ in a background of diffuse interstitial mononuclear cells and fibrosis.

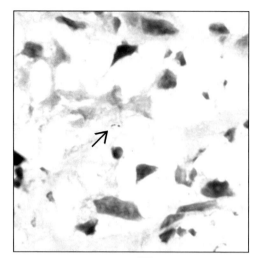

Rare acid-fast organisms ➡ were detected in macrophages in the interstitium of the kidney in a leprosy patient with chronic renal failure.

TERMINOLOGY

Definitions
- Renal manifestations due to immunological host response to *M. leprae* or due to treatment effects

ETIOLOGY/PATHOGENESIS

Mycobacterium leprae
- Obligate intracellular, weakly acid-fast bacillus
- Spectrum of disease from tuberculoid to lepromatous type with intervening borderline categories
- Tuberculoid leprosy
  - Robust cell-mediated immunity with granulomas and paucity of bacilli
  - Preponderance of T-helper-cell (CD4) response
  - Humoral response low
- Lepromatous leprosy
  - Poor cell-mediated immunity with abundant bacilli
  - Predominantly cytotoxic T-cell (CD8) response
  - Robust humoral response with high antibody titers
    - No protective effect but causes immune complex-mediated responses such as erythema nodosum leprosum (ENL), glomerulonephritis

Genetic Factors
- Determine tuberculoid or lepromatous host response

Mechanisms of Glomerular Injury
- Deposition of circulating immune complexes
  - Possible antigens include *M. leprae*, other organisms (coinfection), dapsone
- In situ immune complex deposition
- Cryoglobulinemia

CLINICAL ISSUES

Epidemiology
- Incidence

  - Found worldwide but is endemic in tropics

Presentation
- Renal insufficiency and, rarely, acute renal failure
- Hematuria, proteinuria
- Nephrotic syndrome and edema
- Functional tubular defects of acidification or urinary concentration ability in a few patients

Treatment
- Drugs
  - Antimicrobials: Dapsone, rifampin, clofazimine
  - Steroids and thalidomide helpful in ENL and possibly in glomerulonephritis

MICROSCOPIC PATHOLOGY

Histologic Features
- Tubulointerstitial nephritis
  - Granulomatous nephritis in *M. leprae* infection
    - Associated multinucleated giant cells and lymphocytes
  - Nongranulomatous nephritis due to secondary bacterial infection, antimicrobial therapy
- Glomerulonephritis
  - Mesangial, endocapillary proliferative, or membranoproliferative glomerulonephritis
  - Crescents are rare but can cause acute renal failure
- Amyloidosis (AA type)
  - More common in USA than in endemic areas
  - Often in lepromatous leprosy with recurrent bouts of ENL or trophic skin ulcers
- No histological abnormality in patients with functional tubular defects

ANCILLARY TESTS

Histochemistry
- Modified Ziehl-Neelsen stain (Fite)

LEPROSY

Key Facts

Terminology
- Renal manifestations due to immunological host response to *M. leprae* or due to treatment effects

Etiology/Pathogenesis
- Obligate intracellular, weakly acid-fast bacillus
- Genetic factors determine tuberculoid or lepromatous response to *M. leprae*

Microscopic Pathology
- Tubulointerstitial nephritis, may be granulomatous
- Glomerulonephritis
- Amyloidosis (AA type) common in USA

Ancillary Tests
- Fite stain reveals rod-shaped bacilli
- Granular IgG and C3 deposits in glomerulonephritis
- Congo red stain for amyloid

- o Reactivity: Positive
- o Staining pattern
  - ▪ Rod-like organisms in interstitial nephritis
- Congo red
  - o Reactivity: Positive in presence of amyloid
  - o Staining pattern
    - ▪ Apple-green birefringence under polarized light

Immunofluorescence
- Granular deposits of IgG and C3 in mesangium and capillary walls in glomerulonephritis
- Amyloid subtyping in amyloidosis for amyloid A

Electron Microscopy
- Intracellular degenerated lepra bacilli may be seen within macrophages in interstitial nephritis
- Electron-dense deposits observed in mesangium and subendothelial space in glomerulonephritis
- Randomly oriented amyloid fibrils (8-12 nm thick)

DIFFERENTIAL DIAGNOSIS

Tuberculous Granulomatous Inflammation
- Mycobacterial cultures positive
- Lack of response to dapsone therapy

Drug-induced Interstitial Nephritis
- Clinical history of drug use
- Negative Fite stain

Non-infection-related Glomerulonephritis
- Clinicopathologic correlation and positive serology may be helpful

SELECTED REFERENCES

1. Nakayama EE et al: Renal lesions in leprosy: a retrospective study of 199 autopsies. Am J Kidney Dis. 38(1):26-30, 2001
2. Ahsan N et al: Leprosy-associated renal disease: case report and review of the literature. J Am Soc Nephrol. 5(8):1546-52, 1995
3. Madiwale CV et al: Acute renal failure due to crescentic glomerulonephritis complicating leprosy. Nephrol Dial Transplant. 9(2):178-9, 1994
4. Chopra NK et al: Renal involvement in leprosy. J Assoc Physicians India. 39(2):165-7, 1991
5. Weiner ID et al: Leprosy and glomerulonephritis: case report and review of the literature. Am J Kidney Dis. 13(5):424-9, 1989
6. Jain AP et al: Clinico-pathological study of nephrotic syndrome in leprosy. J Assoc Physicians India. 31(7):437-8, 1983
7. Gupta SC et al: A study of percutaneous renal biopsy in lepromatous leprosy. Lepr India. 53(2):179-84, 1981
8. Ng WL et al: Glomerulonephritis in leprosy. Am J Clin Pathol. 76(3):321-9, 1981
9. Gupta JC et al: Amyloidosis in leprosy. Lepr India. 52(2):260-6, 1980
10. Case records of the Massachusetts General Hospital: Weekly clinicopathological exercises. Case 10-1979. N Engl J Med. 300(10):546-53, 1979
11. Date A et al: Glomerular pathology in leprosy. An electron microscopic study. Am J Trop Med Hyg. 26(2):266-72, 1977

IMAGE GALLERY

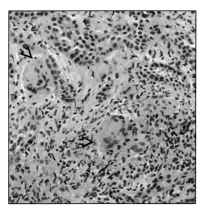 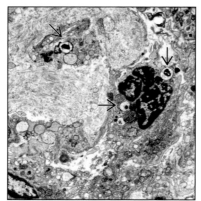 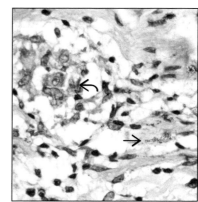

(Left) H&E shows granulomatous interstitial nephritis ⊵ in a patient with chronic renal insufficiency and peripheral nerve involvement by leprosy. Clinical renal involvement is rare in leprosy. *(Center)* EM shows degenerated intracellular mycobacteria ⊅ in the kidney biopsy of a patient with leprosy. *(Right)* Peripheral nerve biopsy in a patient with lepromatous leprosy and renal insufficiency shows abundant acid-fast organisms ⊅ and a granuloma ⊅.

NOCARDIOSIS

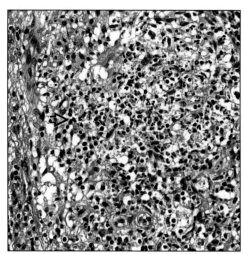

Nocardia infection in the kidney is characterized by multiple necrotizing microabscesses ▷ with associated renal parenchymal damage.

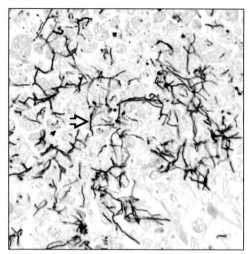

A GMS stain shows slender branching filamentous organisms ▷ characteristic of Nocardia infection within the microabscesses. (Courtesy A. Husain, MD.)

TERMINOLOGY

Definitions
- Acute inflammation of renal parenchyma by bacteria of genus *Nocardia*

ETIOLOGY/PATHOGENESIS

Infectious Agents
- *Nocardia asteroides* is most common agent in temperate climates
- *N. brasiliensis* is more common in tropical climates
- Less common species include *N. caviae*, *N. nova*, and *N. farcinica*
- Ubiquitous organisms in soil
  - Infection due to inhalation of organisms or direct inoculation into skin via trauma or animal bite

Predisposing Factors
- Opportunistic infection in immunocompromised host
  - Renal transplantation
  - Corticosteroid therapy
  - HIV infection
- Can occur in setting of chronic lung disease, carcinoma, or even in healthy individuals

CLINICAL ISSUES

Epidemiology
- Incidence
  - *Nocardia* infection is rare; occurs in ≤ 2% of renal transplant recipients
    - Lungs are most commonly affected organs
    - Kidney involvement is rare and secondary to diffuse hematogenous infection

Site
- Kidney parenchyma and perinephric tissues

Presentation
- Fever, chills
- Pulmonary symptoms with septicemia
- Pain and tenderness in loin or around renal allograft
- Skin involvement with draining sinuses may be present

Laboratory Tests
- Aerobic bacterial cultures of blood, body fluids, or tissue
- Urine cultures positive for *Nocardia* if pyelitis is present

Treatment
- Drugs
  - Sulfonamides are first line of treatment
  - In sulfonamide-resistant cases, alternative agents such as amikacin, imipenem, and 3rd generation cephalosporins may be used
  - Prolonged treatment for 6-12 months required, especially in immunocompromised patients

Prognosis
- Central nervous system involvement is sign of poor prognosis

IMAGE FINDINGS

General Features
- Renal parenchymal or perinephric abscesses may be identified

MICROSCOPIC PATHOLOGY

Histologic Features
- Multiple necrotizing microabscesses with neutrophils
- Acute inflammation may affect glomeruli along with adjacent tubulointerstitium
- Blood vessels are usually spared

NOCARDIOSIS

Key Facts

Etiology/Pathogenesis
- *Nocardia asteroides* is most common agent
- Opportunistic infection in immunocompromised host
- Infection due to inhalation of organisms or direct inoculation into skin via trauma

Clinical Issues
- Kidney involvement is rare and secondary to diffuse hematogenous infection

Microscopic Pathology
- Multiple necrotizing microabscesses with neutrophils

Ancillary Tests
- Grocott-Gomori methenamine-silver stain
- Gram stain
- Branched thin filamentous bacteria seen

- Rare case of mesangiocapillary glomerulonephritis has been reported in a patient with *Nocardia* pneumonia

ANCILLARY TESTS

Histochemistry
- Grocott-Gomori methenamine-silver
  - Reactivity: Positive
  - Staining pattern
    - Branched thin filamentous bacteria
- Gram
  - Reactivity: Positive
  - Staining pattern
    - Branched thin filamentous bacteria
- Periodic acid-Schiff and acid-fast stains
  - Filamentous bacteria are less well seen

DIFFERENTIAL DIAGNOSIS

Non-nocardial Bacterial Pyelonephritis
- Histochemical stains and cultures are useful

Pauci-immune Glomerulonephritis and Vasculitis
- Glomerular crescents identified and vasculocentric inflammation may be seen
- Neutrophils seen, but well-defined abscesses are absent

Acute Tubulointerstitial Nephritis
- Predominantly lymphocytic infiltrate

- Neutrophils seen, but well-defined abscesses are absent

Infectious Granulomatous Pyelonephritis
- Epithelioid histiocytes and multinucleated giant cells present at the periphery of necrosis
- Mycobacterial and fungal infections should be excluded
  - Acid-fast bacilli stain, Grocott-Gomori methenamine-silver stain and cultures are helpful

SELECTED REFERENCES

1. Einollahi B et al: Invasive fungal infections following renal transplantation: a review of 2410 recipients. Ann Transplant. 13(4):55-8, 2008
2. D'Cruz S et al: Isolated nocardial subcapsular and perinephric abscess. Indian J Pathol Microbiol. 47(1):24-6, 2004
3. Frangié C et al: A rare infection in a renal transplant recipient. Nephrol Dial Transplant. 16(6):1285-7, 2001
4. Jose MD et al: Mesangiocapillary glomerulonephritis in a patient with Nocardia pneumonia. Nephrol Dial Transplant. 13(10):2628-9, 1998
5. Salahuddin F et al: Urinary tract infection with an unusual pathogen (Nocardia asteroides). J Urol. 155(2):654-5, 1996
6. Raghavan R et al: Fungal and nocardial infections of the kidney. Histopathology. 11(1):9-20, 1987
7. Presant CA et al: Disseminated extrapulmonary nocardiosis presenting as a renal abscess. Arch Pathol. 89(6):560-4, 1970

IMAGE GALLERY

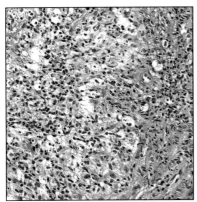 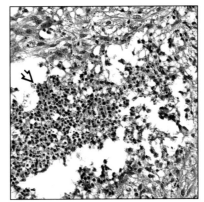 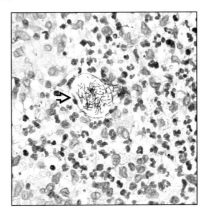

(Left) The glomeruli and tubulointerstitium are replaced by necrotizing inflammation in nocardiosis. No obvious microorganisms are seen on this hematoxylin and eosin stain. *(Center)* The microabscesses seen in Nocardia infection have central collections of neutrophils ⊵ with peripheral lymphohistiocytic inflammation. *(Right)* A Gram stain highlights a small collection of tangled filamentous Nocardia organisms ⊵ within the microabscesses.

LEPTOSPIROSIS

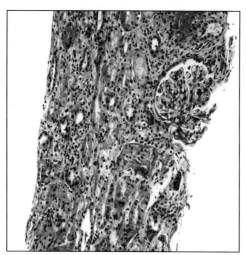

Diffuse interstitial edema with a mononuclear infiltrate and acute tubular injury are apparent in this biopsy specimen from a patient with leptospirosis. The glomerulus is spared. (Courtesy V. Royal, MD.)

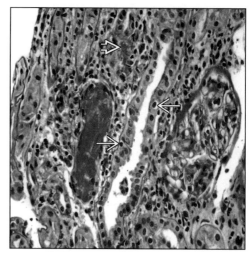

Interstitial mononuclear inflammation, tubulitis ➡, tubular casts, and focal cast extrusion ⟥ are evident in this case of leptospirosis. (Courtesy V. Royal, MD.)

TERMINOLOGY

Definitions
- Zoonotic infectious disease caused by spirochetes of genus *Leptospira*

ETIOLOGY/PATHOGENESIS

Infectious Agents
- *Leptospira interrogans* is a group of spirochetes with several subspecies that are pathogenic for humans
  ○ *L. icterohemorrhagica, L. canicola, L. pomona, L. bataviae, L. grippotyphosa*, and others
- Predominantly tropical disease; zoonosis, with rats as principal reservoir
  ○ Also skunks, foxes, ducks, dogs, and frogs
- *Leptospira* are excreted in urine of animal reservoir
- Contaminated food/water and direct contact with blood/tissue of infected animals are sources of exposure
  ○ Outbreaks often coincide with flooding
- *Leptospira* enter host through abrasions of skin or mucous membranes

Pathogenesis of Infection
- Within 48 hours of infection, there is wide dissemination of these organisms
- Infection has 2 phases
  ○ Early phase: 3-7 days, caused by leptospiremia and direct infection of organs
  ○ Immunological phase: 4-20 days, caused by immunologic reaction to *Leptospira* antigens
- Acute renal failure arises from a number of factors
  ○ Direct tubular injury: Leptospiral outer membrane protein and endotoxin acting via Toll-like receptors
  ○ Immunologic injury: Tubulointerstitial nephritis
  ○ Ischemic injury: Peripheral vasodilation, hypovolemia, myocarditis
  ○ Toxic tubular injury from endogenous toxins

- Hepatic failure: Bilirubin; rhabdomyolysis, myoglobin

CLINICAL ISSUES

Presentation
- Variable spectrum from subclinical infection to self-limited febrile illness to fatal disease
- Disease has sudden onset after incubation period of 7-12 days
- 2 main patterns
  ○ Anicteric form (80-90% of cases)
    ▪ Self-limited fever, chills, myalgia, headache, conjunctivitis, rash
  ○ Icteric form (10-20% of cases): Weil disease
    ▪ Fever, jaundice, acute renal failure
    ▪ Fulminant form has bleeding diathesis with thrombocytopenia and pulmonary hemorrhage
- 40-60% have acute renal failure in course of disease
- Urine has mild proteinuria, granular casts, hematuria, leukocyturia, bile, and heme casts
  ○ *Leptospira* are identifiable on dark field microscopy or by immunofluorescence with antileptospiral antibodies in weeks 1-4
- Isolation is possible using special media (EMcCJH or Fletcher medium) and takes 4 weeks or more
- Microagglutination assay for detection of leptospiral antibodies or *Leptospira* DNA detection by PCR is diagnostic
- Kidneys may be swollen on ultrasonography

Treatment
- Drugs
  ○ Antibiotics: Penicillin, ceftriaxone, cefotaxime
    ▪ Risk of Jarisch-Herxheimer reaction
  ○ Steroids are used in severe illness

Prognosis
- Mortality in Weil disease (*L. icterohemorrhagica*): 10%
- ~ 25% mortality with acute renal failure

LEPTOSPIROSIS

Key Facts

Terminology
- Zoonotic infectious disease caused by spirochetes of genus *Leptospira*

Etiology/Pathogenesis
- Early phase: 3-7 days, caused by leptospiremia and direct infection of organs
- Immunological phase: 4-20 days, caused by immunologic reaction to *Leptospira* antigens

Clinical Issues
- Anicteric form (80-90% of cases)
- Icteric form (10-20% of cases)
  - Weil disease: Fever, jaundice, acute renal failure

Microscopic Pathology
- Tubulointerstitial nephritis is characteristic
- Leptospiral organisms or antigen may be detectable in interstitium and in tubules

---

- 90% of survivors recover renal function

MACROSCOPIC FEATURES

General Features
- Enlarged kidneys with petechial hemorrhages ± ecchymoses on capsular and cut surfaces, calyceal and pelvic mucosa
- In Weil disease, brown-yellow discoloration of kidney

MICROSCOPIC PATHOLOGY

Histologic Features
- Glomeruli, arteries, and arterioles are unremarkable
- Tubulointerstitial nephritis is characteristic
  - Early lesions have acute tubular injury
  - Later lesions have tubulointerstitial inflammation, edema, tubulitis, and possibly hemorrhage
  - Infiltrates are composed of lymphocytes, macrophages, and occasional granulocytes
  - Tubular casts may be hyaline, necrotic, bile, myoglobin, or hemoglobin
- Warthin-Starry, Steiner, or Levaditi stains may allow visualization of helical, 6-20 µm spirochetes in tubules and interstitium
- Immunofluorescence
  - Leptospiral antigen may be detectable in interstitium and in tubules
- Electron microscopy

  - Leptospira may be seen in tubular lumens, epithelium, and capillaries

DIFFERENTIAL DIAGNOSIS

Tubulointerstitial Nephritis
- Infection: Rickettsiae, hantavirus, adenovirus (nuclear inclusions), dengue
  - Microbial antigens detectable by immunohistochemistry
- Drug hypersensitivity

DIAGNOSTIC CHECKLIST

Pathologic Interpretation Pearls
- Acute tubular injury and tubulointerstitial nephritis are characteristic; organisms or leptospiral antigen is detectable in situ

SELECTED REFERENCES

1. Yang CW et al: Leptospirosis renal disease. Nephrol Dial Transplant. 16 Suppl 5:73-7, 2001
2. Arean VM: The pathologic anatomy and pathogenesis of fatal human leptospirosis (Weil's disease). Am J Pathol. 40:393-423, 1962

IMAGE GALLERY

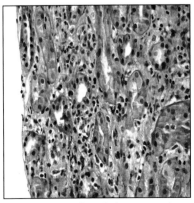 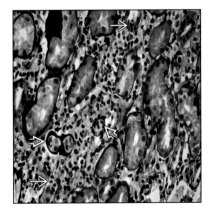 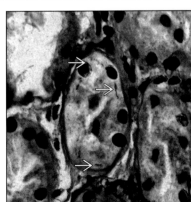

(Left) Mononuclear cells including macrophages and activated lymphoid cells are seen predominantly in the interstitium. (Courtesy V. Royal, MD.) *(Center)* Macrophages and lymphoid cells are associated with atrophic tubules ➡, and there is focal tubulitis ➡ with breaks in the tubular basement membrane. (Courtesy V. Royal, MD.) *(Right)* Silver positive intraepithelial structures ➡ consistent with Leptospira spirochetes are seen using Warthin-Starry or Steiner stains. (Courtesy V. Royal, MD.)

MUCORMYCOSIS

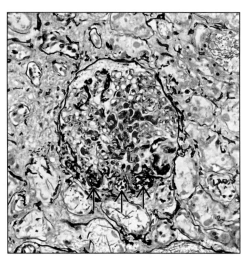

Jones methenamine silver at autopsy of an immunocompromised patient shows numerous fungal hyphae within the glomerulus and hilar arteriole ➔. (Courtesy E. Bracamonte, MD.)

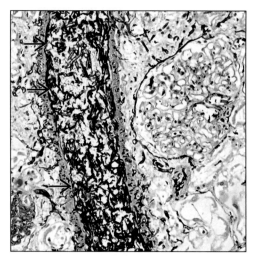

Jones methenamine silver shows numerous fungal nonseptate branching hyphae ➔ invading the arterial lumen in an area with extensive cortical necrosis. (Courtesy E. Bracamonte, MD.)

TERMINOLOGY

Synonyms
- Invasive zygomycosis

Definitions
- Opportunistic infection of typically immunocompromised or immunosuppressed patients

ETIOLOGY/PATHOGENESIS

Infectious Agents
- *Mucor*
  - Class: Zygomycetes
  - Order: Mucorales
    - Most common species is *Rhizopus*
    - Others species (in descending frequency): *Rhizomucor, Cunninghamella, Apophysomyces, Saksenaea, Absidia, Mucor*
  - Ubiquitous organisms found in soil and decaying matter, including moldy bread

CLINICAL ISSUES

Epidemiology
- Incidence
  - Disease generally only caused in immunocompromised patients
    - Poorly controlled diabetics
    - Leukemia
    - Transplant recipients
    - Malnourished

Site
- Sinus and brain (rhinocerebral) ~ 50% of cases
- Pulmonary, cutaneous
- GI, kidney less common

Presentation
- Acute renal failure
- Fever
- Flank pain
- Hematuria

Laboratory Tests
- Fungal cultures
- Biopsy

Treatment
- Surgical approaches
  - Nephrectomy
- Drugs
  - Antifungal therapy
    - Amphotericin B
  - Reduction of immunosuppressive agents

Prognosis
- Poor: > 50% mortality in disseminated disease
  - Mucormycosis isolated to kidney may have better prognosis

MACROSCOPIC FEATURES

General Features
- Arterial thrombosis
  - Main renal artery
  - Arcuate &/or interlobar arteries
- Large infarcts

MICROSCOPIC PATHOLOGY

Histologic Features
- Nonseptate fungal hyphae with 90° branching
  - Found in areas of infarct, granuloma, thrombi, microabscesses
- Cortical necrosis
- Thrombi

MUCORMYCOSIS

Key Facts

Clinical Issues
- Renal involvement in 20% of patients with disseminated disease
- Fever
- Flank pain
- Treat with nephrectomy and amphotericin B

Macroscopic Features
- Large infarcts
- Arterial thrombosis

  ○ Main renal, arcuate, or interlobar artery

Microscopic Pathology
- Nonseptate fungal hyphae with 90° branching
- Cortical necrosis, arterial thrombi
- Microabscesses

Top Differential Diagnoses
- Aspergillosis
- Candidiasis

- Arteritis
- Microabscesses
- Granulomatous interstitial nephritis
  ○ Frequent multinucleated giant cells

DIFFERENTIAL DIAGNOSIS

Aspergillosis
- Septate hyphae with 45° branching

Pseudallescheriasis
- Septate hyphae

Fusariosis
- Septate hyphae

Candidiasis
- Pseudohyphae and budding yeast forms

Tuberculosis
- Caseating necrosis in granulomas with acid-fast bacilli

Bacterial Pyelonephritis
- Prominent neutrophilic infiltrate or abscesses
- No fungal organisms

Sarcoidosis
- Granulomatous inflammation without microorganisms present

DIAGNOSTIC CHECKLIST

Pathologic Interpretation Pearls
- Fungal cultures establish diagnosis
- Distinguishing fungal species based on morphologic evaluation alone is difficult

SELECTED REFERENCES

1. Nalmas S et al: Mucormycosis in a transplanted kidney. Transpl Infect Dis. 10(4):269-71, 2008
2. Tayyebi N et al: Renal allograft mucormycosis: report of two cases. Surg Infect (Larchmt). 8(5):535-8, 2007
3. Ahmad M: Graft mucormycosis in a renal allograft recipient. J Nephrol. 18(6):783-6, 2005
4. Jianhong L et al: Isolated renal mucormycosis in children. J Urol. 171(1):387-8, 2004
5. Keogh CF et al: Renal mucormycosis in an AIDS patient: imaging features and pathologic correlation. AJR Am J Roentgenol. 180(5):1278-80, 2003
6. Chkhotua A et al: Mucormycosis of the renal allograft: case report and review of the literature. Transpl Int. 14(6):438-41, 2001
7. Gupta KL et al: Renal zygomycosis: an under-diagnosed cause of acute renal failure. Nephrol Dial Transplant. 14(11):2720-5, 1999

IMAGE GALLERY

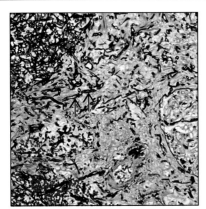 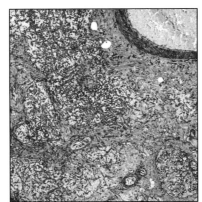 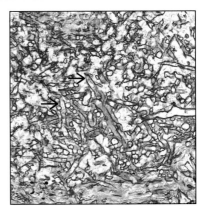

(Left) Jones methenamine silver shows numerous hyphae ➡, typical of mucormycosis in an area of cortical necrosis. (Courtesy E. Bracamonte, MD.) (Center) Periodic acid-Schiff shows fungal hyphae in an area of cortical necrosis in a hematopoietic cell transplant patient. The absence of prominent interstitial inflammation may be due to immunosuppression. (Courtesy E. Bracamonte, MD.) (Right) Periodic acid-Schiff shows numerous, broad, nonseptate hyphae ➡ branching at approximately right angles. (Courtesy E. Bracamonte, MD.)

CANDIDIASIS

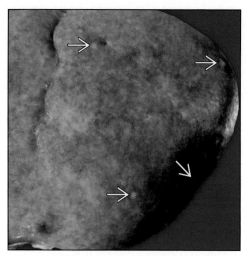

This gross photograph of the capsular surface of this kidney at autopsy shows many small abscesses ⟹ due to disseminated candidiasis from Candida tropicalis.

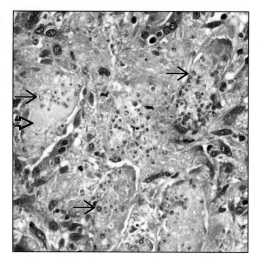

Histology shows numerous yeast forms of Candida tropicalis ⟹ intermixed with Tamm-Horsfall protein (uromodulin) ⊳ within tubular lumens and in the interstitium from ruptured tubules.

TERMINOLOGY

Synonyms
- Oidiomycosis

Definitions
- *Candida* infection of kidney
  - Typically in immunocompromised patient

ETIOLOGY/PATHOGENESIS

Infectious Agents
- *C. albicans*
  - Normal flora of skin, gastrointestinal, and genitourinary tracts
- *C. glabrata*
  - Previously named *Torulopsis glabrata* (also known as torulopsosis)
- *C. parapsilosis*
- *C. tropicalis*
- *C. krusei*

CLINICAL ISSUES

Epidemiology
- Incidence
  - Uncommon
    - 8 cases per 100,000 persons in United States
    - 4th most common nosocomial bloodstream infection
    - Risk factors include diabetes, chemotherapy, immunosuppression
- Age
  - Neonates
    - Very low birth weight babies susceptible to invasive candidiasis
  - Elderly
    - > 65 years of age

- Gender
  - No gender predilection
- Ethnicity
  - Higher incidence among African-Americans

Presentation
- Renal dysfunction
- Acute renal failure
  - May be due to ureteral or bladder obstruction by *Candida*

Laboratory Tests
- Fungal culture
- Direct microscopy

Treatment
- Surgical approaches
  - Renal allograft nephrectomy
- Drugs
  - Fluconazole
  - Echinocandins
    - Caspofungin
    - Anidulafungin
    - Micafungin
  - Voriconazole
  - Amphotericin B
- Reduction of immunosuppression

Prognosis
- Up to 50% mortality in disseminated or invasive candidiasis

IMAGE FINDINGS

CT Findings
- Hypodense lesions correspond to renal abscesses
- Fungus balls
- Papillary necrosis

CANDIDIASIS

Key Facts

Etiology/Pathogenesis
- *C. albicans*
- *C. glabrata*
- *C. parapsilosis*
- *C. tropicalis*

Clinical Issues
- Therapeutic options
  - Fluconazole
  - Amphotericin B
  - Reduction of immunosuppressive agents in transplant patients
  - Transplant nephrectomy

Macroscopic Features
- Cortical abscesses
- Papillary necrosis

- Pyelitis
- Mycotic pseudoaneurysm

Microscopic Pathology
- Acute inflammation
- Fungal organisms
  - Pseudohyphae
  - Budding yeast forms
- Cortical abscesses
  - May be centered around glomeruli
- Rare cortical infarcts

Top Differential Diagnoses
- Aspergillosis
- Mucormycosis
- Histoplasmosis
- Cryptococcosis

MACROSCOPIC FEATURES

General Features
- Abscesses
  - Cortical abscesses
    - Miliary distribution
  - Perinephric abscesses
- Pyelitis
  - Fungus balls
- Papillary necrosis
  - 20% of patients with disseminated candidiasis at autopsy
- Mycotic pseudoaneurysm or occlusion of major renal arteries in allograft

MICROSCOPIC PATHOLOGY

Histologic Features
- Cortical abscesses
  - May be centered around glomeruli
  - Rare cortical infarcts
- Fungal organisms
  - Pseudohyphae
  - Budding yeast forms, 4-6 μm
  - May be present within glomerular capillaries &/or arterioles
- Granulomatous interstitial nephritis
  - Atypical feature
  - May contain predominantly budding yeast forms

DIFFERENTIAL DIAGNOSIS

Aspergillosis
- Septate hyphae with 45° branching

Mucormycosis
- Nonseptate hyphae with 90° branching

Fusariosis
- Septate hyphae

Pseudallescheriasis
- Septate hyphae

Histoplasmosis
- 2-4 μm in diameter

Cryptococcosis
- Capsule-deficient variant mimics *Candida* yeast forms

Blastomycosis
- 8-15 μm ovoid yeast forms with broad-based budding

Tuberculosis
- Caseating granulomas with acid-fast bacilli present

Sarcoidosis
- Noncaseating granulomas without microorganisms

DIAGNOSTIC CHECKLIST

Pathologic Interpretation Pearls
- Budding yeast and pseudohyphae combination characteristic
- Fungal cultures needed for definitive identification

SELECTED REFERENCES

1. Wasi N et al: A rare case of acute renal failure due to massive renal allograft infiltration with Candida glabrata. Nephrol Dial Transplant. 23(1):374-6, 2008
2. Meehan SM et al: Granulomatous tubulointerstitial nephritis in the renal allograft. Am J Kidney Dis. 36(4):E27, 2000
3. Fidel PL Jr et al: Candida glabrata: review of epidemiology, pathogenesis, and clinical disease with comparison to C. albicans. Clin Microbiol Rev. 12(1):80-96, 1999

CANDIDIASIS

Gross and Microscopic Features

(Left) The cut surface of this autopsy kidney shows several discrete white lesions with hemorrhagic rims ⮕ in the cortex ⮕, corresponding to areas of necrosis and active inflammation in a typical appearance of disseminated infection. *(Right)* The cut surface of the kidney has a hemorrhagic pelvic mucosa ⮕, similar to that in the bladder (not shown). Some blunting of a renal papilla ⮕ is noted. Severe cases can develop papillary necrosis. Cortical abscesses are also seen ⮕.

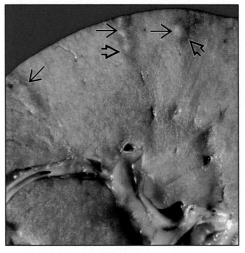 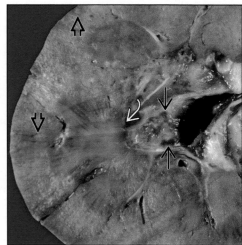

(Left) Gross photograph of prominent small and large green lesions ⮕ on the renal papilla of this autopsy specimen represents colonization by Candida. (Courtesy C. Abrahams, MD.) *(Right)* Microscopic examination shows numerous, round, basophilic yeast forms ⮕ within the tubules of this patient with disseminated candidiasis due to Candida albicans. Significant lymphocytic or granulomatous interstitial inflammation may be seen in candidiasis but is not present in this area.

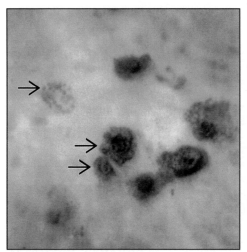 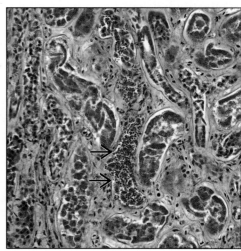

(Left) High power reveals abundant yeast ⮕ and a few pseudohyphae ⮕ consistent with Candida within a tubule and adjacent interstitial regions of this autopsy kidney with scattered interstitial lymphocytes ⮕ and neutrophils. A red blood cell ⮕ (6-8 microns in diameter) is larger than many adjacent yeast bodies. *(Right)* Gomori methenamine-silver stain shows yeast forms ⮕ within the renal tubules and a few pseudohyphae ⮕, a helpful finding in the identification of Candida.

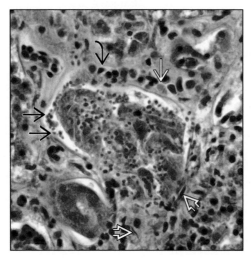 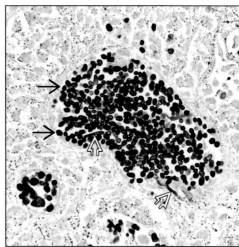

CANDIDIASIS

Microscopic Features

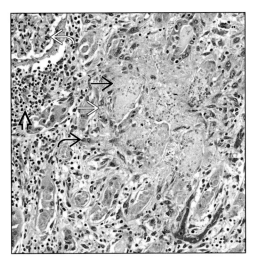

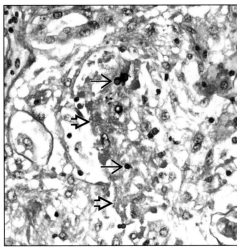

(Left) Hematoxylin & eosin stain shows fungal organisms ➡ intermixed with a Tamm-Horsfall protein (uromodulin) with focal necrosis and rupture of the tubules ⬈ associated with a granulomatous reaction ⬈ and scattered interstitial lymphocytes ⬈. The glomerulus ⬈ is normal. *(Right)* Periodic acid-Schiff stain highlights Candida yeast forms ➡ intermixed with a Tamm-Horsfall protein ⬈ and some sloughed epithelial cells within a tubular lumen.

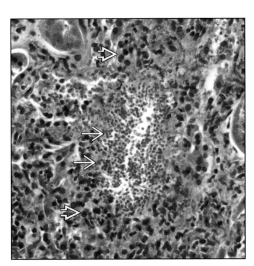

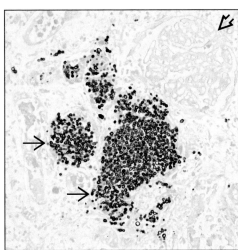

(Left) Hematoxylin & eosin stain shows numerous yeast forms ➡ of Candida albicans within the tubule in the center with prominent interstitial inflammation ⬈. The inflammation may be mononuclear, granulocytic, or granulomatous. *(Right)* Gomori methenamine-silver stain highlights numerous yeast forms of variable size ➡ within the proximal tubules and focal spillage into the interstitium. An adjacent glomerulus ⬈ shows no involvement by fungal organisms.

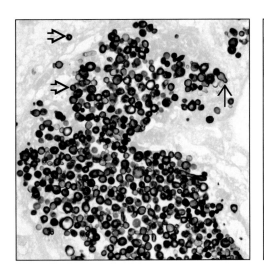

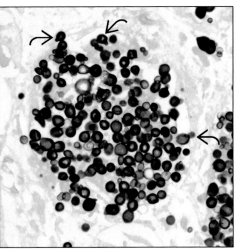

(Left) Gomori methenamine-silver stain shows numerous yeast forms ⬈ and a budding yeast ➡ of Candida tropicalis within a renal tubular lumen. In the proper clinical context, the absence of pseudohyphae may raise the consideration of blastomycosis or cryptococcosis. *(Right)* Gomori methenamine-silver stain at high magnification reveals many yeast forms of Candida, primarily within the renal tubular lumina. Some yeast appear to be forming buds ➡.

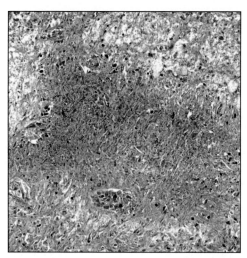

Hematoxylin & eosin shows extensive cortical necrosis at autopsy in a kidney with numerous round Histoplasma organisms due to disseminated disease in a patient with AIDS.

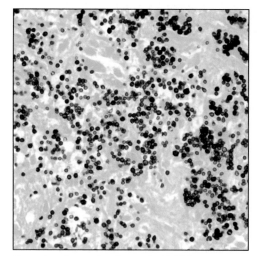

Gomori methenamine-silver stain highlights numerous fungal organisms from a patient with disseminated histoplasmosis within a necrotic area of the renal cortex.

TERMINOLOGY

Synonyms
- Ohio Valley disease, Darling disease

ETIOLOGY/PATHOGENESIS

Environmental Exposure
- Present in soil
  - Bird or bat droppings
- Inhalation of airborne conidia (spores)

Infectious Agents
- *Histoplasma capsulatum*
  - Dimorphic fungus (yeast in body, mycelia in soil)
  - Endemic to Mississippi and Ohio river valleys
  - South and Central America, Africa, Australia, and East Asia

CLINICAL ISSUES

Epidemiology
- Incidence
  - Kidney involved in 40% with disseminated disease
  - AIDS patients in endemic areas at risk (10-25%)
- Age
  - No age predilection
- Gender
  - M:F = 4:1
    - Similar gender exposure based on skin tests

Presentation
- Asymptomatic renal involvement
  - Renal dysfunction unusual
  - Flu-like acute respiratory infection
  - Chronic form mimics tuberculosis

Laboratory Tests
- Radioimmunoassay
  - *Histoplasma capsulatum* polysaccharide antigen
- Complement fixation test
  - More sensitive, less specific than immunodiffusion
  - False-positives from cross-reactivity with antigens from *Blastomyces dermatitidis* and *Coccidioides immitis*
- Immunodiffusion
- Culture
- Biopsy

Treatment
- Drugs
  - Amphotericin B
  - Ketoconazole
  - Itraconazole
  - Fluconazole
  - Decreased immunosuppression

Prognosis
- Disseminated form fatal without treatment
  - May lead to irreversible renal failure
- Self-limited localized form in normal individuals

MACROSCOPIC FEATURES

General Features
- Discrete nodular masses
- Papillary necrosis
- Diffuse inflammation and necrosis

MICROSCOPIC PATHOLOGY

Histologic Features
- Fungi are oval to round, 2-4 µm in diameter
- Granulomatous interstitial nephritis
  - Noncaseating granulomas
  - Occasional intratubular granulomas
  - Absence of granulomatous response in severely immunosuppressed patients
  - Organisms in macrophages

HISTOPLASMOSIS

Etiology/Pathogenesis
- *Histoplasma capsulatum*
  - Dimorphic fungus
  - Endemic to Mississippi and Ohio river valleys

Clinical Issues
- M:F = 4:1

Microscopic Pathology
- Granulomatous interstitial nephritis

Key Facts
- Cortical necrosis
- Thrombotic microangiopathy
- Oval to round fungal organisms, 2-4 μm in diameter
- Mesangial proliferative glomerulonephritis

Top Differential Diagnoses
- Blastomycosis
- Cryptococcosis
- Candidiasis
- Tuberculosis

  - Focal necrosis, medulla
  - Prominent interstitial inflammation
- Cortical necrosis
- Thrombotic microangiopathy
  - Glomerular capillary thrombi with entrapped fungal organisms may be observed
- Mesangial proliferative glomerulonephritis
  - Rare association with disseminated histoplasmosis
  - *H. capsulatum* antigen detected in mesangial areas

DIFFERENTIAL DIAGNOSIS

Blastomycosis
- 8-15 μm in diameter
- Thick wall
- Broad-based budding

Cryptococcosis
- Capsule-deficient variant causes granulomatous inflammation
  - Fontana-Masson silver stain positive

Candidiasis
- Budding yeasts may resemble *Histoplasma*

Coccidioidomycosis
- Endospores resemble *Histoplasma*

Tuberculosis
- Caseating granulomas
- Acid-fast bacilli present

Sarcoidosis
- Noncaseating granulomas
- No microorganisms present

Drug-induced Acute Interstitial Nephritis
- No microorganisms present

DIAGNOSTIC CHECKLIST

Pathologic Interpretation Pearls
- Necrotizing granulomas
- Yeast forms are smaller than erythrocytes

SELECTED REFERENCES

1. Sethi S: Acute renal failure in a renal allograft: an unusual infectious cause of thrombotic microangiopathy. Am J Kidney Dis. 46(1):159-62, 2005
2. Nasr SH et al: Granulomatous interstitial nephritis. Am J Kidney Dis. 41(3):714-9, 2003
3. Burke DG et al: Histoplasmosis and kidney disease in patients with AIDS. Clin Infect Dis. 25(2):281-4, 1997
4. Peddi VR et al: Disseminated histoplasmosis in renal allograft recipients. Clin Transplant. 10(2):160-5, 1996

IMAGE GALLERY

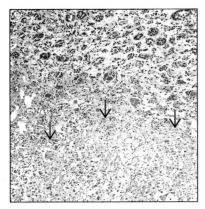 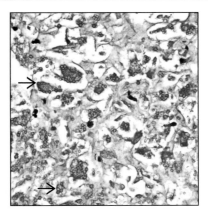 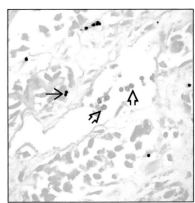

(Left) Hematoxylin & eosin stain shows a necrotic focus ⊒ adjacent to preserved tubules in the renal medulla without significant inflammation in an end-stage AIDS patient. *(Center)* Periodic acid-Schiff stain shows numerous clusters of round organisms ⊒ characteristic of Histoplasma capsulatum within the renal tubules. *(Right)* Gomori methenamine-silver stain confirms scattered Histoplasma organisms ⊒, which are much smaller in size than the red blood cells (6-8 μm in diameter) ⊒ within an adjacent peritubular capillary.

COCCIDIOIDOMYCOSIS

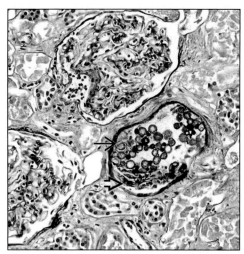

Jones methenamine silver shows numerous immature Coccidioides spherules ⊡ compressing the glomerulus ⊡ within the urinary space in a patient with disseminated disease. (Courtesy E. Bracamonte, MD.)

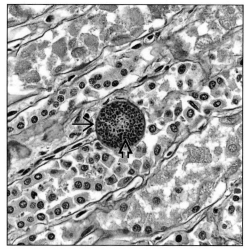

Periodic acid-Schiff shows a thick-walled mature spherule ⊡ with endospores ⊡ characteristic of Coccidioides among the renal tubules of this autopsy kidney. (Courtesy E. Bracamonte, MD.)

TERMINOLOGY

Synonyms
- Valley fever

ETIOLOGY/PATHOGENESIS

Infectious Agents
- *Coccidioides immitis*
  - Geographically limited to California San Joaquin valley, southwestern United States, and Mexico
- *C. posadasii*
  - Geographically limited to southwestern United States, Mexico, and South America
- Acquired through inhalation of fungal spores (arthroconidia) in environment
- Dimorphic fungi

CLINICAL ISSUES

Epidemiology
- Incidence
  - ~ 3% among renal transplant patients in endemic regions
- Gender
  - Pregnancy is risk factor for disseminated coccidioidomycosis
- Ethnicity
  - Persons of African, Asian, and Hispanic descent more likely than Caucasians to develop disseminated disease

Presentation
- Flu-like symptoms
  - Fever
  - Cough
  - Headache
  - Myalgia
  - Rash
- Eosinophilia
- Acute renal failure

Laboratory Tests
- Skin test
  - 10-50% of those in endemic areas test positive
  - Coccidioidin
  - Spherulin
- Enzyme immunoassay
  - IgA
  - IgM
    - Antibodies difficult to detect in immunosuppressed patients
- Immunodiffusion assay
- Complement fixation test
- Culture
  - Sputum
  - Other body fluids
- Direct microscopy

Treatment
- Surgical approaches
  - Surgical resection for some with pulmonary, bone, or joint involvement
- Drugs
  - Fluconazole
  - Amphotericin B
    - 2nd-line agent
    - Used for disseminated disease or azole-resistant strains of *Coccidioides*
  - Reduction of immunosuppressive agents

Prognosis
- Good in limited disease
- Poor in disseminated disease
  - Mortality rate > 50%
  - Up to 75% mortality rate in transplant patients

COCCIDIOIDOMYCOSIS

Key Facts

Etiology/Pathogenesis
- *Coccidioides immitis*
- *C. posadasii*
- Acquired through inhalation of fungal spores (arthroconidia) in environment

Clinical Issues
- Flu-like symptoms
- Surgical resection for some with pulmonary, bone, or joint involvement

- Fluconazole: First-line agent

Macroscopic Features
- Perinephric abscess

Microscopic Pathology
- *Coccidioides* spherules

Top Differential Diagnoses
- Blastomycosis
- Cryptococcosis

IMAGE FINDINGS

Radiographic Findings
- Pyelocalyceal alterations similar to tuberculosis in transplant kidneys

MACROSCOPIC FEATURES

General Features
- Perinephric abscess: Compression of renal transplant artery may be detected by angiogram

MICROSCOPIC PATHOLOGY

Histologic Features
- *Coccidioides* spherules
  o Round and thick walled (PAS and methenamine silver positive)
  o 10-80 μm in diameter
  o Contain numerous endospores (2-5 μm in diameter)
- Necrotic nodules
  o Septate hyphae seen in transitional form
- Granulomatous interstitial inflammation
  o Absent in severely immunocompromised patients

DIFFERENTIAL DIAGNOSIS

Blastomycosis
- 8-15 μm in diameter

Cryptococcosis
- Capsule-deficient variant, silver stain positive
- No endospores

DIAGNOSTIC CHECKLIST

Pathologic Interpretation Pearls
- Spherules and endospores characteristic for *Coccidioides*
- Renal involvement rare
- Fungal cultures and serologic tests confirm presence of coccidioidomycosis

SELECTED REFERENCES

1. Braddy CM et al: Coccidioidomycosis after renal transplantation in an endemic area. Am J Transplant. 6(2):340-5, 2006
2. Yoshino MT et al: Coccidioidomycosis in renal dialysis and transplant patients: radiologic findings in 30 patients. AJR Am J Roentgenol. 149(5):989-92, 1987
3. Conner WT et al: Genitourinary aspects of disseminated coccidioidomycosis. J Urol. 113(1):82-8, 1975

IMAGE GALLERY

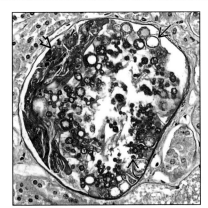 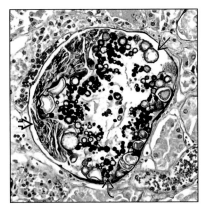 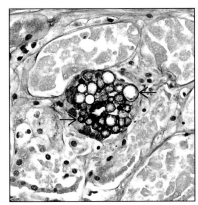

(Left) Periodic acid-Schiff shows numerous immature spherules ➡ and endospores ➡ that are characteristic of Coccidioides immitis within Bowman space compressing the adjacent glomerulus ➡. *(Courtesy E. Bracamonte, MD.)* *(Center)* Jones methenamine silver shows immature spherules ➡ and endospores ➡ of Coccidioides within the urinary space of a compressed glomerulus ➡. *(Courtesy E. Bracamonte, MD.)* *(Right)* Jones methenamine silver shows the immature spherules ➡ of Coccidioides with variable diameters. *(Courtesy E. Bracamonte, MD.)*

BLASTOMYCOSIS

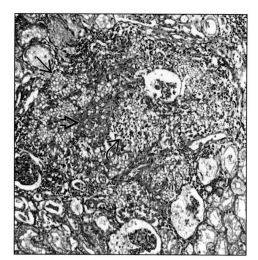

Hematoxylin & eosin shows a microabscess with necrosis ⊡, neutrophils ➡, and numerous round yeast forms ➡ in the renal cortex of this kidney involved by disseminated blastomycosis.

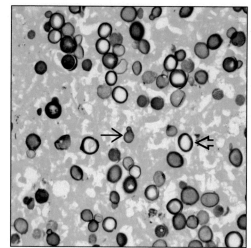

GMS (Gomori methenamine-silver) reveals Blastomyces with a broad-based budding yeast form ➡. The thick capsules ⊡ can resemble those of Cryptococcus and Coccidioides.

TERMINOLOGY

Synonyms
- North American blastomycosis
- Gilchrist disease
- Chicago disease

ETIOLOGY/PATHOGENESIS

Environmental Exposure
- Ubiquitous fungus in environment
  - Acquired by inhalation

Infectious Agents
- *Blastomyces dermatitidis*
  - Endemic to central and southern United States and Canada
  - Reported in parts of Central and South America, Europe, and Africa
  - Dimorphic fungus

CLINICAL ISSUES

Epidemiology
- Incidence
  - 1-2 per 100,000 in endemic areas
- Age
  - 30-50 years old
- Gender
  - Male predilection
    - M:F = 2-15:1
- Ethnicity
  - African-American predilection

Site
- Lungs
- Skin
- Genitourinary tract
  - Prostate
  - Epididymis
  - Kidney
    - < 10% involvement in disseminated disease

Presentation
- Asymptomatic
  - 50% of cases
- Fever
- Malaise

Laboratory Tests
- Fungal culture
  - Slow growth
- Direct microscopy

Treatment
- Drugs
  - Itraconazole
  - Amphotericin B
  - Ketoconazole
  - Fluconazole
  - Voriconazole

Prognosis
- Overall mortality rate of 4-22%
  - Mortality rate of 90% with kidney involvement
  - Mortality rate of 50% in AIDS patients

MACROSCOPIC FEATURES

General Features
- Bilateral involvement common
- Abscesses
  - More cortical than medullary involvement
  - Perinephric and sinus

MICROSCOPIC PATHOLOGY

Histologic Features
- Fungal organisms

BLASTOMYCOSIS

Key Facts

Etiology/Pathogenesis

- *Blastomyces dermatitidis*
  - Endemic to central/southern United States, Canada
  - Reported in Central/South America, Europe, and Africa
  - Ubiquitous dimorphic fungus acquired by inhalation

Macroscopic Features

- Abscesses

Microscopic Pathology

- Microorganisms, fungus
  - Thick wall, 8-15 μm in diameter
  - Broad-based budding
- Granulomatous inflammation

Top Differential Diagnoses

- Cryptococcosis
- Coccidioidomycosis

- Thick wall, 8-15 μm in diameter
- Broad-based budding
- Some yeast forms are < 8 μm in diameter
- May be surrounded by or located within multinucleated giant cells
- Granulomatous inflammation
- Neutrophilic inflammation

DIFFERENTIAL DIAGNOSIS

Cryptococcosis

- Capsule or clear halo, mucicarmine positive
- Capsule-deficient variant, silver stain positive

Coccidioidomycosis

- Spherules with characteristic endospores

Paracoccidioidomycosis

- Characteristic clear halos, 12-14 μm in diameter

Candidiasis

- Pseudohyphae and yeasts

Tuberculosis

- Caseating granulomata with acid-fast bacilli

Sarcoidosis

- Granulomatous inflammation without microorganisms

Drug-induced Acute Interstitial Nephritis

- Granulomatous inflammation without microorganisms

DIAGNOSTIC CHECKLIST

Pathologic Interpretation Pearls

- Coinfection with other fungal or viral organisms common

SELECTED REFERENCES

1. Bruce Light R et al: Seasonal variations in the clinical presentation of pulmonary and extrapulmonary blastomycosis. Med Mycol. 46(8):835-41, 2008
2. Taxy JB: Blastomycosis: contributions of morphology to diagnosis: a surgical pathology, cytopathology, and autopsy pathology study. Am J Surg Pathol. 31(4):615-23, 2007
3. Dworkin MS et al: The epidemiology of blastomycosis in Illinois and factors associated with death. Clin Infect Dis. 41(12):e107-11, 2005
4. Lemos LB et al: Blastomycosis: organ involvement and etiologic diagnosis. A review of 123 patients from Mississippi. Ann Diagn Pathol. 4(6):391-406, 2000
5. Sekhon AS et al: Blastomycosis: report of three cases from Alberta with a review of Canadian cases. Mycopathologia. 68(1):53-63, 1979

IMAGE GALLERY

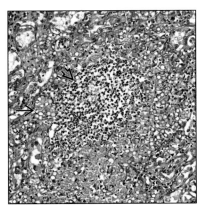 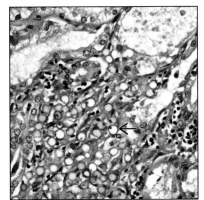 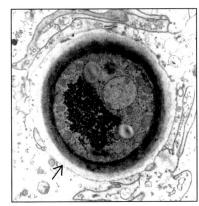

(Left) Periodic acid-Schiff highlights numerous thick-walled yeast forms ⊡ of Blastomyces surrounding a microabscess ⊡ in the renal cortex. *(Center)* Periodic acid-Schiff demonstrates the characteristic thick capsule ⊡ of Blastomyces, which ranges in diameter from 8-15 μm but may be as large as 30 μm. *(Right)* Electron micrograph shows the yeast form of Blastomyces with the outer electron-lucent capsule ⊡ and other internal structures entirely engulfed within a macrophage. *(Courtesy J. Taxy, MD.)*

PARACOCCIDIOIDOMYCOSIS

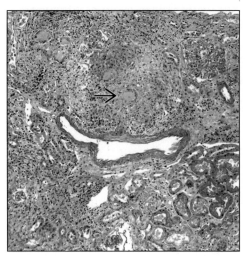

Light microscopy shows a granuloma in the cortex with prominent Langhans giant cells ⇨ surrounded by mononuclear cells in a Brazilian male with renal failure. (Courtesy A. Billis, MD.)

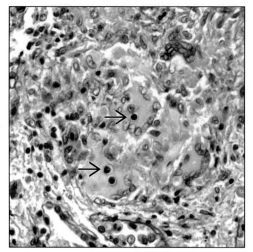

Periodic acid-Schiff highlights Paracoccidioides organisms with a pale halo ⇨ within a granuloma in the cortex with prominent Langhans giant cells. (Courtesy A. Billis, MD.)

TERMINOLOGY

Abbreviations
- Paracoccidioidomycosis (PCM)

Synonyms
- South American blastomycosis
- Brazilian blastomycosis
- Lutz-Splendore-Almeida disease

ETIOLOGY/PATHOGENESIS

Environmental Exposure
- Agricultural workers
- Construction workers

Infectious Agents
- *Paracoccidioides brasiliensis*
  - Endemic to South America and Brazil
  - Dimorphic fungus
    - Septate hyphae at room temperature
    - Yeast forms at body temperature
  - Acquired through inhalation

CLINICAL ISSUES

Epidemiology
- Incidence
  - Rare
- Age
  - Rare in children or teenagers
  - Affects those older than 30 years of age
- Gender
  - Male predilection
    - M:F = 15-78:1
    - Similar exposure rates between males and females based on skin testing results
- Ethnicity
  - No ethnic predilection

Presentation
- Asymptomatic
- Acute renal failure

Laboratory Tests
- Skin test
  - Positive result indicates exposure not active disease
- Enzyme-linked immunoassay
  - Detects antibodies to gp43
  - High sensitivity and specificity
- Complement fixation test
  - May cross-react with *Histoplasma capsulatum* antigen
- Immunodiffusion
- Western blot
  - High sensitivity and specificity
- Fungal culture
  - Sabouraud dextrose agar
  - May require up to 30 days of growth
  - Growth of yeast form at 37°C confirms diagnosis
- Direct microscopy
  - Wet mount with potassium hydroxide
    - 1 large yeast with budding forms resembles "pilot wheel"
- Biopsy

Natural History
- Generally asymptomatic in immunocompetent hosts

Treatment
- Drugs
  - Itraconazole
    - Low rate of relapse
  - Ketoconazole
  - Sulfonamides
    - Sulfadiazine
    - Sulfadimethoxine
  - Amphotericin B
  - Reduction of immunosuppressive agents in transplant patients

PARACOCCIDIOIDOMYCOSIS

Key Facts

Terminology
- Synonyms
  - South American blastomycosis
  - Brazilian blastomycosis
  - Lutz-Splendore-Almeida disease

Etiology/Pathogenesis
- *Paracoccidioides brasiliensis*
  - Endemic to South America and Brazil

Clinical Issues
- Male predilection
- Laboratory testing
  - Enzyme-linked immunoassay
  - Complement fixation test
  - Culture
  - Biopsy

- Drugs
  - Itraconazole: First-line agent

Microscopic Pathology
- Granulomatous interstitial nephritis
- Glomerular granulomas
- Glomerular capillary thrombi
- Glomerular fibrinoid necrosis
- Yeast forms with clear halos

Top Differential Diagnoses
- Cryptococcosis
- Lobomycosis
- Blastomycosis
- Tuberculosis
- Sarcoidosis
- Drug-induced acute interstitial nephritis

Prognosis
- If untreated: Up to 25% mortality rate
- If treated: Good prognosis
- Poor prognosis in rare juvenile form of disease

MICROSCOPIC PATHOLOGY

Histologic Features
- Granulomatous interstitial nephritis
  - Associated with *Paracoccidioides* organisms
  - Central caseation or caseating necrosis occasionally present
  - Multinucleated giant cells
- Glomerular granulomas
  - May resemble cellular crescents
- Thrombotic microangiopathy
  - Glomerular capillary thrombi
- Glomerular fibrinoid necrosis
- Prominent acute inflammation
  - Pyogenic abscesses
- Fungal organisms
  - Characteristic clear halos
  - Budding yeast forms, 12-14 μm in diameter

DIFFERENTIAL DIAGNOSIS

Cryptococcosis
- Capsule positive for mucicarmine stain

Lobomycosis
- Endemic to Central and South America
- Round intracellular yeast, 6-12 μm in diameter

Blastomycosis
- 8-15 μm in diameter
- DNA confirmation probe may cross-react with *Paracoccidioides*

Histoplasmosis
- 2-4 μm in diameter

Tuberculosis
- Caseating granulomas
- Acid-fast bacilli present
- Coinfection with PCM reported

Sarcoidosis
- No microorganisms present
- Diagnosis of exclusion

Drug-induced Acute Interstitial Nephritis
- No microorganisms present

DIAGNOSTIC CHECKLIST

Pathologic Interpretation Pearls
- Fungal culture or serologic tests confirm infection by *Paracoccidioides brasiliensis*

SELECTED REFERENCES

1. Zavascki AP et al: Paracoccidioidomycosis in organ transplant recipient: case report. Rev Inst Med Trop Sao Paulo. 46(5):279-81, 2004
2. Bethlem EP et al: Paracoccidioidomycosis. Curr Opin Pulm Med. 5(5):319-25, 1999
3. Shikanai-Yasuda MA et al: Paracoccidioidomycosis in a renal transplant recipient. J Med Vet Mycol. 33(6):411-4, 1995
4. Sugar AM et al: Paracoccidioidomycosis in the immunosuppressed host: report of a case and review of the literature. Am Rev Respir Dis. 129(2):340-2, 1984

Microscopic Features

(Left) Periodic acid-Schiff shows interstitial and glomerular granulomas ➡️ with glomerular destruction ⮈ in a severe case with a miliary pattern of systemic involvement. Lungs, lymph nodes, and oral mucosa are commonly involved, and less commonly the kidney, spleen, bones, and meninges. *(Courtesy A. Billis, MD.)* *(Right)* Periodic acid-Schiff shows a glomerulus with remnants of Bowman capsule ➡️ occupied by a granuloma consisting of epithelioid giant cells. *(Courtesy A. Billis, MD.)*

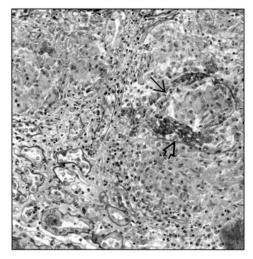
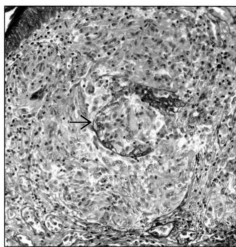

(Left) Trichrome shows granulomas ➡️ distributed throughout the cortex and medulla with surrounding fibrosis and mononuclear inflammation. One granuloma involves a glomerulus, which has segmental fibrinoid necrosis ➡️. *(Courtesy A. Billis, MD.)* *(Right)* Trichrome stain shows 2 Langhans giant cells surrounded by mononuclear cells. The differential diagnosis includes tuberculosis, sarcoidosis, and other fungal infections. *(Courtesy A. Billis, MD.)*

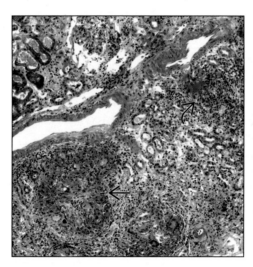
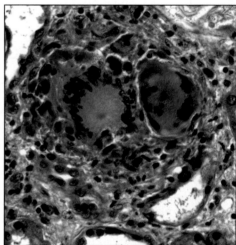

(Left) Periodic acid-Schiff shows 3 Paracoccidioides fungi ➡️ in macrophages, surrounded by clear halos. *(Courtesy A. Billis, MD.)* *(Right)* Grocott-Gomori methenamine-silver stain of granulomas containing fungal bodies shows strong peripheral silver uptake ➡️. An adjacent glomerulus contains a granuloma ⮈. The mechanism of glomerular involvement is believed to be embolic lodging of fungi in the capillaries with subsequent thrombus and inflammation. *(Courtesy A. Billis, MD.)*

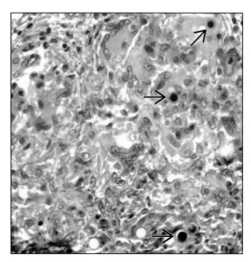
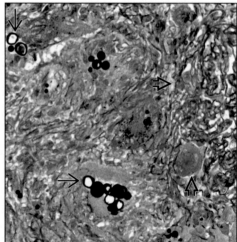

Light and Electron Microscopy

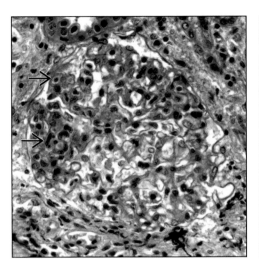

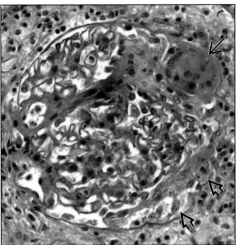

(Left) Masson trichrome stain shows mononuclear cells ➡ segmentally in a few glomerular capillary loops. This is a minimal and probably early lesion that may evolve to a full-blown granuloma. (Courtesy A. Billis, MD.) *(Right)* Hematoxylin & eosin of a glomerulus shows segmental injury with a multinucleated giant cell ➡ and florid granulomatous inflammation, which resembles a cellular crescent ➡. Many glomeruli showed isolated granulomas or giant cells. (Courtesy A. Billis, MD.)

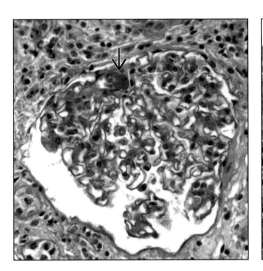

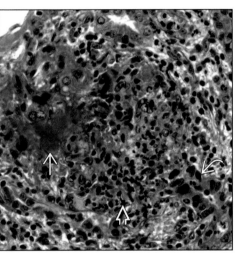

(Left) Hematoxylin & eosin shows a single fibrin thrombus ➡ within a glomerular capillary loop near the hilum of an otherwise unremarkable glomerulus. (Courtesy A. Billis, MD.) *(Right)* Masson trichrome stain of a glomerulus shows segmental fibrinoid necrosis ➡ and a prominent mixed inflammatory infiltrate with abundant neutrophils ➡ in Bowman space extending into the tubule ➡. (Courtesy A. Billis, MD.)

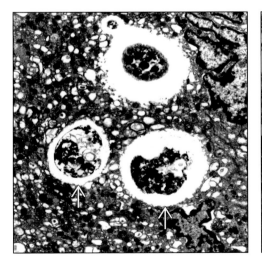

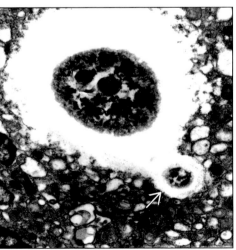

(Left) Electron micrograph of mononuclear giant cells shows 3 Paracoccidioides brasiliensis fungal organisms ➡ with a clear halo. (Courtesy A. Billis, MD.) *(Right)* Electron micrograph of a mononuclear giant cell shows a budding Paracoccidioides braziliensis fungal organism ➡ surrounded by a clear halo. (Courtesy A. Billis, MD.)

ASPERGILLOSIS

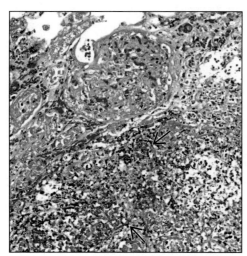

Hematoxylin & eosin shows a necrotic area of renal cortex with prominent neutrophilic inflammation and many acute angle branching hyphae ⊟ that are characteristic of Aspergillus.

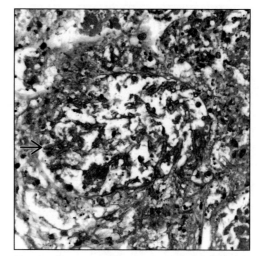

Hematoxylin & eosin shows septate hyphae ⊟ with 45° angle branching, which has entirely replaced a glomerulus in an autopsied kidney of a patient with disseminated aspergillosis.

TERMINOLOGY

Definitions
- *Aspergillus* infection of kidney in immunosuppressed or immunocompromised patients

ETIOLOGY/PATHOGENESIS

Environmental Exposure
- Ubiquitous fungus in environment

Infectious Agents
- *Aspergillus*
  - *A. fumigatus*
  - *A. flavus*
  - *A. niger*
  - *A. terreus*
  - *A. nidulans*

CLINICAL ISSUES

Epidemiology
- Incidence
  - 0.1% in kidney transplant patients after 1 year
- Age
  - No age predilection
- Gender
  - M:F = 4:1
- Ethnicity
  - No ethnic predilection

Site
- Lungs
  - Most common site of involvement
- Kidneys
  - 30-40% involvement in disseminated aspergillosis
  - Isolated involvement in some deceased donor kidney allografts

- Probable transmission from deceased donor or during organ procurement
- Fungi account for up to 2.5% of isolates cultured from perfusion solutions used for kidney preservation

Presentation
- Fever
- Flank pain
- Hematuria

Laboratory Tests
- Serologic tests
  - Enzyme-linked immunoassay
    - Detection of galactomannan antigen of *Aspergillus*
  - Immunodiffusion
  - Complement fixation
- Cultures
- Direct microscopy

Treatment
- Surgical approaches
  - Renal allograft nephrectomy
  - Nephrostomy drainage and systemic antifungal therapy
- Drugs
  - Voriconazole
    - 1st-line agent for invasive aspergillosis
  - Itraconazole
  - Amphotericin B
- Reduction of immunosuppressive agents in transplant patients

Prognosis
- Poor
  - 50-100% mortality rate for invasive aspergillosis

ASPERGILLOSIS

Key Facts

Etiology/Pathogenesis
- *A. fumigatus*
- *A. flavus*
- *A. niger*

Clinical Issues
- Treatment
  - Renal allograft nephrectomy
  - Nephrostomy drainage and systemic antifungal therapy
  - Voriconazole
- Incidence
  - 0.1% in kidney transplant patients after 1 year
- Presentation
  - Fever
  - Flank pain
  - Hematuria

- Laboratory tests
  - Cultures

Macroscopic Features
- Abscesses, cortical or perinephric

Microscopic Pathology
- Microorganisms, fungus
  - Septate hyphae with 45° angle branching
  - Vascular invasion
- Tubulointerstitial inflammation, neutrophil rich

Top Differential Diagnoses
- Candidiasis
- Mucormycosis
- Pseudallescheriasis
- Fusariosis
- Bacterial pyelonephritis

IMAGE FINDINGS

CT Findings
- Hypodense lesions in kidney

MACROSCOPIC FEATURES

General Features
- Abscesses
  - Cortical
  - Perinephric

MICROSCOPIC PATHOLOGY

Histologic Features
- Necrosis
- Suppurative inflammation
- Fungal organisms
  - Septate hyphae with 45° angle branching
  - 3-4 μm uniform diameter of hyphae
  - Vascular invasion
- Thrombosis
  - Hemorrhagic infarcts

DIFFERENTIAL DIAGNOSIS

Candidiasis
- Pseudohyphae and budding yeast forms

Mucormycosis
- Nonseptate hyphae with 90° angle branching

Pseudallescheriasis
- *Pseudallescheria boydii*
- Septate hyphae
- Culture or PCR needed

Fusariosis
- Septate hyphae
- Culture or PCR needed

Tuberculosis
- Caseating granulomas
- Acid-fast bacilli present

Bacterial Pyelonephritis
- Abscesses
- No fungal organisms

DIAGNOSTIC CHECKLIST

Pathologic Interpretation Pearls
- Fungal cultures useful to confirm diagnosis

SELECTED REFERENCES

1. Keven K et al: Fatal outcome of disseminated invasive aspergillosis in kidney allograft recipients. Med Mycol. 46(7):713-7, 2008
2. Oosten AW et al: Bilateral renal aspergillosis in a patient with AIDS: a case report and review of reported cases. AIDS Patient Care STDS. 22(1):1-6, 2008
3. Jung SI et al: Surgical treatment of invasive renal aspergillosis after chemotherapy. J Pediatr Urol. 3(3):250-2, 2007
4. Van Meensel B et al: Fatal right-sided endocarditis due to Aspergillus in a kidney transplant recipient. Med Mycol. 45(6):565-8, 2007
5. Veroux M et al: Voriconazole in the treatment of invasive aspergillosis in kidney transplant recipients. Transplant Proc. 39(6):1838-40, 2007
6. Gottfredsson M et al: Disseminated invasive aspergillosis in a patient with acute leukaemia. Acta Biomed. 77 Suppl 2:10-3, 2006
7. Linden E et al: Aspergillus infection limited to renal allograft: case report and review of literature. Transpl Infect Dis. 8(3):177-81, 2006
8. Halpern M et al: Renal aspergilloma: an unusual cause of infection in a patient with the acquired immunodeficiency syndrome. Am J Med. 92(4):437-40, 1992

Microscopic Features

(Left) A necrotic region in the renal cortex with septate hyphae ⇨ is seen with acute angle branching, which is associated with active inflammation. The diameter of Aspergillus hyphae is uniform, which contrasts with mucormycosis or Pseudallescheria. *(Right)* Periodic acid-Schiff highlights septate hyphae ⇨ with acute angle branching that are characteristic of Aspergillus, which is present in a necrotic region of renal cortex with prominent active interstitial inflammation.

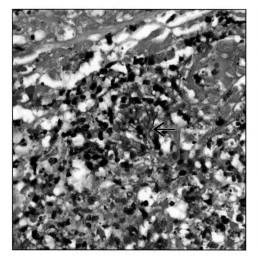 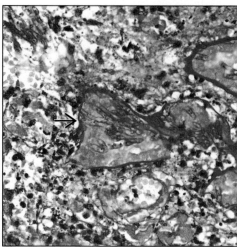

(Left) Periodic acid-Schiff reveals a few Aspergillus hyphae within a glomerulus ⇨ and an arteriole ⇨ in the autopsy examination of an immunocompromised patient with widely disseminated aspergillosis. *(Right)* Gomori methenamine-silver shows a fungus ball consisting of numerous septate hyphae ⇨ with acute angle branching in the renal medulla of a patient with disseminated aspergillosis.

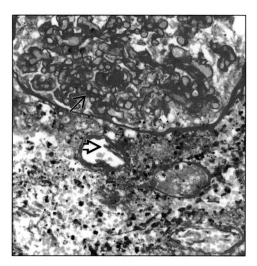 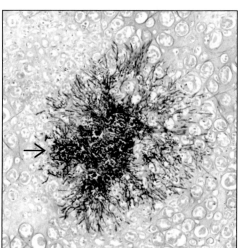

(Left) Gomori methenamine-silver highlights septate hyphae of Aspergillus throughout the renal cortex in tubules ⇨, a glomerulus ⇨, and arterioles ⇨. *(Right)* Gomori methenamine-silver reveals hyphal elements characteristic of Aspergillus ⇨ within a glomerulus. The diameter of Aspergillus hyphae is uniform and less broad than those of pseudallescheriasis or mucormycosis. Septate hyphae with acute angle branching help to exclude mucormycosis.

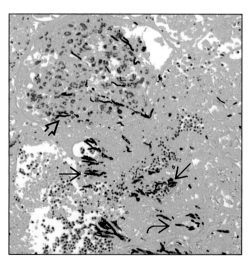 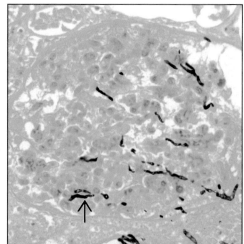

Differential Diagnosis

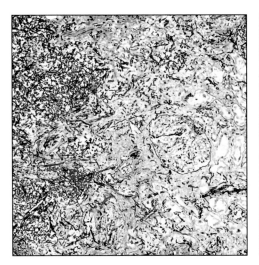

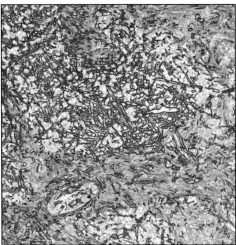

(Left) Jones methenamine silver highlights numerous nonseptate hyphae of mucormycosis in the renal cortex. (Courtesy E. Bracamonte, MD.) (Right) Periodic acid-Schiff shows many broad nonseptate hyphae with right angle branching throughout the kidney of a hematopoietic cell transplant patient with disseminated mucormycosis. The severe immunosuppressive state may account for the absence of significant interstitial inflammation. (Courtesy E. Bracamonte, MD.)

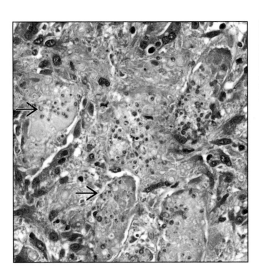

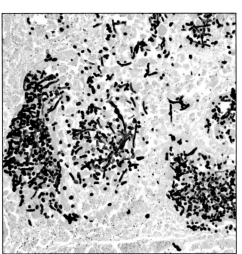

(Left) Hematoxylin & eosin shows round fungal organisms within the tubular lumina in an area with necrosis and rupture of the tubular basement membranes. The abundance of smaller yeast forms ⊟ raises the consideration of histoplasmosis as a differential diagnosis. (Right) Gomori methenamine-silver reveals numerous budding yeasts of Candida. The additional presence of pseudohyphae can occasionally be abundant, and rarely, septate hyphae may be seen.

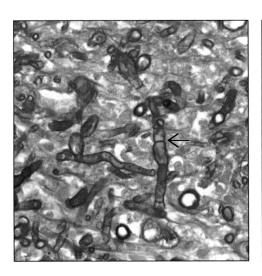

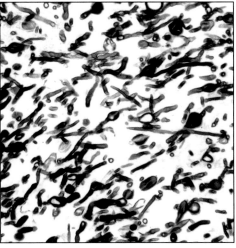

(Left) Periodic acid-Schiff shows septate hyphae ⊟ of Fusarium with varying hyphal diameter that can help distinguish this infection from Aspergillus. Pseudallescheria boydii also morphologically resembles Fusarium and rarely involves the kidneys of patients with disseminated disease. (Right) Gomori methenamine-silver highlights numerous septate hyphae in an immunocompromised patient with fusariosis.

CRYPTOCOCCOSIS

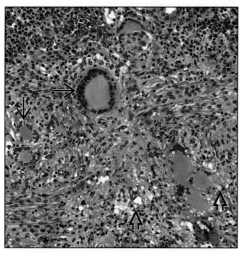

Hematoxylin & eosin shows large multinucleated giant cells ➡ and Cryptococci with characteristic clear halos ➡, which are distinct from the adjacent foamy macrophages in this kidney allograft.

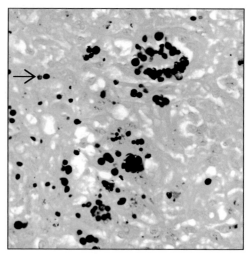

Gomori methenamine-silver shows strong staining of numerous round Cryptococcal organisms ➡ within the prominent granulomatous inflammation.

TERMINOLOGY

Synonyms
- European blastomycosis
- Torulosis

Definitions
- Cryptococcal infection, typically in immunocompromised patients

ETIOLOGY/PATHOGENESIS

Environmental Exposure
- Present in soil
- Inhalation of airborne fungal forms

Infectious Agents
- *Cryptococcus neoformans*
- *C. gattii*
  - Found in Pacific Northwest of United States and Canada
  - Isolated from eucalyptus trees in the subtropical and tropical regions
- *C. laurentii*
  - Rare isolate
- *C. albidus*
  - Rare isolate

CLINICAL ISSUES

Epidemiology
- Incidence
  - 1/100,000 in general population
    - 2-7/1,000 in AIDS patients
  - 2.8-5% in solid organ transplant patients
    - 0.8-5.8% in renal transplant patients
- Age
  - Rare in children before puberty
- Gender

- Male predilection

Presentation
- Acute renal failure
- Proteinuria

Laboratory Tests
- Cryptococcal antigen test
- Fungal culture
- Direct microscopy

Treatment
- Drugs
  - Antifungal agents
    - Amphotericin B
    - Fluconazole
- Reduction of immunosuppressive agents in transplant patients

Prognosis
- Graft loss in 9% of renal transplant patients

MACROSCOPIC FEATURES

General Features
- Papillary necrosis
  - May be present in cryptococcal pyelonephritis

MICROSCOPIC PATHOLOGY

Histologic Features
- Granulomatous interstitial inflammation
  - Absence of significant granulomatous or inflammatory response in severely immunocompromised patients
- Fungal organisms
  - Capsule is mucicarmine, PAS, and silver stain positive
  - Capsule-deficient variant of *Cryptococcus* (all silver stains)

CRYPTOCOCCOSIS

Key Facts

Etiology/Pathogenesis
- *Cryptococcus neoformans*
- *C. gattii*

Clinical Issues
- Rare in children before puberty
- Male predilection
- Amphotericin B
- Fluconazole

Microscopic Pathology
- Granulomatous interstitial inflammation
- Fungal organisms
  - Clear halo; mucicarmine, PAS, and silver stain positive
  - 5-10 μm in diameter
- Tubulointerstitial inflammation with tubulitis

Top Differential Diagnoses
- Blastomycosis

- 5-10 μm in diameter
- Narrow-based budding
- May be present in glomerular capillaries within macrophages
- Prominent tubulointerstitial inflammation
- Tubulitis
- Necrotizing and crescentic glomerulonephritis
  - Single report in association with pulmonary cryptococcosis with resolution after antifungal therapy

DIFFERENTIAL DIAGNOSIS

Blastomycosis
- 8-15 μm in diameter
- Broad-based budding

Candidiasis
- Budding yeasts
- Pseudohyphae

Histoplasmosis
- 2-4 μm in diameter
- Endemic to Mississippi and Ohio river valleys

Coccidioidomycosis
- Spherules with characteristic endospores
- Endemic to southwest United States, Mexico, and South America

Tuberculosis
- Caseating necrosis
- Acid-fast bacilli present

Paracoccidioidomycosis
- Endemic to South America and Brazil
- Clear halo, Gomori methenamine-silver positive

Sarcoidosis
- No microorganisms present
- Tight noncaseating granulomas

Drug-induced Acute Interstitial Nephritis
- No microorganisms present

SELECTED REFERENCES

1. Silveira FP et al: Cryptococcosis in liver and kidney transplant recipients receiving anti-thymocyte globulin or alemtuzumab. Transpl Infect Dis. 9(1):22-7, 2007
2. Iglesias JI et al: AIDS, nephrotic-range proteinuria, and renal failure. Kidney Int. 69(11):2107-10, 2006
3. Nakayama M et al: A case of necrotizing glomerulonephritis presenting with nephrotic syndrome associated with pulmonary cryptococcosis. Clin Exp Nephrol. 9(1):74-8, 2005

IMAGE GALLERY

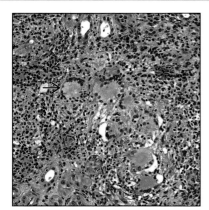 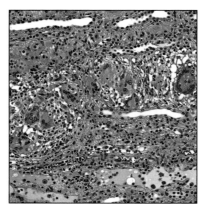 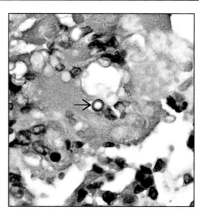

(Left) Hematoxylin & eosin shows numerous multinucleated giant cells ➔ without necrosis and a prominent granulomatous interstitial nephritis with many lymphocytes and plasma cells. Careful inspection reveals round microorganisms with thick outer capsules, which are not apparent at this magnification. *(Center)* Hematoxylin & eosin shows prominent granulomatous interstitial inflammation that involves primarily the renal medulla. *(Right)* Mucicarmine stain highlights the thick outer capsule ➔ that characterizes Cryptococcus.

MICROSPORIDIOSIS

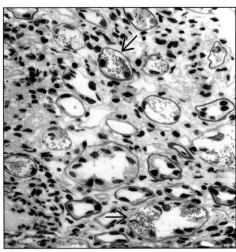

PAS stain of active interstitial nephritis in an HIV-positive patient with microsporidiosis shows that the organisms in tubules ⇨ are not strongly stained, which allows differentiation from usual fungi.

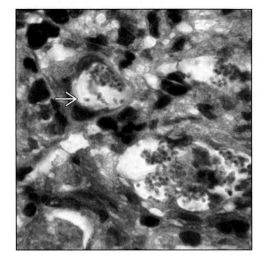

Giemsa stain viewed under oil reveals the characteristic morphology of Microsporidia, which are oval organisms with a central, densely stained nucleus ⇨. These may be confused with Toxoplasma.

TERMINOLOGY

Definitions
- Infection by one of many species of Microsporidia particularly affecting immunocompromised hosts

ETIOLOGY/PATHOGENESIS

Infectious Agents
- Microsporidia
  - Ubiquitous obligate intracellular eukaryotic pathogens
    - Unique group of fungi with reduced cell organelles (no mitochondria, Golgi)
  - Infects all phyla of organisms
    - Initially identified as silkworm pathogen in 1857 and as human pathogen 50 years ago
  - 14 species infect humans
    - Most common: *Enterocytozoon bieneusi*, *Encephalitozoon intestinalis*, and *Encephalitozoon cuniculi*
  - Unique method of inserting spore contents into cell via a polar tube that behaves like a hypodermic needle
- Kidney involved in minority of cases, typically as part of systemic infection
  - *E. intestinalis* and *E. cuniculi* most common organisms in disseminated cases
  - *E. cuniculi* infects dogs and cats
- *E. bieneusi* limited to GI tract and hepatobiliary system
- Immunodeficiency predisposes to disease
  - HIV patients (CD4 < 100/mm³), transplant recipients (3 weeks to 7 years post transplant)

CLINICAL ISSUES

Presentation
- Acute renal failure

- Chronic renal failure
- Renal allograft dysfunction
  - Kidney involved in ~ 40% of recipients with microsporidiosis
- Fever
- Diarrhea
- Weight loss
- Other sites: Lung, brain, heart, liver, eye

Treatment
- Drugs
  - Fumagillin, albendazole
  - Tapering immunosuppressive drugs

Prognosis
- Good if treated with antibiotics and immunocompetence can be improved

MICROSCOPIC PATHOLOGY

Histologic Features
- Acute and chronic interstitial nephritis
- Tubules
  - Severe tubular injury, disruption, and destruction
  - Intraluminal and intracellular 1 x 2 μm ovoid spores in aggregates
    - No budding or pseudohyphae
  - Purple with Gram stain (Brown-Hopps, Brown-Brenn)
  - Giemsa stains central body (nucleus)
  - PAS and silver positivity in punctate pattern (posterior body)
  - Positive acid-fast stain (red with Ziehl-Neelsen)
  - Calcofluor white fluorochrome stains cell wall polysaccharide (fluoresces blue with DAPI filter)
- Interstitium
  - Acute and chronic inflammation
  - Neutrophils, eosinophils, monocytes, lymphocytes, plasma cells
- Glomeruli

MICROSPORIDIOSIS

Key Facts

Terminology
- Microsporidia obligate intracellular fungi

Etiology/Pathogenesis
- Kidney involved as part of systemic infection

Clinical Issues
- Diarrhea usual presentation
- Acute or chronic renal failure

Microscopic Pathology
- Acute &/or chronic interstitial inflammation
- Oval 1 x 2 μm intracellular spores in tubules
  - Purple with Brown-Hopps stain
  - Giemsa-positive central body
- EM identification by unique polar tube

Top Differential Diagnoses
- Toxoplasmosis
- Candidiasis and other fungal infections

  - No specific feature
  - HIV-associated glomerular disease may be present
- Vessels
  - No specific feature

ANCILLARY TESTS

Immunohistochemistry
- Negative for *Toxoplasma gondii* antigens

PCR
- Identification of species in paraffin-embedded tissues

Electron Microscopy
- Intracellular spores
  - Distinctive and pathognomonic coiled polar tube in spore
    - Allows speciation

DIFFERENTIAL DIAGNOSIS

Toxoplasmosis
- Similar size
- Negative on Brown-Brenn or Brown-Hopps stain
- Positive for anti-*Toxoplasma* antigens by IHC

Candidiasis and Infection by Other Fungi
- PAS-positive cell walls
- Budding spores, pseudohyphae

SELECTED REFERENCES

1. Kradin RL: Diagnostic Pathology of Infectious Disease. Philadelphia: Saunders-Elsevier, 2010
2. Lanternier F et al: Microsporidiosis in solid organ transplant recipients: two Enterocytozoon bieneusi cases and review. Transpl Infect Dis. 11(1):83-8, 2009
3. Viriyavejakul P et al: High prevalence of Microsporidium infection in HIV-infected patients. Southeast Asian J Trop Med Public Health. 40(2):223-8, 2009
4. Chan KS et al: Extraction of microsporidial DNA from modified trichrome-stained clinical slides and subsequent species identification using PCR sequencing. Parasitology. 135(6):701-3, 2008
5. Orenstein JM et al: Fatal pulmonary microsporidiosis due to encephalitozoon cuniculi following allogeneic bone marrow transplantation for acute myelogenous leukemia. Ultrastruct Pathol. 29(3-4):269-76, 2005
6. Orenstein JM: Diagnostic pathology of microsporidiosis. Ultrastruct Pathol. 27(3):141-9, 2003
7. Keeling PJ et al: Microsporidia: biology and evolution of highly reduced intracellular parasites. Annu Rev Microbiol. 56:93-116, 2002
8. Aarons EJ et al: Reversible renal failure caused by a microsporidian infection. AIDS. 8(8):1119-21, 1994

IMAGE GALLERY

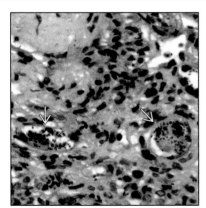 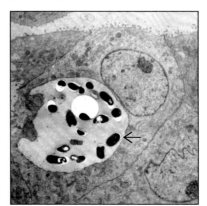 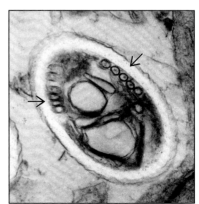

(Left) Brown-Hopps (modified Gram) stains Microsporidia blue/purple. Here the organisms are seen as aggregates in tubules ➡ in a case of acute and chronic interstitial nephritis. *(Center)* Electron micrograph shows intracellular Microsporidia spores ➡ in tubular epithelium. *(Right)* High-power electron micrograph shows the pathognomonic polar tube coils ➡, a unique structure of Microsporidia spores. Here, 5 coils are present, typical of E. intestinalis.

RICKETTSIAL INFECTIONS

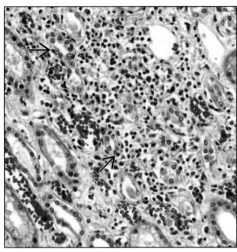

Hematoxylin & eosin reveals nodular interstitial mononuclear inflammation, which tends to be multifocal. Tubulitis is mild and focal ➡. Vessels are congested. (Courtesy J. Olano, MD.)

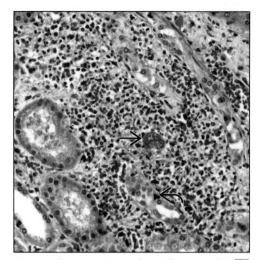

Hematoxylin & eosin reveals capillary vasculitis ➡ with interstitial hemorrhage and a predominantly mononuclear inflammatory infiltrate. Focal tubulitis is also evident ➡. (Courtesy J. Olano, MD.)

TERMINOLOGY

Abbreviations
- Rocky mountain spotted fever (RMSF), Mediterranean spotted fever (MSF), scrub typhus (ST), epidemic typhus (ET)

Synonyms
- Rickettsial diseases, Boutonneuse fever (MSF), typhus

Definitions
- Systemic infection by rickettsial microorganisms with direct infection of kidney

ETIOLOGY/PATHOGENESIS

Arthropod-borne Zoonoses
- Transmitted to humans via arthropod bites
  - RMSF: *Rickettsia rickettsii* infection, transmitted by ticks
  - MSF: *R. conorii* infection, transmitted by ticks
  - ST: *Orientia tsutsugamushi* infection, transmitted by mites
  - ET: *R. prowazekii* infection, transmitted by body lice
- Rickettsial organisms directly infect vascular endothelium and tubular epithelium
- Uptake into endothelium is by cholesterol receptor-mediated endocytosis
- Smooth muscle cells of vessel walls are also infected
- Endothelial injury causes
  - Loss of adhesion, detachment, increased permeability, hemorrhage, and thrombosis
- Intrarenal vasculitis, acute tubular injury, and tubulointerstitial inflammation contribute to acute renal failure

CLINICAL ISSUES

Presentation
- Incidence is ~ 5.6 per 1,000,000 in USA for RMSF; higher in hyperendemic areas (e.g., 18 per 1,000,000 in children in Arizona)
- Symptoms: Fever, headache, myalgia, and rash
  - RMSF: Fever, rash, and history of tick exposure is classic triad
    - Peak incidence in spring and early summer
    - Latency of 2-14 days
    - Rash in 3-5 days; maculopapular &/or purpuric (45% of cases), involves palms and soles of feet
    - Also nausea, vomiting, abdominal pain, and cough
  - MSF: Eschar, maculopapular rash
  - ST: Eschar, influenza-like illness, lymphadenopathy
  - ET: Influenza-like illness, jaundice, petechiae, hypotension, proteinuria, and hematuria
- Acute renal failure, ± hypovolemic shock, may be associated with any of these infections
- Diagnosis
  - Blood or tissue culture: Cell culture with immunofluorescent antibody detection of early antigens (results in 48-72 hours)
  - Identification of rickettsial antigen by immunohistochemistry (IHC) in tissue
  - PCR assay used to detect *htrA* antigen gene
  - Serologic evidence of rising antirickettsial titers (antibodies take 7-10 days to appear)

Treatment
- Tetracycline or chloramphenicol

Prognosis
- Overall ~ 5% fatality, even with treatment
- Fatality rates vary from 2-25%, and fatality tends to occur in 9-15 days
- In fulminant cases, death may occur as early as 3-5 days

RICKETTSIAL INFECTIONS

Key Facts

Terminology
- Systemic infection by rickettsial microorganisms with direct infection of kidney

Etiology/Pathogenesis
- Organisms directly infect vascular endothelium

Clinical Issues
- Symptoms: Fever, headache, myalgia, rash, acute renal failure

Microscopic Pathology
- Vasculitis, perivascular tubulointerstitial nephritis, acute tubular injury

Diagnostic Checklist
- Acute renal failure from acute tubular injury, tubulointerstitial inflammation, and vasculitis
- Rickettsial antigen identified by IHC, cell culture, or PCR

- Risk factors for increased severity of disease
  - Delayed diagnosis
  - Older age, especially in males
  - Glucose-6-phosphate dehydrogenase deficiency
  - Alcoholism

MACROSCOPIC FEATURES

Gross Features
- Enlarged heavy kidneys with petechial hemorrhages, most notable in outer medulla

MICROSCOPIC PATHOLOGY

Histologic Features
- Tubulointerstitial nephritis: Corticomedullary junction and outer medulla
  - Lymphoid cells (T cells abundant, few B cells), macrophages, rare eosinophils, edema, tubulitis
  - Nodular perivascular infiltrates
  - May be interstitial hemorrhage
- Acute tubular injury
- Vasculitis
  - Endothelial infection primarily involves peritubular capillaries, venules, and occasionally arteries and arterioles
  - Endothelial necrosis and thrombosis
  - Rickettsia in endothelium on Giemsa stain (low sensitivity)

- Glomeruli may have capillary thrombi and, rarely, glomerulonephritis
- IHC for rickettsial antigen positive in endothelium and occasionally in tubules
- Membrane-bound ovoid organisms by electron microscopy

DIFFERENTIAL DIAGNOSIS

Tubulointerstitial Nephritis with Hemorrhage or Vasculitis
- Hantavirus: Viral antigens in vasculature by IHC
- Adenovirus: Tubular nuclear inclusions; viral antigens in tubules by IHC

DIAGNOSTIC CHECKLIST

Pathologic Interpretation Pearls
- Vasculitis, nodular tubulointerstitial inflammation, hemorrhage, acute tubular injury
- Detectable rickettsial antigen by IHC

SELECTED REFERENCES
1. Walker DH et al: Acute renal failure in Rocky Mountain spotted fever. Arch Intern Med. 139(4):443-8, 1979

IMAGE GALLERY

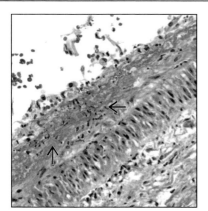 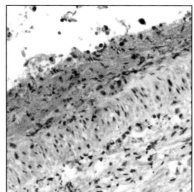 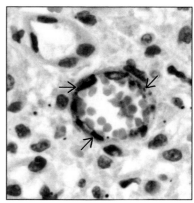

(Left) Hematoxylin & eosin reveals fibrinoid necrosis with leukocytoclasis ➡ in the arterial intima with reactive endothelium. *(Courtesy J. Olano, MD.)* *(Center)* Immunohistochemical staining using a specific anti-rickettsial antibody reveals rickettsial antigen in the arterial intima in an area of fibrinoid change and leukocytoclasis. *(Courtesy J. Olano, MD.)* *(Right)* Immunohistochemical staining using a specific anti-rickettsial antibody reveals rickettsial antigen in the endothelium of a congested interstitial capillary ➡ with perivascular inflammation. *(Courtesy J. Olano, MD.)*

TOXOPLASMOSIS

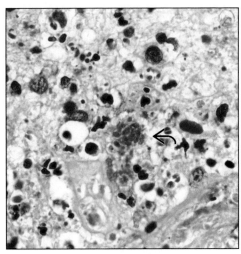

Toxoplasma gondii tachyzoites ⤳ are seen within foci of extensive necrosis in an immunocompromised patient with encephalitis and disseminated toxoplasma infection. (Courtesy J. Karamchandani, MD.)

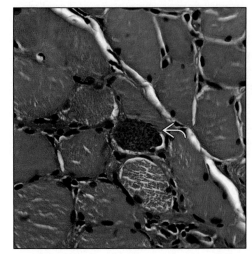

H&E stained section of cardiac muscle from a kidney transplantation recipient shows Toxoplasma gondii pseudocysts ⤳. These cysts range from 5-50 μm in diameter. (Courtesy J. Montoya, MD.)

TERMINOLOGY

Definitions
- Renal manifestations due to protozoan *Toxoplasma gondii* infection

ETIOLOGY/PATHOGENESIS

Infectious Agents
- *Toxoplasma gondii* is an obligate intracellular parasite
  - Primary host is house cat, but it can also be transmitted by dogs, rabbits, and guinea pigs
  - Parasite grows in gastrointestinal mucosal cells of the cat
  - Oocysts shed in cat feces are source of human infection
  - Parasites elicit cellular and humoral host responses

Congenital Infection
- Transplacental transmission is known
- Often fatal form of disease with encephalomyelitis, chorioretinitis, and cerebral calcifications
- Preterm low birth weight infants in endemic areas

Acquired Infection
- Primary infection or reactivation of latent infection
  - Immunocompetent host often has febrile illness with lymphadenopathy and rash
  - Immunocompromised hosts more susceptible
    - Renal transplantation of seronegative recipients from seropositive donors a risk factor
    - Organ involvement may be extensive including myocarditis, myositis, and encephalitis

CLINICAL ISSUES

Epidemiology
- Incidence
  - Worldwide distribution
  - Prevalence ranges from 20-60%

Site
- Kidney involvement can occur occasionally
- Transplanted kidney usually not affected

Presentation
- Often mild proteinuria with normal renal function
- Nephritic syndrome with hematuria, edema, and hypertension in some patients
- Nephrotic syndrome in infants with congenital toxoplasmosis or adults with disseminated disease

Laboratory Tests
- Detection of circulating *Toxoplasma* antigens by IgG immunoassay or PCR DNA amplification
- Increased titers of specific IgG anti-*Toxoplasma* antibodies
- Parasite isolation from infected tissues or body fluids

Treatment
- Drugs
  - Pyrimethamine, sulfadiazine, or clindamycin for treatment of toxoplasmosis

Prognosis
- If untreated, disseminated toxoplasmosis is lethal
- Nephrotic syndrome remits after treatment of toxoplasmosis

MICROSCOPIC PATHOLOGY

Histologic Features
- Glomerular mesangial and endocapillary proliferation
- Karyorrhectic debris may be seen in glomeruli
- Interstitial inflammation, tubular atrophy, and interstitial fibrosis
- Toxoplasma pseudocysts can be rarely seen
  - Pseudocysts are packed with round or piriform organisms with distinct cell membranes and homogeneous cytoplasm

TOXOPLASMOSIS

Key Facts

Terminology
- Renal manifestations due to protozoan *Toxoplasma gondii* infection

Etiology/Pathogenesis
- Parasites elicit cellular and humoral host responses
- Immunocompromised hosts are more susceptible

Clinical Issues
- Kidney involvement presents with mild proteinuria

- Detection of circulating *Toxoplasma* antigens
- Parasite isolation from infected tissues or body fluids

Microscopic Pathology
- Glomerular mesangial and endocapillary proliferation
- Mesangial and segmental capillary wall deposits

Ancillary Tests
- Wright-Giemsa stain or *Toxoplasma* immunostain highlights organisms

---

- Renal manifestations in congenital toxoplasmosis include pseudocysts in glomeruli or tubules, extensive global glomerulosclerosis, and mesangial proliferative glomerulonephritis

ANCILLARY TESTS

Histochemistry
- Wright-Giemsa stain
  - Reactivity: Positive
  - Staining pattern
    - Highlights the pseudocysts and tachyzoites of Toxoplasma

Immunohistochemistry
- Toxoplasma immunostain can highlight organisms

Immunofluorescence
- Granular mesangial and segmental capillary wall deposits with IgG, IgA, IgM, and C3
- Presence of Toxoplasma antigen has been demonstrated in deposits

Electron Microscopy
- Mesangial and subendothelial deposits may be seen
- Mesangial sclerosis and podocyte foot process effacement may be observed

DIFFERENTIAL DIAGNOSIS

Non-Toxoplasma-related Immune Complex-mediated Glomerulonephritis
- Clinical history may be most helpful
- Laboratory tests to exclude active Toxoplasma infection

SELECTED REFERENCES

1. Segall L et al: Toxoplasmosis-associated hemophagocytic syndrome in renal transplantation. Transpl Int. 19(1):78-80, 2006
2. Haskell L et al: Disseminated toxoplasmosis presenting as symptomatic orchitis and nephrotic syndrome. Am J Med Sci. 298(3):185-90, 1989
3. Beale MG et al: Congenital glomerulosclerosis and nephrotic syndrome in two infants. Speculations and pathogenesis. Am J Dis Child. 133(8):842-5, 1979
4. Krick JA et al: Toxoplasmosis in the adult--an overview. N Engl J Med. 298(10):550-3, 1978
5. Ginsburg BE et al: Case of glomerulonephritis associated with acute toxoplasmosis. Br Med J. 3(5932):664-5, 1974
6. Shahin B et al: Congenital nephrotic syndrome associated with congenital toxoplasmosis. J Pediatr. 85(3):366-70, 1974
7. Wickbom B et al: Coincidence of congenital toxoplasmosis and acute nephritis with nephrotic syndrome. Acta Paediatr Scand. 61(4):470-2, 1972
8. Cohen SN: Toxoplasmosis in patients receiving immunosuppressive therapy. JAMA. 211(4):657-60, 1970

IMAGE GALLERY

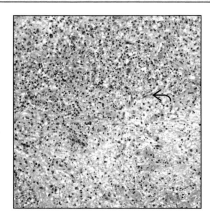
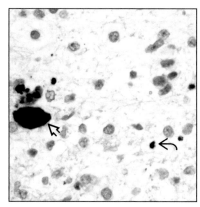
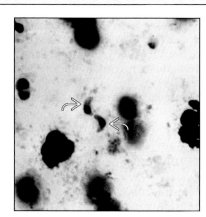

(Left) Extensive brain necrosis ➡ in a patient with disseminated toxoplasma infection is shown. *(Courtesy J. Karamchandani, MD.)* *(Center)* The toxoplasma immunostain highlights a pseudocyst filled with bradyzoites ➡ as well as tachyzoites ➡ in a patient with encephalitis. *(Courtesy J. Karamchandani, MD.)* *(Right)* Wright-Giemsa stain highlights T. gondii tachyzoites ➡ in a bronchoalveolar lavage specimen from an AIDS patient with pneumonia. *(Courtesy J. Montoya, MD.)*

HYDATIDOSIS

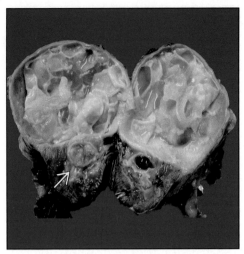

This kidney is largely replaced by a large dominant hydatid cyst. The cyst has a very thick, fibrous wall with attached brood capsules. There is also a 2nd small cyst ➡ adjacent to the large cyst.

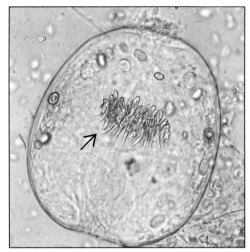

Wet preparation of cyst contents shows a scolex, the infective agent of Echinococcus granulosus. In this scolex, the rostellum, or ring of hooks ➡, is visible along with several other organelles.

TERMINOLOGY

Synonyms
- Hydatid cyst
- Hydatid disease
- Echinococcosis

Definitions
- Cystic parasitic disease caused by larval form of cestode *Echinococcus granulosus*

ETIOLOGY/PATHOGENESIS

Infectious Agents
- Adult worm (6 mm) lives in small intestine of dog, sheep, and cattle
  - Excreted eggs ingested by humans, who are an intermediate host
  - Oncospheres
    - Hatch from eggs in duodenum
    - Penetrate mucosa and enter portal vein
    - Reach liver (60%), lungs (5-15%), and kidney (2-4%)
- Each oncosphere develops into hydatid cyst
  - Brood capsules
    - Develop from inner germinal membrane
    - Contain 5-20 scolices, the infective agent
    - Detach from wall to form daughter cysts
  - Hydatid cysts contain hundreds to thousands of scolices
- Kidneys may be involved by direct extension

CLINICAL ISSUES

Epidemiology
- Incidence
  - Endemic: Africa, Mediterranean, Eurasia, Canada, South America

- Age
  - Affects adults in 3rd to 5th decades of life
- Gender
  - M:F = 1:1

Presentation
- Chronic dull flank pain most common: 40% of patients
- Systemic symptoms of fever and malaise
- Hydatiduria: Less than 10-20%
- Hematuria or nephrotic syndrome: Rare

Laboratory Tests
- Laboratory tests
  - ELISA positive in 80%
- Hydatiduria
  - Grape-like daughter cysts enter urine following cyst rupture into collecting system
- Eosinophilia in 20-50%

Treatment
- Surgical approaches
  - Complete or partial nephrectomy
  - Percutaneous drainage not recommended
  - Antihelminthics
    - Cysts disappear in 33%
    - Cyst size reduced in 30-50%

Prognosis
- Depends upon number of organs affected
- Rare fatal anaphylactic reaction during surgery
- Complications: Cyst rupture, infection, and abscess

IMAGE FINDINGS

Radiographic Findings
- Ring-shaped, amorphous, or curvilinear calcification

Ultrasonographic Findings
- Unilocular or multilocular cystic lesion

HYDATIDOSIS

Key Facts

Terminology
- Hydatid disease
- Hydatid cyst
- Echinococcosis

Etiology/Pathogenesis
- Cystic parasitic disease caused by larval form of echinococcus granulosus

Clinical Issues
- Chronic dull flank pain or mass
- Systemic symptoms of fever and malaise
- Hydatiduria, hematuria, nephrotic syndrome

Image Findings
- Radiograph: Ring-shaped curvilinear calcification
- US/CT: Unicystic to multivesicular lesion

Macroscopic Features
- Thick-walled cyst with brood capsules

Microscopic Pathology
- 3-layered hydatid cyst wall
- Brood capsules composed of laminated membrane
  - Contains 5-20 scolices
- Wet prep or Papanicolaou stain
  - Scolices with crown or rostellum of hooks
  - Hooks are acid-fast, stain positive

Ancillary Tests
- EIA or ELISA assay

Top Differential Diagnoses
- Cystic nephroma
- Multilocular cystic renal cell carcinoma

CT Findings
- Unilocular cyst with calcification
- Multivesicular cyst containing daughter cysts

MACROSCOPIC FEATURES

General Features
- Usually fluid-filled, thick-walled cyst containing daughter cysts
  - Unilocular cyst typical in children
  - Multivesicular cyst typical in adults

MICROSCOPIC PATHOLOGY

Histologic Features
- Hydatid cyst wall has 3 layers
  - Pericyst: Outer fibrous layer of host tissue
  - Ectocyst: Acellular laminated membrane
  - Endocyst: Inner germinal membrane
- Closed cyst
  - All 3 layers intact
- Exposed cyst
  - Pericyst layer absent
- Open or ruptured cyst
  - All 3 layers are absent
- Brood capsules bud from inner cyst wall
  - Rupture releases scolices into cyst ("hydatid sand")
- Scolex
  - 4 suckers and rostellum of hooks
  - Hooks are acid-fast, stain positive
- Glomerulonephritis: Rare complication of extrarenal disease
  - Membranoproliferative glomerulonephritis
  - Membranous glomerulonephritis

Cytologic Features
- Identifying scoleces in cyst contents by wet prep or Papanicolaou stain

DIFFERENTIAL DIAGNOSIS

Cystic Neoplasms
- Cystic nephroma
- Multilocular cystic renal cell carcinoma

DIAGNOSTIC CHECKLIST

Pathologic Interpretation Pearls
- Cyst containing free-floating cysts is infectious, not neoplastic

SELECTED REFERENCES

1. da Silva AM: Human echinococcosis: a neglected disease. Gastroenterol Res Pract. pii: 583297, 2010
2. Gargah T et al: Reversible nephrotic syndrome secondary to pulmonary hydatid disease. S Afr Med J. 100(7):424-5, 2010
3. Ishimitsu DN et al: Best cases from the AFIP: renal hydatid disease. Radiographics. 30(2):334-7, 2010
4. Sayilir K et al: A case of isolated renal hydatid disease. Int J Infect Dis. 13(1):110-2, 2009
5. Mongha R et al: Primary hydatid cyst of kidney and ureter with gross hydatiduria: A case report and evaluation of radiological features. Indian J Urol. 24(1):116-7, 2008
6. Kaya K et al: Isolated renal and retroperitoneal hydatid cysts: a report of 23 cases. Trop Doct. 36(4):243-6, 2006
7. Yaycioglu O et al: Isolated renal hydatid disease causing ureteropelvic junction obstruction and massive destruction of kidney parenchyma. Urology. 67(6):1290, 2006
8. Yilmaz Y et al: Our experience in eight cases with urinary hydatid disease: a series of 372 cases held in nine different clinics. Int J Urol. 13(9):1162-5, 2006
9. Göğüş C et al: Isolated renal hydatidosis: experience with 20 cases. J Urol. 169(1):186-9, 2003
10. Horchani A et al: Hydatid cyst of the kidney. A report of 147 controlled cases. Eur Urol. 38(4):461-7, 2000

HYDATIDOSIS

Gross Features

(Left) This kidney is largely replaced by a hydatid cyst that has a thick fibrous wall ⊅. Its 3 cyst layers are not discernible grossly. Both opened ⊡ and unopened ⊞ brood capsules are present. Within the brood capsules, the infective scolices reside. *(Right)* This kidney is also largely replaced by a large hydatid cyst. Several unopened brood capsules ⊞ are visible. The remaining kidney shows mild hydronephrosis with expanded calyces ⊳ and blunted renal pyramids.

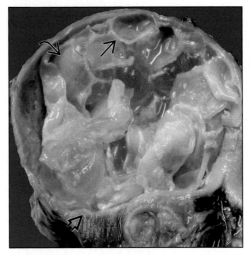
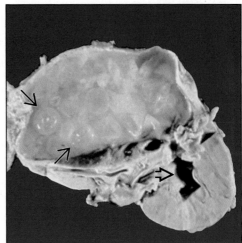

(Left) This bivalved nephrectomy specimen has been entirely converted into a massive hydatid cyst without visible residual parenchyma. The cyst is packed with daughter cysts and brood capsules. *(Right)* This field consists entirely of daughter cysts ⊞ that vary in size. Their cyst wall is known as the acellular laminated membrane. The contents of the daughter cyst range from clear to opaque. Within the cysts are scolices, the infective form of the disease.

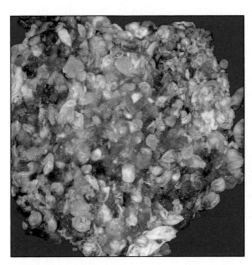
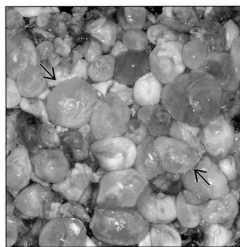

(Left) This is a cystic nephroma, which the WHO defines as a benign cystic neoplasm composed of epithelial and stromal elements. It consists entirely of cystic spaces and cyst septae without solid areas or freely mobile cysts. *(Right)* This is a multilocular cystic renal cell carcinoma. The WHO defines this lesion as a tumor composed entirely of numerous cysts, the septa of which contain small groups of clear cells indistinguishable from grade 1 clear cell carcinoma.

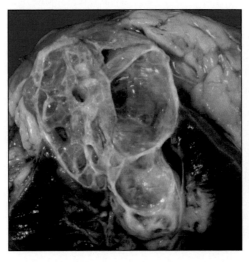
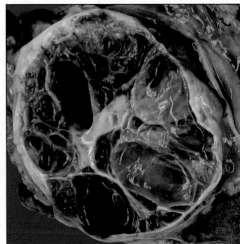

Microscopic Features

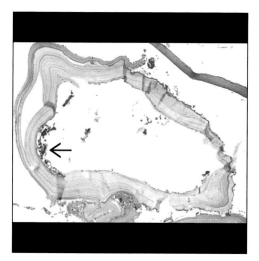

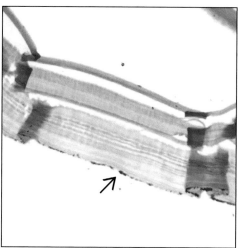

(Left) This is a daughter cyst. The cyst wall consists of the ectocyst layer, also known as the acellular laminated membrane. Fragments of the internal germinal membrane ➡ are visible along the inside of a portion of this daughter cyst. (Right) This is the ectocyst or acellular laminated membrane. It lacks the pericyst fibrotic membrane formed from atrophic host tissue. A thin remnant of the germinal membrane ➡ where brood capsules form is barely visible along its inner surface.

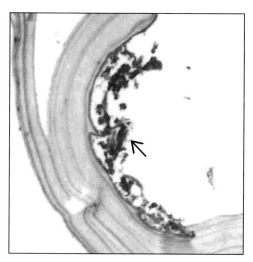

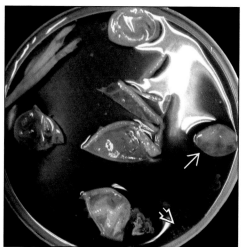

(Left) Along the inner aspect of the acellular laminated membrane of this daughter cyst is the endocyst or germinal membrane layer. Some of the rounded structures ➡ are likely the infective agents, the scolices. (Right) Several daughter cysts have been placed in this dish. Notice the translucent nature of the cyst wall ➡ and the small amount of hydatid sand ➡. These cysts would need careful handling since they each harbor from 5-20 infective scolices.

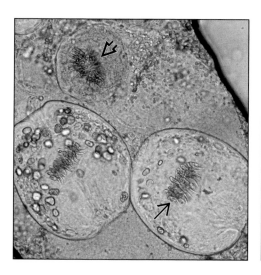

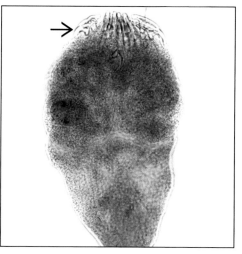

(Left) In this wet preparation, 3 scolices are visible. In each scolex, a characteristic ring of hooks ➡ is visible. The radial arrangement of the hooks is discernible in 1 scolex ➡. The other 2 are viewed laterally. (Right) This Pap-stained pleural effusion shows a scolex. Each scolex is approximately 100 μm in size. The rostellum, or crown of hooklets, is easily visible at the top of the larva. Each hook ➡ is sickle-shaped and approximately 20-40 μm in size.

POLYOMAVIRUS NEPHRITIS

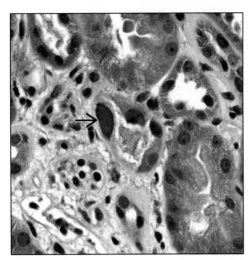

Hematoxylin & eosin shows an intranuclear inclusion ➡ with a "ground-glass" appearance in this distal tubule. The adjacent interstitium shows edema and scattered lymphocytes.

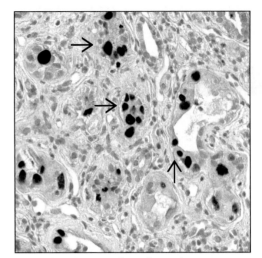

Immunohistochemistry for polyoma large T antigen (SV40) stains polyomavirus ➡ in many tubular epithelial cell nuclei accompanied by prominent interstitial inflammation.

TERMINOLOGY

Abbreviations
- Polyomavirus nephritis (PVN)

Synonyms
- Polyomavirus tubulointerstitial nephritis
- Polyomavirus nephropathy
- BK virus nephropathy

Definitions
- Polyomavirus infection of the kidney, usually in an immunocompromised host
  - Renal allograft
  - Native kidney
    - Recipients of other organ transplants (rare)
    - Hematopoietic cell transplantation
    - AIDS patients
    - Inherited immunodeficiency

ETIOLOGY/PATHOGENESIS

Infectious Agents
- Human polyomavirus
  - BK virus
    - High seroprevalence in adults (80%)
    - Causes pathology only in immunocompromised patients
    - Causes ~ 80% of PVN
    - Tropism for the genitourinary tract epithelium
  - JC virus
    - Causes ~ 20% of PVN, usually milder than BK
    - Causes progressive multifocal leukoencephalopathy
  - Simian virus 40 (SV40)
    - Rarely, if ever, causes interstitial nephritis in humans

Pathogenesis
- Reactivation of latent virus

- Transplanted kidney a risk factor (vs. other organs)
  - Renal injury promotes viral replication
  - Rejection contributes to pathogenesis
- Higher risk of PVN with the use of tacrolimus/ mycophenolate vs. cyclosporine/azathioprine

CLINICAL ISSUES

Epidemiology
- Incidence
  - ~ 5% in kidney transplant patients on tacrolimus and mycophenolate mofetil

Presentation
- Acute renal failure
- Hemorrhagic cystitis
- Ureteral obstruction

Laboratory Tests
- Urine cytology
  - Decoy cells
    - Not specific for PVN, but indicate polyoma infection of urinary tract
  - Polyomavirus aggregates ("Haufen") by negative staining EM
    - High sensitivity and specificity for PVN (> 98%)
- Viral culture (shell vial)
- Polymerase chain reaction (PCR)
  - Urine
    - High viral loads raise suspicion of PVN
  - Blood
    - Rare PVN in absence of BK viremia

Treatment
- Drugs
  - Current antivirals not highly effective
  - Cidofovir
  - Leflunomide
- Reduce or alter immunosuppressive agents

POLYOMAVIRUS NEPHRITIS

Terminology
- Polyomavirus infection in kidney allografts or native kidneys of immunosuppressed or immunocompromised patients

Etiology/Pathogenesis
- Human polyomavirus
  - BK virus usual, 80%
  - JC virus ~ 20%, milder

Clinical Issues
- Acute renal failure
- ~ 5% prevalence in kidney transplant patients

Microscopic Pathology
- Interstitial inflammation, mononuclear
- Tubulitis
- Nuclear inclusions

Key Facts
- TBM immune complex deposition

Ancillary Tests
- IHC for polyoma large T antigen
- EM for viral particles

Top Differential Diagnoses
- Acute tubulointerstitial (type I) rejection
- Adenovirus tubulointerstitial nephritis
- Acute tubular necrosis
- Acute interstitial nephritis

Diagnostic Checklist
- Concurrent PVN and acute rejection can occur, but infrequently
- Endarteritis or C4d in peritubular capillaries indicates rejection also present

Prognosis
- Graft loss depends on stage at diagnosis (13-100%)
  - Poorer prognosis with interstitial fibrosis and tubular atrophy
- Residual impairment of renal function common
- Rare graft loss with JC

MICROSCOPIC PATHOLOGY

Histologic Features
- Interstitial mononuclear inflammation
  - Lymphocytes and eosinophils
  - Plasma cells usually prominent
  - Associated with viral-infected epithelial cells
  - Interstitial edema
- Intranuclear inclusions in tubular epithelium
  - "Ground-glass" nuclear appearance
  - Nuclear enlargement and hyperchromatism
  - Nuclear inclusions may be present in sloughed cells in tubular lumina
  - No inclusions in inflammatory cells
  - Inclusions may not be evident in early PVN
- Tubulitis and tubular injury
  - Plasma cells occasionally in tubules
  - Apoptosis common
- Distal nephron involved more than proximal nephron
  - May involve only renal medulla in early stages, especially collecting ducts
  - Advanced stages involve parietal epithelial cells of glomeruli
- Late changes
  - Interstitial fibrosis and tubular atrophy
  - Extent of tubulointerstitial scarring often correlates with duration of viral infection
  - Correlates with graft survival
  - Dedifferentiated pattern of tubular epithelial cells; appear spindled, possibly reflecting epithelial-mesenchymal transition (EMT)

ANCILLARY TESTS

Immunohistochemistry
- Polyomavirus large T antigen IHC diagnostic
  - Strong nuclear staining of epithelial cells
    - Tubular epithelial cells, often more distal than proximal tubules
    - Commonly clustered positive cells
    - Infrequent glomerular parietal epithelial cells
  - Protein of early phase of polyomavirus infection
  - Usual antibody to SV40 large T antigen detects both BK and JC virus

Immunofluorescence
- Granular staining of tubular basement membranes (TBM) for IgG, C3, and C4d
  - Subset of PVN (~ 50%)
  - May persist despite disappearance of polyomavirus by IHC or EM
  - Significance unknown, associated with higher Cr
  - SV40 antigen detected in TBM deposits by Aviv Hever and Cynthia Nast
- Granular TBM C4d in atrophic tubules may mimic linear staining of peritubular capillaries seen in antibody-mediated rejection

Electron Microscopy
- Transmission
  - Polyomavirus particles present within epithelial cells
    - Viral particles in paracrystalline arrays or loose clusters
    - Predominantly nuclear and occasionally cytoplasmic location
    - 40-50 nm in diameter
  - Discrete electron-dense deposits within tubular basement membranes
    - May be present in atrophic tubules
    - Use IF to confirm that electron-dense deposits represent immune complexes

POLYOMAVIRUS NEPHRITIS

Histologic Patterns of PVN

Grade	Viral Cytopathic Effect	Interstitial Inflammation/Tubular Atrophy	Graft Loss at 3 Years
A	Present	None/minimal	13%
B1	Present	< 25%	40%
B2	Present	25-50%	60%
B3	Present	> 50%	77%
C	Rare in atrophic tubules	Extensive	100%

DIFFERENTIAL DIAGNOSIS

Acute Tubulointerstitial (Type I) Rejection
- Prominent interstitial inflammation with tubulitis
- IHC negative for polyoma large T antigen (SV40)
- Rare cases of concurrent acute rejection and PVN

Adenovirus Tubulointerstitial Nephritis
- Prominent interstitial inflammation
- Viral cytopathic effect
- Necrosis
- IHC negative for polyoma large T antigen (SV40)

Acute Tubular Necrosis
- Nuclear enlargement and reactive atypia of tubular epithelial cells
- No prominent interstitial inflammation or intranuclear inclusions
- IHC negative for polyoma large T antigen (SV40)

Acute Interstitial Nephritis
- Marked interstitial inflammation
  - May be prominent in renal medulla
- No intranuclear inclusions
- IHC negative for polyoma large T antigen (SV40)

DIAGNOSTIC CHECKLIST

Clinically Relevant Pathologic Features
- Stages of disease correlate with outcome
  - Early stage (A): Minimal inflammation, rare viral cytopathic effect
  - Active stage (B): Prominent inflammation, tubular injury, inclusions
  - Inactive stage (C): Extensive fibrosis, tubular atrophy, little or no demonstrable virus

Pathologic Interpretation Pearls
- Interstitial inflammation that predominantly involves or is entirely limited to renal medulla should raise diagnostic suspicion for PVN
- When borderline inflammatory infiltrate is considered, SV40 immunohistochemistry study should always be ordered
  - Early PVN may **NOT** demonstrate nuclear enlargement or apparent viral cytopathic changes
- Tubular basement membrane immune complex deposition may persist after resolution of PVN
- Detection of SV40 staining in 1 tubular epithelial cell nucleus is diagnostic of PVN

  - Prominent interstitial inflammation in setting of sparse SV40 staining raises consideration of concurrent acute rejection
- Concurrent PVN and acute rejection can occur, but infrequently

SELECTED REFERENCES

1. Prince O et al: Risk factors for polyoma virus nephropathy. Nephrol Dial Transplant. 24(3):1024-33, 2009
2. Singh HK et al: Presence of urinary Haufen accurately predicts polyomavirus nephropathy. J Am Soc Nephrol. 20(2):416-27, 2009
3. Dall A et al: BK virus nephritis after renal transplantation. Clin J Am Soc Nephrol. 3 Suppl 2:S68-75, 2008
4. Hever A et al: Polyoma virus nephropathy with simian virus 40 antigen-containing tubular basement membrane immune complex deposition. Hum Pathol. 39(1):73-9, 2008
5. Seemayer CA et al: BK virus large T and VP-1 expression in infected human renal allografts. Nephrol Dial Transplant. 23(12):3752-61, 2008
6. Bracamonte E et al: Tubular basement membrane immune deposits in association with BK polyomavirus nephropathy. Am J Transplant. 7(6):1552-60, 2007
7. Chang A et al: Spectrum of renal pathology in hematopoietic cell transplantation: a series of 20 patients and review of the literature. Clin J Am Soc Nephrol. 2(5):1014-23, 2007
8. Drachenberg CB et al: Histologic versus molecular diagnosis of BK polyomavirus-associated nephropathy: a shifting paradigm?. Clin J Am Soc Nephrol. 1(3):374-9, 2006
9. Meehan SM et al: Nephron segment localization of polyoma virus large T antigen in renal allografts. Hum Pathol. 37(11):1400-6, 2006
10. Limaye AP et al: Polyomavirus nephropathy in native kidneys of non-renal transplant recipients. Am J Transplant. 5(3):614-20, 2005
11. Drachenberg CB et al: Histological patterns of polyomavirus nephropathy: correlation with graft outcome and viral load. Am J Transplant. 4(12):2082-92, 2004
12. Gardner SD et al: New human papovavirus (B.K.) isolated from urine after renal transplantation. Lancet. 1(7712):1253-7, 1971

Microscopic Features

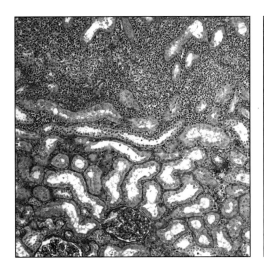 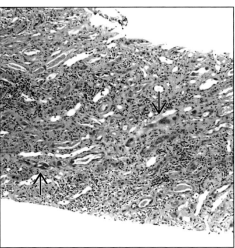

(Left) *Periodic acid-Schiff demonstrates dense zonal or regional interstitial inflammation, which emphasizes the importance of sufficiently sampling an allograft. The diagnosis of PVN would be missed if only the lower 1/2 of this renal cortex were biopsied.* *(Right)* *Light microscopy of PVN shows widespread tubular changes with large, atypical epithelial cells with spindle shapes and enlarged nuclei ➡️. The inflammation is confined to areas with viral cytopathic changes.*

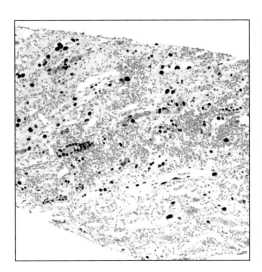 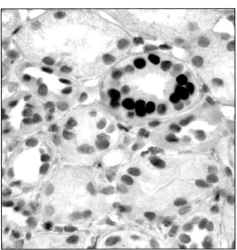

(Left) *IHC for polyoma large T antigen (SV40) shows widespread infection of tubules, with a characteristic clustering of positive cells within individual tubules. The inflammatory infiltrate is typically in the same area as the virus, arguing that the virus causes the inflammation.* *(Right)* *SV40 shows polyoma large T antigen in a cortical collecting duct. Almost every cell in this cross section is infected, suggesting that the virus spreads to adjacent cells.*

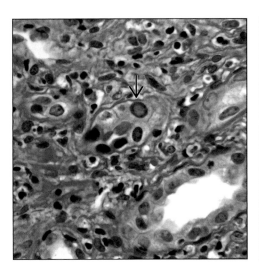 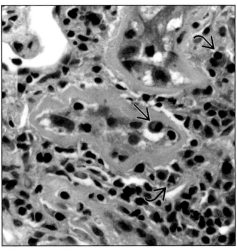

(Left) *Light microscopy at high power shows a characteristic inclusion in a cortical tubular epithelial cell ➡️.* *(Right)* *This tubule has largely dedifferentiated or missing epithelium. A plasma cell is present in the tubule ➡️, a distinctive finding in PVN. Many plasma cells are in the interstitium, which is also typical of PVN ➡️.*

POLYOMAVIRUS NEPHRITIS

Polyomavirus Inclusions

(Left) Hematoxylin & eosin shows several nuclei ➡ with characteristic cytopathic effect of polyomavirus infection. Nucleoli are often pushed to the nuclear membrane. These features correlate with electron microscopic findings. *(Right)* A nucleus of a tubular epithelial cell is enlarged with a "ground-glass" appearance ➡. There is associated interstitial edema and inflammation with tubulitis ➡. Such characteristic inclusions may not always be present.

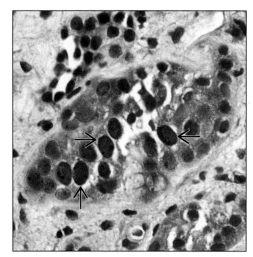
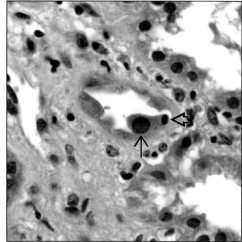

(Left) Periodic acid-Schiff shows severe interstitial inflammation and a typical, lavender, homogeneous intranuclear inclusion ➡ of polyomavirus. Lymphocytes and plasma cells are in the interstitial infiltrate. *(Right)* In this biopsy from a patient with an advanced stage of PVN, tubular atrophy, interstitial fibrosis, and a focal mononuclear infiltrate are present, which are all nonspecific findings. Only 1 nuclear inclusion was found as a clue to the etiology ➡.

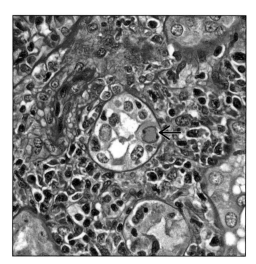
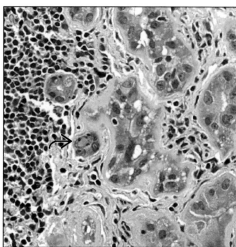

(Left) Spindle-shaped (dedifferentiated) tubular cells show viral inclusions in nuclei ➡. *(Right)* Periodic acid-Schiff reveals several tubular epithelial cells with "ground-glass" intranuclear inclusions ➡ and nucleoli displaced against the nuclear membrane. Tubulitis ➡ (or lymphocytes between tubular epithelial cells and tubular basement membrane) is a common finding that mimics acute rejection when viral cytopathic changes are not prominent.

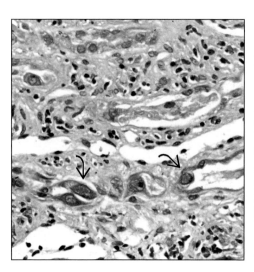
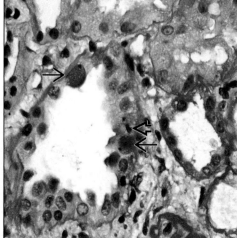

Microscopic Features

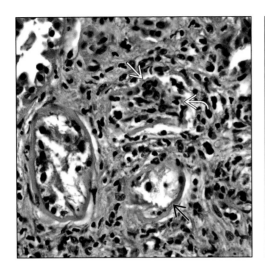

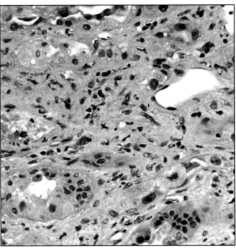

(Left) Severe destruction of tubules is evident ➡, with loss of normal structure and infiltration by inflammatory cells, including occasional eosinophils ➡. Some tubules have little if any remaining epithelium ➡, the residue of viral cytolysis. (Right) An advanced stage of PVN may show only nonspecific tubular loss, atrophy, and interstitial fibrosis, a.k.a. "chronic allograft nephropathy." Without a prior diagnosis of PVN, the cause would be unknown in this patient.

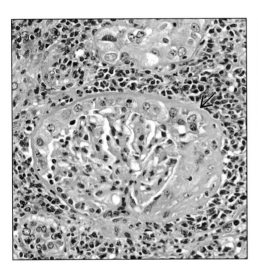

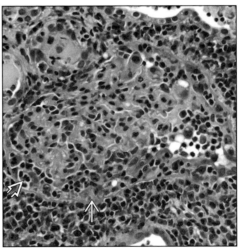

(Left) Hematoxylin & eosin shows prominence of the parietal epithelial cells ➡, which may be seen in a small subset of PVN and may occasionally mimic cellular crescents. Glomerular fibrinoid necrosis is absent. (Right) Hematoxylin & eosin shows prominent infiltration by lymphocytes ➡ between the Bowman capsule and the parietal epithelial cells ➡. Large aggregates of interstitial plasma cells and lymphocytes are present surrounding the glomerulus.

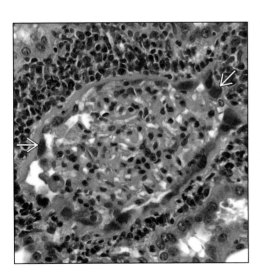

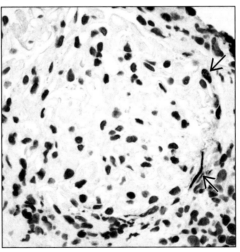

(Left) Hematoxylin & eosin shows several parietal epithelial cells with enlarged and smudged nuclei ➡ and scattered lymphocytes between the Bowman capsule and epithelial cells (or "capsulitis"), which is an uncommon histologic feature of severe PVN. (Right) SV40 immunohistochemistry shows several parietal epithelial cells ➡ infected by polyomavirus without nuclear enlargement. Scattered interstitial inflammation is present adjacent to this glomerulus.

Electron Microscopy

(Left) *Electron micrograph of a severely altered tubule shows large aggregates of polyoma virions in the tubular epithelial nuclei ➡, as well as an intratubular plasma cell ➡ and lymphocyte ➡. The tubular basement membrane is unremarkable ➡. **(Right)** Electron micrograph demonstrates numerous individual viral particles ➡ within the nucleus ➡ of a tubular epithelial cell. Nucleoli ➡ are pushed aside against the nuclear membrane. This can also be appreciated on light microscopy.*

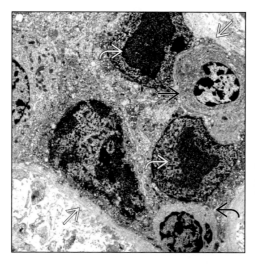
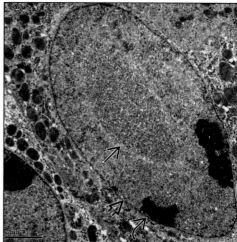

(Left) *EM shows numerous polyomavirus virions ➡ clustered together within the center of the nucleus in a tubular epithelial cell of a renal allograft. EM does not distinguish species of polyomavirus, but it separates the polyoma group from herpes viruses and adenoviruses. **(Right)** High-power electron micrograph of a tubular epithelial cell nucleus shows a cluster of polyoma virions that measure about 50 nm. These are significantly smaller than adenovirus or herpes viruses.*

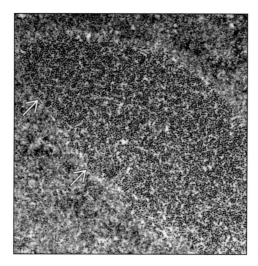
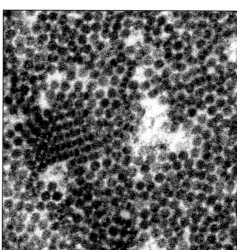

(Left) *Electron micrograph shows an aggregate of virions within the cytoplasm next to the nucleus of this infected tubular epithelial cell. The viral particles can be closely grouped together or occasionally arranged in a paracrystalline array (not shown). **(Right)** Electron micrograph of a tubular epithelial cell shows shedding of polyomavirus into the lumen ➡ and formation of cast-like aggregates ➡, which can be detected in the urine as "Haufen" by negative-staining EM.*

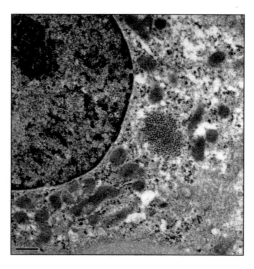
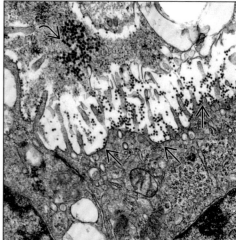

Tubular Basement Membrane Deposits

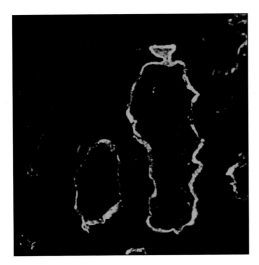

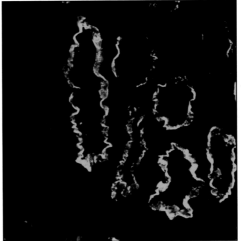

(Left) Immunofluorescence in a case of PVN shows intense granular deposition of IgG in some but not all tubular basement membranes. Granular IgG in the TBM is indicative of immune complex deposition and is not a nonspecific finding. *(Right)* Immunofluorescence in a case of PVN shows intense granular to broad linear deposition of C3 in some but not all tubular basement membranes. Broad linear C3 in the TBM is a common nonspecific finding in renal biopsies of any diagnosis.

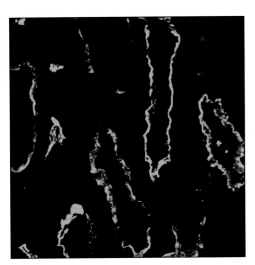

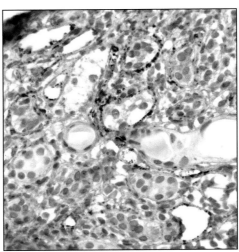

(Left) Immunofluorescence in a case of PVN shows intense granular deposition of C4d in some but not all tubular basement membranes. C4d is not commonly seen in the TBM (vs. C3) and, here, is part of an immune complex. This pattern may be confused with the C4d deposition in peritubular capillaries; the latter are usually smaller. *(Right)* Immunohistochemistry for C4d shows granular deposits along the TBM of a subset of the tubules. The peritubular capillaries are negative.

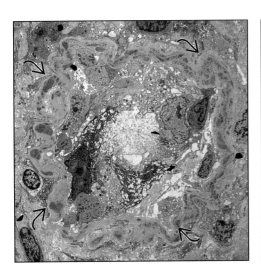

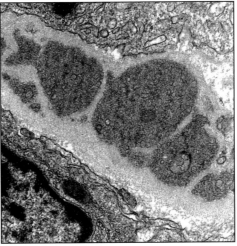

(Left) Low-power electron micrograph of a cross section of a tubule reveals widespread electron-dense amorphous deposits in the TBM ⮥. *(Right)* Electron micrograph of the tubular basement membrane deposits at high power shows that the deposits are amorphous and contain scattered membranous debris. No viral particles are evident. SV40 antigen has been detected in these deposits using indirect IF microscopy (not shown).

Urothelium and Urine

(Left) Stain for SV40 large T antigen reveals positive (red) nuclear staining in scattered urothelial cells within the renal pelvis of an allograft nephrectomy specimen.
(Right) This is the original case of polyomavirus infection from an allograft, reported by S.D. Gardner (St. Mary's Hospital, London). The ureter shows intense inflammation and ulceration. The patient's initials were BK, and the then novel polyomavirus was named accordingly. Ureteral stenosis occurs in 5-10% of patients with BK PVN. (Courtesy E. Ramos, MD.)

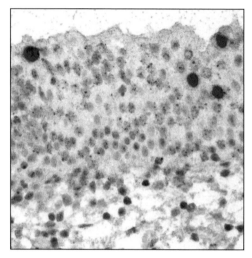
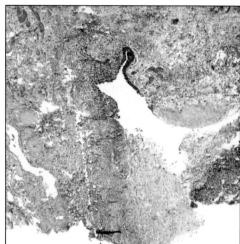

(Left) Ureter from an allograft nephrectomy with PVN stained for SV40 large T antigen shows numerous positive urothelial cells ➔. The mucosa shows marked inflammation, with scattered lymphocytes invading the epithelium ➔.
(Right) Composite image of urine cytology from patients with PVN shows decoy cells with inclusions. These cells, which resemble malignant cells, are not diagnostic of PVN but only of polyoma infection of the urinary tract, which may be asymptomatic.

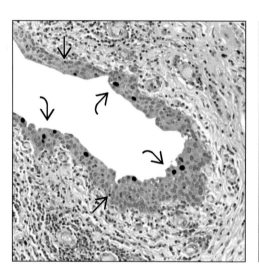
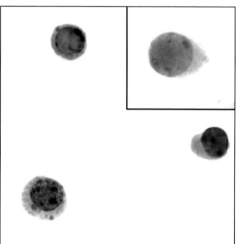

(Left) Antibody to SV40 large T antigen shows prominent staining of debris in a collected duct cast. When shed in the urine, these are the origin of the "Haufen" detected by EM. (Courtesy V. Nickeleit, MD.) (Right) Urine sediment examined by negative staining electron microscopy from a patient with PVN shows an aggregate of virions about 50 nm in diameter, typical of polyomavirus. These aggregates are found almost exclusively in patients with PVN. (Courtesy V. Nickeleit, MD.)

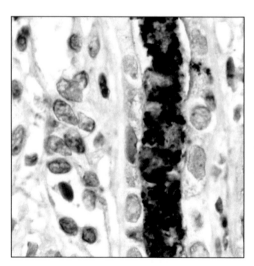
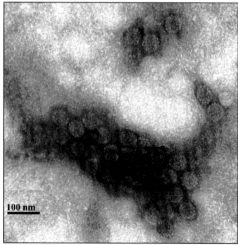

POLYOMAVIRUS NEPHRITIS

JC Virus Nephropathy

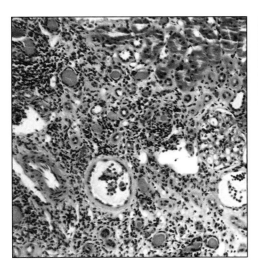

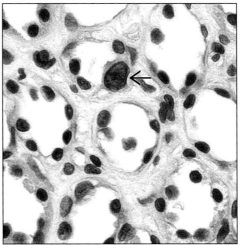

(Left) Hematoxylin & eosin shows marked interstitial inflammation associated with interstitial fibrosis and tubular atrophy in an allograft with JC virus infection. Scarce viral cytopathic changes are typical of JC virus infection of kidney allografts. (Courtesy C. Drachenberg, MD.) (Right) SV40 IHC shows nuclear staining in 1 tubular epithelial cell ➡ with an intranuclear inclusion. Blood PCR testing confirmed the presence of JC virus. (Courtesy C. Drachenberg, MD.)

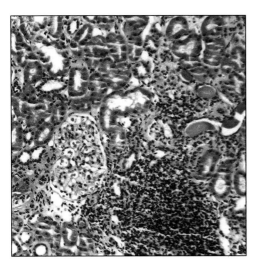

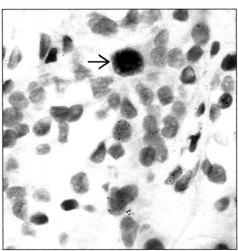

(Left) Hematoxylin & eosin shows focally prominent interstitial inflammation in the renal cortex of an allograft with JC virus infection, which is indistinguishable from BK virus infection by light microscopy. (Courtesy C. Drachenberg, MD.) (Right) SV40 IHC shows strong nuclear staining ➡ in a tubular epithelial cell from a patient with JC viremia. The number of infected epithelial cells is decreased in JC virus infection compared to BK virus nephropathy. (Courtesy C. Drachenberg, MD.)

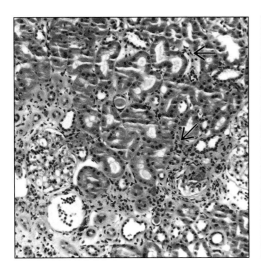

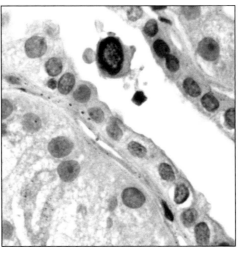

(Left) Hematoxylin & eosin shows patchy mild interstitial inflammation in the renal cortex ➡, which can mimic acute tubulointerstitial rejection or a borderline inflammatory infiltrate. (Courtesy C. Drachenberg, MD.) (Right) SV40 IHC shows staining of an intranuclear inclusion within a sloughed tubular cell from an allograft in a patient with JC viremia. JC virus shows similar cytopathic changes to those of BK virus but with a tendency to infect fewer cells. (Courtesy C. Drachenberg, MD.)

CYTOMEGALOVIRUS INFECTION

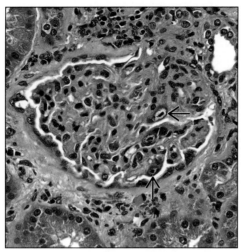

Hematoxylin & eosin shows characteristic intranuclear ("owl-eye") inclusions ➡ of CMV infection within the glomerular endothelial cells.

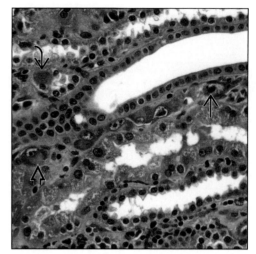

Hematoxylin & eosin shows CMV intranuclear inclusions ➡ in endothelial cells of a peritubular capillary with basophilic cytoplasmic changes ➤ that are also present in a tubular epithelial cell ➡.

TERMINOLOGY

Abbreviations
- Cytomegalovirus nephritis (CMV nephritis)

Synonyms
- CMV tubulointerstitial nephritis (TIN), CMV nephropathy, CMV glomerulonephritis

Definitions
- Direct CMV infection of kidneys, usually associated with systemic CMV involvement and immunocompromise
  - CMV may promote indirect effects on kidney, particularly in renal transplants, including acute allograft glomerulopathy

ETIOLOGY/PATHOGENESIS

Infectious Agents
- Cytomegalovirus
  - *Herpesviridae*
    - β-subfamily
    - Double-stranded DNA virus
  - Human herpesvirus-5 (HHV-5)

Risk Factors
- Immunocompromised patients at risk for systemic CMV
  - Transplant recipients on immunosuppression
    - Transplant CMV from donor organ or reactivation in recipient
    - Matching CMV serologic status in renal transplant patients has minimized incidence of CMV TIN
  - Infants
    - Neonatal CMV infection from maternal transmission
  - HIV-infected patients
- Causes benign, self-limited mononucleosis syndrome in normal individuals

Site of Infection
- Epithelium, endothelium, monocytes
- Renal involvement almost always associated with systemic infection
  - Lungs, liver, adrenals, retina, GI tract, epididymitis, pancreas, bone marrow

Latent Virus
- Most individuals infected before adulthood
  - Benign self-limited disease in normal individuals
  - Seroprevalence (90%)
  - Virus remains present in latent state lifelong

Effects on Immune System
- Increased IL-6 and IL-10, decreased Th1 cytokines (γ-interferon)
- Decreased expression of HLA antigens

CLINICAL ISSUES

Epidemiology
- Incidence
  - Neonatal CMV
    - Most common neonatal infection
    - 0.2-2% of live births in USA
    - 9.4 per 100,000 infants ages 1-4 years in Australia
  - Transplant CMV
    - ~ 20% incidence of CMV disease with ganciclovir prophylaxis
    - ~ 45% incidence without prophylaxis
    - Frequency of CMV infection in renal transplant biopsies < 1%
- Age
  - Neonatal, intrauterine
  - Immunocompromised adults
- Gender
  - Male predilection
- Ethnicity
  - No ethnic predilection

CYTOMEGALOVIRUS INFECTION

Key Facts

Terminology
- CMV infection in kidneys, usually associated with systemic CMV in immunocompromised patient

Etiology/Pathogenesis
- Cytomegalovirus
- Immunocompromised patients at risk

Clinical Issues
- Presentation
  - Renal dysfunction
  - Flu-like symptoms
- Antiviral agents
  - Ganciclovir or valganciclovir
  - CMV immune globulin
- Reduce or alter immunosuppressive agents

Microscopic Pathology
- Nuclear inclusions
  - Most prominent in tubular epithelium
  - Glomerular capillary &/or peritubular capillary endothelial cells
- Interstitial inflammation, mononuclear
- Acute glomerulonephritis (rare)

Top Differential Diagnoses
- Polyomavirus nephropathy
- Adenovirus tubulointerstitial nephritis
- Acute cellular rejection
- Acute allograft glomerulopathy (form of rejection)

Diagnostic Checklist
- Coinfection with other fungal or viral organisms may occur

Presentation
- Fever
- Malaise
- Leukopenia
- Renal dysfunction
- Acute renal failure
- Proteinuria

Laboratory Tests
- CMV IgM antibodies
  - Suggest recent or active infection
  - False-positives due to rheumatoid factor
- CMV IgG antibodies
- CMV antigen test
  - Indirect IF test to detect pp65 protein of CMV in peripheral blood leukocytes
- CMV polymerase chain reaction (PCR)
- Viral culture
  - Shell vial assay

Treatment
- Drugs
  - Ganciclovir or valganciclovir
    - Prophylaxis
    - Intravenous therapy
  - Foscarnet
    - Side effects include crystal formation leading to glomerulopathy
    - Multinucleation of tubular epithelial cell nuclei may persist after foscarnet therapy
  - Cidofovir
  - CMV intravenous immune globulin (IVIG)
- Reduce or alter immunosuppressive agents
- Vaccination to prevent maternal transmission

Prognosis
- Neonatal CMV
  - 30% mortality among symptomatic infants
  - Survivors commonly have neurologic deficits
- CMV disease in transplant recipient
  - Increased graft loss in past (10-20%)
  - Less adverse effect of CMV in patients on current immunosuppressive protocols

MICROSCOPIC PATHOLOGY

Histologic Features
- Pattern I: Large intranuclear inclusions in tubular epithelial cells with interstitial nephritis
  - Variable interstitial inflammation
  - Occasional granulomatous inflammation
  - Rare or no intranuclear inclusions in endothelial cells
  - Monocyte inclusions in interstitial infiltrate
- Pattern II: Large eosinophilic intranuclear inclusions in endothelial cells
  - Glomerular and peritubular capillary endothelial cells may be infected
  - When endothelial cells are predominant cell infected by CMV, epithelial cells tend to be spared
  - Interstitial inflammation **not** prominent in cases with primarily endothelial cell infection
- Pattern III: Acute glomerulonephritis (rare)
  - Endocapillary hypercellularity
  - Inclusions in glomerular endothelial cells or in circulating monocytes
  - Crescents may be present
  - Scant deposits by EM

ANCILLARY TESTS

In Situ Hybridization
- In situ hybridization for CMV positive

Electron Microscopy
- Virions in nucleus and cytoplasm
- 150-200 nm in diameter
- Dense core surrounded by thick capsule

CYTOMEGALOVIRUS INFECTION

Immunohistochemistry

Antibody	Reactivity	Staining Pattern	Comment
CMV	Positive	Nuclear & cytoplasmic	Epithelial or endothelial cells
SV40	Negative	Not applicable	
Adenovirus	Negative	Not applicable	
EBV-LMP	Negative	Not applicable	
HSV1/2	Negative	Not applicable	

DIFFERENTIAL DIAGNOSIS

Polyoma Virus Nephropathy
- Intranuclear inclusions with "ground-glass" appearance in tubular epithelial cells
- Immunohistochemical for SV40 large T antigen positive
- Prominent interstitial plasmacytic inflammation with tubulitis
- No endothelial inclusions

Adenovirus Tubulointerstitial Nephritis
- Prominent interstitial inflammation and tubular necrosis
- Granulomatous inflammation
- Viral cytopathic effect in tubular epithelial cells
- Immunohistochemical confirmation of adenovirus infection

Acute Cellular Rejection
- Prominent interstitial inflammation with tubulitis
- No viral cytopathic effect
- Endarteritis helpful if present

Acute Allograft Glomerulopathy (Form of Rejection)
- Marked glomerular cell endothelial swelling and activation
- Mesangiolysis: Webs of PAS(+) material
- CD8 T cells in glomeruli
- No inclusions or viral antigens in glomeruli
- May be indirect effect of CMV in some patients
- Endarteritis common
- C4d negative

Acute Glomerulonephritis
- No CMV inclusions or antigens
- Deposits in GBM

DIAGNOSTIC CHECKLIST

Pathologic Interpretation Pearls
- Inclusions readily evident at low power (10x)
- CMV intranuclear inclusions present in predominantly endothelial cells or epithelial cells
- Coinfection with other fungal or viral organisms may occur
- Features of foscarnet toxicity may be present in patients treated for CMV infection

SELECTED REFERENCES

1. Humar A et al: An assessment of herpesvirus co-infections in patients with CMV disease: correlation with clinical and virologic outcomes. Am J Transplant. 9(2):374-81, 2009
2. Pass RF et al: Vaccine prevention of maternal cytomegalovirus infection. N Engl J Med. 360(12):1191-9, 2009
3. Seale H et al: Trends in hospitalizations for diagnosed congenital cytomegalovirus in infants and children in Australia. BMC Pediatr. 9:7, 2009
4. Cathro HP et al: Cytomegalovirus glomerulitis in a renal allograft. Am J Kidney Dis. 52(1):188-92, 2008
5. Kliem V et al: Improvement in long-term renal graft survival due to CMV prophylaxis with oral ganciclovir: results of a randomized clinical trial. Am J Transplant. 8(5):975-83, 2008
6. Luo X et al: Two rare forms of renal allograft glomerulopathy during cytomegalovirus infection and treatment. Am J Kidney Dis. 51(6):1047-51, 2008
7. Romanelli RM et al: Prognostic markers of symptomatic congenital cytomegalovirus infection. Braz J Infect Dis. 12(1):38-43, 2008
8. Sadeghi M et al: Dysregulated cytokine responses during cytomegalovirus infection in renal transplant recipients. Transplantation. 86(2):275-85, 2008
9. Suneja M et al: Cytomegalovirus glomerulopathy in a kidney allograft with response to oral valganciclovir. Am J Kidney Dis. 52(1):e1-4, 2008
10. Carstens J et al: Cytomegalovirus infection in renal transplant recipients. Transpl Infect Dis. 8(4):203-12, 2006
11. Joshi K et al: Pathological spectrum of cytomegalovirus infection of renal allograft recipients-an autopsy study from north India. Indian J Pathol Microbiol. 47(3):327-32, 2004
12. Onuigbo M et al: Cytomegalovirus-induced glomerular vasculopathy in renal allografts: a report of two cases. Am J Transplant. 2(7):684-8, 2002
13. Giral M et al: Mycophenolate mofetil does not modify the incidence of cytomegalovirus (CMV) disease after kidney transplantation but prevents CMV-induced chronic graft dysfunction. J Am Soc Nephrol. 12(8):1758-63, 2001
14. Wong KM et al: Cytomegalovirus-induced tubulointerstitial nephritis in a renal allograft treated by foscarnet therapy. Am J Nephrol. 20(3):222-4, 2000
15. Detwiler RK et al: Cytomegalovirus-induced necrotizing and crescentic glomerulonephritis in a renal transplant patient. Am J Kidney Dis. 32(5):820-4, 1998

CYTOMEGALOVIRUS INFECTION

Neonatal CMV Infection

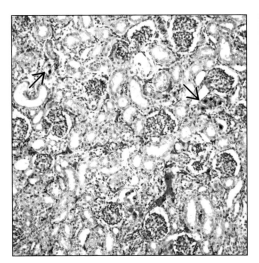

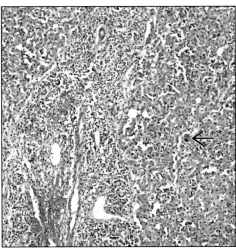

(Left) Hematoxylin & eosin shows clusters of tubular epithelial cells with large eosinophilic intranuclear inclusions ➡ characteristic of CMV, which are apparent even at low magnification. The glomeruli are normal with an immature appearance in this neonatal kidney. (Courtesy J. Taxy, MD.) (Right) Hematoxylin & eosin shows diffuse and severe interstitial inflammation. Scattered inclusions are seen in epithelial cells ➡ but not in endothelial cells. (Courtesy J. Taxy, MD.)

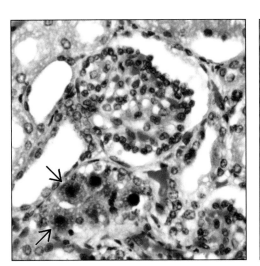

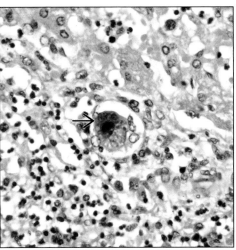

(Left) Hematoxylin & eosin shows prominent intranuclear inclusions ➡ within several tubular epithelial cells in a neonate with CMV infection. An adjacent glomerulus is uninvolved by CMV infection. (Courtesy J. Taxy, MD.) (Right) Hematoxylin & eosin shows diffuse interstitial inflammation with primarily lymphocytes and plasma cells and a large intranuclear inclusion ➡ in an epithelial cell that is characteristic of CMV. (Courtesy J. Taxy, MD.)

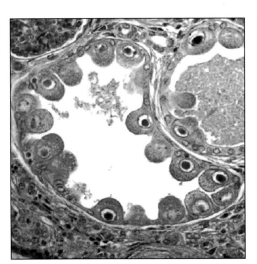

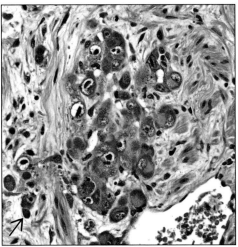

(Left) Hematoxylin & eosin of an autopsy from an infant who died from systemic CMV disease shows frequent large eosinophilic inclusions in the tubular epithelial cells, which have a "hobnail" pattern. (Right) CMV "owl-eye" intranuclear inclusions in endothelial cells of a renal transplant obscure the vessel lumina, but a few red blood cells are noted. Prominent basophilic changes are noted in the cell cytoplasm of the CMV-infected cells with focal eosinophilic granules ➡.

Renal Transplant CMV

(Left) Hematoxylin & eosin shows numerous CMV intranuclear inclusions ➡ within endothelial cells in small vessels within the renal sinus of this transplant nephrectomy specimen. (Right) Hematoxylin & eosin of a renal transplant biopsy shows a moderately intense mononuclear infiltrate, edema, and tubular injury, resembling acute cellular rejection. Inclusions typical of CMV, however, are seen in the tubules, even at low power ➡.

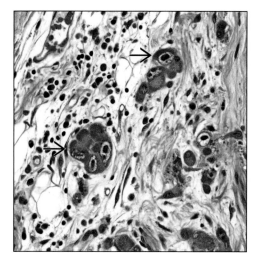 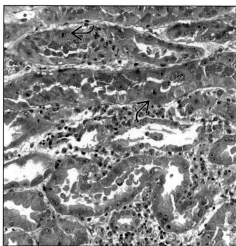

(Left) Hematoxylin & eosin of a glomerulus from a renal transplant patient with systemic CMV disease shows prominent inclusions ➡ in the capillaries, presumably glomerular endothelial cells. (Courtesy S. Singh, MD.) (Right) Hematoxylin & eosin shows a glomerulus from a renal transplant patient with systemic CMV disease with prominent inclusions in the capillaries, presumably glomerular endothelial cells; these may also be seen in circulating monocytes. (Courtesy H. Cathro, MBBCh.)

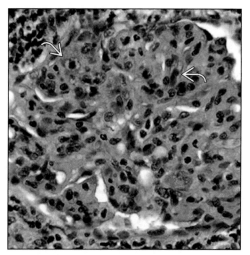 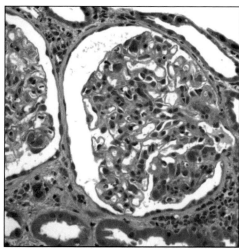

(Left) Jones methenamine silver stain from a renal transplant recipient with systemic CMV disease is shown. Inclusions are evident in intracapillary endothelial cells or monocytes ➡. (Courtesy H. Cathro, MBBCh.) (Right) Acute allograft glomerulopathy, a form of humoral rejection, in a renal transplant recipient with systemic CMV shows endothelial swelling and scattered mononuclear cells in capillary loops. The PAS(+) webs are indicative of mesangiolysis ➡. No CMV inclusions were present.

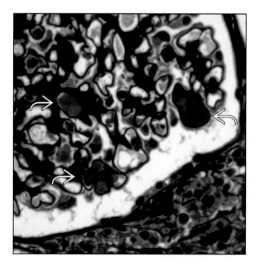 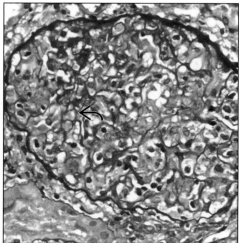

Immunohistochemistry and Electron Microscopy

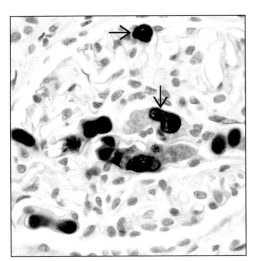

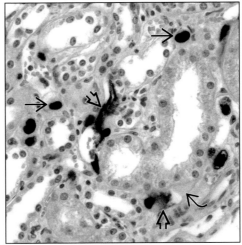

(Left) CMV immunohistochemistry demonstrates strong nuclear staining ⇨ and a blush of cytoplasmic staining within several glomerular endothelial cells. *(Right)* CMV immunohistochemistry shows strong nuclear ⇨ and some cytoplasmic ⇨ staining of many peritubular capillary endothelial cells ⇨ with marked nuclear enlargement. No CMV staining of the tubular epithelial cells is noted in this photomicrograph.

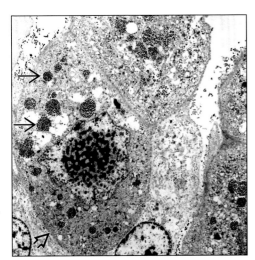

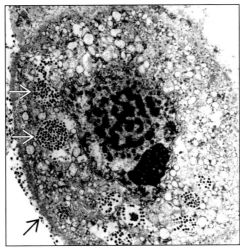

(Left) Electron microscopy shows several prominent aggregates of CMV viral particles ⇨ within the nucleus ⇨ of this infected epithelial cell. Scattered individual virions are also present throughout the nucleus and cell cytoplasm. (Courtesy J. Taxy, MD.) *(Right)* This electron micrograph demonstrates aggregates of CMV viral particles within the nucleus ⇨ and many scattered CMV virions within the cytoplasm ⇨ of this tubular epithelial cell. (Courtesy J. Taxy, MD.)

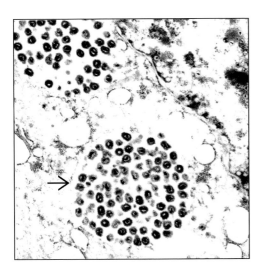

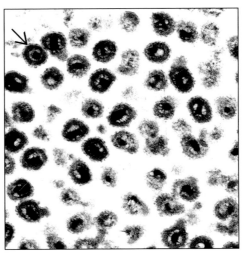

(Left) This electron micrograph reveals several clusters of CMV virions that are contained within an electron lucent membrane ⇨ in the nucleus of this infected epithelial cell. (Courtesy J. Taxy, MD.) *(Right)* Electron microscopy shows individual viral particles ⇨ measuring approximately 150-200 nm in diameter with dense central cores surrounded by a thick capsule, which is characteristic of Cytomegalovirus. (Courtesy J. Taxy, MD.)

ADENOVIRUS INFECTION

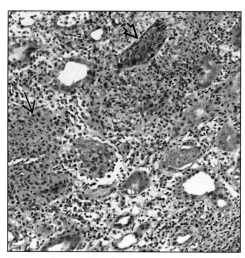

Hematoxylin & eosin demonstrates severe interstitial inflammation, granulomas ➡, tubular necrosis ➡, and interstitial edema in this renal allograft with adenovirus infection.

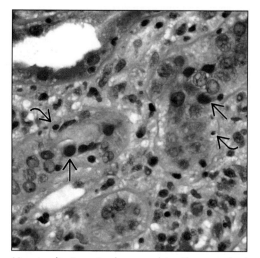

Hematoxylin & eosin shows nuclei with a smudged appearance ➡ in several tubular epithelial cells, which are characteristic of an adenovirus infection. There is frequent tubulitis ➡.

TERMINOLOGY

Abbreviations
- Adenovirus (AdV)

Synonyms
- Adenovirus tubulointerstitial nephritis
- Adenovirus nephritis

Definitions
- Adenovirus infection of kidney

ETIOLOGY/PATHOGENESIS

Infectious Agents
- Adenovirus
  - Nonenveloped, double-stranded DNA virus
  - Possible routes of infection
    - Reactivation of endogenous latent infection
    - Transplanted organ or tissue
- Other organs affected: Bladder, lung, liver, GI tract

CLINICAL ISSUES

Epidemiology
- Incidence
  - Rare in kidney transplant recipients (< 1%)
    - Onset typically in 1st 3 months post transplant
  - AdV infection more common in bone marrow and stem cell recipients (3-7%)
    - Native kidney occasionally involved
- Age
  - Children more susceptible (< 5 years)

Presentation
- Hemorrhagic cystitis
- Gross hematuria
- Acute renal failure
- Fever

- Diarrhea
- Graft tenderness

Laboratory Tests
- Real-time polymerase chain reaction (RT-PCR)
  - AdV in blood precedes symptoms by > 3 weeks
- Shell vial assay (culture)
- Serology
  - Enzyme immunoassay for AdV antigen
  - Complement fixation

Treatment
- Drugs
  - Cidofovir, ribavirin
  - Valganciclovir or ganciclovir
  - Intravenous immunoglobulin (IVIG)
- Reduction of immunosuppressive agents

Prognosis
- Disseminated disease often fatal (> 60%)
- Recovery common if localized

MACROSCOPIC FEATURES

General Features
- White-yellowish streaks with hemorrhagic rim primarily in renal medulla
- Hemorrhagic mucosal surface in renal pelvis and ureters
- Bladder and ureter involvement may cause obstructive uropathy

MICROSCOPIC PATHOLOGY

Histologic Features
- Acute tubular injury and interstitial nephritis
  - Granulomas associated with viral-infected tubular epithelial cells and tubular destruction
  - Focal necrosis of tubules

ADENOVIRUS INFECTION

Key Facts

Terminology
- Synonym
  - Adenovirus tubulointerstitial nephritis

Etiology/Pathogenesis
- Nonenveloped, double-stranded DNA virus

Clinical Issues
- Fever
- Graft tenderness
- Gross hematuria
- Acute renal failure
- Blood RT-PCR for diagnosis and surveillance
- Cidofovir, ribavirin, IVIG

Microscopic Pathology
- Granulomatous inflammation
- Necrosis of tubules

- Interstitial hemorrhage
- Smudgy, basophilic, intranuclear inclusions in tubular cells

Ancillary Tests
- Positive for AdV by immunohistochemistry
- EM shows characteristic 75-80 nm virions

Top Differential Diagnoses
- Acute cellular rejection
- Polyomavirus nephritis
- Aspergillosis
- Tuberculosis

Diagnostic Checklist
- Coinfection with other organisms common
- Antiviral antibody panel valuable in differential diagnosis (AdV, SV40, CMV)

  - Hemorrhage
  - Edema
- Viral cytopathic effect
  - Basophilic intranuclear inclusions with smudged appearance in tubular epithelial cells
  - Detached infected cells may be within tubular lumina
  - Distal tubules more commonly infected than proximal tubules
  - Occasional glomerular (visceral and parietal) epithelial cells may be infected
- Ureter &/or bladder commonly involved

ANCILLARY TESTS

Immunohistochemistry
- Nuclear and cytoplasmic staining for adenovirus
- Negative for polyoma large T antigen (SV40)

Electron Microscopy
- Viral particles 75-80 nm in diameter

In Situ Hybridization
- Nuclear and cytoplasmic staining

DIFFERENTIAL DIAGNOSIS

Acute Cellular Rejection
- Reactive atypia of tubular nuclei may mimic viral inclusions
- No viral antigen present
- Less severe hemorrhage and tubular necrosis than AdV
- Endarteritis

Polyomavirus Nephritis
- Positive SV40 immunohistochemistry
- Less severe hemorrhage and tubular necrosis than AdV
- More plasmacellular and less granulomatous inflammation

Tuberculosis
- Acid-fast bacilli, no hemorrhage

Bacterial Pyelonephritis
- Intratubular and interstitial neutrophils

Aspergillosis
- Septate hyphae with 45° angle branching

Drug-induced Acute Interstitial Nephritis
- Hemorrhage and necrosis minimal
- No viral antigen present
- More prominent eosinophils

DIAGNOSTIC CHECKLIST

Pathologic Interpretation Pearls
- Coinfection with other fungal or viral organisms may occur
- Panel of antiviral antibodies valuable in differential diagnosis (AdV, SV40, CMV, HSV)
- AdV rarely causes renal infection in absence of cystitis
- Necrotizing granuloma is distinctive feature

SELECTED REFERENCES

1. Varma MC et al: Early onset adenovirus infection after simultaneous kidney-pancreas transplant. Am J Transplant. 11(3):623-7, 2011
2. Mazoyer E et al: A case report of adenovirus-related acute interstitial nephritis in a patient with AIDS. Am J Kidney Dis. 51(1):121-6, 2008
3. Lim AK et al: Adenovirus tubulointerstitial nephritis presenting as a renal allograft space occupying lesion. Am J Transplant. 5(8):2062-6, 2005
4. Asim M et al: Adenovirus infection of a renal allograft. Am J Kidney Dis. 41(3):696-701, 2003
5. Kim SS et al: Adenovirus pyelonephritis in a pediatric renal transplant patient. Pediatr Nephrol. 18(5):457-61, 2003
6. Mori K et al: Acute renal failure due to adenovirus-associated obstructive uropathy and necrotizing tubulointerstitial nephritis in a bone marrow transplant recipient. Bone Marrow Transplant. 31(12):1173-6, 2003
7. Ito M et al: Necrotizing tubulointerstitial nephritis associated with adenovirus infection. Hum Pathol. 22(12):1225-31, 1991

ADENOVIRUS INFECTION

Microscopic Features

(Left) Necrotizing granulomata are typical of adenovirus infection, with neutrophils, plasma cells, and lymphocytes in this renal allograft. Viral cytopathic effect ➡ and tubulitis ⇨ are noted. *(Courtesy L. Novoa-Takara, MD.)* *(Right)* Periodic acid-Schiff reveals prominent interstitial inflammation and frequent tubulitis in the renal medulla, which is common for adenovirus but atypical for acute rejection. Patchy involvement of the renal cortex (not shown) is also present.

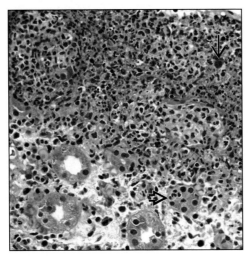
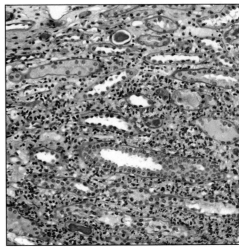

(Left) Hematoxylin & eosin shows viral cytopathic effect ➡ in several tubular epithelial cell nuclei within a tubule with tubulitis ➡ and necrosis ⇨, which is surrounded by abundant interstitial inflammation. *(Right)* Periodic acid-Schiff shows enlarged, tubular epithelial cell nuclei with a "smudged" appearance ➡, which resemble polyomavirus, but the presence of tubular degeneration/necrosis ⇨ and granulomatous inflammation favors adenovirus nephritis.

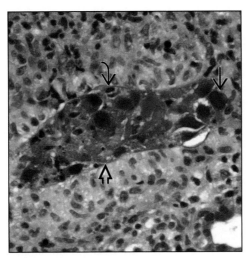
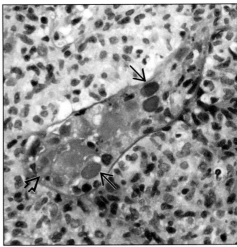

(Left) Hematoxylin & eosin reveals 2 giant cells ➡ surrounding a severely injured tubule with necrosis ⇨. Interstitial inflammatory cells consist of epithelioid macrophages, lymphocytes, plasma cells, and rare eosinophils. *(Right)* Periodic acid-Schiff highlights multinucleated giant cells ➡ closely associated with an injured tubule, which contains necrotic and sloughed epithelial cells that are intermixed with lymphocytes in a renal allograft infected with adenovirus.

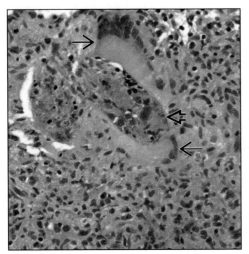
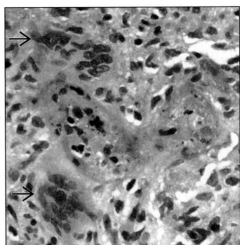

ADENOVIRUS INFECTION

Ancillary Techniques

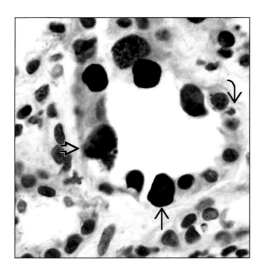
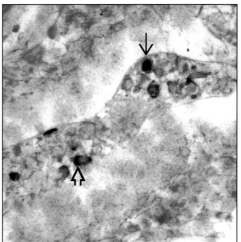

(Left) Adenovirus immunohistochemistry shows both strong staining ➡ and faint staining ⊃ in the nuclei of several tubular epithelial cells in a renal allograft biopsy. Note the scattered interstitial inflammatory cells and focal tubulitis ➡. (Right) In situ hybridization for adenovirus highlights a few tubular epithelial cell nuclei ➡ and cell cytoplasm ⊃ within this tubule with extensive injury and necrosis.

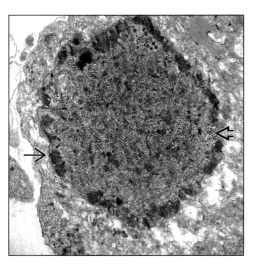
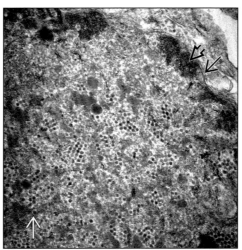

(Left) Electron microscopy reveals numerous adenovirus virions ⊃ that have displaced the nuclear chromatin ➡ against the nuclear membrane within this infected epithelial cell nucleus. The nucleus corresponds with a nuclear inclusion that is observed by light microscopy. (Right) Electron microscopy demonstrates numerous individual adenovirus virions ➡ within this nucleus, which has displaced the nuclear chromatin ⊃ against the nuclear membrane ➡.

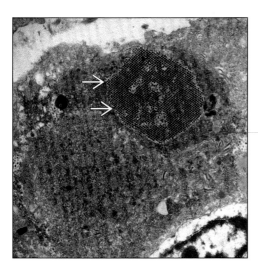
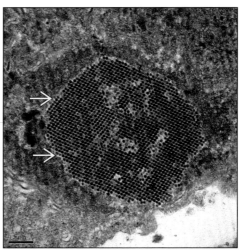

(Left) Electron microscopy shows numerous adenovirus viral particles forming a paracrystalline array ➡ within the nucleus of this infected epithelial cell. (Right) Electron microscopy shows adenovirus virions ➡ in a paracrystalline array within an infected epithelial cell nucleus. The individual virions measure approximately 80 nm in diameter, which is nearly twice the size of human polyomavirus. The scale bar in the bottom left corner measures 500 nm.

HERPES SIMPLEX ACUTE NEPHRITIS

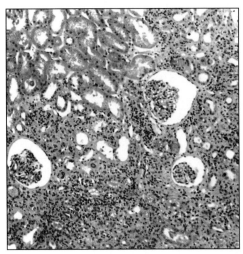

H&E shows marked interstitial inflammation without apparent viral cytopathic effect in a kidney transplant patient with disseminated herpes simplex virus. (Courtesy K-K. Park, MD, PhD.)

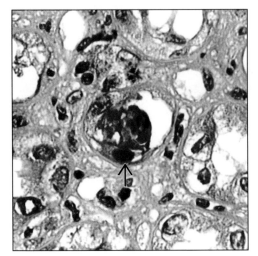

H&E shows viral cytopathic effect ➡ in tubular epithelial cells with scattered interstitial inflammation in a kidney transplant patient infected by herpes simplex virus. (Courtesy K-K. Park, MD, PhD.)

TERMINOLOGY

Abbreviations
- Herpes simplex virus (HSV) nephritis

Definitions
- HSV infection in renal allografts

ETIOLOGY/PATHOGENESIS

Infectious Agents
- HSV-1
- HSV-2
  - No documented cases of HSV-2 nephritis

CLINICAL ISSUES

Epidemiology
- Incidence
  - Rare
- Age
  - No age predilection
- Gender
  - No gender predilection
- Ethnicity
  - No ethnic predilection

Presentation
- Acute renal failure
- HSV infection in other sites

Laboratory Tests
- Polymerase chain reaction
- Serologic tests
  - Enzyme-linked immunoassay
  - Western blot
    - Anti-gpG1 glycoprotein for HSV-1
    - Anti-gpG2 glycoprotein for HSV-2
  - Immunofluorescence assays

- Viral culture
  - Shell vial assay

Treatment
- Drugs
  - Acyclovir
- Reduction of immunosuppressive agents

Prognosis
- Good
  - Worse if HSV hepatitis present

MICROSCOPIC PATHOLOGY

Histologic Features
- Prominent interstitial inflammation
- Tubulitis
- Viral cytopathic effect
  - Tubular epithelial cell nuclei
  - HSV virions measure approximately 110 nm in diameter
- Acute tubular injury
- Interstitial hemorrhage

DIFFERENTIAL DIAGNOSIS

Polyomavirus Nephritis
- Prominent interstitial inflammation with tubulitis
- Positive SV40 immunohistochemistry
- Individual virions measure 45 nm in diameter

Adenovirus Nephritis
- Prominent interstitial granulomatous inflammation with tubulitis
- Viral cytopathic effect with smudged nuclei
  - Positive adenovirus immunohistochemistry
  - Individual virions measure approximately 90 nm in diameter
- Tubular necrosis

HERPES SIMPLEX ACUTE NEPHRITIS

Key Facts

Etiology/Pathogenesis
- HSV-1

Clinical Issues
- Acute renal failure
  - Rare kidney involvement
- Acyclovir

Microscopic Pathology
- Prominent interstitial inflammation

- Viral cytopathic effect
- Tubulitis
- Acute tubular injury &/or necrosis
- Interstitial hemorrhage

Top Differential Diagnoses
- Polyomavirus nephritis
- Adenovirus nephritis
- Acute cellular rejection
- Cytomegalovirus tubulointerstitial nephritis

Immunohistochemistry

Antibody	Reactivity	Staining Pattern	Comment
HSV1/2	Positive	Nuclear & cytoplasmic	Tubular epithelial cells
SV40	Negative	Not applicable	
Adenovirus	Negative	Not applicable	
CMV	Negative	Not applicable	
EBV-LMP	Negative	Not applicable	

Cytomegalovirus Tubulointerstitial Nephritis
- Enlarged tubular epithelial cell nuclei with characteristic "owl-eye" nuclear inclusions and basophilic cytoplasmic inclusions
- Prominent interstitial inflammation with tubulitis

Acute Cellular Rejection
- Prominent interstitial inflammation with tubulitis
- No viral cytopathic effect
- Endarteritis

DIAGNOSTIC CHECKLIST

Pathologic Interpretation Pearls
- Coinfection with other viral or fungal microorganisms can occur

SELECTED REFERENCES

1. Kang YN et al: Systemic herpes simplex virus infection following cadaveric renal transplantation: a case report. Transplant Proc. 38(5):1346-7, 2006
2. Sachdeva MU et al: Viral infections of renal allografts--an immunohistochemical and ultrastructural study. Indian J Pathol Microbiol. 47(2):189-94, 2004
3. Silbert PL et al: Herpes simplex virus interstitial nephritis in a renal allograft. Clin Nephrol. 33(6):264-8, 1990

IMAGE GALLERY

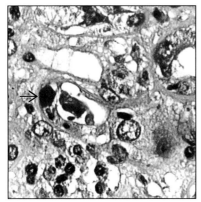 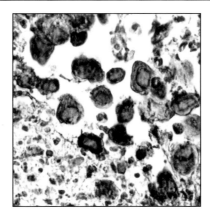 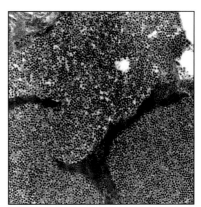

(Left) Hematoxylin & eosin shows enlarged nuclei with smudged appearance ⇨ in a renal transplant patient with disseminated herpes simplex virus infection. (Courtesy K-K. Park, MD, PhD.) *(Center)* HSV1/2 shows strong nuclear and cytoplasmic staining in many sloughed urothelial cells in this renal allograft. (Courtesy K-K. Park, MD, PhD.) *(Right)* Electron microscopy shows numerous herpes simplex viral particles measuring 105-110 nm in diameter in an infected tubular epithelial cell of a kidney transplant patient. (Courtesy K-K. Park, MD, PhD.)

EPSTEIN-BARR VIRUS NEPHRITIS

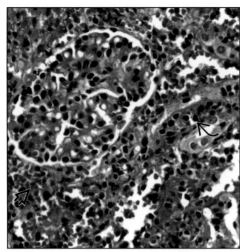

Hematoxylin & eosin reveals prominent diffuse interstitial mononuclear cell inflammation ⮑ and hemorrhage ⮕ in the kidney of a 16-month-old boy with an acute EBV infection. (Courtesy H. Cathro, MD.)

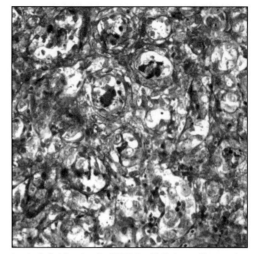

In situ hybridization for EBER-1 mRNA is usually negative in tubular epithelial cells. Rare interstitial lymphocytes may stain positive, but none are present. (Courtesy H. Cathro, MD.)

TERMINOLOGY

Abbreviations
- Epstein-Barr virus (EBV)

Definitions
- Primary EBV infection in pediatric population can result in acute kidney injury

ETIOLOGY/PATHOGENESIS

Infectious Agents
- Epstein-Barr virus
  - a.k.a human herpes virus 4 (HHV4)
  - 95% of adults infected by age 40
- EBV can infect proximal tubular epithelial cells, which express CD21

CLINICAL ISSUES

Epidemiology
- Incidence
  - EBV infections are commonly asymptomatic
  - Infectious mononucleosis
    - Renal involvement in up to 15%
- Age
  - Usually < 18 years old
- Gender
  - Male predilection for EBV nephritis
    - M:F = 3:1

Presentation
- Asymptomatic
  - Majority of cases
- Infectious mononucleosis
  - Proteinuria (14%)
  - Hematuria (11%)
- Acute renal failure
  - Oliguria (rare)

- May be associated with hepatic failure or rhabdomyolysis

Laboratory Tests
- EBV polymerase chain reaction
  - Blood
- Enzyme-linked immunoassay
  - EBV capsid antigen (VCA)-IgM
  - EBV capsid antigen: IgG
  - EBV nuclear antigen (EBNA)
  - Early antigen (EA)
- Mononucleosis ("monospot") or heterophile antibody test
  - Often negative in children < 10 years old

Treatment
- Drugs
  - Acyclovir
  - Corticosteroids: Variable efficacy

Prognosis
- Good, usually rapid resolution

MICROSCOPIC PATHOLOGY

Histologic Features
- Interstitial inflammation
  - Lymphocyte predominant
- Tubulitis
- Nuclear atypia of tubular epithelial cells (viral cytopathic effect)
- Interstitial edema
- Glomerular alterations
  - Occasional mesangial hypercellularity
  - Glomerular capillary thrombi (rare)
  - Podocyte injury; minimal change disease (rare)
  - Immune complex-mediated glomerulonephritis (rare)

EPSTEIN-BARR VIRUS NEPHRITIS

Key Facts

Etiology/Pathogenesis
- Epstein-Barr virus
  - a.k.a human herpes virus 4 (HHV4)

Clinical Issues
- EBV infections are commonly asymptomatic
- Infectious mononucleosis
  - 60% with subclinical renal involvement
- Observed mostly in male pediatric patients

Microscopic Pathology
- Interstitial inflammation and edema
- Tubulitis
- Negative immunohistochemistry for EBV-LMP, SV40, or adenovirus

Top Differential Diagnoses
- Acute interstitial nephritis
- Polyomavirus nephritis

ANCILLARY TESTS

Immunohistochemistry
- Negative
  - EBV latent membrane protein (LMP)
  - EBNA
  - EBV-VCA in tubular epithelial cells
    - Positive staining in occasional circulating or interstitial leukocytes
  - Simian virus 40 (SV40)
  - Cytomegalovirus
  - Adenovirus

In Situ Hybridization
- EBV-encoded small RNA1 (EBER-1) mRNA
  - Positive staining in rare circulating or interstitial leukocytes

DIFFERENTIAL DIAGNOSIS

Acute Interstitial Nephritis
- Prominent interstitial inflammation
- No viral cytopathic effect
- Absence of acute EBV infection

Acute Tubular Necrosis
- Prominent injury of tubular epithelial cells
- Interstitial inflammation not prominent

Polyomavirus Nephritis
- Prominent plasmacytic interstitial inflammation with tubulitis
- Viral cytopathic effect
- Positive SV40 immunohistochemistry

DIAGNOSTIC CHECKLIST

Pathologic Interpretation Pearls
- Clinical correlation and serologic testing needed to confirm diagnosis

SELECTED REFERENCES

1. Tsai JD et al: Epstein-Barr virus-associated acute renal failure: diagnosis, treatment, and follow-up. Pediatr Nephrol. 18(7):667-74, 2003
2. Cataudella JA et al: Epstein-Barr virus-associated acute interstitial nephritis: infection or immunologic phenomenon?. Nephron. 92(2):437-9, 2002
3. Norwood VF et al: Unexplained acute renal failure in a toddler: a rare complication of Epstein-Barr virus. Pediatr Nephrol. 17(8):628-32, 2002
4. Okada H et al: An atypical pattern of Epstein-Barr virus infection in a case with idiopathic tubulointerstitial nephritis. Nephron. 92(2):440-4, 2002
5. Lei PS et al: Acute renal failure: unusual complication of Epstein-Barr virus-induced infectious mononucleosis. Clin Infect Dis. 31(6):1519-24, 2000
6. Becker JL et al: Epstein-Barr virus infection of renal proximal tubule cells: possible role in chronic interstitial nephritis. J Clin Invest. 104(12):1673-81, 1999

IMAGE GALLERY

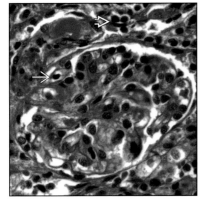 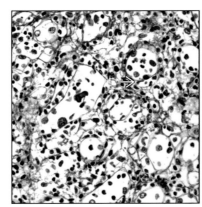 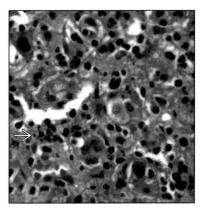

(Left) Occasional circulating leukocytes ⇨ in glomerular capillaries are present in a male toddler with an acute EBV infection. Interstitial inflammation ⇨ surrounds a normal glomerulus. (Courtesy H. Cathro, MD.) *(Center)* EBV-LMP shows a lymphocyte ⇨ in a peritubular capillary with faint positive (brown) staining, but most cells are negative. (Courtesy H. Cathro, MD.) *(Right)* Diffuse interstitial inflammation and nuclear atypia in tubular cells ⇨ are seen in a male toddler with acute EBV infection. (Courtesy H. Cathro, MD.)

HANTAVIRUS NEPHROPATHY

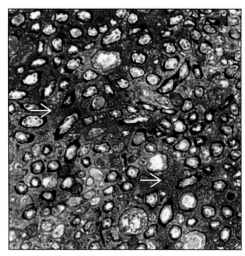

Periodic acid-Schiff of a case of Puumala hantavirus infection shows abundant interstitial hemorrhage ➡ spreading apart the renal tubules. (Courtesy D. Ferluga, MD.)

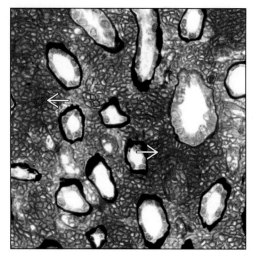

Periodic acid-Schiff of a case of Puumala hantavirus infection shows abundant interstitial hemorrhage ➡. (Courtesy D. Ferluga, MD.)

TERMINOLOGY

Abbreviations
- Hantavirus pulmonary syndrome (HPS)
- Hantavirus nephropathy (HVN)

Synonyms
- Hemorrhagic fever with renal syndrome (HFRS)
- *Nephropathia epidemica*: Milder form of HFRS

Definitions
- Acute renal failure caused by HVN
- HVN or HVN-like syndrome caused by Old World (Hantaan, Dobra, Seoul, and Puumala) and New World (Sin Nombre) viruses

ETIOLOGY/PATHOGENESIS

Environmental Exposure
- Humans infected by inhaling aerosolized host rodent excreta

Infectious Agents
- ~ 30 strains (> 20 of which are pathogenic) of hantaviruses
  - Belong to Bunyaviridae family
- Hantaan virus
  - From striped field mouse (*Apodemus agrarius*)
  - Severe HFRS in Far East Russia, China, and Korea
- Seoul virus
  - From gray rat (*Rattus norvegicus*)
  - Moderate HFRS seen worldwide and most common HVN in United States
- Dobravirus
  - Carried by yellow-necked field mouse (*Apodemus flavicollis*)
  - Genetically and serologically related virus initially isolated in Slovenia
  - Severe HFRS in central and southeastern Europe (Balkans)

- Puumala virus
  - Carried by black vole (*Clethrionomys glareolus*)
  - 5,000 people annually with milder form of HFRS with lower mortality (< 1%)
  - Throughout Europe (Balkans, Scandinavia, and Russia)
- Sin Nombre virus
  - Western USA
  - Carried by deer mouse (*Peromyscus maniculatus*)
  - Causes hantavirus pulmonary syndrome (HPS), primarily affecting lungs

Microvascular/Immune System Interaction
- Endothelial cells, macrophages, and dendritic cells are infected
- Cytokine release (interleukins, tumor necrosis factor [TNF]-α, vascular endothelial growth factor [VEGF], and γ-interferon)
- Severe microvascular injury and hemorrhage

CLINICAL ISSUES

Epidemiology
- Incidence
  - ~ 150,000/year worldwide
  - Rare in USA, positive Seoul virus serum antibodies in urban USA residents is < 1%

Presentation
- HFRS has several phases
  - Febrile (3-5 days) with fever/chills, hypotensive (hours to 2 days), oliguric (few days to weeks), polyuric (diuretic, occurs in some cases), and convalescent
- Proteinuria
  - Severe tubular proteinuria with low urine specific gravity
- Hematologic abnormalities: Disseminated intravascular coagulation (DIC) with thrombocytopenia and petechiae

HANTAVIRUS NEPHROPATHY

Key Facts

Terminology
- Old World and New World viruses syndromes
- Hantaan virus and Dobravirus types are primary examples
- Hemorrhagic renal failure syndrome (HFRS) seen in kidney involvement

Etiology/Pathogenesis
- Humans typically infected by inhaling aerosolized rodent excreta

- Flu-like syndrome leads to severe multiorgan hemorrhagic microvascular involvement with shock

Microscopic Pathology
- Interstitial inflammation, hemorrhage, or fibrosis
- Acute tubular injury/necrosis
- Membranoproliferative or diffuse proliferative glomerulonephritis
- EM may be useful in demonstrating viral nucleocapsid or ultrastructural injury

- Edema
  - Vascular leak syndrome leads to periorbital edema, retroperitoneal fluid accumulation, hemoconcentration, and postural hypotension
- Nausea/vomiting
- Abdominal/back pain and myalgias
- Photophobia

Prognosis
- Mortality rate of 5-15% for Hantaan and Dobravirus, 1-5% for Seoul, 0.1-1% for Puumala, and > 50% for Sin Nombre

MICROSCOPIC PATHOLOGY

Histologic Features
- Interstitium
  - Acute interstitial nephritis with predominance of lymphocytic inflammation and admixed neutrophils
  - Interstitial inflammation and tubular atrophy occurs 1st with interstitial fibrosis being a late finding
  - Interstitial hemorrhage
- Necrosis
  - Acute tubular injury/necrosis is often present
- Glomerulonephritis, diffuse
  - Mesangial hypercellularity may first be observed
  - Diffuse proliferative or membranoproliferative glomerulonephritis in small number of cases

ANCILLARY TESTS

Electron Microscopy
- Transmission
  - Bunyaviridae are 100 nm in diameter, round or oval viruses with double-layered lipid envelopes with protruding spikes
  - Nucleocapsid composed of hollow microfilaments or dense granules
  - Golgi apparatus enlarged in infected cells
  - Peritubular capillaries engorged with red blood cells
  - Necrotizing endothelial injury and destruction with extravasated red blood cells in interstitium

SELECTED REFERENCES

1. Ferluga D et al: Hantavirus nephropathy. J Am Soc Nephrol. 19(9):1653-8, 2008
2. Weiss M et al: Pyelonephritis and other infections, reflux nephropathy, hydronephrosis, and nephrolithiasis. In Jennette JC et al: Heptinstall's Pathology of the Kidney. 6th ed. Philadelphia: Lippincott Williams & Wilkins. 991-1081, 2007
3. Tai PW et al: Hanta hemorrhagic fever with renal syndrome: a case report and review. J Microbiol Immunol Infect. 38(3):221-3, 2005
4. Peters CJ et al: Spectrum of hantavirus infection: hemorrhagic fever with renal syndrome and hantavirus pulmonary syndrome. Annu Rev Med. 50:531-45, 1999

IMAGE GALLERY

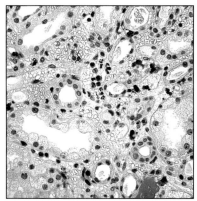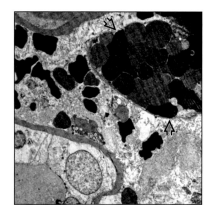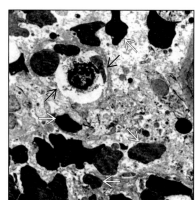

(Left) A mixed interstitial inflammatory infiltrate in Puumala hantavirus infection is shown with a dual immunohistochemical staining for CD8(+) T cells (brown) and CD68(+) (KP-1) (red) monocytes/macrophages. (Courtesy D. Ferluga, MD.) *(Center)* EM shows a congested peritubular capillary with hemorrhage of red blood cells into the interstitium. (Courtesy D. Ferluga, MD.) *(Right)* EM shows necrotizing destruction of the endothelium of peritubular capillaries with hemorrhage of red blood cells into the interstitium. (Courtesy D. Ferluga, MD.)

Developmental and Cystic Diseases

Disease of Development

Cystic Diseases

CLASSIFICATION OF CONGENITAL ANOMALIES OF THE KIDNEY AND URINARY TRACT

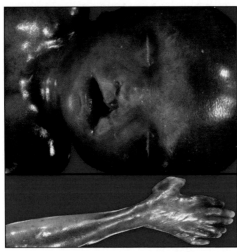

Gross images depict extrarenal manifestations of Spitz-Lemli-Opitz syndrome. Note the dysmorphic facial features (cleft palate), syndactyly, and polydactyl.

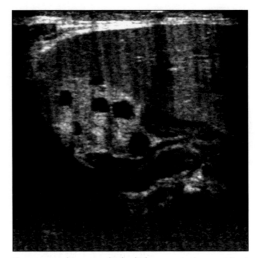

Sonogram shows multiple kidney cysts in a patient with prune belly syndrome (cryptorchidism, abdominal muscle maldevelopment, CAKUT).

TERMINOLOGY

Definitions
- Defective development of kidney and urinary tract, often referred to as congenital anomalies of kidney or lower urinary tract (CAKUT)

ETIOLOGY/PATHOGENESIS

Developmental Anomaly
- CAKUT can occur singly or in combinations as a syndrome
  - Categories
    - Renal hypoplasia: Small, architecturally normal kidneys
    - Renal agenesis or aplasia: No kidney formation or involution after early branching
    - Renal dysplasia: Architecturally abnormal kidneys with blastema elements and immature nephrons
    - Duplicated collecting system: Partial or complete duplication of ureter with distinct orifices into bladder
    - Ectopic kidneys or malrotation: Abnormal location
    - Multicystic dysplasia: Cysts of various sizes across kidney parenchyma and renal dysplasia
    - Duplex or multiple kidneys: Initiation of more than 1 kidney
    - Horseshoe or fused kidneys: Joining in the midline, complete or partial
    - Ureteropelvic junctional (UPJ) abnormalities and hydronephrosis: Proximal narrowing of ureter, dilatation of pelvis
    - Megaureter: Large, tortuous, dilated
    - Hydroureter: Dilated ureter
    - Vesicoureteral reflux (VUR): Backflow of urine from bladder to ureter
    - Ureterovesicle junction (UVJ) abnormalities: Narrowing or obstruction of distal ureter-bladder junction
    - Ureterocele: Ureter ending blindly into bladder
    - Posterior urethral valves (PUV): Malpositioned or abnormally developed urethral valves, leads to urinary reflux
- Multisystem involvement due to genes important in developmental processes of multiple organs
- Causes
  - Toxins or environmental exposure
    - Dioxins (agent orange): Hydronephrosis
  - Medications
  - Familial or inherited; inheritance may be simple or complex
    - Mendelian: Autosomal recessive or dominant, X-linked
    - Non-Mendelian: Epigenetic, modifier genes with incomplete penetrance and variable expressivity
  - Spontaneous or de novo mutations
- Etiological classification according to different steps in early kidney development
  - Pronephros and mesonephros defects
    - Nephric duct growth and maturation defects: Renal agenesis, ureter and collecting system defects, male gonadal duct (vas deferens)
    - Failure to repress anterior buds: Supernumerary ureters, gonadal descent defects
  - Metanephros defects
    - Ureteric bud (UB) induction: Renal agenesis, hypoplasia
    - Branching morphogenesis: Hypoplasia, dysplasia, cysts, tubulogenesis defects, glomerulogenesis defects; encompasses reciprocal interactions among all 3 major components: UB, mesenchyme, and stroma
  - Ureter or UGS maturation defects
    - Proximal or upper ureter: UPJ, hydronephrosis, bifid ureters

- Distal or lower urinary tract: UVJ, VUR, megaureter, hydroureter, ureterocele, PUV
  - ○ Position abnormalities
    - Failure to ascend or rotate: Ectopic kidneys, horseshoe kidneys, crossed renal ectopy
  - ○ Factors extrinsic to kidney primordia
    - Lateral mesoderm and notochord: Ectopic kidneys, fusion, WD maturation, horseshoe kidneys

Genes and Syndromes Associated with CAKUT and Extrarenal Manifestations

- Townes-Brocks syndrome: *SAL1*; limb, sensorineural hearing loss, anal atresia, CAKUT
- CAKUT-Hirschsprung disease or MEN2A: *RET*; intestinal aganglionosis, medullary thyroid carcinoma, pheochromocytoma, CAKUT
- Hypothyroidism deafness, renal (HDR) syndrome: *GATA3*
- Renal cyst and diabetes syndrome (RCAD): *TCF2*, *HNF1B*; glomerulocystic kidney disease, CAKUT, *MODY5* diabetes, genital defects
- Fraser syndrome: *FRAS1*, *FREM2*; syndactyly, cryptophthalmos, renal agenesis, hypoplasia/dysplasia
- Meckel-Gruber: *MKS1*, *MKS3*; polydactyly, liver malformations, encephalocele, renal dysplasia, cysts
- Simpson Golabi Behmel: *GPC3*; somatic overgrowth, tumors, CAKUT
- Kallmann syndrome: *KAL1*; hypogonadotropic hypogonadism, anosmia, renal agenesis
- RHD: *BMP4*, *SIX2*; microphthalmia, cleft lip, renal hypo/dysplasia
- Prune belly syndrome: Gene not known; cryptorchidism, abdominal muscle maldevelopment, CAKUT
- Wolf-Hirschhorn or 4p deletion syndrome: Deletion of end of 4p; dysmorphic facial features, delayed growth, intellectual disability, CAKUT
- Bardet-Biedl syndrome: Many cilia genes; retinopathy, digital anomalies, obesity, male hypogonadism, renal dysplasia
- Fanconi anemia: DNA repair pathway genes *FANCA-M*; anemia, AML, limb malformations, CAKUT
- Smith-Lemli-Opitz syndrome: Cholesterol biosynthesis (*DHCR7*); dysmorphic facial features, microcephaly, syndactyly, mental retardation, dysplastic kidneys
- Branchio-oto-renal syndrome (BOR): *EYA1*, *SIX1*, *SIX5*, *MYOG*; deafness, branchial cysts, CAKUT
- Renal coloboma syndrome: *PAX2*; retinal coloboma, CAKUT

EPIDEMIOLOGY

Incidence
- Reported in 0.5-1% live births; likely an underestimation
- Incidence varies by malformation type
- 25% of ESRD patients have CAKUT

Age Range
- Most diagnosed in utero or perinatally

- Subtle defects may go undetected and present later in life

Gender
- Some malformations have gender preferences
  - ○ PUV only in males
  - ○ VUR more common in females

Ethnicity Relationship
- Affects individuals of any race or ethnicity

CLINICAL IMPLICATIONS

Clinical Presentation
- In utero
  - ○ Oligohydramnios
  - ○ IUGR
  - ○ Routine imaging
- Postnatal
  - ○ Multiple UTI
  - ○ Uremia
  - ○ Renal failure
  - ○ Hypertension
  - ○ Stones
- Clinical issues
  - ○ Spontaneous resolution
  - ○ Surgical/urologic correction
  - ○ Genetic counseling
  - ○ Stricture, scarring, recurrence
  - ○ Medical: Dialysis

MACROSCOPIC FINDINGS

General Features
- Various depending on phenotype
- Upper tract may be secondarily affected due to lower tract anomaly or may be affected independent of lower tract defects

MICROSCOPIC FINDINGS

General Features
- Various depending on phenotype

SELECTED REFERENCES

1. Song R et al: Genetics of congenital anomalies of the kidney and urinary tract. Pediatr Nephrol. 26(3):353-64, 2011
2. Hildebrandt F: Genetic kidney diseases. Lancet. 375(9722):1287-95, 2010
3. Kerecuk L et al: Renal tract malformations: perspectives for nephrologists. Nat Clin Pract Nephrol. 4(6):312-25, 2008
4. Winyard P et al: Dysplastic kidneys. Semin Fetal Neonatal Med. 13(3):142-51, 2008
5. Vize PD et al: The Kidney: From Normal Development to Congenital Disease. London: Academic Press. 2003

CLASSIFICATION OF CONGENITAL ANOMALIES OF THE KIDNEY AND URINARY TRACT

CAKUT Classification Based on Embryology

(Left) Illustration shows renal malformations due to Wolffian duct (WD) or mesonephros maturation defects. Increased net signaling from the WD can result in supernumerary ureteric buds (UBs) or duplicated collecting systems. *(Right)* Induction defects or net decreased WD maturation or growth can lead to renal agenesis or hypoplasia. Main reasons include failure of distal WD growth, UB induction defects causing failure of UB induction, or malpositioning of UB.

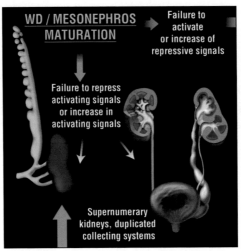

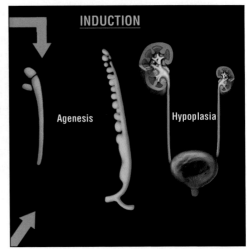

(Left) Illustration summarizes normal kidney development stages: Pronephros, caudal extension of WD during mesonephros, induction of ureteric bud (UB) in metanephros followed by branching morphogenesis and ascent. Distal ureter maturation also ensures its normal entry into the bladder. *(Right)* Branching morphogenesis defects can cause hypoplasia (reduced nephrons) or dysplasia (abnormally patterned) due to aberrant reciprocal interactions and differentiation defects.

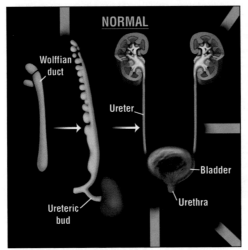

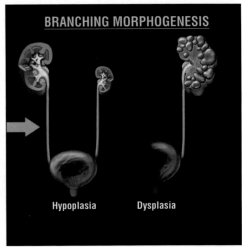

(Left) Graphic shows the spectrum of malformations that can result from ureter or urogenital sinus (UGS) maturation defects affecting both the upper and lower urinary tract. Megaureter may result from any of the lower tract abnormalities. *(Right)* Graphic shows renal malformations resulting from defects in ascent or malrotation during kidney development.

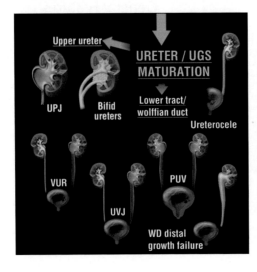

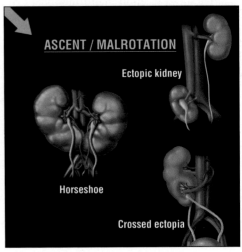

6

Renal Malformation Syndromes

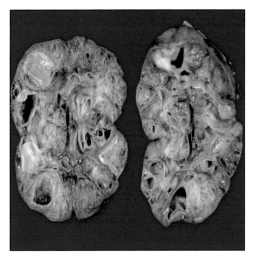
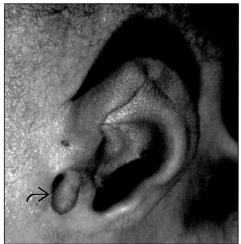

(Left) Cut surface of kidneys depict macroscopic features of Meckel-Gruber Syndrome. Note enlarged kidney with multiple cysts, histologically confirmed to be multicystic dysplasia. *(Right)* Preauricular tag ⮡ can be seen frequently in renal malformation syndromes such as branchio-oto-renal and 4p deletion syndrome.

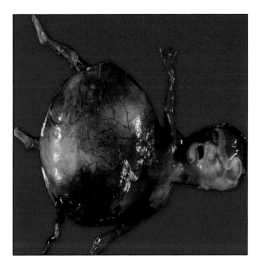
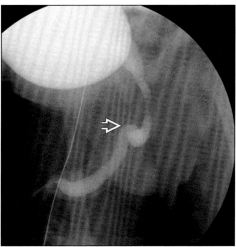

(Left) Fetopsy shows massively distended abdomen in prune belly syndrome. Normally these patients have a shriveled appearance of abdomen due to muscle maldevelopment; however, this fetus had dilated bladder distending the abdomen, thus masking the typical abdomen appearance. Other features such as cryptorchidism and renal dysplasia were also seen in this case. *(Right)* Voiding cystoureterogram shows tortuous urethra ⮞ and distended bladder in prune belly syndrome.

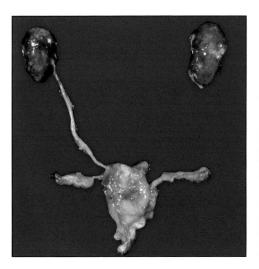
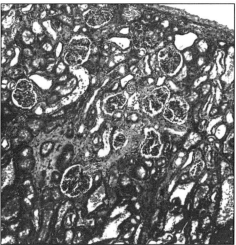

(Left) Gross dissection of the urogenital system from a patient with chromosome 4p deletion syndrome shows bilateral hypoplastic kidneys. The ureter on the right was removed before the photograph. *(Right)* Histology of hypoplastic kidney from a 4p deletion syndrome patient shows normal kidney architecture but fewer glomerular generations (3-4), as opposed to 13-14 in a normal kidney.

6

DYSPLASIA/HYPOPLASIA/AGENESIS

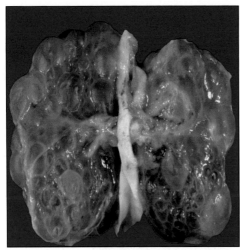

Gross photograph shows massively enlarged, bilateral dysplastic kidneys. Dysplastic kidneys may be diffusely cystic (multicystic), as apparent in this example, and present as abdominal masses.

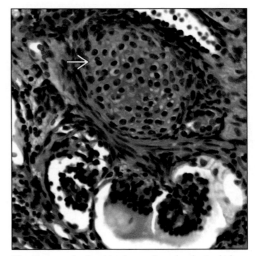

Shown here is the histology of a dysplastic kidney with metaplastic cartilage ➡, bordering an area with immature glomeruli in a case with focal dysplasia.

TERMINOLOGY

Abbreviations
• Metanephric mesenchyme (MM)
• Ureteric bud (UB)

Definitions
• Renal hypoplasia: Small, architecturally normal kidneys with decreased number of nephrons below 2 standard deviations of age-matched normal kidneys
• Renal agenesis: Absent kidney due to abolished kidney induction
• Renal aplasia: Absent or rudimentary kidneys, initially induced but involuted after early branching
• Renal dysplasia: Architecturally abnormal kidneys with immature nephrons, incompletely branched ducts, and undifferentiated stroma, occasionally with metaplastic cartilage

ETIOLOGY/PATHOGENESIS

Developmental Anomaly
• Defects during different steps of kidney development

Genetic
• Familial or inherited
• Spontaneous or de novo mutations

In Utero Urinary Obstruction
• Mechanical: UPJ, ureter obstruction, posterior urethral valves, ectopic distal ureter orifice, abnormal insertion into urinary bladder, prune belly syndrome (thick bladder wall muscle in absence of physical obstruction)
• Functional (e.g., reflux)

Toxins, Environmental Exposure, Drugs
• Vitamin A deficiency or increase
• ACE-1 inhibitors
• Maternal malnutrition
• Maternal iron deficiency

Renal Agenesis
• Pronephros and mesonephros defects
  ○ Nephric duct growth and maturation defects
• Metanephros defects
  ○ UB induction: Failure to form UB or invade MM, early branching
  ○ UB position: Rostral or caudal to normal budding site, inability to invade MM

Renal Hypoplasia
• UB induction: Slow
• UB position: Rostral or caudal, partly invades MM
• Branching morphogenesis: Slow

Renal Dysplasia and Aplasia
• Branching morphogenesis: Inadequate, disorganized, disrupted reciprocal interactions between MM, stroma, and UB

CLINICAL ISSUES

Presentation
• Bilateral agenesis
  ○ Oligohydramnios or ahydramnios by ultrasound
• Unilateral agenesis
  ○ Asymptomatic
  ○ Later secondary FSGS with hypertension, proteinuria
• Dysplasia
  ○ Identified by routine antenatal ultrasound as increased echogenicity
  ○ Abdominal mass
  ○ Entire kidney or only part may be affected
  ○ Multicystic dysplastic kidneys are nonfunctional, often with underdeveloped ureters or ureteral stenosis
• Bilateral hypoplasia may be idiopathic or associated with oligomeganephronia

DYSPLASIA/HYPOPLASIA/AGENESIS

Key Facts

Terminology
- Renal hypoplasia: Small, architecturally normal kidneys, reduced number of nephrons
- Renal agenesis or aplasia: No kidney formation or involution after early branching
- Renal dysplasia: Architecturally abnormal kidneys with varying degree of undifferentiated mesenchyme, stroma, and epithelium

Etiology/Pathogenesis
- Nephric duct growth and maturation defects: Renal agenesis
- UB induction defects: Renal agenesis, hypoplasia
- UB position defects: Renal agenesis, hypoplasia, dysplasia
- Branching morphogenesis defects: Hypoplasia, aplasia, dysplasia

Clinical Issues
- Bilateral renal agenesis: Incompatible with life
- Unilateral renal agenesis: Incidentally identified in adults, document presence of 2 kidneys before nephrectomy
  - Moderate risk of hypertension, proteinuria
  - 50-70% associated with other genitourinary anomalies
  - May show compensatory hypertrophy
- Bilateral small kidneys may be dysplastic

Top Differential Diagnoses
- Renal aplasia
- Renal cystic disease

- The term "hypoplasia" is often loosely used in radiological exams for small kidneys
  - Kidneys that appear grossly or radiographically small may have glomerular cysts and tubular dysgenesis microscopically; may not be truly hypoplastic
- Symptoms and signs in bilateral renal hypoplasia or dysplasia
  - Failure to thrive
  - Growth retardation
  - Hypertension
  - Excessive thirst
  - Increased urine output
  - Kidney failure
  - Salt wasting
- Syndromes associated with renal agenesis or dysplasia or hypoplasia
  - Branchio-oto-renal syndrome (BOR)
  - Renal cysts and diabetes syndrome (RCAD)
  - Fanconi syndrome
  - Kallmann syndrome
  - DiGeorge syndrome
  - Smith-Lemli-Opitz syndrome
  - Hereditary renal adysplasia (unilateral agenesis with contralateral dysplasia)
  - Caudal regression syndrome (imperforate anus, absent bladder, absent urethra)
  - Down syndrome
- Potter sequence
  - Due to oligohydramnios or anhydramnios in some of these conditions, lung hypoplasia ensues, causing neonatal death
  - Musculoskeletal anomalies
    - Wide-set eyes
    - Prominent epicanthal folds
    - Flat nose, ears
    - Limb defects

Prognosis
- Bilateral renal agenesis
  - Stillborn or perinatal death
- Unilateral renal agenesis

- Generally good with no consequences in isolated disease
- Moderate risk of hypertension and proteinuria due to FSGS
- Hypoplasia
  - Bilateral hypoplasia: Most develop end-stage renal disease (ESRD) in mid to late childhood
  - Increased risk of hypertension and heart disease (oligomeganephronia)
- Dysplasia
  - Unilateral: Good prognosis, treat infections and hypertension
  - Routine surgical removal not recommended

MACROSCOPIC FEATURES

Bilateral Agenesis
- Absent kidneys
- Ureters may be absent or truncated
- Hypoplastic lungs

Unilateral Agenesis
- Contralateral kidney may show hypertrophy
- Affected side may have normal, truncated, or absent ureter
- 50-70% associated with other genitourinary anomalies
  - Ureteral ectopia, renal dysplasia, absence of vas deferens, reflux nephropathy

Renal Dysplasia
- Small, normal, or slightly enlarged kidneys with randomly distributed cysts (multicystic)
- Loss of reniform shape
- 50-70% may have contralateral kidney defects
- Often associated with other lower urinary tract anomalies (ureterocele, posterior urethral valves, hydronephrosis)

Renal Hypoplasia
- Weight usually less than 50%
- Normal architecture
- Decreased renal lobes

- May accompany renal artery hypoplasia
- Simple hypoplasia
  - Bilateral greater than unilateral
  - Usually no hypertrophy
  - Reduced kidney volume
- Oligomeganephronia
  - Hypertrophy of nephrons, which are decreased in number

MICROSCOPIC PATHOLOGY

Histologic Features

- Histology is gold standard to correctly classify these anomalies; however, biopsies are rarely done and diagnosis is mainly from radiological studies, nephrectomies, and autopsies
- Unilateral renal agenesis
  - Normal or compensatory hypertrophy
- Renal hypoplasia
  - Normal organization into cortex, medulla, and papillae
  - Simple hypoplasia: Normal histology
    - May see secondary glomerulosclerosis in severe cases
  - Oligomeganephronia: Glomeruli may be 3x larger than normal
- Renal dysplasia
  - Dysplasia may be segmental (more frequently in adults), diffuse (almost always in children), or zonal (affecting outer cortex, most recently formed)
    - Reduced number of nephrons
    - Thinned cortex (zonal dysplasia)
  - Dysplastic areas have little or no proximal nephron components (glomeruli, proximal, distal tubules), only primitive collecting ducts/cysts (ureteric bud)
    - Disorganized architecture with no definitive cortex or medulla
    - Undifferentiated mesenchyme
    - Focal or diffuse cysts
    - Smooth muscle collarettes surrounding primitive collecting ducts
    - Nodules of cartilage in 30%
    - Immature and disorganized tubules may be present, adjacent to dysplastic areas

Cytologic Features

- Reduced epithelial proliferation
- Increased apoptosis
- Cell differentiation defects

DIFFERENTIAL DIAGNOSIS

Renal Agenesis

- Renal aplasia: Solitary kidneys may have contralateral renal aplasia (not true agenesis); kidneys were induced but regressed or involuted with time
- Renal dysplasia: Dysplastic kidneys may regress over time, making it difficult to differentiate from agenesis
  - Need radiology evaluation during embryogenesis and perinatally to rule out dysplasia in child or adult with solitary kidney

Renal Dysplasia

- Renal cystic diseases: May show dysplastic features (glomerulocystic, multicystic dysplasia)
  - Correlate with histological pattern, kidney size, other organ involvement, and genetics
  - Polycystic kidney disease (early onset ADPKD, ARPKD)
  - Primary glomerulocystic kidney disease (autosomal dominant)
- Reflux nephropathy
  - Medulla more affected than cortex
  - Uretero pelvic junction obstruction (UPJO), uretero vesicle junction obstruction (UVJO), ureterocele, posterior urethral valves, vesico ureteral reflux (VUR)

Renal Hypoplasia

- Acquired kidney disease
- Aplastic kidney
- Secondary damage: If radiographic exam with contrast shows scarring, calyceal clubbing
- Small kidneys due to dysplasia or atrophy

SELECTED REFERENCES

1. Kerecuk L et al: Renal tract malformations: perspectives for nephrologists. Nat Clin Pract Nephrol. 4(6):312-25, 2008
2. Liapis H et al: Cystic diseases and developmental kidney defects. In Jennette JC et al: Heptinstall's Pathology of the Kidney. 6th ed. Philadelphia: Lippincott Williams & Wilkins. 1257-1306, 2007
3. Jain S et al: Mice expressing a dominant-negative Ret mutation phenocopy human Hirschsprung disease and delineate a direct role of Ret in spermatogenesis. Development. 131(21):5503-13, 2004
4. Vize P et al: The Kidney: From Normal Development to Congenital Disease. London: Academic Press. 2003
5. Hiraoka M et al: Renal aplasia is the predominant cause of congenital solitary kidneys. Kidney Int. 61(5):1840-4, 2002

Main Characteristics of Dysplasia, Hypoplasia, and Agenesis

	Dysplasia	Hypoplasia	Agenesis
Definition	Disorganized architecture, undifferentiated mesenchyme and stroma, abnormal branching	Small, architecturally normal kidney; reduced nephrons	Absent kidney
Incidence	1:7,500 (unilateral), 1:7,500 (bilateral)	1:1,000 (unilateral), 1:4,000 (bilateral)	1:1,000 male = female, left > right (unilateral); 1:10,000 male > female (bilateral)
Mechanism	Defective branching morphogenesis	Slow UB induction, reduced branching, incorrect UB position	WD development defect, UB induction failure
Ultrasonogram findings	Noncommunicating hypoechogenic cysts, small kidney	Small kidney	Absent kidney
Prognosis	Perinatal death or ESRD (if bilateral), normal outcome if unilateral (risk of FSGS)	Most ESRD (bilateral), normal outcome if unilateral (risk of FSGS)	Perinatal death (bilateral), normal outcome if unilateral (risk of FSGS)
Macroscopic	Nonreniform, multicystic; small, normal, or large size	Small, normally shaped kidneys, reduced number of pyramids	No kidneys, earlobe shape, elongated adrenals
Microscopic	Disorganized parenchyma, immature glomeruli and tubules, smooth muscle collarettes around collecting ducts, metaplastic cartilage (30%)	Normal organization, large nephrons in oligomeganephronia	Normal or compensatory hypertrophy in unilateral agenesis

Gross and Histologic Features of Hypoplasia, Agenesis

(Left) This is the gross appearance of the urinary tract from a 4-month-old baby, showing the left unilateral agenesis ➡ and right hydronephrosis ➡. *(Right)* Gross appearance of urinary tract depicts left renal agenesis and right small dysplastic cystic kidney ➡.

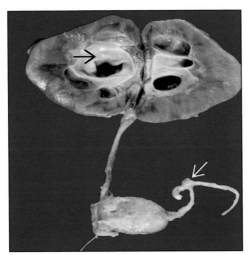 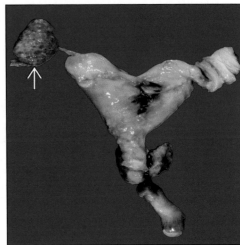

(Left) Adrenal glands from a baby with bilateral renal agenesis are shown. Note the elongated "ear-shaped" large adrenal glands due to the absence of caudal resistance by the kidneys. *(Right)* Shown here are severely hypoplastic lungs ➡ in a baby due to oligohydramnios resulting from bilateral renal agenesis.

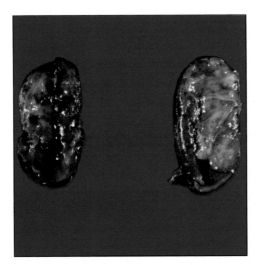 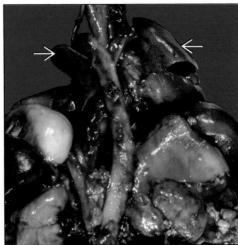

(Left) Urinary tract of a mutant mouse with reduced receptor tyrosine kinase Ret signaling shows unilateral agenesis ➡ and a hypoplastic kidney ➡. Ret is expressed in the ureteric bud and is involved with ureteric branching. Mutations in Ret are found in 35% of patients with renal agenesis. *(Right)* Histological section of hypoplastic kidney from a mouse with decreased Ret signaling shows preserved organization of cortex, medulla, and papilla. An adrenal gland is seen lying on top of the kidney.

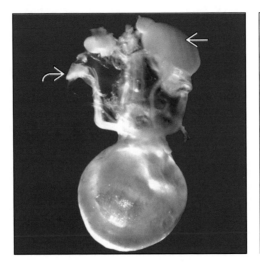 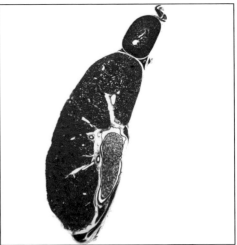

Gross and Histological Features of Dysplasia

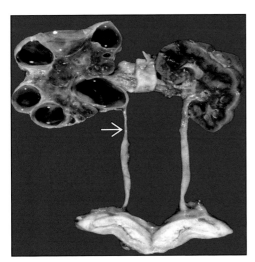
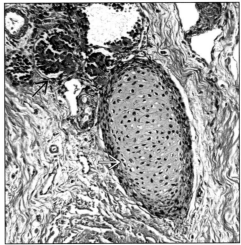

(Left) Shown is the coronal section of the urinary tract from a patient with right multicystic dysplasia and proximal ureter stenosis ➡. The left kidney section shows normal architecture with a well-formed cortex and medulla and a normal ureter. Intrauterine obstruction is a common cause of dysplasia. (Right) Dysplastic kidney with metaplastic cartilage ➡ and an adjacent primitive glomerulus ➡ is shown.

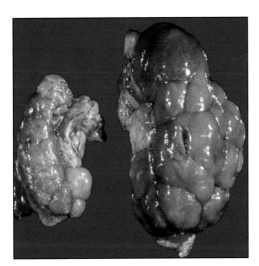
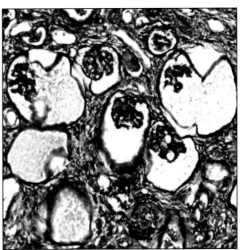

(Left) Gross photograph shows a small right kidney compared to the normal left kidney. The small kidney showed histological changes of glomerulocystic dysplasia and had UPJ obstruction. (Right) Histological section of small kidney shows glomerulocystic dysplasia. Note that cyst size inversely correlates with the cellular component of the glomeruli, eventually leading to complete cystic replacement of the glomerulus.

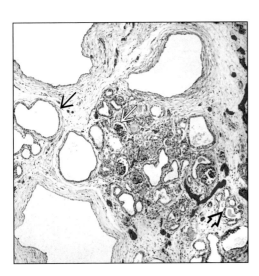
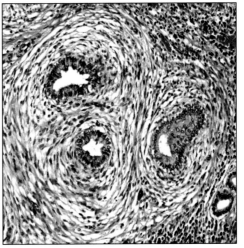

(Left) Histological section of a dysplastic kidney shows a lack of organization of kidney parenchyma into cortex, medulla, and papilla. Note the random arrangement of immature kidney elements with scattered dilated and atrophic tubules ➡, immature glomeruli ➡, and undifferentiated collecting ducts ➡. (Right) Dysplastic kidney shows underdeveloped collecting ducts surrounded by smooth muscle-like collarettes.

OLIGOMEGANEPHRONIA

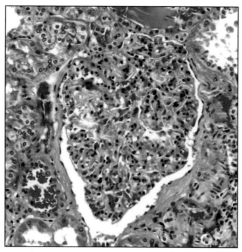

The hallmark of oligomeganephronia (OMN) is hypertrophy of the glomeruli due to a compensatory response to a congenital deficiency of nephrons. Glomeruli also have mesangial hypercellularity.

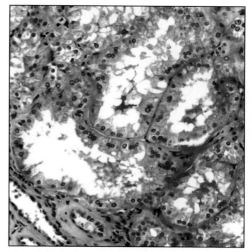

The tubules in OMN respond to congenitally decreased nephron numbers by increasing their diameter, as shown in these hypertrophied proximal tubules.

TERMINOLOGY

Abbreviations
- Oligomeganephronia (OMN)

Synonyms
- Oligomeganephronic hypoplasia

Definitions
- Renal hypoplasia with marked compensatory nephron hypertrophy occurring both sporadically and due to specific genetic disorders

ETIOLOGY/PATHOGENESIS

Sporadic (Most Common)
- Occasional *PAX2* mutations, but in most cases etiology is unknown
- Prematurity and low birth weight

Genetic Disorders (Rare)
- Papillorenal syndrome (OMIM 120330), a.k.a. renal-coloboma syndrome
  - *PAX2* mutation in 50%
    - Associated with optic disc/nerve abnormality
    - Autosomal dominant, chromosome 10q
- Wolf-Hirschhorn syndrome (OMIM 194190)
  - Monosomy 4p, multiple congenital anomalies
- Branchio-oto-renal syndrome (OMIM 113650, 610896, and 600963), a.k.a. Melnick-Fraser syndrome
  - Brachial fistulae/clefts, ear malformations, and OMN
  - *EYA1* (40%), *SIX5*, and *SIX1* genes combined are involved in about 50% of all cases
  - Autosomal dominant
- *HNF-1B* mutations
- Acrorenal syndrome (OMIM 102520)

Pathogenesis
- Abnormal nephron development

- *PAX2, EYA1, SIX* transcription factors and *HNF-1B* are necessary for normal kidney development
- Reduced branching morphogenesis and induction of nephrons
- Secondary FSGS and progression to ESRD

CLINICAL ISSUES

Presentation
- Growth retardation
- Vomiting
- Polydipsia, polyuria
- Enuresis

Natural History
- Renal function is usually stable for a few years, but later deteriorates to ESRD
  - May present as ESRD at birth
- Proteinuria, a consequence of secondary FSGS

Treatment
- ACE inhibitors may slow progression
- Transplantation

Prognosis
- Poor: Renal failure in late childhood to early adulthood

IMAGE FINDINGS

Ultrasonographic Findings
- Small, hyperechoic kidneys, most often bilateral

MACROSCOPIC FEATURES

General Features
- Number of renal lobes is reduced (1-5)
- Surface is smooth to finely granular
- Parenchyma is pale and firm

OLIGOMEGANEPHRONIA

Key Facts

Etiology/Pathogenesis

- Reduced nephron formation during development leads to nephron hypertrophy, secondary FSGS, and eventually ESRD
- Most cases sporadic, some related to mutations in *PAX2*, *EYA1*, *SIX1*, *SIX5*, or *HNF-1B*

Macroscopic Features

- Small, dense kidneys with reduced number of renal lobes

Microscopic Pathology

- Fewer than normal glomeruli
- Hypertrophy of remaining glomeruli and proximal tubules
- Focal interstitial fibrosis and tubular atrophy
- Secondary FSGS

Top Differential Diagnoses

- Nephronophthisis
- Dysplasia

---

   o Overall shape may be rounded

Size

- < 50% of expected weight, bilateral

MICROSCOPIC PATHOLOGY

Histologic Features

- Reduced nephron number with little atrophy or scarring
- Glomerular hypertrophy (increased diameter, cell number)
- Proximal tubule hypertrophy (increased diameter, cell size, cell number)
- Interstitial fibrosis and tubular atrophy are usually only focal
- Secondary FSGS lesions may be evident

Predominant Pattern/Injury Type

- Nephron hypertrophy

Predominant Cell/Compartment Type

- Multiple

DIFFERENTIAL DIAGNOSIS

Nephronophthisis

- OMN does not have prominent cysts or TBM duplication
- Autosomal recessive inheritance of nephronophthisis

Dysplasia

- OMN lacks dysplastic elements (cartilage, smooth muscle, immature tubules)

DIAGNOSTIC CHECKLIST

Clinically Relevant Pathologic Features

- FSGS lesions
- Underlying molecular defects

SELECTED REFERENCES

1. Bohn S et al: Distinct molecular and morphogenetic properties of mutations in the human HNF1beta gene that lead to defective kidney development. J Am Soc Nephrol. 14(8):2033-41, 2003
2. Sagen JV et al: Enlarged nephrons and severe nondiabetic nephropathy in hepatocyte nuclear factor-1beta (HNF-1beta) mutation carriers. Kidney Int. 64(3):793-800, 2003
3. Salomon R et al: PAX2 mutations in oligomeganephronia. Kidney Int. 59(2):457-62, 2001
4. Park SH et al: Oligomeganephronia associated with 4p deletion type chromosomal anomaly. Pediatr Pathol. 13(6):731-40, 1993
5. Miltényi M et al: A new variant of the acrorenal syndrome associated with bilateral oligomeganephronic hypoplasia. Eur J Pediatr. 142(1):40-3, 1984

IMAGE GALLERY

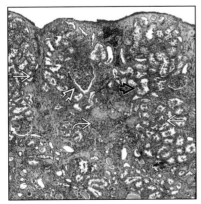 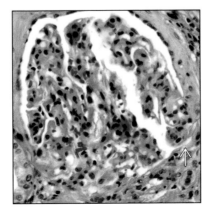 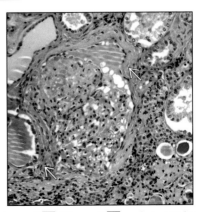

(Left) In OMN the number of glomeruli is low, as shown here by the presence of just 2 levels of glomeruli ➤. Glomeruli ➤ are hypertrophied. Tubules have an increased diameter ➤. Patchy fibrosis and atrophy ➤ become prominent as secondary FSGS develops. *(Center)* Secondary FSGS in OMN is shown. This glomerulus has a focal adhesion to Bowman capsule ➤. *(Right)* A glomerulus with secondary FSGS in OMN is shown. Evidence of proteinuria can be seen in Bowman space and the tubules ➤.

ECTOPIA, MALROTATION, DUPLICATION, FUSION, SUPERNUMERARY KIDNEY

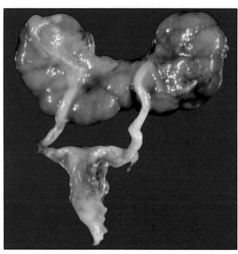

Gross photograph shows horseshoe kidney. Note the fusion of the 2 kidneys at the lower pole.

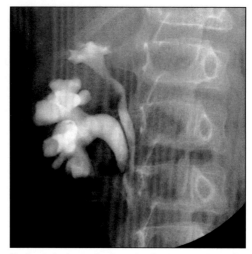

Radiograph shows duplicated collecting system, in this case arising from bifid ureters. The lower ureter shows hydronephrosis.

TERMINOLOGY

Definitions

- Ectopia: Kidneys not located in renal fossa
- Malrotation: Normally located but abnormally rotated on its long axis
- Fusion: Fusion of renal parenchyma, including capsule
- Duplication: Duplication of ureter or entire collecting system
- Supernumerary kidney: Extra kidney or ureteric buds

ETIOLOGY/PATHOGENESIS

Developmental Anomaly

- Failure to ascend
  - Ectopia
    - Simple ectopia: Ipsilateral to pelvis
    - Crossed ectopia: Contralateral to ureter entering bladder
  - Malrotation
- Fusion anomalies
  - Horseshoe kidneys: Usually lower pole fused, fibrous tissue at midline
  - Crossed fused renal ectopia: Crosses over and fuses with the contralateral kidney
  - Fused pelvic kidney: Ectopic kidney and fused; may have horseshoe shape
- Nephric duct (ND) or ureter bud (UB)
  - Duplication
    - Partial ureter duplication: Ureter or UB bifurcate before reaching metanephric mesenchyme or prior to branching of UB ampulla
    - Complete ureter or collecting system duplication: 2 UBs from the ND will give 2 ureters and 2 kidneys
  - Supernumerary kidneys
    - Multiple kidneys budding separately or due to growth of multiple UBs into metanephric mesenchyme

Mechanism

- Simple ectopia
  - Ascent failure
- Crossed ectopia
  - Presence of only 1 nephrogenic cord
  - Abnormal ureter migration to contralateral side
  - Abnormal umbilical artery development may prevent ascent, leading to contralateral deviation
- Fusion
  - Abnormal positioning of mesenchyme or nephric ducts (Wolffian ducts); in crossed fused ectopia mesenchyme on only 1 side
- Duplication or supernumerary ureters
  - Failure to repress extra UB outgrowths from nephric duct
  - Overactivity of pathways involved in UB and ureter growth
- Malrotation
  - Failure of medial rotation during ascent, usually resulting in hilum facing anteriorly

CLINICAL ISSUES

Epidemiology

- Incidence
  - Ectopia
    - Simple: 1 in 1,000 (autopsy); 1 in 10,000 (clinical)
    - Solitary crossed renal ectopia: 1 in 1,500,000
  - Fusion
    - Horseshoe: Most common fusion, 1 in 400
    - Crossed fused renal ectopia: 2nd most common, 1 in 2,000
  - Duplication: 1 in 125 in clinical setting; 1 in 25 in postmortem studies
  - Malrotation: 1 in 500
- Age
  - Antenatally, perinatally, or in adulthood
- Gender
  - Duplication: 65% females; 35% males

Key Facts

Etiology/Pathogenesis
- Simple ectopia: Ipsilateral to pelvis
- Crossed ectopia: Contralateral to ureter entering bladder
- Horseshoe kidneys: Usually lower pole fused, fibrous tissue at midline
- Malrotation: Failure of medial rotation during ascent
- Duplication or supernumerary ureters
  - Failure to repress extra ureteric bud (UB) outgrowths from nephric duct
  - Overactivity of pathways involved in UB and ureter growth

Clinical Issues
- Duplication
  - 40% complete
  - 80% with upper pole dilation and ureterocele

- Ectopia, malrotation, fusion anomalies, duplication
  - Usually asymptomatic

Macroscopic Features
- Weigert-Meyer law for duplicated systems
  - Upper ureter enters lower or more distal in outflow tract (inferomedially) in bladder, urethra, or vagina; drains upper pole if kidneys fused
  - Lower ureter (often the normal site) enters superolaterally (higher or more proximal in outflow tract) into bladder; drains lower pole if kidneys fused
- VUR commonly seen, usually lower pole/kidney
- Ureterocele often present in ureter draining upper pole or kidney

Presentation
- Antenatal screening
- Incidentally discovered
- Hydronephrosis
- Vesicoureteral reflux (VUR)
  - 20% could be in ectopic kidney
- Pyelonephritis
- Abdominal pain, cramps
- Mass
- With other syndromes
  - Ectopia
    - Mayer-Rokitansky-Küsher-Hauser syndrome: Female reproductive tract, skeletal, cardiac, urinary, and otologic defects
    - Goldenhar syndrome: Craniofacial, cardiac, pulmonary, or renal defects
    - Treacher Collins syndrome: Craniofacial defects, hearing loss, malformed ears, drooping lower eyelids
- Duplication
  - 20% bilateral
  - 60% bifid ureters
  - 40% complete
  - 80% with upper pole dilation and ureterocele
- Ectopia, malrotation, fusion anomalies, duplication
  - Usually asymptomatic unless other anomalies develop

Treatment
- Possible options
  - Pyeloplasty if VUR present
  - Reconstruction for fused pelvic kidney
  - Antibiotics to reduce UTIs
  - Nephrectomy of ectopic nonfunctional kidney

Prognosis
- Usually no clinical significance
  - Ectopia
    - Blood pressure is usually normal in childhood
    - Ectopic kidney function is reduced, overall function may be normal

- Reflux may resolve if lower grade, but monitor if duplication and high grade
- Duplication
  - Ureteropelvic junction (UPJ)
  - Complete duplication has higher VUR incidence and higher VUR grade
  - Some may develop transitional cell carcinoma

MACROSCOPIC FEATURES

Ectopia
- Simple
  - Kidney usually in pelvis
  - Ureter may be short
- Crossed
  - Ureter crossing to contralateral side from where it enters bladder
  - Ectopic kidney may be fused with orthotopic kidney
- Solitary crossed
  - Single crossed ectopic kidney
- May see VUR or hydronephrosis
- May have anomalous blood supply, derived from distal branches of aorta

Fusion Anomalies
- Many variations
- May see VUR or hydronephrosis
- Horseshoe
  - Frequently lower pole is fused
  - Ureters enter laterally into bladder
  - Fibrous tissue in middle
- Crossed fused renal ectopia
  - Mesenchyme contralateral to ureter bladder insertion and kidney fused
- Fused pelvic kidney

Duplication
- Many variations
  - May see bifid ureters that split into 2 before pelvis
    - Single orifice in bladder
  - Complete duplication: 2 ureters and 2 kidneys
  - Ureter may terminate ectopically (e.g., vagina)

Main Characteristics of Ectopia, Fusion, Malrotation, Duplication, and Supernumerary Kidneys

	Ectopia	Fusion	Malrotation	Duplication	Supernumerary
Definition	Outside renal fossa	Meeting of 2 kidney anlages	Abnormal rotation	More than 1 ureter or collecting system	Extra kidneys or ectopic UBs
Types	Simple, crossed, solitary crossed	Horseshoe, crossed fused, fused pelvic	Not applicable	Bifid ureters, complete duplication	Separate or multiplexed
Incidence	1:1,000 (autopsy); 1:10,000 (clinical)	1:400 (horseshoe); 1:2,000 (crossed fused)	1:500	1:25 (autopsy); 1:125 (clinical)	Rare
Mechanism	Failure to ascent, absence of metanephric mesenchyme on 1 side (crossed), abnormal ureter migration	Abnormal ND or mesenchyme position	Failure of medial rotation during ascent	Failure to repress extra UB from ND, overactivity of ND or UB	Failure to repress extra UB from ND, overactivity of ND or UB
Presentation/ prognosis/ treatment	Usually asymptomatic; may have reflux	Follow if associated UPJ, VUR, pyeloplasty, or reconstruction	Asymptomatic, some hydronephrosis and other anomalies	Follow if VUR or ureterocele, else most may be asymptomatic	Most asymptomatic, evaluate for reflux or hydroureter
Macroscopic	Pelvic kidney, ureter crossing over to contralateral kidney	Lower poles fused, fusion of pelvic kidneys, crossing over and fusing	Posteriorly facing kidneys	Upper UVJ drains lower kidney/pole (may have VUR), ureter from upper kidney/pole enters inferomedially (most have ureterocele)	Extra kidneys, may be fused with normal kidneys

- o May be more than 2 (triplicate)
- Weigert-Meyer law
  - o Upper ureter enters lower or more distally in outflow tract (inferomedially) in bladder, urethra, or vagina; drains upper pole if kidneys fused
  - o Lower ureter (often normal site) enters superolaterally (higher or more proximal in outflow tract) into bladder, drains lower pole if kidneys fused
- Duplex kidney may be more elongated
- VUR commonly seen, usually lower pole/kidney
- Ureterocele often present in ureter, draining upper pole or kidney
- UPJ may be present

Supernumerary Buds
- Extra kidney ectopically located or can fuse with normally located kidney
- Hydroureter or megaureter or VUR may be present

MICROSCOPIC PATHOLOGY

Histologic Features
- Duplex kidneys or supernumerary kidneys may show hypoplasia or dysplasia
- Horseshoe-fused kidneys may show capsule fusion and fibrous septa; parenchyma histologically normal unless associated hydronephrosis or VUR

DIFFERENTIAL DIAGNOSIS

Duplications
- Hydronephrosis
- VUR
- UPJ obstruction
- Solitary renal cyst
- Polycystic kidney disease

DIAGNOSTIC CHECKLIST

Pathologic Interpretation Pearls
- Most cases may be asymptomatic, a reason why incidence in autopsy is higher
- VUR and hydronephrosis may be associated independent anomalies or should be considered as top differential diagnoses

SELECTED REFERENCES

1. Song R et al: Genetics of congenital anomalies of the kidney and urinary tract. Pediatr Nephrol. Epub ahead of print, 2010
2. van den Bosch CM et al: Urological and nephrological findings of renal ectopia. J Urol. 183(4):1574-8, 2010
3. Chen F: Genetic and developmental basis for urinary tract obstruction. Pediatr Nephrol. 24(9):1621-32, 2009
4. Liapis H et al: Cystic diseases and developmental kidney defects. In Jennette JC et al: Heptinstall's Pathology of the Kidney. 6th ed. Philadelphia: Lippincott Williams & Wilkins. 1286-1306, 2007
5. Ichikawa I et al: Paradigm shift from classic anatomic theories to contemporary cell biological views of CAKUT. Kidney Int. 61(3):889-98, 2002
6. Stephens FD et al: Congenital Anomalies of the Kidney, Urinary and Genital Tracts. 2nd ed. New York: Informa Healthcare. 2002
7. Whitten SM et al: Duplex systems. Prenat Diagn. 21(11):952-7, 2001
8. Haddad et al: The Weigert-Meyer Law demystified. JIMA. 28:16-19, 1996
9. N'Guessan G et al: Supernumerary kidney. J Urol. 130(4):649-53, 1983

ECTOPIA, MALROTATION, DUPLICATION, FUSION, SUPERNUMERARY KIDNEY

Ascent, Rotation, and Number Defects

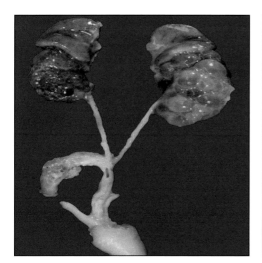

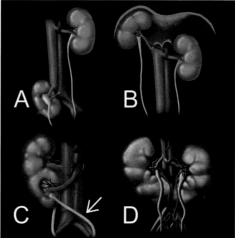

(Left) Gross photograph shows an example of ureter ectopy where 2 ureters are from the same side. Note that both kidneys are small and multicystic. *(Right)* Graphic shows ascent and fusion defects: (A) malrotated ectopic right kidney, (B) ectopic right kidney in thoracic cavity, (C) crossed fused ectopy in which left ureter ⮕ crosses over and the corresponding kidney is small and fused to the orthotopic kidney, and (D) horseshoe kidney with fused lower poles.

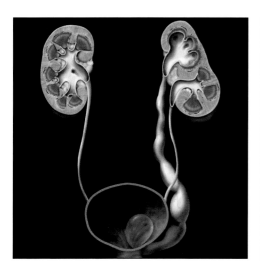

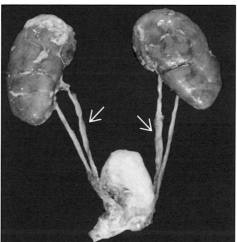

(Left) Illustration depicts complete duplication of the ureters. Note that the ureter attached to the lower pole of the kidney inserts superomedially into the bladder, as predicted by the Weigert-Meyer rule. The ureter attached to the upper pole of the fused kidney is dilated (megaureter). Hydronephrosis is present in the corresponding upper pole of the kidney. *(Right)* Complete bilateral ureteral duplication is shown. The 2 upper pole ureters ⮕ are moderately dilated.

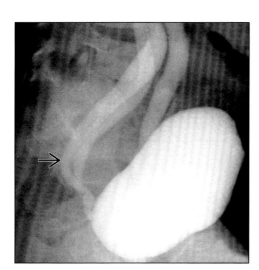

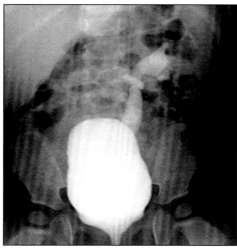

(Left) Radiograph with contrast material in collecting system shows complete bilateral duplication ⮕ in dilated ureters. *(Right)* Voiding cystoureterogram shows massively dilated ureter with reflux of dye, indicative of an incompetent ureterovesicle valve and VUR.

ASK-UPMARK KIDNEY

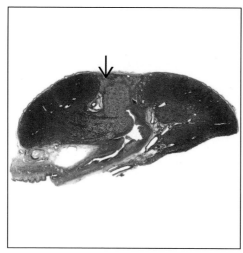

Light microscopy of a whole cross section of a kidney shows a central scar ➡ characteristic of the Ask-Upmark kidney.

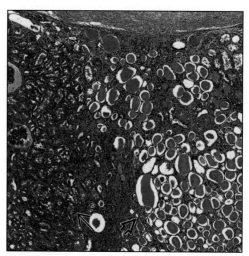

Section of an Ask-Upmark kidney shows the abrupt transition from normal cortex ➡ to the atrophic cortex with thyroidization of tubules and lack of glomeruli ➡ in the central scar.

TERMINOLOGY

Synonyms
- Segmental renal hypoplasia

Definitions
- Congenital or acquired kidney lesion characterized by sharply defined segmental parenchymal hypoplasia of uncertain pathogenesis

ETIOLOGY/PATHOGENESIS

Developmental Anomaly
- Ask-Upmark kidney was originally regarded as a developmental anomaly
  - Absence of glomeruli (as opposed to glomerular scarring) in affected segments argues for developmental nature of disorder (glomeruli are never formed or minimally produced)
  - Challenged by natural history studies suggesting degenerative nature of process

Reflux Hypothesis
- Longitudinal studies showed progressive nature of disease where reflux preceded onset of segmental scar by a few years
- If disease is due to reflux, disease process may begin in utero (would explain morphology)
  - Atrophic cystic tubules and markedly reduced glomeruli are also observed in dysplasia secondary to in utero urinary obstruction

Ischemic Hypothesis
- Segmental renal artery abnormality is shown in cases of Ask-Upmark kidney
- Similar to reflux, hypoperfusion might occur early enough in development to result in absent glomeruli
  - Glomerulogenesis is known to be dependent on intact vascular blood flow during nephrogenesis

CLINICAL ISSUES

Epidemiology
- Age
  - Usually identified in children or young adults
- Gender
  - Female predilection

Presentation
- Hypertension
  - Elevated renin levels in some but not all patients
  - Hypertension often severe, especially in pediatric cases
  - Usually cured by nephrectomy
- Usually normal renal function, but can also be decreased
- Recurrent UTI or proteinuria may complicate presentation

IMAGE FINDINGS

Radiographic Findings
- Renal hypoplasia
- Segmental renal artery stenosis or aneurism may be seen

MACROSCOPIC FEATURES

General Features
- Kidney is small
- One or more hypoplastic segments are sharply delineated
  - Thinned parenchyma
  - Dilated, deep calyces underlying parenchymal lesion
- Central groove (hypoplastic area) from cortex to a dilated calyx

Key Facts

Terminology
- Congenital or acquired kidney lesion characterized by sharply defined segmental parenchymal hypoplasia of uncertain pathogenesis

Clinical Issues
- Hypertension often severe, especially in pediatric cases
  - Usually cured by nephrectomy

Macroscopic Features
- One or more hypoplastic segments are sharply delineated

Microscopic Pathology
- Central groove (hypoplastic area) from cortex to a dilated calyx
- Abrupt transition from normal to atrophic cortex with thyroidization of tubules and lack of glomeruli

MICROSCOPIC PATHOLOGY

Histologic Features
- Glomeruli
  - Absence of glomeruli is characteristic of Ask-Upmark kidney
- Tubules and interstitium
  - Abrupt transition from normal to atrophic cortex with thyroidization of tubules and lack of glomeruli
    - Pattern is characteristic of Ask-Upmark kidney and can also be seen in cases of focal chronic pyelonephritis
  - Many atrophic tubules are in contrast to lack of sclerotic glomeruli
  - Sparse interstitial inflammation
- Arteries
  - Thickened media and intimal fibrosis
- Electron microscopy and immunofluorescence noncontributory

DIFFERENTIAL DIAGNOSIS

Chronic Obstruction and Reflux Nephropathy/Pyelonephritis
- Ask-Upmark kidney may be a form of reflux nephropathy
- Sclerosed rather than absent glomeruli

Renal Dysplasia
- Dysplastic elements including cysts, immature tubules, collecting ducts, and abnormally formed glomeruli
- Presence of cartilage especially helpful in diagnosis
- Renal dysplasia may be focal

Renal Hypoplasia
- Hypoplasia/oligomeganephronia is normally not segmental in nature
- Overall nephron number is reduced, but ratio of glomeruli to tubules is intact

SELECTED REFERENCES

1. Babin J et al: The Ask-Upmark kidney: a curable cause of hypertension in young patients. J Hum Hypertens. 19(4):315-6, 2005
2. Marwali MR et al: Ask-Upmark kidney associated with renal and extrarenal arterial aneurysms. Am J Kidney Dis. 33(4):e4, 1999
3. Shindo S et al: Evolution of renal segmental atrophy (Ask-Upmark kidney) in children with vesicoureteric reflux: radiographic and morphologic studies. J Pediatr. 102(6):847-54, 1983
4. Arant BS Jr et al: Segmental "hypoplasia" of the kidney (Ask-Upmark). J Pediatr. 95(6):931-9, 1979
5. Ask-Upmark E: One-sided kidney affections and arterial hypertension. Acta Med Scand. 173:141-6, 1963
6. Ask-Upmark E: Uber juvenile maligne nephrosclerose und ihr verhaltris zu storunger in der nierenentwicklung. Acta Path Microbiol Scand. 6:383–442, 1929

IMAGE GALLERY

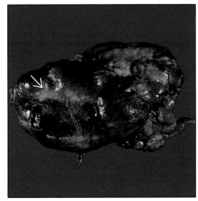 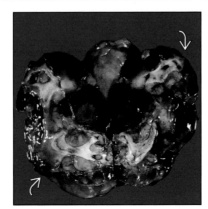 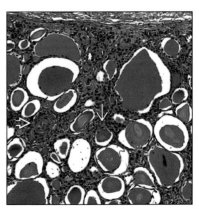

(Left) Ask-Upmark kidney removed from a 38-year-old woman with recurrent urinary tract infections and nephrolithiasis is shown. Segmental scars can be seen on kidney surface ➡. (Center) Cross sectioning reveals segmental hypoplasia is in several areas ➡. (Right) Typical histology shows atrophic, focally dilated tubules with 'thyroidization" ➡, stromal fibrosis, and no glomeruli. A hypertrophic small artery ➡ is also seen, another characteristic feature.

RENAL TUBULAR DYSGENESIS

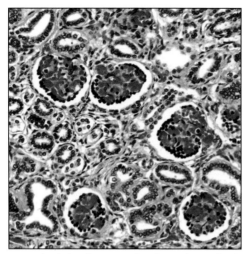

In renal tubular dysgenesis the glomeruli are closely packed and the tubules appear immature and small, resembling distal tubules. No mature proximal tubules with a brush border can be identified.

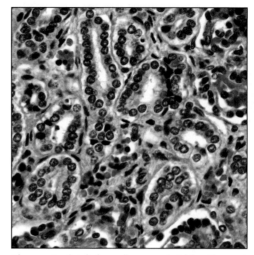

The proximal tubular cells are cuboidal with scant cytoplasm and closely spaced nuclei resembling distal tubules. They express distal tubular markers (EMA) but not proximal tubular markers (CD10).

TERMINOLOGY

Abbreviations
- Renal tubular dysgenesis (RTD)

Synonyms
- Isolated congenital renal tubular immaturity
- Congenital hypernephronic nephromegaly with tubular dysgenesis

Definitions
- Congenital absence or incomplete differentiation of proximal tubules related to defects in the renin-angiotensin system

ETIOLOGY/PATHOGENESIS

Autosomal Recessive
- Homozygous or compound heterozygous mutation of renin-angiotensin system genes
  - Renin
  - Angiotensinogen
  - Angiotensin converting enzyme
  - Angiotensin II type 1 receptor

Twin-Twin Transfusion Syndrome
- Donor fetus develops RTD

Complication of Maternal Drug Use
- Angiotensin converting enzyme inhibitors
- Angiotensin II receptor antagonists
- Nonsteroidal anti-inflammatory drugs

CLINICAL ISSUES

Epidemiology
- Incidence
  - Rare but probably under recognized
    - No definitive data

Presentation
- Oligohydramnios after 20-22 weeks gestation
- Respiratory failure at birth
- Renal failure at birth
- Intractable hypotension in surviving neonates
- Skull ossification defects with autosomal recessive form

Treatment
- Drugs
  - Mineralocorticoids and inotrope have been used in childhood survivors

Prognosis
- Most neonates die from respiratory failure soon after birth
- Rare childhood survivors

IMAGE FINDINGS

Radiographic Findings
- Skull ossification defects with large sutures and fontanelles

Ultrasonographic Findings
- Mild echogenicity with poor corticomedullary differentiation

MACROSCOPIC FEATURES

Potter Sequence Due to Oligohydramnios
- Facial dysmorphia with low-set ears
- Pulmonary hypoplasia
- Limb positioning defects with arthrogryposis

Normal or Moderately Enlarged Kidneys
- Poor corticomedullary differentiation

RENAL TUBULAR DYSGENESIS

Key Facts

Terminology
- Absent or incomplete proximal tubule differentiation

Etiology/Pathogenesis
- Autosomal recessive due to mutation of renin-angiotensin genes
- Maternal drug use
- Twin-twin transfusion

Clinical Issues
- Oligohydramnios
- Renal failure at birth
- Respiratory failure at birth

Macroscopic Features
- Potter oligohydramnios sequence
- Normal or enlarged kidneys
- Skull ossification defects

Microscopic Pathology
- Cortical tubules small and immature

Ancillary Tests
- Failure to express immunohistochemical markers of proximal tubular differentiation
- Express immunohistochemical markers of distal tubular differentiation

Top Differential Diagnoses
- Chronic renal artery stenosis
- Bilateral cystic renal diseases and agenesis
  - Autosomal recessive polycystic kidney disease
  - Cystic renal dysplasias
  - Potter sequence bilateral renal agenesis

MICROSCOPIC PATHOLOGY

Histologic Features
- Proximal tubules are short, straight, and lined by small cuboidal cells, resembling distal tubules
- Limited medullary ray-cortical labyrinth differentiation
- Glomeruli normal but closely spaced

ANCILLARY TESTS

Histochemistry
- Periodic acid-Schiff
  - Reactivity: Proximal tubules
  - Staining pattern
    - Negative: No brush border to stain

Immunohistochemistry
- Increased expression of renin in juxtaglomerular apparatus
- Failure to express proximal tubule markers
  - CD10 negative
  - Winged pea lectin negative
  - Angiotensin converting enzyme negative
- Expression of distal tubule/collecting duct markers
  - Epithelial membrane antigen (EMA) positive
  - Cytokeratin 7 positive
  - *Arachis hypogaea* (peanut lectin) positive

DIFFERENTIAL DIAGNOSIS

Renal Artery Stenosis
- Diffuse tubular atrophy with glomerular clustering
- Occlusive renal artery lesion
  - Fibromuscular dysplasia in a child

Oligohydramnios and Respiratory Failure
- Autosomal recessive polycystic kidney disease
  - Bilateral massive enlarged kidneys
- Bilateral cystic renal dysplasias

- Enlarged cystic kidneys with lower urinary tract malformations
- Extrarenal malformations may be present
- Potter sequence of bilateral renal agenesis

DIAGNOSTIC CHECKLIST

Pathologic Interpretation Pearls
- Consider RTD when oligohydramnios & respiratory failure present in neonate with normal-sized kidneys

SELECTED REFERENCES

1. Gubler MC et al: Renin-angiotensin system in kidney development: renal tubular dysgenesis. Kidney Int. 77(5):400-6, 2010
2. Schreiber R et al: Inherited renal tubular dysgenesis may not be universally fatal. Pediatr Nephrol. 25(12):2531-4, 2010
3. Delaney D et al: Congenital unilateral renal tubular dysgenesis and severe neonatal hypertension. Pediatr Nephrol. 24(4):863-7, 2009
4. Uematsu M et al: A further case of renal tubular dysgenesis surviving the neonatal period. Eur J Pediatr. 168(2):207-9, 2009
5. Daïkha-Dahmane F et al: Foetal kidney maldevelopment in maternal use of angiotensin II type I receptor antagonists. Pediatr Nephrol. 21(5):729-32, 2006
6. Lacoste M et al: Renal tubular dysgenesis, a not uncommon autosomal recessive disorder leading to oligohydramnios: Role of the Renin-Angiotensin system. J Am Soc Nephrol. 17(8):2253-63, 2006
7. Gribouval O et al: Mutations in genes in the renin-angiotensin system are associated with autosomal recessive renal tubular dysgenesis. Nat Genet. 37(9):964-8, 2005
8. Ariel I et al: Familial renal tubular dysgenesis: a disorder not isolated to proximal convoluted tubules. Pediatr Pathol Lab Med. 15(6):915-22, 1995
9. Bernstein J et al: Renal tubular dysgenesis: evidence of abnormality in the renin-angiotensin system. J Am Soc Nephrol. 5(2):224-7, 1994
10. Landing BH et al: Labeled lectin studies of renal tubular dysgenesis and renal tubular atrophy of postnatal renal ischemia and end-stage kidney disease. Pediatr Pathol. 14(1):87-99, 1994

Microscopic Features

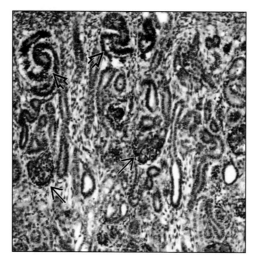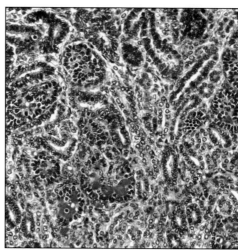

(Left) This fetal kidney shows the nephrogenic zone. There are glomeruli in the S-phase ⇗ of formation and well-differentiated glomeruli ➡. However, no proximal tubular differentiation is evident. All tubules are small and lined by small cells with little cytoplasm. (Right) This fetal kidney with RTD shows normal glomeruli. The tubules are all small and contain cells with scant cytoplasm rather than the abundant eosinophilic cytoplasm characteristic of normal proximal tubules.

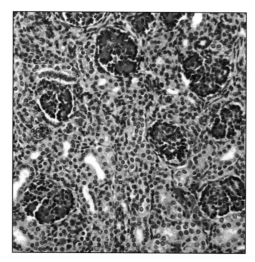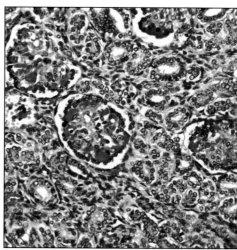

(Left) The kidney of this newborn with RTD shows tubular profiles that are all similar in appearance. There is no delineation between proximal tubules and distal tubules. The cells in all tubules are small and lack a brush border. (Right) In this newborn with RTD, the glomeruli are closely spaced. The podocytes are prominent and cuboidal-appearing, which is normal at this age. All of the proximal tubules are small and lined by cells with little cytoplasm that are indistinguishable from distal tubular cells.

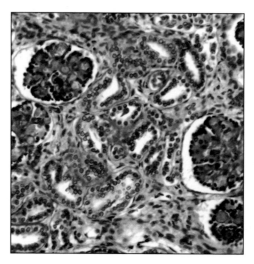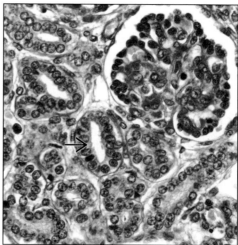

(Left) This is a kidney from a newborn with renal tubular dysgenesis. A PAS stain demonstrates no evidence of staining along the luminal surface, indicating that there is no brush border characteristic of proximal tubular differentiation. (Right) This kidney is from a newborn with renal tubular dysgenesis. All of the tubules ➡ lack the luminal PAS-positive brush border that is characteristic of proximal tubular differentiation. All tubules resemble distal tubules.

RENAL TUBULAR DYSGENESIS

Immunohistochemistry and Electron Microscopy

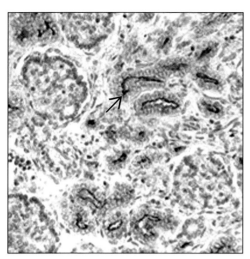

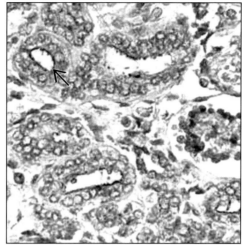

(Left) The biopsy from a neonate with renal tubular dysgenesis shows that the proximal tubules exhibit a distal tubule immunophenotype when stained for epithelial membrane antigen ➡. Proximal tubules in a normal kidney would not stain. *(Right)* Epithelial membrane antigen, a distal tubule/collecting duct marker, stains the luminal surface of all tubular cells ➡ indicating failure of proximal tubular differentiation. Normal proximal tubules would not stain with EMA.

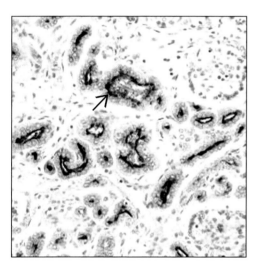

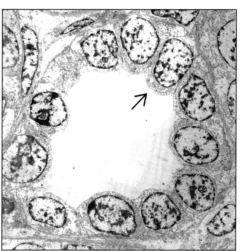

(Left) The kidney of a neonate with RTD shows that the distal tubule/collecting duct marker *Arachis hypogaea* lectin (peanut agglutinin) stains ➡ the apical cytoplasm of all proximal tubules. This indicates distal tubule/collecting duct differentiation. *(Right)* The cells lining this tubule in a patient with renal tubular dysgenesis appear identical to a distal tubule cells. They have little cytoplasm, no luminal microvilli ➡, and lack complex basal-lateral membrane infolding.

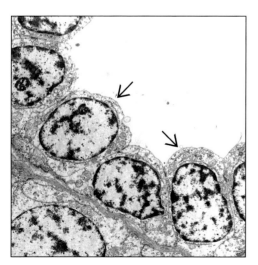

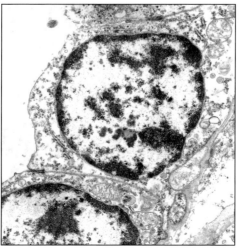

(Left) This is a typical proximal tubule in renal tubular dysgenesis. It shows little cytoplasm and few intracellular organelles. There are no basal-lateral membrane infolding or luminal microvilli (brush border) ➡ present. *(Right)* This proximal tubule cell in renal tubular dysgenesis has scant cytoplasm, few organelles, and no luminal microvilli. The normal proximal tubule cell contains numerous organelles, especially mitochondria, and has a luminal surface covered with microvilli.

CLASSIFICATION OF CYSTIC DISEASES

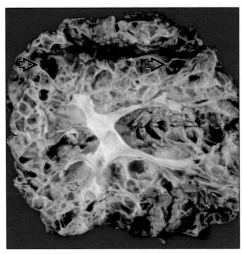

Adult ADPKD kidneys are massively enlarged and contain numerous oval/spherical cysts dispersed throughout the cortex and medulla. Cysts are lined by thin walls; some contain hemorrhagic fluid ⮆.

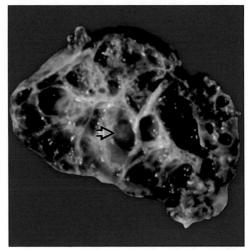

Early onset ADPKD in a young child shows oval cysts varying in size, filled with turbid gelatinous fluid ⮆. Overall size of the kidney is moderately large for age.

PATHOGENETIC CLASSIFICATION

Definition
- Renal diseases characterized predominately by cysts
  - Cyst: Closed cavity in a previously noncystic structure
    - Cysts may arise in any part of nephron, but most frequently in tubules
    - Cysts may be found in renal cortex, medulla, or both
    - Cysts may be diffuse, focal, unilateral, or bilateral
    - Bilateral cysts are most commonly hereditary
    - Cysts can be randomly or uniformly distributed (e.g., along corticomedullary junction)
    - Sometimes ectasia is present rather than a closed cyst
  - Cysts arising in glomeruli are called glomerular cysts
  - Term "polycystic" should only be used for autosomal dominant and autosomal recessive polycystic kidney disease (ADPKD, ARPKD)
  - Location and shape of renal cysts are important for classification
  - No universally accepted classification scheme
  - Features considered
    - Genetic basis
    - Cystic anatomic structure (tubule, glomerulus, other)
    - Distribution of cysts (cortex, medulla)

Categories
- Hereditary cystic diseases
  - Autosomal dominant polycystic kidney disease (ADPKD)
  - Autosomal recessive polycystic kidney disease (ARPKD)
  - Medullary cystic kidney disease (MCKD)
  - Nephronophthisis (NPH)
  - Tuberous sclerosis (TSC)
  - von Hippel-Lindau (VHL) disease
  - Primary glomerulocystic kidney disease (GCKD)
- Acquired cystic diseases
  - Secondary GCKD
  - Acquired cystic disease (end-stage kidney)
  - Medullary sponge kidney
  - Multilocular renal cyst
  - Simple cortical cyst
- Non-nephron renal cystic diseases
  - Pyelocalyceal diverticula
  - Perinephric pseudocyst
  - Lymphangiectasis/lymphangiomatosis

EPIDEMIOLOGY

Incidence
- ADPKD: 1 in 500 live births
- ARPKD: 1 in 20,000 live births
- NPH: 1 in 8,000,000 in USA, 1 in 50,000 in Canada
- TSC: 1 in 10,000-15,000 live births

ETIOLOGY/PATHOGENESIS

Histogenesis
- Cystogenesis: Process involving aberrant formation or maintenance of a normally noncystic structure
- Causes of tubular cysts
  - Epithelial cell proliferation
  - Apoptosis and defective clearance of apoptotic cells causing tubular obstruction
  - Scarring of tubule due to inflammation, injury and fibrosis with consequent obstruction
  - Expansion of luminal contents by vectorial fluid/solute shift
    - Electrolyte contents reveal distal or proximal tubular transport function
  - May begin as an ectatic tubule that later becomes a closed cystic space
- Causes of glomerular cysts unclear
  - May involve scarring of outlet
  - Failure of normal proximal tubule formation

CLASSIFICATION OF CYSTIC DISEASES

MACROSCOPIC FINDINGS

Differential Diagnostic Features
- Spherical cysts in bilaterally enlarged kidneys are diagnostic of ADPKD
- Cylindrical cysts (really ectatic collecting ducts) in enlarged pediatric kidneys are diagnostic of ARPKD
- A few small cysts at corticomedullary junction are characteristic of NPH
- Isolated cortical cysts, usually unilateral, are nonhereditary, simple cysts seen in elderly patients with no renal disease

MICROSCOPIC FINDINGS

Differential Diagnostic Features
- Cysts contain abundant eosinophilic fluid and micropapillary proliferations characteristic of ADPKD
- Cylindrical cysts are characteristic of ARPKD
- Glomerular cysts affecting > 5% of glomeruli define glomerulocystic kidney disease as being either primary or secondary
- Secondary GCKD is more common than primary and presents in children with ADPKD, ARPKD, or TSC
  - Glomerular cysts are defined as Bowman capsule dilation > 3x normal
- Cysts containing renal cell carcinoma are characteristic of hereditary neoplasia syndromes (TSC, von Hippel-Lindau disease) ADPKD, or hemodialysis-induced cysts
- Cysts in NPHP/MCDK form are ex vacuo (degenerative); may contain Tamm-Horsfall protein and show tubular basement membrane duplication
- Incidental, simple cysts are also degenerative and often lack epithelial lining

HEREDITARY CYSTIC DISEASES

ADPKD
- Classic ADPKD in adults
- Early onset ADPKD in children

ARPKD
- Classic ARPKD in neonates and infants
- Late onset ARPKD in adolescents presenting with medullary ectasia and hepatic fibrosis

GCKD, Primary
- Hereditary GCKD due to *UMOD* or *HNF1B* mutations
- Familial GCKD with unknown gene mutations

Nephronophthisis
- Nephronophthisis, autosomal recessive
- Juvenile/adult nephronophthisis *NPHP1, 3*
- *NPHP4-11* variable age of onset
- *NPHP1, NPHP5* associated with Senior-Loken syndrome
- Infantile *NPHP2*

Medullary Cystic Kidney Disease
- Autosomal dominant MCKD
- MCKD associated with hyperuricemia

von Hippel-Lindau Disease
- Lined by clear cells
- Associated with renal cell carcinoma, clear cell type

Tuberous Sclerosis
- Cysts lined by large plump cells with deeply eosinophilic cytoplasm
  - Nuclear pleomorphism of cyst lining epithelium
- Associated with angiomyolipoma and renal cell carcinoma

NON-HEREDITARY CYSTIC DISEASES

Acquired Cystic Disease
- > 50% of dialysis patients develop cysts within 5 years
  - Cysts may appear even before initiation of dialysis
- 3 or more cysts in dialysis patient are required for diagnosis
- Typically proliferative (Ki67) and hobnailed cells
- Increased risk for intracystic renal cell carcinoma

Multilocular Renal Cyst
- Also known as multilocular cystic nephroma
- Most cases are sporadic; some congenital
- Tumor usually encapsulated with noncommunicating cysts filled with gelatinous fluid
- Infrequent lesion; occurs in both children and adults

Localized Cystic Disease
- May be mistaken for ADPKD
- Overall kidney size not increased, unlike ADPKD
- Cysts are naked; intervening renal parenchyma normal
- Uncommon presentation of unilateral, segmental, or bilateral multiple cysts nonhereditary

Simple Cortical Cysts
- Oval or round with smooth outline, located in renal cortex
- Randomly distributed
- 12-15% of adults and a common autopsy finding

GCKD, Secondary and Sporadic
- Associated with numerous syndromes
- Can be secondary to other diseases such as ADPKD, ARPKD or tuberous sclerosis
- Due to vascular ischemia such as HUS and renal artery branch stenosis
- Sporadic GCKD

Medullary Sponge Kidney
- Disease of adults
- Genetic basis, if any, unknown
- Characterized by calcium-filled cysts in medullary collecting ducts
- Usually diagnosed radiologically as incidental finding
  - Retention of filtered contrast dye in medullary pyramids

6

CLASSIFICATION OF CYSTIC DISEASES

Pathogenetic Classification of Renal Cystic Diseases

Hereditary

Polycystic kidney disease

ADPKD

Early onset ADPKD in children

ARPKD

Classic ARPKD in neonates and infants

Late onset ARPKD in older children with hepatic fibrosis

GCKD

Primary

Familial GCKD with unknown gene mutations

Hereditary GCKD due to *UMOD* or *HNF1B* mutations

Secondary GCKD

Associated with ADPKD/ARPKD/TSC

Cysts in hereditary cancer syndromes

Tuberous sclerosis

von Hippel-Lindau disease

Renal medullary cysts

Nephronophthisis

Juvenile/adult *NPHP1, NPHP3*

Infantile *NPHP2*

NPHP4-11 variable onset

NPHP1, NPHP5 associated with Senior-Loken syndrome

Medullary cystic diseases

Autosomal dominant MCKD

MCKD associated with hyperuricemia

Nonhereditary

GCKD

Secondary

Associated with numerous syndromes

Due to ischemia, e.g., HUS and renal artery branch stenosis

Sporadic GCKD

Simple cortical cysts

Localized cystic disease

Acquired cystic disease (end-stage renal disease)

Typically dialysis related

Multilocular renal cyst

Medullary sponge kidney

Non-nephron renal cystic diseases

Pyelocalyceal diverticula

Perinephric pseudocyst

Lymphangiectasis/lymphangiomatosis

NON-NEPHRON CYSTIC DISEASE

Pyelocalyceal Diverticulum
- Associated with nephrolithiasis
- Lined by urothelium
- Echogenic and mobile material within cyst-like lesion

Perinephric Pseudocyst
- No epithelial lining
- May arise from a urine leak

Lymphangiectasis/Lymphangiomatosis
- Dilated lymphatics and accumulation of lymph fluid around kidney
  - Hygroma renalis
- May have systemic lymphangiectasis
- Some may be low-grade neoplasms

MIMICS OF CYSTIC DISEASES

Renal Dysplasia
- May be strikingly multicystic
- Cartilage and smooth muscle present
- Absent glomeruli in sites of dysplasia

Pancreatic Pseudocyst
- Sometimes abuts kidney

Perinephric Abscess
- Other signs of abscess evident

SELECTED REFERENCES

1. Bonsib SM: The classification of renal cystic diseases and other congenital malformations of the kidney and urinary tract. Arch Pathol Lab Med. 134(4):554-68, 2010
2. Katabathina VS et al: Adult renal cystic disease: a genetic, biological, and developmental primer. Radiographics. 30(6):1509-23, 2010
3. Lennerz JK et al: Glomerulocystic kidney: one hundred-year perspective. Arch Pathol Lab Med. 134(4):583-605, 2010
4. Liapis H et al: Cystic diseases and developmental kidney defects. In Jennette JC et al: Heptinstall's Pathology of the Kidney. 6th ed. Philadelphia: Lippincott Williams & Wilkins. 1286-1306, 2007
5. Wilson PD et al: Cystic disease of the kidney. Annu Rev Pathol. 2:341-68, 2007
6. Bisceglia M et al: Renal cystic diseases: a review. Adv Anat Pathol. 13(1):26-56, 2006

Gross and Microscopic Features

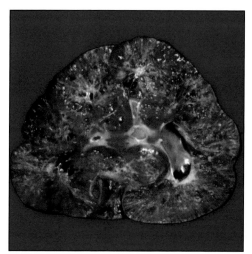

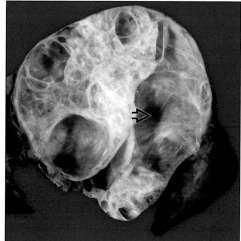

(Left) Newborn kidney is shown with cylindrical cysts characteristic of ARPKD. Most of the "cysts" are really ectatic collecting ducts, which later become cystic. *(Right)* Nephrectomy from a young infant shows a well-encapsulated cystic mass with variably sized cysts containing gelatinous fluid ➡. These findings are characteristic of multilocular renal cyst, also called cystic nephroma.

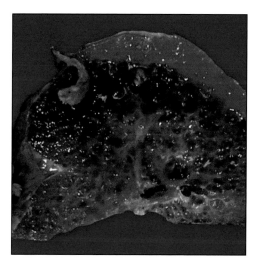

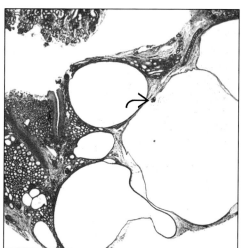

(Left) Nephrectomy specimen from a newborn with bilateral kidney cysts detected by ultrasound contains numerous small cysts. Microscopically, the majority of the glomerular cysts are of glomerular origin. *(Right)* There are variably size cysts, most of which are empty, not lined by epithelium. However, small nubs of retracted glomerular tufts are apparent in some cysts ➡, demonstrating a glomerular orgin.

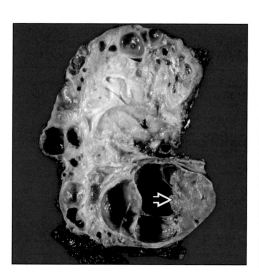

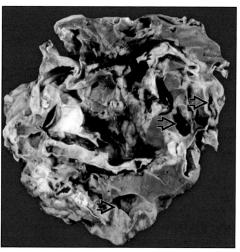

(Left) This nephrectomy specimen from a patient with dialysis-induced cysts is complicated by renal cell carcinoma ➡. The extensive cysts can mimic ADPKD, but usually the kidneys are not as large. *(Right)* Note the multiple collapsed, empty cysts ➡ with normal intervening renal parenchyma in this normal-sized kidney from a patient with localized cystic kidney disease.

6

AUTOSOMAL DOMINANT POLYCYSTIC KIDNEY DISEASE

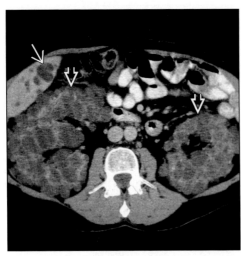

Contrast-enhanced CT shows multiple cysts of varying size essentially replacing the renal parenchyma ➡. Cysts are also seen in the liver ➡.

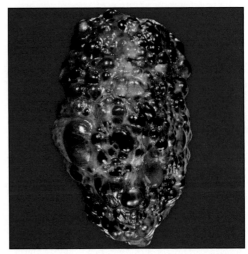

Numerous cysts are present in this kidney that weighs 2.5 kg and measures 28 cm in length. Only ADPKD leads to such massive enlargement of the kidneys. (Courtesy J. Steinmetz, MD.)

TERMINOLOGY

Abbreviations
- Autosomal dominant polycystic kidney disease (ADPKD)

Synonyms
- Adult-type PKD

ETIOLOGY/PATHOGENESIS

Genetic Disease
- Classified as "ciliopathy"
- Autosomal dominant
  - Random somatic mutation of normal allele in individual cells

PKD-1 (Polycystin-1) Mutation
- Located on chromosome 16
- Accounts for 85% of ADPKD
- Component of primary cilium
  - Interacts with and regulates polycystin-2
  - Mechanosensor for flow

PKD-2 (Polycystin-2) Mutation
- Located on chromosome 4
- Accounts for 15% of ADPKD
- May act as cation channel for calcium entry into cell

Possible Pathogenic Mechanisms Related to Cilium
- Abnormal cell proliferation
- Deregulated apoptosis
- Defective cellular polarity
- Increased secretion of fluids into tubular lumens

CLINICAL ISSUES

Epidemiology
- Incidence
  - 1 in 500 live births
- Age
  - Cysts develop progressively
    - Usual clinical presentation is 30-40 years old
    - Can rarely present in childhood
- Gender
  - Women have more cysts in liver and develop them at earlier age than men

Presentation
- Abdominal pain/discomfort
- Hematuria
- Urinary tract infections
- Hypertension
  - Cerebral arterial aneurysms with intracranial hemorrhage in 5-10%

Laboratory Tests
- Genetic tests for *PKD-1* or *PKD-2* mutations
  - Mutation detection rate of 65-70% for *PKD-1*
  - Mutation detection rate of nearly 90% for *PKD-2*

Treatment
- None effective to slow progression
  - Clinical trials of mTOR inhibitors, vasopressin receptor antagonists
- Bilateral nephrectomy if kidneys are too enlarged, or repeat episodes of pyelonephritis

Prognosis
- Approximately 50% of patients will require dialysis or kidney transplant by age of 50
- *PKD-2* mutations result in milder clinical course compared to *PKD-1* mutations

AUTOSOMAL DOMINANT POLYCYSTIC KIDNEY DISEASE

Key Facts

Terminology
- Autosomal dominant polycystic kidney disease (ADPKD)

Etiology/Pathogenesis
- Genetic disease, autosomal dominant
- Ciliopathy involving proteins of primary cilium
  - *PKD-1* (Polycystin-1) 85%
  - *PKD-2* (Polycystin-2) 15%

Clinical Issues
- 1 in 400-1,000 individuals
- Symptoms
  - Hypertension
  - Renal failure
  - Abdominal pain/discomfort
  - Hematuria, infections
- No known preventive treatment
- ~ 50% require dialysis or kidney transplant by age 50

Macroscopic Features
- Numerous cysts throughout both kidneys
- Kidneys weigh up to 3 or 4 kg

Microscopic Pathology
- Numerous cysts at all levels of nephron; bilateral
- May be renal cell tumors
- Cysts in multiple other organs
  - Liver, pancreas, arachnoid, pineal, seminal vesicle

Top Differential Diagnoses
- Acquired cystic disease
- Autosomal recessive PKD

IMAGE FINDINGS

Radiographic Findings
- Numerous cysts throughout kidney

MACROSCOPIC FEATURES

General Features
- Numerous randomly distributed cysts throughout both kidneys
  - Rare cases of "1-sided" ADPKD
- Kidneys weigh up to 3 or 4 kg

MICROSCOPIC PATHOLOGY

Histologic Features
- Cysts in cortex and medulla up to several cm in diameter
  - Can arise from any segment of nephron or collecting duct
  - Glomerular, tubular cysts
  - Lined by single layer of flattened to cuboidal epithelial cells
  - Hemorrhage may be present
  - May be normal intervening parenchyma, depending on stage
- Diffuse interstitial fibrosis and tubular atrophy
- Renal cell tumors sometimes present

Extrarenal Pathology
- Liver cysts (> 90%)
  - Can predominate over renal disease rarely
  - Termed polycystic liver disease
- Cysts in pancreas (10%), seminal vesicles (39%), pineal gland (< 5%), arachnoid, and ovaries
- Mitral valve prolapse or aortic regurgitation in 25%
- Diverticulosis
- Inguinal, ventral, hiatal hernias
- Cerebral (berry) aneurysms

DIFFERENTIAL DIAGNOSIS

Acquired Cystic Disease
- Usually < 1 kg, cysts not as widespread
- Underlying renal disease evident
- Hyperplastic tubular epithelium
- May be present in ADPKD

Simple Cysts
- Isolated cysts and much normal parenchyma
- Difficult to distinguish from early stage ADPKD

Autosomal Recessive PKD
- Congenital or childhood onset
- Ectatic collecting ducts and bile ducts

DIAGNOSTIC CHECKLIST

Pathologic Interpretation Pearls
- Careful examination of nephrectomy specimens to exclude neoplasia
  - Bread loaf at 1 cm

SELECTED REFERENCES

1. Bae KT et al: Imaging for the prognosis of autosomal dominant polycystic kidney disease. Nat Rev Nephrol. 6(2):96-106, 2010
2. Deltas C et al: Cystic diseases of the kidney: molecular biology and genetics. Arch Pathol Lab Med. 134(4):569-82, 2010
3. Perico N et al: Sirolimus therapy to halt the progression of ADPKD. J Am Soc Nephrol. 21(6):1031-40, 2010
4. Bonsib SM: Renal cystic diseases and renal neoplasms: a mini-review. Clin J Am Soc Nephrol. 4(12):1998-2007, 2009
5. Gunay-Aygun M: Liver and kidney disease in ciliopathies. Am J Med Genet C Semin Med Genet. 151C(4):296-306, 2009
6. Torres VE et al: Autosomal dominant polycystic kidney disease: the last 3 years. Kidney Int. 76(2):149-68, 2009
7. Grantham JJ: Clinical practice. Autosomal dominant polycystic kidney disease. N Engl J Med. 359(14):1477-85, 2008

6

AUTOSOMAL DOMINANT POLYCYSTIC KIDNEY DISEASE

Imaging, Gross, and Microscopic Features

(Left) Contrast-enhanced CT shows relatively normal size and function of the kidneys, but with innumerable small cortical and medullary cysts ➡. This is an example of type 2 ADPKD. *(Right)* Numerous cysts are present throughout this kidney from a patient with ADPKD. Due to the marked enlargement, only half of the kidney is framed within this image. Very little identifiable residual renal parenchyma is seen. Focal hemorrhage is noted within a cyst ⧁. *(Courtesy J. Moore, MD.)*

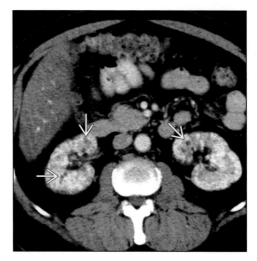
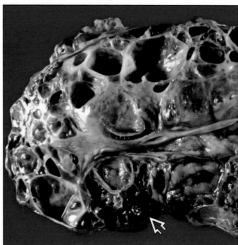

(Left) This is a kidney from a patient with ADPKD (bivalved). Kidney architecture is severely distorted by numerous cysts distributed throughout the parenchyma. *(Right)* Several cysts from a polycystic kidney contain proteinaceous fluid. A globally sclerotic glomerulus ➡ is compressed between several cysts that have mostly replaced the renal parenchyma and resulted in marked and diffuse interstitial fibrosis and tubular atrophy.

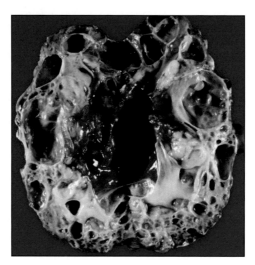
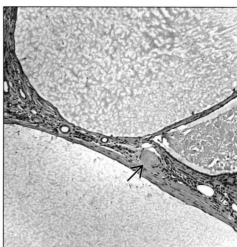

(Left) This enlarged cyst is lined by cuboidal to flattened epithelial cells ⧁. Diffuse tubular atrophy and interstitial fibrosis with an associated nonspecific inflammatory cell infiltrate are noted. *(Right)* These cysts demonstrate the spectrum of findings that may be present within cyst contents. One cyst demonstrates hemorrhage with numerous red blood cells ⧁. The other 2 adjacent cysts ➡ contain proteinaceous material that show varying degrees of eosinophilia.

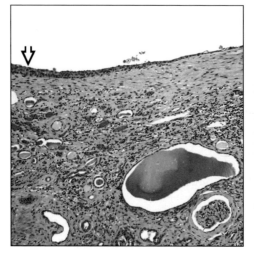
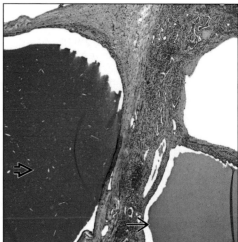

AUTOSOMAL DOMINANT POLYCYSTIC KIDNEY DISEASE

Microscopic Features

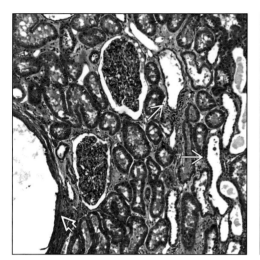

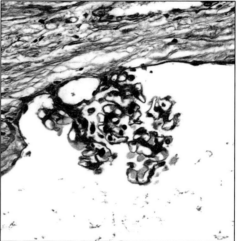

(Left) In this micrograph of the polycystic kidney, a single cyst lined by flattened epithelium ➡ is adjacent to a relatively intact renal cortical tissue. Some tubules show flattening of the epithelium indicating tubular injury ➡. **(Right)** Glomerular cysts are a common feature of ADPKD. This should not be confused with GCKD.

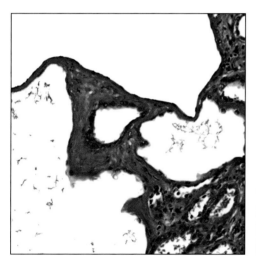

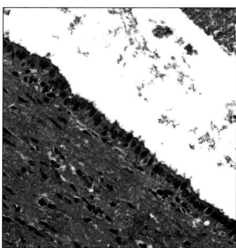

(Left) Most cysts are lined by flattened epithelia as shown in this micrograph. Cysts affect all levels of the nephron, from the glomerulus to the collecting ducts. **(Right)** Some cysts are lined by epithelia with columnar morphology. This is quite distinct from the enlarged, hyperplastic hobnailed cells seen in acquired cystic disease.

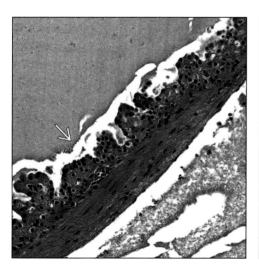

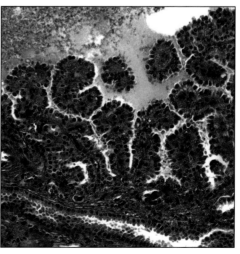

(Left) A minority of cysts in ADPKD kidneys may be lined by epithelia showing papillary proliferation ➡. **(Right)** The papillary proliferation of cyst-lining epithelium can be quite exuberant as shown in this micrograph of polycystic kidney. ADPKD kidneys are believed to have an increased probability of developing papillary renal cell carcinoma. Tumors can usually be detected on gross examination after breadloafing at 1 cm, and appear as solid yellow or white nodules.

AUTOSOMAL RECESSIVE POLYCYSTIC KIDNEY DISEASE

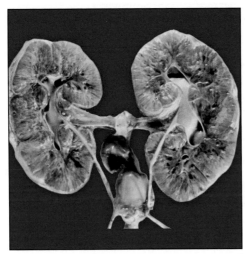

These bivalved kidneys in a case of neonatal autosomal recessive polycystic kidney disease show diffuse, radially arrayed cortical and medullary collecting duct cysts with normal ureters and bladder.

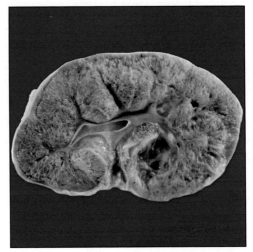

The cystic change in this neonatal case of autosomal recessive polycystic kidney disease is very uniform. The corticomedullary distinction is lost. The "cysts" represent ectatic collecting ducts.

TERMINOLOGY

Abbreviations
- Autosomal recessive polycystic kidney disease (ARPKD)

Synonyms
- Infantile polycystic kidney disease
  - Terminology not recommended because of childhood and adult presentations
- Sponge kidney
  - Descriptive term, not to be confused with medullary sponge kidney

Definitions
- Cystic kidney disease/congenital hepatic fibrosis due to mutation of *PKHD1*, chromosome 6p12

ETIOLOGY/PATHOGENESIS

Genetic Factors
- *PKHD1* encodes for polyductin/fibrocystin protein
- Polyductin/fibrocystin protein located in primary cilium
  - Primary cilium is a sensory organ
  - Controls tubular cell differentiation
- > 300 *PKHD1* mutations have been identified
- Poor genotype-phenotype correlation
  - Presence of 2 truncating mutations has been associated with severe neonatal disease

CLINICAL ISSUES

Presentation
- Autosomal recessive
- 1:20,000 live births
- Newborn
  - Respiratory failure from pulmonary hypoplasia
  - Renal failure
  - Abdominal mass
- Childhood
  - Systemic hypertension and renal insufficiency in 50%
  - Portal hypertension in 10%
  - Renal concentrating defects ± medullary cysts

Treatment
- Renal transplantation in children and adults

Prognosis
- Lethal outcome in 40% of neonates
- If neonate survives the 1st month of life, 90% 1-year and 5-year survival

IMAGE FINDINGS

Radiographic Findings
- Hypoplastic thorax in neonatal presentation
- Bilateral diffusely cystic kidneys in neonates
  - Absence of lower urinary tract abnormalities

Ultrasonographic Findings
- Bilateral enlarged echogenic kidneys in neonates
- Normal-sized or enlarged kidney with echogenicity limited to medulla ± focal cortical involvement

MACROSCOPIC FEATURES

General Features
- Lethal neonatal form
  - Kidneys massively enlarged
  - Diffuse radially oriented cysts in cortex and medulla
  - Small hypoplastic lungs
  - Portal fibrosis/bile duct malformation
- Infantile and childhood form
  - Smaller kidneys and larger lungs
  - Medullary cysts and few or no rounded cortical cysts
  - Congenital hepatic fibrosis

AUTOSOMAL RECESSIVE POLYCYSTIC KIDNEY DISEASE

Key Facts

Terminology
- Cystic kidney disease/congenital hepatic fibrosis

Etiology/Pathogenesis
- Mutation of *PKHD1* gene on chromosome 6p12

Clinical Issues
- Neonates present with respiratory failure
- Older children
  - Portal hypertension
  - Renal insufficiency or concentrating defects

Image Findings
- Echogenic large kidneys on ultrasound in neonates
- Normal size ± medullary cysts in older patients

Macroscopic Features
- Massive, diffusely cystic kidneys in neonates

- Bilateral hypoplastic lungs
- Medullary cysts ± cortical cysts in older patients
  - Congenital hepatic fibrosis

Microscopic Pathology
- Radially dilated collecting ducts in neonates
  - Bile duct plate malformation in liver
- Medullary collecting duct ectasia in older patients
  - Congenital hepatic fibrosis in children and adults

Ancillary Tests
- Test for *PKHD1* mutation

Top Differential Diagnoses
- Cystic renal dysplasia
- Medullary sponge kidney

MICROSCOPIC PATHOLOGY

Histologic Features
- Nonobstructive fusiform dilatation of cortical and medullary collecting ducts in neonatal cases
  - Nephrons are normal without dysgenetic features
- Smaller rounded collecting duct cysts separated by focally atrophic tissue in childhood
- Occasional medullary cysts in older children and adults
- Mild ectasia of proximal tubules is an early lesion

Liver
- Congenital hepatic fibrosis is bile duct plate abnormality (retention of embryonic plate configuration)
  - Abnormally shaped and distributed bile ducts
  - Periportal fibrosis and portal-portal bridging without inflammation
  - Abnormal portal vein branching
  - When associated with dilatation of intrahepatic bile, known as Caroli syndrome

ANCILLARY TESTS

Molecular Genetics
- Test for *PKHD1* mutations
  - Identified in 80-85% of cases

DIFFERENTIAL DIAGNOSIS

Cystic Renal Dysplasia
- Lower urinary tract usually abnormal
- May be associated with extrarenal malformations

Medullary Sponge Kidney
- Distal papillary collecting ducts affected
- Papillary tip calcification
- Nephrolithiasis

SELECTED REFERENCES

1. Denamur E et al: Genotype-phenotype correlations in fetuses and neonates with autosomal recessive polycystic kidney disease. Kidney Int. 77(4):350-8, 2010
2. Gunay-Aygun M et al: Correlation of kidney function, volume and imaging findings, and PKHD1 mutations in 73 patients with autosomal recessive polycystic kidney disease. Clin J Am Soc Nephrol. 5(6):972-84, 2010
3. Guay-Woodford LM et al: Genetic testing: considerations for pediatric nephrologists. Semin Nephrol. 29(4):338-48, 2009
4. Gunay-Aygun M: Liver and kidney disease in ciliopathies. Am J Med Genet C Semin Med Genet. 151C(4):296-306, 2009
5. Al-Bhalal L et al: Molecular basis of autosomal recessive polycystic kidney disease (ARPKD). Adv Anat Pathol. 15(1):54-8, 2008
6. Gunay-Aygun M et al: Congenital hepatic fibrosis overview. In Pagon RA et al (eds.): GeneReviews [Internet]. Seattle: University of Washington. Posted December 9, 2008
7. Guay-Woodford LM: Autosomal recessive PKD in the early years. Nephrol News Issues. 21(12):39, 2007
8. Rossetti S et al: Genotype-phenotype correlations in autosomal dominant and autosomal recessive polycystic kidney disease. J Am Soc Nephrol. 18(5):1374-80, 2007
9. Adeva M et al: Clinical and molecular characterization defines a broadened spectrum of autosomal recessive polycystic kidney disease (ARPKD). Medicine (Baltimore). 85(1):1-21, 2006
10. Bisceglia M et al: Renal cystic diseases: a review. Adv Anat Pathol. 13(1):26-56, 2006
11. Gunay-Aygun M et al: Autosomal recessive polycystic kidney disease and congenital hepatic fibrosis: summary statement of a first National Institutes of Health/Office of Rare Diseases conference. J Pediatr. 149(2):159-64, 2006
12. Bergmann C et al: Clinical consequences of PKHD1 mutations in 164 patients with autosomal-recessive polycystic kidney disease (ARPKD). Kidney Int. 67(3):829-48, 2005
13. Parfrey PS: Autosomal-recessive polycystic kidney disease. Kidney Int. 67(4):1638-48, 2005
14. Wang S et al: The autosomal recessive polycystic kidney disease protein is localized to primary cilia, with concentration in the basal body area. J Am Soc Nephrol. 15(3):592-602, 2004

AUTOSOMAL RECESSIVE POLYCYSTIC KIDNEY DISEASE

Gross Features

(Left) This is a lethal neonatal case of ARPKD. The neonate presented with respiratory failure and massive abdominal enlargement due to bilateral cystic kidneys. The kidneys have retained a reniform shape. *(Right)* This is a lethal neonatal case of ARPKD. It shows massively enlarged kidneys with persistent fetal lobation. The diffuse cysts are tiny and not visible through the renal capsule. The ureters are anterior and nonrotated but are of normal caliber ➡.

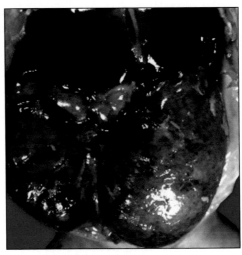 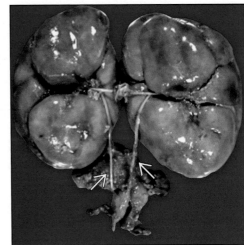

(Left) This bivalved kidney in a case of lethal neonatal ARPKD shows radial cortical cysts ➢. The medullary cysts ➡ can appear rounded dependent upon the plane of sectioning. *(Right)* This is a lethal neonatal case of ARPKD. The radial arrangement of the cortical cysts is apparent ➡. Since most renal pyramids angle toward the collecting system from an anterior or posterior direction, rounded medullary cysts ➢ are often seen. The collecting system is completely normal ➥.

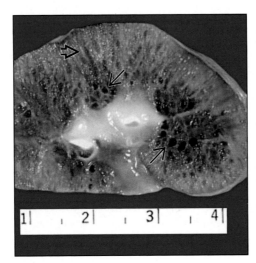 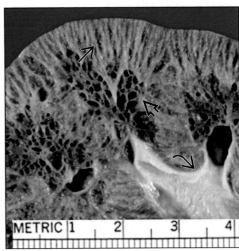

(Left) This is a childhood case of autosomal recessive PKD. There are cysts in both the cortex and the medulla. Compared to a lethal neonatal case, both the cortical cysts and medullary cysts are larger ➡, fewer in number, and more rounded ➢ in contour. *(Right)* This is a childhood case of autosomal recessive PKD; it shows a normal-sized kidney. Cortical cysts are not grossly apparent. The cysts present ➡ are infrequent, rounded, and predominately located within the renal medulla.

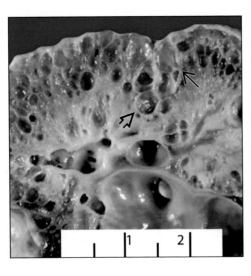 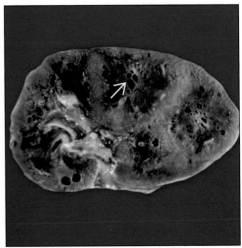

AUTOSOMAL RECESSIVE POLYCYSTIC KIDNEY DISEASE

Microscopic Features

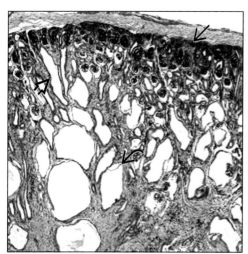

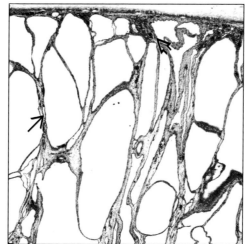

(Left) This is an autopsy kidney from a 2nd trimester elective termination for ARPKD. It shows the subcapsular nephrogenic zone ➡. There are both cortical ⊇ and medullary cysts ➡. The medullary cysts are larger than the cortical cysts. *(Right)* This is an autopsy kidney from a term neonate. There is no nephrogenic zone present. There is massive fusiform dilatation of cortical collecting ducts ➡. There are normally shaped nephron elements ⊇ in between the cortical cysts.

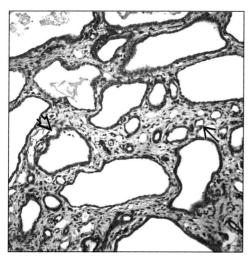

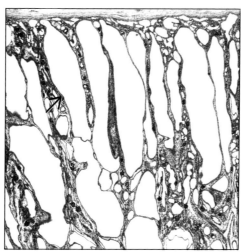

(Left) This is renal medulla from a term neonate. It shows dilated medullary collecting ducts ⊇ lined by a low cuboidal epithelium. The interstitium is loose and paucicellular with thin loops of Henle ➡ present. *(Right)* This is an autopsy kidney from a term neonate. The kidney shows massive fusiform dilation of cortical collecting ducts ➡. The intervening nephrons are normally formed. The number of nephrons appear reduced because the kidney volume is markedly increased.

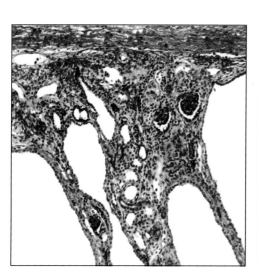

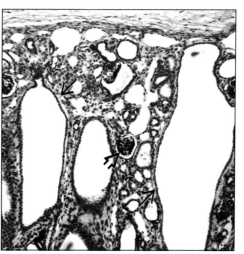

(Left) In cases of autosomal recessive PKD, the nephron elements are normally formed and are most numerous beneath the renal capsule. Abnormalities of metanephric differentiation as occurs in dysplastic kidneys are not present. *(Right)* The cystic collecting ducts ➡ are lined by low cuboidal epithelium. Some of the smaller cysts likely affect proximal tubules, regarded as a secondary process. The glomerulus ⊇ in the center is normal. No dysplastic elements are present.

AUTOSOMAL RECESSIVE POLYCYSTIC KIDNEY DISEASE

Microscopic Features

(Left) This is a newborn kidney with autosomal recessive PKD. The glomeruli, proximal ⊳ and distal tubules ⟿ appear normal. The collecting ducts ⊳ are dilated and lined by low cuboidal epithelium. No interstitial fibrosis is present. *(Right)* This is a kidney from a 7 month old with autosomal recessive PKD. The glomeruli are normal. There is moderate collecting duct ⊳ dilatation and mild proximal tubule dilation ⟿. The cortical interstitium is expanded by fibrosis.

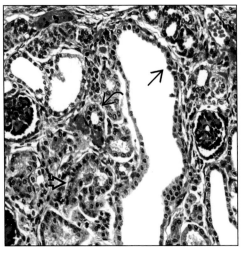 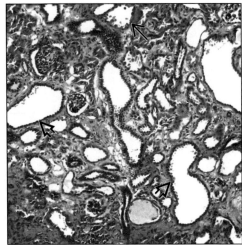

(Left) This kidney from a 2.5 year old with autosomal recessive PKD shows marked variability in cortical collecting duct dilatation. The collecting duct ranges from severely ⊳ to mildly ⊳ cystic. There is also interstitial fibrosis. *(Right)* This kidney from a 2.5 year old with autosomal recessive PKD shows glomerulosclerosis ⟿, tubular atrophy, and interstitial fibrosis. Notice the normal caliber collecting duct in the center ⊳ between 2 dilated collecting ducts ⟿.

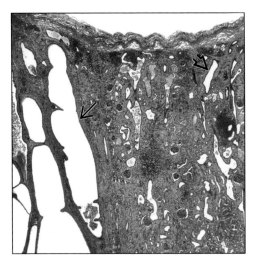 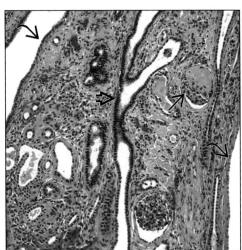

(Left) This kidney is from a 3 year old with autosomal recessive PKD kidney. It shows well-preserved cortex with ectasia of proximal tubules ⟿. There are several rounded ectatic collecting ducts in the cortex and the medulla ⊳. *(Right)* This kidney is from a 3 year old with autosomal recessive PKD. It shows mild tubular ectasia ⟿ in an otherwise largely normal superficial cortex. However, there is marked dilation of deep cortex and medullary collecting ducts ⊳.

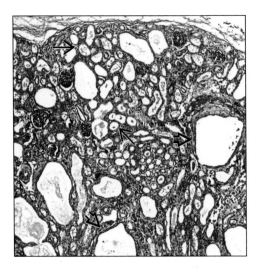 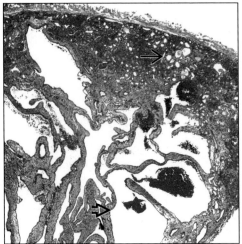

Congenital Hepatic Fibrosis

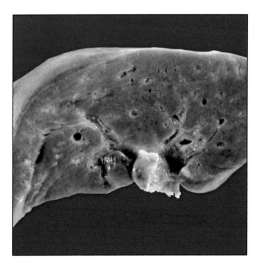

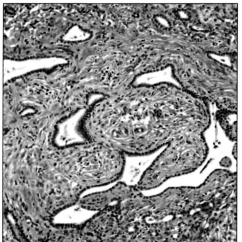

(Left) This is the liver from a neonate with autosomal recessive PKD. The cut surface is somewhat pale, rather than red, and felt firmer than normal. There is subtle portal tract expansion visible. *(Right)* This is a portal triad in a neonate with autosomal recessive PKD with severe renal involvement. It shows the characteristic bile duct plate malformation. The number of bile ducts is increased with a peripheral location within the triad. There is also fibrous portal triad expansion.

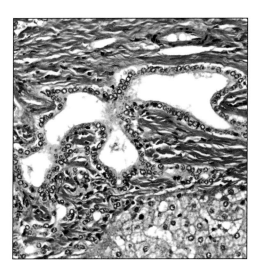

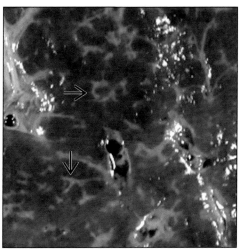

(Left) The bile duct plate malformation in autosomal recessive PKD refers to the elongated, curved, and branched bile ducts. The bile ducts are lined by low cuboidal epithelium like the collecting duct cysts in the kidney. The bile ducts are surrounded by dense fibrosis but portal inflammation is absent. *(Right)* This autopsy liver is from a 3 year old with autosomal recessive PKD and congenital hepatic fibrosis. The cut surface shows portal triad to portal triad bridging fibrosis ➡.

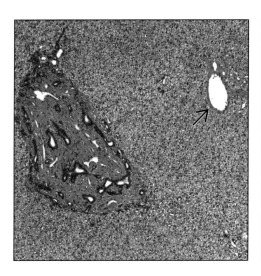

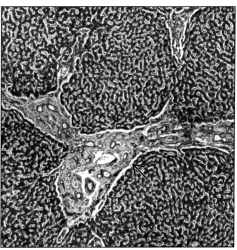

(Left) This is an autopsy liver from a 3 year old with congenital hepatic fibrosis. It shows the characteristic portal triad changes with dense fibrosis and peripheral abnormally contoured bile ducts with sparing of the central vein ➡. *(Right)* This is the liver of a 3 year old with autosomal recessive PKD and congenital hepatic fibrosis. It shows portal triad to portal triad bridging fibrosis ➡. There is an increased number of bile ducts throughout the fibrous tissues.

GLOMERULOCYSTIC DISEASE

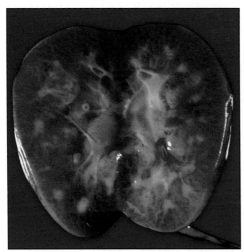

Bisected kidney with GCKD from 20-week-old fetus is shown. There are numerous small cysts throughout the cortical renal parenchyma.

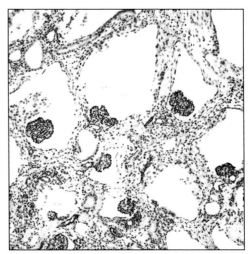

Glomerulocystic kidney has markedly dilated Bowman capsules containing glomerular tufts separated by small tubules. No connection to the proximal tubules is evident. Little or no inflammation is present.

TERMINOLOGY

Abbreviations
- Glomerulocystic kidney disease (GCKD)
- Glomerulocystic kidney (GCK) refers to pattern of injury irrespective of cause

Synonyms
- Autosomal dominant glomerulocystic kidney disease (ADGCKD)

Definitions
- Cystic dilatation of Bowman space to 2-3x normal, > 5% of glomeruli in absence of other kidney diseases
- Glomerulocystic kidneys are divided into 5 clinicopathologic categories
  - 1: Familial
  - 2: Associated with other hereditary diseases
  - 3: Syndromic nonhereditary
  - 4: Sporadic
  - 5: Acquired
- GCKD reserved for diseases caused by mutations in uromodulin or *HNF1β* genes

ETIOLOGY/PATHOGENESIS

Glomerulocystic Kidney Disease
- Familial hypoplastic GCKD (OMIM 137920)
  - *HNF1β* mutation (*TCF1*)
  - Autosomal dominant
  - Can also result in oligomeganephronia and renal dysplasia
  - Renal cysts and diabetes syndrome (RCAD), maturity onset diabetes of the young (MODY)
- Uromodulin mutation (*UMOD*)
  - Autosomal dominant
  - Uromodulin mutation also in autosomal dominant medullary cystic kidney disease (MCKD), which can be manifested by GCK

- Oro-facial-digital syndrome type 1 (OMIM 311200)
  - X-linked dominant (*Xp22*) mutation in *CXORF5*
  - Abnormalities of face, teeth, cystic kidneys
  - Lethal in males
- Renal-hepatic-pancreatic dysplasia syndrome (OMIM 208540), due to *NPHP3* mutation
- Not otherwise specified (genetic basis unknown)

Secondary Glomerular Cysts
- Atubular glomeruli formed secondary to destruction of proximal tubule
- Many causes

CLINICAL ISSUES

Epidemiology
- Incidence
  - Extremely rare diseases
    - *TCF1* GCKD > 40 cases
    - *UMOD* GCKD = 3 cases

Presentation
- Polydipsia/polyuria
- Renal insufficiency
- Findings vary considerably

Prognosis
- Course is variable, may progress to ESRD

MACROSCOPIC FEATURES

General Features
- Kidneys are usually enlarged, but may be normal in size or small
- Cortical cysts may be grossly evident

GLOMERULOCYSTIC DISEASE

Key Facts

Terminology

- 2-3x dilatation of Bowman space, > 5% of glomeruli in absence of other kidney diseases
- GCKD reserved for uromodulin or *HNF1β* mutations

Etiology/Pathogenesis

- GCKD
  - *HNF1β* mutation (*TCF1*)
  - Uromodulin mutation (*UMOD*)
- Secondary glomerular cysts in many diseases

Microscopic Pathology

- Dilation of Bowman capsule
- Glomerulus on side of cyst (atubular glomeruli)
- No connection with proximal tubule

Top Differential Diagnoses

- ADPKD and ARPKD
- Nephronophthisis
- Cystic renal dysplasia

MICROSCOPIC PATHOLOGY

Histologic Features

- Cortical cysts lined by flattened or cuboidal epithelium
- Serial sectioning reveals glomerular tufts present in most cysts
- Little inflammation
- Poorly developed proximal tubules
- Abnormal distal tubules with focal crowded nuclei (similar to macula densa) (*UMOD*)
- EM may show dilated intracellular protein vacuoles in distal tubules (*UMOD*)

DIFFERENTIAL DIAGNOSIS

ADPKD and ARPKD

- Less likely if kidneys are small
- ARPKD dilated collecting ducts
- ADPKD rarely presents in infants

Nephronophthisis: MCKD

- Closely related uromodulin mutations
- May have similar presentation, gross and microscopic appearance

Cystic Renal Dysplasia

- Immature tubules with fibromuscular collars, cartilage

Obstruction, Tuberous Sclerosis

- Clinical history is important to differentiate

DIAGNOSTIC CHECKLIST

Pathologic Interpretation Pearls

- Genetic testing needed for definitive diagnosis
- Rare diseases with limited pathologic analysis

SELECTED REFERENCES

1. Lennerz JK et al: Glomerulocystic kidney: one hundred-year perspective. Arch Pathol Lab Med. 134(4):583-605, 2010
2. Bergmann C et al: Loss of nephrocystin-3 function can cause embryonic lethality, Meckel-Gruber-like syndrome, situs inversus, and renal-hepatic-pancreatic dysplasia. Am J Hum Genet. 82(4):959-70, 2008
3. Bingham C et al: Mutations in the hepatocyte nuclear factor-1beta gene are associated with familial hypoplastic glomerulocystic kidney disease. Am J Hum Genet. 68(1):219-24, 2001
4. Feather SA et al: Oral-facial-digital syndrome type 1 is another dominant polycystic kidney disease: clinical, radiological and histopathological features of a new kindred. Nephrol Dial Transplant. 12(7):1354-61, 1997
5. Sharp CK et al: Dominantly transmitted glomerulocystic kidney disease: a distinct genetic entity. J Am Soc Nephrol. 8(1):77-84, 1997

IMAGE GALLERY

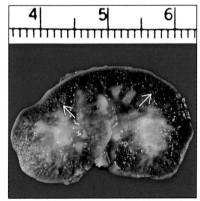
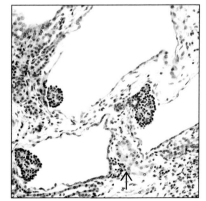
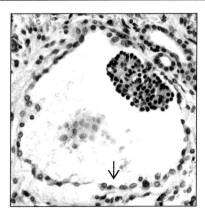

(Left) Gross photograph shows a formalin fixed kidney from a 20-week fetus with glomerulocystic disease. Small cortical cysts are seen ➡. *(Center)* Normal fetal glomerular tufts within markedly dilated urinary spaces and Bowman capsules are shown. The interstitium has few proximal tubules ➡. *(Right)* In this cystic glomerulus, the Bowman capsule is lined by squamous to low cuboidal epithelium ➡, without a connection to the proximal tubule. These are also known as atubular glomeruli.

MEDULLARY CYSTIC KIDNEY DISEASE/NEPHRONOPHTHISIS

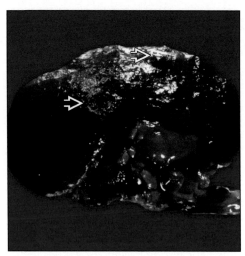

This kidney is from a 17-year-old man who presented with polydipsia and polyuria and was subsequently diagnosed with nephronophthisis. A few small cortical cysts < 1 cm in size are noted ➡. Kidney size is normal.

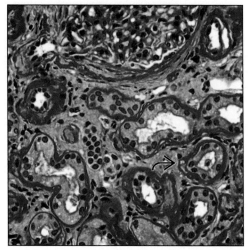

Biopsy from a child with Joubert syndrome shows prominent focal tubular atrophy with segmental thickening and duplication ➔ of the tubular basement membrane and nonspecific interstitial fibrosis.

TERMINOLOGY

Abbreviations
- Medullary cystic kidney disease (MCKD)
- Nephronophthisis (NPHP or NPH)

Definitions
- Inherited group of renal disorders characterized by presence of corticomedullary cysts secondary to mutations in ciliary proteins

ETIOLOGY/PATHOGENESIS

Genetics
- *NPHP1*
  - ○ Encodes nephrocystin-1
  - ○ Mutations account for ~ 85% of NPHP type I (juvenile) cases
  - ○ Autosomal recessive inheritance
  - ○ Maps to chromosome 2q13
- *NPHP2*
  - ○ Encodes inversin
    - Involved in determining left-right axis
  - ○ Infantile form or NPHP type II
  - ○ Maps to chromosome 9p22-31
- *NPHP3*
  - ○ Encodes nephrocystin-3
  - ○ Adolescent form or NPHP type III
  - ○ Truncation mutations associated with infantile form and Meckel-Gruber syndrome
- *NPHP4-11, NPHP1L*
  - ○ Multiple genes encoding nephrocystins 4-11 and nephrocystin 1L
  - ○ *NPHP4* mutations associated with 2% of cases; median age of ESRD = 21 years
  - ○ *NPHP5* mutations associated with 3.6% of cases; early onset retinitis pigmentosa; median age of ESRD = 13 years

- ○ *NPHP6, 8,* and *11* mutations are rare; associated with Joubert and Meckel-Gruber syndromes
- *MCKD1*
  - ○ Maps to chromosome 1q21
  - ○ Autosomal dominant inheritance
- *MCKD2*
  - ○ Encodes uromodulin
  - ○ Maps to chromosome 16p12
  - ○ Autosomal dominant inheritance

CLINICAL ISSUES

Epidemiology
- Incidence
  - ○ NPHP
    - 1:50,000 (Canada) to 1:1,000,000 live births (USA)
  - ○ MCKD: Rare
- Age
  - ○ NPHP type II (infantile form): Median age of ESRD < 5 years of age
  - ○ NPHP type I (juvenile): Median age of ESRD = 12 years
  - ○ NPHP type III (adolescent form): Median age of ESRD = 19 years
  - ○ MCKD type I: Median age of ESRD = 61 years
  - ○ MCKD type II: Median age of ESRD = 32 years

Presentation
- NPHP type I
  - ○ Polyuria, polydipsia, decreased urine concentrating ability, growth retardation, and enuresis
  - ○ Hyperuricemia and gout
  - ○ 10-15% retinitis pigmentosa (Senior-Loken syndrome)
  - ○ 2% oculomotor apraxia (Cogan syndrome)
  - ○ Rare mental retardation, optic nerve coloboma, and cerebellar vermis ataxia (Joubert syndrome)
  - ○ Rare hepatic fibrosis and epiphyseal bone defects (Mainzer-Saldino syndrome)

MEDULLARY CYSTIC KIDNEY DISEASE/NEPHRONOPHTHISIS

Key Facts

Clinical Issues
- NPHP patients develop ESRD < 5 to 19 years
- MCKD patients develop ESRD as adults
- NPHP is due to mutations in nephrocystin genes
- MCKD is due to mutations in *MCKD1* and *MCKD2* genes
- Gene sequencing *NPHP* and *MCKD* genes

Image Findings
- Ultrasound
  - Corticomedullary cysts
  - Absence of cysts does not rule out MCKD/NPH
  - Loss of corticomedullary differentiation
  - Increased echogenicity

Microscopic Pathology
- Tubular basement membrane disruption and thickening
- Dilatation of distal tubules and collecting ducts
- Diffuse interstitial fibrosis and chronic inflammation

Ancillary Tests
- Electron microscopy
  - Thickening, splitting, and duplication of tubular basement membrane

Top Differential Diagnoses
- ADPKD
- ARPKD
- Bardet-Biedl syndrome

- NPHP type II (infantile)
  - Oligohydramnios, hypertension, ventricular septal defect, situs inversus, hepatic fibrosis
- NPHP type III (adolescent)
  - Similar to NPHP type I
- Meckel-Gruber syndrome
  - Occipital meningoencephalocele, polydactyly
  - Associated with *NPHP* mutations
- MCKD types I and II
  - Polyuria, polydipsia, decreased concentrating ability
  - Hyperuricemia and gout

Laboratory Tests
- Gene sequencing NPHP and MCKD genes

Treatment
- Dialysis and renal transplantation

IMAGE FINDINGS

Ultrasonographic Findings
- Corticomedullary cysts
  - Absence of cysts does not rule out MCKD/NPH
- Loss of corticomedullary differentiation
- Increased echogenicity

MICROSCOPIC PATHOLOGY

Histologic Features
- Predominately a tubulointerstitial disease
- Glomeruli
  - 20-50% glomerulosclerosis
- Tubules
  - Tubular basement membrane disruption with duplication and thickening
  - Dilation of distal tubules and collecting ducts
  - Atrophy
- Interstitium
  - Diffuse fibrosis and mild inflammation
- No histologic features distinguish NPHP from MCKD

ANCILLARY TESTS

Electron Microscopy
- Thickening, splitting, and duplication of tubular basement membrane
- Tubular dilation

DIFFERENTIAL DIAGNOSIS

Autosomal Dominant Polycystic Kidney Disease
- Bilateral renal cysts and hepatic cysts
- Markedly enlarged kidneys
- Due to mutations in *PKD1* encoding polycystin 1

Autosomal Recessive Polycystic Kidney Disease
- Bilaterally enlarged kidneys (infant)
- Cylindrical cysts in collecting ducts and distal tubules
  - Radially arranged in cross section of cortex
- Hepatic fibrosis
- Due to mutations in *PKHD1* encoding fibrocystin/polyductin

Bardet-Biedl Syndrome
- Renal dysplasia
- Retinopathy, digit abnormalities, obesity, diabetes, male hypogonadism

SELECTED REFERENCES

1. Hurd TW et al: Mechanisms of nephronophthisis and related ciliopathies. Nephron Exp Nephrol. 118(1):e9-14, 2011
2. Wolf MT et al: Nephronophthisis. Pediatr Nephrol. 26(2):181-94, 2011
3. Hildebrandt F et al: Nephronophthisis: disease mechanisms of a ciliopathy. J Am Soc Nephrol. 20(1):23-35, 2009
4. Stavrou C et al: Autosomal-dominant medullary cystic kidney disease type 1: clinical and molecular findings in six large Cypriot families. Kidney Int. 62(4):1385-94, 2002

Nephronophthisis and Joubert Syndrome

(Left) Kidney ultrasound from a patient with nephronophthisis shows small cortical and corticomedullary cysts ⮑. *(Courtesy C. Menias, MD.)* *(Right)* Patient with Joubert syndrome has tubular basement membrane duplication highlighted with Jones silver stain ⮑. While this is not a specific finding, it is characteristic of this group of diseases.

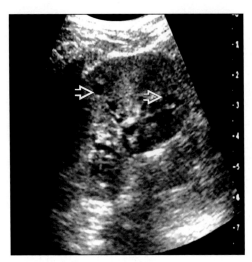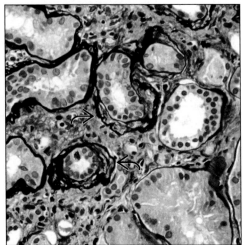

(Left) Focal segmental, global sclerosis and periglomerular fibrosis are frequent findings in biopsies of patients with nephronophthisis. This example shows focal sclerosis (Jones silver). *(Right)* This kidney is from a child with ESRD due to nephronophthisis. Sections show markedly dilated tubules filled with intensely eosinophilic Tamm-Horsfall protein, now known as uromodulin. Interstitial extrusion of uromodulin is evident by the irregular space without an epithelial lining ⮑.

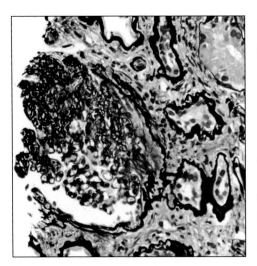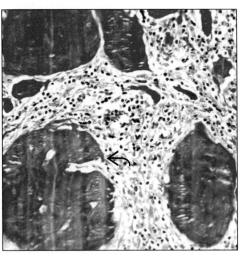

(Left) Shown is tubular dilatation, epithelial cell detachment and thinning ⮑, and multilayering ⮑ of the basement membrane in a child with nephronophthisis. *(Right)* Dilated tubule denuded of epithelial lining shows basement membrane multilayering ⮑ evident by electron microscopy in a patient with nephronophthisis.

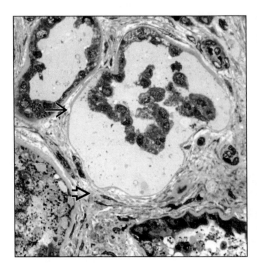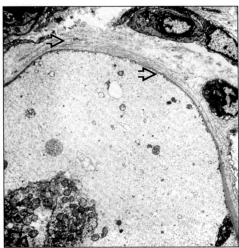

MCKD and Meckel-Gruber Syndrome

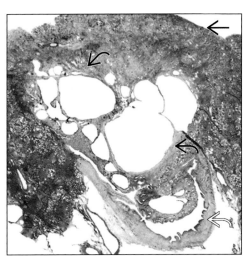

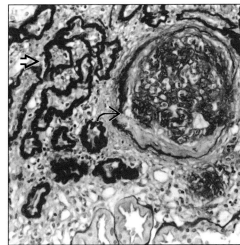

(Left) Medullary cystic kidney disease at low power shows the predominance of the cysts in the medulla and corticomedullary junction ⤵. A full cross section of a renal lobe is shown with the calyx at the bottom ⮕ and the capsule at the top ⮕. *(Right)* Biopsy from 56-year-old man with MCKD shows tubular atrophy with typical basement membrane thickening ⮕. The glomerulus shows periglomerular fibrosis ⮕ (PAS). (Courtesy I. Zouvani, MD et al.)

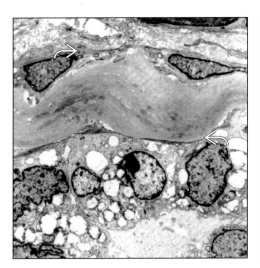

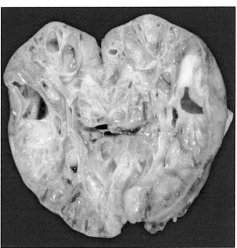

(Left) Tubular basement membrane thickening ⮕ is evident on electron microscopy in this 56-year-old patient with MCKD. (Courtesy A. Pieridis, MD et al.) *(Right)* This kidney was resected from a 2-day-old female infant with Meckel-Gruber syndrome, born with multiple anomalies including CNS abnormalities and polydactyly. Both kidneys were enlarged with multiple cortical and medullary cysts. Fixed specimen.

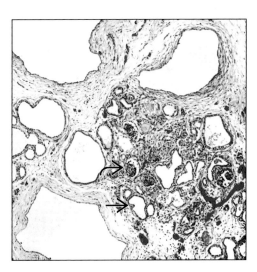

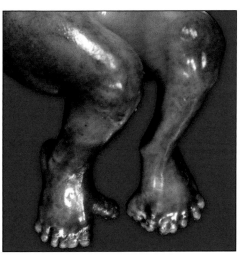

(Left) Histologic findings in Meckel-Gruber kidneys are unlike those seen in MCKD/NPHP. Typically, there is disorganized renal parenchyma with multiple cysts and immature glomeruli ⮕ and tubules ⮕, characteristic of renal dysplasia. *(Right)* Bilateral polydactyly is one of the complex malformations in Meckel-Gruber syndrome.

VON HIPPEL-LINDAU DISEASE

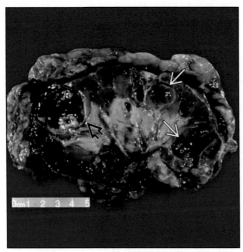

This nephrectomy in VHL contains several variably sized renal cysts ➡ and a cystic clear cell renal cell carcinoma ⧐. The carcinoma is yellow with extensive intracystic hemorrhage.

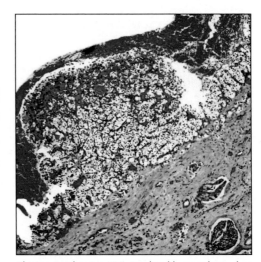

This is a renal cyst in VHL. It is lined by neoplastic clear cells and contains a small mural nodule of clear cell renal cell carcinoma. The nuclear grade of the tumor is low, typical of this disease.

TERMINOLOGY

Abbreviations
- von Hippel-Lindau (VHL) disease

Definitions
- Germline mutation of *VHL* tumor suppressor gene
- Member of phacomatosis familial cancer syndromes
- Cardinal manifestations: Hemangioblastoma, clear cell renal cell carcinoma, pheochromocytoma, epididymal papillary cystadenoma, renal and pancreatic cysts
  - If no family history
    - Diagnosis requires 2 cardinal manifestations, including retinal or CNS involvement and excluding cysts
  - With positive family history
    - 1 cardinal manifestation excluding cysts

ETIOLOGY/PATHOGENESIS

Molecular Genetics
- Autosomal dominant
- Germline mutation of *VHL* gene, 3p25-26
  - *VHL* mutation in 50% of sporadic renal cell carcinoma (RCC)
  - 2nd inactivating event predisposes to neoplasms
- VHL protein
  - Promotes destruction of hypoxia inducible factor 1 alpha (HIF-1-α) via ubiquitin pathway
    - Loss of function leads to increased levels of vascular endothelial growth factor (VEGF)
  - HIF independent regulation of the primary cilium and apoptosis via factors NF-kB
    - Loss of function promotes renal cysts
- Genotype-phenotype correlations
  - Type 1 VHL (truncating and exon deletions)
    - Low risk of pheochromocytoma
  - Type 2 VHL (missense mutations)
    - High risk of pheochromocytoma

- Type 2a: Low risk of RCC
- Type 2b: High risk of RCC
- Type 2c: Familial pheochromocytoma without hemangioblastoma or RCC

CLINICAL ISSUES

Epidemiology
- Incidence
  - 1:36,000 live births
  - 90% penetrance by age 65
  - Mean age of renal involvement = 35-40 years

Presentation
- Clear cell renal cell carcinoma
  - Bilateral and multifocal in 40-60%
  - Likely arise from atypical clear cell cysts
    - Carcinoma and cyst lining cells are euploid
  - Hematuria ± back pain
- Renal cysts
  - Bilateral and multifocal in 70-80%
  - Usually fewer than in autosomal dominant polycystic kidney disease (ADPKD)
- Hemangioblastoma most frequent lesion in VHL
  - Cerebellum in 60-80%
  - Retina in 50-60%
  - Spinal cord in 15-60%
- Pheochromocytoma in 10-25%
- Pancreatic cysts in 60-80%
- Epididymal papillary cystadenoma in 20-50%
- Pancreatic neuroendocrine neoplasms uncommon
- Pancreatic epithelial neoplasms uncommon

Treatment
- Surgical approaches
  - Nephron-sparing surgery
  - Tumor resection when other organs affected

Prognosis
- Death due to renal cell carcinoma in 50%

VON HIPPEL-LINDAU DISEASE

Key Facts

Terminology
- Familial cancer syndrome (phacomatosis)

Etiology/Pathogenesis
- Germline mutation *VHL* gene on chr 3p25-26
- 2nd inactivating event predisposes to neoplasms

Clinical Issues
- Neoplastic diathesis involving multiple organs
- Death from renal cell carcinoma in 50%

Image Findings
- Multiple and bilateral renal cysts
- Multiple and bilateral renal cell carcinomas

Macroscopic Features
- Cysts are multiple and have thin yellow lining
- Solid and cystic yellow renal cell carcinomas

Microscopic Pathology
- Cysts are lined by clear cells
- Clear cell renal cell carcinoma, usually cystic

Top Differential Diagnoses
- Acquired cystic kidney disease
  - Cysts lined by flattened to hyperplastic epithelium
  - Diverse array of renal neoplasms
- Tuberous sclerosis/autosomal dominant polycystic kidney disease contiguous gene syndrome
  - Diffusely cystic kidneys
  - Angiomyolipoma
  - Rarely, clear cell renal cell carcinoma
- Dominant polycystic kidney disease
  - Risk of renal neoplasms controversial

  - Metastases to liver, lung, and bone

MACROSCOPIC FEATURES

General Features
- Multiple and bilateral cysts
- Multiple and bilateral cystic renal cell carcinomas
- Solid renal cell carcinomas

MICROSCOPIC PATHOLOGY

Histologic Features
- Cysts
  - Lined by large cells with cleared-out cytoplasm
  - Benign cyst lined by single cell layer
  - Atypical cysts lined by piled up or stratified cells
- Clear cell renal cell carcinoma
  - Multicystic or solid tumors
  - Composed of cells with cleared-out cytoplasm
  - Microscopic to macroscopic lesions
  - Early lesion
    - Intratubular proliferation of clear cells

DIFFERENTIAL DIAGNOSIS

Cystic Renal Diseases Associated with Renal Neoplasms
- Acquired cystic kidney disease
  - Cyst frequency proportional to duration of ESRD
  - Diverse array of renal cell carcinomas
- Tuberous sclerosis complex/autosomal dominant polycystic kidney disease contiguous gene syndrome
  - Diffusely cystic kidneys identical to ADPKD
  - Multiple and bilateral angiomyolipomas
  - Rarely, clear cell renal cell carcinoma
- Autosomal dominant polycystic kidney disease
  - Risk of renal cell carcinoma may be increased but controversial
  - Far more numerous cysts than in VHL

DIAGNOSTIC CHECKLIST

Pathologic Interpretation Pearls
- Bilateral renal cysts and liver cysts: Think ADPKD
- Bilateral renal cysts and pancreatic cysts: Think VHL

SELECTED REFERENCES

1. Calzada MJ: Von Hippel-Lindau syndrome: molecular mechanisms of the disease. Clin Transl Oncol. 12(3):160-5, 2010
2. Kim JJ et al: Von Hippel Lindau syndrome. Adv Exp Med Biol. 685:228-49, 2010
3. Moch H: Cystic renal tumors: new entities and novel concepts. Adv Anat Pathol. 17(3):209-14, 2010
4. Bonsib SM: Renal cystic diseases and renal neoplasms: a mini-review. Clin J Am Soc Nephrol. 4(12):1998-2007, 2009
5. Reed AB et al: Surgical management of von Hippel-Lindau disease: urologic considerations. Surg Oncol Clin N Am. 18(1):157-74, x, 2009
6. Shehata BM et al: Von Hippel-Lindau (VHL) disease: an update on the clinico-pathologic and genetic aspects. Adv Anat Pathol. 15(3):165-71, 2008
7. Esteban MA et al: Formation of primary cilia in the renal epithelium is regulated by the von Hippel-Lindau tumor suppressor protein. J Am Soc Nephrol. 17(7):1801-6, 2006
8. Truong LD et al: Renal cystic neoplasms and renal neoplasms associated with cystic renal diseases: pathogenetic and molecular links. Adv Anat Pathol. 10(3):135-59, 2003
9. Paraf F et al: Renal lesions in von Hippel-Lindau disease: immunohistochemical expression of nephron differentiation molecules, adhesion molecules and apoptosis proteins. Histopathology. 36(5):457-65, 2000
10. Salomé F et al: Renal lesions in Von Hippel-Lindau disease: the benign, the malignant, the unknown. Eur Urol. 34(5):383-92, 1998
11. Neumann HP et al: Renal cysts, renal cancer and von Hippel-Lindau disease. Kidney Int. 51(1):16-26, 1997
12. Chauveau D et al: Renal involvement in von Hippel-Lindau disease. Kidney Int. 50(3):944-51, 1996
13. Solomon D et al: Renal pathology in von Hippel-Lindau disease. Hum Pathol. 19(9):1072-9, 1988

VON HIPPEL-LINDAU DISEASE

Gross and Microscopic Features

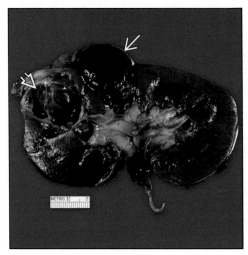 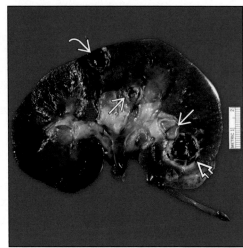

(Left) *This bivalved kidney is from a patient with VHL disease. It contains 2 cystic lesions. One has a thin, yellow lining* ⮫. *The other is filled with hemorrhage* ➡ *and likely harbors a carcinoma.* **(Right)** *Kidney shows 2 cystic lesions and 2 small solid renal cell carcinomas* ➡. *The smaller cyst* ⮫ *is benign and contains blood. The larger cyst* ⮫ *contains blood but also has yellow nodules representing a clear cell renal cell carcinoma.*

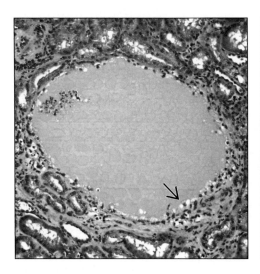 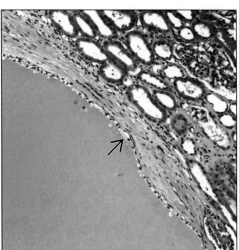

(Left) *This is a small (1 mm) benign cyst. In contrast to simple cortical cysts common in adult kidneys, this cyst is lined by cells* ➡ *with complete cytoplasmic clearing and low-grade nuclear features. The lack of stratification qualifies this cyst as a benign cyst.* **(Right)** *This is a portion of a benign 2 cm cyst in VHL. The cyst is lined by a single layer of clear cells* ➡. *The cells have low-grade nuclear features. Additional cysts and several carcinomas were present elsewhere.*

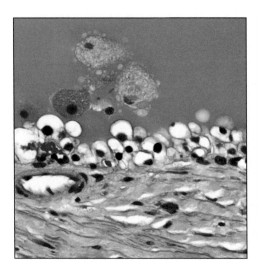 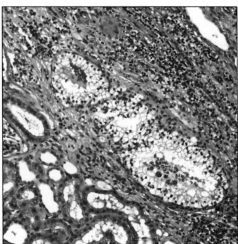

(Left) *This is a cyst from a VHL disease case. This cyst is also lined by clear cells that are stratified with grade 2 nuclear features. The cyst wall is fibrotic. Because of this and similar changes elsewhere in this cyst, it is classified as atypical, possibly destined to become a renal cell carcinoma.* **(Right)** *A small clear cell renal cell carcinoma is present in this field. It consists of several small, confluent acinar structures with centrally located red blood cells.*

Gross Features

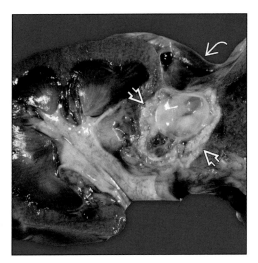

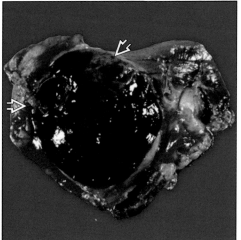

(Left) *This VHL patient has 2 cystic lesions. One is a large, superficial, collapsed cyst ⊅. The other lesion is associated with prominent sclerosis ⊃ and contains a central cyst. The sclerotic areas harbored nests of clear cell, indicating the presence of clear cell renal cell carcinoma.* *(Right)* *This is a nephron-sparing, partial nephrectomy in VHL disease. It contains a renal cell carcinoma. There are small yellow nodules of tumor ⊅ associated with extensive hemorrhage.*

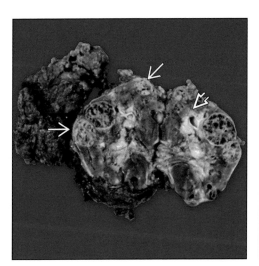

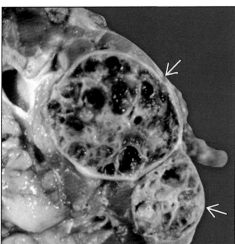

(Left) *This bivalved kidney in VHL disease contains multiple renal cell carcinomas and benign renal cysts. 2 of the carcinomas ➡ have both solid and cystic areas and appear yellow. The 3rd carcinoma ➡ is also cystic and yellow but contains hemorrhage.* *(Right)* *These 2 clear cell renal cell carcinomas ➡ appear yellow because they have high lipid content. Both carcinomas are very cystic, and the larger carcinoma shows more hemorrhage. All tumors in this case were renal limited.*

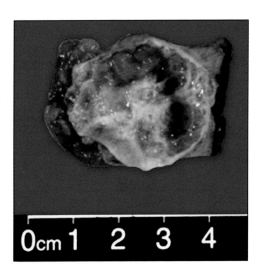

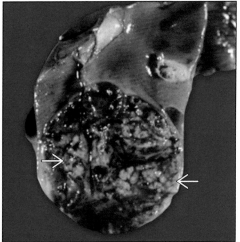

(Left) *This is a partial nephrectomy in a patient with VHL and multiple renal cell carcinomas elsewhere. This particular carcinoma is cystic with sclerotic areas. The sclerosis is a regressive feature and correlates with a low volume of tumor cells.* *(Right)* *This is from another VHL patient treated with a partial nephrectomy for multiple renal tumors. Multiple small nodules of clear cell renal cell carcinoma are visible within this hemorrhagic tumor. There is also a small cyst ➡.*

VON HIPPEL-LINDAU DISEASE

Pancreas

(Left) This is a clear cell renal cell carcinoma of several centimeters in VHL disease. The carcinoma is composed of cystic areas and solid areas all populated by similar appearing low-grade clear cells. The presence of solid areas qualifies the lesion as a carcinoma. *(Right)* The cells lining the cystic spaces ⇨ and the cells within the solid areas ⇛ or cyst septae appear identical, with low-grade nuclear features. The solid areas qualify this lesion as a renal cell carcinoma.

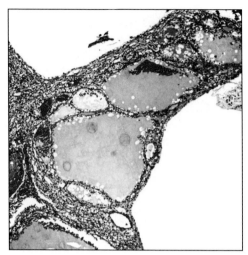
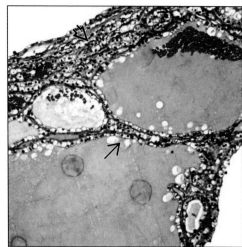

(Left) The clear cell renal cell carcinomas that develop in patients with VHL disease are often low grade with Fuhrman nuclear 1 or 2. The cytoplasmic clearing results from extraction of abundant lipid and glycogen, characteristic of clear cell carcinomas. *(Right)* This kidney contained a clear cell carcinoma of several centimeters. In this section, distant from the main tumor, is a clear cell-lined cyst ⇨ and 2 small solid nests of clear cell carcinoma ⇛. All cells exhibit a low nuclear grade.

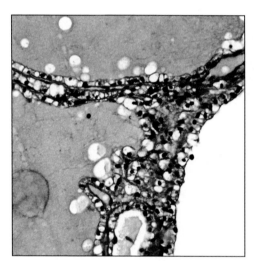
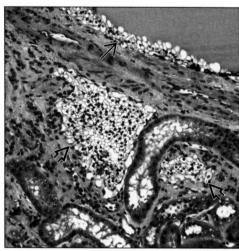

(Left) This solid nodule of clear cell renal cell carcinoma was present within a tumor that was otherwise extensively cystic. Notice the low nuclear grade with uniform-appearing nuclei. *(Right)* Clear cell renal cell carcinoma in VHL is indistinguishable from sporadic clear cell renal cell carcinoma. The delicate capillary lattice present here ⇨ is a characteristic feature of all clear cell renal cell carcinomas and comprises an essential component of their WHO definition.

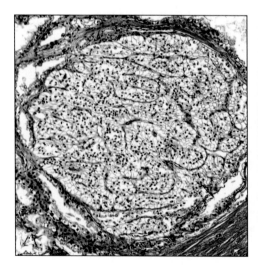
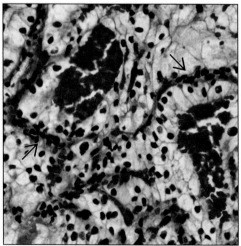

Pancreatic Lesions in VHL Disease

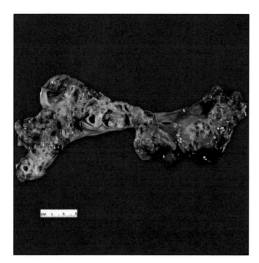

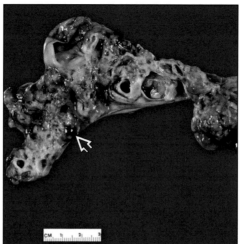

(Left) This is the pancreas from an autopsy in a patient with VHL disease. The pancreas is diffusely affected by benign cysts. The endocrine function of this gland is unaffected by the cysts. There are no solid tumor nodules present. (Right) The cysts in this pancreas vary greatly in size. In contrast to many renal cysts in VHL, these cysts do not have a yellow lining and also lack hemorrhage, a feature characteristic of renal cysts. One hemorrhagic cyst is present ➡.

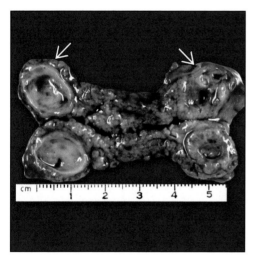

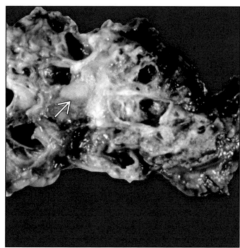

(Left) This is a bivalved pancreas from an autopsied patient with VHL disease. It contains 2 dominant cysts ➡. There are also several smaller cysts, more difficult to appreciate in this photograph. The central portions of the pancreas appear grossly normal. (Right) This is the pancreas from an autopsied patient with VHL disease. It is severely affected. It shows numerous variably sized cysts and extensive areas of sclerosis ➡; however, no neoplasms were present.

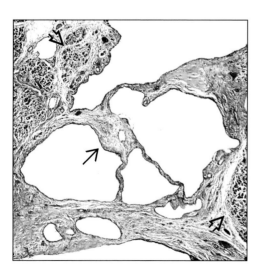

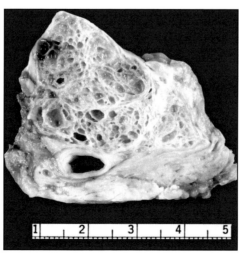

(Left) This is the pancreas from an autopsied patient with VHL disease. The normal pancreatic parenchyma is visible at the edges ➡. The cysts are derived from the pancreatic duct system and lined by a single layer of benign cuboidal duct epithelium ➡. (Right) This pancreas from an autopsied patient with VHL disease shows a single multicystic lesion known as a serous cystadenoma, a benign neoplasm. The cysts are lined by a single layer of clear cells similar to the renal cysts.

TUBEROUS SCLEROSIS

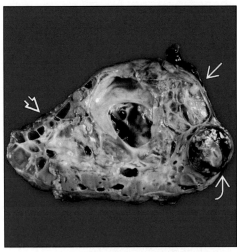

Cross section of a kidney from a patient with tuberous sclerosis is shown. An angiomyolipoma ➡, many cysts of various sizes ⬌, and a renal cell carcinoma ➡ are all typical lesions in TSC.

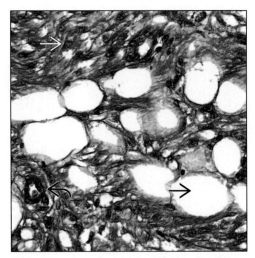

High-power view of an angiomyolipoma in tuberous sclerosis is shown with all 3 histological components of the tumor: Fat ➡, smooth muscle ➡, and blood vessels ➡.

TERMINOLOGY

Abbreviations
- Tuberous sclerosis (TSC)

Synonyms
- Tuberous sclerosis complex

Definitions
- Molecular disorder of hamartin of tuberin proteins resulting in hamartomatous lesions in skin, CNS, kidney, and other organs

ETIOLOGY/PATHOGENESIS

Molecular Pathology
- *TSC1* gene, chromosome 9q34: Hamartin
- *TSC2* gene, chromosome 16p13: Tuberin
- Abnormal Pi3K: AKT, mTOR signaling
- Hamartin and tuberin normally interact and inhibit cell growth/proliferation
- Pi3K plays role in dissociation of hamartin/tuberin complex
- Chromosome 16p deletion may result in *TSC2/PKD1* contiguous gene syndrome with early onset polycystic kidney disease

CLINICAL ISSUES

Epidemiology
- Incidence
  o 1 in 10,000 to 1 in 15,000
  o Autosomal dominant mode of inheritance
  o 60% of cases are sporadic
  o *TSC2* mutations account for majority of sporadic cases

Presentation
- Facial angiofibromas and other skin abnormalities, mucosal fibromas
- Retinal hamartomas
- Seizures
- Mental retardation
- Brain cortical defects including tubers: Abnormal accumulations of glial cells
- Cardiac rhabdomyomas
- Kidney angiomyolipomas, cysts, and renal cell carcinomas
- Diagnosis requires either 2 major, or 1 major and 2 minor features
  o Major features
    ▪ Facial angiofibromas, ungual or periungual fibromas
    ▪ More than 3 hypomelanotic macules, shagreen patch
    ▪ Retinal hamartomas, cortical tuber, subependymal nodule or astrocytoma
    ▪ Cardiac rhabdomyoma, lymphangioleiomyomatosis, renal angiomyolipoma
  o Minor features
    ▪ Multiple renal cysts, hamartomatous rectal polyps
    ▪ Retinal achromic patch, white matter radial migration tracts
    ▪ Bone cysts, gingival fibromas, "confetti" skin lesions, enamel pits

Treatment
- Annual monitoring with kidney ultrasound
- Nephrectomy if non-remitting pain and hemorrhage or presence of renal cell carcinoma
- Rapamycin is being tested as experimental drug
- Control of hypertension
- Renal transplantation in ESRD: Bilateral nephrectomy should be considered

TUBEROUS SCLEROSIS

Key Facts

Etiology/Pathogenesis
- *TSC1* gene, chromosome 9q34: Hamartin
- *TSC2* gene, chromosome 16p13: Tuberin
- Chromosome 16p deletion may result in *TSC2/PKD1* contiguous gene syndrome with early onset PKD

Clinical Issues
- Major features
  - Facial angiofibromas, ungual or periungual fibromas
  - More than 3 hypomelanotic macules, shagreen patch
  - Retinal hamartomas, cortical tuber, subependymal nodule or astrocytoma
  - Cardiac rhabdomyoma, lymphangioleiomyomatosis, renal angiomyolipoma

- Minor features
  - Multiple renal cysts, hamartomatous rectal polyps, retinal achromic patch, white matter radial migration tracts, bone cysts, gingival fibromas, "confetti" skin lesions, enamel pits

Microscopic Pathology
- Angiomyolipomas and angiomyolipomatous change of renal parenchyma is most common finding
- Cysts lined by large plump cells with deeply eosinophilic cytoplasm are characteristic of TSC
- Renal cell carcinomas

Top Differential Diagnoses
- ADPKD
- VHL
- Multicystic dysplasia

Prognosis
- Progressive decline of renal function due to progression of angiomyolipomas and cystic disease
- CNS and kidney lesions are main causes of mortality

IMAGE FINDINGS

Radiographic Findings
- MR will show both bright intensities (cysts) and dark areas (fat in angiomyolipomas)
- Ultrasound is used to follow-up progression of lesions

MACROSCOPIC FEATURES

General Features
- Kidneys are enlarged
- External surface is often distorted by cortical cysts
- Firm to fleshy, tan to yellow angiomyolipomas can be identified
  - Larger lesions are usually well demarcated
- Cysts of various sizes are randomly distributed throughout cortex and medulla

MICROSCOPIC PATHOLOGY

Histologic Features
- Angiomyolipomas and angiomyolipomatous change of renal parenchyma is most common finding
- Multiple cysts involving both cortex and medulla
  - Cysts lined by large plump cells with deeply eosinophilic cytoplasm are characteristic of TSC
  - Cysts with deeply eosinophilic luminal content
  - Nuclear pleomorphism of cyst lining epithelium
- Glomerular microhamartomas can sometimes be seen
  - Glomerular mass lesions featuring polygonal epithelial cells containing lipid vacuoles
- FSGS lesions may develop
- Renal cell carcinomas and oncocytomas
  - Most common: Clear cell renal cell carcinoma

- Chromophobe renal cell carcinoma and oncocytomas are also common
- Papillary and collecting duct carcinomas are rare

DIFFERENTIAL DIAGNOSIS

Autosomal Dominant Polycystic Kidney Disease (ADPKD)
- If angiomyolipomas are present, that favors tuberous sclerosis
- Clinical history is important
- The presence of *TSC2/PKD1* contiguous gene syndrome complicates the diagnosis, particularly in juvenile cases

von Hippel-Lindau Disease (VHL)
- Both TSC and VHL may present with kidney cysts and renal cell carcinoma
- VHL does not have angiomyolipomas
- Molecular diagnosis may be required in difficult cases

Multicystic Dysplasia
- Presence of dysplastic elements (immature tubules with loose fibrous collars, cartilage) should favor dysplasia

SELECTED REFERENCES

1. Bonsib SM: Renal cystic diseases and renal neoplasms: a mini-review. Clin J Am Soc Nephrol. 4(12):1998-2007, 2009
2. Rosser T et al: The diverse clinical manifestations of tuberous sclerosis complex: a review. Semin Pediatr Neurol. 13(1):27-36, 2006
3. Henske EP: Tuberous sclerosis and the kidney: from mesenchyme to epithelium, and beyond. Pediatr Nephrol. 20(7):854-7, 2005
4. Lendvay TS et al: The tuberous sclerosis complex and its highly variable manifestations. J Urol. 169(5):1635-42, 2003
5. Martignoni G et al: Renal pathology in the tuberous sclerosis complex. Pathology. 35(6):505-12, 2003

TUBEROUS SCLEROSIS

Gross and Microscopic Features

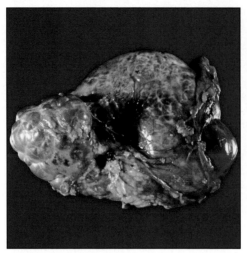
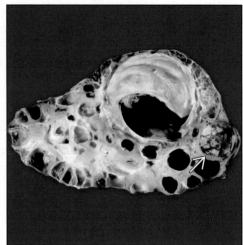

(Left) External surface of a kidney from a patient with tuberous sclerosis shows multiple cysts of various sizes. This resembles the external appearance of kidneys in autosomal dominant polycystic disease (ADPKD). **(Right)** Cross section of a fixed nephrectomy specimen from a patient with tuberous sclerosis shows the extent of the parenchymal involvement by cystic change and an angiomyolipoma ➡.

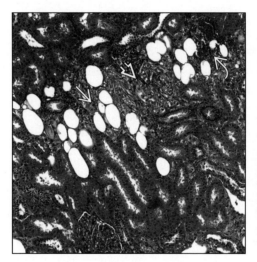
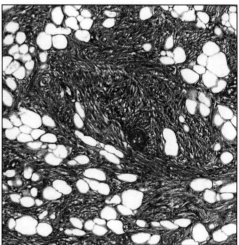

(Left) Angiomyolipomatous change can be seen throughout the kidney in tuberous sclerosis. In this micrograph the abnormal tissue consisting of fat ➡, smooth muscle ⧐, and small blood vessels ➢ percolates through the renal cortex. **(Right)** Low-power view of an angiomyolipoma is shown. Lipomatous and smooth muscle components are most prominent in this view. Angiomyolipomas are the most common finding in TSC.

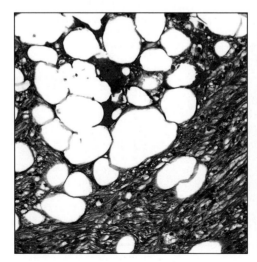
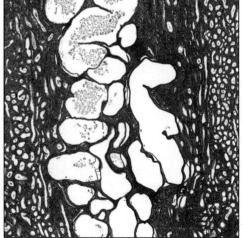

(Left) Shown here is a high-power view of an angiomyolipoma. Small vascular channels are engorged with blood between adipocytes. **(Right)** Kidney cysts are seen throughout the kidney parenchyma in this patient with tuberous sclerosis, involving both the cortex and the medulla. In this micrograph, cysts involving the collecting segment are linearly arranged and are probably ectatic tubules rather than true cysts.

Microscopic Features

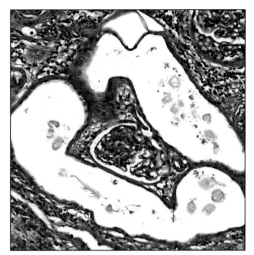 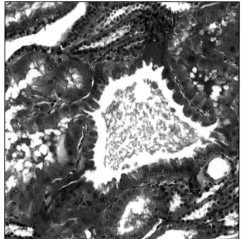

(Left) A small cortical tubular cyst shown here surrounds a glomerulus. In addition to tubular cysts, glomerular cysts can be commonly seen in TSC. *(Right)* A characteristic appearance of kidney cysts in TSC is shown. The cells comprising the cystic epithelium have plump eosinophilic cytoplasm with a hobnail pattern, and are much larger than cells in noncystic tubules.

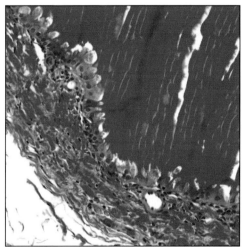 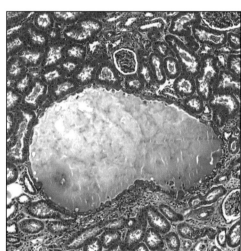

(Left) Many cysts show, in addition to characteristic epithelial cellular changes, an accumulation of deeply eosinophilic material in the cyst lumen. Nuclear pleomorphism is also evident. *(Right)* This is another example of a cortical cyst in TSC. Even at this low power, one can appreciate how large the cells lining the cyst lumen are.

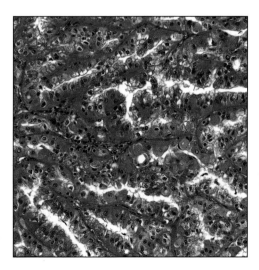 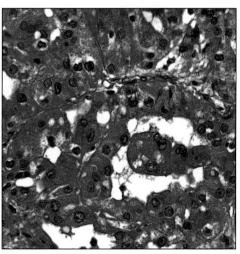

(Left) The most common renal cell carcinoma in TSC is the clear cell type, followed by the chromophobe type. The papillary renal cell carcinoma shown here is only rarely observed. *(Right)* High-power view of a papillary renal cell carcinoma in tuberous sclerosis is shown forming tubular structures that resemble normal proximal tubules.

ZELLWEGER SYNDROME

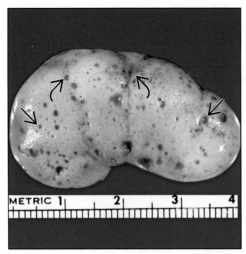

This autopsy kidney from a patient with Zellweger syndrome is developmentally normal. There is subtle persistence of fetal lobation ⇨. Multiple small, superficial cortical cysts are present ⇨.

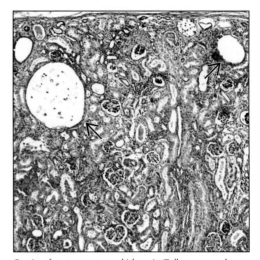

Section from an autopsy kidney in Zellweger syndrome illustrates that most nephrons are usually normal but associated with scattered small cysts ⇨ lined by a thin epithelial cell layer.

TERMINOLOGY

Abbreviations
- Zellweger syndrome (ZS)

Synonyms
- Cerebrohepatorenal syndrome (CHRS)

Definitions
- Autosomal recessive multisystem disease
- Most severe form of 3 peroxisome synthesis disorders
  - Zellweger syndrome
  - Neonatal adrenoleukodystrophy
  - Infantile Refsum syndrome

ETIOLOGY/PATHOGENESIS

PEX Mutations
- *PEX* encodes for peroxins, proteins required for peroxisome assembly
  - Cytoplasmic peroxidase enzymes fail to be incorporated into peroxisomes
- 12 mutations identified
  - *PEX1* mutation most common (70% of cases)
- Absent or reduced peroxisomes in kidney, liver, and other organs

CLINICAL ISSUES

Epidemiology
- Incidence
  - 1 in 50,000

Presentation
- Neonatal presentation
  - Craniofacial dysmorphism
    - High forehead
    - Large fontanelles
    - Hypotelorism
  - Limb dysmorphism
  - Central nervous system disease
    - Seizures
    - Hypotonia
    - Difficulty feeding
  - Liver dysfunction
    - Neonatal jaundice
    - Elevated liver function tests
  - Renal dysfunction
    - Mild azotemia
    - Proteinuria (25%)
    - Aminoaciduria (25%)

Laboratory Tests
- Elevated plasma and tissue very long-chain fatty acids
- Biochemical testing of cultured fetal fibroblasts

Prognosis
- Most patients die within 1st year of life

IMAGE FINDINGS

Radiographic Findings
- Chondroplasia puncta (stippled epiphyses)
  - Patellae and long bones

MACROSCOPIC FEATURES

General Features
- Kidney
  - Cortical cysts in > 90%
    - Subcapsular
    - Range < 0.01-1 cm in size
- Central nervous system
  - Macrogyria
  - Cerebellar hypoplasia
- Liver
  - Hepatomegaly at birth
  - Micronodular cirrhosis later

ZELLWEGER SYNDROME

Key Facts

Terminology
- Autosomal recessive multisystem disease

Etiology/Pathogenesis
- *PEX* mutations (12 identified)
- Peroxisome synthesis defect

Clinical Issues
- Craniofacial and limb dysmorphism
- Central nervous system malformations
- Liver dysfunction
- Usually asymptomatic renal cystic disease

Image Findings
- Stippled epiphyses

Macroscopic Features
- Cortical cysts, usually < 1 cm

- CNS macrogyria and cerebellar hypoplasia

Microscopic Pathology
- Subcapsular renal cysts
- Hepatic hemosiderosis
- Abnormal neuronal migration and myelination with cortical heterotopia
- Adrenal cytomegaly

Ancillary Tests
- Increase very long-chain fatty acids in plasma and tissues
- Biochemical testing of cultured fetal fibroblasts

Top Differential Diagnoses
- Enzyme defects of peroxisomal metabolism
  - Acyl-CoA oxidase deficiency
  - Carnitine palmitoyltransferase II deficiency

MICROSCOPIC PATHOLOGY

Histologic Features
- Kidneys
  - Glomerular and tubular microcysts
    - Pericystic fibrosis
  - Rarely, altered metanephric differentiation
    - Immature tubules
    - Dysgenetic glomeruli
    - Poorly formed medulla
- Liver
  - Hemosiderin in hepatocytes, preferentially periportal, and Kupffer cells
  - Micronodular cirrhosis
- Central nervous system
  - Abnormal neuronal migration and myelination
  - Cortical heteropsia

ANCILLARY TESTS

Electron Microscopy
- Absent peroxisomes in organs affected

DIFFERENTIAL DIAGNOSIS

Clinical ZS Phenotype
- May result from enzyme defects of peroxisome metabolism
- Acyl-CoA oxidase deficiency (glutaric acidemia type II)
  - Dysmorphic features, cystic dysplasia of kidneys, CNS abnormalities, diffuse lipid infiltration of organs
- Carnitine palmitoyltransferase II deficiency
  - Dysmorphic features, cystic dysplasia kidneys and brain, cardiomyopathy, fatty infiltration of organs

SELECTED REFERENCES

1. Ebberink MS et al: Genetic classification and mutational spectrum of more than 600 patients with a Zellweger syndrome spectrum disorder. Hum Mutat. 32(1):59-69, 2011
2. Steinberg SJ et al: Peroxisome biogenesis disorders, Zellweger syndrome spectrum. In Pago RA et al (eds.): GeneReviews [Internet]. Seattle: University of Washington. Posted December 12, 2003; updated January 18, 2011
3. Ebberink MS et al: Spectrum of PEX6 mutations in Zellweger syndrome spectrum patients. Hum Mutat. 31(1):E1058-70, 2010
4. Takenouchi T et al: Germinal matrix hemorrhage in zellweger syndrome. J Child Neurol. 25(11):1398-400, 2010
5. Al-Dirbashi OY et al: Zellweger syndrome caused by PEX13 deficiency: report of two novel mutations. Am J Med Genet A. 149A(6):1219-23, 2009
6. Lindhard A et al: Postmortem findings and prenatal diagnosis of Zellweger syndrome. Case report. APMIS. 101(3):226-8, 1993
7. Poll-The BT et al: Infantile Refsum disease: an inherited peroxisomal disorder. Comparison with Zellweger syndrome and neonatal adrenoleukodystrophy. Eur J Pediatr. 146(5):477-83, 1987
8. Zellweger H: The cerebro-hepato-renal (Zellweger) syndrome and other peroxisomal disorders. Dev Med Child Neurol. 29(6):821-9, 1987
9. Nakamura K et al: Cerebro-hepato-renal syndrome of Zellweger. Clinical and autopsy findings and a review of previous cases in Japan. Acta Pathol Jpn. 36(11):1727-35, 1986
10. Powers JM et al: Fetal cerebrohepatorenal (Zellweger) syndrome: dysmorphic, radiologic, biochemical, and pathologic findings in four affected fetuses. Hum Pathol. 16(6):610-20, 1985
11. Carlson BR et al: Giant cell transformation cerebrohepatorenal syndrome. Arch Pathol Lab Med. 102(11):596-9, 1978
12. Sommer A et al: The cerebro-hepato-renal syndrome (Zellweger's syndrome). Biol Neonate. 25(3-4):219-29, 1974
13. Passarge E et al: Cerebro-hepato-renal syndrome. A newly recognized hereditary disorder of multiple congenital defects, including sudanophilic leukodystrophy, cirrhosis of the liver, and polycystic kidneys. J Pediatr. 71(5):691-702, 1967

ZELLWEGER SYNDROME

Microscopic and Gross Features

(**Left**) Section of kidney from an autopsy in Zellweger syndrome shows that the majority of nephrons are normal. Several microcysts are present. Most of the cysts are glomerular cysts since a glomerular tuft ➡ is present in the majority. (**Right**) Glomerular cyst in Zellweger syndrome is shown. Although Bowman capsule is dilated ⧉ and much larger than normal, the glomerular tuft ➡ appears completely normal. The capillary loops are open and the mesangium is inconspicuous.

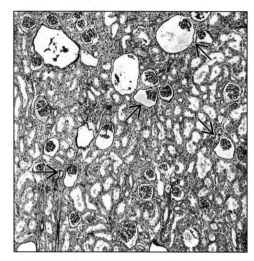
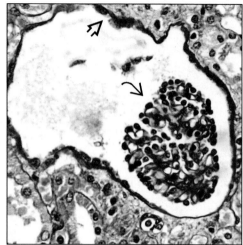

(**Left**) Autopsy kidneys in a patient with Zellweger syndrome are diffusely altered by cysts. The cysts are small, less than a centimeter each. The kidneys are reniform and their cut surface showed corticomedullary differentiation with cysts throughout the cortex. (**Right**) A bivalved, severely cystic kidney in Zellweger syndrome is shown. A portion of the collecting system ⧉ is present. Both the cortex and medulla contain small cysts with the renal medulla ➡ most severely affected.

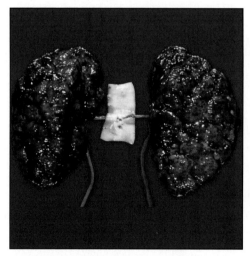
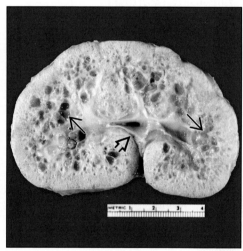

(**Left**) This autopsy kidney in Zellweger syndrome demonstrates the pericystic rim of fibrosis ⧉ and the characteristic subcapsular location of most cysts ➡. The nephrons in the deeper cortex appear progressively more normal. (**Right**) Section from an autopsy in a patient with Zellweger syndrome shows cysts with a pericystic layer of fibrosis ➡. One cyst is glomerular with a tiny glomerular tuft ➡ visible. The other cysts are likely glomerular with tufts out of the plane.

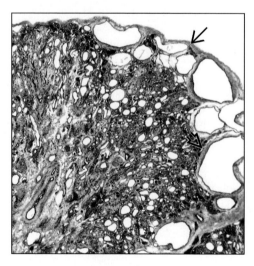
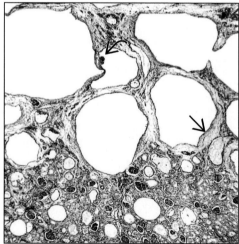

ZELLWEGER SYNDROME

Microscopic Features of Kidney and Liver

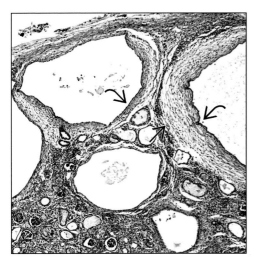

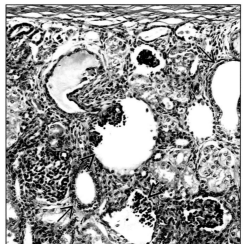

(Left) At this higher magnification, the pericystic fibrous layer ➡ is more clearly illustrated. The cysts are lined by a flattened epithelium ➡. No dysplastic features are noted in the noncystic cortex. *(Right)* Section from an autopsy in Zellweger syndrome shows both glomerular cysts ➡ and microcystic change in renal tubules ➡. The cystic tubules have a shallow, cuboidal cell lining in contrast to the flattened cell lining of the glomerular cysts.

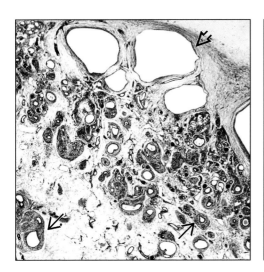

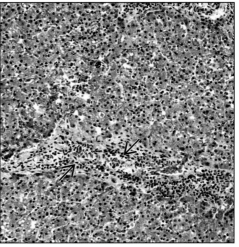

(Left) Severely affected kidney in Zellweger syndrome is shown. There are subcapsular cysts ➡ and marked failure of metanephric differentiation with very few nephron elements present. There are dysplastic ducts with collarettes of spindle cells ➡. *(Right)* Section of liver from an autopsy in a patient with ZS shows bile duct proliferation ➡. The hepatocytes appear normal; however, hemosiderin pigment is present in hepatocytes, visible at higher magnification.

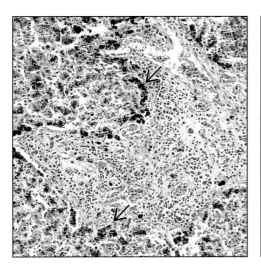

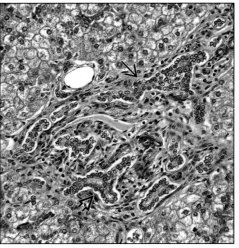

(Left) Iron stain shows hepatocytes laden with blue-stained hemosiderin granules. The iron in Zellweger syndrome is within all hepatocytes but characteristically most heavily deposited in periportal hepatocytes ➡. *(Right)* This liver is from a neonate with Zellweger syndrome. There is a marked increase of portal triad bile ducts ➡. Some bile ducts are abnormally branched ➡. There is no fibrous expansion of the portal tract, inflammation, or sinusoidal fibrosis present.

MEDULLARY SPONGE KIDNEY

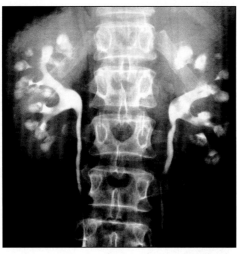

Excretory urogram shows classic "paintbrush" appearance of tubular ectasia bilaterally in a patient with medullary sponge kidney (MSK).

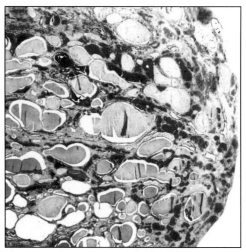

Renal papilla shows multiple ectatic medullary papillary ducts in MSK. This was an incidental finding at autopsy.

TERMINOLOGY

Abbreviations
- Medullary sponge kidney (MSK)

Synonyms
- Cystic disease of renal pyramids
- Precalyceal canalicular ectasia
- Lenarduzzi-Cacchi-Ricci disease

Definitions
- Cystic disease of renal medulla characterized by ectasia of terminal collecting ducts

ETIOLOGY/PATHOGENESIS

Developmental Anomaly
- Developmental defect of collecting system
  - Despite manifesting in 2nd-3rd decades of life, MSK is thought to originate as developmental abnormality of collecting system
- Most cases are sporadic

Genetics
- About 5% of all cases are hereditary, autosomal-dominant mode of inheritance
- RET oncogene is implicated in MSK and plays important role in development of kidney collecting system
- Associated with hemihypertrophy, Ehlers-Danlos syndrome, Beckwith-Wiedemann syndrome, pyloric stenosis, Wilms tumors, multiple endocrine neoplasia type 2 (MEN2), Marfan syndrome

CLINICAL ISSUES

Epidemiology
- Incidence
  - 1/5,000-1/20,000 adults

- Accounts for up to 1/4 of nephrolithiasis cases
- Gender
  - Both sexes equally affected

Presentation
- Hematuria
- Obstruction and stone formation (calcium salts)
- Urinary tract infection
  - MSK greatly increases risk of developing pyelonephritis
- Distal renal tubular acidosis may be present in ~ 1/3 of patients with MSK

Treatment
- Prevention and control of infection and stone formation
  - Hydration
  - Thiazide diuretics
  - Chronic antibiotics in repeated infections

Prognosis
- If infections and stone formation are controlled, course is benign
- ESRD is rare

IMAGE FINDINGS

Radiographic Findings
- Excretory urogram
  - "Paintbrush" ureteral ectasia also sometimes referred to as "bouquet of flowers"
- Urinary stones can be frequently detected, usually bilateral

MACROSCOPIC FEATURES

Size
- Most kidneys are normal in size
- Slight enlargement is observed in ~ 1/3 of cases

MEDULLARY SPONGE KIDNEY

Key Facts

Terminology

- Medullary sponge kidney (MSK)
- Cystic disease of medulla characterized by ectasia of terminal collecting ducts

Clinical Issues

- If infections and stone formation are controlled, course is benign

Image Findings

- "Paintbrush" ureteral ectasia also sometimes referred to as "bouquet of flowers"

Macroscopic Features

- Cysts of various sizes (most < 10 mm) are observed in medullary pyramids
- Renal papillae are most affected

Gross Cysts

- Cysts of various sizes (most less than a few millimeters) are observed in medullary pyramids
- Renal papillae are most affected
- Degree of involvement of 2 kidneys varies, but disease is usually bilateral
- Calculi may be observed associated with cysts

MICROSCOPIC PATHOLOGY

Histologic Features

- Cysts in medullary pyramids lined by cuboidal to columnar epithelium
- Stratification of epithelium may be observed in proximity to urothelial surface (transitional or metaplastic squamous)
- Cyst lumens may contain calculi, RBCs, or inflammatory cells
- Stroma may be expanded with increased cellularity
- Stone formation of infection may lead to stromal inflammation
- Cysts outside of medullary pyramids are normally not observed

DIFFERENTIAL DIAGNOSIS

Medullary Cystic Disease

- MCD rarely involves deep medulla (commonly involves medullary rays) while in MSK, papillary tips are most involved
- Calcifications are associated with MSK but not MCD

Autosomal Dominant Polycystic Kidney Disease

- May exhibit pericaliceal canalicular ectasia
- Presence of cortical cysts and family history separates ADPKD since most cases of MSK are sporadic

SELECTED REFERENCES

1. Pritchard MJ: Medullary sponge kidney: causes and treatments. Br J Nurs. 19(15):972-6, 2010
2. Bisceglia M et al: Renal cystic diseases: a review. Adv Anat Pathol. 13(1):26-56, 2006
3. Diouf B et al: Association of medullary sponge kidney disease and multiple endocrine neoplasia type IIA due to RET gene mutation: is there a causal relationship? Nephrol Dial Transplant. 15(12):2062-3, 2000
4. Indridason OS et al: Medullary sponge kidney associated with congenital hemihypertrophy. J Am Soc Nephrol. 7(8):1123-30, 1996
5. Ginalski JM et al: Medullary sponge kidney on axial computed tomography: comparison with excretory urography. Eur J Radiol. 12(2):104-7, 1991

IMAGE GALLERY

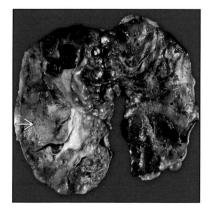 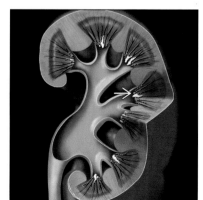 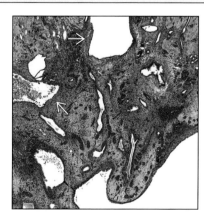

(Left) Gross photograph of an autopsy kidney specimen shows lesions of medullary sponge kidney. Cysts of various sizes can be seen in the medulla ➡. *(Center)* Diagram of the lesions in MSK shows dilation of the renal tubules within the medulla and the presence of numerous small calculi ➡ at the pyramid tips. These calculi may lead to repeated bouts of renal colic. *(Right)* The medullary cysts ➡ are accompanied by marked stromal fibrosis, hypercellularity, and inflammation.

MULTILOCULAR CYSTIC NEPHROMA

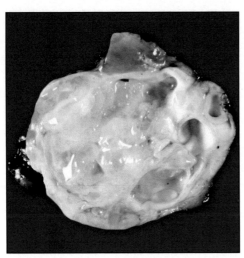

Gross photograph shows a multilocular cystic nephroma (MCN). The multicystic mass is well circumscribed. The cysts contain clear, thin to gelatinous fluid.

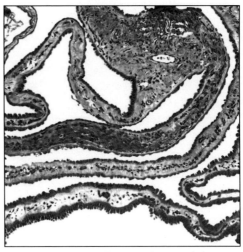

Representative section shows cyst lining epithelium in a MCN. The cyst lining epithelium is flat to low columnar. The stroma of the cyst wall has varied thickness and cellularity.

TERMINOLOGY

Abbreviations
- Multilocular cystic nephroma (MCN)

Synonyms
- Cystic nephroma (CN), multilocular cyst

Definitions
- Benign multicystic neoplasm of renal parenchyma overlapping with mixed epithelial and stromal tumor (MEST) of kidney

ETIOLOGY/PATHOGENESIS

Adult Cystic Nephromas
- Relationship to sex hormones is suggested
  - Female preponderance
  - Estrogen and progesterone receptor (ER/PR) immunopositivity
  - Associated with sex hormone exposure in both males and females

Pediatric Cystic Nephromas
- Thought to be etiologically different from adult CN
- ER/PR are negative
- Considered to be fully differentiated form of nephroblastoma

CLINICAL ISSUES

Epidemiology
- Age
  - Adult population, wide age distribution
    - Usually > 30 years
  - Children
    - Usually < 4 years
    - Accounts for ~ 5% of pediatric tumors
- Gender
  - Female:male ratio is 8:1 in adult cases and 2:1 in pediatric cases

Presentation
- Most commonly an incidental finding
- Can present with pain, hematuria

Treatment
- Conservative surgical excision is curative
- Very rare cases of local recurrence after surgical excision

Prognosis
- Excellent prognosis after surgical excision

IMAGE FINDINGS

Ultrasound, CT, or MR Studies
- While useful, these studies do not allow one to discriminate between MCN and other entities in differential diagnosis in both adult and pediatric cases

MACROSCOPIC FEATURES

General Features
- Well-circumscribed, encapsulated, multicystic mass
- Cysts contain clear or gelatinous fluid
- Often near hilum but may involve cortex in larger lesions

MICROSCOPIC PATHOLOGY

Histologic Features
- Epithelial lining of cysts ranges from flat to cuboidal to hobnailed to columnar
- Cytoplasmic clearing of lining epithelium can be seen
- Fibrous septae show range of cellularity, from paucicellular and hyalinized to highly cellular, reminiscent of ovarian stroma

MULTILOCULAR CYSTIC NEPHROMA

Key Facts

Terminology
- Multilocular cystic nephroma (MCN)
- Cystic nephroma (CN), multilocular cyst

Etiology/Pathogenesis
- Relationship to sex hormones is suggested

Clinical Issues
- Female:male ratio is 8:1 in adult cases and 2:1 in pediatric cases
- Conservative surgical excision is curative

Microscopic Pathology
- Epithelial lining of cysts ranges from flat to cuboidal to hobnailed to columnar
- Fibrous septae show range of cellularity, from paucicellular and hyalinized to highly cellular, reminiscent of ovarian stroma

- Cytoplasmic clearing of lining epithelium can be seen
- Fibrous pseudocapsule surrounds lesion

Ancillary Tests
- ER, PR stains are commonly positive in stroma

Top Differential Diagnoses
- Cystic renal cell carcinoma
- Tubulocystic carcinoma
- Wilms tumor
- MEST
  - If solid nodules are present or if septae are beyond a few millimeters in thickness, MEST diagnosis should be considered
- Cystic dysplasia
- Polycystic kidney disease

- Focal calcifications and atrophic renal tubules can be seen in septae
- Foamy histiocytes may be present
- Fibrous pseudocapsule surrounds lesion

ANCILLARY TESTS

Immunohistochemistry
- ER, PR stains are commonly positive in stroma
- Inhibin, calretinin, CD10 can also be positive in stroma

DIFFERENTIAL DIAGNOSIS

Cystic Carcinomas
- In adult cases, cystic carcinomas need to be excluded
- Cystic renal cell carcinoma (RCC)
  - Careful examination of tumor for collections of clear cells in septae is required
  - ER/PR staining is negative
- Tubulocystic carcinoma
  - High-grade lining epithelial cells
  - Incomplete septae with fibrotic or desmoplastic stroma
  - ER/PR staining is negative

Wilms Tumor
- In pediatric cases, Wilms tumor is a top differential diagnosis
- MCN should not have blastema or other components of Wilms Tumor

Mixed Epithelial and Stromal Tumor of Kidney (MEST)
- MEST and MCN are likely 2 variants of the same etiological entity
- Gene expression, treatment, and prognosis are very similar
- MCN should not contain significant solid component

- If solid nodules are present or if septae are beyond a few millimeters in thickness, MEST diagnosis should be considered
- MEST can rarely show malignant (more commonly sarcomatous) transformation
- It has been proposed to unify MCN and MEST as single entity: Renal epithelial and stromal tumor (REST)

Other Cystic Kidney Diseases
- Cystic dysplasia
- Polycystic kidney disease
- These should be relatively easy to differentiate based on combination of gross and microscopic findings

SELECTED REFERENCES

1. Zhou M et al: Adult cystic nephroma and mixed epithelial and stromal tumor of the kidney are the same disease entity: molecular and histologic evidence. Am J Surg Pathol. 33(1):72-80, 2009
2. Lane BR et al: Adult cystic nephroma and mixed epithelial and stromal tumor of the kidney: clinical, radiographic, and pathologic characteristics. Urology. 71(6):1142-8, 2008
3. Turbiner J et al: Cystic nephroma and mixed epithelial and stromal tumor of kidney: a detailed clinicopathologic analysis of 34 cases and proposal for renal epithelial and stromal tumor (REST) as a unifying term. Am J Surg Pathol. 31(4):489-500, 2007
4. Bastian PJ et al: Local recurrence of a unilateral cystic nephroma. Int J Urol. 11(5):329-31, 2004
5. Eble JN et al: Extensively cystic renal neoplasms: cystic nephroma, cystic partially differentiated nephroblastoma, multilocular cystic renal cell carcinoma, and cystic hamartoma of renal pelvis. Semin Diagn Pathol. 15(1):2-20, 1998
6. Castillo OA et al: Multilocular cysts of kidney. A study of 29 patients and review of literature. Urology. 37(2):156-62, 1991
7. Boggs LK et al: Benign multilocular cystic nephroma: report of two cases of so-called multilocular cyst of the kidney. J Urol. 76(5):530-41, 1956

Microscopic Features

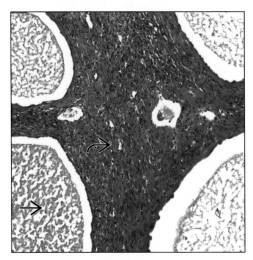
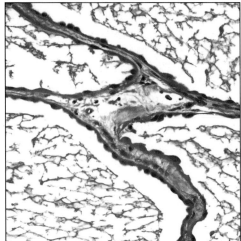

(Left) The cysts in MCN are separated by septae with cellular stroma ⮕, reminiscent of ovarian tissue. The cells in the stroma are ER/PR positive. Abundant proteinaceous material can be seen in the cyst lumina ⮕, accounting for the gelatinous gross appearance. (Right) Most cysts in MCN are separated by thin-walled septae with minimal stroma. Variable amounts of edema can also be seen.

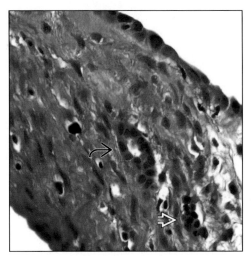
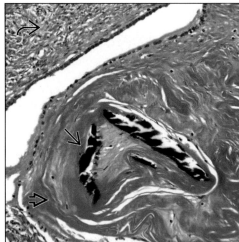

(Left) In the cyst septae, one commonly finds atrophic tubules ⮕ and inflammatory cells ⮕. (Right) The stroma varies in the septae of MCN. The cellular stroma ⮕ and hyalinized stroma ⮕ are present on 2 sides of a single cyst. Calcifications ⮕ are commonly observed in septae of MCN.

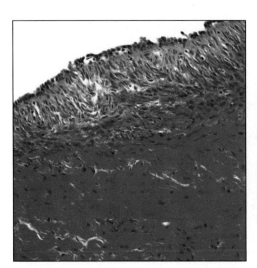
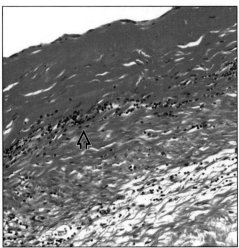

(Left) MCN has a juxtaposition of highly cellular stroma and paucicellular, fibrotic stroma. ER/PR staining is usually positive in both stromal components. (Right) The stromal cellularity varies as well as the inflammatory infiltrate in MCN ⮕. Septal wall thickness is increased. If the septal thickness is > 5 mm, a diagnosis of mixed epithelial and stromal tumor (MEST) should be considered, even in the absence of stromal nodules.

MULTILOCULAR CYSTIC NEPHROMA

Microscopic Features

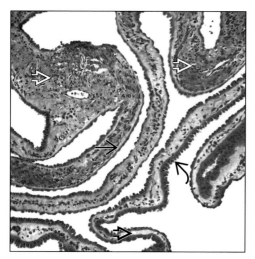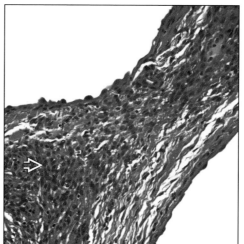

(Left) Epithelial and stromal morphology in MCN is shown. The epithelial lining varies from flat ➡ to low columnar ⬈ with significant "hobnailing." The septal stroma also varies from thin and relatively paucicellular ⮊ to thicker with increased cellularity ⮊. *(Right)* H&E shows an area of densely cellular stroma ⮊ in MCN.

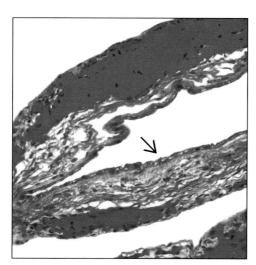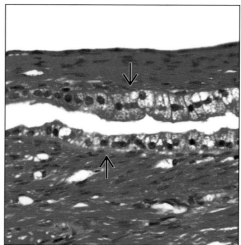

(Left) In this micrograph of MCN, the surface epithelium shows some clear cell change ➡. *(Right)* Clear cell change of cyst lining epithelium in MCN ➡ is shown. One should be careful not to miss the diagnosis of multilocular cystic renal cell carcinoma. Stromal ER/PR positivity and absence of clear cell nests in the septae are reassuring signs.

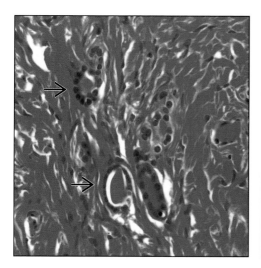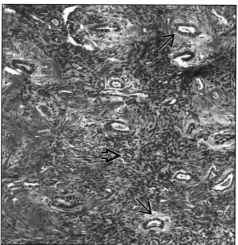

(Left) H&E shows atrophic tubules ➡ in collagenous stroma of the septae in MCN. *(Right)* When nodular stromal proliferation is observed, a diagnosis of mixed epithelial and stromal tumor (MEST) should be considered. Here, atrophic-appearing tubules with hyaline collars ➡ are embedded in variably cellular stroma, resembling ovarian stroma ⮊.

ACQUIRED CYSTIC DISEASE

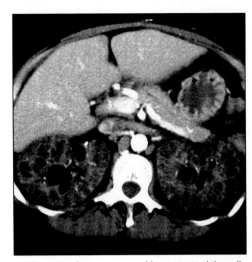

Axial CECT shows innumerable cysts in bilaterally enlarged kidneys of a patient who has been on dialysis for many years.

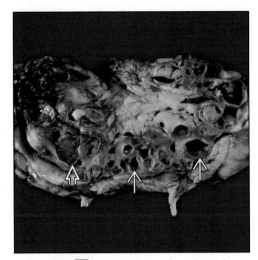

Multiple cysts ➡ are located throughout this end-stage kidney from a dialysis patient. This native kidney was removed for a suspicious mass ➡, which demonstrated both clear cell and papillary features.

TERMINOLOGY

Abbreviations
- Acquired cystic disease (ACD)

Synonyms
- Acquired cystic kidney disease
- Acquired cystic renal disease

Definitions
- Presence of 3 or more cysts in native kidneys of patients with end-stage renal disease satisfies clinical diagnosis of ACD

ETIOLOGY/PATHOGENESIS

Unknown Pathogenesis
- Believed to involve physiologic response to chronic renal failure
  - Possible uncharacterized humoral factor
    - Successful renal transplantation may decrease size of cysts
  - Increased proliferation of cyst-lining epithelium
- Unclear role of calcium oxalate crystals
- Not necessarily secondary to dialysis
  - Cyst formation occurs in some patients even before dialysis therapy

CLINICAL ISSUES

Epidemiology
- Incidence
  - 60-80% of patients on dialysis for more than 4 years may be diagnosed with ACD
- Age
  - All ages
- Gender
  - Male predilection
- Ethnicity

- Africans may be more likely than Caucasians to develop ACD

Presentation
- Asymptomatic
  - Cysts
- Back pain
  - Possible infection of kidney cysts
- Hematuria
  - Possible bleeding into kidney cysts

Natural History
- No difference between peritoneal dialysis or hemodialysis
- Increased risk of developing renal cell carcinoma

Treatment
- Options, risks, complications
  - If asymptomatic, no treatment is necessary
  - Diagnosis of ACD is established by radiologic findings
    - Careful monitoring of cyst size may be sufficient for small cysts and when few in number
  - If cysts become infected, antibiotics may be necessary
  - Large cysts may be painful and require drainage
- Surgical approaches
  - Nephrectomy
    - Rapid change in cyst size warrants this treatment option for potential renal cell carcinoma of cystic type
- Renal transplantation
  - ACD usually improves or resolves after transplantation

Prognosis
- 2-7% of patients with ACD will develop cystic renal cell carcinoma
  - 40-100x increased risk for renal cell carcinoma compared to general population

ACQUIRED CYSTIC DISEASE

Key Facts

Terminology
- Presence of 3 or more cysts in native kidneys of patients with end-stage renal disease satisfies clinical diagnosis of ACD

Clinical Issues
- 60-80% of patients on dialysis for more than 4 years may be diagnosed with ACD
  - Increased risk of developing renal cell carcinoma
  - 2-7% of patients with ACD will develop cystic renal cell carcinoma
- Rapid change in cyst size warrants nephrectomy
- Renal transplantation may decrease cyst size

Macroscopic Features
- ACD kidney weights range from 5-800 grams with an average of 130 grams

- Bilateral involvement
- Masses or nodules that may represent carcinoma are common

Microscopic Pathology
- Tubular cysts
  - Present throughout cortex and medulla
  - Lined by flat cuboidal epithelial cells
  - Most stain for proximal tubular markers
  - Intracystic hemorrhage may be present
- Diffuse interstitial fibrosis and tubular atrophy
- Calcium oxalate crystal deposition

Top Differential Diagnoses
- Autosomal dominant polycystic kidney disease
- Autosomal recessive polycystic kidney disease
- Medullary cystic disease/juvenile nephronophthisis

MACROSCOPIC FEATURES

General Features
- Enlarged kidneys with multiple cysts, from mm to several cm in diameter
  - Weights range from 5-800 grams with an average of 130 grams
- Sometimes new or old hemorrhage
- Solid areas common, suggests neoplasm

MICROSCOPIC PATHOLOGY

Histologic Features
- Tubular cysts
  - Present throughout cortex and medulla
  - Lined by flat cuboidal epithelial cells
    - Most stain for proximal tubular markers
    - May stain for Arachis hypogaea, a marker of distal tubules
  - Some lined by columnar epithelial cells
    - Tufts of epithelial cells may be present
  - Occasional cysts lined by clear cells
    - Positive immunohistochemical staining for carbonic anhydrase IX
    - May represent an early lesion of clear cell carcinoma of kidney
  - Intracystic hemorrhage may be present
- Diffuse interstitial fibrosis and tubular atrophy
  - Features of end-stage kidney
- Tubular loss
- Calcium oxalate crystal deposition
- Extensive global glomerulosclerosis
- Renal cell carcinoma may be present
- Severe arteriosclerosis

ANCILLARY TESTS

Immunohistochemistry
- May be useful to characterize epithelial cell lining of cysts and their nephron segment origin
- Ki-67 demonstrates increased proliferation of cyst lining cells

DIFFERENTIAL DIAGNOSIS

Autosomal Dominant Polycystic Kidney Disease
- Kidney size and both number and size of cysts typically much larger than ACD

Autosomal Recessive Polycystic Kidney Disease
- Cysts may be largely in medulla
- Absence of long-term dialysis (> 4 years) helpful

Medullary Cystic Disease/Juvenile Nephronophthisis
- Cysts largely in medulla or cortico-medullary junction
- Nonproliferative

DIAGNOSTIC CHECKLIST

Pathologic Interpretation Pearls
- Careful macroscopic evaluation of kidney is essential to exclude presence of renal cell carcinoma
  - Gross examination of slices through kidney at 1 cm recommended

SELECTED REFERENCES

1. Costa MZ et al: Histogenesis of the acquired cystic kidney disease: an immunohistochemical study. Appl Immunohistochem Mol Morphol. 14(3):348-52, 2006
2. Tickoo SK et al: Spectrum of epithelial neoplasms in end-stage renal disease: an experience from 66 tumor-bearing kidneys with emphasis on histologic patterns distinct from those in sporadic adult renal neoplasia. Am J Surg Pathol. 30(2):141-53, 2006
3. Nadasdy T et al: Proliferative activity of cyst epithelium in human renal cystic diseases. J Am Soc Nephrol. 5(7):1462-8, 1995

ACQUIRED CYSTIC DISEASE

Gross and Microscopic Features

(Left) Axial NECT shows a high-density area representing spontaneous hemorrhage within one of many renal cysts due to acquired cystic kidney disease. *(Right)* Numerous cysts ➡ are present in this kidney with acquired cystic disease. Nephrectomy of the native kidney is usually performed when imaging studies identify potential renal neoplasms, such as these suspicious nodules ➡.

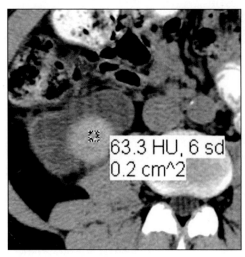 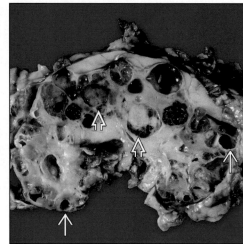

(Left) Numerous cysts ➡ are present throughout this bisected kidney with ACD. In addition, multiple solid tumor nodules ➡ are present, which can be a common finding in this pathologic setting. *(Right)* Numerous cysts lined by flattened epithelial cells are shown. Some epithelial cells have a foamy cytoplasm. The cysts contain eosinophilic proteinaceous material. There is marked and diffuse interstitial fibrosis and tubular atrophy between the large cysts, consistent with an end-stage kidney.

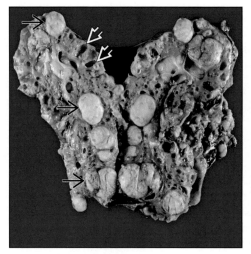 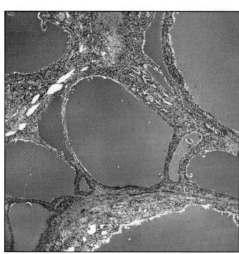

(Left) These 2 cysts are lined by a single layer of epithelial cells, which show a hobnail appearance ➡ with granular cytoplasm. *(Right)* These cysts are lined by a single layer of epithelial cells with eosinophilic cytoplasm ➡. These cysts may be derived from the proximal segments of the nephron. Occasional tufts of epithelial cells may be noted (not shown) and have been termed atypical cysts in the literature.

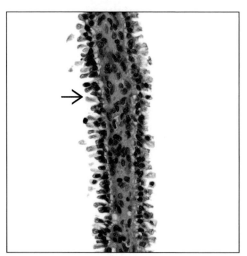 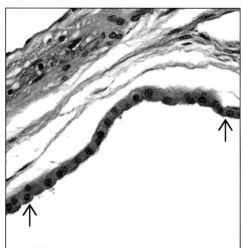

ACQUIRED CYSTIC DISEASE

Microscopic Features

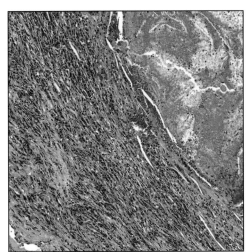

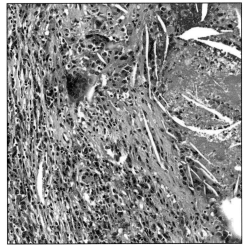

(Left) Rupture of the cysts may lead to nonspecific secondary changes, including accumulation of hemosiderin-laden macrophages. *(Right)* Rupture of the cysts may lead to nonspecific secondary changes in the parenchyma adjacent to and within the ruptured cysts. These can include accumulation of hemosiderin-laden macrophages, foreign body giant cell reaction, and cholesterol cleft formation.

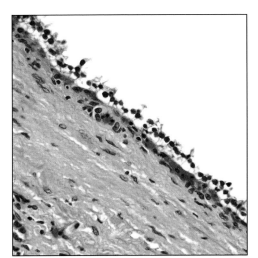

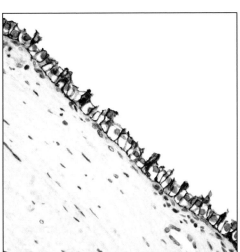

(Left) This cyst is lined by a single layer of epithelial cells with clear cytoplasm. This finding may represent the earliest lesion of clear cell carcinoma. ACD patients have up to a 100x increased risk of developing renal cell carcinoma. *(Right)* Immunohistochemistry for carbonic anhydrase IX demonstrates strong membranous staining of the clear cells, which is a marker of clear cell carcinoma. The cysts that are lined by eosinophilic, granular, or foamy cytoplasm do not show positive staining.

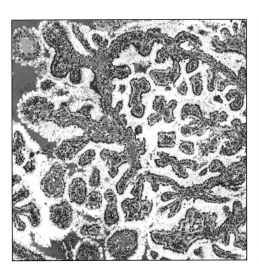

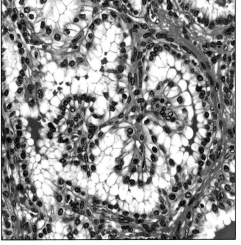

(Left) The combination of a papillary architecture lined by clear cells is a common characteristic of tumors arising from kidneys with ACD, but can also occur sporadically. Other neoplasms may demonstrate eosinophilic cytoplasm with marked nuclear atypia and have been termed ACD-associated renal cell carcinoma (not shown). *(Right)* Fibrovascular cores lined by epithelial cells with abundant clear cytoplasm characterize a subset of neoplasms associated with ACD.

6

SIMPLE AND MISCELLANEOUS CYSTS

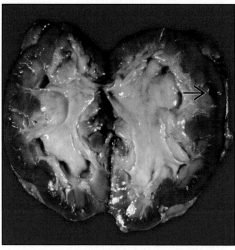

Most simple cysts are incidental findings. This kidney was removed due to hydronephrosis and recurrent infections. A solitary simple deep cortical cyst can be seen in the specimen ➡.

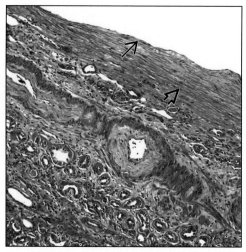

Typical histology of a simple cortical cyst is shown. The cyst lining epithelium is attenuated ➡ and is often absent. A dense fibrous tissue surrounds the cyst ➡.

TERMINOLOGY

Synonyms
- Simple cortical cyst

Definitions
- Sporadic, self-limited cystic nephron dilatation

ETIOLOGY/PATHOGENESIS

Acquired Defect
- Simple cysts are thought to originate from diverticula of cortical tubules and ducts secondary to weakened basement membrane

CLINICAL ISSUES

Epidemiology
- Incidence
  - Occur in ~ 12% of adult population (5% overall)
- Age
  - Incidence increases with age (found in ~ 1/3 of people > 80 years old)
  - Cyst size and number also increase with age
- Gender
  - More common in men (M:F = 2:1)

Presentation
- Most commonly an incidental finding on radiography or in autopsy
- May present with pain, hematuria, infection
- Hypertension may develop, presumably due to pressure effects of cyst on renal circulation

Treatment
- None required in most cases
- Cyst drainage and marsupialization in symptomatic cases
- Excision may be considered if malignancy is suspected

Prognosis
- No significant health consequences

MACROSCOPIC FEATURES

General Features
- Single or multiple, predominantly unilocular, smooth-walled cortical cyst filled with clear fluid
- Randomly distributed

MICROSCOPIC PATHOLOGY

Histologic Features
- Epithelial lining is attenuated and is commonly absent
- Dense fibrous tissue surrounds cyst

DIFFERENTIAL DIAGNOSIS

Cystic Nephroma
- Simple cysts are rarely septated with incomplete septa
- Variability of stroma and presence of cellular stroma in septae strongly favors cystic nephroma

Cystic Renal Cell Carcinoma
- Radiographic discrimination can sometimes be impossible

Autosomal Dominant Polycystic Kidney Disease (ADPKD)
- Multiple simple cysts raise possibility of ADPKD
- Family history and other manifestations, such as liver cysts, are important to consider

Localized/Unilateral Renal Cystic Disease
- Rare benign condition; perhaps an extreme form of multiple simple cysts
- Cysts are innumerable and usually replace normal kidney architecture

SIMPLE AND MISCELLANEOUS CYSTS

Key Facts

Clinical Issues
- Occur in ~ 12% of adult population (5% overall)
- Incidence increases with age (~ 33% of those > 80 years old)
- Cyst size and number increase with age
- More common in men (M:F = 2:1)

Macroscopic Features
- Single or multiple, predominantly unilocular, smooth-walled cortical cyst filled with clear fluid

Microscopic Pathology
- Epithelial lining is attenuated and is commonly absent
- Dense fibrous tissue surrounds cyst

Top Differential Diagnoses
- ADPKD
- Cystic renal cell carcinoma
- Acquired cystic kidney disease

Other Localized Cystic Kidney Diseases

Name	Etiology	Clinical Considerations	Pathology
Perinephric pseudocyst	Traumatic	Localized, often painful condition that may sometimes cause mass effect; history of blunt trauma or recent abdominal surgery	No lining epithelium; fat and fibrous tissue with variable amounts of inflammation
Renal calyceal diverticulum	Believed to originate from developmental defect in collecting system	May be an incidental radiographic finding; may produce pain, hematuria due to urinary stone formation, UTI	Cyst wall lined by flat urothelium and smooth muscle; inflammation and calcifications may be present in complicated cases
Localized/unilateral cystic kidney disease	Etiology is not clear	Rare disease, perhaps a variant of multiple simple cysts; clinical course is usually nonprogressive, necessitating differentiation from ADPKD	1 kidney is globally or segmentally replaced by innumerable cysts; other kidney may show simple cysts

Acquired Cystic Kidney Disease
- Epithelial proliferation, "hobnailing," and papillary projections
- Arises in end-stage kidney disease

SELECTED REFERENCES

1. Bisceglia M et al: Renal cystic diseases: a review. Adv Anat Pathol. 13(1):26-56, 2006
2. Bisceglia M et al: AMR series unilateral (localized) renal cystic disease. Adv Anat Pathol. 12(4):227-32, 2005
3. Terada N et al: The natural history of simple renal cysts. J Urol. 167(1):21-3, 2002
4. Caglioti A et al: Prevalence of symptoms in patients with simple renal cysts. BMJ. 306(6875):430-1, 1993
5. Wulfsohn MA: Pyelocaliceal diverticula. J Urol. 123(1):1-8, 1980
6. Cho KJ et al: Localized cystic disease of the kidney: angiographic-pathologic correlation. AJR Am J Roentgenol. 132(6):891-5, 1979
7. Baert L et al: Is the diverticulum of the distal and collecting tubules a preliminary stage of the simple cyst in the adult? J Urol. 118(5):707-10, 1977

IMAGE GALLERY

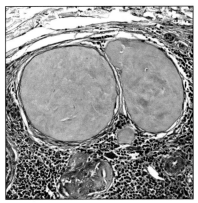 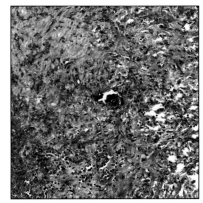 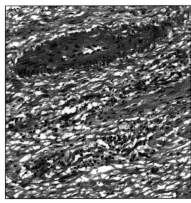

(Left) A small subcapsular cortical cyst is shown. *(Center)* This micrograph shows histology of a renal calyceal diverticulum complicated by nephrolithiasis, showing fibrosis, inflammation, and histiocytic reaction to calcified material. *(Right)* This frozen section micrograph shows typical histology of a perinephric pseudocyst. Fibrous connective tissue and an inflammatory infiltrate dominate the histology. No epithelial or endothelial lining was present.

RENAL LYMPHANGIECTASIS

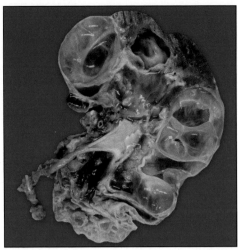

Kidney with lymphangiectasis shows multiple thin-walled cysts with clear fluid content. The cysts displace renal parenchyma, making it difficult to distinguish lymphangiectasis from other cystic diseases.

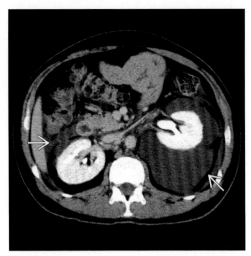

CT scan of a patient with renal lymphangiectasis shows perinephric accumulations of fluid bilaterally ➡, although there is significant asymmetry in the degree of cystic change.

TERMINOLOGY

Synonyms
- Renal lymphangioma, hygroma renalis, renal lymphangiectasis pericalyceal lymphangiectasis, peripylic lymphangiectasis

Definitions
- Hamartomatous or acquired obstructive lesion resulting in cystic dilatation of kidney lymphatics

ETIOLOGY/PATHOGENESIS

Developmental Anomaly
- Malformation of kidney lymphatic drainage system has been suggested

Lymphatic Obstruction
- Lymphatic obstruction secondary to trauma or inflammation in renal pelvis has also been suggested

Additional Associations
- Rare occurrence in siblings suggests genetic component
- Sometimes found in association with generalized lymphangiomatosis
- Reported in a case of tuberous sclerosis

CLINICAL ISSUES

Epidemiology
- Incidence
  - Rare disorder; only ~ 60 cases are reported in the literature
  - No age or gender predilection
    - May be exacerbated by pregnancy

Presentation
- May be asymptomatic

- Flank pain
- Abdominal mass or ascites
- Hematuria &/or proteinuria
- Hypertension (renin-dependent) and, sometimes, polycythemia due to mass effect of lesion and decreased kidney perfusion
- Renal vein thrombosis may develop, perhaps due to combination of polycythemia and mass effect of dilated lymphatics on kidney circulation

Treatment
- Observation is sufficient in most cases
- Cyst aspiration and marsupialization in complicated cases
- Nephrectomy may be considered in refractory cases

Prognosis
- Most cases are stable or slowly progressive; partial regression had also being reported

IMAGE FINDINGS

Radiographic Findings
- Most cases show perinephric cysts but intrarenal or renal sinus (peripelvic) cysts are also common
  - If predominantly peripelvic, may resemble hydronephrosis
- Kidney size is usually normal; nephromegaly may be present if significant intrarenal component exists
- Most (> 90%) cases are bilateral; distribution may vary significantly

MACROSCOPIC FEATURES

General Features
- Normal in size or somewhat enlarged kidney
- Multiple subcapsular and peripelvic cysts
  - Clear or focally hemorrhagic cyst fluid

RENAL LYMPHANGIECTASIS

Key Facts

Terminology
- Hamartomatous or acquired obstructive lesion resulting in cystic dilatation of kidney lymphatics

Clinical Issues
- No age or gender predilection; may be exacerbated by pregnancy
- May present with flank pain, abdominal mass or ascites, hematuria &/or proteinuria, hypertension, polycythemia, renal vein thrombosis

Microscopic Pathology
- Cyst lining is negative for epithelial markers and positive for vascular &/or lymphatic markers: CD31, CD34, podoplanin (D2-40)

Top Differential Diagnoses
- Polycystic kidney disease
- Cystic dysplasia
- Cystic nephroma
- Wilms tumor

- Fluid content is similar in ion composition to blood plasma

MICROSCOPIC PATHOLOGY

Histologic Features
- Thin-walled subcapsular or perihilar cysts are lined by endothelial cells
  - Cyst lining is negative for epithelial markers and positive for vascular &/or lymphatic markers: CD31, CD34, podoplanin (D2-40)
  - Dilated lymphatics can also be seen in parenchyma
- Lymphatic channels, normally absent from cortical parenchyma (outside the vasculature), may be seen intermixed with glomeruli and tubules
- Parenchymal edema may be pronounced, creating parenchymal spaces on histology (not lined by epithelial or endothelial cells)
  - Marked edema should raise suspicion of potential renal vein thrombosis, which is one complication
  - In case of renal vein thrombosis, characteristic glomerular changes will also be observed (such as marked glomerular capillary congestion)

DIFFERENTIAL DIAGNOSIS

Polycystic Kidney Disease
- Cysts are epithelial in origin in polycystic kidney
- Keratin vs. lymphovascular markers should be helpful

Cystic Dysplasia
- Presence of dysplastic elements: Characteristic immature tubules with loose fibrous collars and cartilage

Cystic Nephroma
- Cysts are epithelial in origin, cellular stroma in septae

Wilms Tumor
- Other tumor elements are present (blastema)

SELECTED REFERENCES

1. Bazari H et al: Case records of the Massachusetts General Hospital. Case 23-2010. A 49-year-old man with erythrocytosis, perinephric fluid collections, and renal failure. N Engl J Med. 363(5):463-75, 2010
2. Upreti L et al: Imaging in renal lymphangiectasia: report of two cases and review of literature. Clin Radiol. 63(9):1057-62, 2008
3. Torres VE et al: Extrapulmonary lymphangioleiomyomatosis and lymphangiomatous cysts in tuberous sclerosis complex. Mayo Clin Proc. 70(7):641-8, 1995
4. Younathan CM et al: Renal peripelvic lymphatic cysts (lymphangiomas) associated with generalized lymphangiomatosis. Urol Radiol. 14(3):161-4, 1992
5. Meredith WT et al: Exacerbation of familial renal lymphangiomatosis during pregnancy. AJR Am J Roentgenol. 151(5):965-6, 1988

IMAGE GALLERY

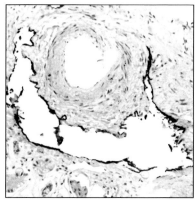 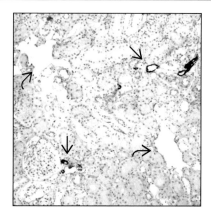 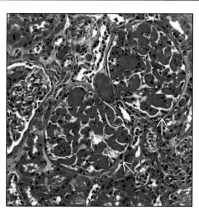

(Left) D2-40 stain of a biopsy specimen in a case of renal lymphangiectasis shows dilated lymphatic channel. *(Center)* Cortical biopsy in a case of renal lymphangiectasia stained for podoplanin (D2-40 antibody) shows lymphatic channels in abnormal locations (adjacent to a glomerulus and intermixed with renal tubules ➡). Marked dissection of the tissue spaces is evident ➢. *(Right)* Marked glomerular congestion ➡ should raise suspicion of renal vein thrombosis.

Diseases of the Collecting System

Obstruction, Reflux, and Stones

INTRODUCTION TO IMPEDIMENTS TO URINE FLOW

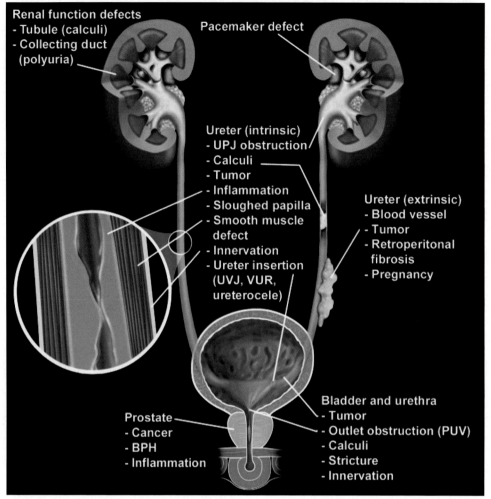

Renal function defects
- Tubule (calculi)
- Collecting duct (polyuria)

Pacemaker defect

Ureter (intrinsic)
- UPJ obstruction
- Calculi
- Tumor
- Inflammation
- Sloughed papilla
- Smooth muscle defect
- Innervation
- Ureter insertion (UVJ, VUR, ureterocele)

Ureter (extrinsic)
- Blood vessel
- Tumor
- Retroperitonal fibrosis
- Pregnancy

Prostate
- Cancer
- BPH
- Inflammation

Bladder and urethra
- Tumor
- Outlet obstruction (PUV)
- Calculi
- Stricture
- Innervation

This illustration depicts the different causes (urinary tract intrinsic or extrinsic) of impediments to urine flow. The lesions can arise anywhere along the path of urine flow, beginning in the kidney and extending through the ureters to the bladder and urethra. The major consequences on the kidney are obstructive or reflux nephropathy, which is manifested by dilation of the pelvis and calyces (hydronephrosis), loss of the medullary pyramids, and secondary atrophy of the cortex. These conditions increase the risk of urinary tract infection, which leads to further injury in the form of acute and chronic pyelonephritis.

TERMINOLOGY

Definitions
- Impediment to urine flow: Retrograde or hindered urine flow due to obstructive or nonobstructive causes
- Reflux: Retrograde urine flow from bladder into ureters or kidney due to functional or physical defects of lower tract
- Hydronephrosis: Dilatation of renal pelvis due to functional or physical impediment of urine flow
- Obstructive nephropathy: Damage to kidney due to obstruction
- Reflux nephropathy: Damage to kidney due to urine reflux

CLASSIFICATION

Type of Impediment
- Obstructive

- Physical
  - Internal urinary system obstruction: Stones, tumors of urinary tract, infections
  - External compression of urinary system: Tumors, pregnancy, retroperitoneal fibrosis, endometriosis, crossing vessels
- Functional
  - Ureter or collecting duct dysfunction
- Congenital
  - Ureteropelvic junction obstruction (UPJO)
  - Primary obstructive megaureter or ureterovesical junction obstruction (UVJO)
  - Ureterocele
  - Posterior urethral valves (PUV)
- Acquired
- Nonobstructive: Vesicoureteral reflux (VUR)
  - Primary VUR
  - Secondary VUR

INTRODUCTION TO IMPEDIMENTS TO URINE FLOW

Region of Impediment and Associated Major Abnormalities
- Upper urinary tract
  - Kidney (tubules, collecting duct)
    - UPJO
- Lower urinary tract
  - Ureter
    - UPJO
    - UVJO or megaureter
    - Ureterocele
  - Bladder and ureter
    - VUR
  - Bladder and urethra
    - PUV

ETIOLOGY/PATHOGENESIS

Developmental Mechanisms
- UPJO
  - Most common cause of obstructive nephropathy
  - Kidney
    - Abnormal water absorption or collecting duct cell function (functional obstruction)
    - Abnormal pacemaker function regulating peristalsis (functional obstruction)
  - Ureter
    - Abnormal ureter or pelvic wall development (increased extracellular matrix, disorganized smooth muscle) leading to defective peristalsis (functional obstruction)
  - Extrinsic
    - Crossing by lower pole renal vessels (physical obstruction)
    - Nervous system (pyeloureteral innervation) mediated defects in peristalsis (functional obstruction)
- Megaureter
  - UVJO, abnormal muscular development or stricture, ureter insertion into bladder may be normal
  - Supernumerary ureters ectopically inserted into bladder
  - Refluxing megaureter due to primary or secondary reflux
- Ureterocele
  - Distal blind-ending ureter often in completely duplicated collecting system
- Primary VUR
  - Distal Wolffian duct (WD) &/or ureter maturation
    - Abnormal ureteric bud (UB) budding site
    - Failure of ureter insertion into bladder, abnormality of vesicoureteral junction
    - Failure of ureter to separate from WD
    - Abnormal common nephric duct (CND) degeneration
  - Most common congenital anomalies of kidney and urinary tract (CAKUT)
    - 50% of children with UTIs may have VUR
    - 15-34% of children with asymptomatic bacteriuria may have VUR
- PUV
  - Failure of urogenital membrane disintegration

Genetic Mechanisms
- UPJO
  - Families exhibiting autosomal dominant inheritance have been reported; cannot rule out other modes of inheritance
  - Genes associated or mutated
    - *Shh, Bmp4, Tshz3, Adamts1, Dlgh1, Calcineurin, renin-angiotensin system (RAS), Tbx18, Id2, Limp2*
- Primary VUR
  - Genetically heterogeneous
  - Inheritance patterns include autosomal dominant, autosomal recessive, polygenic, sporadic, recessive X-linked with incomplete penetrance and variable expressivity
  - Not unusual to skip generations
  - Individuals in same family may have VUR or other CAKUT
  - Modifier genes or epigenetics can affect phenotype
  - 80% chance in monozygotic twin
  - 32% in siblings
  - Known genetic mutations account for only small number of cases
    - Genome-wide association studies (GWAS) identified several common variants of primary VUR; however, in most cases it is unknown if the associated genes are causal
    - Long-range effects of common variants
    - Rare deleterious variant burden in coding, splice junctions, or insertions/deletions may underlie genetic causes
  - Genes associated and mutated
    - *UPK3A, ROBO2, RET,* HLA complex, *ACE, AGTR2, UPK1A,* ABO blood group, *TNFα, TGFβ, PTGS2, IGF1, IGF1R, EGF, CCL2*
- PUV
  - Autosomal dominant, incomplete penetrance, variable expressivity, compound recessive with modifier genes, de novo
  - No known genes

Nongenetic Mechanisms
- Environmental: Toxins, drugs, nutrition
- Epigenetic: Methylation, acetylation

CLINICAL IMPLICATIONS

Clinical Presentation
- Lung hypoplasia, oligohydramnios
- Acute pyelonephritis
- Chronic pyelonephritis
- Cystitis
- Hypertension
- Nausea and vomiting
- Failure to thrive
- Flank pain
- Abdominal distension
- Weak stream
- Proteinuria

Characteristics of Major Congenital Impediments to Urine Flow

	UPJ	Megaureter	VUR	PUV
Definition	Severe narrowing of ureter at junction of ureter and pelvis	Large, dilated, and often tortuous ureter	Retrograde urine flow from bladder to kidneys	Abnormal persistence of urogenital membrane causing severe narrowing of proximal urethra
Incidence	1:500 (left > right)	1:10,000 (left > right)	At least 1:100	1:5,000 males
Mechanism	Kidney collecting duct defect, pacemaker abnormality, ureter smooth muscle defect	Abnormal lower ureter wall (UVJ), abnormal insertion of ectopic ureters, secondary to reflux	Distal WD/ureter maturation or developmental defects leading to failure of valve mechanism	Abnormal mesenchymal development resulting in failure of urogenital membrane disintegration
Radiological findings	Hydronephrosis	Dilated, tortuous ureter	Different grades of VUR	Narrow to obliterated distal urethral lumen, dilated proximal urethra, huge irregular bladder shape, reflux
Pathological outcome	Obstructive nephropathy	Obstructive or reflux nephropathy depending on etiology	Reflux nephropathy	Obstructive or reflux nephropathy
Macroscopic	Dilatation of pelvis, calyceal blunting, compression of cortex	Large ureteral lumen; dilated, tortuous, long ureter	Different degrees of ureter dilatation with renal parenchymal compression in grade 5; abnormal entry of ureter into bladder or intravesicular tunnel	Large trabeculated bladder in addition to dilated urethra and reflux
Microscopic	Ureter smooth muscle disorganization (if ureter etiology); obstructive nephropathy changes including tubular atrophy, tubulointerstitial inflammation, fibrosis, atubular glomeruli, glomerulosclerosis, compressed cortex, dysplasia (if congenital)	Similar changes as UPJ; if megaureter due to primary reflux, then reflux nephropathy changes such as segmental renal scarring	Reflux nephropathy changes in primary or secondary VUR including renal scarring, tubulointerstitial inflammation, chronic or acute pyelonephritis, cortical thinning; may see dysplasia if congenital	Thick bladder muscle wall, histopathological changes of obstructive or reflux nephropathy

MACROSCOPIC FINDINGS

General Features
- UPJO
  - Dilatation of pelvis, blunting of calyces
  - Compression of cortex
  - Compensatory hypertrophy in contralateral kidney
- Megaureter
  - Segmental or complete ureteral dilatation
  - Tortuous ureter
- VUR
  - Different grades of reflux causing ureter and pelvicalyceal dilatation
- Other CAKUT may be present
- Defects in other organ systems in syndromic cases
- Enlarged trabeculated bladder in PUV
- Segmental or diffuse scarring if progresses to nephropathy and cortical thinning

MICROSCOPIC FINDINGS

General Features
- Primary UPJO or UVJO ureter histology
  - Disorganized smooth muscle layer
  - Increased extracellular matrix
  - Reduced innervation
  - Increased fibrosis
  - Lumen narrow and irregular
  - Intravesicle tunnel is typically normal in UVJ unless coexisting reflux
- VUR
  - Intravesicular tunnel typically not evaluated for histology
- PUV
  - Thick-walled bladder
- If severe, histopathological changes of reflux or obstructive nephropathy in kidney

SELECTED REFERENCES

1. Klein J et al: Congenital ureteropelvic junction obstruction: human disease and animal models. Int J Exp Pathol. Epub ahead of print, 2010
2. Chen F: Genetic and developmental basis for urinary tract obstruction. Pediatr Nephrol. 24(9):1621-32, 2009
3. Uetani N et al: Plumbing in the embryo: developmental defects of the urinary tracts. Clin Genet. 75(4):307-17, 2009
4. Murawski IJ et al: Gene discovery and vesicoureteric reflux. Pediatr Nephrol. 23(7):1021-7, 2008
5. Rosen S et al: The kidney in congenital ureteropelvic junction obstruction: a spectrum from normal to nephrectomy. J Urol. 179(4):1257-63, 2008
6. Williams G et al: Vesicoureteral reflux. J Am Soc Nephrol. 19(5):847-62, 2008

INTRODUCTION TO IMPEDIMENTS TO URINE FLOW

Different Types of Lower Urinary Tract Abnormalities

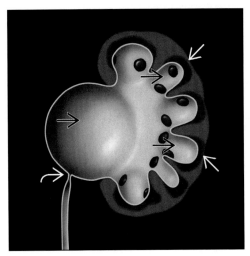
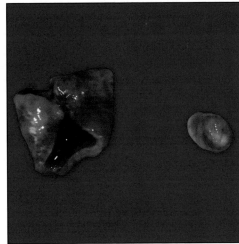

(Left) This diagram illustrates typical features of UPJO ➡, including hydronephrosis with dilatation of the pelvis and calyces ➡ due to increased back pressure. This leads to secondary thinning of the cortex ➡. *(Right)* This case depicts the appearance of the cross sections of the ureter in a child with UPJO. Note the massively dilated ureter (left) proximal to obstruction and ureter with narrow lumen distal to the obstruction (right).

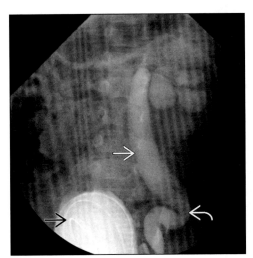
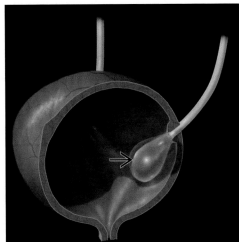

(Left) This voiding cystourethrogram shows primary reflux of urine from the bladder ➡ into the ureter ➡, resulting in a massively dilated and tortuous ureter ➡. Vesicoureteral reflux (VUR) is one of the most common kidney anomalies; however, it is a rare cause of end-stage renal disease. *(Right)* Illustration shows a ureterocele ➡ (blind-ending ureter) that can cause obstruction to urine flow. Ureteroceles are rare and are typically seen in ectopic ureters.

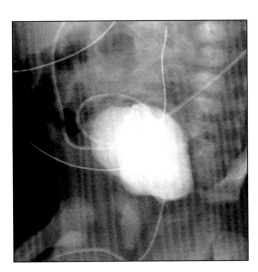
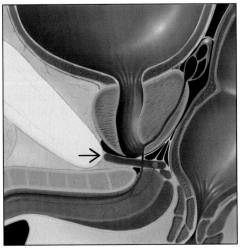

(Left) Voiding cystourethrogram shows an enlarged bladder with trabeculations in a patient with posterior urethral valves (PUV). PUVs are a major cause of renal insufficiency in male children. *(Right)* This diagram shows an anatomical defect in PUV. There is narrowing of the prostatic urethra ➡ (keyhole sign) due to abnormal development of the mesenchymal component of the urogenital sinus causing obstruction. The result is bladder hypertrophy and reflux.

OBSTRUCTIVE NEPHROPATHY

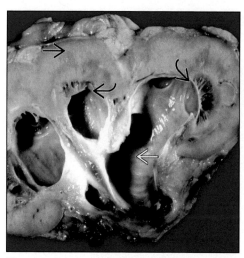

The typical features of chronic obstruction include dilation of the pelvis and calyces (hydronephrosis) ➡️, loss of the medullary pyramids ➡️, and secondary thinning of the cortex ➡️.

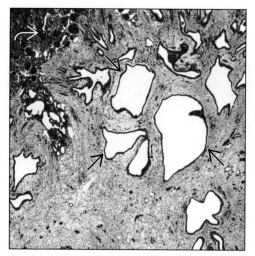

A section of the medulla from a child with UPJO shows dilation of the larger medullary collecting ducts ➡️ due to increased urine back-pressure. The cortex is relatively spared ➡️.

TERMINOLOGY

Definitions
- Obstructive nephropathy
  - Damage to kidney due to urine flow obstruction
- Hydronephrosis
  - Dilatation of renal pelvis due to functional or physical impediment to urine flow

ETIOLOGY/PATHOGENESIS

Causes
- Physical obstruction
  - Stone
  - Tumors of the urinary tract
    - Prostate, bladder, ureter
  - Benign prostate hyperplasia (BPH)
  - External compression (tumors, pregnancy, retroperitoneal fibrosis, endometriosis, crossing vessels)
- Functional obstruction
  - Developmental anomalies: Posterior urethral valves (PUV), ureterocele, ureteropelvic junction obstruction (UPJO), primary megaureter
    - UPJO is most common cause of obstructive nephropathy

Pathophysiology
- Impediment to urine flow causes increase in back-pressure into collecting system and tubules
- Increased back-pressure and retention of urine causes dilatation of collecting system and alterations in transporters and channels
- Compression of renal parenchyma accompanies vascular compromise and inflammatory response
- Cellular changes in interstitium and nephrons lead to varying degrees of scarring
- Intrauterine obstruction during nephrogenesis can cause renal dysplasia

Animal Models
- Unilateral ureteral obstruction (UUO)
  - Commonly used in rodents, marsupials
- Genetic models
  - Provide evidence for functional defects rather than physical causes of obstructive nephropathy (*Aqp2* mutations)

CLINICAL ISSUES

Presentation
- Acute obstruction
  - Flank pain, nausea, and vomiting
  - Renal failure if bilateral
- Chronic obstruction
  - Recurrent episodes of pyelonephritis
  - Hypertension
  - Renal failure if bilateral

Treatment
- Surgical repair
- Decompression

Prognosis
- Prognostic criteria for congenital impediments to urine flow are not well defined; therefore, management criteria are debatable
- Kidney failure may ensue if accompanied by dysplasia due to congenital obstruction
- Correction of congenital obstruction may not resolve kidney damage; children should be followed into adulthood
- High propensity to develop renal insufficiency in PUV patients

IMAGE FINDINGS

Ultrasonographic Findings
- Dilated pelvis

OBSTRUCTIVE NEPHROPATHY

Key Facts

Terminology
- Acute or chronic damage to kidney due to obstruction of urine flow

Etiology/Pathogenesis
- Many causes, congenital and acquired
  - Developmental defect
  - Neoplasia
  - Stones
- UPJO most common cause

Clinical Issues
- Chronic or repeated pyelonephritis
- Flank pain
- Hypertension
- Renal failure (bilateral)

Macroscopic Features
- Dilatation of pelvis (hydronephrosis), blunting of calyces
- Marked loss of medulla, cortical thinning

Microscopic Pathology
- Marked loss of tubules
- Global and segmental glomerulosclerosis
- Interstitial fibrosis, chronic inflammation
- Dilation of collecting ducts
- Dysplasia indicates congenital origin

Top Differential Diagnoses
- Reflux nephropathy
- Tubulointerstitial diseases

MACROSCOPIC FEATURES

General Features
- Dilatation of pelvis (hydronephrosis), blunting of calyces
- Compression of the cortex
- Irregular kidney surface due to scarring
- Other anomalies or syndromes may be present: Hydronephrosis, small kidneys, duplicated collecting system, megaureter, hydroureter, dysplastic kidneys
- Compensatory hypertrophy in contralateral kidney

MICROSCOPIC PATHOLOGY

Histologic Features
- Glomeruli
  - Glomeruli relatively spared but eventually become globally sclerotic
    - Periglomerular fibrosis prominent
    - Global glomerulosclerosis, obsolescent glomeruli, glomerular cysts
    - Atubular glomeruli (cystic dilation of Bowman space)
  - Crescents seen rarely
  - Increased glomerular size in contralateral kidney
- Tubules
  - Tubular atrophy, apoptosis
  - Thyroidization of tubules (end-stage atrophy)
  - Microcystic dilatation of distal nephron segments
  - Dilation of tubules may be more prominent in subcapsular collecting ducts
  - Rupture with leakage of Tamm-Horsfall protein
- Interstitium
  - Fibrosis, diffuse
  - Mononuclear inflammation, plasma cells
  - Sometimes intense in sites of tubular rupture
  - Presence of cartilage or smooth muscle indicative of dysplasia
    - Segmental (lobar) or zonal (outer cortex) distribution
- Vessels
  - Arterial medial hypertrophy and intimal fibroelastosis are indicative of hypertension
- Pelvis and ureter
  - Pelvic dilatation, papillae effacement
  - Hypertrophy and dilation of ureter
  - Chronic inflammation mucosa of pelvis and ureter

Acute Obstruction
- May have few pathologic findings
- Interstitial edema, mild inflammation
- Dilation of subcapsular collecting ducts
- Dilated lymphatics contain Tamm-Horsfall protein

DIFFERENTIAL DIAGNOSIS

Reflux Nephropathy
- Generally less hydronephrosis
- Correlate with clinical and radiological information

Ask-Upmark Kidney
- Segmental scar with atrophic tubules and no glomeruli

Chronic Tubulointerstitial Diseases
- No calyceal dilation or hydronephrosis
- Medulla shows less severe destruction

SELECTED REFERENCES

1. Chevalier RL et al: Mechanisms of renal injury and progression of renal disease in congenital obstructive nephropathy. Pediatr Nephrol. 25(4):687-97, 2010
2. Klein J et al: Congenital ureteropelvic junction obstruction: human disease and animal models. Int J Exp Pathol. Epub ahead of print, 2010

OBSTRUCTIVE NEPHROPATHY

Gross Features

(Left) Extreme hydronephrosis results in a kidney with a bag-like appearance and almost complete loss of parenchyma. In this case, the cortex and medulla in the lobes are just a few millimeters thick ➡. *(Right)* This case of chronic obstructive nephropathy depicts severe dilatation of the ureter ➡ indicative of distal obstruction. Note several areas of cortical thinning and absent pyramids ➡ with marked dilation of the pelvis ➡.

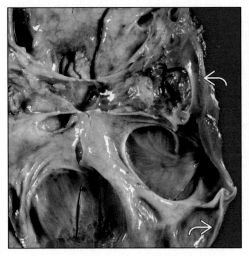
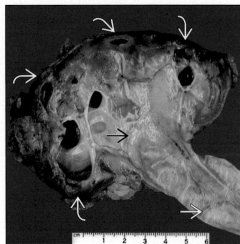

(Left) Primary megaureter in a child is highlighted by overall ureter dilation with a segment with marked dilation ➡. The kidney does not have a normal reniform shape due to abnormal development. Intrauterine obstruction is a known cause of renal dysplasia. *(Right)* Gross image of a kidney shows features of obstructive nephropathy. There are varying degrees of corticomedullary thinning ➡. There are regions of papillae flattening ➡ and scarring ➡.

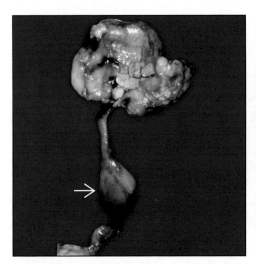
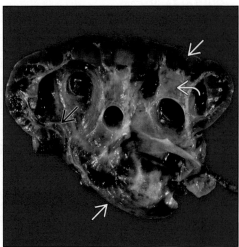

(Left) Xanthogranulomatous pyelonephritis and staghorn calculi can complicate obstructive nephropathy. This pelvicaliceal system is dilated and filled with staghorn calculi ➡. The yellow chronic infection can be seen in the medullary areas ➡. *(Right)* Section of a kidney with ureteropelvic junction obstruction (UPJO) causing hydronephrosis demonstrates marked dilatation of the pelvis ➡.

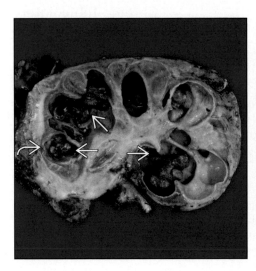
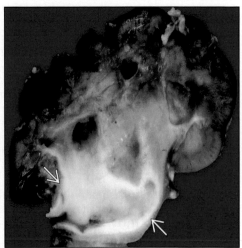

OBSTRUCTIVE NEPHROPATHY

Imaging and Microscopic Features

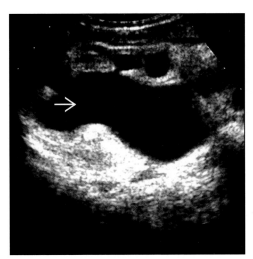
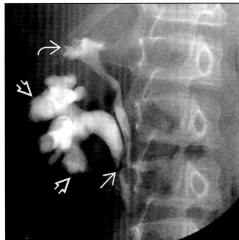

(Left) Ultrasound can demonstrate hydronephrosis in revealing a dilated pelvis ➡, here shown in a child with UPJO. *(Right)* In this image of duplicated ureters, the lower ureter has UPJO ➡ causing urine backflow and hydronephrosis, as revealed by contrast material in the clubbed calyces ➡. The calyces drained by the other ureter are relatively normal and have sharp fornices ➡.

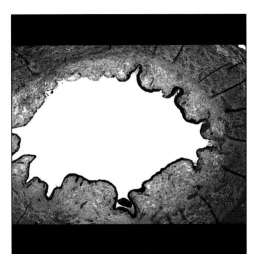
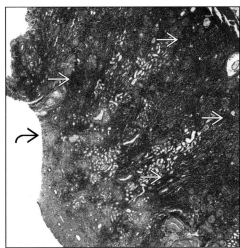

(Left) This ureter cross section is dilated, moderately inflamed, and hypertrophied, an appearance typical of chronic obstruction. *(Right)* Histopathological changes of obstructive nephropathy due to UPJO are highlighted in this low-power image. Note that pelvicalyceal expansion causes effacement of the papillae ➡ and diffuse inflammation involving the entire cortex ➡. No dysplasia is present, consistent with postnatal onset of obstruction.

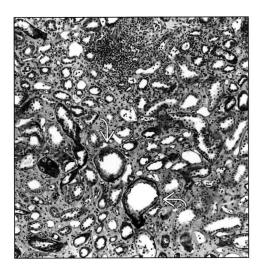
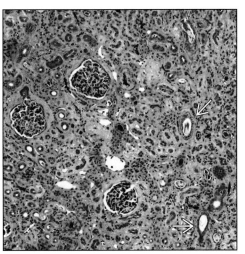

(Left) Histologic evidence of obstruction on biopsy can be subtle. Here, there is diffuse edema, mild mononuclear inflammation, and dilation of the medullary collecting ducts ➡. *(Right)* Trichrome stain in a chronically obstructed kidney shows marked loss and atrophy of tubules, with diffuse fine interstitial fibrosis. The glomeruli are relatively spared although they are probably "atubular" glomeruli. A few residual collecting ducts are seen ➡.

OBSTRUCTIVE NEPHROPATHY

Microscopic Features

(Left) Leakage of Tamm-Horsfall protein (THP), which is produced in the distal tubule, occurs as a consequence of obstruction and elicits an inflammatory response. Here THP can be seen in the interstitium around a collecting duct ➡ and in the lymphatics ➡. *(Right)* This kidney section shows globally sclerosed glomeruli ▣ and extensive cortical interstitial inflammation in the cortex in a patient with urinary tract obstruction.

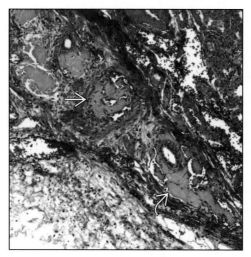
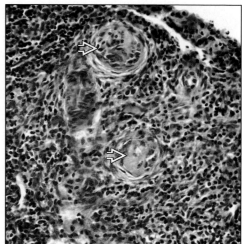

(Left) Occasionally in chronic obstruction, especially in children, cellular crescents are found, here with a squamous appearance ➡. This was initially described in UPJO by Seymour Rosen et al. and should not be mistaken for a coincidental glomerulonephritis. *(Right)* Obstruction in utero not uncommonly leads to dysplasia in the developing kidney. One form it takes is zonal dysplasia, where the outer cortex (subcapsular and in the columns of Bertin) show cartilage ➡ or smooth muscle.

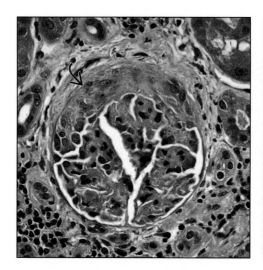
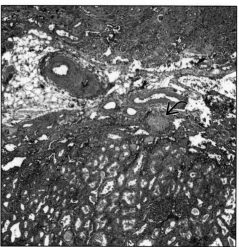

(Left) Secondary focal glomerulosclerosis occurs in patients with chronic obstruction. The glomeruli are hypertrophied, and one has a segmental adhesion ➡ in a region of periglomerular fibrosis. *(Right)* EM image shows a glomerulus from a patient with 2.8 g/d proteinuria due to secondary focal segmental glomerulosclerosis from chronic obstruction. The GBM is moderately thickened ➡, indicative of glomerular hypertrophy, and podocytes have patchy effacement of foot processes ➡.

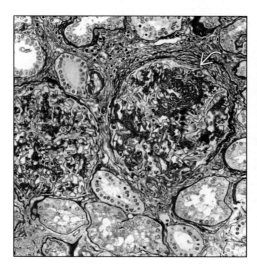
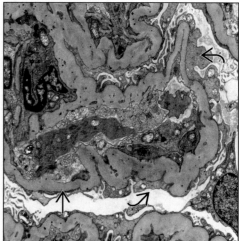

Animal Models of Obstruction

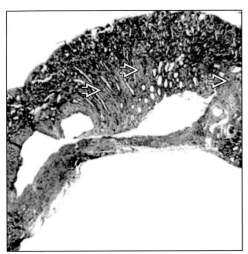

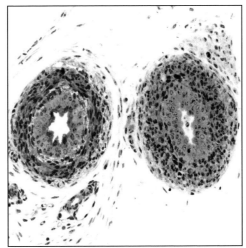

(Left) Increased fibrosis ⇨ is highlighted by trichrome stain in a opossum model of ureteral obstruction. Note the hydronephrosis. (Right) Section shows ureter wall abnormalities in UPJO in a Dlg1 knockout mouse. Left image from a normal mouse shows normal ureter with a well-formed lumen and well-organized inner longitudinal and outer circular smooth muscles. Right image from Dlg1 knockout mouse shows a narrow lumen and disorganized smooth muscle. (Courtesy J. Miner, PhD.)

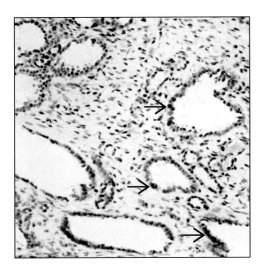

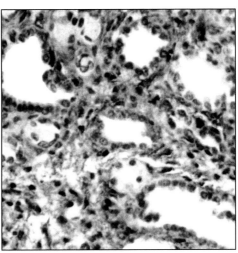

(Left) Apoptosis (TUNEL) stain of a kidney section shows increased apoptosis ⇨ in obstructive nephropathy in a opossum. Tubular epithelial apoptosis is an early response to acute obstruction. (Right) Immunoperoxidase staining of kidney sections with anti-smooth muscle actin (SMA) antibody shows increased labeling in interstitial cells in ureteral obstruction in the opossum. Some of these cells are believed to derive from epithelial or endothelial mesenchymal transition.

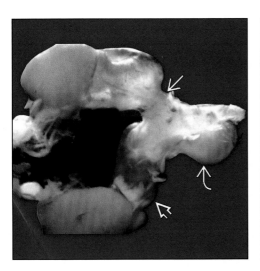

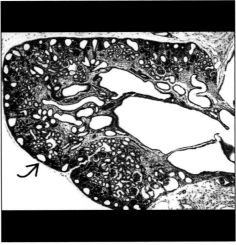

(Left) The urinary tract from a mouse lacking Ret-activated Plc-γ signaling shows lower ureter obstruction ⇨ near the bladder ⇨, which caused megaureter ⇨. (Right) Kidney from a mouse with ureteral obstruction due to lack of Ret-activated Plc-γ signaling during development shows pelvicaliceal dilation and cystic dysplasia, a consequence of obstruction in utero. Subcapsular dilation of collecting ducts ⇨ is also a characteristic of obstruction in humans.

REFLUX NEPHROPATHY

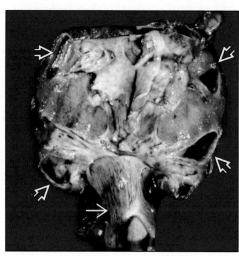

Reflux nephropathy with megaureter ➡ shows marked thinning of the cortex and loss of the medulla, especially at the poles ⮞.

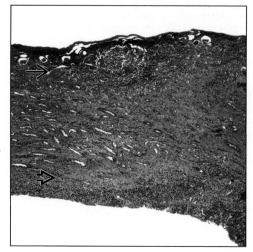

Cross-section through full-thickness of cortex ➱ and medulla ⮞ in a 7-year-old boy with reflux nephropathy shows the markedly thin parenchyma corresponding to the gross appearance.

TERMINOLOGY

Definitions
- Reflux: Retrograde urine flow from bladder into ureters or kidney due to functional or physical lower tract defects
- Reflux nephropathy: Renal parenchymal scarring due to urine reflux

ETIOLOGY/PATHOGENESIS

Causes
- Vesicoureteral reflux (VUR)
  - Primary VUR
    - Congenital anomaly, unilateral or bilateral
    - Abnormal insertion of ureter into bladder, abnormal intravesicular tunnel length of ureter
    - Incompetent valve
  - Secondary VUR
    - Distal obstruction, neurogenic bladder: Posterior urethral valves (PUV), multiple sclerosis, spinal cord injury, stroke, diabetic neuropathy, pelvic surgery, B12 deficiency
    - Dysfunctional elimination syndrome: Abnormal holding of urine and voiding pattern
- Acquired: Urinary tract infections

Pathophysiology Points
- Reflux due to VUR or lower tract obstruction
- Reflux nephropathy develops in some patients with VUR
- Reflux urine enters renal parenchyma via compound papillae (2-3 fused papillae at poles that have round orifice)
- Reflux gives bacteria access to kidney
- Continued exposure of kidneys to high-pressure urine reflux or bacteria causes acute or chronic immune response

- Tubulointerstitial damage ensues with these events leading to edema, ischemia, necrosis, inflammation, tubular atrophy, fibrosis, and scar formation
  - Focal scars in compound papillae
  - Ongoing damage can alter anatomy of simple papillae (dome-shaped with slit-like orifice and drain single lobe) to compound type and cause more diffuse scars
- Glomerulosclerosis
- Renin-angiotensin system is activated and causes hypertension
- Etiology of scar formation is not fully understood
  - Reflux may not be a prerequisite for scar formation as scar can develop in kidneys without intrarenal reflux
  - Bacterial colonization of kidneys may not be necessary to induce kidney damage as scars have been observed in patients without history of urinary tract infection (UTI)
  - New renal scars can develop in presence of reflux and pyelonephritis
- Intrarenal reflux during development can lead to partial or complete maturation and developmental arrest of developing kidney
- Genes causing reflux may be similar to those important in kidney development
  - Genes tested and found to be associated with VUR phenotype in humans
    - HLA complex (DNA analysis and serotyping)
    - TNFα (DNA analysis)
    - TGFβ1 (DNA analysis)
    - ACE (DNA analysis, protein and mRNA studies)
    - PTGS2 (protein and mRNA studies)
    - IGF1 (protein and mRNA studies)
    - IGF1R (protein and mRNA studies)
    - EGF (protein and mRNA studies)
    - CCL2 (protein and mRNA studies)
    - ROBO2 (DNA analysis)
    - UPK3A (DNA analysis)
    - UPK1A (DNA analysis)

REFLUX NEPHROPATHY

Key Facts

Terminology
- Reflux nephropathy: Renal parenchymal scarring due to urine reflux

Etiology/Pathogenesis
- Vesicoureteral reflux (VUR), UTIs
- Exposure of kidneys to high-pressure urine reflux or bacteria causes tubulointerstitial damage and scarring
- Intrarenal reflux in utero affects kidney development

Clinical Issues
- Most common cause of severe hypertension in children
- Manage UTIs, acute pyelonephritis, chronic pyelonephritis, and VUR
- Diagnosis: DMSA scan; depends on adequate renal blood flow and cellular uptake

- Prophylactic antibiotics and monitoring for nephropathy may be advisable for higher grades of reflux (4 and 5)

Microscopic Pathology
- Tubulointerstitial inflammation, fibrosis, atrophy, and global glomerulosclerosis
- Dysplasia indicates congenital component leading to reflux
- Histological features in primary and secondary urine reflux may be similar and overlap with many features of obstructive nephropathy
- Clinical and radiological correlation necessary

Top Differential Diagnoses
- Obstructive nephropathy
- Tubulointerstitial nephritis

- *GNB3* (DNA analysis)
- *AGTR2* (DNA analysis)
- *ABO* blood group (serotyping)
- Finding of progression to kidney failure even after correction of reflux suggests ongoing irreversible damage

CLINICAL ISSUES

Epidemiology
- Incidence
  - Reflux nephropathy is a cause of renal failure in 3-5% of renal dialysis or transplant patients
  - Most common cause of severe hypertension in children

Presentation
- Hypertension
- Proteinuria
- UTI, acute pyelonephritis, chronic pyelonephritis
  - 50-80% of children with febrile UTI have renal scarring
- Primary or secondary VUR

Laboratory Tests
- Renal parenchyma scintigraphy: Tc-99m dimercaptosuccinic acid (DMSA) scan; depends on adequate renal blood flow and cellular uptake
- Voiding cystourethrogram (VCUG) for lower urinary tract disorder
- Renal function test, urinalysis

Treatment
- Surgical repair
- Antibiotics

Prognosis
- High-grade reflux more likely to cause nephropathy than low grade; 5% of renal failure in children due to reflux nephropathy
- Proteinuria, reduced creatinine clearance and GFR, hypertension, high-grade reflux, and bilateral VUR

increase likelihood of progression to chronic kidney disease
- Management criteria are debatable; prophylactic antibiotics and monitoring for nephropathy may be advisable for higher grades of reflux (4 and 5)
- Functional development of kidney may be affected if reflux in early embryogenesis
- 20% of renal failure in boys with reflux due to PUV

Urine Reflux Grading
- 5 grades depending on degree of anatomical changes in the collecting system due to reflux
  - Grade 1: Confined to ureter
  - Grade 2: Involves ureter and pelvis
  - Grade 3: More severe ureter and pelvis involvement with increased tortuosity
  - Grade 4: Grade 3 with blunting of calyces
  - Grade 5: Marked dilatation of pelvis and calyces, tortuosity of ureter

MACROSCOPIC FEATURES

Key Findings
- Different grades of reflux may be present
- Irregular kidney surface due to scarring
- Segmental or diffuse cortical scarring
- Other congenital anomalies of kidney and urinary tract (CAKUT) may be present

MICROSCOPIC PATHOLOGY

Histologic Features
- Reflux nephropathy
  - Segmental or diffuse scarring, chronic pyelonephritis
    - Tubular atrophy
    - Sclerotic glomeruli
    - Thyroidization of tubules
    - Thinning of cortex
    - Interstitial fibrosis
    - Reduced number of nephrons

REFLUX NEPHROPATHY

VUR Grading

Grade	Extent of Reflux	Reflux Nephropathy Risk
Grade 1	Confined to ureter	None
Grade 2	Ureter and into pelvis	None
Grade 3	Grade 2 and mild increase in tortuosity of ureter	Minimal
Grade 4	Grade 3, moderate tortuosity, and blunting of calyces	Moderate
Grade 5	Grade IV with marked collecting system tortuosity and compression of renal parenchyma	High

Reflux nephropathy risk increases if there is accompanying UTI or high back-flow pressure.

Etiology of Reflux Nephropathy

Primary VUR (Congenital)	Secondary VUR (Congenital)	Secondary VUR (Acquired)
Abnormal ureter intravesicular tunnel	PUV	Neurogenic bladder
Ectopic ureter	Ureterocele	Multiple sclerosis
Primary ureter	Diverticula	Diabetic neuropathy
	Urethral stricture	Spinal cord injury
	Primary megaureter	Pelvic surgery
		Vitamin B12 deficiency
		Urinary tract infections
		Dysfunctional elimination syndrome
		Cancer
		Benign prostate hyperplasia

- ■ Mixed inflammatory infiltrate consisting of lymphocytes, plasma cells, and neutrophils may be present if there is concurrent acute infection
- ■ Dysplasia indicates congenital component leading to reflux
- ■ Glomerulosclerosis
- ■ Compensatory hypertrophy of viable glomeruli
- ○ Acute pyelonephritis: Neutrophils in tubular lumen or interstitium may be present
- • Histological features in primary and secondary urine reflux may be similar and overlap with many features of obstructive nephropathy

DIFFERENTIAL DIAGNOSIS

Obstructive Nephropathy
- • Clinical and radiological correlation necessary

Tubulointerstitial Nephritis
- • Renal intrinsic causes of tubulointerstitial diseases
- • Rule out lower urinary tract abnormalities; however, may coexist in some cases

Ask-Upmark Kidney
- • Segmental well-demarcated scar without glomeruli
- • Lack of glomeruli is a key feature

DIAGNOSTIC CHECKLIST

Pathologic Interpretation Pearls
- • Dysplasia suggests congenital VUR as a cause of nephropathy

SELECTED REFERENCES

1. Peters C et al: Vesicoureteral reflux associated renal damage: congenital reflux nephropathy and acquired renal scarring. J Urol. 184(1):265-73, 2010
2. Uetani N et al: Plumbing in the embryo: developmental defects of the urinary tracts. Clin Genet. 75(4):307-17, 2009
3. Brakeman P: Vesicoureteral reflux, reflux nephropathy, and end-stage renal disease. Adv Urol. PubMed Central PMCID:PMC2478704, 2008
4. Murawski IJ et al: Gene discovery and vesicoureteric reflux. Pediatr Nephrol. 23(7):1021-7, 2008
5. Smith EA: Pyelonephritis, renal scarring, and reflux nephropathy: a pediatric urologist's perspective. Pediatr Radiol. 38 Suppl 1:S76-82, 2008
6. Williams G et al: Vesicoureteral reflux. J Am Soc Nephrol. 19(5):847-62, 2008
7. Liapis H et al: Cystic diseases and developmental kidney defects. In Jennette JC et al: Heptinstall's Pathology of the Kidney. Philadelphia: Lippincott Williams and Wilkins. 1257-1306, 2007

REFLUX NEPHROPATHY

Gross and Diagrammatic Features

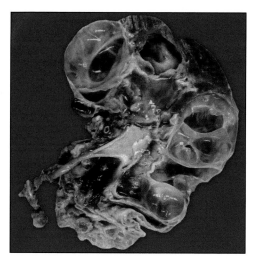

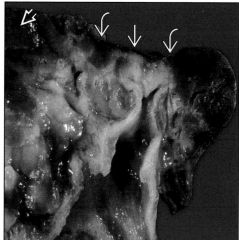

(Left) Gross image depicts multiple cysts and malformed kidney consistent with cystic dysplasia and vesicoureteral reflux in utero. Dysplasia in this setting indicates congenital etiology of reflux nephropathy. *(Right)* Gross image depicts a segmental scar ⮡ overlying the dilated calyx in reflux nephropathy. Note the thinning of cortex ➡ and adjoining normal parenchyma ⮡.

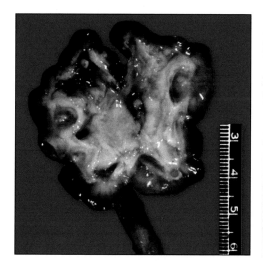

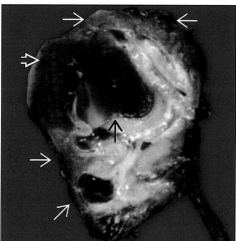

(Left) Gross image from a 23-month-old boy with reflux nephropathy shows moderate thinning of the cortex and a dilated ureter and pelvis. *(Right)* Image depicts both upper and lower lobe cortical thinning ➡ and obliteration of the medulla in a reflux nephropathy patient. The middle lobe cortex ⮡ is relatively normal. The middle lobe simple papillae are on the verge of being deformed by encroachment from the scarred upper and lower lobes ⮡.

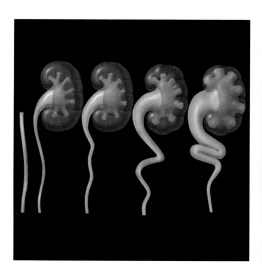

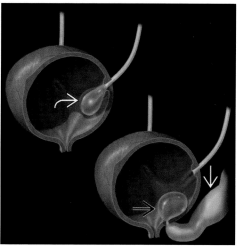

(Left) Schematic depicts different grades of VUR (1-5). The leftmost image depicts grade 1, and the rightmost image depicts grade 5. *(Right)* Illustration shows a ureterocele as an example of a lower tract obstruction causing reflux. The graphic on top shows a ureterocele ➡ in a single ureter, and the bottom depicts a ureterocele ⮡ in an ectopic ureter ➡ causing reflux.

REFLUX NEPHROPATHY

Microscopic Features

(Left) In reflux, the damage to the kidney can be quite segmental, as illustrated here at low power, with a band of almost completely destroyed tubules ⮞ adjacent to a relatively normal cortex ⮞. The outer cortex is preferentially involved ➡. *(Right)* Kidney section shows segmental scar with dysplastic tubules (left of the dashed line) as a result of high-grade VUR. Relatively unaffected parenchyma is on the right.

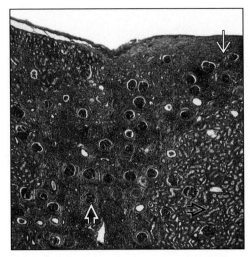
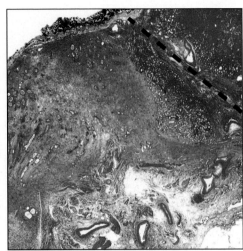

(Left) With the loss of nephrons due to reflux nephropathy, the remaining glomeruli hypertrophy, as shown here in a 25-year-old woman with end-stage disease after onset of reflux in childhood. *(Right)* Glomerular hypertrophy ⮞ and secondary FSGS are commonly present in the late stages of bilateral reflux nephropathy. The adhesion and hyaline are typically in a perihilar location ➡.

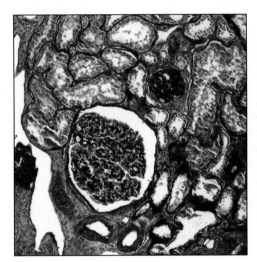
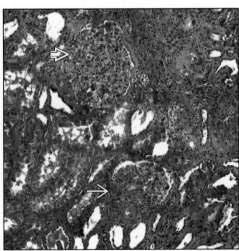

(Left) Reflux nephropathy characteristically has atrophic tubules with a microcystic appearance (thyroidization) and loss of epithelium ➡. There are several globally sclerosed glomeruli ⮞. *(Right)* Rupture and leakage of tubular contents, including PAS(+) Tamm-Horsfall protein ➡, is characteristic of reflux nephropathy and commonly elicits local inflammation, sometimes granulomatous.

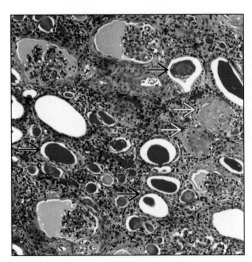
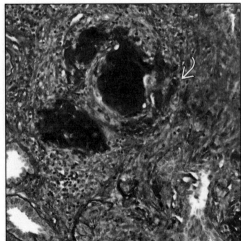

Radiologic Features

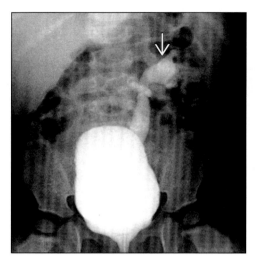
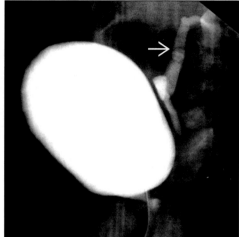

(Left) Voiding cystourethrogram shows a megaureter due to vesicoureteral reflux. The presence of dye in the pelvis ➥ denotes grade 3 reflux. *(Right)* Voiding cystourethrogram shows vesicoureteral reflux. Note reflux from the bladder into the ureter ➥.

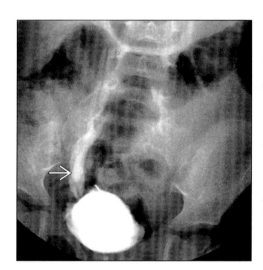
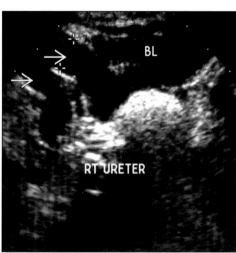

(Left) Radiologic image shows vesicoureteral reflux in a patient with a duplicated collecting system ➥. *(Right)* Ultrasound image shows a tortuous megaureter ➥ in a patient with primary high-grade VUR. BL = bladder.

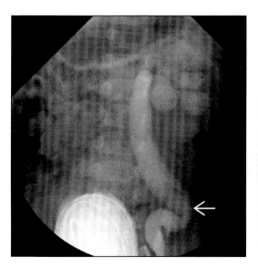
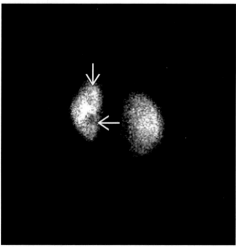

(Left) Radiologic image shows grade 5 reflux in a 4-year-old child. Note the extreme tortuosity of the ureter ➥. *(Right)* DMSA scan from a 2-year-old child with a urinary tract infection shows 2 areas of low uptake ➥ suggestive of scarring in the lower and upper poles of the left kidney.

NEPHROLITHIASIS

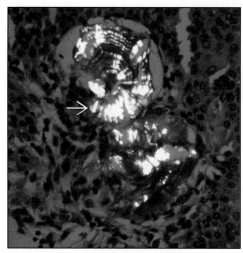

Polarized light reveals spiderweb-like organic stone matrix with calcium oxalate in radial arrays ➡ located in the suburothelium of the renal pelvis.

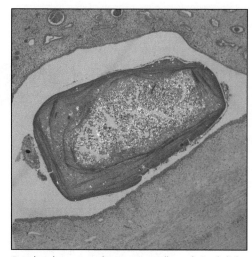

Renal calyx, viewed using partially polarized light, contains refractile crystalline material embedded in organic matrix with an irregular laminated structure.

TERMINOLOGY

Synonyms
- Kidney stone disease, renal stone disease, renal calculi, urolithiasis, lithiasis

Definitions
- Concretion of urinary mineral or inorganic crystals in collecting system of kidney

ETIOLOGY/PATHOGENESIS

Stone Types by Mineral Content
- Calcium-containing stones (~ 80% of all stones) are composed of the following compounds
  - Calcium oxalate (30%)
  - Calcium oxalate and calcium phosphate (35-45%)
  - Calcium phosphate: Hydroxyapatite (3.75-6%)
  - Calcium monohydrogen phosphate: Brushite (1.25-2%)
- Struvite (magnesium-ammonium phosphate and calcium carbonate-apatite) (5-10%)
- Uric acid (5-10%)
- Cystine (1-2%)
- Miscellaneous: Xanthine, 2,8-dihydroxyadenine, drugs (e.g., indinavir, sulphadiazine, silica-containing antacids), melamine

Predisposing Factors
- Calcium stones
  - Hypercalciuria (defined as > 4 mg Ca/kg/day in urine) without hypercalcemia
    - Idiopathic
    - Renal tubular acidosis
    - Medullary sponge kidney
    - Cadmium and beryllium nephrotoxicity
  - Hypercalcemia and hypercalciuria: Primary and secondary hyperparathyroidism
  - Hyperoxaluria

- Primary: Autosomal recessive, types I and II
- Secondary: Enteric, due to small intestinal malabsorption or excess intake; dietary, due to poisoning (ethylene glycol)
- Struvite stones
  - Infection by urea-splitting organisms: *Proteus*, *Pseudomonas*, *Providencia* species and others
  - Alkaline urine increases risk
- Uric acid stones
  - Hyperuricosuria
    - Associated with uric acid lithiasis and with ~ 40% of calcium oxalate lithiasis
  - Acidic urine with pH < 5.5
- Cystine stones
  - Hereditary disorders of tubular transport with mutations of solute-linked carriers *3A1* and *7A9* genes
- General
  - Low urine volume

Pathophysiology of Stone Formation
- Urine is supersaturated with stone constituents
- Nucleation is condensation of dissolved salts to solid phase crystals
  - Homogeneous nucleation: When solubility limits are exceeded
  - Heterogeneous nucleation: Cell membranes, cell debris, or other types of crystal form a nidus
  - Heterogeneous nucleation occurs at lower supersaturation than homogeneous nucleation
- Randall plaque
  - Deposition of calcium phosphate as hydroxyapatite (apatite) in renal papillae
  - Apatite deposits grow beneath papillary urothelium and around Bellini ducts forming Randall plaque
  - Randall plaque is thought to be heterogeneous nucleation site for calcium oxalate stone formation
- Brushite, hydroxyapatite, and cystine stones can develop from deposits within Bellini ducts

NEPHROLITHIASIS

Key Facts

Terminology
- Concretion of urinary mineral or inorganic crystals in kidney

Etiology/Pathogenesis
- Causes
  - 25% known cause
  - 50% idiopathic hypercalciuria
  - 25% unknown cause

Clinical Issues
- Frequency: 5% of females and 12% of males in USA
- Symptoms include renal colic and hematuria
- Stones recur in ~ 50% of instances
- Treatment includes hydration, thiazide diuretics, shock wave lithotripsy, and nephrolithotomy

- Stone mineral content (stone type) is determined by infrared spectroscopy or x-ray diffraction

Diagnostic Checklist
- Stones grow at papillary tip from Randall plaques or from crystal plugs in Bellini ducts
- Randall plaque is observed in idiopathic calcium oxalate, calcium phosphate (brushite), mixed oxalate and phosphate (hyperparathyroidism), and cystine lithiasis
- Bellini duct dilation and stone protrusion at papillary tip seen in calcium phosphate, uric acid, cystine, and some oxalate (enteric) lithiasis
- Cortical scarring may occur as a result of obstruction, infection, lithotripsy, or surgical intervention

---

- Stone composition: About 95% aggregated crystals and 5% organic mucoprotein matrix
  - Cut surface of stone has concentrically laminated appearance
  - Concentric layers are organic matrix skeleton, and crystalline aggregates are in radial arrays

Causes of Nephrolithiasis
- 25% known causes
  - Primary hyperparathyroidism and other causes of hypercalcemia
  - Renal tubular acidosis
  - Hyperoxaluria
  - Medullary sponge kidney
  - Drugs: Antivirals (acyclovir, ganciclovir, indinavir), sulfonamide derivatives, triamterene, glafenine, pyridoxylate
- 50% idiopathic hypercalciuria
- 25% unknown cause

CLINICAL ISSUES

Presentation
- Frequency: 5% of females and 12% of males in USA
- Nonobstructive stones have only hematuria without other symptoms or signs
- Renal colic is associated with stone passage, which is dependent on stone size
  - < 5 mm: High chance of passage
  - 5-7 mm: ~ 50% chance of passage
  - > 7 mm: Requires intervention for removal

Treatment
- Extracorporeal shock wave lithotripsy utilizes ultrasonic waves to break up stones
- Endoscopic laser-guided stone disruption
- Percutaneous nephrostomy permits removal of larger stones
- Medical treatment includes hydration to increase urinary volume and thiazide diuretics to reduce calcium excretion

Prognosis
- Stones recur in ~ 50% of instances
- Stone formers have higher blood pressure than nonstone formers
- Stone formers with high body mass index (> 27) have lower GFR than matched nonstone formers
- Almost any stone type can be complicated by urinary obstruction or infection

MACROSCOPIC FEATURES

Morphology of Common Stone Types
- Calcium oxalate and apatite
  - Solitary or multiple; hard, radiopaque; yellow-brown
- Struvite
  - Large and branched ("staghorn"); hard, gray-white, radiopacity dependent on calcium content
- Uric acid
  - Multiple; seldom > 2 cm; hard, smooth surface, yellow-brown; mainly radiolucent
- Cystine
  - Multiple; small, smooth, rounded (rarely "staghorn"); yellow, waxy, radiopaque
- 80% of stones are unilateral
- Stones protrude from Bellini ducts in calcium phosphate, uric acid, cystine, and some cases of enteric oxaluria associated lithiasis

MICROSCOPIC PATHOLOGY

Histologic Features
- Mineral deposits
  - Calcium oxalate forms pale yellow, refractile, sheaves: Birefringent by polarization microscopy
  - Apatite is basophilic, laminated, and angulate: Confirmed by von Kossa or Yasue staining
  - Accurate identification of tissue mineral deposits requires infrared spectroscopy
- Medullary histology

NEPHROLITHIASIS

Kidney Stones

Composition	Frequency	Predisposing Factors	Kidney Histology
Calcium stones	80%	Hypercalciuria	Randall plaque
Calcium oxalate	30%	Hypercalcemia	Collecting and Bellini duct apatite
Calcium oxalate and phosphate	35-45%	Hyperoxaluria	Medullary inflammation and fibrosis
Calcium phosphate	5-8%		Cortical scarring and calcification
Magnesium ammonium phosphate (struvite)	5-10%	Urea-splitting bacterial infection (e.g., Proteus)	Pyelonephritis (may be xanthogranulomatous) "staghorn" calculus
Uric acid	5-10%	Hyperuricosuria	Medullary urate deposits
Cystine	1-2%	Cystinuria	Randall plaque, collecting duct apatite, Bellini duct cystine

- o Papillary suburothelial and periductal apatite deposits correspond to Randall plaque
- o Apatite deposit in basement membranes of loops of Henle are thought to be earliest lesions of Randall plaque
- o Bellini ducts and medullary collecting ducts are dilated and plugged with mineral in most calcium phosphate, cystine, and some oxalate stone formers
- o Collecting ductal epithelial injury, dilation, medullary inflammation, and fibrosis are evident in most stone formers, with the exception of idiopathic calcium oxalate lithiasis
- o Uric acid lithiasis is associated with intratubular and interstitial sodium urate deposits with giant cell reaction (gouty tophus)
- o Struvite stones are associated with changes of acute, chronic, or xanthogranulomatous pyelonephritis
- o Small medullary apatite deposits may be seen in nonstone formers
- Cortical histology
  - o Cortical calcium phosphate deposits are evident in hypercalcemia and in cystine lithiasis
  - o Cortical interstitial fibrosis, tubular atrophy, and glomerular sclerosis are prominent in brushite and cystine lithiasis
- Most stone disease can be complicated by obstruction and infection (acute, chronic, and xanthogranulomatous pyelonephritis)
- Cortical scarring may occur as a result of obstruction, infection, lithotripsy, or surgical intervention

ANCILLARY TESTS

Histochemistry
- von Kossa
  - o Reactivity: Positive reaction with phosphate
  - o Staining pattern
    - Black precipitate in areas of calcium phosphate deposits
- Yasue
  - o Reactivity: Positive reaction with calcium deposit
  - o Staining pattern
    - Black precipitate in areas of calcium deposits

DIFFERENTIAL DIAGNOSIS

Stone Identification
- Stone mineral content and, therefore, stone type are determined by infrared spectroscopy or x-ray diffraction

Cause of Lithiasis
- Stone type determines investigation of secondary causes

DIAGNOSTIC CHECKLIST

Clinically Relevant Pathologic Features
- Stones grow at papillary tip from Randall plaques or from crystal plugs in Bellini ducts
- Randall plaque is observed in idiopathic calcium oxalate, calcium phosphate (brushite), mixed oxalate and phosphate (hyperparathyroidism), and cystine lithiasis
- Bellini duct dilation and stone protrusion seen in calcium phosphate, uric acid, cystine, and some oxalate (enteric) lithiasis

Pathologic Interpretation Pearls
- Randall plaque is medullary subepithelial apatite deposit
- Cortical scarring is most prominent in brushite stone formers
- Cortical scarring may occur as a result of obstruction, infection, lithotripsy, or surgical intervention

SELECTED REFERENCES

1. Miller NL et al: A formal test of the hypothesis that idiopathic calcium oxalate stones grow on Randall's plaque. BJU Int. 103(7):966-71, 2009
2. Evan AP et al: Role of interstitial apatite plaque in the pathogenesis of the common calcium oxalate stone. Semin Nephrol. 28(2):111-9, 2008
3. Miller NL et al: Pathogenesis of renal calculi. Urol Clin North Am. 34(3):295-313, 2007
4. Coe FL et al: Kidney stone disease. J Clin Invest. 115(10):2598-608, 2005

NEPHROLITHIASIS

Microscopic and Endoscopic Features

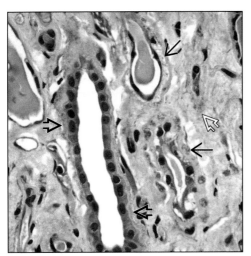

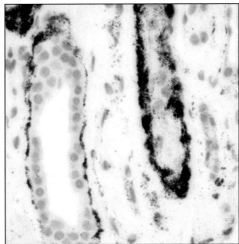

(Left) The earliest recognizable lesions of Randall plaque have apatite deposits seen as basophilic dust-like particles along the basement membranes of the loops of Henle ⇨ and the collecting duct ⇨ and in the interstitium ⇨. *(Right)* von Kossa histochemical stain for phosphate deposition highlights peritubular and interstitial calcium phosphate (apatite) deposits with a brown-black appearance in this image of an early Randall plaque.

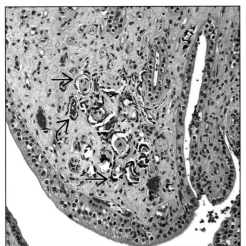

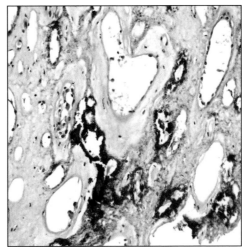

(Left) Apatite deposits are shown around loops of Henle ⇨ and vasa recta ⇨ at the papillary tip in a nonstone former. Note that the suburothelium is devoid of apatite. *(Right)* Peritubular, perivascular, and interstitial basophilic apatite deposits in Randall plaque from an idiopathic calcium oxalate stone former are shown. In this specimen, the papillary urothelium is absent (lower right).

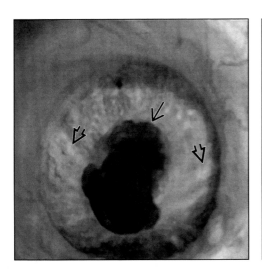

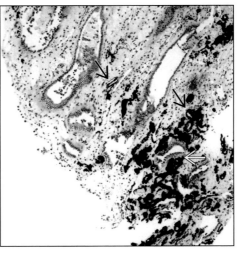

(Left) Endoscopic gross photograph shows a calcium oxalate stone attached at the papillary tip ⇨. The sides of the papilla have white suburothelial (Randall) plaque ⇨. (Courtesy A. Evan, MD.) *(Right)* A papillary biopsy stained for calcium (Yasue) reveals abundant apatite around the loops of Henle ⇨ and the collecting ducts ⇨ and in the interstitium, forming part of a Randall plaque. The papillary urothelium is not sampled in this biopsy. (Courtesy A. Evan, MD.)

NEPHROLITHIASIS

Ultrastructural, Endoscopic, and Microscopic Features

(Left) Electron micrograph reveals spherical electron-dense apatite particles ⬌ in the thickened and lamellated basement membrane of a loop of Henle. The epithelium appears intact. These are thought to be the earliest lesions of Randall plaque. (Courtesy A. Evan, MD.)
(Right) Electron micrograph reveals a mixture of matrix material and spherical apatite deposit ⬌ in the medullary interstitium in early Randall plaque formation. (Courtesy A. Evan, MD.)

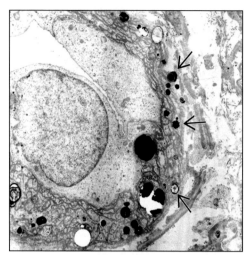
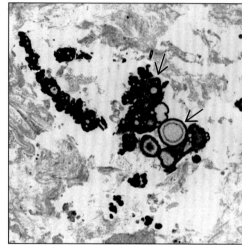

(Left) Electron micrograph reveals the multilayered structure of the spherical deposit. The crystalline material is apatite. The matrix is electron dense. (Courtesy A. Evan, MD.) (Right) Flattened medullary papilla with dilated Bellini and collecting ducts ⬌ is shown. Tubules are plugged with apatite ⬌ and oxalate ⬌. The interstitium has extensive inflammation and fibrosis in this tissue from a mixed oxalate and apatite stone former, viewed using partially polarized light.

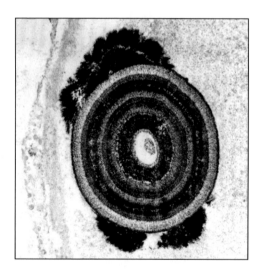
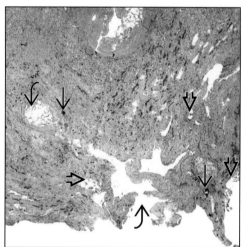

(Left) Endoscopic gross photograph shows a cystine stone protruding from the opening of a Bellini duct ⬌. Dilated openings of the ducts of Bellini are also evident ⬌. (Courtesy A. Evan, MD.)
(Right) A stain for calcium (Yasue) reveals a tubule plugged with apatite ⬌ in a fibrotic medullary papilla in a papillary biopsy from a cystine stone former. Cystine deposits typically fill the ducts of Bellini (not shown). (Courtesy A. Evan, MD.)

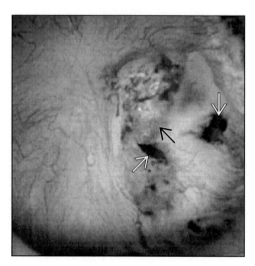
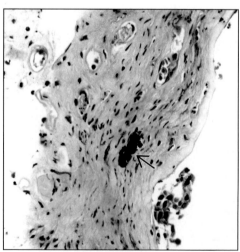

Endoscopic and Microscopic Features

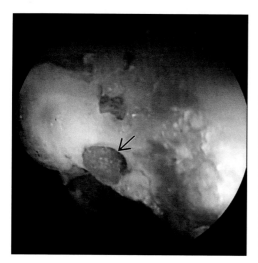

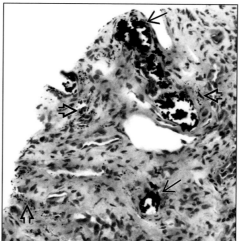

(Left) Endoscopic gross photograph from a patient with primary hyperparathyroidism demonstrates a protruding brown calcium stone ⇨ in a flattened medullary papilla. (Courtesy A. Evan, MD.) *(Right)* A stain for calcium (Yasue) reveals intratubular calcium containing apatite plugs ⇨ and fine interstitial deposits ⇨ in a papillary biopsy from a patient with primary hyperparathyroidism. (Courtesy A. Evan, MD.)

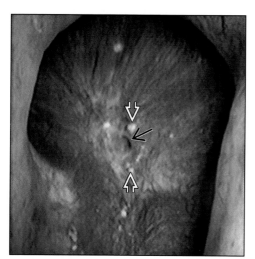

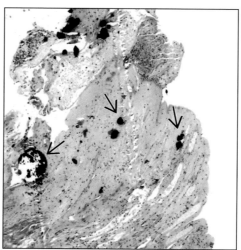

(Left) Endoscopic gross photograph from a patient with intestinal bypass surgery for obesity reveals a dilated duct of Bellini at the papillary tip ⇨. Small yellow deposits of apatite are also evident ⇨. (Courtesy A. Evan, MD.) *(Right)* A calcium stain (Yasue) reveals tubular plugging with apatite ⇨ and medullary fibrosis in a papillary biopsy specimen from a patient with intestinal bypass surgery for obesity and calcium oxalate kidney stones. (Courtesy A. Evan, MD.)

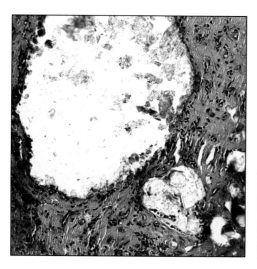

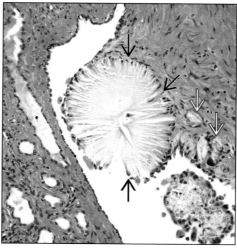

(Left) Fractured, refractile, clear yellow crystals in a scarred papilla are shown in this patient with Crohn disease and a history of small intestinal resection and calcium oxalate lithiasis. *(Right)* A calyceal uric acid deposit at the fornix is shown. An epithelial-lined, radially clefted, organic matrix is highlighted ⇨. The uric acid crystals are dissolved by aqueous fixative. Other smaller deposits are also evident ⇨.

LOIN PAIN HEMATURIA SYNDROME

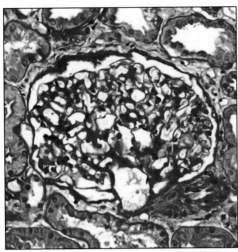

In general, kidney biopsies from LPHS patients do not reveal specific pathology. This image shows a normal glomerulus with patent capillary loops and delicate walls. The mesangium is inconspicuous.

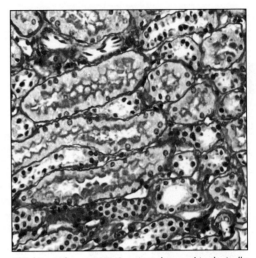

This biopsy from an LPHS patient shows a histologically normal cortical tubulointerstitium. The proximal tubules show preserved brush borders. The tubules are back-to-back, and the interstitium is inconspicuous.

TERMINOLOGY

Abbreviations
- Loin pain hematuria syndrome (LPHS)

Definitions
- Recurrent pain in lower flanks and intermittent hematuria without identifiable cause

ETIOLOGY/PATHOGENESIS

Unclear
- Proposed classification: Idiopathic disease vs. clinical mimics
- LPHS: Idiopathic disease
  - Possible etiology: Glomerular capillary hemorrhage
    - RBC and RBC casts obstruct tubules, leading to backleak of glomerular filtration
    - Tubular injury and interstitial edema lead to capsular distension and pain
- Clinical mimics of LPHS
  - IgA nephropathy
  - Thin basement membrane nephropathy
  - Occult nephrolithiasis
  - Vascular malformation
  - Inflammatory renal vascular diseases
  - Vascular spasm

CLINICAL ISSUES

Epidemiology
- Incidence
  - Diagnosis of exclusion, so incidence cannot be estimated from population-based studies
- Age
  - Children and adults from 1st to 6th decade
  - Median age: Mid 30s
- Gender

- More common in females (70%) than in males (30%)

Presentation
- Severe recurrent lower flank pain and hematuria
  - Pain is unilateral at initial presentation
    - Radiates to abdomen, inguinal and inner thigh
  - Eventually may develop bilateral flank pain
  - Hematuria may be gross or microscopic
    - Pain may not always be associated with hematuria
- Physical examination is unremarkable and nonspecific
  - Costovertebral angle tenderness
  - Low-grade fever may be present
  - No hypertension, except preexisting

Laboratory Tests
- Urine analysis may show RBCs and RBC casts

Treatment
- Options, risks, complications
  - Multidisciplinary pain management
    - Analgesia: NSAIDs and opioids
    - Intraureteric capsaicin
    - Nerve blockade
    - Antidepressants
    - Nephrectomy with autotransplantation

Prognosis
- Long-term prognosis is excellent
  - Renal function is well preserved
  - Spontaneous resolution in 30% after conservative treatment

IMAGE FINDINGS

Radiographic Findings
- Normal or nonspecific
- Minor vascular alterations may present

LOIN PAIN HEMATURIA SYNDROME

Key Facts

Etiology/Pathogenesis
- Unknown or tubular obstruction from intranephron hemorrhage

Clinical Issues
- LPHS is a diagnosis of exclusion

Microscopic Pathology
- Normal or nonspecific
  - Arteriolar sclerosis and isolated glomerulosclerosis
  - Focal interstitial fibrosis or edema
  - RBCs and RBC casts in tubules
- Immunofluorescence
  - Mesangial IgM/C3 reaction, arteriolar C3
- Electron microscopy
  - Segmental thinning of GBM

Top Differential Diagnoses
- Urologic causes
  - Neoplasms
  - Occult renal lithiasis
  - Kidney or bladder infection
  - Cystic renal disease
- Glomerular diseases
  - IgA nephropathy
  - Thin basement membrane nephropathy
  - Glomerular diseases with nephritic presentation
- Renal vascular diseases
  - Isolated polyarteritis nodosa
  - Vascular malformations

Diagnostic Checklist
- Biopsy important to exclude specific causes

MICROSCOPIC PATHOLOGY

Histologic Features
- Normal or nonspecific
  - Subcapsular glomerulosclerosis
  - Focal interstitial scarring
  - Arterial and arteriolar sclerosis
  - Focal interstitial edema
  - RBCs and RBC casts in tubules

ANCILLARY TESTS

Immunofluorescence
- Negative or nonspecific reactions
  - Nonspecific mesangial IgM and C3 due to trapping
  - Arteriolar C3 deposition

Electron Microscopy
- Normal or minor GBM alterations
- Segmental thinning of GBM

DIFFERENTIAL DIAGNOSIS

Urologic Causes of Hematuria
- Neoplasms
- Occult renal lithiasis
- Infection of kidney or bladder
- Cystic kidney disease

Renal Glomerular Diseases
- IgA nephropathy
  - 20% of LPHS show IgA nephropathy
- Thin basement membrane nephropathy
- Glomerulonephritis of various types with nephritic presentation

Renal Vascular Diseases
- Isolated polyarteritis nodosa
- Vascular malformations

DIAGNOSTIC CHECKLIST

Clinically Relevant Pathologic Features
- No identifiable urologic causes
- No evidence of specific medical renal disease
- Negative or nonspecific renal biopsy findings

Pathologic Interpretation Pearls
- Importance of biopsy: Excludes other diagnoses

SELECTED REFERENCES

1. Dube GK et al: Loin pain hematuria syndrome. Kidney Int. 70(12):2152-5, 2006
2. Kolhe N et al: Renal artery dissection secondary to medial hyperplasia presenting as loin pain haematuria syndrome. Nephrol Dial Transplant. 19(2):495-7, 2004
3. Ghanem AN: Intra-ureteric capsaicin in loin pain haematuria syndrome: efficacy and complications. BJU Int. 91(4):429-30, 2003
4. Bultitude M et al: Loin pain haematuria syndrome: distress resolved by pain relief. Pain. 76(1-2):209-13, 1998
5. Praga M et al: Association of thin basement membrane nephropathy with hypercalciuria, hyperuricosuria and nephrolithiasis. Kidney Int. 54(3):915-20, 1998
6. Sheil AG et al: Evaluation of the loin pain/hematuria syndrome treated by renal autotransplantation or radical renal neurectomy. Am J Kidney Dis. 32(2):215-20, 1998
7. Górriz JL et al: Renal-limited polyarteritis nodosa presenting with loin pain and haematuria. Nephrol Dial Transplant. 12(12):2737-9, 1997
8. Hebert LA et al: Loin pain-hematuria syndrome associated with thin glomerular basement membrane disease and hemorrhage into renal tubules. Kidney Int. 49(1):168-73, 1996
9. Lucas PA et al: Loin pain and haematuria syndrome: a somatoform disorder. QJM. 88(10):703-9, 1995

LOIN PAIN HEMATURIA SYNDROME

Microscopic Features

(Left) A wide spectrum of nonspecific microscopic changes may be encountered in kidney biopsies from patients with LPHS. Nonsenescent or isolated glomerular sclerosis ⮕ in the subcapsular region or cortex may be seen in young patients. **(Right)** Focal arteriolosclerosis ⮕, ischemia-induced glomerular capillary changes, and tubulointerstitial scarring may be present in patients with no history of hypertension. A localized vascular malformation may be the cause for this phenomenon.

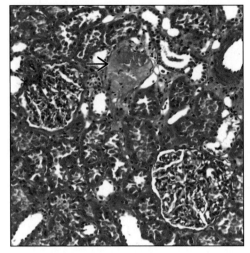
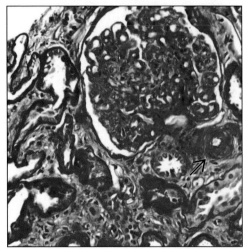

(Left) In this case, light microscopy revealed red blood cells within tubules leading to obstruction of tubular lumens ⮕. The tubules otherwise appear unaffected. **(Right)** Light microscopy shows RBC casts and obstructed tubules with attenuated epithelium in the medulla ⮕. This form of tubular obstruction may cause backleak of glomerular filtration, acute tubular injury, and interstitial edema. Distension of the renal capsule due to interstitial edema may result in loin pain.

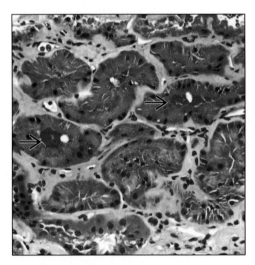
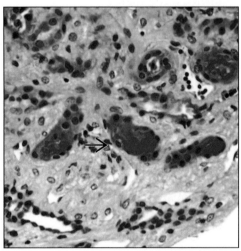

(Left) In this example, immunofluorescence revealed the nonspecific trapping of IgM in the mesangium ⮕. Mesangial C3 staining due to nonspecific trapping may also present. IgG, IgA, kappa, and lambda stains were all negative. **(Right)** The immunofluorescence in this case demonstrated arteriolar C3 deposition ⮕ without immune deposits. Arteriolar C3 deposition is not a marker of any specific disease and is commonly encountered in renal biopsies, especially in adults.

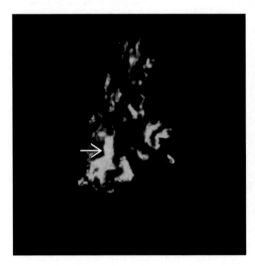
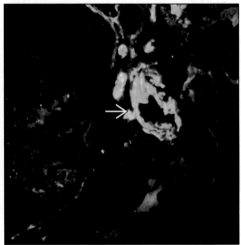

EM Features and Differential Diagnosis

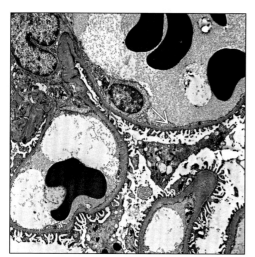

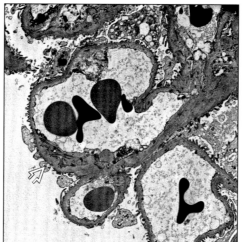

(Left) Minor GBM ultrastructural changes may be seen in LPHS. The most common alteration is focal thinning of the GBM ➡, as seen in this glomerulus where most GBMs are of normal thickness. In general, foot processes are preserved, and electron-dense material is not present. (Right) Focal thickening and irregularity of the GBM and widening of the subendothelial space may also be identified ➡. However, lamellation and widespread thinning of the GBM are, by definition, absent.

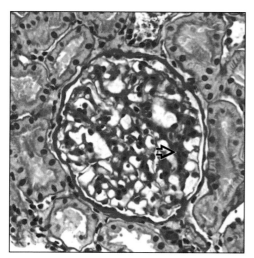

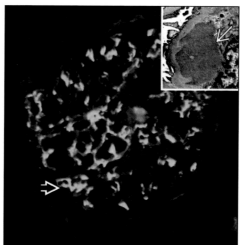

(Left) LPHS needs to be differentiated from IgAN, seen in 20% of kidney biopsies from clinically diagnosed LPHS. Although IgAN characteristically reveals mesangial hypercellularity ➡, a wide spectrum of histologic phenotypes may be seen, from no lesion, as in this case, to endocapillary proliferation to crescentic glomerulonephritis. (Right) Here is granular mesangial deposition of IgA ➡, characteristic of IgAN. The EM inset shows mesangial electron-dense deposits ➡.

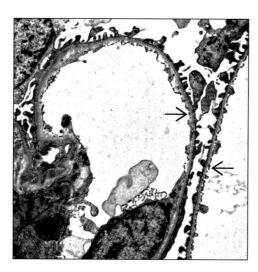

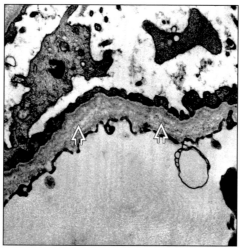

(Left) LPHS needs to be differentiated from thin basement membrane nephropathy and from Alport syndrome. This example of TBMN shows widespread thinning of the GBM ➡. No lamellations characteristic of Alport syndrome are present. (Right) In Alport syndrome, there are diffuse alterations of the GBM with irregular thickening and thinning with lamellations ➡. In early stages, these characteristic features may not present, and IF for collagen IV α-chains may be required.

Diseases of the Renal Allograft

PATHOLOGICAL CLASSIFICATION OF RENAL ALLOGRAFT DISEASES

TERMINOLOGY

Pathogenetic Classification
- Based on pathogenesis, divided into broad categories of alloimmune, drug-related, nonalloimmune, and donor-derived diseases

Abbreviations
- Acute cellular rejection (ACR)
  - Acute T-cell-mediated rejection
- Acute humoral rejection (AHR)
  - Acute antibody-mediated rejection
- Chronic humoral rejection (CHR)
  - Chronic active antibody-mediated rejection
- Peritubular capillaries (PTC)
- Focal segmental glomerulosclerosis (FSGS)
- Membranous glomerulonephritis (MGN)
- Membranoproliferative glomerulonephritis (MPGN)
- Interstitial fibrosis and tubular atrophy (IFTA), not otherwise specified (NOS)
- Epstein-Barr virus (EBV)
- Thrombotic microangiopathy (TMA)
- Mammalian target of rapamycin (mTOR)

DEFINITIONS

T-cell-mediated Rejection
- Target antigens expressed on cell surfaces of endothelial and parenchymal cells
- Accessory cells, such as macrophages participate
- Alloimmune reaction of T cells to donor alloantigens, predominantly those of the major histocompatibility complex (MHC), in humans termed HLA

Antibody-mediated Rejection
- Alloantibody mediated injury to cells expressing donor alloantigens, predominantly HLA class I and II antigens
- Accessory mechanisms includes complement activation and cells with Fc receptors

HLA Molecules
- Polymorphic antigens encoded in the MHC locus on chromosome 6
  - Class I molecules (A, B, C) widely expressed on all nucleated cells
  - Class II molecules (DR, DQ, DP), limited expression, B cells, dendritic cells, endothelial cells, macrophages, and activated T cells
- Increased expression by interferon-γ

Minor Histocompatibility Antigens
- Non-MHC antigens that are polymorphic
- Able to trigger allograft rejection in MHC identical recipients

C4d
- Fragment of C4 produced by complement activation that binds covalently to nearby molecules

Multilamination
- Multilayered basement membranes, typically > 4 layers

Transplant Glomerulopathy
- Glomerular disease seen in transplants defined by presence of duplication of GBM
- Has several causes, including CHR, TMA, and recurrent MPGN

Transplant Glomerulitis
- Mononuclear or polymorphonuclear cells in glomerular capillary loops
- Glomerular endothelial swelling and mesangiolysis in more severe cases

Endarteritis/Endothelialitis
- Mononuclear cell infiltration under arterial endothelium

Tubulitis
- Mononuclear infiltration in tubules

ALLOIMMUNE RESPONSE

T-cell-mediated Rejection
- Acute T-cell-mediated rejection (acute cellular rejection)
  - Tubulointerstitial (Banff type I)
  - Endarteritis/endothelialitis (Banff type II)
  - Arterial transmural inflammation or fibrinoid necrosis (Banff type III)
  - Transplant glomerulitis (no Banff type)
- Chronic T-cell-mediated rejection
  - Tubulointerstitial (Banff I + fibrosis and tubular atrophy)
  - Transplant arteriopathy (Banff II + intimal fibrosis/ foam cells)

Antibody-mediated Rejection
- Hyperacute rejection
  - Usually C4d(+) PTC (early samples may be negative)
  - Pathology similar to AHR, but occurring < 24 hours post transplant
- Acute antibody-mediated rejection (acute humoral rejection)
  - Tubular injury (Banff type I)
  - Capillaritis with neutrophils (Banff type II)
  - Arterial fibrinoid necrosis (Banff type III)
  - C4d(+) PTC
- Chronic antibody-mediated rejection (chronic humoral rejection)
  - Transplant glomerulopathy and glomerulitis
  - PTC multilamination and capillaritis
  - Transplant arteriopathy
  - Usually C4d(+) PTC, may be C4d(-)

Alloreactivity without Pathologic Evidence of Rejection
- Accommodation
  - C4d(+) PTC without evidence of active rejection (Banff)
  - Donor reactive antibody without graft injury or C4d deposition

Auto-/Alloantibody-mediated Diseases
- De novo membranous glomerulonephritis

PATHOLOGICAL CLASSIFICATION OF RENAL ALLOGRAFT DISEASES

- Anti-angiotensin type II receptor autoantibody syndrome

Recipient-specific Alloantibody-mediated Diseases

- Anti-GBM disease in Alport syndrome
- Nephrotic syndrome in nephrin-deficient recipients
- Anti-TBM disease in TBM antigen-deficient recipients

DRUG TOXICITY AND HYPERSENSITIVITY

Calcineurin Inhibitor Toxicity

- e.g., cyclosporine, tacrolimus
- Chronic (hyaline arteriolopathy, fibrosis, tubular atrophy, FSGS, TMA)
- Functional (vacuolar vasospasm)
- Acute (tubulopathy, TMA)

mTOR Inhibitor Toxicity

- e.g., rapamycin, sirolimus
- Acute tubular injury
- FSGS
- TMA

Antiviral Tubular Toxicity

- Crystal formation (foscarnet)
- Mitochondrial toxicity (adefovir, tenovir)

Drug-associated Acute Interstitial Nephritis

- Antibiotics and others

NONALLOIMMUNE DISEASES

Acute Ischemic Injury

- Donor derived
- Harvest related
- Post transplant

Viral Infection

- Polyomavirus
- Cytomegalovirus
- Adenovirus
- Herpes simplex

Bacterial and Fungal Infection (Partial List)

- Acute pyelonephritis
- Chronic pyelonephritis
- Tuberculosis
- Malacoplakia

Major Vessel Disease

- Arterial thrombosis
- Venous thrombosis
- Arterial dissection
- Arterial stenosis
- Arteriosclerosis (small vessels also)

Pelvis/Ureter

- Urine leak
- Obstruction
- Ureteral rejection
- Ureteral polyomavirus infection

De Novo Glomerular Disease (Partial List)

- FSGS
- Diabetic nephropathy

Recurrent Primary Disease (Partial List)

- FSGS
- Hemolytic-uremic syndrome
- MPGN, type I
- IgA nephropathy
- Oxalosis

Neoplasia

- Post-transplant lymphoproliferative disease
  - EBV and non-EBV-related

Idiopathic

- Interstitial fibrosis and tubular atrophy, not otherwise specified (IFTA, NOS)

DONOR DISEASE (PARTIAL LIST)

Present at Time of Transplant

- Acute tubular injury (ischemia)
- Arteriosclerosis
- Thrombotic microangiopathy
- Rhabdomyolysis (trauma)
- Pyelonephritis
- Glomerular disease
  - Global glomerulosclerosis due to hypertension/aging
  - IgA nephropathy, MGN, and others
- Neoplasia
  - Primary (renal cell carcinoma)
  - Metastatic tumor

NOTES

Comments

- Rejection may be manifested by clinical signs or be subclinical (normal renal function)
- Biopsy specimens often show combinations of diseases

SELECTED REFERENCES

1. Solez K et al: Banff 07 classification of renal allograft pathology: updates and future directions. Am J Transplant. 8(4):753-60, 2008
2. Colvin RB et al: Renal transplant pathology. In Jennette JC et al: Heptinstall's Pathology of the Kidney. 6th ed. Philadelphia: Lippincott Williams & Wilkins. 1347-1490, 2006

EVALUATION OF THE ALLOGRAFT KIDNEY

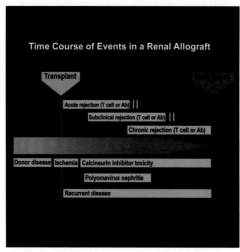

Timeline of major potential diseases in the transplanted kidney begins with donor disease and progresses through rejection (above) and nonrejection categories (below). (Courtesy J. Chapman, MD.)

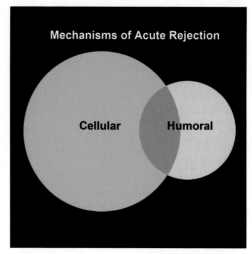

Diagram represents the 2 major mechanisms of acute renal allograft rejection: T-cell- and antibody-mediated rejection (cellular and humoral rejection, respectively). These overlap in a substantial number of cases.

TERMINOLOGY

Definitions

- Major histocompatibility complex (MHC)
  - Locus on chromosome 6 that contains genes encoding class I and class II human leukocyte antigens (HLA); MHC antigens are primary target of graft rejection
- Minor histocompatibility antigens
  - Molecules other than MHC antigens that are polymorphic and can elicit immune response in same species
- Class I MHC antigens
  - Heterodimeric protein universally expressed by nucleated cells, consisting of polymorphic α chain and monomorphic β2-microglobulin
    - Recognized by CD8(+) T cells and NK cells
    - Encoded by 3 loci (A, B, C)
- Class II MHC antigens
  - Heterodimeric protein expressed constitutively by dendritic cells, B cells, monocytes, and endothelial cells, consisting of polymorphic α chain and a β chain
    - Recognized by CD4(+) T cells
    - Encoded by 3 loci (DR, DP, DQ)
    - Increased by interferon gamma on many cell types

ETIOLOGY/PATHOGENESIS

Afferent Phase

- Donor MHC antigens elicit immune response by recipient T cells and B cells
  - On donor cells (direct pathway)
  - Processed and presented by recipient dendritic cells (indirect pathway)

Efferent Phase

- Donor-reactive T cells infiltrate graft

- Direct injury to donor cells (cytotoxicity)
- Indirect injury (via secreted cytokines and other mediators)
- Other cells recruited and participate
  - Macrophages, granulocytes, NK cells
- Target cells include arterial and capillary endothelium, tubular epithelium, and others
- Antibodies to donor HLA antigens bind to graft endothelium
  - Complement fixation
    - Release of chemotactic and vasoconstrictive mediators
    - Lysis and loss of endothelial cells
    - Activation of endothelial cells
  - Non-complement-dependent mechanisms possible
    - Activation of endothelial cells
    - Induction of proliferation
  - Cellular participation via Fc receptors
    - Monocytes, NK cells, granulocytes

Effects Determined by Many Variables

- Cellular target (endothelium of arteries, tubular epithelium, glomeruli)
- Type of immune response (antibodies vs. T cells)
- Intensity of immune response
- Resistance of graft to injury
- Immunosuppressive drug therapy

Consequences

- Ischemia
- Loss of nephron integrity
- Promotion of fibrosis
- Repair and recovery

CLINICAL IMPLICATIONS

Clinical Risk Factors

- HLA mismatch
  - HLA identical sibling graft half-life = 29 years

EVALUATION OF THE ALLOGRAFT KIDNEY

- o HLA haplo-identical living donor graft half-life = 19 years
- Deceased vs. living donor kidneys
  - o Deceased
    - Graft half-life = 10 years
    - 1-year graft survival = 89%
  - o Living unrelated
    - Graft half-life = 18 years
    - 1-year graft survival = 95%
- Older vs. younger donor
- Presensitization
- Delayed graft function
- Certain recipient diseases that recur
- Inadequate or over-immunosuppression

Current Drug Therapy
- Induction
  - o Anti-T-cell antibody (thymoglobulin, alemtuzumab)
  - o Anti-CD25 antibody (basiliximab, daclizumab)
- Maintenance
  - o Calcineurin inhibitors (cyclosporine, tacrolimus)
  - o Corticosteroids (prednisone)
  - o Antiproliferative agent (azathioprine, mycophenolate mofitel)
  - o Alternatives
    - Inhibitors of mTOR (rapamycin, everolimus)
    - Steroid-free regimens
    - CTLA4-Ig based therapy (belatacept)
- Acute rejection treatment
  - o Pulse steroids
  - o Anti-T-cell antibody
  - o Plasmapheresis
  - o IVIg

BIOPSY PROCESSING

Sample
- 16-gauge needle better than 18-gauge for sample adequacy; no great complication rate
  - o 47% of 18-gauge single cores are inadequate (< 7 glomeruli and 1 artery) vs. 24% for 16-gauge
- 2 cores needed for adequacy
  - o Single core has ~ 90% sensitivity for acute rejection; 2 cores approach 99% sensitivity

Adequacy
- Minimum 7 glomeruli, 2 arteries (Banff)
- Depends on disease to be identified
  - o Some diagnoses can be made in medulla (antibody-mediated rejection, polyomavirus infection)

Routine Pathology Techniques
- Light microscopy: Multiple levels (2-3 microns); stained with H&E, PAS, trichrome, and other stains
  - o IHC for viruses, cell phenotype as needed
  - o IHC for C4d on paraffin if no frozen tissue
- Immunofluorescence microscopy on frozen tissue: C4d, full panel if glomerular disease suspected
- Electron microscopy, especially if glomerular disease suspected

EVALUATION OF BIOPSY

Careful Examination of All Four Components as in Native Kidney Biopsies
- Glomeruli, tubules, interstitium, and vessels
- Multiple levels important, since most processes are focal (e.g., endarteritis)

Assess and Report Extent of Changes
- Give number of glomeruli, arteries, cores
- Quantitate pathologic features (% affected)
  - o Cortex (fibrosis, infiltrate)
  - o Glomeruli (sclerosis, glomerulitis, glomerular basement membrane [GBM] duplication)
  - o Tubules (atrophy, tubulitis)
  - o Arteries (endarteritis, fibrinoid necrosis, intimal fibrosis)
- Compare with previous biopsy if any
- Report diagnostic findings according to current consensus definitions
  - o Banff recommended and widely used
- Interpretation of findings needs to be made in conjunction with clinical information

SPECIAL CONSIDERATIONS IN TRANSPLANT BIOPSIES

Important Clinical Information
- Donor source
- Time post transplant
- Whether kidney had good initial function
- Drug therapy
- Original disease
- Renal function
- Anti-donor HLA antibodies

Multiple Diseases May Be Present
- Rejection, drug toxicity, viral infection, donor disease

Important to Compare with Previous Biopsies
- Progression or resolution of process
- Late samples may be nondiagnostic of cause

NEW APPROACHES

Insights Emerging from Research Studies May Have Future Application
- Gene expression in tissue, blood, and urine
- Proteomics urine, blood, tissue
- Systems analysis of pathologic data ("pathomics")
  - o Morphometry
  - o Active pathways (e.g., phosphorylation of signaling molecules)

Expected Added Value
- Assessment of drug effects
- Measurement of activity
- Assessment of pathways involved in tissue injury

PROTOCOL BIOPSIES (SURVEILLANCE BIOPSIES)

Definition
- Biopsies taken according to plan, not for abnormal renal function

Purpose
- Used to monitor status of graft in high-risk patients
  - Some centers use surveillance biopsies in routine care
- Common in clinical trials to assess efficacy and toxicity
- Provides insights into mechanisms and prevalence of graft pathology

Value
- Identification of subclinical graft pathology
  - Cellular or humoral rejection
    - Subclinical cellular rejection varies by therapy; 1-43% at 1-2 months and 0-15% at 1 year
  - Polyoma infection
  - Drug toxicity
- Appreciation that accepted grafts can have benign infiltrates
  - Pathology of accepted grafts not well characterized
- Necessary to trace evolution of chronic progressive diseases

BANFF CLASSIFICATION

Background
- Classification is currently based on light microscopy, immunofluorescence, or immunohistochemistry, and in some instances, electron microscopy
  - Diagnostic categories defined by semiquantitative scores
  - Opportunity to add other modalities, e.g., gene expression
- Refinement occurs through biannual open meetings to reach consensus on additions/changes based on published, confirmed evidence
- Widely used in drug trials
- Adequacy is 7 glomeruli and 2 arteries and should be noted

Banff Categories
- **1: Normal**
- **2: Antibody-mediated rejection (C4d[+])**
  - Requires acute or chronic tissue injury or inflammation, evidence of antibody interaction with tissue (usually C4d in peritubular capillaries [PTC]), and circulating antibodies reactive to donor endothelium
  - Acute antibody-mediated rejection
    - I: Acute tubular injury
    - II: Peritubular &/or glomerular capillary inflammation (neutrophils), ± thrombi
    - III: Arterial involvement by transmural arteritis, &/or arterial fibrinoid necrosis and medial smooth muscle necrosis with inflammatory infiltrate in vessel

  - Chronic antibody-mediated rejection
    - Chronic tissue injury includes GBM duplication without immune complex deposition (transplant glomerulopathy), PTC basement membrane multilamination (usually seen by electron microscopy), transplant arteriopathy, and interstitial fibrosis and tubular atrophy
    - Often manifested by mononuclear cells in PTC (capillaritis) &/or glomeruli (transplant glomerulitis)
  - Hyperacute rejection
    - Usually due to preformed antibody, e.g., antibodies to HLA or ABO antigens
  - C4d deposition without evidence of active rejection
- **3: Borderline or suspicious for acute cellular rejection**
  - Defined by t > 0 and i1 or t1 and i > 0
- **4: T-cell-mediated rejection**
  - Requires > i1 and ≥ t2 or > v0; C4d negative for pure T-cell-mediated rejection
  - Acute T-cell-mediated rejection
    - IA: Interstitial inflammation (> 25% of unscarred cortex) and foci of moderate tubulitis (> 4 mononuclear cells per tubular cross section)
    - IB: Interstitial inflammation (> 25% of unscarred cortex) and foci of severe tubulitis (> 10 mononuclear cells per tubular cross section)
    - IIA: Mild to moderate intimal arteritis (< 25% of luminal area) (v1)
    - IIB: Severe intimal arteritis (> 25% of luminal area) (v2)
    - III: Transmural arteritis &/or fibrinoid necrosis of medial smooth muscle (v3)
  - Chronic active T-cell-mediated rejection
    - Chronic allograft arteriopathy (arterial intimal fibrosis with mononuclear cell infiltration in fibrosis, formation of neo-intima)
- **5: Interstitial fibrosis and tubular atrophy, no evidence of any specific etiology**
  - Use only when etiology of IF/TA is unknown
  - Formerly known as chronic allograft nephropathy (CAN)
- **6: Other**
  - Changes considered not due to rejection
    - Calcineurin inhibitor toxicity, polyomavirus infection, and others

Caveats
- Biopsies may meet criteria for 2 or more diagnoses
- Detailed criteria established only for rejection categories
- Reproducibility of certain categories and features is limited

BANFF SCORING CATEGORIES

Interstitial Inflammation (i)
- Mononuclear inflammation in nonfibrotic areas; excludes subcapsular cortex and perivascular infiltrates
  - i0: < 10% of nonfibrotic cortex
  - i1: 10-25%
  - i2: 26-50%

- i3: > 50%
- Do not include fibrotic areas in denominator

Tubulitis (t)

- Mononuclear cells in tubules; for longitudinal sections count per 10 tubular epithelial nuclei
  - t0: No mononuclear cells in tubules
  - t1: Foci with 1-4 cells/tubular cross section
  - t2: Foci with 5-10 cells/tubular cross section
  - t3: Foci with > 10 cells/tubular cross section
- Need at least 2 foci of tubulitis to be present

Vascular Inflammation (v)

- Mononuclear cells in intima or media of arteries or medial necrosis
  - v0: No arteritis
  - v1: Intimal arteritis in < 25% of lumen (minimum = 1 cell, 1 artery)
  - v2: Intimal arteritis in ≥ 25% of lumen in ≥ 1 artery
  - v3: Transmural arteritis &/or medial smooth muscle necrosis (fibrinoid necrosis)

Glomerulitis (g)

- % of glomeruli with increased mononuclear cells in capillaries
  - g0: No glomerulitis
  - g1: < 25% of glomeruli
  - g2: 25-75% of glomeruli
  - g3: > 75% of glomeruli

Interstitial Fibrosis (ci)

- % of cortex with fibrosis
  - ci0: ≤ 5%
  - ci1: 6-25%
  - ci2: 26-50%
  - ci3: > 50%

Tubular Atrophy (ct)

- % of cortex with atrophic tubules
  - ct0: 0%
  - ct1: ≤ 25%
  - ct2: 26-50%
  - ct3: > 50%

Arterial Fibrointimal Thickening (cv)

- % of narrowing of lumen of most severely affected artery
  - cv0: 0%
  - cv1: ≤ 25%
  - cv2: 26-50%
  - cv3: > 50%
- Note if lesions characteristic of chronic cellular rejection are present (inflammatory cells in intima, foam cells, breaks in internal elastica or lack of fibroelastosis in intima)

Transplant Glomerulopathy (cg)

- % of glomerular capillary loops with duplication of GBM in most affected glomerulus
  - cg0: < 10%
  - cg1: 10-25%
  - cg2: 26-50%
  - cg3: > 50%

Mesangial Matrix Increase (mm)

- % of glomeruli with mesangial increase, defined as > 2 mesangial cells in width in at least 2 glomerular lobules
  - mm0: 0%
  - mm1: ≤ 25%
  - mm2: 26-50%
  - mm3: > 50%

Arteriolar Hyalinosis (ah)

- Circumferential or noncircumferential (focal) hyaline
  - ah0: No arterioles with hyaline
  - ah1: 1 arteriole with noncircumferential hyaline
  - ah2: ≥ 1 arteriole with noncircumferential hyaline
  - ah3: ≥ 1 arteriole with circumferential hyaline
- Note if peripheral nodules are present

Peritubular Capillary Inflammation (ptc)

- % of cortical PTC with neutrophils or mononuclear cells
  - ptc0: < 10% PTC with cells
  - ptc1: > 10% with < 5 cells/PTC
  - ptc2: > 10% with 5-10 cells/PTC
  - ptc3: > 10% with > 10 cells/PTC
- Note whether only mononuclear cells, < 50% neutrophils, or > 50% neutrophils

C4d Score in PTC (C4d)

- % of PTC with C4d deposition scored in at least 5 HPF
  - C4d0: 0%
  - C4d1: 1-9%
  - C4d2: 10-50%
  - C4d3: > 50%
- Note technique used (frozen vs. paraffin)

Total Inflammation (ti)

- Includes all cortical inflammation, even subcapsular, perivascular, nodular, and fibrotic areas
  - ti0: < 10% of cortex
  - ti1: 10-25%
  - ti2: 26-50%
  - ti3: > 50%

SELECTED REFERENCES

1. Sis B et al: Banff '09 meeting report: antibody mediated graft deterioration and implementation of Banff working groups. Am J Transplant. 10(3):464-71, 2010
2. Solez K et al: Banff '05 Meeting Report: differential diagnosis of chronic allograft injury and elimination of chronic allograft nephropathy ('CAN'). Am J Transplant. 7(3):518-26, 2007
3. Colvin RB et al: Renal transplant pathology. In Jennette JC et al: Heptinstall's Pathology of the Kidney. Philadelphia: Lippincott Williams & Wilkins. 1347-1490, 2006
4. Furness PN et al: International variation in histologic grading is large, and persistent feedback does not improve reproducibility. Am J Surg Pathol. 27(6):805-10, 2003
5. Racusen LC et al: Antibody-mediated rejection criteria - an addition to the Banff 97 classification of renal allograft rejection. Am J Transplant. 3(6):708-14, 2003
6. Racusen LC et al: The Banff 97 working classification of renal allograft pathology. Kidney Int. 55(2):713-23, 1999

EVALUATION OF THE DONOR KIDNEY

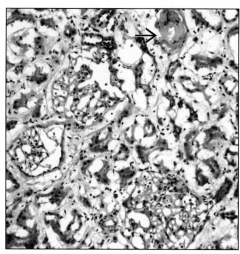

This deceased donor kidney biopsy appears edematous and the glomeruli appear hypercellular, common artifacts of frozen sections. The percentage of globally sclerotic glomeruli ⇒ is routinely reported.

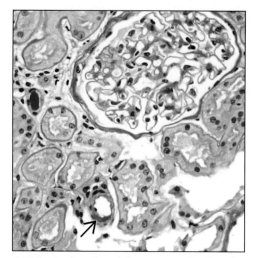

A PAS-stained section of the corresponding formalin-fixed, paraffin-embedded section reveals a normal-appearing glomerulus and mild intimal hyalinosis of an arteriole ⇒.

TERMINOLOGY

Definitions
- Donor biopsy
  - Biopsy performed prior to implantation, evaluated by frozen section
  - Used in attempt to determine suitability of kidney for transplantation
  - Performed on deceased donor kidneys
- Implantation biopsy, zero-hour biopsy
  - Biopsy performed just after or just prior to implantation, evaluated on permanent sections
  - Used in clinical trials to determine baseline histologic features of donor kidney or subclinical renal disease
  - May be performed on either deceased or living donor kidneys
- Expanded criteria donor (ECD)
  - Donor age > 60 years
  - Donor age 50-60 years and at least 2 of the following
    - Death from cerebrovascular accident
    - Hypertension
    - Serum creatinine (Cr) > 1.5 mg/dL
  - Increased risk of graft failure (relative hazard ratio 1.70) and delayed graft function compared to standard-criteria donor
    - Survival benefit for recipients of ECD kidneys compared to continued dialysis
- Donation after cardiac death
  - Donors do not meet criteria for brain death
  - Absence of cardiac function prior to organ procurement

CLINICAL ISSUES

Purpose of Donor Biopsy
- Suitability of ECD kidney
  - ~ 40% of ECD kidneys are discarded
- Suspected donor disease

- Evaluation of neoplasm

Kidney Acceptance Criteria
- Judgment of clinician based on pathological report and patient
  - Older patient or highly sensitized may benefit from marginal kidney
  - No absolute cut-off has been established for any pathologic criteria
    - Risk of overestimating damage and discarding useful kidneys
  - Can do double transplant

Purpose of Implantation Biopsy
- Baseline for clinical trials
- Evidence of antibody-mediated injury in presensitized recipient

MICROSCOPIC PATHOLOGY

Evaluation of Donor Biopsy on Frozen Section
- Sample adequacy
  - On donor biopsy, at least 25 glomeruli should be present, including from deep cortex
  - At least 2 arteries should be present
- Some degree of chronic changes are present in most time-zero or donor kidney biopsies
- Chronic changes are usually mild in living donors and increase with donor age
- Percentage of globally sclerotic glomeruli
  - If > 20% globally sclerotic glomeruli, higher incidence of delayed graft function (DGF) requiring transient dialysis, higher Cr at 3-24 months, variable effect on graft survival
  - > 20% global sclerosis has minimal effect on 1-year graft survival and only if donor Cr clearance is ≤ 80 mL/min (83% vs. 79%)

EVALUATION OF THE DONOR KIDNEY

Key Facts

Clinical Issues
- Suitability of ECD kidney
  - Judgment of clinician based on pathological report and patient
  - No absolute cutoff has been established for any pathologic criteria
- Baseline for clinical trials

Microscopic Pathology
- Sample adequacy
  - ≥ 25 glomeruli including deep cortex
  - ≥ 2 arteries should be present
- > 20% globally sclerotic glomeruli often cited
  - Higher incidence of DGF
  - Higher Cr at 3-24 months
  - Variable effect on graft survival
  - No effect if donor Cr clearance is > 80 mL/min

- Moderate arteriosclerosis (> 25% luminal narrowing) predictor of worse graft outcome (graft loss, DGF, higher Cr)
- Many donor diseases have full recovery
  - IgA nephropathy
  - Thrombotic microangiopathy

Diagnostic Checklist
- Difficulties in interpretation of frozen sections
  - Interstitium looks edematous, resembles fibrosis
  - Glomeruli appear hypercellular
  - Difficult to appreciate acute tubular injury
- Globally sclerotic glomeruli overestimated with wedge biopsies
- Risk of overestimating renal pathology and discarding potentially beneficial donor kidneys

---

  - No absolute cutoff point for percent global glomerulosclerosis has been determined
  - Sclerotic glomeruli predominately in subcapsular cortex in arteriosclerosis, overestimated in wedge biopsies
  - Strong correlation with age
- Arteriosclerosis
  - Moderate arteriosclerosis (> 25% luminal narrowing) a predictor of worse graft outcome (graft loss, DGF, higher Cr)
- Interstitial fibrosis and tubular atrophy
  - Not consistently predictive
- Thrombi in glomeruli, arteries
  - Head trauma in donor can precipitate TMA
  - Even with glomerular thrombi, good outcome possible
  - Cholesterol emboli may be contraindication

Implantation Biopsy
- Process and score same as indication transplant biopsies on paraffin process material
- C4d in presensitized recipient
- Immunofluorescence and EM if considering donor glomerular disease

Donor Diseases with Documented Full Recovery
- IgA nephropathy
  - IgA present in ~ 10% of donor biopsies
- Membranous glomerulonephritis
- Lupus nephritis
- Acute post-streptococcal infection glomerulonephritis
- Membranoproliferative glomerulonephritis
- Thrombotic microangiopathy
- Preeclampsia
- Hepatorenal syndrome

Maryland Aggregate Pathology Index
- Aggregate score predictive of graft survival (glomerulosclerosis ≥ 15%, hyalinosis, increased wall/lumen ratio of arteries, periglomerular fibrosis, and scar)

DIAGNOSTIC CHECKLIST

Pathologic Interpretation Pearls
- Sclerotic glomeruli overestimated in wedge biopsies
- Difficulties in interpretation of frozen sections
  - Interstitium looks edematous, resembles fibrosis
  - Glomeruli appear hypercellular
  - Difficult to appreciate acute tubular injury
  - Red cell casts lyse on freezing

REPORTING CRITERIA

Donor Biopsy (Frozen or Permanent)
- Site/type of biopsy (cortex, medulla/wedge, needle)
- Number of glomeruli and arteries
- Number of globally sclerotic glomeruli
- Intimal fibrosis and arteriolar hyalinosis
- Percentage fibrosis/tubular atrophy
- Thrombi in glomeruli or vessels
- Any other notable features

Implantation Biopsy
- Standard scoring of transplant biopsies (Banff)

SELECTED REFERENCES

1. Nickeleit V: Pathology: donor biopsy evaluation at time of renal grafting. Nat Rev Nephrol. 5(5):249-51, 2009
2. Rao PS et al: The alphabet soup of kidney transplantation: SCD, DCD, ECD--fundamentals for the practicing nephrologist. Clin J Am Soc Nephrol. 4(11):1827-31, 2009
3. Kayler LK et al: Correlation of histologic findings on preimplant biopsy with kidney graft survival. Transpl Int. 21(9):892-8, 2008
4. Munivenkatappa RB et al: The Maryland aggregate pathology index: a deceased donor kidney biopsy scoring system for predicting graft failure. Am J Transplant. 8(11):2316-24, 2008
5. Colvin RB et al: Renal transplant pathology. In Jennette JC et al: Heptinstall's Pathology of the Kidney 2006. Philadelphia: Lippincott Williams & Wilkins. 1347-1490, 2006

Comparison of Frozen and Permanent Sections

(Left) Frozen section of a donor biopsy shows apparent interstitial edema, likely the "normal" state of the kidney before dehydration during processing for permanent sections. Tubular morphology is uninterpretable. *(Right)* Periodic acid-Schiff on the corresponding permanent section shows intimal arteriolar hyalinosis ⊇, a feature difficult to identify on a frozen section. This feature was seen in several arterioles on the permanent section.

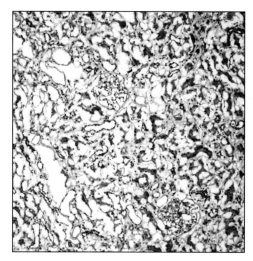 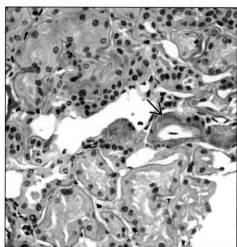

(Left) Glomeruli normally appear hypercellular on frozen sections, as illustrated in this donor kidney biopsy; glomeruli were not hypercellular on permanent sections. The interstitium appears edematous. *(Right)* After routine permanent processing, the kidney shows only focal fine interstitial edema and normal glomeruli.

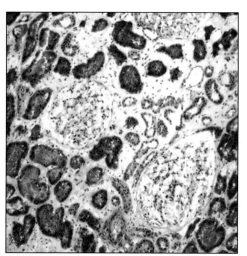 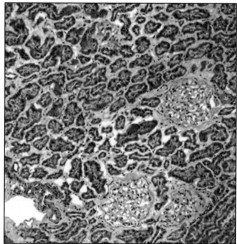

(Left) Frozen section of a donor biopsy shows eosinophilic material in 2 capillary loops, which are fibrin thrombi ⊇. These can be easily overlooked, especially if they are focal. *(Right)* Light microscopy shows glomerular thrombi ⊇ in a donor biopsy specimen from a 52-year-old woman who died from a subarachnoid hemorrhage. Thrombi are common in donors who died from stroke or head injury. Scattered thrombi do not contraindicate use of the kidney.

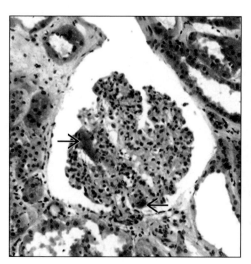 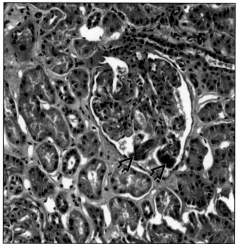

EVALUATION OF THE DONOR KIDNEY

Donor Diseases

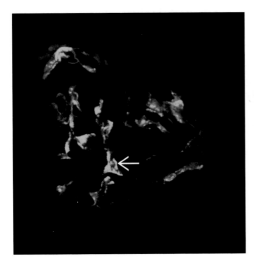
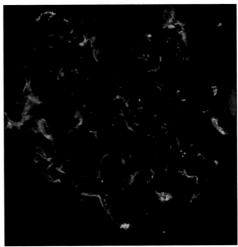

(Left) Immunofluorescence of a living donor kidney shows prominent IgA in the mesangium ➡. The ABO-incompatible donor had no clinical or laboratory evidence of glomerular disease. (Right) Immunofluorescence of a protocol biopsy taken 3 months after transplant of an ABO-incompatible living donor kidney with prominent IgA in the mesangium shows complete loss of the mesangial IgA deposits. The recipient had no clinical evidence of glomerular disease.

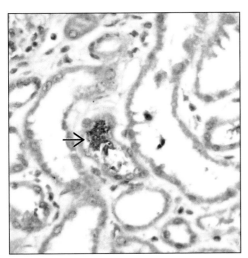
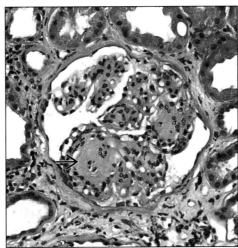

(Left) The donor of this kidney died from trauma and the kidney had severe tubular injury, with granular eosinophilic casts that stained for myoglobin ➡. (Right) Transplant biopsy taken 17 days after transplant shows prominent nodular diabetic glomerulopathy ➡. The donor and the recipient were diabetic. The nodules were not apparent in a donor frozen section, even in retrospect. The graft was eventually lost. Donation to a nondiabetic recipient might have been more salutary.

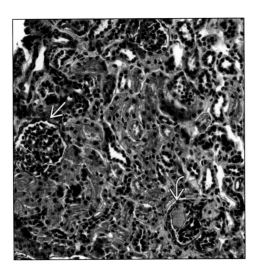
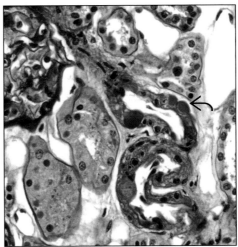

(Left) Donor kidney biopsy from a child shows immature glomeruli ➡ with crowded podocytes and one glomerulus with focal segmental glomerulosclerosis ➡, probably developmental. (Right) Nodular peripheral arteriolar hyalinosis ➡ in a donor biopsy looks exactly like the hyalinosis commonly found in chronic calcineurin inhibitor (CNI) toxicity and once thought to be specific for CNI. This feature, however, is uncommonly seen in the absence of CNI administration.

ACUTE CELLULAR REJECTION

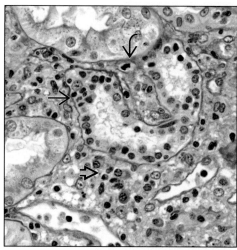

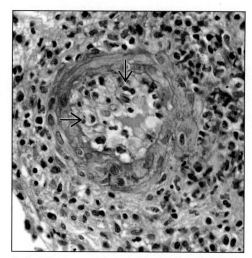

Tubulitis ➡ and interstitial mononuclear inflammation ➡ are the defining features of type I acute cellular rejection. The infiltrating cells appear activated, and mitotic figures are present ➡.

Endarteritis in a renal transplant biopsy, the defining feature of type II acute cellular rejection, is shown. Many mononuclear cells ➡ are in the intima. The cells are primarily T cells and monocytes.

TERMINOLOGY

Abbreviations
- Acute cellular rejection (ACR)

Synonyms
- Acute T-cell-mediated rejection

Definitions
- Acute immunologic reaction to renal alloantigens mediated by T cells
  - Type I: Tubulointerstitial
  - Type II: Endarteritis
  - Type III: Fibrinoid arterial necrosis or transmural inflammation

ETIOLOGY/PATHOGENESIS

T-cell-mediated Rejection
- Alloreactive T cells against donor antigens
  - MHC (HLA) or non-MHC
- Target varies and includes capillary and arterial endothelium, tubules, and glomeruli

CLINICAL ISSUES

Epidemiology
- Incidence
  - 5-10% in 1st year post transplant in conventional transplants
    - Type I: ~ 65%
    - Type II: ~ 30%
    - Type III: < 5%

Presentation
- Acute renal failure
- Oliguria or decreased urine output
- Graft tenderness (severe cases)

Treatment
- Drugs
  - Type I and cases borderline/suspicious for ACR are usually responsive to pulse steroid therapy
  - Type II usually resistant to pulse steroid therapy; additional treatment may consist of anti-T-cell agent
  - Type III resistant to current therapies

Prognosis
- 1-year graft survival
  - Type I: ~ 95%
  - Type II: ~ 75%
  - Type III: ~ 15%

MICROSCOPIC PATHOLOGY

Histologic Features
- Glomeruli
  - Usually spared
  - Occasional cases show glomerulitis with mononuclear cells in glomerular capillaries
    - Primarily T cells
    - Glomerulitis more commonly found in humoral rejection and macrophages predominate
    - Not currently included as criterion for ACR
  - Acute allograft glomerulopathy in < 5%
    - Markedly swollen endothelial cells occluding capillary lumen
    - Mesangiolysis with PAS-positive webs
    - When present, usually associated with type II ACR
- Interstitium
  - Mononuclear cell inflammation in interstitium
    - Diagnosis of rejection by Banff criteria requires > 25% of nonscarred cortex to have mononuclear infiltrate
    - Lesser degrees of inflammation considered "suspicious" or "borderline" for rejection
    - Cells mostly CD4(+) and CD8(+) T cells and CD68(+) macrophages

ACUTE CELLULAR REJECTION

Key Facts

Etiology/Pathogenesis
- Alloreactive T cells against donor antigens

Clinical Issues
- Acute renal failure
- 5-10% in 1st year post transplant in conventional transplants
- Oliguria or decreased urine output
- ACR type I and borderline/suspicious for ACR cases are usually responsive to pulse steroid therapy
- ACR type II usually resistant to pulse steroid therapy; additional treatment may consist of anti-T-cell agent

Microscopic Pathology
- Mixed mononuclear interstitial inflammation and tubulitis (type I ACR)

- Mononuclear cell accumulation under endothelium of arteries (type II ACR)
- Fibrinoid necrosis of arteries (type III ACR)
- Interstitial edema and sometimes hemorrhage
- Glomerular involvement is usually mild, but glomerulitis can be pronounced
- C4d is negative in pure T-cell-mediated rejection, but positive if combined with humoral rejection

Top Differential Diagnoses
- Acute humoral rejection (AHR)
- BK polyomavirus interstitial nephritis
- Pyelonephritis
- Acute allergic tubulointerstitial nephritis
- Post-transplant lymphoproliferative disorder

- B cells usually not prominent
  o Eosinophils, plasma cells, and a few neutrophils may also be present in infiltrate
    - Plasma cell-rich rejection has worse prognosis
    - Some studies show that eosinophils portend worse outcome
  o Interstitial edema
  o Hemorrhage in more severe cases
- Tubules
  o T cells and macrophages within tubule ("tubulitis")
    - Only nonatrophic tubules are evaluated for Banff criteria
  o Tubular cell injury (loss of brush border, apoptosis)
  o Tubular basement membranes sometimes rupture with severe tubulitis
    - May form granulomas
- Arteries
  o Mononuclear inflammatory cells beneath endothelium in arteries ("endarteritis" or "endothelialitis")
    - CD3(+) T cells and CD68(+) monocytes/ macrophages
    - Focal process, affecting ~ 25% of cross sections of arteries and ~ 12% of arterioles
    - Larger vessels affected more than arterioles
    - Endothelialitis in arterioles sometimes seen in conjunction with endothelialitis in arteries; has same significance
  o Marginated mononuclear cells along endothelial surface
    - Does not count for endarteritis, but associated with it
  o Venulitis found in some cases of ACR, but not prognostically significant
  o Endothelium may develop signs of "activation," with basophilic cytoplasm, enlarged active nuclei
  o Transmural inflammation in more severe cases
    - Fibrinoid necrosis also occasionally seen in severe cases, but more commonly associated with antibody-mediated rejection

ANCILLARY TESTS

Immunofluorescence
- Generally little or no immunoglobulin or C3 deposition in glomeruli or interstitium
  o Fibrin diffusely present in edematous interstitium
  o Fibrinoid necrosis typically has IgM/IgG and C3 in deposits
- C4d negative in pure T-cell-mediated rejection
- ACR cases with C4d deposition have superimposed acute &/or chronic humoral rejection

Electron Microscopy
- Not generally used for diagnosis
- Glomeruli in acute allograft glomerulopathy show marked endothelial reaction (swollen cytoplasm, loss of fenestrations)
- Lymphocytes between tubular cells and under arterial endothelium

DIFFERENTIAL DIAGNOSIS

BK Polyomavirus Interstitial Nephritis
- Plasma cells in infiltrate
- Intranuclear inclusions in tubular epithelial cells
- Inflammation primarily in sites with viral infection (IHC)

Pyelonephritis
- Neutrophilic casts and abscesses
- Positive urine culture for bacterial infection

Thrombotic Microangiopathy (TMA)
- Endothelialitis and luminal fibrin may be present
- Fragmented erythrocytes in intima favor TMA
- Thrombi with minimal endothelial inflammation and mucoid intimal thickening favor TMA

Acute Allergic Tubulointerstitial Nephritis
- May represent an allergic drug reaction
- Difficult or impossible to distinguish from tubulointerstitial acute cellular rejection (type I)

ACUTE CELLULAR REJECTION

Obstruction

- Edema and collecting duct dilation may be present
- Usually not more than "borderline" infiltrates (< 25% of cortex)
- Dilated lymphatics, sometimes containing Tamm-Horsfall protein
- Can never rule out by morphology

Resolving/Partially Treated ACR

- More severe tubulitis present compared to interstitial inflammation
- Inflammation in areas of interstitial fibrosis

Acute Humoral Rejection (AHR)

- C4d deposition in peritubular capillaries, circulating anti-donor antibodies
- May be superimposed on acute cellular rejection

Peritubular Capillaritis

- Marginated mononuclear cells and a few neutrophils in peritubular capillaries
- Common finding on protocol biopsy in patients with donor-specific anti-HLA antibody
  - No tubulitis
  - C4d stain usually negative
- Significance remains to be defined, may be precursor to chronic humoral rejection

Post-transplant Lymphoproliferative Disorder (PTLD)

- Little edema and predominance of atypical B cells rather than T cells
  - Monoclonal B cell infiltrate most common
- Most cases are EBER positive
- Necrosis of infiltrating cells

Atheromatous Embolism

- Endothelialitis and luminal fibrin may be present
- Unusual finding; thorough examination of tissue levels should reveal cholesterol clefts in arteries with inflammation

Acute Transient Arteriopathy

- Rare lesion (< 1%); occurs in very early post-transplant period (< 2 weeks) in deceased donor transplants
- Markedly reactive endothelial cells
  - Endothelial cell swelling, lifting, and vacuolization
  - No endothelialitis or thrombi
  - C4(-)
- Usually occurs with acute tubular injury
- May represent acute reactive endothelial changes analogous to acute tubular injury
- Lesion resolves on follow-up biopsy

DIAGNOSTIC CHECKLIST

Pathologic Interpretation Pearls

- Multiple levels need to be examined to detect focal lesions, such as endarteritis, which are more specific for ACR
- 1 biopsy core has false-negative rate of about 10%

- Biopsies may meet criteria for ACR and antibody-mediated rejection (C4d[+]), in which case outcome is dominated by latter

GRADING

Banff Grading of ACR

- Borderline/suspicious for acute cellular rejection
  - Interstitial inflammation in 10-25% of unscarred cortex and foci of mild tubulitis
- Tubulointerstitial ACR (type I)
  - Banff type IA: Interstitial inflammation in > 25% of unscarred cortex and foci of moderate tubulitis (4-10 mononuclear cells per tubular cross section)
  - Banff type IB: Interstitial inflammation in > 25% of unscarred cortex and foci of severe tubulitis (> 10 mononuclear cells per tubular cross section)
- ACR with endothelialitis (type II)
  - Banff type IIA: Mild to moderate endothelialitis
  - Banff type IIB: Severe endothelialitis
- ACR with transmural arterial inflammation (type III)
  - Banff type III: Transmural arteritis, &/or arterial fibrinoid change and necrosis of medial smooth muscle

SELECTED REFERENCES

1. Sis B et al: Banff '09 meeting report: antibody mediated graft deterioration and implementation of Banff working groups. Am J Transplant. 10(3):464-71, 2010
2. Cornell LD et al: Kidney transplantation: mechanisms of rejection and acceptance. Annu Rev Pathol. 3:189-220, 2008
3. Solez K et al: Banff 07 classification of renal allograft pathology: updates and future directions. Am J Transplant. 8(4):753-60, 2008
4. Colvin RB et al: Renal transplant pathology. In Jennette JC et al: Heptinstall's Pathology of the Kidney. Philadelphia: Lippincott Williams & Wilkins. 1347-1490, 2006
5. Hirsch HH et al: Polyomavirus-associated nephropathy in renal transplantation: interdisciplinary analyses and recommendations. Transplantation. 79(10):1277-86, 2005
6. Nickeleit V et al: Polyomavirus allograft nephropathy and concurrent acute rejection: a diagnostic and therapeutic challenge. Am J Transplant. 4(5):838-9, 2004
7. Emovon OE et al: Clinical significance of eosinophils in suspicious or borderline renal allograft biopsies. Clin Nephrol. 59(5):367-72, 2003
8. McCarthy GP et al: Diagnosis of acute renal allograft rejection: evaluation of the Banff 97 Guidelines for Slide Preparation. Transplantation. 73(9):1518-21, 2002
9. Meehan SM et al: The clinical and pathologic implications of plasmacytic infiltrates in percutaneous renal allograft biopsies. Hum Pathol. 32(2):205-15, 2001
10. Meehan SM et al: The relationship of untreated borderline infiltrates by the Banff criteria to acute rejection in renal allograft biopsies. J Am Soc Nephrol. 10(8):1806-14, 1999
11. Racusen LC et al: The Banff 97 working classification of renal allograft pathology. Kidney Int. 55(2):713-23, 1999
12. Nickeleit V et al: The prognostic significance of specific arterial lesions in acute renal allograft rejection. J Am Soc Nephrol. 9(7):1301-8, 1998

Acute Cellular Rejection, Type I (Tubulointerstitial)

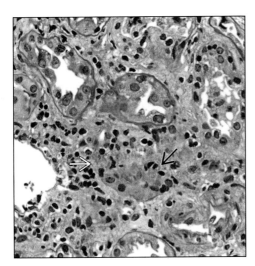 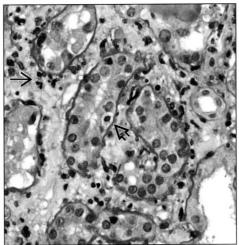

(Left) Interstitial mononuclear cell infiltrate and tubulitis ➡️, a tubulointerstitial lesion of ACR, are shown. Part of the tubular basement membrane is disrupted ➡️. *(Right)* Mild tubulitis (t1 lesion) in ACR type IA is shown. A mononuclear inflammatory cell ➡️ can be recognized by its dark nucleus and surrounding halo. Interstitial inflammation is also present ➡️.

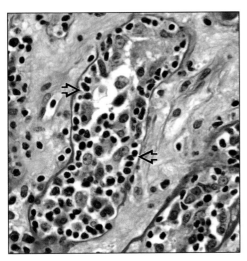 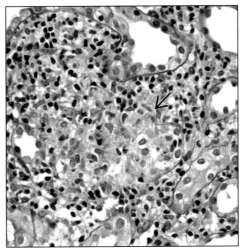

(Left) Severe tubulitis (t3 lesion) in a case of ACR type IB shows numerous mononuclear cells ➡️ within the tubule. The tubular epithelium is displaced from the tubular basement membrane. This is not uncommonly seen in grafts after withdrawal of immunosuppressive drugs. *(Right)* In tubulitis, tubular basement membrane rupture ➡️ is associated with a poorer outcome. A granulomatous response to rupture may develop and should not be confused with an infection.

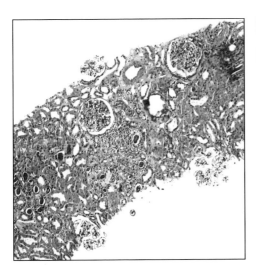 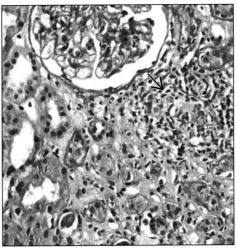

(Left) Findings are borderline/suspicious for ACR. Note patchy interstitial inflammation in ≤ 25% of the cortex, with associated tubulitis. This is a 4-month transplant protocol biopsy in a patient on a steroid-free immunosuppressive protocol and with normal renal function. *(Right)* Focally severe tubulitis ➡️ in tubules that are nonatrophic or no more than mildly atrophic are borderline/suspicious for ACR.

Acute Cellular Rejection, Type II (Endarteritis)

(Left) *Endarteritis in a small artery can be seen at low power. Subendothelial mononuclear cells are focally under the endothelium ➡. Multiple levels need to be examined to detect this lesion, which is focal and on average affects only ~ 25% of arterial cross sections.* **(Right)** *Endothelialitis: A few mononuclear cells ⇒ are present beneath the arterial endothelium.*

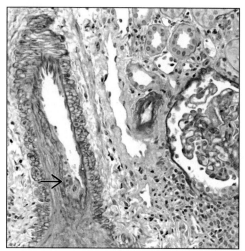
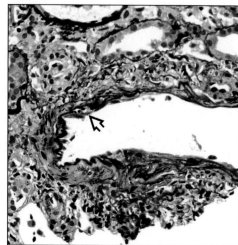

(Left) *Occasionally, mononuclear cells ➡ are adherent to or marginated along the surface of the endothelium. If this finding occurs alone, it is a clue to look carefully for endothelialitis, and perhaps look at deeper tissue levels.* **(Right)** *Endothelialitis lesion with several foamy cells ⇒ is shown. This is a more chronic lesion, usually not seen in early rejection, and may be associated with hyperlipidemia.*

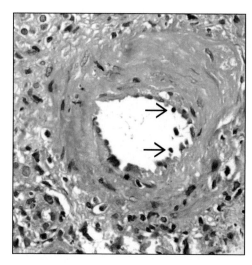
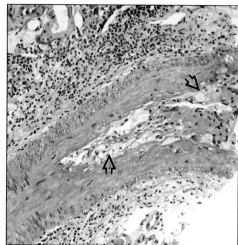

(Left) *Endothelialitis ⇒ along with inflammation in a thickened arterial intima ⇒ due to donor arteriosclerosis is shown. This may be confused with chronic transplant arteriopathy.* **(Right)** *A stain for CD3 reveals CD3(+) T cells in endothelialitis ➡. The majority of the T cells in these lesions are CD8(+).*

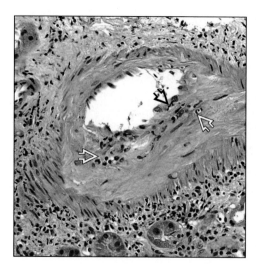
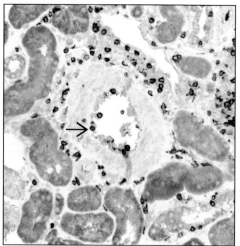

Acute Cellular Rejection, Type III

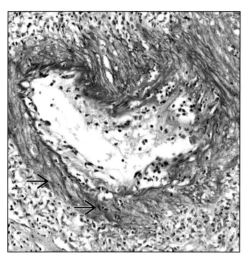
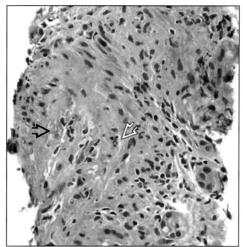

(Left) Type III acute cellular rejection with transmural inflammation of an arcuate-sized artery is shown. Inflammatory cells can be seen in the media as round dark nuclei ➡. *(Right)* ACR type III with transmural inflammation ➡ is seen on this biopsy. Fibrin was also present within the arterial lumen ➡ (not fibrinoid necrosis of the artery in this case). A C4d stain was negative. This graft was lost due to rejection after several months.

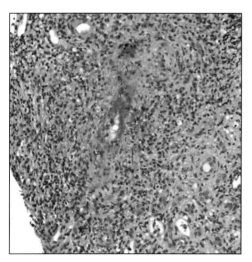
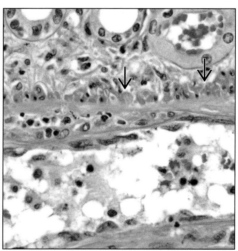

(Left) Fibrinoid necrosis is seen in a small artery in an allograft 10 years post transplant. Immunosuppression was reduced 4 months previously due to T-cell PTLD. While fibrinoid necrosis is more commonly associated with humoral rejection, this biopsy was C4d(-). *(Right)* Early necrosis or apoptosis of the smooth muscle of the media of a small artery ➡ is shown. Other arteries in this sample had typical type III arterial lesions.

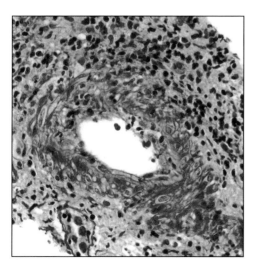
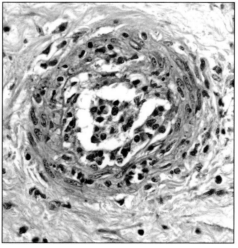

(Left) This shows transmural inflammation in a small artery in an allograft 10 years post transplant. Immunosuppression was reduced 4 months previously due to T-cell PTLD. C4d was negative. *(Right)* Transmural inflammation in an artery in the pelvic fat from a patient who developed graft dysfunction 12 hours post transplant and lost the graft. There was no evidence of antibody-mediated rejection (C4d negative and cross match negative). Similar arterial lesions were in the cortex.

ACUTE CELLULAR REJECTION

Variant Microscopic Features

(Left) Resolving/ongoing ACR is seen on biopsy 1 month following an episode of ACR. The follow-up biopsy shows continued interstitial inflammation, here in areas of fibrosis. Up to 50% of biopsies taken within 1-2 months after ACR show continued inflammation. (Right) Continued interstitial inflammation within areas of fibrosis ⊡ is shown. Those grafts that show continued inflammation after an ACR episode have a worse prognosis. A stain for BK polyomavirus was negative in this case.

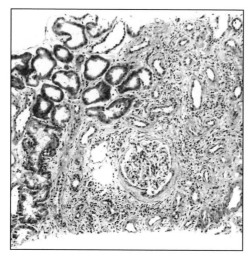
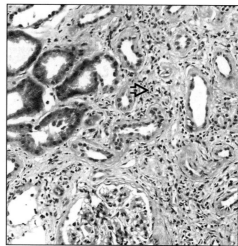

(Left) Resolving ACR type II shows a few inflammatory cells within a "loose" intima ⊡, likely representing early transplant arteriopathy. A biopsy from this patient 2 months earlier showed endothelialitis. (Right) A case of ACR with AHR shows diffuse interstitial inflammation with tubulitis, diagnostic of ACR. Immunofluorescence staining (inset) reveals diffuse, bright PTC staining for C4d, indicative of humoral rejection. The patient had anti-HLA class II donor-specific antibody.

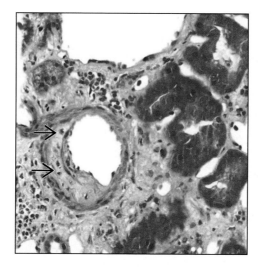
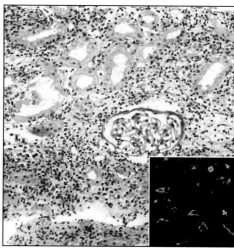

(Left) Plasma-cell-rich ACR and AHR show numerous plasma cells ⊡ and interstitial edema in this variant of acute rejection. Most cases of plasma cell-rich acute rejection are C4d positive. A BK polyomavirus stain in this case was negative. (Right) An immunohistochemical stain for CD3 shows numerous infiltrating T cells, typical of ACR. A C4d stain was also positive, indicative of humoral rejection.

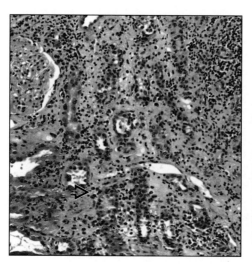
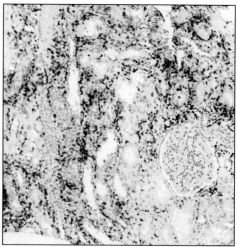

Variants and Electron Microscopy

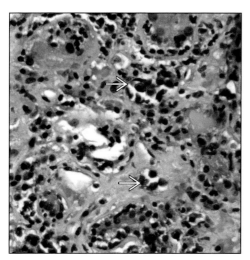
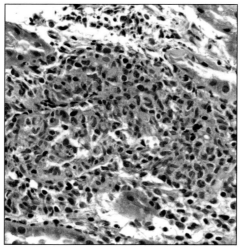

(Left) ACR, type I, is rich in plasma cells. The plasma cells are prominent in interstitium and the peritubular capillaries ➡. This biopsy was taken 2 years after transplant. The C4d stain was negative at this time but became positive 2 years later with development of transplant glomerulopathy. *(Right)* ACR, type II, has a prominent granulomatous response to a ruptured tubule. This may be confused with an infectious process, particularly adenovirus infection.

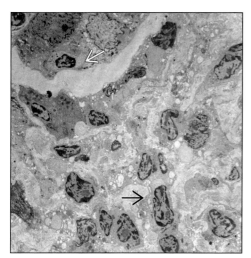
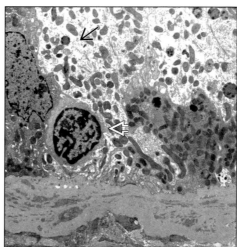

(Left) Interstitial inflammatory cells ➡ are seen by electron microscopy. A lymphocyte is also seen within a tubule ➡. *(Right)* Tubulitis with an infiltrating mononuclear cell ➡ is seen by electron microscopy. The loss of cytoplasmic density indicates injury of the adjacent tubular epithelium ➡.

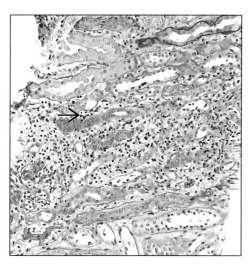
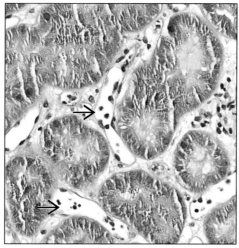

(Left) In the differential diagnosis of ACR is subclinical peritubular capillaritis in patients with donor-specific antibody. From low magnification, the infiltrate appears to be interstitial, but inflammatory cells are within the peritubular capillaries ➡, or are within areas of fibrotic interstitium. *(Right)* On higher magnification, the inflammatory cells are within peritubular capillaries ➡. No tubulitis is present.

ACUTE CELLULAR REJECTION

Glomerular Lesions

(Left) Mild glomerulitis is not uncommon in acute cellular rejection. The cells are primarily T cells rather than monocytes. *(Right)* Acute cellular rejection can affect glomeruli, as shown in this capillary loop with pronounced endothelial reaction and loss of fenestrae ➡. Podocytes also show segmental foot process effacement ➡, which rarely can be extreme, resembling minimal change disease.

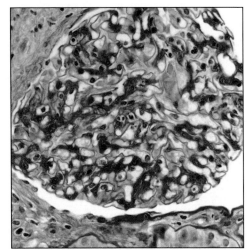
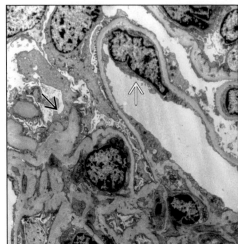

(Left) PAS shows acute allograft glomerulopathy in a patient with Cytomegalovirus (CMV) pneumonia. Type II ACR was also present; C4d was negative. This lesion is associated with type II rejection and variably with CMV. It is believed to be a form of rejection, as CMV is not detected in the glomeruli. *(Right)* Marked accumulation of mononuclear cells ➡ is evident in this glomerulus from a biopsy with ACR. When severe, glomerulitis is associated with type II rejection and graft loss.

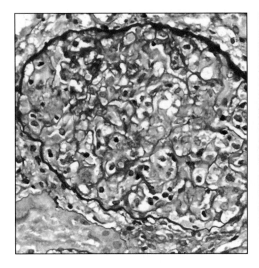
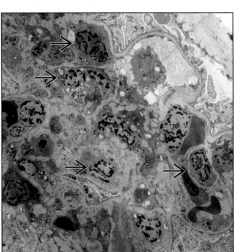

(Left) This glomerular capillary is filled with mononuclear cells ➡ and the endothelium is reactive. Podocytes show little change. *(Right)* Glomerulitis associated with ACR typically has predominately T cells in the capillaries, as seen on this immunohistochemical stain for CD3. Monocytes predominate in humoral rejection.

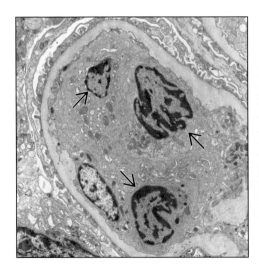
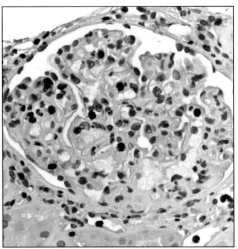

Differential Diagnosis: Interstitial Infiltrates

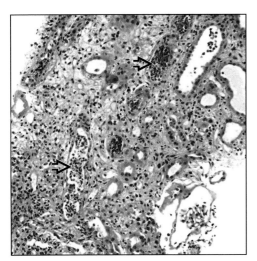

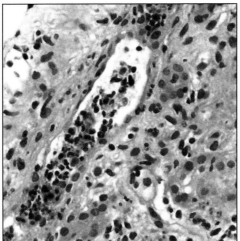

(Left) H&E shows acute pyelonephritis. Tubulointerstitial inflammation is present in this transplant biopsy, similar to ACR. The presence of neutrophilic casts ⧐ is a clue to the diagnosis of acute pyelonephritis. This patient had a positive urine culture, and bacteria were seen on urine microscopy. (Right) A neutrophilic cast is seen in acute pyelonephritis in an allograft.

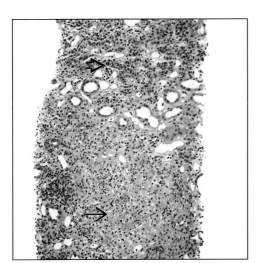

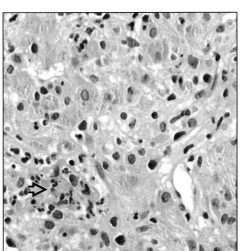

(Left) Malakoplakia is seen in a transplant biopsy, where there is a diffuse infiltrate of large macrophages ➔, along with lymphocytes and plasma cells ⧐. (Right) In this transplant biopsy with malakoplakia there is a diffuse infiltrate of large eosinophilic macrophages. Neutrophils ⧐ are present as well, raising the possibility of a bacterial infection. A follow-up biopsy 3 months later, after antibiotic therapy, showed resolution.

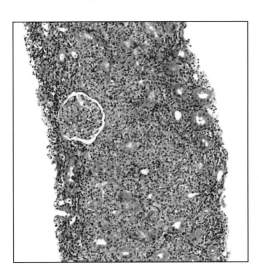

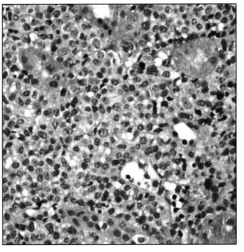

(Left) PTLD is in the differential diagnosis of ACR. This biopsy shows a dense lymphoid infiltrate. (Right) The infiltrating cells of PTLD are atypical, including some large cells. Immunostaining revealed atypical CD20(+) B cells; the patient had a post-transplant marginal zone lymphoma. This case also showed tubulitis with CD3(+) T cells, and so a component of ACR may have been present. PTLD treatment usually includes decreased immunosuppression.

Differential Diagnosis: Polyomavirus

(Left) In BK polyomavirus infection, the presence of plasma cells in the infiltrate, including plasma cell tubulitis ➡, raises the possibility of BK infection. In situ hybridization or immunohistochemistry studies confirm BK infection. *(Right)* In another case of BK polyomavirus infection, viral inclusions can be seen within tubular epithelial cell nuclei ➡.

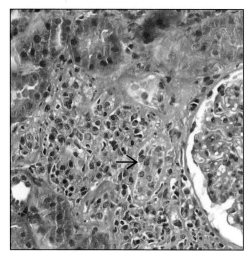
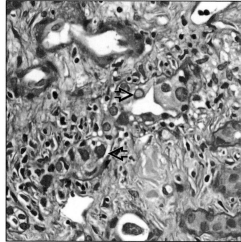

(Left) In ACR and BK polyomavirus infection, interstitial inflammatory cell infiltrate can be seen within the cortex. *(Right)* On higher magnification of ACR and BK polyomavirus infection, mononuclear cell tubulitis is apparent ➡. No viral inclusions are identified in this area. Of note, this patient had low-level BK viremia.

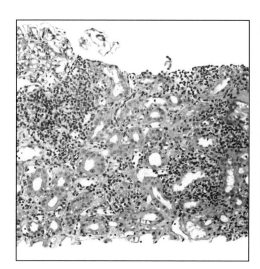
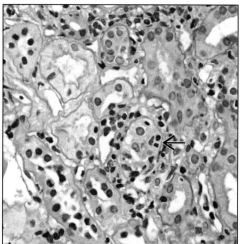

(Left) In ACR and BK polyomavirus infection, a focal plasma cell infiltrate is present in the medulla ➡. *(Right)* In situ hybridization reveals BK-positive cells ➡ in focal tubules within the medulla, remote from an area of ACR in the cortex. ACR type I with concurrent BK infection may be difficult to diagnose, but the presence of the physically remote BK virus from the area of BK-negative tubulointerstitial inflammation is a helpful feature.

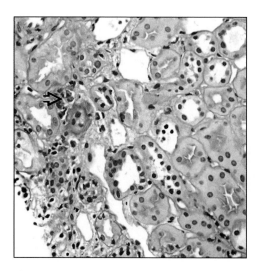
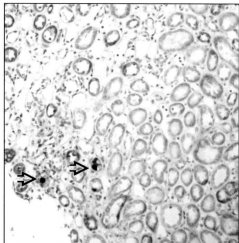

Differential Diagnosis: Arterial Lesions

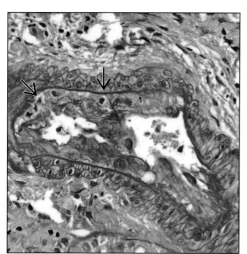

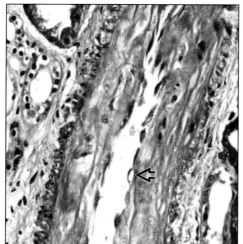

(Left) Periodic acid-Schiff shows thrombotic microangiopathy in a native kidney due to factor H deficiency. The intimal inflammation ➡ resembles endarteritis due to rejection. Endothelial cells are markedly reactive. (Right) In acute transient arteriopathy, endothelial cells are enlarged and show areas of vacuolization ⮧ without endothelialitis. The biopsy also showed acute tubular injury. The patient was 1 week post deceased donor transplant and had delayed graft function.

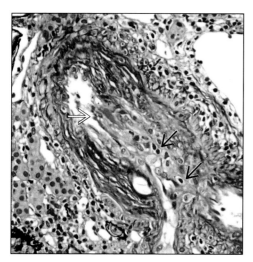

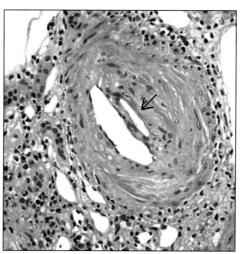

(Left) Endothelialitis ➡ and intimal fibrin ➡ are associated with atheromatous embolism; these features may be confused for endothelialitis of acute cellular rejection. (Right) Other tissue levels on this case of atheromatous embolism revealed cholesterol clefts ➡, confirming a diagnosis of atheromatous embolism rather than acute cellular rejection, type II.

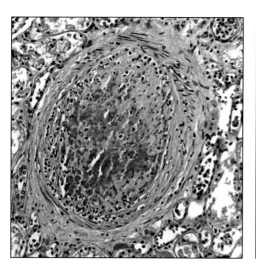

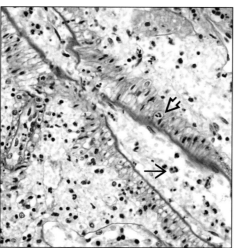

(Left) Arterial inflammation resembles endarteritis in a renal transplant with acute renal vein thrombosis. (Right) An artery from a graft lost to major vascular thrombosis shows neutrophils in the lumen ➡ and along the endothelium, as well as within the vessel wall ⮧, and is not diagnostic of rejection. This lesion seen in areas of necrosis is in the differential diagnosis of transmural arteritis (v3 lesion).

CHRONIC CELLULAR REJECTION

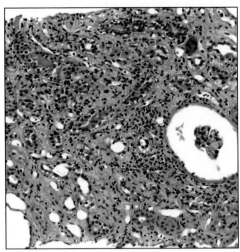

A late graft biopsy with chronic cellular rejection shows a diffuse infiltrate of mononuclear cells in areas with interstitial fibrosis, a combination that has a poor prognosis.

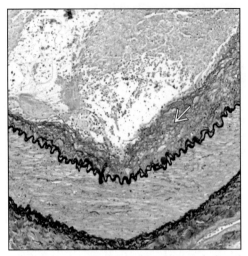

Arteries with chronic cellular rejection have a thickened intima with fibrosis and a sparse infiltrate ➡. In contrast to intimal fibrosis due to hypertension, duplication of the elastica is not prominent.

TERMINOLOGY

Abbreviations
- Chronic cellular rejection (CCR)

Synonyms
- Chronic T-cell-mediated rejection
- Chronic active T-cell-mediated rejection

Definitions
- Persistent or recurrent T-cell-mediated rejection leading to chronic changes in allograft
  - e.g., transplant arteriopathy, interstitial fibrosis, and tubular atrophy

ETIOLOGY/PATHOGENESIS

T-cell-mediated Injury to Arteries, Tubules, and Vasculature
- Alloresponse to HLA antigens
- Other antigens, including autoantigens, may be relevant
- Other cells participate
  - Macrophages, mast cells

Stimulation of Fibrosis
- Epithelial and endothelial mesenchymal transition postulated but not proved in humans

CLINICAL ISSUES

Presentation
- Chronic renal failure
- Hypertension
- Proteinuria
- May be asymptomatic
  - Subclinical rejection

Prognosis
- Interstitial fibrosis with inflammation shortens graft survival more than either alone
- Presence of chronic transplant arteriopathy also shortens graft survival

MICROSCOPIC PATHOLOGY

Histologic Features
- Glomeruli
  - Global glomerulosclerosis
  - Focal, segmental glomerulosclerosis
- Interstitium
  - Mononuclear infiltrate meeting criteria of acute cellular rejection
  - Interstitial fibrosis
  - Inflammation in areas of fibrosis
    - Not counted in standard Banff i score
  - Plasma cells often prominent
- Tubules
  - Tubulitis in nonatrophic tubules
  - Tubulitis also in atrophic tubules
    - Not counted in Banff t score
- Arteries
  - Intimal fibrosis
    - Lacks duplication of elastica in intima, typical of hypertension
  - Mononuclear cells in intima
    - Typically most concentrated under intima
    - Also present in media and adventitia
  - Foam cells in intima
    - Typically lined up against internal elastica

ANCILLARY TESTS

Immunofluorescence
- No significant immunofluorescence findings

CHRONIC CELLULAR REJECTION

Key Facts

Clinical Issues
- Presents as chronic renal failure, often with proteinuria and hypertension
- May be asymptomatic

Microscopic Pathology
- Mononuclear infiltrate and tubulitis
- Inflammation in areas of fibrosis
- Intimal fibrosis and mononuclear cells in arteries

Ancillary Tests
- Negative stain for C4d in PTCs

Top Differential Diagnoses
- Chronic antibody-mediated rejection
- Chronic calcineurin inhibitor toxicity

Diagnostic Checklist
- Inflammation in areas of fibrosis correlates with progressive graft injury

---

o Negative stain for C4d in peritubular capillaries (PTCs)

DIFFERENTIAL DIAGNOSIS

Chronic Antibody-mediated Rejection
- C4d positive in PTCs
  o Some cases may be C4d negative; correlate with presence of circulating donor-specific antibody and history of humoral (C4d[+]) rejection
- Transplant glomerulopathy often present
- Multilamination of basement membrane of PTCs typical

Chronic Calcineurin Inhibitor Toxicity
- Severe arteriolar hyalinosis
  o Peripheral nodular hyalinosis
- "Striped" fibrosis pattern generally not discriminatory

Late Stage of BK Polyoma Virus Nephropathy
- Prior biopsies showing polyoma virus infection give best clue

Hypertensive Arteriosclerosis
- Abundant duplication of elastica in intima
- Minimal or no mononuclear infiltrate

DIAGNOSTIC CHECKLIST

Pathologic Interpretation Pearls
- Chronic cellular and humoral rejection may coexist

- Tubulitis in atrophic tubules is not specific but may be responsible for tubular damage
- Inflammation in areas of fibrosis is not counted in standard Banff i score, but it correlates with progressive graft injury and is therefore likely to be relevant
  o Proposed Banff "total inflammation (ti)" score to account for inflammation in areas of fibrosis
- Late stages of diseases often lose their specific diagnostic features

SELECTED REFERENCES

1. Sis B et al: Banff '09 meeting report: antibody mediated graft deterioration and implementation of Banff working groups. Am J Transplant. 10(3):464-71, 2010
2. Cornell LD et al: Kidney transplantation: mechanisms of rejection and acceptance. Annu Rev Pathol. 3:189-220, 2008
3. Solez K et al: Banff '05 Meeting Report: differential diagnosis of chronic allograft injury and elimination of chronic allograft nephropathy ('CAN'). Am J Transplant. 7(3):518-26, 2007
4. Colvin RB et al: Renal transplant pathology. In Jennette JC et al: Heptinstall's Pathology of the Kidney. Philadelphia: Lippincott Williams & Wilkins. 1347-1490, 2006
5. Moreso F et al: Subclinical rejection associated with chronic allograft nephropathy in protocol biopsies as a risk factor for late graft loss. Am J Transplant. 6(4):747-52, 2006
6. Shishido S et al: The impact of repeated subclinical acute rejection on the progression of chronic allograft nephropathy. J Am Soc Nephrol. 14(4):1046-52, 2003

IMAGE GALLERY

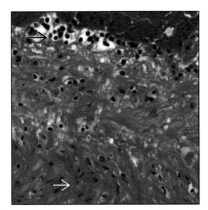 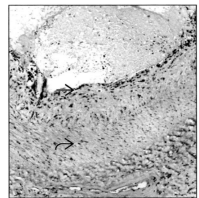 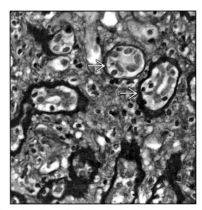

(Left) High-power view of an artery with transplant arteriopathy demonstrates mononuclear cells under the endothelium ➡. The internal elastic is seen ➡. *(Center)* CD3 stain reveals an infiltrate of T cells in an artery. T cells typically accumulate under the endothelium ➡ but are also found throughout the intima and media ➡. *(Right)* Tubulitis in atrophic tubules ➡ in allografts with late dysfunction is often associated with tubulitis in nonatrophic tubules.

HYPERACUTE REJECTION

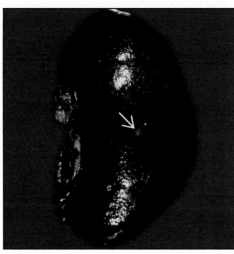

Nephrectomy of a transplanted kidney with hyperacute rejection is shown. The kidney is swollen, hemorrhagic, dusky, and has pale focal areas of necrosis ➡.

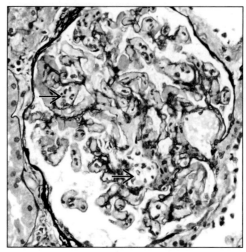

Numerous neutrophils ➡ are seen within glomerular capillaries on this biopsy taken several hours after implantation. This patient had preformed donor-specific HLA antibodies.

TERMINOLOGY

Definitions
- Rejection immediately (minutes to hours) upon implantation and perfusion of graft

ETIOLOGY/PATHOGENESIS

Antibody Mediated (Usual)
- Preexisting antibodies to donor endothelium at time of implantation
  - May be due to anti-donor ABO blood group or HLA antibody (class I or class II)
    - Rare cases of non-HLA or non-blood group antibody-mediated hyperacute rejection
  - Anti-donor antibody titers high enough to cause immediate rejection
    - Lower levels may have delayed onset as acute humoral rejection (days)
- Complement activation by antibody, endothelial activation, platelet activation

T-cell Mediated (Rare)
- Primed cytotoxic T cells

CLINICAL ISSUES

Epidemiology
- Incidence
  - < 0.5% of transplants
  - Decreased incidence due to improved pretransplant testing for antibody against donor

Presentation
- Anuria
- Graft primary nonfunction
  - Or within hours after graft implantation
- Fever
- Lack of graft perfusion by imaging studies

Treatment
- No effective treatment currently
- Preventive therapy in ABO-incompatible or positive crossmatch transplants
  - Plasmapheresis to remove donor-specific antibody
  - Intravenous immunoglobulin (IVIG)
  - Rituximab (anti-CD20)
  - Splenectomy
  - Anti-complement drug (experimental)

Prognosis
- Usually results in rapid graft loss

MACROSCOPIC FEATURES

Gross Pathology
- Cyanosis of graft minutes to hours after perfusion, then becomes swollen, hemorrhagic with focal necrosis over 12-24 hours

MICROSCOPIC PATHOLOGY

Histologic Features
- Early (1-12 hours)
  - Platelet and neutrophil margination in glomerular or peritubular capillaries
  - Congested glomerular and peritubular capillaries with compacted red blood cells
  - Scattered thrombi in glomeruli and arterioles
- Later (12-24 hours)
  - Interstitial edema and hemorrhage
  - Widespread thrombi in glomeruli and arteries
  - Fibrinoid necrosis of arteries
    - Larger arteries may be spared (e.g., HLA-DR antibodies)
  - Cortical and medullary necrosis
- Histologic features resemble severe acute humoral rejection

HYPERACUTE REJECTION

Key Facts

Terminology
- Rejection immediately upon implantation and perfusion of graft

Etiology/Pathogenesis
- Preexisting donor reactive HLA or blood group antibodies at time of implantation

Clinical Issues
- Graft primary nonfunction
- Rare; < 0.5% of transplants
- Decreased incidence due to improved pre-transplant testing for antibody
- Becomes apparent hours to few days after graft implantation
- No effective treatment currently

Macroscopic Features
- Cyanosis of graft minutes to hours after perfusion; then becomes swollen, hemorrhagic, and necrotic

Microscopic Pathology
- Resemble severe acute humoral rejection
- Platelet and neutrophil margination in capillaries
- Thrombi in glomeruli and arterioles
- Interstitial edema and hemorrhage
- Cortical necrosis in 12-24 hours
- Usually C4d positive peritubular capillaries
  - May be negative

Top Differential Diagnoses
- Major vascular thrombosis (renal artery &/or vein)
- Perfusion nephropathy
- Donor thrombotic microangiopathy

ANCILLARY TESTS

Immunohistochemistry
- PTC and glomeruli
  - C4d and CD61 (platelets)

Immunofluorescence
- Most cases show C4d positive peritubular capillaries
  - Negative or granular luminal PTC C4d staining does not exclude diagnosis of hyperacute rejection
    - Technical staining difficulties due to poor perfusion early and lack of viable tissue late
    - Possible C4d negative antibody-mediated hyperacute rejection
    - Possible T-cell-mediated hyperacute rejection
- IgG, IgM, &/or C3 may be present in capillaries
  - IgM most common in ABO-incompatible grafts
- Fibrin staining of thrombi

Electron Microscopy
- Glomeruli
  - Swollen, enlarged endothelial cells
  - Subendothelial lucency
  - Loss of endothelium
    - Bare basement membranes in glomeruli
  - Fibrin tactoids, platelet aggregates, neutrophils
- PTC
  - Similar changes to glomerular capillaries

DIFFERENTIAL DIAGNOSIS

Major Vascular Thrombosis (Renal Artery or Vein)
- May be due to technical problems of vascular anastomosis or to hypercoagulable state
- Infarction may be present
- Thrombi due to technical problems are usually limited to larger vessels
- C4d negative in viable tissue

Perfusion Nephropathy
- Extensive loss of endothelium
- Thrombi and congestion within capillaries
- C4d negative

Donor Thrombotic Microangiopathy
- C4d negative

DIAGNOSTIC CHECKLIST

Pathologic Interpretation Pearls
- C4d(+) peritubular capillaries
- Cortical necrosis with widespread thrombosis in glomeruli and arterioles
- Can see TMA pattern early

SELECTED REFERENCES

1. Colvin RB et al: Renal transplant pathology. In Jennette JC et al: Heptinstall's Pathology of the Kidney. Philadelphia: Lippincott Williams & Wilkins. 1347-1490, 2006
2. Racusen LC et al: Antibody-mediated rejection in renal allografts: lessons from pathology. Clin J Am Soc Nephrol. 1(3):415-20, 2006
3. Gaber LW et al: Successful reversal of hyperacute renal allograft rejection with the anti-CD3 monoclonal OKT3. Transplantation. 54(5):930-2, 1992
4. Ahern AT et al: Hyperacute rejection of HLA-AB-identical renal allografts associated with B lymphocyte and endothelial reactive antibodies. Transplantation. 33(1):103-6, 1982
5. Kirkman RL et al: Transplantation in miniature swine. VII. Evidence for cellular immune mechanisms in hyperacute rejection of renal allografts. Transplantation. 28(1):24-30, 1979
6. Spector D et al: Perfusion nephropathy in human transplants. N Engl J Med. 295(22):1217-21, 1976
7. Kissmeyer-Nielsen F et al: Hyperacute rejection of kidney allografts, associated with pre-existing humoral antibodies against donor cells. Lancet. 2(7465):662-5, 1966

Hyperacute Rejection, Early Changes

(Left) H&E shows neutrophils within peritubular capillaries (PTC) in hyperacute rejection ➔. This biopsy was taken a few hours after implantation. The PTC are markedly congested. **(Right)** H&E shows higher magnification of glomerular thrombi ➔ in hyperacute rejection. The differential is between a thrombotic microangiopathy, possibly donor disease, or a consequence of preservation. C4d stains are helpful in the differential diagnosis, as well as testing for anti-donor antibodies.

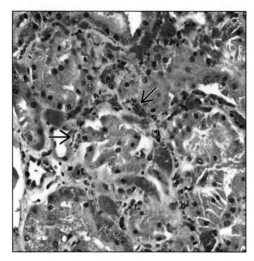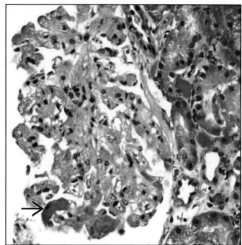

(Left) Hyperacute rejection, post-perfusion biopsy, shows a 3rd kidney in a patient who received a 6-antigen deceased donor match and was crossmatch negative. Neutrophils are prominent in glomeruli ➔. **(Right)** Shown here are neutrophils ➔ within glomerular capillaries within a few hours post implantation in hyperacute rejection. Capillaries are congested and some have lost endothelial nuclei ➔. These are the first histological signs of hyperacute rejection.

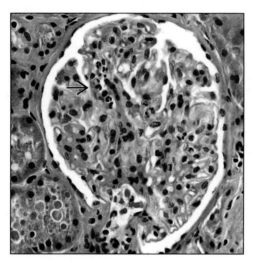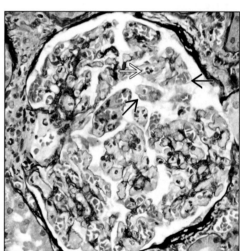

(Left) Post-perfusion biopsy (hours) in a patient shows patchy C4d staining in peritubular capillaries ➔. Several capillaries are negative ➔. Immunofluorescence on frozen tissue was nondiagnostic. **(Right)** Post-perfusion biopsy in a patient shows prominent CD61 staining in peritubular capillaries, indicating the presence of platelets ➔. CD61 detects the platelet receptor for fibrinogen (IIb/IIIa) and may be a useful test to detect hyperacute rejection.

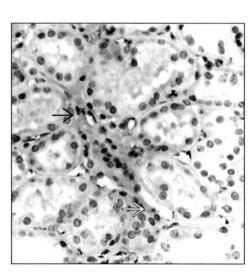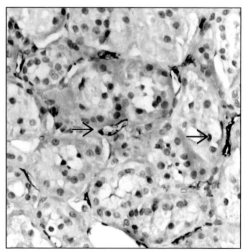

Hyperacute Rejection, Later Changes

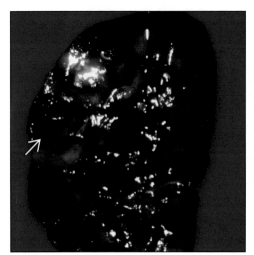
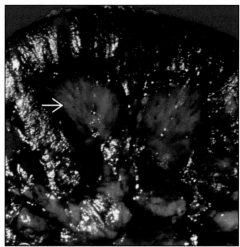

(Left) Nephrectomy specimen with hyperacute rejection shows edema, as indicated by the glistening cut surface, and hemorrhage. The dark zones at the corticomedullary junction are due to marked congestion ➡. The medullary areas are pale due to ischemia. (Right) Gross photo shows nephrectomy specimen from an allograft with hyperacute rejection. The medullary pyramids are pale and necrotic ➡, surrounded by congestion at the corticomedullary junction.

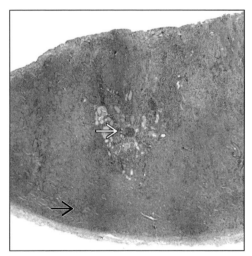
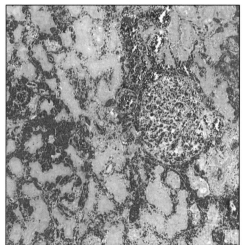

(Left) H&E shows low-magnification view of a renal allograft with hyperacute rejection. Cortical necrosis and hemorrhage are widespread ➡. C4d stain was negative in the necrotic areas, comprising 95% of the sample. Nonnecrotic areas were selected from the paraffin-embedded material for C4d staining ➡. (Right) This nephrectomy specimen from a patient with hyperacute rejection, 3 days post transplant, shows congestion and necrosis involving all elements of the kidney.

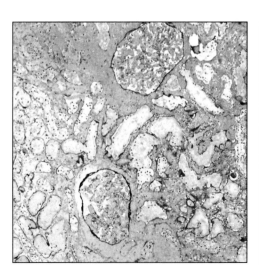
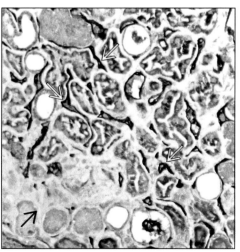

(Left) This nephrectomy specimen was removed from a patient with hyperacute rejection, 3 days post transplant. Low power shows diffuse cortical necrosis. (Right) Shown is an immunoperoxidase stain for C4d in a wedge biopsy from a patient with hyperacute rejection. C4d(+) PTC are seen focally ➡. Necrotic areas are C4d(-) ➡. C4d can be negative in early biopsies of hyperacute rejection, probably due to poor perfusion.

ACUTE HUMORAL REJECTION

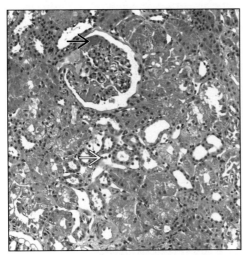

Glomerular intracapillary thrombi are present in this ABO blood group-incompatible allograft ➔. Dilated peritubular capillaries containing marginated mononuclear cells and neutrophils are also seen ➔.

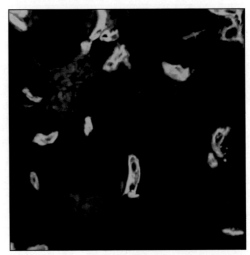

Diffuse, bright staining of peritubular capillaries for C4d by immunofluorescence is shown. A positive C4d stain is defined as linear and diffuse PTC staining, usually taken as > 50%.

TERMINOLOGY

Abbreviations
- Acute humoral rejection (AHR)

Synonyms
- Acute antibody-mediated rejection (acute AMR)

ETIOLOGY/PATHOGENESIS

Donor-specific Antibody (DSA)
- DSA usually directed against HLA class I or II on endothelium
  - ABO blood group antigen in ABO-incompatible grafts
  - Other, unknown, non-MHC antigens on endothelium
- DSA activates complement via classical pathway
  - C4d is an inactive fragment of C4b of classical complement pathway
  - C4d is covalently bound at site of complement activation on endothelium
  - Complement-fixing DSA associated with greater acute graft injury

CLINICAL ISSUES

Epidemiology
- Incidence
  - ~ 25% of acute rejection episodes are due to antibody

Presentation
- Acute renal failure
- Oliguria

Laboratory Tests
- Circulating donor-specific anti-HLA class I or II antibody in 88-95% of AHR with C4d deposition

- Minority (5-10%) have undetectable DSA
  - May be due to non-HLA antibody
  - Possible antibody absorption by graft

Treatment
- Plasmapheresis
- Increased immunosuppression
- Intravenous immunoglobulin (IVIG)
- Rituximab (anti-CD20, B cell)
- Anti-plasma cell therapy (experimental)
  - Bortezomib, proteosome inhibitor
- Complement inhibition (experimental)
  - Eculizumab, inhibitor of C5 and others

Prognosis
- Worse allograft survival in AHR compared to C4d-negative acute cellular rejection (ACR)
  - ~ 30% graft loss within 1 year, vs. 4% graft loss for ACR
- Increased risk of developing transplant glomerulopathy (CHR)
- Plasma cell-rich variant resistant to treatment; poor clinical outcome

MICROSCOPIC PATHOLOGY

Histologic Features
- Glomeruli
  - Glomerulitis, neutrophils, monocytes, fibrin
  - Glomerular thrombi or mesangiolysis, particularly in ABO blood group-incompatible grafts
- Peritubular capillaries
  - Dilated
  - Neutrophils and mononuclear cells, termed "peritubular capillaritis"
- Arteries
  - Fibrinoid necrosis in minority of cases
- Interstitium
  - Edema, sparse infiltrate
  - Hemorrhage occasionally

ACUTE HUMORAL REJECTION

Key Facts

Etiology/Pathogenesis
- DSA usually directed against HLA class I or II on endothelium; may be against ABO blood group antigen in ABO-incompatible grafts

Clinical Issues
- Acute renal failure
- Oliguria
- Serum donor-specific antibody (DSA)
  - Usually donor specific anti-HLA antibody; AHR may also occur in ABO blood group-incompatible allografts
- Worse allograft survival in AHR compared to C4d negative ACR
- Increased risk of developing transplant glomerulopathy (CHR) after AHR

Microscopic Pathology
- Glomerulitis, neutrophils, monocytes, fibrin
- Glomerular thrombi or mesangiolysis
- Peritubular capillary neutrophils
- Dilated peritubular capillaries
- Diffuse, bright positive staining of peritubular capillaries for C4d

Top Differential Diagnoses
- Acute cellular rejection
- Pyelonephritis
- Acute tubular necrosis
- Accommodation
  - C4d deposition without histologic injury or graft dysfunction

---

- Plasma cell rich variant
  - Associated with edema and high interferon-γ
- Tubules
  - Acute tubular injury
  - Little or no tubulitis
  - Sometimes neutrophils in lumen

Banff Classification of AHR
- Histologic patterns
  - Type I: Acute tubular injury, minimal inflammation
  - Type II: Peritubular capillary &/or glomerular capillary inflammation, &/or thromboses
  - Type III: Arterial fibrinoid necrosis or transmural inflammation (v3 lesion)
- In addition to these histologic patterns, cases should show peritubular capillary (PTC) C4d deposition and serologic evidence of DSA; if only 1 of these 2 criteria is present with histologic changes, then biopsy is "suspicious" for AHR

ANCILLARY TESTS

Immunohistochemistry
- Diffuse PTC staining by immunohistochemistry (IHC)
  - IHC less sensitive than immunofluorescence (IF)

Immunofluorescence
- Diffuse, bright positive staining of peritubular capillaries for C4d by IF
  - Small minority of probable AHR cases are C4d negative
  - Focal C4d (10-50%) less commonly has detectable DSA
  - C4d staining remains positive ~ 5-7 days after removal of antibody from circulation

Electron Microscopy
- Peritubular and glomerular capillary endothelial changes
  - Cell enlargement, loss of fenestrations, microvillous changes, detachment from the basement membrane, lysis, apoptosis

DIFFERENTIAL DIAGNOSIS

Chronic Humoral Rejection
- Chronic rejection features: Transplant glomerulopathy, peritubular capillaropathy, transplant arteriopathy
- Usually a stable or slowly declining clinical course
- Mononuclear cells in capillaries vs. neutrophils

Acute Cellular Rejection
- 20-30% of ACR cases are C4d positive, indicative of concurrent antibody-mediated rejection

Accommodation
- C4d deposition without histologic evidence of graft injury and without graft dysfunction
- Commonly seen in ABO blood group-incompatible grafts

Acute Pyelonephritis
- Neutrophils and neutrophilic tubulitis may be seen in AHR or in pyelonephritis
- Neutrophilic casts on biopsy and positive urine culture for bacterial infection favor pyelonephritis
- C4d negative

Acute Tubular Necrosis/Injury
- C4d negative

SELECTED REFERENCES

1. Lipták P et al: Peritubular capillary damage in acute humoral rejection: an ultrastructural study on human renal allografts. Am J Transplant. 5(12):2870-6, 2005
2. Desvaux D et al: Acute renal allograft rejections with major interstitial oedema and plasma cell-rich infiltrates: high gamma-interferon expression and poor clinical outcome. Nephrol Dial Transplant. 19(4):933-9, 2004
3. Racusen LC et al: Antibody-mediated rejection criteria - an addition to the Banff 97 classification of renal allograft rejection. Am J Transplant. 3(6):708-14, 2003
4. Mauiyyedi S et al: Acute humoral rejection in kidney transplantation: II. Morphology, immunopathology, and pathologic classification. J Am Soc Nephrol. 13(3):779-87, 2002

ACUTE HUMORAL REJECTION

Microscopic Features

(Left) Glomerular intracapillary thrombi ⇨ are present in this case of severe AHR. Glomeruli are commonly affected, with neutrophils and monocytes in capillaries, thrombi, and even segmental necrosis. The differential includes thrombotic microangiopathy. *(Right)* Pure AHR commonly shows accumulation of neutrophils in PTC ⇨ with little mononuclear inflammation. Patient was highly sensitized due to 3 prior transplants. The histological changes of AHR can be subtle.

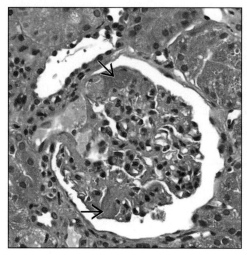
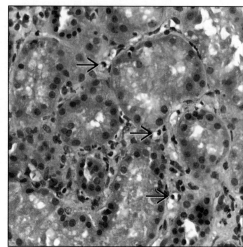

(Left) Immunohistochemical stain for C4d reveals diffusely positive peritubular capillaries ⇨ and glomerular capillaries ⇨. A positive stain must be linear, circumferential, and not in the lumen. Luminal staining is an artifact of fixing plasma C4 in the vessels, not seen in frozen sections. *(Right)* Diffuse, bright staining of peritubular capillaries for C4d by IF is shown. IF using frozen sections is more sensitive and has fewer artifacts than immunohistochemistry.

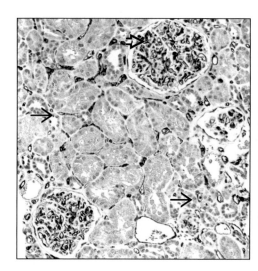
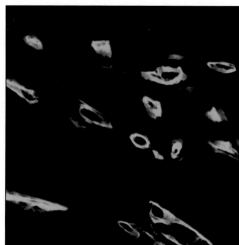

(Left) Numerous neutrophils ⇨ are seen marginated within peritubular capillaries and within the interstitium in this case of AHR 1 week post transplant. Recurrent oxalosis was present as well (note calcium oxalate crystal ⇨), which likely contributed to the patient's renal failure and oliguria. *(Right)* Marginated inflammatory cells are present within peritubular capillaries ⇨. This case also shows acute tubular injury with dilated tubules and flattened epithelium ⇨.

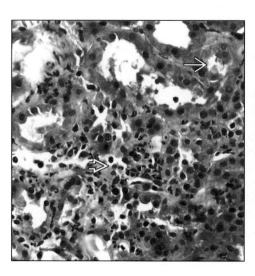
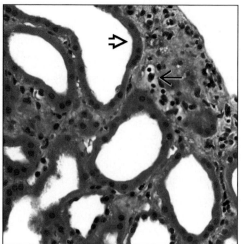

ACUTE HUMORAL REJECTION

Variant Microscopic Features

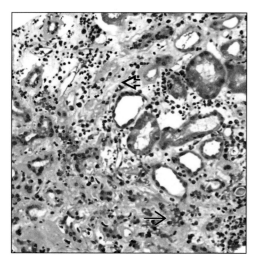

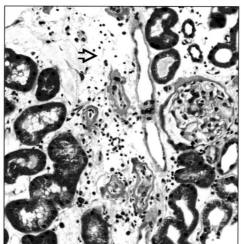

(Left) H&E shows plasma-cell-rich acute humoral rejection, with interstitial hemorrhage ⇒ and marked interstitial edge ⇒. This case was C4d positive by immunofluorescence. **(Right)** Plasma cell-rich acute humoral rejection is shown with marked interstitial edema ⇒. This type of rejection typically arises later after transplantation and has a poor prognosis. Plasma cells are sometimes found in PTCs.

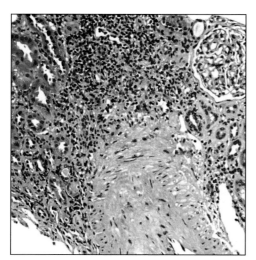

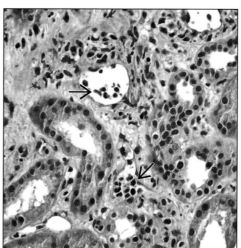

(Left) H&E shows a biopsy with both acute cellular rejection and acute humoral rejection. Interstitial inflammation with tubulitis is present; a C4d stain was positive. Combined AHR and ACR may be seen last post-transplant, particularly in patients who are nonadherent to immunosuppression therapy. **(Right)** H&E shows AHR in an HLA-identical graft. By light microscopy, there is PTC inflammation ⇒ and interstitial edema, and a C4d stain was positive by IF, features typical of AHR.

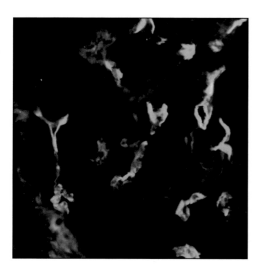

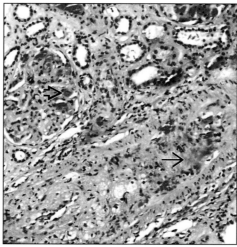

(Left) AHR in an HLA-identical graft shows diffuse, bright staining for C4d by IF. This patient's sibling donor was HLA-identical, even by molecular typing methods. Rare cases of AHR in HLA-identical sibling patients have been reported, with rejection presumably due to non-HLA antigens. **(Right)** AHR in an HLA-identical graft with fibrinoid necrosis of an artery ⇒ and glomerular thrombi ⇒ is shown in a patient with relentless acute humoral rejection.

Resolution of Acute Humoral Rejection

(Left) H&E shows acute humoral rejection that arose 2 weeks post transplant. Congestion of peritubular capillaries that contain scattered neutrophils is evident, as well as loss of open glomerular capillary loops. **(Right)** A C4d stain is positive in a case of acute humoral rejection that arose 2 weeks post transplant. A frozen section at high power shows widespread peritubular capillary deposition of C4d.

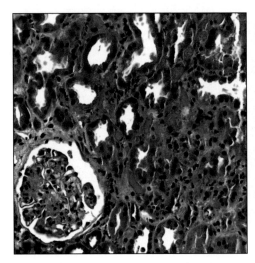
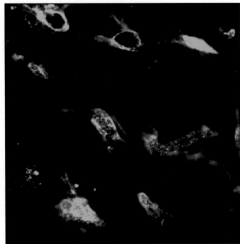

(Left) Acute humoral rejection arising 2 weeks post transplant is depicted. Electron microscopy shows marked endothelial swelling in glomerular capillaries, corresponding to the lack of open capillary loops by light microscopy. **(Right)** This case of acute humoral rejection was treated with plasmapheresis, rituximab, and IVIG. C4d has largely disappeared from peritubular capillaries 7 days after a biopsy showed widespread C4d. If antibodies are removed, C4d deposition resolves over ~1 week.

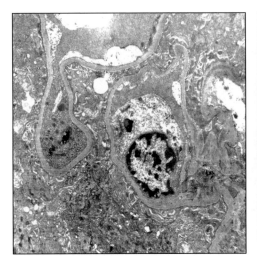
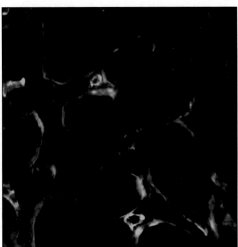

(Left) Follow-up biopsy was performed 90 days post transplant, after an episode of AHR at 2 weeks. The congestion and neutrophils in peritubular capillaries have disappeared since the 14-day biopsy. Glomeruli appear normal. Full recovery can be observed in AHR. **(Right)** Follow-up biopsy occurred 90 days post transplant, after an episode of AHR at 2 weeks. Glomeruli appear normal. The endothelium has recovered from the previous biopsy with AHR. No GBM duplication or subendothelial lucency was observed.

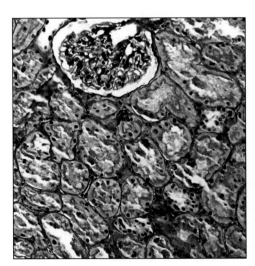
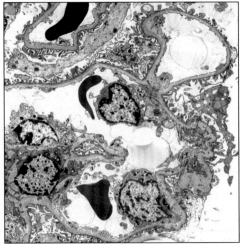

Evolution of Acute to Chronic Humoral Rejection

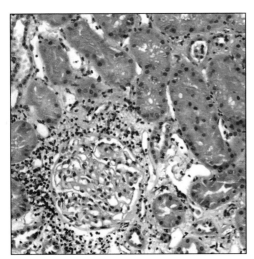

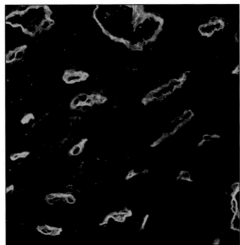

(Left) H&E shows acute humoral and cellular rejection at 6 months after transplantation. Edema, a sparse infiltrate, and intracapillary cells are seen in this patient treated with bolus steroids before biopsy. Patient had high-titer anti-donor HLA class II antibody. (Right) Acute humoral and cellular rejection arising 6 months after transplantation is shown. Widespread intense staining for C4d is in the peritubular capillaries. Patient had a high-titer anti-donor HLA class II antibody.

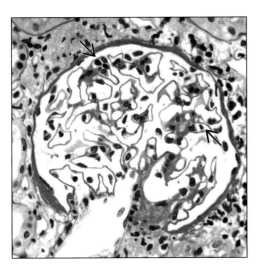

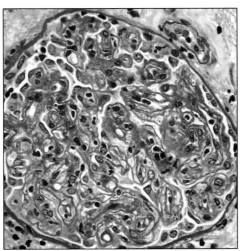

(Left) Acute humoral and cellular rejection arising 6 months after transplantation is shown. The glomeruli are normal, aside from an occasional intracapillary cell ➔. (Right) CHR developed 6 years after an episode of AHR. Glomerular capillaries have numerous mononuclear leukocytes, the GBM is duplicated, and podocytes are reactive. Tacrolimus had been decreased. Anti-donor class II antibodies were present. AHR increases the likelihood of later CHR.

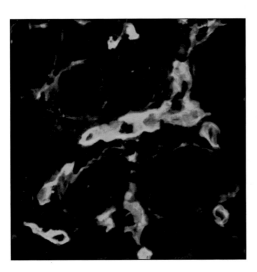

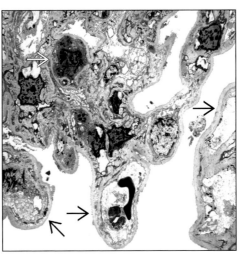

(Left) Chronic humoral rejection developed 6 years later in a patient who had had AHR 6 months after transplantation. C4d is present in peritubular capillaries, less extensive than on the 6-month biopsy. Anti-donor HLA class II antibodies were present. (Right) Transplant glomerulopathy developed 6 years after an episode of AHR. The GBM is duplicated ➔. Neutrophils ➔ are in capillaries. C4d was positive and anti-donor antibodies (class II) were present.

CHRONIC HUMORAL REJECTION

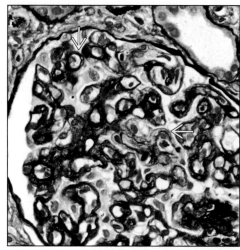

Transplant glomerulopathy, defined by glomerular basement membrane duplication ➡, is a common manifestation of chronic humoral rejection but is not specific for that condition.

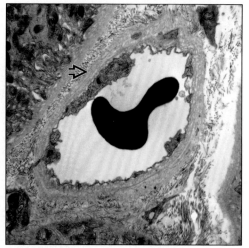

Circumferential peritubular capillary basement membrane multilamination (PTCBMML) ➳ in a case of CHR is shown. This feature, especially when severe (> 6 layers), is highly associated with CHR.

TERMINOLOGY

Abbreviations
- Chronic humoral rejection (CHR)

Synonyms
- Chronic antibody-mediated rejection (chronic AMR)

ETIOLOGY/PATHOGENESIS

Donor-specific Antibody
- Episodic antibody-mediated endothelial injury/activation/repair
- Antibody activates complement by classical pathway
  - C4d deposition in graft is marker of complement activation
- Potential endothelial damage by antibody without complement activation
  - In vitro studies and animal models
- Donor-specific antibody (DSA) against HLA class II most common

Transplant Arteriopathy as Manifestation of CHR
- Mouse model
  - RAG-1 knockout mice with passive transfer of complement-fixing, anti-MHC antibody develop C4d deposition and transplant arteriopathy (TA)
    - Antibody is sufficient for development of TA in absence of functioning B and T cells
    - TA remains after administration of alloantibody and after disappearance of C4d
  - Non-complement-fixing, anti-MHC antibody can also produce TA
    - May explain some cases of C4d(-) CHR

CLINICAL ISSUES

Presentation
- Chronic renal failure
- Proteinuria
- Hypertension

Laboratory Tests
- Serum donor-specific antibody
  - Usually DSA directed against HLA class I or class II
  - May not be detectable in serum at time of biopsy

Treatment
- Drugs
  - No known effective treatments
  - Rituximab (anti-CD20)
  - Intravenous immunoglobulin (IVIG)
  - Bortezomib (proteosome inhibitor) to deplete plasma cells that produce alloantibody

Prognosis
- 50% graft loss rate at 5 years after diagnosis of transplant glomerulopathy (TG)
  - C4d(+) cases have poorer survival
  - Subset of cases with molecular markers of endothelial activation show poorer survival, even if C4d(-)

Diagnostic Criteria for CHR
- Histologic evidence of tissue injury
  - Transplant arteriopathy
  - Transplant glomerulopathy
  - Peritubular capillary basement membrane multilamination
  - Interstitial fibrosis and tubular atrophy
- Immunopathologic evidence for antibody-mediated injury in tissue (usually demonstrated by C4d in peritubular capillaries [PTCs])
- Serologic evidence of DSA

CHRONIC HUMORAL REJECTION

Key Facts

Etiology/Pathogenesis
- Episodic antibody-mediated endothelial injury/activation/repair
- C4d deposition in graft is marker of complement activation
- DSA against HLA class II most common

Clinical Issues
- Chronic renal failure
- No known effective treatments for CHR
- Diagnostic criteria for CHR
  - Histologic evidence of chronic tissue injury
  - Evidence for antibody-mediated injury in tissue
  - Serologic evidence of DSA

Microscopic Pathology
- Transplant glomerulopathy

- Transplant arteriopathy
- Peritubular capillaropathy
- Interstitial fibrosis and tubular atrophy (nonspecific)
- PTC C4d may be diffuse, focal, or negative

Top Differential Diagnoses
- Pattern of transplant glomerulopathy
  - Chronic thrombotic microangiopathy
  - Immune complex glomerulonephritis (recurrent or de novo)
- Pattern of transplant arteriopathy
  - Chronic T-cell-mediated rejection
  - Arteriosclerosis
- Accommodation
  - C4d deposition or circulating DSA in absence of histologic changes and graft dysfunction

---

- If only 2 of these 3 criteria are present, diagnosis is "suspicious" for CHR

MICROSCOPIC PATHOLOGY

Histologic Features
- Transplant glomerulopathy (chronic allograft glomerulopathy)
  - Duplication of glomerular basement membrane (GBM)
  - Absence of evidence of immune complex glomerulonephritis or chronic thrombotic microangiopathy
  - Glomerulitis may be present
    - CD68(+) monocytes (majority)
    - CD3(+) T cells (minority)
- Transplant arteriopathy (chronic allograft arteriopathy)
  - Fibrous intimal thickening of arteries
  - Inflammatory cells present within thickened intima
    - CD3(+) T cells &/or CD68(+) monocytes/macrophages
- Peritubular capillaropathy
  - Best seen as peritubular capillary basement membrane (PTCBMML) by electron microscopy
  - PTC basement membrane duplication or multilamination may be seen by light microscopy
  - Disappearance of PTCs over time
    - Loss of PTCs may be appreciated with stain for endothelial cells (e.g., CD34)
    - PTC loss correlates with increasing serum creatinine
- Peritubular capillaritis
  - Mononuclear cells in PTCs, particularly moderate to severe (Banff ptc score > 1), is often seen in CHR
  - May precede development of TG or other CHR features in presensitized patients with normal graft function
    - Often seen on protocol biopsy of presensitized patients
  - C4d deposition in some cases

- Interstitial fibrosis and tubular atrophy
  - Nonspecific feature; may be seen in CHR
  - Correlates with loss of PTCs
  - If present, C4d deposition may be diagnostic clue of CHR

ANCILLARY TESTS

Immunohistochemistry
- Evidence of C4d deposition in PTCs
- Glomerular C4d may be seen by immunohistochemistry (IHC)
  - Glomerular staining for C4d in paraffin sections suggestive of CHR, but also seen in other causes
    - Immune complex disease
    - Thrombotic microangiopathy

Immunofluorescence
- Evidence of C4d deposition
  - PTC C4d may be diffuse, focal, or negative
  - > 40% of TG cases may not be C4d(+) on biopsy
    - Antibody levels vary with time; may be below threshold for C4d(+) at time of biopsy
    - GBM duplication represents previous active endothelial injury by antibody
    - C4d(-) cases may represent non-complement-fixing DSA
- Immunofluorescence more sensitive and easier to interpret than paraffin-embedded IHC
  - Formalin fixed paraffin embedded tissue may have artifact due to fixation of plasma C4 in lumen of capillaries
  - Glomerular mesangium normally positive for C4d in frozen tissue, not fixed tissue

Electron Microscopy
- EM more sensitive for TG than light microscopy
- Early changes seen by EM before development of TG
  - Hypertrophied endothelium and vacuolization
  - Expanded lamina rara interna
  - Subendothelial serration of GBM with early GBM duplication

CHRONIC HUMORAL REJECTION

- Circumferential PTCBMML
  - Grading: Mild, 2-4 layers; moderate, 5-6; severe, 7 or more
  - Greater sensitivity for CHR with higher PTCBMML grade
- Endothelial gene expression
  - Can detect CHR in absence of C4d when DSA present

DIFFERENTIAL DIAGNOSIS

Transplant Glomerulopathy
- Chronic thrombotic microangiopathy
  - Sometimes associated with calcineurin inhibitor toxicity
- Immune complex glomerulonephritis (recurrent or de novo), chronic or acute
  - Membranoproliferative glomerulonephritis or other
  - Cause of GBM duplication related to immune deposits, not antibody-mediated injury
  - GBM immune deposits seen by immunofluorescence and electron microscopy

Transplant Arteriopathy
- Arteriosclerosis
  - Related to hypertension; may be donor disease
  - Fibroelastic intimal thickening
    - Elastic fibers can be identified on elastic stain
  - Absence of inflammatory cells within thickened intima in arteriosclerosis
  - May coexist with transplant arteriopathy
- Chronic T-cell-mediated rejection
  - Transplant arteriopathy may be result of humoral rejection, T-cell-mediated rejection, or both
  - C4d staining and presence of serum donor-specific antibody may help distinguish humoral and T-cell-mediated rejection
- Atheromatous embolism
  - Uncommon finding in allograft
  - Atheromatous embolism may show inflammatory response and fibrin
  - Cholesterol clefts may be visible on deeper tissue sections
- Thrombotic microangiopathy
  - Arteries may show endothelialitis and intimal thickening

Peritubular Capillaropathy
- Mild or segmental PTC basement membrane multilamination may be seen in various nonspecific causes, e.g., acute tubular injury

Peritubular Capillary Cell Margination
- Acute cellular rejection, type I (ACR)
  - ACR shows tubulointerstitial inflammation, while CHR may show peritubular capillary inflammation
- Acute humoral rejection (AHR)
  - AHR usually shows more neutrophils and less severe PTC margination (lower PTC score)
  - Clinical presentation of acute renal failure
  - AHR may be superimposed on CHR

Accommodation
- C4d deposition or circulating DSA in absence of histologic changes and graft dysfunction
  - Common in ABO incompatible grafts
  - Present in 2-6% of protocol biopsies of HLA incompatible grafts
- Long-term stability unknown

DIAGNOSTIC CHECKLIST

Pathologic Interpretation Pearls
- CHR typically has less extensive C4d PTC deposition than AHR and may be CD4(-)
- Mononuclear cells in PTC indicative of activity

SELECTED REFERENCES

1. Hirohashi T et al: Complement independent antibody-mediated endarteritis and transplant arteriopathy in mice. Am J Transplant. 10(3):510-7, 2010
2. Colvin RB: Pathology of chronic humoral rejection. Contrib Nephrol. 162:75-86, 2009
3. Loupy A et al: Outcome of subclinical antibody-mediated rejection in kidney transplant recipients with preformed donor-specific antibodies. Am J Transplant. 9(11):2561-70, 2009
4. Sis B et al: Endothelial gene expression in kidney transplants with alloantibody indicates antibody-mediated damage despite lack of C4d staining. Am J Transplant. 9(10):2312-23, 2009
5. Cornell LD et al: Kidney transplantation: mechanisms of rejection and acceptance. Annu Rev Pathol. 3:189-220, 2008
6. Issa N et al: Transplant glomerulopathy: risk and prognosis related to anti-human leukocyte antigen class II antibody levels. Transplantation. 86(5):681-5, 2008
7. Gloor JM et al: Transplant glomerulopathy: subclinical incidence and association with alloantibody. Am J Transplant. 7(9):2124-32, 2007
8. Solez K et al: Banff '05 Meeting Report: differential diagnosis of chronic allograft injury and elimination of chronic allograft nephropathy ('CAN'). Am J Transplant. 7(3):518-26, 2007
9. Uehara S et al: Chronic cardiac transplant arteriopathy in mice: relationship of alloantibody, C4d deposition and neointimal fibrosis. Am J Transplant. 7(1):57-65, 2007
10. Wavamunno MD et al: Transplant glomerulopathy: ultrastructural abnormalities occur early in longitudinal analysis of protocol biopsies. Am J Transplant. 7(12):2757-68, 2007
11. Ishii Y et al: Injury and progressive loss of peritubular capillaries in the development of chronic allograft nephropathy. Kidney Int. 67(1):321-32, 2005
12. Racusen LC et al: Antibody-mediated rejection criteria - an addition to the Banff 97 classification of renal allograft rejection. Am J Transplant. 3(6):708-14, 2003
13. Ivanyi B et al: The value of electron microscopy in the diagnosis of chronic renal allograft rejection. Mod Pathol. 14(12):1200-8, 2001
14. Mauiyyedi S et al: Chronic humoral rejection: identification of antibody-mediated chronic renal allograft rejection by C4d deposits in peritubular capillaries. J Am Soc Nephrol. 12(3):574-82, 2001
15. Iványi B et al: Peritubular capillaries in chronic renal allograft rejection: a quantitative ultrastructural study. Hum Pathol. 31(9):1129-38, 2000

CHRONIC HUMORAL REJECTION

Transplant Glomerulopathy

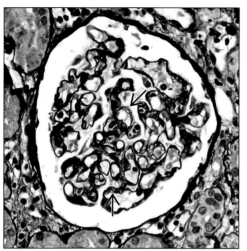

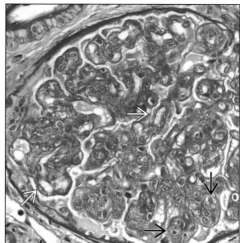

(Left) Segmental glomerular basement membrane duplication ➡ in a glomerulus with TG is shown. *(Right)* PAS shows TG with prominent intracapillary mononuclear inflammatory cells (glomerulitis) ➡, a common feature associated with C4d(+). Duplication of the GBM is also evident ➡. Patient had class II DSA and PTCs were positive for C4d.

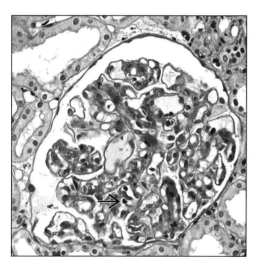

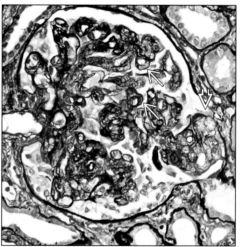

(Left) Glomerulitis ➡, with marginated mononuclear cells within glomerular capillaries, was present in this case that showed TG. *(Right)* Many areas of glomerular basement membrane duplication ➡ appear in this glomerulus showing TG. A segmental scar, representing secondary focal segmental glomerulosclerosis, is also seen ➡. Immunofluorescence staining was negative for an immune complex glomerulonephritis.

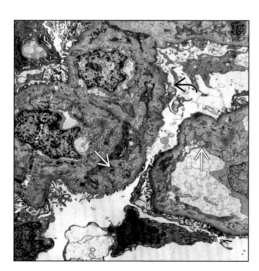

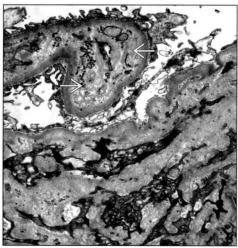

(Left) Glomerular basement membrane duplication with intervening lucent material ➡ is shown. Podocyte foot process effacement is also present ➡. *(Right)* Glomerular basement membrane duplication with marked luminal narrowing and subendothelial lucent material ➡ is seen by electron microscopy. No immune-type, electron-dense deposits are present.

Peritubular Capillaries

(Left) *Peritubular* ➢ *and glomerular* ➢ *capillaries show marginated mononuclear cells (mostly monocytes/macrophages) with occasional neutrophils.* **(Right)** *Peritubular capillaries are dilated* ➔ *and show numerous marginated mononuclear cells* ➢. *Note that inflammatory cells are largely within the capillaries, not in the interstitium, and thus do not imply acute cellular rejection.*

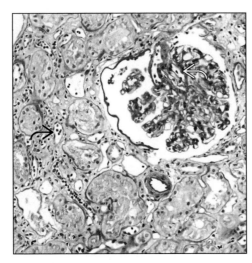
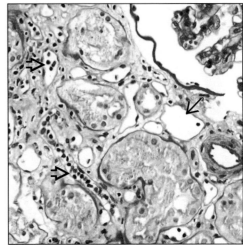

(Left) *This case shows circumferential PTCBMML* ➢ *along with activated-appearing endothelial cells and marginated leukocytes* ➧ *within the capillary. The endothelial cells here are enlarged and show loss of fenestrations and microvillous changes* ➔. **(Right)** *Rarely in peritubular capillaropathy, PTC basement membrane duplication or multilamination* ➔ *can be seen by light microscopy.*

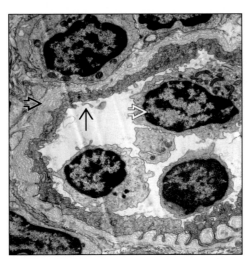
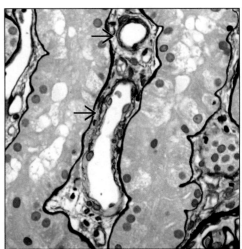

(Left) *Mild PTCBMML is shown with a few circumferential basement membrane layers. Some basement membrane layers are fragmented* ➔. **(Right)** *Severe multilayering of the glomerular basement membranes in a case of TG is shown; the basement membranes in this case narrow and nearly occlude the capillary lumen.*

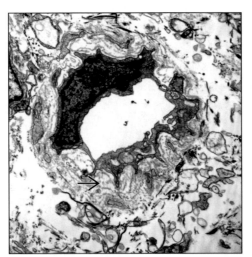
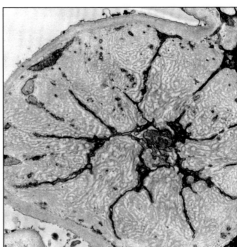

Peritubular Capillaries

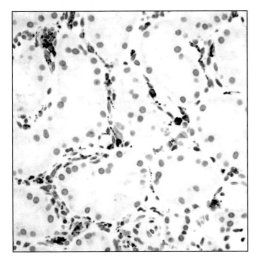

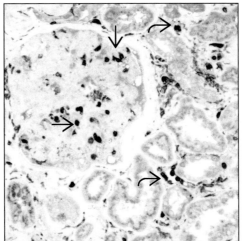

(Left) Immunohistochemical stain shows CD68(+) monocytes/macrophages within peritubular capillaries. PTCs also contain CD3(+) T cells. (Right) IHC stain for the FcγRIII receptor (CD16) shows numerous cells in glomerular capillaries ➡ and PTCs ⤳ in a case of CHR in this haploidentical living related graft 23 years post transplant. Monocytes and NK cells express CD16 and may mediate endothelial injury independent of complement.

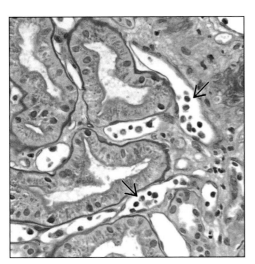

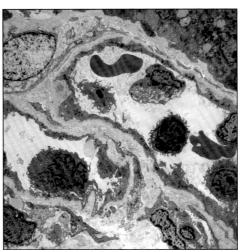

(Left) Intracapillary mononuclear cells ➡ are typically prominent in CHR, while neutrophils are more common in AHR. This patient was 4 years status post kidney/liver transplantation and had TG and positive C4d. (Right) Mononuclear cells in PTC are associated with reactive endothelium. This patient presented with proteinuria (2.8 g/day) and elevated Cr (2 mg/dL) 6 years post transplant. C4d was positive.

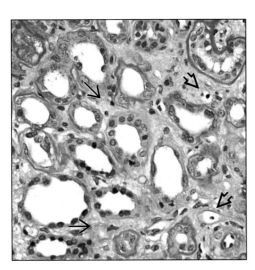

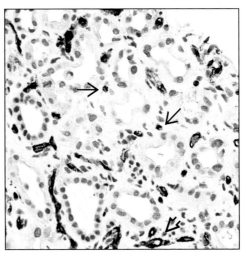

(Left) In this case of CHR, peritubular capillaries are inconspicuous in areas where they would be expected ➡. Some PTCs are seen ⤳. (Right) A CD34 stain demonstrates loss of peritubular capillaries with staining of scattered residual endothelial cells without associated lumens ➡. A few residual PTCs are also seen ⤳. This phenomenon may explain focal staining for C4d in biopsies with few residual PTCs.

CHRONIC HUMORAL REJECTION

C4d Stains in CHR

(Left) Immunoperoxidase stain of case with CHR shows extensive staining of PTCs for C4d; > 90% were positive. Cells in PTC were also evident ➡. *(Right)* Immunoperoxidase stain of case with CHR shows focal staining of PTCs for C4d. 13% of PTCs were positive. There is a wide variation in the percent of positive PTC for C4d in biopsies from patients with presumptive CHR (DSA + TG or PTCBMML), possibly related to variation in complement fixation or resistance of the endothelial cells.

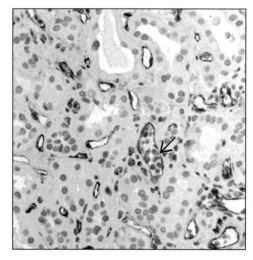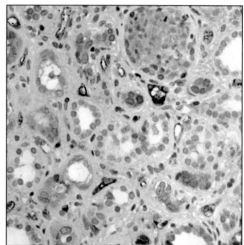

(Left) Double IHC stain with anti-C4d (blue) followed by anti-CD34 (brown) is shown. Many PTCs stain for CD34 but not C4d. In these studies, the 1st antibody reaction product blocks the 2nd. (Courtesy A. B. Collins, BS.) *(Right)* An immunofluorescence stain for C4d reveals focal positive peritubular capillaries ➡. In CHR, PTCs may show diffuse, focal, or negative staining for C4d.

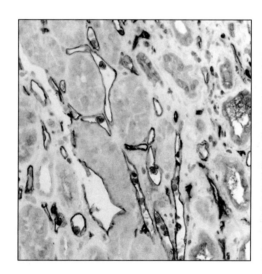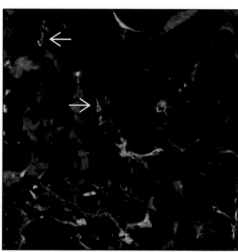

(Left) Immunoperoxidase stain in paraffin-embedded tissue from a patient with TG and DSA shows rare PTCs positive for C4d ➡. In contrast, the frozen tissue, which is usually more sensitive, was more extensively positive. *(Right)* Immunofluorescence stains in frozen tissue from a patient with TG and DSA show many PTCs positive for C4d ➡, in contrast to the corresponding IHC stain illustrated. CHR can occur with little or no C4d staining, but criteria for C4d(-) CHR have not been established.

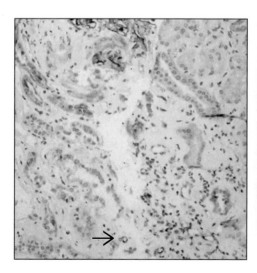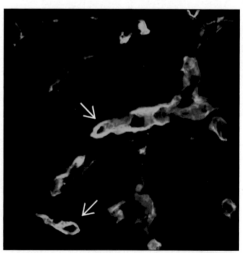

Arterial Lesions

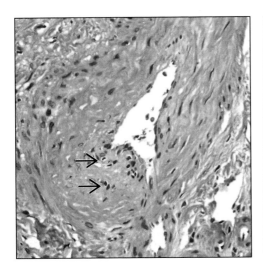 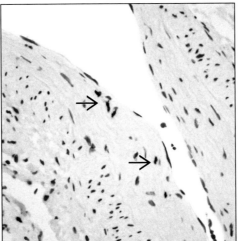

(Left) This artery shows a thickened intima with embedded mononuclear inflammatory cells ➡. This patient has known donor-specific antibody. This biopsy was negative for C4d, but previous biopsies from this allograft showed C4d deposition. *(Right)* An immunohistochemical stain for CD3 reveals T cells ➡ within the thickened intima. The presence of inflammatory cells confirms that the intimal thickening is related to rejection rather than hypertension. Some cases show CD68(+) cells.

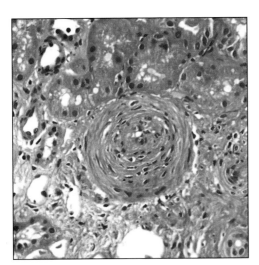 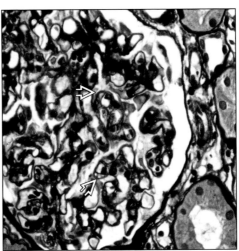

(Left) Transplant arteriopathy has severe narrowing of the arterial lumen. This biopsy also showed transplant glomerulopathy. The C4d was negative; the patient had a donor-specific HLA class II antibody. *(Right)* Transplant glomerulopathy, with glomerular basement membrane duplication ➡, is seen in a case that also showed transplant arteriopathy. Both TG and TA lesions can be seen in CHR, but do not necessarily occur together.

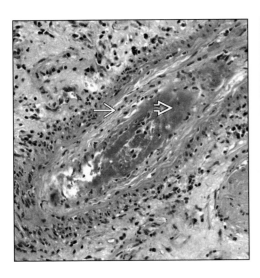 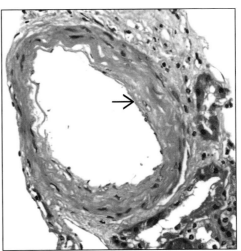

(Left) This case shows features of acute and chronic rejection, with T-cell-mediated and humoral rejection. Intimal thickening with inflammatory cells ➡ is a lesion of chronic rejection, while fibrin ➡ is a feature seen in acute humoral rejection. A C4d stain was positive. *(Right)* A typical lesion of arteriosclerosis shows intimal thickening ➡, but without inflammation.

CHRONIC HUMORAL REJECTION

Stages of CHR

(Left) Postulated stages in the evolution of CHR are given, beginning with the production of DSA and progressing to clinically evident CHR. C4d and DSA may be intermittently present during this time. The time between stages is unknown and progression is not necessarily inevitable. *(Right)* Electron microscopy can reveal early features predictive of later development of TG: Subendothelial lucency ⮕, enlarged endothelial cells ⮕, and corrugation of the GBM ⮎ are seen here.

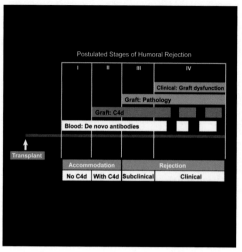
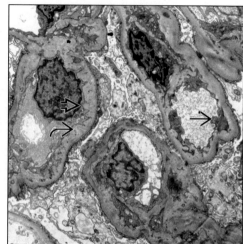

(Left) A normal glomerulus is seen on biopsy 6 months post transplant from a patient with graft dysfunction due to AHR. There was class II DSA and C4d deposition. *(Right)* Evolution of glomerular changes is seen 6 years after an AHR episode. The patient presented with elevated Cr, proteinuria, persistent class II DSA, and positive C4d. Glomerulitis ⮕ and GBM duplication ⮎ are prominent in this hypertrophied glomerulus. The graft was lost 18 months later.

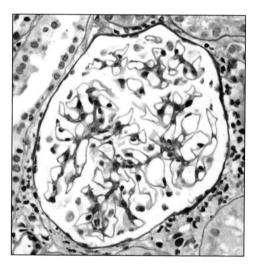
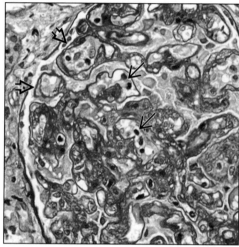

(Left) A 4-month protocol biopsy from a positive-crossmatch transplant patient with stable renal function is shown. Mononuclear cells are marginated within peritubular capillaries ⮕. Glomeruli show no evidence of TG. A C4d stain was negative. *(Right)* By 7 months post transplant, this patient developed renal insufficiency (SCr 3.1 mg/dL). A biopsy shows TG with GBM duplication ⮎. Peritubular capillaritis is present ⮕, as was on the 4-month biopsy. There was no history of AHR.

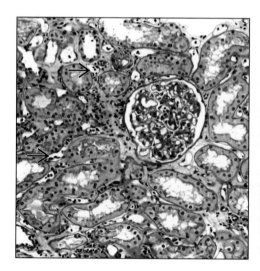
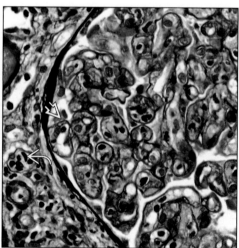

Differential Diagnosis

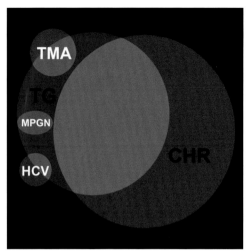

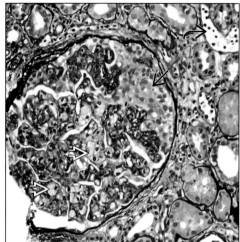

(Left) Venn diagram shows differential diagnosis of TG. Most cases are due to CHR (57% C4d positive, DSA), but other causes include chronic TMA (13%), hepatitis C virus (4%), MPGN (2%), and idiopathic (24%). This is based on 137 cases of TG, 1999-2009 (RB Colvin, unpublished). **(Right)** An unusual case of TG shows numerous foam cells ⮞ within glomerular capillaries, with podocyte hyperplasia ⮞, a feature of collapsing glomerulopathy. Peritubular capillaritis is also present ⮞.

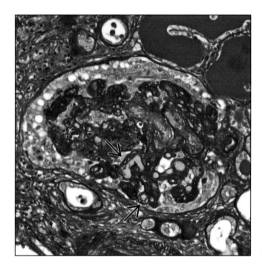

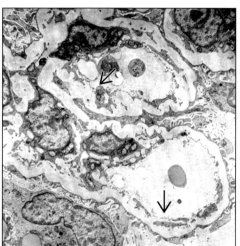

(Left) Collapsing glomerulopathy and thrombotic microangiopathy in an allograft with chronic calcineurin inhibitor toxicity. GBM duplication ⮞ due to TMA can resemble CHR and is one of the causes of transplant glomerulopathy. **(Right)** Duplication of the GBM ⮞ due to subclinical thrombotic microangiopathy is seen in a native kidney from a heart transplant recipient. This resembles the TG seen in allograft kidneys, due to CHR.

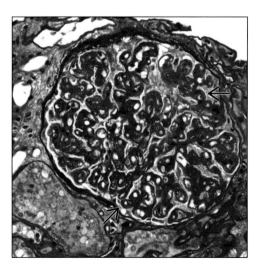

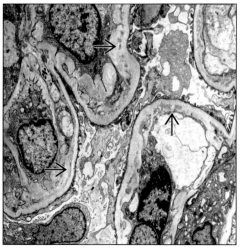

(Left) Recurrent membranoproliferative glomerulonephritis (MPGN, type I) causes duplication of the GBM ⮞ and a pattern of transplant glomerulopathy. However, MPGN can usually be distinguished from CHR by the presence of immunoglobulin and C3 deposits by IF, prominent electron dense subendothelial deposits by EM, and negative C4d in PTC. **(Right)** MPGN, which may mimic transplant glomerulopathy, shows prominent subendothelial deposits by EM ⮞.

Recurrent Disease After Kidney Transplantation

Renal Disease	Recurrence Rate	5-10 Year Graft Loss	Additional Features
Immune Complex Mediated			
MGN	30%	10-15% (10 year)	IgG4 is dominant subclass compared to IgG1 in de novo MGN
IgA nephropathy/Henoch-Schönlein purpura	13-50%	10% (10 year)	Crescentic GN may be unusual manifestation of recurrent disease
MPGN type I	20-50%	10-40%	Recurrence rate increases with successive allografts
Dense deposit disease (MPGN type II)	> 80%	10-20%	Living-related grafts do better than deceased donor grafts
Lupus nephritis	Up to 30%	< 5%	Podocytopathy or FSGS may represent unusual manifestation of recurrent lupus nephritis
Nonimmune Complex Mediated			
FSGS	20-40%	15-20% (10 year)	May recur with features of collapsing glomerulopathy
Diabetic nephropathy	> 50%	5%	
Atypical or non-Shiga toxin HUS	33-82%	40-50%	High recurrence rate for *CFH* and *FI* mutations; 20% recurrence for *CD46* mutation
Deposits with Substructure			
Amyloidosis, AL type	10-30%	35%	
Amyloidosis, AA type	< 10%	Rare	
Fibrillary GN	50%	20%	
Immunotactoid glomerulopathy	Rare reports	Not available	
Monoclonal immunoglobulin deposition disease	70-85%	> 50%	
Crescentic GN			
Anti-GBM disease	< 5%	Rare	
Pauci-immune (ANCA-associated) crescentic GN	0-20%	10% (10 year)	Recurrent disease may spare kidney allograft
Genetic/Metabolic Disorders			
Primary hyperoxaluria	90-100% if kidney transplant alone	80-100%	Liver transplantation is curative and may obviate need for kidney transplantation; excretion of oxalate may simulate disease recurrence
Fabry disease	Low	Rare	Decreasing recurrence with advent of enzyme replacement therapy
Cystinosis	Rare	0%	Macrophages with cystine crystals may deposit in interstitium or glomerular mesangium; cystine accumulates in other organs
Sickle cell nephropathy	Rare reports	Not available	Sickle cell crisis common within 1st year of transplantation

All percentages are approximate, based on combined large reported series.

6. Casquero A et al: Recurrent acute postinfectious glomerulonephritis. Clin Nephrol. 66(1):51-3, 2006
7. Choy BY et al: Recurrent glomerulonephritis after kidney transplantation. Am J Transplant. 6(11):2535-42, 2006
8. Little MA et al: Severity of primary MPGN, rather than MPGN type, determines renal survival and post-transplantation recurrence risk. Kidney Int. 69(3):504-11, 2006
9. Braun MC et al: Recurrence of membranoproliferative glomerulonephritis type II in renal allografts: The North American Pediatric Renal Transplant Cooperative Study experience. J Am Soc Nephrol. 16(7):2225-33, 2005
10. Couser W: Recurrent glomerulonephritis in the renal allograft: an update of selected areas. Exp Clin Transplant. 3(1):283-8, 2005
11. Kowalewska J et al: IgA nephropathy with crescents in kidney transplant recipients. Am J Kidney Dis. 45(1):167-75, 2005
12. Soler MJ et al: Recurrence of IgA nephropathy and Henoch-Schönlein purpura after kidney transplantation: risk factors and graft survival. Transplant Proc. 37(9):3705-9, 2005
13. Floege J: Recurrent glomerulonephritis following renal transplantation: an update. Nephrol Dial Transplant. 18(7):1260-5, 2003
14. Briganti EM et al: Risk of renal allograft loss from recurrent glomerulonephritis. N Engl J Med. 347(2):103-9, 2002

Recurrent FSGS

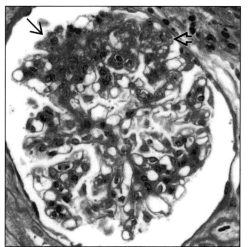

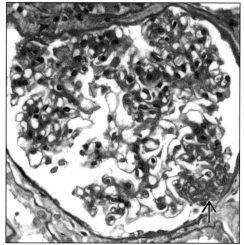

(Left) Periodic acid-Schiff highlights segmental sclerosis ⊡, characterized by segmental accumulation of the matrix and obliteration of the capillary lumina with prominence of adjacent podocytes ➡ in the biopsy of an 11-year-old boy with recurrent FSGS. *(Right)* Periodic acid-Schiff demonstrates sclerosis involving a portion of a glomerular tuft ➡ with loss of the capillary lumina and an adhesion to a Bowman capsule in this allograft with recurrent FSGS.

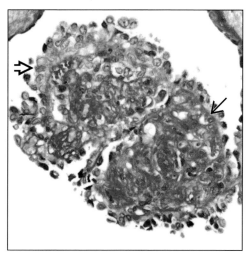

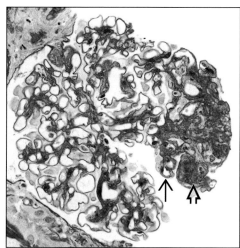

(Left) Periodic acid-Schiff highlights collapsed glomerular tufts ➡ with prominence of podocytes ⊡. Recurrence of collapsing FSGS may manifest with either collapsing or noncollapsing segmental sclerosis. *(Right)* Periodic acid-Schiff shows segmental occlusion of glomerular capillaries by hyaline and matrix ⊡ in this allograft with recurrent FSGS 6 years after transplantation. Focal duplication of GBM ➡ suggests chronic transplant glomerulopathy.

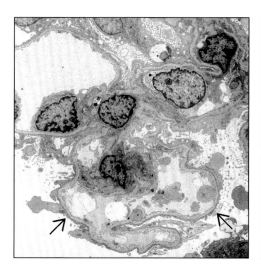

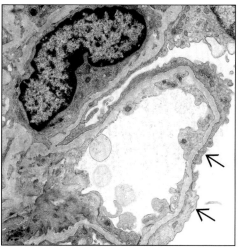

(Left) Electron microscopy reveals diffuse effacement of the podocyte foot processes ➡ along the glomerular basement membranes, which correlates with the clinical history of severe proteinuria. This ultrastructural feature precedes the finding of segmental sclerosis by light microscopy by weeks or months. *(Right)* Electron microscopy shows extensive effacement of the podocyte foot processes ➡ in this biopsy with recurrence of FSGS within 2 weeks after renal transplantation.

DISEASES THAT RECUR IN ALLOGRAFTS

Recurrent MGN and MPGN

(Left) Periodic acid-Schiff reveals thick GBMs, characteristic of MGN, in an allograft with recurrent disease. Duplicated GBMs ⇨ indicate chronic transplant glomerulopathy. (Right) Periodic acid-Schiff shows marked thickening of the GBMs ⇨ with a vacuolated appearance, characteristic of MGN. Other injuries include segmental glomerular scarring ⇨ with a fibrous attachment ⇨ to the Bowman capsule and marked arteriolar hyalinosis ⇨ in this 7-year-old allograft.

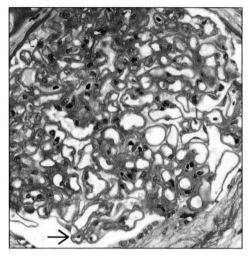
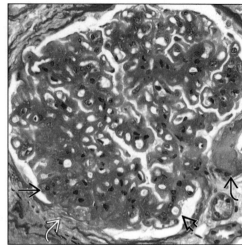

(Left) Immunofluorescence microscopy for C4d reveals strong granular staining of the glomerular capillary walls. This may be the 1st clue to establish the diagnosis of recurrent MGN when C4d is the only antibody routinely used to evaluate kidney allograft biopsies. (Right) Immunofluorescence microscopy for IgG shows strong granular staining of the glomerular capillary walls ⇨ in an allograft with recurrent MGN.

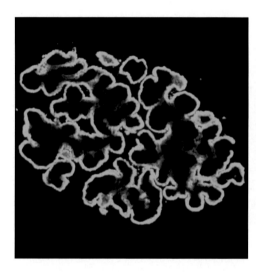
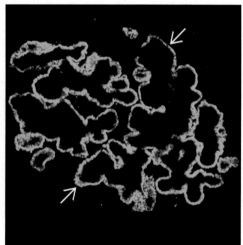

(Left) Periodic acid-Schiff shows severe infiltration by inflammatory cells within this glomerulus and duplication of the glomerular basement membranes ⇨ in an allograft with recurrence of MPGN type I. (Right) Periodic acid-Schiff reveals a cellular crescent ⇨ that accompanies marked endocapillary hypercellularity with numerous inflammatory cells ⇨ and duplication of the GBM in an allograft with recurrent MPGN type I.

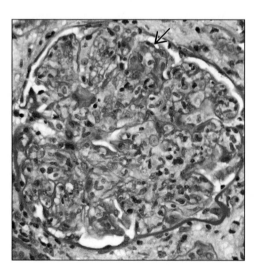
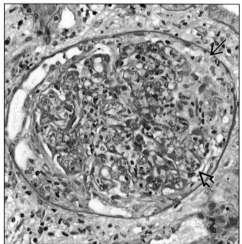

DISEASES THAT RECUR IN ALLOGRAFTS

Recurrent IgA Nephropathy

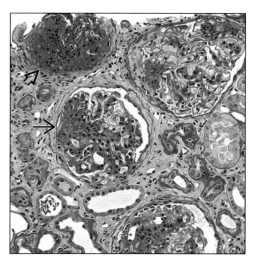
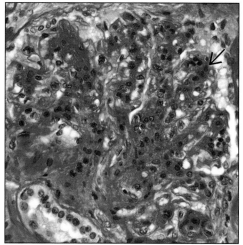

(Left) Periodic acid-Schiff reveals severe cortical fibrosis as shown in this allograft with recurrent IgA nephropathy 9 years after transplantation. The close clustering of glomeruli indicates substantial tubular loss. Segmental ⮕ and near global ⮚ glomerular scarring are also present. *(Right)* Periodic acid-Schiff demonstrates marked mesangial hypercellularity ⮕ in this glomerulus with recurrent IgA nephropathy, which is a common feature of recurrent disease.

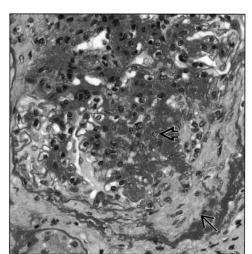
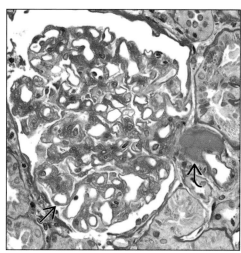

(Left) Periodic acid-Schiff of a glomerulus from an allograft with recurrent IgA nephropathy shows mesangial hypercellularity ⮚ and a fibrocellular crescent ⮕. *(Right)* Periodic acid-Schiff of this glomerulus with recurrent IgA nephropathy from an allograft 18 years after transplantation shows duplication of the GBM ⮕ that is consistent with chronic transplant glomerulopathy and arteriolar hyalinosis ⮺, suggesting chronic calcineurin inhibitor toxicity.

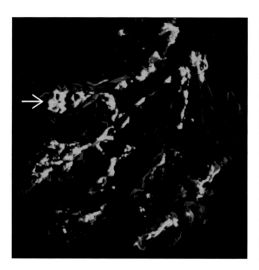
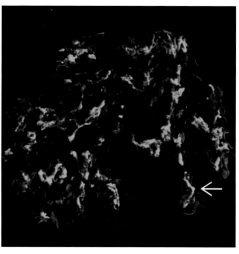

(Left) Immunofluorescence microscopy for IgA shows strong granular mesangial ⮕ staining in a kidney allograft with recurrent IgA nephropathy, which is identical to the pattern of involvement in the native kidneys. *(Right)* Immunofluorescence microscopy for lambda light chains reveals strong granular mesangial ⮕ staining. The intensity of lambda light chain staining is greater than kappa light chains (not shown), which is a characteristic feature of IgA nephropathy.

Recurrent Lupus Nephritis

(Left) Periodic acid-Schiff shows focal mesangial hypercellularity ➡ and mesangial sclerosis ⊳, which are common alterations in the early phase of recurrent lupus nephritis. When glomeruli are normal on light microscopy, immunofluorescence microscopy may detect the presence of immune complexes in patients with lupus. *(Right)* Segmental fibrinoid necrosis ➡ and endocapillary hypercellularity ⊳ are present in this case of recurrent lupus nephritis.

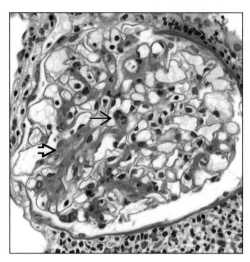

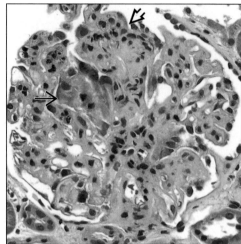

(Left) Periodic acid-Schiff demonstrates a cellular crescent ➡ intimately associated with a glomerular tuft that exhibits prominent endocapillary hypercellularity ⊳ from an allograft with recurrent lupus nephritis. *(Right)* Immunofluorescence microscopy for IgG reveals discrete granular and confluent staining along the capillary walls and some mesangial regions in this kidney allograft with lupus nephritis, class IV and V.

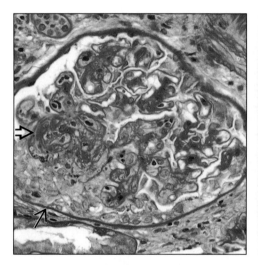

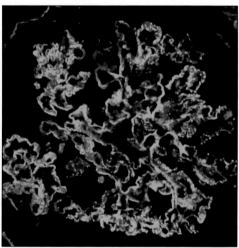

(Left) Immunofluorescence shows granular C4d staining along the GBM, which is suggestive of lupus MGN. This staining pattern is distinct from the mesangial C4d staining that may be present in normal glomeruli. *(Right)* Immunofluorescence microscopy for C3 in a biopsy with recurrent lupus nephritis shows granular capillary wall and mesangial ⊳ deposits, which is less intense than IgG or C4d (not shown). The cluster of round deposits is probably podocyte reabsorption droplets ➡.

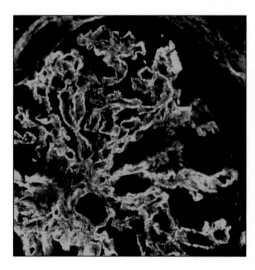

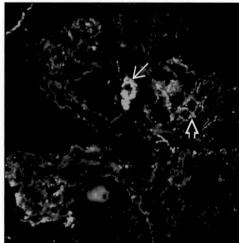

DISEASES THAT RECUR IN ALLOGRAFTS

Recurrence of Other Diseases

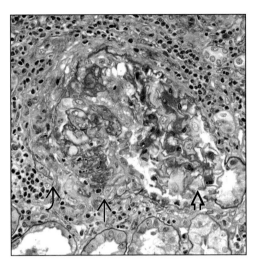

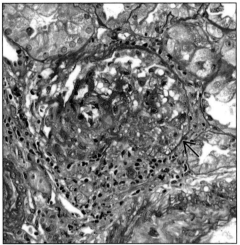

(Left) Recurrent ANCA-associated disease has a fibrocellular crescent ⇒ and a spared segment of the glomerulus ⊇. The patient had post-transplant pulmonary hemorrhage, positive myeloperoxidase antibody, and recurrent pauci-immune crescentic GN. The Bowman capsule is disrupted ⇒, a useful sign of crescents. *(Right)* Periodic acid-Schiff reveals a cellular crescent ⇒ in this allograft from a 57-year-old female with recurrent ANCA-associated pauci-immune crescentic GN.

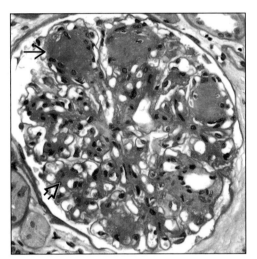

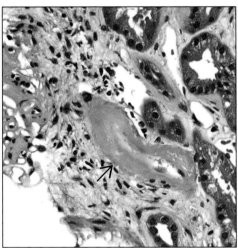

(Left) Periodic acid-Schiff shows diffuse mesangial ⊇ and nodular sclerosis ⇒, which characterizes recurrence of diabetic nephropathy in an allograft. *(Right)* Severe arteriolar hyalinosis is present ⇒ in this allograft with recurrent diabetic nephropathy 6 years after transplantation. Calcineurin inhibitor toxicity and hypertension may also contribute, as their histologic features can be indistinguishable from diabetic vascular injury.

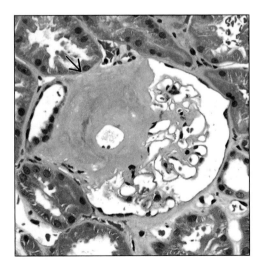

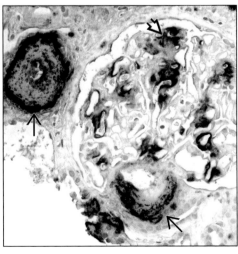

(Left) Hematoxylin & eosin shows prominent deposition of amorphous eosinophilic material in a hilar arteriole ⇒, suggestive of recurrent amyloidosis in this 9-year-old allograft from a 47-year-old man with ankylosing spondylitis. *(Right)* IHC confirms the presence of AA deposits in a 47-year-old man with ankylosing spondylitis. Note the prominent amyloid deposition within the arterioles ⇒ and much less involvement of mesangial areas ⊇ in the glomeruli.

DE NOVO FOCAL SEGMENTAL GLOMERULOSCLEROSIS

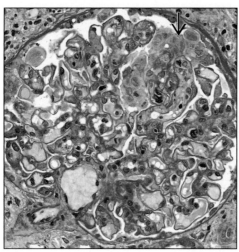

Collapsing type de novo focal segmental glomerulosclerosis (FSGS) in a renal transplant patient with nephrotic-range proteinuria shows prominent adjacent visceral epithelial cells (podocytes) ⊡.

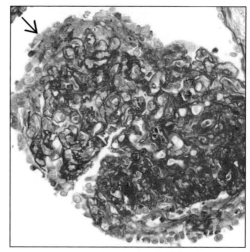

Prominent podocytes ⊡ overlie a collapsed tuft in this case of de novo collapsing glomerulopathy in a transplant patient with severe proteinuria whose original disease was diabetic nephropathy.

TERMINOLOGY

Abbreviations
- Focal segmental glomerulosclerosis (FSGS)

Synonyms
- Collapsing glomerulopathy (CG)
  - Variant of FSGS

Definitions
- FSGS or its variants in kidney transplant patients with original disease **not** due to FSGS

ETIOLOGY/PATHOGENESIS

Hyperfiltration
- Pediatric kidneys transplanted into adult recipients
- Longstanding allografts with severe nephron loss
- Severe vascular disease

Severe Vascular Disease
- De novo CG associated with deceased donor kidneys
- Zonal distribution of CG

Drug Induced
- Higher frequency with calcineurin inhibitors (CNI)
  - CNI may contribute via microvascular disease
- Mammalian target of rapamycin (mTOR) inhibitors

CLINICAL ISSUES

Presentation
- Proteinuria
  - Variable, unlike recurrent FSGS
- Chronic renal failure

Laboratory Tests
- Urinalysis
- 24 hour urine protein collection

Treatment
- Not well defined
- If CNI implicated, alter drug regimen

Prognosis
- De novo FSGS: 60% graft survival within 5 years of diagnosis
- De novo CG: 50% loss of graft within 1 year of diagnosis

MICROSCOPIC PATHOLOGY

Histologic Features
- Segmental glomerulosclerosis with any of the following findings
  - Synechial or fibrous attachments to Bowman capsules
  - Obliteration of glomerular capillary lumina by foam cells &/or hyaline
  - Segmental accumulation of mesangial matrix
  - Prominence of visceral epithelial cells (podocytes)
  - Protein reabsorption droplets in podocytes
  - Foot process effacement
- Collapsing glomerulopathy (variant of FSGS)
  - Collapse of glomerulus with podocyte hypercellularity
  - Associated with severe vascular disease and CNI toxicity
  - Zonal distribution
- Global glomerulosclerosis
- Interstitial fibrosis and tubular atrophy
  - Often severe
- Occasionally, interstitial foam cells is correlate of severe proteinuria
- Arteriolar hyalinosis
  - Subendothelial hyalinosis
  - Adventitial hyaline nodules may be present

DE NOVO FOCAL SEGMENTAL GLOMERULOSCLEROSIS

Key Facts

Etiology/Pathogenesis
- Hyperfiltration
  - Observed in longstanding allografts with severe nephron loss
- Severe vascular disease
- New-onset FSGS

Clinical Issues
- Proteinuria, nephrotic range
- Chronic renal failure

Microscopic Pathology
- Focal, segmental glomerulosclerosis or collapsing glomerulopathy
- Arterial or arteriolar sclerosis

Top Differential Diagnoses
- Recurrent FSGS
- Chronic transplant glomerulopathy
- Calcineurin inhibitor toxicity

ANCILLARY TESTS

Immunofluorescence
- IgM and C3 in segmental scars

Electron Microscopy
- Podocyte foot process effacement
- Separation of podocytes from GBM if CG

DIFFERENTIAL DIAGNOSIS

Recurrent FSGS
- Usually presents earlier (< 1 year)

Chronic Transplant Glomerulopathy
- Duplication of GBM without immune complex deposition
- Variable C4d peritubular capillary deposition
- May occur concurrently with de novo FSGS

Immune Complex-mediated Glomerulonephritis, De Novo or Recurrent
- Positive immunofluorescence staining for immunoglobulins (immune complex deposition)

DIAGNOSTIC CHECKLIST

Pathologic Interpretation Pearls
- FSGS should trigger IF and EM workup
- CG may mimic crescentic glomerulonephritis

SELECTED REFERENCES

1. Goes NB et al: Case records of the Massachusetts General Hospital. Case 12-2007. A 56-year-old woman with renal failure after heart-lung transplantation. N Engl J Med. 356(16):1657-65, 2007
2. Swaminathan S et al: Collapsing and non-collapsing focal segmental glomerulosclerosis in kidney transplants. Nephrol Dial Transplant. 21(9):2607-14, 2006
3. Nadasdy T et al: Zonal distribution of glomerular collapse in renal allografts: possible role of vascular changes. Hum Pathol. 33(4):437-41, 2002
4. Cosio FG et al: Focal segmental glomerulosclerosis in renal allografts with chronic nephropathy: implications for graft survival. Am J Kidney Dis. 34(4):731-8, 1999
5. Trimarchi HM et al: Focal segmental glomerulosclerosis in a 32-year-old kidney allograft after 7 years without immunosuppression. Nephron. 82(3):270-3, 1999
6. Meehan SM et al: De novo collapsing glomerulopathy in renal allografts. Transplantation. 65(9):1192-7, 1998
7. Barama A et al: Focal segmental glomerulosclerosis in one of two "en bloc" pediatric transplanted kidneys. Am J Kidney Dis. 30(2):271-4, 1997
8. Woolley AC et al: De novo focal glomerulosclerosis after kidney transplantation. Am J Med. 84(2):310-4, 1988

IMAGE GALLERY

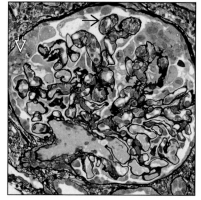 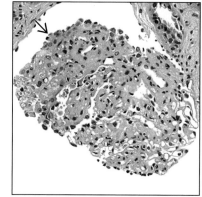 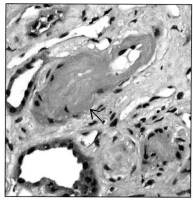

(Left) Protein reabsorption droplets ⬗ accentuate a few prominent podocytes, which correlate with proteinuria. Duplication of the glomerular basement membranes is present ➡, which raises the consideration of chronic transplant glomerulopathy (Jones methenamine silver). *(Center)* The podocytes ➡ are prominent in this glomerulus with features of collapsing glomerulopathy. *(Right)* Prominent subendothelial hyalinosis ➡ of an arteriole is present in an allograft biopsy with collapsing glomerulopathy, implying that it may be related to calcineurin inhibitor toxicity.

DE NOVO MEMBRANOUS GLOMERULONEPHRITIS

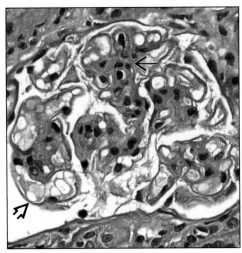

Periodic acid-Schiff shows thickening of the glomerular basement membranes ⮥ and focal mild mesangial hypercellularity ⮥.

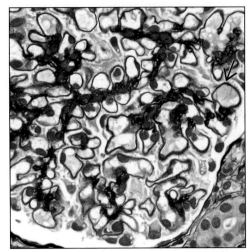

Jones methenamine silver shows a hint of subepithelial "spike" formation ⮥ along some of the glomerular basement membranes.

TERMINOLOGY

Abbreviations
- Membranous glomerulonephritis (MGN)

Synonyms
- Membranous glomerulopathy, de novo
- Membranous nephropathy, de novo
- Membranous glomerulonephropathy, de novo

Definitions
- MGN in kidney allograft when primary cause of end-stage renal disease is **not** MGN

ETIOLOGY/PATHOGENESIS

Allo/Auto Antibody
- May represent unusual manifestation of chronic humoral rejection
- Can occur in HLA identical grafts, presumably due to non-HLA antigen
  - Rat model of de novo MGN occurs only in transplant not native kidney
- 1 autopsy showed de novo MGN involving only kidney allograft **without** MGN in native kidneys
- 1 de novo MGN case with donor specific antibodies against HLA-DQ7
- Association with C4d deposition in peritubular capillaries and anti-HLA-DQ
- No auto-antibodies to DLA2R

CLINICAL ISSUES

Epidemiology
- Incidence
  - 0.5-9% of kidney transplant patients

Presentation
- Typically manifests late (> 3 years)

- Renal dysfunction
- Proteinuria
  - 2nd most common cause of proteinuria in renal allograft patients
  - Often nephrotic range (> 3 g/24 hours), may be intermittent or persistent

Treatment
- Not well defined

Prognosis
- Unfavorable
  - 5-year graft loss of 50% or more
  - 2/3 eventually proceed to renal failure
- De novo MGN may recur in subsequent renal allografts

MACROSCOPIC FEATURES

General Features
- Renal vein thrombosis occasional present
  - Less common than idiopathic MGN in native kidneys

MICROSCOPIC PATHOLOGY

Histologic Features
- GBM thickening
  - Focal &/or segmental thickening common
- Glomerular capillaritis in ~ 50%
  - Increased leukocytes within glomerular capillaries
- Mesangial hypercellularity in ~ 33%
- Double contours or duplication of GBM in 50%
  - Possibly due to concurrent chronic transplant glomerulopathy (chronic humoral rejection)
- Prominent interstitial inflammation
  - Often sufficient for diagnosis of acute (cell-mediated) rejection
- Intimal arteritis

DE NOVO MEMBRANOUS GLOMERULONEPHRITIS

Key Facts

Clinical Issues
- 0.5-9% of kidney transplant patients
- Proteinuria
- Renal dysfunction
- Unfavorable prognosis
  - 2/3 of patients eventually require renal replacement therapy

Microscopic Pathology
- Glomerular basement membrane thickening, diffuse or segmental
  - GBM "spike" formation
- Granular IgG staining in glomerular capillary walls
  - C4d and C3 may also stain glomerular capillaries in similar pattern

- Careful evaluation of C4d glomerular staining pattern is critical if this is only antibody tested in transplant kidney biopsies
- C4d in peritubular capillaries found in ~ 70% of cases
- Subepithelial electron dense deposits seen by electron microscopy ± basement membrane "spike" formation
- Mesangial hypercellularity in 1/3 of cases
- Spikes of GBM on silver or PAS stains, ± "Swiss cheese" appearance depending on stage of MGN

Top Differential Diagnoses
- Recurrent MGN
- Chronic transplant glomerulopathy

- Acute (type 2) rejection found in subset

ANCILLARY TESTS

Immunofluorescence
- Positive granular capillary wall staining for IgG, kappa and lambda light chains
  - IgG1 is predominant subclass
    - IgG4 is predominant subclass in primary MGN
  - Variable capillary wall staining for C4d, C3, C1q, and IgM
- C4d(+) PTC in ~ 70%

Electron Microscopy
- Transmission
  - Subepithelial amorphous electron-dense deposits
    - Often small and relatively sparse
    - Stage I (Ehrenreich-Churg) deposits common
  - Duplication of GBMs
    - Subendothelial space widening when injured endothelial cells detach from GBM

DIFFERENTIAL DIAGNOSIS

Recurrent MGN
- Clinical history that original disease was MGN
- Earlier onset (< 3 months)
- IgG4 predominant

Donor-derived MGN
- Present in donor biopsy, disappears in a few months

Chronic Transplant Glomerulopathy
- Duplication of GBM without immune complexes
- Occurs concurrently in 50% of de novo MGN cases
- C4d(+) in peritubular capillaries
- Multilamination of peritubular capillaries on EM

DIAGNOSTIC CHECKLIST

Pathologic Interpretation Pearls
- Significant proteinuria should trigger additional evaluation by IF &/or EM
- Thickening or duplication of GBMs or segmental glomerular sclerosis should trigger additional IF &/or EM
- C4d immunofluorescence microscopy may reveal granular glomerular capillary wall staining
  - Useful finding for those that stain kidney transplant biopsies for C4d only

SELECTED REFERENCES

1. Lal SM: De novo membranous nephropathy in renal allografts with unusual histology. Arch Pathol Lab Med. 131(1):17, 2007
2. Sebire NJ et al: Posttransplant de novo membranous nephropathy in childhood. Fetal Pediatr Pathol. 24(2):95-103, 2005
3. Poduval RD et al: Treatment of de novo and recurrent membranous nephropathy in renal transplant patients. Semin Nephrol. 23(4):392-9, 2003
4. Heidet L et al: Recurrence of de novo membranous glomerulonephritis on renal grafts. Clin Nephrol. 41(5):314-8, 1994
5. Schwarz A et al: Impact of de novo membranous glomerulonephritis on the clinical course after kidney transplantation. Transplantation. 58(6):650-4, 1994
6. Monga G et al: Membranous glomerulonephritis (MGN) in transplanted kidneys: morphologic investigation on 256 renal allografts. Mod Pathol. 6(3):249-58, 1993
7. Truong L et al: De novo membranous glomerulonephropathy in renal allografts: a report of ten cases and review of the literature. Am J Kidney Dis. 14(2):131-44, 1989
8. Pirson Y et al: Aetiology and prognosis of de novo graft membranous nephropathy. Proc Eur Dial Transplant Assoc Eur Ren Assoc. 21:672-6, 1985
9. Collins AB et al: De novo MGN is immunologically distinct from idiopathic MGN and associated with C4d deposition. J Am Soc Nephrol, In Press

DE NOVO MEMBRANOUS GLOMERULONEPHRITIS

Microscopic Features

(Left) Duplication of the GBMs ⮕ may be frequent in de novo MGN, as demonstrated in this glomerulus from a pediatric patient with renal transplant due to renal dysplasia (Jones methenamine silver). *(Right)* Periodic acid-Schiff reveals duplication of the GBMs ⮕, which is consistent with chronic transplant glomerulopathy and a common finding in de novo MGN. The glomerulus also demonstrates segmental sclerosis ⮕. The peritubular capillaries did not reveal C4d deposition, ruling out chronic humoral rejection.

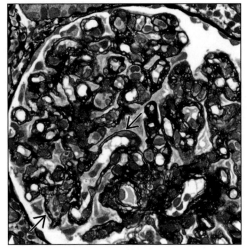
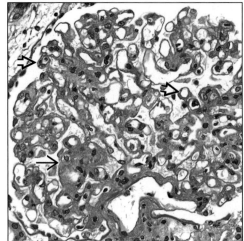

(Left) This renal allograft with de novo MGN shows a glomerulus with segmental mesangial hypercellularity and loss of some capillary lumina, which is consistent with segmental sclerosis ⮕ (Jones methenamine silver). *(Right)* Periodic acid-Schiff of a biopsy with de novo MGN reveals thick GBMs with a vacuolated appearance ⮕ in a glomerulus with segmental accumulation of matrix and hyaline ⮕, which obscures the capillary lumina.

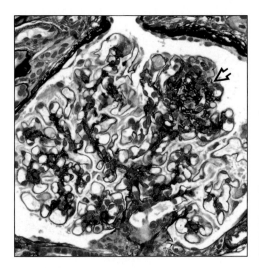
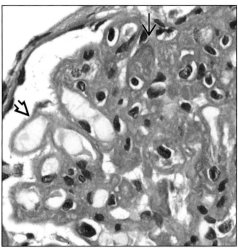

(Left) Immunofluorescence microscopy for IgG demonstrates granular staining of all glomerular capillaries. Clinical correlation is necessary to confirm whether this represents recurrent or de novo MGN. *(Right)* Immunofluorescence microscopy shows granular C4d staining along the glomerular basement membranes. This finding may be the 1st indication of a diagnosis of MGN, which should trigger additional IF and EM studies to confirm the diagnosis.

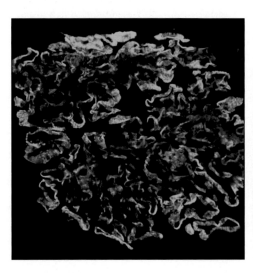
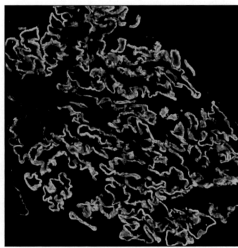

DE NOVO MEMBRANOUS GLOMERULONEPHRITIS

Immunofluorescence and Electron Microscopy Features

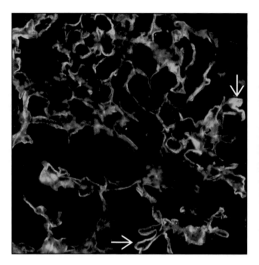

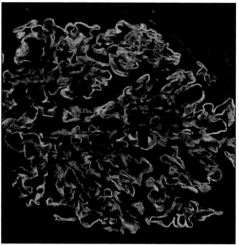

(Left) Immunofluorescence reveals segmental granular IgG in the glomerular capillaries ⮕ in a patient transplanted for renal dysplasia. *(Right)* Immunofluorescence microscopy shows granular kappa light chain staining of the glomerular capillary walls, which is characteristic of MGN. This biopsy was obtained from a patient 9 years after transplantation.

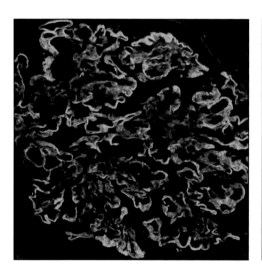

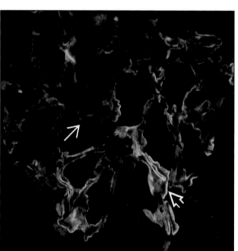

(Left) Immunofluorescence for lambda light chains shows a similar but less intense staining pattern as IgG and kappa light chain along the glomerular capillaries. *(Right)* Immunofluorescence for IgG highlights the segmental distribution of immune complex deposition along the glomerular capillaries ⮕. Several glomerular capillaries or segments of GBM show no significant staining ⮕. A similar pattern but less intense staining was also seen with kappa and lambda light chains.

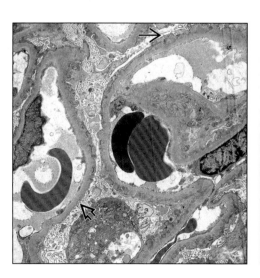

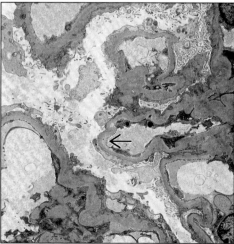

(Left) Electron microscopy reveals segmental distribution of many small subepithelial electron-dense deposits ⮕. The podocyte foot processes demonstrate diffuse effacement ⮕. *(Right)* Electron microscopy reveals many discrete electron dense deposits in subepithelial locations. Focal separation of the endothelial cell from the GBM ⮕ is noted, but duplication of the GBM is not apparent in this or other glomerular capillaries.

Electron Microscopy and Immunofluorescence

(Left) Prominent granular deposits along the GBM are revealed in this patient with de novo MGN transplanted 6 years ago for FSGS. The deposits tend to be more segmental than in MGN involving native kidneys. *(Right)* EM of a glomerulus with de novo MGN from a patient transplanted 6 years ago for FSGS shows subepithelial deposits ⊡→ surrounded by GBM spikes ⊟→, typical of stage II MGN.

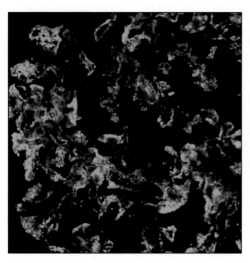
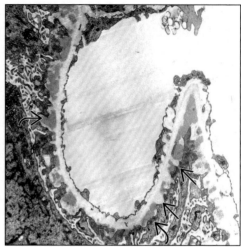

(Left) EM of a glomerulus with de novo MGN shows very small deposits in contact with the podocyte ⊟→ with only minimal spike formation, typical of early and mild MGN. The patient was transplanted 4 years previously for diabetic nephropathy. *(Right)* Electron micrograph of a glomerulus with de novo MGN shows very small deposits in contact with the podocyte ⊟→ with only minimal spike formation, typical of early and mild MGN. This pattern is not uncommon in de novo MGN.

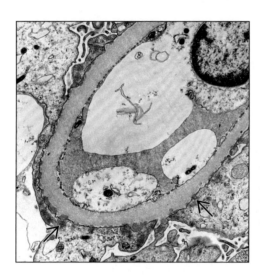
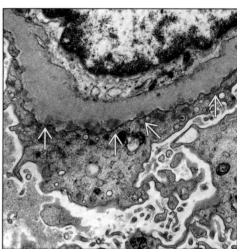

(Left) Sparse granules in the GBM stain for IgG in this patient with de novo MGN 13 years after transplantation for interstitial nephritis. The patient had 10 g/day proteinuria and a Cr of 2.3 mg/dL. C4d was present in peritubular capillaries (not shown). *(Right)* Peritubular capillary C4d deposits are noted in a patient with de novo MGN 13 years after transplantation for interstitial nephritis. Chronic humoral rejection and de novo MGN may be related, as both are thought to be due to alloantibodies.

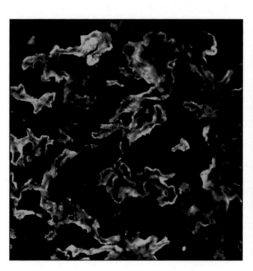
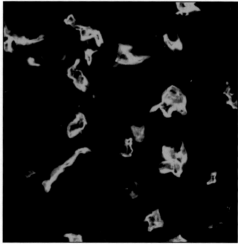

Association with Chronic Humoral Rejection

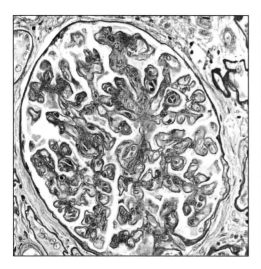

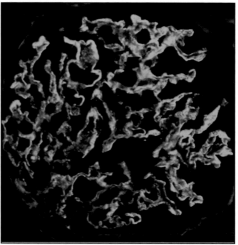

(Left) *Glomerulus with de novo MGN and chronic humoral rejection shows prominent and widespread duplication of the GBM. (Right) Granular IgG deposits in the GBM in a patient with C4d deposition in peritubular capillaries and donor reactive HLA antibodies. De novo MGN is associated with chronic humoral rejection and may be a manifestation of alloantibody reacting to glomerular antigens.*

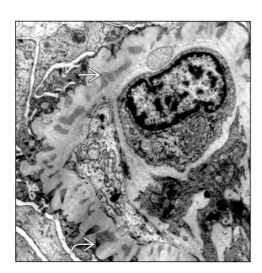

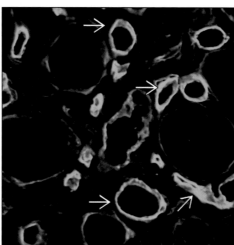

(Left) *Electron micrograph of a glomerulus from a patient with both chronic humoral rejection and de novo MGN shows duplication of the GBM and amorphous electron dense deposits within the GBM ➡ and in subepithelial locations ➡. (Right) C4d deposition is present in the peritubular capillaries in a patient with donor reactive HLA antibodies and de novo MGN. The peritubular capillaries have widespread linear deposits of C4d, typical of antibody-mediated rejection ➡.*

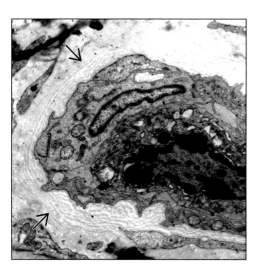

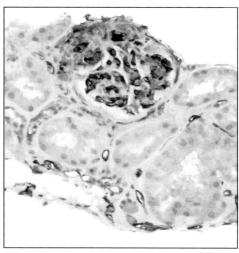

(Left) *Electron micrograph shows multilamination of the peritubular capillary basement membrane ➡ in a patient with donor reactive HLA antibodies and de novo MGN. (Right) C4d deposits are detected in the GBM and in peritubular capillaries in this patient with de novo MGN in a 2nd transplant. The 1st graft was lost to de novo MGN and chronic humoral rejection. Prior de novo MGN is a risk factor for a 2nd episode.*

ANTI-GBM DISEASE IN ALPORT SYNDROME

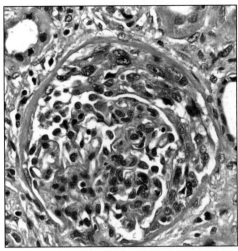

Hematoxylin & eosin stained tissue section from a patient with de novo anti-GBM disease 18 months after transplantation for Alport syndrome shows a cellular crescent compressing the glomerulus.

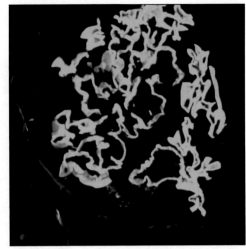

Immunofluorescence microscopy from the same patient 3 months earlier shows bright linear staining of the GBM for IgG. Kappa, lambda, C4d, and C3 were similar with focal staining of the tubular basement membranes.

TERMINOLOGY

Abbreviations
- Anti-glomerular basement membrane (anti-GBM) disease in Alport syndrome (AS)

Synonyms
- De novo anti-GBM nephritis

Definitions
- Glomerulonephritis mediated by anti-GBM antibodies in renal transplant recipients with AS

ETIOLOGY/PATHOGENESIS

Exposure to Nonendogenous GBM Antigens After Kidney Transplantation
- Antibodies develop against α-3, α-4, or α-5 chains of collagen IV of transplant kidney in AS patients due to genetic absence of endogenous antigen
  - AS patients with large deletions of COL4A5 are at higher risk
  - X-linked AS patients target NC1 domain of COL4A5 in intact type IV collagen hexamer
  - Autosomal recessive AS patients target NC1 domain of COL4A3 or COL4A4, distinct from that of Goodpasture syndrome

CLINICAL ISSUES

Epidemiology
- Incidence
  - 3-5% of AS patients develop de novo anti-GBM disease after kidney transplantation
- Gender
  - Male predominance

- Females with X-linked AS have 1 normal allele of α chains of collagen IV and rarely develop anti-GBM disease
  - Only 2 reports of anti-GBM disease involving females with autosomal recessive AS

Presentation
- Acute renal failure
  - 75% of cases occur within 1st year after kidney transplantation
- Hematuria

Laboratory Tests
- Serum anti-GBM assay by western blot

Treatment
- Drugs
  - Cyclophosphamide
  - High-dose corticosteroids
  - Anti-thymocyte globulin
  - Mycophenolate mofetil
- Plasmapheresis

Prognosis
- 90% of kidney allografts fail within weeks to months after disease onset
  - Anti-GBM disease often recurs in subsequent allografts with accelerated course

MICROSCOPIC PATHOLOGY

Histologic Features
- Cellular crescents &/or fibrinoid necrosis, typically affects > 80% of glomeruli
  - Glomerular tufts not involved by crescent formation or fibrinoid necrosis appear normal
- Acute tubular injury
- Red blood cell casts
- Finding of cellular or humoral rejection may also be present

ANTI-GBM DISEASE IN ALPORT SYNDROME

Key Facts

Etiology/Pathogenesis

- Antibodies develop against α-3, α-4, or α-5 chains of collagen IV of transplant kidney
  - AS patients with large deletions of *COL4A5* may be more susceptible to developing anti-GBM disease
- X-linked AS patients target NC1 domain of *COL4A5*
- Autosomal recessive AS patients target NC1 domain of *COL4A3* or *COL4A4*

Clinical Issues

- Acute renal failure
  - 75% of cases occur in 1st post-transplant year
  - 3-5% of AS patients develop de novo anti-GBM disease after kidney transplantation
- Hematuria
- Male predominance
- 90% of grafts fail within months after onset

- Anti-GBM disease often recurs in subsequent allografts with an accelerated course
- Plasmapheresis

Microscopic Pathology

- Cellular crescents &/or fibrinoid necrosis, typically > 80% of glomeruli
- Strong linear IgG immunofluorescence staining of GBM
- Intratubular red blood cell casts
- Acute tubular injury

Top Differential Diagnoses

- Pauci-immune (ANCA-associated) crescentic glomerulonephritis
- Diabetic nephropathy
- Polyomavirus nephritis

ANCILLARY TESTS

Immunofluorescence

- Strong, linear, IgG immunofluorescence staining of GBMs
  - Observed in up to 15% of AS patients after kidney transplantation
  - Kappa and lambda light chains and often C3 stain GBMs in similar pattern with lower intensity
  - Intensity of linear IgG staining substantially greater than albumin
  - Bowman capsules and distal tubular basement membranes may also show linear staining

DIFFERENTIAL DIAGNOSIS

Pauci-Immune (ANCA-associated) Crescentic Glomerulonephritis

- Lacks strong linear immunoglobulin deposition in GBM

Immune-Complex-associated Crescentic Glomerulonephritis

- Granular (nonlinear)

Diabetic Nephropathy

- Strong linear immunofluorescence of GBM for albumin as well as IgG
  - Cellular crescents rarely present

Polyomavirus Nephritis

- Glomerular crescents in minority of cases
  - Viral nuclear inclusions and positive SV40 IHC of nuclei of epithelium of tubules or Bowman capsule

DIAGNOSTIC CHECKLIST

Pathologic Interpretation Pearls

- Linear IgG GBM staining may be present in absence of glomerular inflammation

SELECTED REFERENCES

1. Pedchenko V et al: Molecular architecture of the Goodpasture autoantigen in anti-GBM nephritis. N Engl J Med. 363(4):343-54, 2010
2. Kashtan CE: Renal transplantation in patients with Alport syndrome. Pediatr Transplant. 10(6):651-7, 2006
3. Wang XP et al: Distinct epitopes for anti-glomerular basement membrane alport alloantibodies and goodpasture autoantibodies within the noncollagenous domain of alpha3(IV) collagen: a janus-faced antigen. J Am Soc Nephrol. 16(12):3563-71, 2005
4. Browne G et al: Retransplantation in Alport post-transplant anti-GBM disease. Kidney Int. 65(2):675-81, 2004
5. Hudson BG: The molecular basis of Goodpasture and Alport syndromes: beacons for the discovery of the collagen IV family. J Am Soc Nephrol. 15(10):2514-27, 2004
6. Byrne MC et al: Renal transplant in patients with Alport's syndrome. Am J Kidney Dis. 39(4):769-75, 2002
7. Kalluri R et al: Identification of alpha3, alpha4, and alpha5 chains of type IV collagen as alloantigens for Alport posttransplant anti-glomerular basement membrane antibodies. Transplantation. 69(4):679-83, 2000
8. Rutgers A et al: High affinity of anti-GBM antibodies from Goodpasture and transplanted Alport patients to alpha3(IV)NC1 collagen. Kidney Int. 58(1):115-22, 2000
9. Ding J et al: COL4A5 deletions in three patients with Alport syndrome and posttransplant antiglomerular basement membrane nephritis. J Am Soc Nephrol. 5(2):161-8, 1994
10. Göbel J et al: Kidney transplantation in Alport's syndrome: long-term outcome and allograft anti-GBM nephritis. Clin Nephrol. 38(6):299-304, 1992
11. Peten E et al: Outcome of thirty patients with Alport's syndrome after renal transplantation. Transplantation. 52(5):823-6, 1991
12. Kashtan CE et al: Posttransplant anti-glomerular basement membrane nephritis in related males with Alport syndrome. J Lab Clin Med. 116(4):508-15, 1990

ANTI-GBM DISEASE IN ALPORT SYNDROME

Gross and Microscopic Features

(Left) Gross photograph of an allograft nephrectomy from a 37-year-old woman with ESRD due to X-linked Alport syndrome. Eighteen months post transplant, the patient presented with allograft tenderness and renal failure. Anti-GBM titers were equivocal by ELISA and western blot. *(Right)* Gross photograph from the same patient at higher power shows classic gray glomeruli typical of crescentic glomerulonephritis ➡. The gray color is due to bloodless glomeruli.

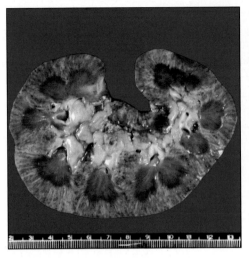
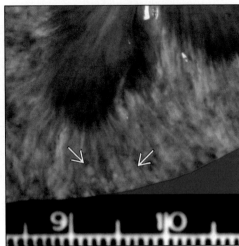

(Left) Hematoxylin & eosin of the same patient shows red cell and pigmented casts ➡ in the cortex, widespread interstitial fibrosis, and tubular injury. *(Right)* Hematoxylin & eosin of the same patient at high magnification shows a small cellular crescent ➡ in the upper right corner of this glomerulus, which appears bloodless.

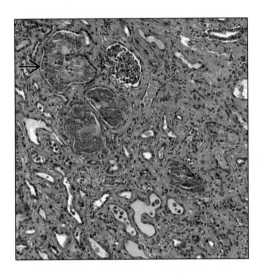
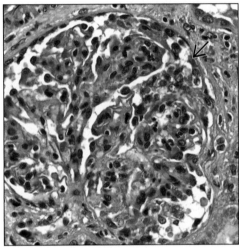

(Left) Immunofluorescence microscopy of a glomerulus from a nephrectomy shows bright linear staining of the glomerular basement membrane, typical of anti-GBM nephritis. C3, C4d, kappa, and lambda light chains showed similar staining patterns. *(Right)* Electron micrograph of a glomerulus shows evidence of past injury of the GBM, where it appears thin and disrupted ➡, probably a site of past rupture and ongoing repair. This is a feature of crescentic glomerulonephritis of any cause.

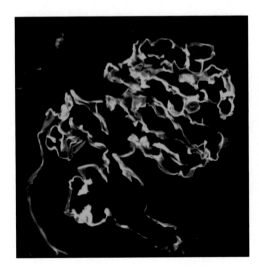
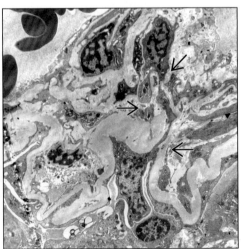

ANTI-GBM DISEASE IN ALPORT SYNDROME

Ancillary Techniques

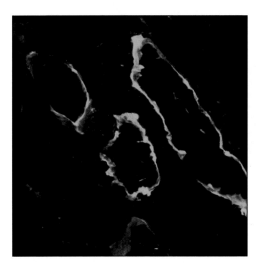

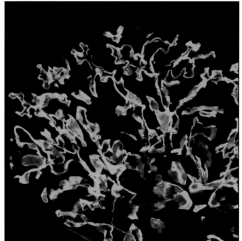

(Left) Immunofluorescence microscopy from a prior biopsy shows focal linear staining of the tubular basement membranes. Anti-GBM antibodies typically stain α-5 chains of type IV collagen, normally expressed in the distal tubules. *(Right)* Immunofluorescence microscopy of a glomerulus with de novo anti-GBM disease shows bright linear staining of the GBM for IgG. The excess IgG staining vs. albumin is typical of anti-GBM nephritis.

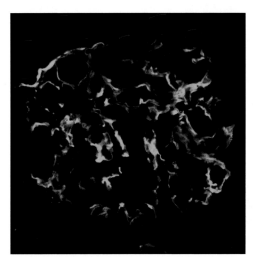

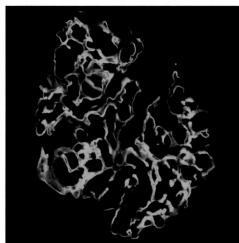

(Left) Immunofluorescence microscopy for C3 of the same patient shows interrupted linear GBM staining that is less intense than IgG, which is not an uncommon finding in anti-GBM nephritis. *(Right)* Immunofluorescence microscopy of the nephrectomy for C4d shows bright linear staining of the GBMs, which is distinct from the deposits of C4d in the mesangium of normal glomeruli. No staining of peritubular capillaries for C4d was seen.

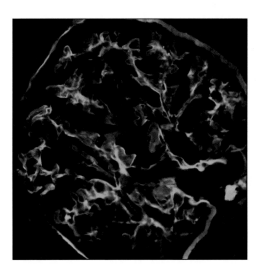

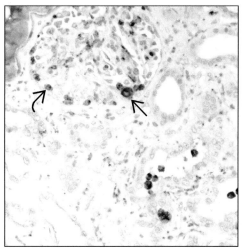

(Left) Immunofluorescence microscopy of a glomerulus shows weak linear staining for albumin, less intense than that for IgG when photographed at the same exposure. *(Right)* CD68 stains of a glomerulus with de novo anti-GBM disease shows CD68-positive cells in Bowman space consisting of macrophages ⇾ and neutrophils ⇗. Macrophages are a common component of cellular crescents in addition to parietal epithelial cells.

HYPERPERFUSION INJURY

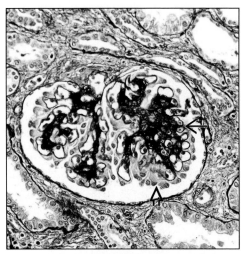

Jones methenamine silver stain shows mesangial sclerosis ➡ with prominence of the adjacent visceral epithelial cells ➢. (Courtesy T. Nadasdy, MD.)

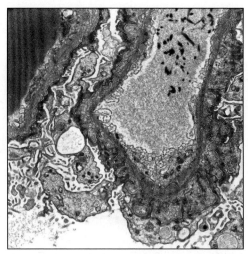

Electron micrograph shows prominent lamellation and splitting of the GBM with diffuse effacement of the overlying podocyte foot processes. (Courtesy T. Nadasdy, MD.)

TERMINOLOGY

Synonyms
- Hyperfiltration injury

Definitions
- Acute and chronic glomerular injury caused by transplantation of very young pediatric kidneys into adult recipients

ETIOLOGY/PATHOGENESIS

Hyperperfusion Injury
- 10% of pediatric kidneys (< 10 years of age) develop hyperperfusion injury when transplanted into adult recipients
  - Infant kidneys (< 1 year of age) more susceptible
  - En bloc (2 kidneys) transplantation may be less susceptible
- Possible contributing factors
  - Greater blood volume in adults compared with children
  - Higher systemic blood pressure in adults compared with children
  - Smaller glomeruli in children compared to adults
  - Thinner glomerular basement membrane (GBM) in children compared to adults
    - GBM thickness reaches maximum thickness at age 12-13
  - Altered composition of α chains of collagen IV in pediatric glomeruli
    - Embryonic GBM consists of α-1 and α-2 chains of collagen IV, gradually replaced by α-3, α-4, and α-5 chains as glomerulus matures

CLINICAL ISSUES

Epidemiology
- Incidence
  - Rare

Presentation
- Renal dysfunction
- Proteinuria
  - Often nephrotic range
- May develop as early as 10 weeks after transplantation

Laboratory Tests
- None
  - Kidney biopsy with electron microscopy is only method to establish this diagnosis

Treatment
- None

Prognosis
- Poor
  - Infant donor kidneys often fail within 1 year of transplantation

MICROSCOPIC PATHOLOGY

Histologic Features
- Global &/or segmental glomerulosclerosis
  - Variable diffuse mesangial sclerosis
- Diffuse lamellation and splitting of glomerular basement membranes seen by electron microscopy (EM)
  - Foot process effacement and microvillous transformation of podocytes
- Indirect IF for α-3 and α-5 chains of collagen IV demonstrates strong linear staining of GBM (normal)
- Interstitial fibrosis and tubular atrophy

HYPERPERFUSION INJURY

Key Facts

Etiology/Pathogenesis
- 10% of pediatric kidneys (< 10 years of age) develop this injury
- Higher blood volume and systemic blood pressure in adults compared with children
- Smaller glomeruli and thinner glomerular basement membrane thickness in children compared to adults

Clinical Issues
- Renal dysfunction
- Proteinuria

Microscopic Pathology
- Global &/or segmental glomerulosclerosis
- Variable diffuse mesangial sclerosis
- Diffuse lamellation and splitting of GBMs seen by EM

Top Differential Diagnoses
- Alport syndrome
- Recurrent focal segmental glomerulosclerosis

DIFFERENTIAL DIAGNOSIS

Alport Syndrome
- Full thickness diffuse lamellation and splitting of GBM with no normal GBM by EM
- Indirect IF shows absence of GBM α-3 &/or α-5 chains of collagen IV
- Extensive donor work-up minimizes this clinical scenario

Recurrent Focal Segmental Glomerulosclerosis
- Normal GBM by EM
- History of primary focal segmental glomerulosclerosis as original native renal disease

DIAGNOSTIC CHECKLIST

Pathologic Interpretation Pearls
- Clinical information of kidney donor is necessary to raise diagnostic consideration of hyperperfusion injury
- EM is essential for diagnosis
- Without EM finding of GBM alterations, light microscopy (LM) features with glomerular and tubulointerstitial scarring is nonspecific

SELECTED REFERENCES

1. Mohanka R et al: Single versus en bloc kidney transplantation from pediatric donors less than or equal to 15 kg. Transplantation. 86(2):264-8, 2008
2. Keitel E et al: Results of en bloc renal transplants of pediatric deceased donors into adult recipients. Transplant Proc. 39(2):441-2, 2007
3. Mahdavi R et al: En bloc kidney transplantation from pediatric cadaveric donors to adult recipients. Urol J. 3(2):82-6, 2006
4. El-Sabrout R et al: Outcome of renal transplants from pediatric donors <5 yr of age. Clin Transplant. 19(3):316-20, 2005
5. Borboroglu PG et al: Solitary renal allografts from pediatric cadaver donors less than 2 years of age transplanted into adult recipients. Transplantation. 77(5):698-702, 2004
6. Nadasdy T et al: Diffuse glomerular basement membrane lamellation in renal allografts from pediatric donors to adult recipients. Am J Surg Pathol. 23(4):437-42, 1999
7. Ratner LE et al: Transplantation of single and paired pediatric kidneys into adult recipients. J Am Coll Surg. 185(5):437-45, 1997
8. Satterthwaite R et al: Outcome of en bloc and single kidney transplantation from very young cadaveric donors. Transplantation. 63(10):1405-10, 1997
9. Hayes JM et al: The development of proteinuria and focal-segmental glomerulosclerosis in recipients of pediatric donor kidneys. Transplantation. 52(5):813-7, 1991
10. Truong LD et al: Electron microscopic study of an unusual posttransplant glomerular lesion. Arch Pathol Lab Med. 115(4):382-5, 1991

IMAGE GALLERY

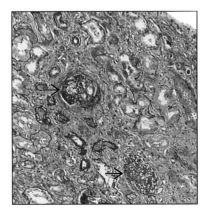 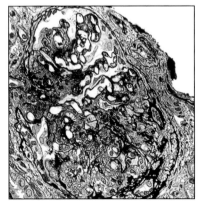 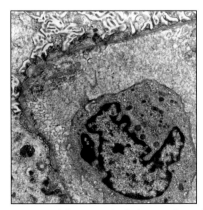

(Left) Periodic acid-Schiff shows 2 globally sclerotic glomeruli ➡ surrounded by severe and diffuse interstitial fibrosis and tubular atrophy in this pediatric kidney allograft. (Courtesy T. Nadasdy, MD.) *(Center)* Jones methenamine silver stain shows a segmentally sclerotic glomerulus with accumulation of the matrix, loss of capillary lumina, and fibrous adhesions to Bowman capsule. (Courtesy T. Nadasdy, MD.) *(Right)* Electron micrograph shows extensive thinning and focal splitting along this segment of the GBM. (Courtesy T. Nadasdy, MD.)

ACUTE ALLOGRAFT ISCHEMIA

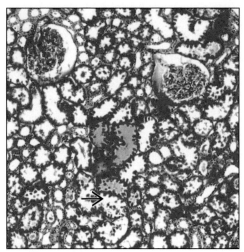

A low-power view shows a kidney with ischemic injury, possessing dilated tubules & epithelial injury in a hobnail pattern ➡.

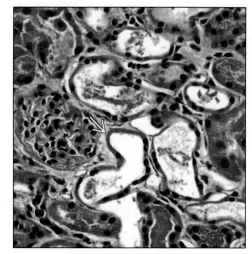

In a deceased donor renal allograft with oliguria on day 2, there is acute tubular injury with marked tubular cytoplasmic thinning, cellular loss, and debris, showing loss of tubular nuclei ➡.

TERMINOLOGY

Synonyms
- Acute tubular injury (ATI)
- Acute tubular necrosis (ATN)
- Ischemia-reperfusion injury (IRI)

Definitions
- Ischemic graft injury in early post-transplant period
- Delayed graft function (DGF): Requires transient dialysis post transplant
- Primary nonfunction (PNF): Graft never functions

ETIOLOGY/PATHOGENESIS

Acute Ischemic Injury
- Decreased oxygen delivery/perfusion
  - Risk higher with increased warm (> 40 min) and cold (> 24 hour) ischemia times
  - May occur in donor before harvest or during harvesting or preservation
- NK- and T-cells produce mediators such as IFN-γ leading to upregulation of adhesion molecules
  - May explain increased rejection risk after DGF
- Complement activation
  - Colocalization of mannose binding lectins (MBL) with complement in IRI
  - Complement regulators reduce IRI damage in animals
- Calcineurin inhibitor toxicity may augment ATI
- Compromised vascular anastomosis
- Renal artery dissection

CLINICAL ISSUES

Epidemiology
- Incidence

  - DGF in 2-25% of deceased donor grafts and PNF in 1-2%; varies with center
  - Asystolic donors have higher rate of DGF (19-84%) and PNF (4-18%)
  - Higher risk from deceased cardiac death (DCD) donors as opposed to heart-beating donation after brain death (DBD)

Treatment
- Transient dialysis
- Reduce calcineurin inhibitors
- Complement inhibitors under investigation

Prognosis
- 95-98% of grafts with DGF recover
  - DGF typically lasts 10-15 days; < 2% last more than 4 weeks
- DGF associated with increased incidence of acute rejection and later fibrosis

MACROSCOPIC FEATURES

General Features
- Blotchy, mottled appearance with darker areas that are poorly perfused

MICROSCOPIC PATHOLOGY

Histologic Features
- Tubules
  - Loss of brush border, thinning, dilation, loss of nuclei, particularly in the proximal tubules
    - Nonisometric tubular cell vacuolization
    - Intratubular cellular debris and neutrophils
    - In severe cases, there is bare tubular basement membrane (TBM) from desquamation of tubular epithelial cells ("nonreplacement phenomenon")
  - Regeneration features (later): Basophilic cytoplasm, prominent nucleoli, mitosis

ACUTE ALLOGRAFT ISCHEMIA

Key Facts

Etiology/Pathogenesis

- Higher risk from deceased cardiac death (DCD) donors as opposed to heart-beating donation after brain death (DBD)
- Glomerular and other microvascular injury through various mediators and complement activation
- Anastomotic site complications and other causes of ischemia such as poor preservation

Clinical Issues

- 95-98% of grafts with DGF recover
- Rejection risk increased
- Drug toxicity (e.g., calcineurin inhibitors) a compounding factor

Microscopic Pathology

- ATI with tubular epithelial cell flattening, vacuolization, and mitoses
- Glomerular injury with variable intracapillary endothelial swelling, neutrophils, and fibrin thrombi
- Interstitial edema and minimal inflammation
- Medullary vessels dilated and filled with mononuclear cells, erythrocytes, and neutrophils

Top Differential Diagnoses

- Calcineurin inhibitor toxicity
- Acute cellular or humoral rejection
- Acute obstruction

Diagnostic Checklist

- Biopsy necessary to determine cause (e.g., rejection vs. ischemia) and recommended after 10 days of DGF

- Interstitium
  - Edema and minimal inflammation with a few neutrophils and mononuclear cells
- Vessels
  - Dilated medullary vessels filled with mononuclear cells and erythroid precursors
  - Negative C4d in peritubular capillaries
  - Arteries unaffected
- Glomeruli variably affected
  - Endothelial swelling and vacuolization, capillary collapse
  - Neutrophils correlate with cold ischemia time and subsequent graft loss
  - Fibrin thrombi do not affect overall outcome

ANCILLARY TESTS

Immunohistochemistry

- Markers of proliferation positive in tubular cells (PCNA, Ki-67)

DIFFERENTIAL DIAGNOSIS

Calcineurin Inhibitor Toxicity (CNIT)

- Difficult to distinguish on histologic grounds alone
- Classically, isometric vacuolization plus ATI
- Associated with high levels of CNI

Acute Humoral Rejection (AHR)

- AHR can present as ATI
- C4d deposition positive in peritubular capillaries
- Donor-specific antibody (DSA) assays positive in > 90%

Acute Cellular Rejection (ACR)

- Interstitial mononuclear inflammation, tubulitis, &/or endarteritis

Pyelonephritis

- Neutrophil casts abundant and densely packed
- Microabscesses in interstitium
- Positive urine cultures

Acute Obstruction

- Collection ducts dilated
- Little tubular necrosis
- Tamm-Horsfall protein in lymphatics

DIAGNOSTIC CHECKLIST

Pathologic Interpretation Pearls

- Biopsy necessary to determine cause (e.g., rejection vs. ischemia) and recommended after 10 days of DGF

SELECTED REFERENCES

1. Colvin RB et al: Renal transplant pathology. In Jennette JC et al: Heptinstall's Pathology of the Kidney. 6th ed. Philadelphia: Lippincott Williams & Wilkins. 1347-1490, 2007
2. Burne-Taney MJ et al: Persistent renal and extrarenal immune changes after severe ischemic injury. Kidney Int. 67(3):1002-9, 2005
3. Keizer KM et al: Non-heart-beating donor kidneys in the Netherlands: allocation and outcome of transplantation. Transplantation. 79(9):1195-9, 2005
4. Basile DP: Rarefaction of peritubular capillaries following ischemic acute renal failure: a potential factor predisposing to progressive nephropathy. Curr Opin Nephrol Hypertens. 13(1):1-7, 2004
5. de Vries B et al: The mannose-binding lectin-pathway is involved in complement activation in the course of renal ischemia-reperfusion injury. Am J Pathol. 165(5):1677-88, 2004
6. Perico N et al: Delayed graft function in kidney transplantation. Lancet. 364(9447):1814-27, 2004
7. Nadasdy T et al: Human acute tubular necrosis: a lectin and immunohistochemical study. Hum Pathol. 26(2):230-9, 1995
8. Olsen S et al: Primary acute renal failure ("acute tubular necrosis") in the transplanted kidney: morphology and pathogenesis. Medicine (Baltimore). 68(3):173-87, 1989
9. Rohr MS: Renal allograft acute tubular necrosis. II. A light and electron microscopic study of biopsies taken at procurement and after revascularization. Ann Surg. 197(6):663-71, 1983

ACUTE ALLOGRAFT ISCHEMIA

Microscopic Features

(Left) High-power view shows a focus of interstitial inflammation ➡ amid tubules with varying degrees of injury. *(Right)* A trichrome stain shows fibrinous clot material ➡ in a glomerulus, a finding that can be observed in acute allograft ischemia or other causes of TMA.

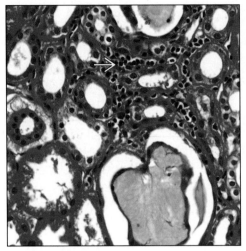
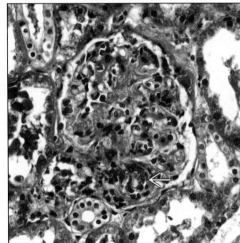

(Left) In this case of acute allograft ischemia, a trichrome stain shows focal edema ➡, naked basement membranes ➡, and hobnailed tubular epithelial cells ➡. *(Right)* Even at low power, injured epithelium with a hobnail pattern ➡ and focal epithelial loss ➡ can be appreciated in this case of acute allograft ischemia (trichrome stain). There is only a thin connective tissue framework between tubules, confirming the lack of appreciable fibrosis.

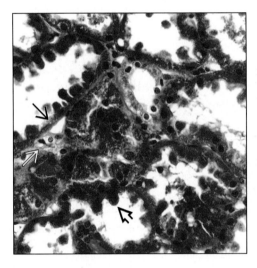
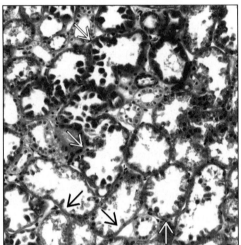

(Left) This H&E of a section taken close to the renal pelvis demonstrates an inflammatory infiltrate, including neutrophils ➡, and adjacent injured tubular epithelium with nuclear loss ➡. *(Right)* Acute tubular injury in a renal allograft with delayed graft function day 5 shows frequent tubular nuclei that stain for Ki-67, a marker of proliferating cells ➡. One study showed that, on average, about 8% of the tubular cells are positive, higher than in native kidney ATI (4%).

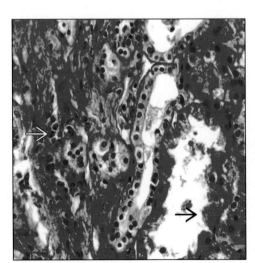
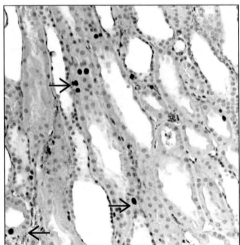

Variant Microscopic Features

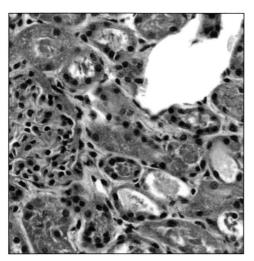

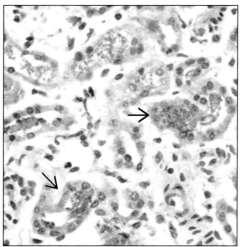

(Left) Renal biopsy for DGF 2 days post transplant. The donor was a 2 year old who died from trauma. Acute tubular injury is present with prominent eosinophilic granular casts, which stained for myoglobin; thus, this is renal failure due to rhabdomyolysis. *(Right)* Renal biopsy for DGF 2 days post transplant. The donor was a 2 year old who died from trauma. Many of the tubular granular casts stain for myoglobin ➡; thus, this is renal failure due to rhabdomyolysis.

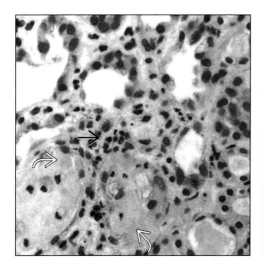

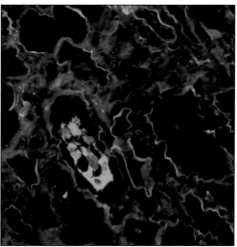

(Left) Asystolic donor transplant biopsy for DGF at day 10. Severe tubular necrosis ➡ is present with neutrophils in the interstitium ➡ & tubules, resembling acute humoral rejection. However, the C4d stain was negative, & the patient recovered graft function. *(Right)* Asystolic donor transplant biopsy for DGF at day 10 shows severe tubular necrosis with neutrophils, resembling acute humoral rejection. However, C4d is negative except for weak staining of necrotic cells in tubules.

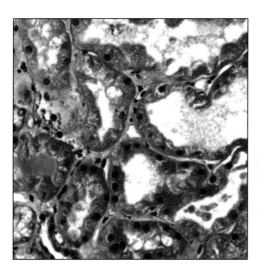

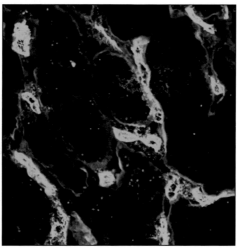

(Left) This renal allograft reveals acute tubular injury with little inflammation, suggesting ischemic injury. However, the C4d stain was positive in the peritubular capillaries and the recipient had anti-donor HLA antibodies, meeting criteria for acute humoral rejection. *(Right)* The C4d stain is positive in the peritubular capillaries in this day 9 biopsy for oliguria in a renal transplant patient who had anti-donor HLA antibodies, meeting criteria of acute humoral rejection.

URINE LEAK

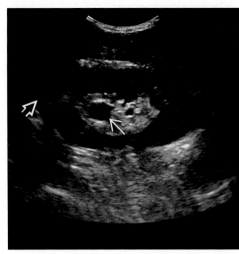

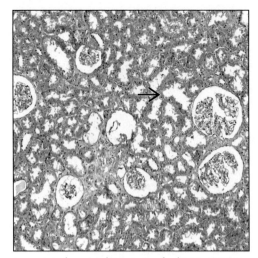

Ultrasound image 7 days post transplant of a graft that developed a urine leak. A collection of perinephric fluid ➡ is seen along 1 pole. The dilated pelvis ➡ is a sign of obstruction.

Low-power hematoxylin & eosin of a biopsy specimen from a patient with urine leak shows irregular, dilated renal tubules ➡ with mild tubular injury.

TERMINOLOGY

Definitions
- Urine collection due to numerous causes, often as anastomotic "leak" in setting of transplantation

ETIOLOGY/PATHOGENESIS

Dysfunctional Anastomosis
- Dysfunctional anastomosis may cause reflux/leakage
- Surgical technical error may be cause
  - Misplacement of ureteral sutures (often at ureterovesical location)
  - Insufficient ureteral length
  - Ureter or renal pelvis laceration
  - Often becomes evident within 24 hours

Ureteral Ischemic Injury
- Risk of proximal ureter devascularization since renal pelvic vessels provide its blood supply
- Ureter ischemic more distally from kidney
- Renal pelvis allograft placement allows minimal length of transplant ureter
  - Special techniques: "Psoas hitch," Boari flap, ureteroureterostomy, pyelovesicostomy, and ileal ureter
- Lowest risk when "golden triangle" of perirenal fat bordered by ureter and lower renal pole is preserved
- Ischemic necrosis leaks usually occur within 1st 14 days after transplantation

Rejection Episodes
- With transplant endarteritis, may involve ureteral graft vessels

Laparoscopic Technique
- Laparoscopic living donor procurement initially associated with high incidence
- Complication rate now lower (almost as good as open donors)

CLINICAL ISSUES

Epidemiology
- Incidence
  - 1-15% of renal transplant recipients have urologic complications
    - e.g., large study with 6.8% of 1,183 renal transplants
  - 1-3% of renal transplant recipients have ureteral leak

Site
- Renal calyx, bladder, or ureter

Presentation
- Oliguria
  - Sudden decrease in urinary output
- Hematuria
- Urinary fistula
  - May result from necrosis of distal ureter
- Creatinine (Cr) and plasma urea increase
  - Due to solute resorption across peritoneum
- Scrotal swelling
- Wound drain
  - Fluid seepage with Cr several times current serum Cr
  - Difficult to determine if fluid production is from preexisting seroma or lymph draining

Laboratory Tests
- Provided good renal excretory function, Cr concentration in leak fluid exceeds plasma Cr

Natural History
- Postoperative period: 1st 4 months (84%)

Treatment
- Surgical approaches
  - Percutaneous nephrostomy
  - Dilatation/stent placement
  - Urgent surgical exploration/reanastomosis
  - Endoscopic methods

URINE LEAK

Key Facts

Etiology/Pathogenesis
- Dysfunctional ureterovesical anastomosis, ischemic injury, or rejection episodes

Clinical Issues
- ~ 1% of renal transplants
- Presentation in postoperative period: 4 months (84%)
  - Hematuria, renal dysfunction, and fistulas

Image Findings
- Radiology may demonstrate fluid leak (urinoma)

Microscopic Pathology
- Interstitial inflammation and tubular injury may be present
- Vascular thrombosis of periureteral vessels (80%)
  - Productive CMV (15%) or BK virus (98%) infection

  - 3-way Foley catheter with irrigation that can intermittently fill and empty bladder

Prognosis
- Does not typically impact 10-year patient or graft survival

IMAGE FINDINGS

General Features
- Ultrasound shows fluid collection but not its source
- Renal scintigraphy tracer urinary extravasation
- Antegrade pyelograph may allow leak localization

MACROSCOPIC FEATURES

General Features
- Fluid leak (urinoma) may be appreciated

MICROSCOPIC PATHOLOGY

Histologic Features
- Limited data on histopathologic changes
  - Renal parenchymal interstitial inflammation and tubular injury may be present
  - Inflammation in surrounding soft tissue
  - Edema in renal parenchyma and in soft tissue surrounding urine leak

- In a study of 25 surgically removed, necrotic, ureteral segments
  - Vascular thrombosis of periureteral vessels (80%), productive CMV (15%), or BK virus (8%)

DIFFERENTIAL DIAGNOSIS

Lymphocele
- Cr and potassium concentrations lower and sodium concentration higher

SELECTED REFERENCES

1. Shoskes D et al: Urological complications after kidney transplantation. In Morris PJ et al: Kidney Transplantation: Principles and Practice. 6th ed. Philadelphia: Saunders Elsevier. 462-468, 2008
2. Colvin RB et al: Renal transplant pathology. In Jennette JC et al: Heptinstall's Pathology of the Kidney. 6th ed. Philadelphia: Lippincott Williams & Wilkins. 1347-1490, 2007
3. Wieczorek G et al: Acute and chronic vascular rejection in nonhuman primate kidney transplantation. Am J Transplant. 6(6):1285-96, 2006
4. Karam G et al: Ureteral necrosis after kidney transplantation: risk factors and impact on graft and patient survival. Transplantation. 78(5):725-9, 2004
5. Jefferson RH et al: Urological evaluation of adult renal transplant recipients. J Urol. 153(3 Pt 1):615-8, 1995
6. Hakim NS et al: Complications of ureterovesical anastomosis in kidney transplant patients: the Minnesota experience. Clin Transplant. 8(6):504-7, 1994

IMAGE GALLERY

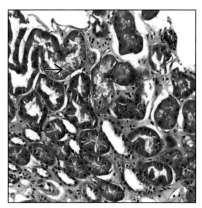 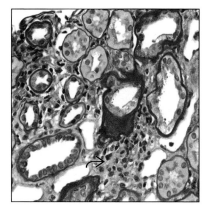 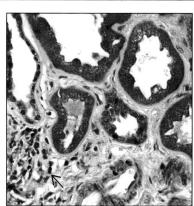

(Left) Medium power of a biopsy specimen from a patient with urine leak shows focal nuclear loss ⇨ and tubular irregularities, both of which are findings of mild tubular injury. (Center) Medium power of a PAS stain in a case of urine leak shows a focal lymphoid infiltrate ⇨. (Right) Medium-power trichome shows a focal lymphoid infiltrate ⇨ amidst an edematous stroma and irregular tubules in a urine leak (trichrome stain).

LYMPHOCELE

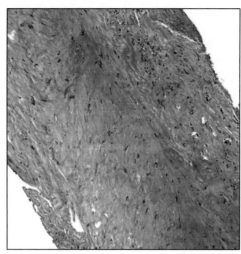

Light microscopy of a lymphocele wall shows that it is composed of fibrous tissue with a focus of mononuclear chronic inflammatory cells.

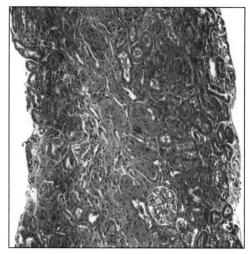

A kidney biopsy at low power shows a minimal focal interstitial inflammation and tubular injury in a case with a lymphocele.

TERMINOLOGY

Definitions
- Collection of lymphatic fluid in nonepithelialized cavity in the perinephric space, typically in the postoperative field

ETIOLOGY/PATHOGENESIS

Incomplete Lymphatic Anastomoses
- Donor renal lymphatics at hilum fail to anastomose with recipient lymphatics
- Normally lymphatics spontaneously reconnect
- Normal sheep kidney makes ~ 0.5-3 mL/hr of lymph, transplanted kidney makes much more (~ 16 mL/hr)
- Careful surgical ligation of lymphatic vessels is necessary to prevent lymphocele formation

Rejection Episodes
- Lead to increased vascular permeability, edema, lymph fluid, and promote lymphocele formation

CLINICAL ISSUES

Epidemiology
- Incidence
  o Large series indicated incidence is around 2%
    ▪ 2-11 years post-transplantation
    ▪ 1/3 had rejection episodes
    ▪ Another series revealed that some lymphoceles are subclinical and indicated 35/386 (9%) of renal transplant recipients → lymphoceles > 50 mL detected on ultrasound
  o 34% of recipients with lymphoceles > 2.5 cm in diameter
    ▪ Higher in patients on rapamycin (45%)
    ▪ May require surgical intervention (16%)
    ▪ Frequency of symptomatic lymphoceles much lower (~ 3-4%)
  o Obesity a risk factor

Presentation
- Infection
  o If large, can lead to obstruction and infectious complications

Treatment
- Surgical approaches
  o Laparoscopic or open drainage
- Ultrasound-guided or CT-guided drainage

Prognosis
- 5-10% recur but does not affect graft survival

IMAGE FINDINGS

Ultrasonographic Findings
- Most are small and detected only on ultrasound
- Some are large and may be multilocular or multiple in number
- Hydronephrosis with dilated calyces due to obstruction of ureter may be present

MACROSCOPIC FEATURES

General Features
- Perinephric nonsanguinous and nonpurulent fluid collection

MICROSCOPIC PATHOLOGY

Histologic Features
- Typically fibrous tissue with internal cystic formation with inflammatory cells in wall
- Predominantly composed of mononuclear lymphoid cells

LYMPHOCELE

Key Facts

Terminology
- Collections of lymphatic fluid in perinephric space

Etiology/Pathogenesis
- Incomplete lymphatic anastomosis
- Rejection
- Normally lymphatics spontaneously reconnect

Clinical Issues
- Around 34% of transplant patients have clinically significant lymphocele

Diagnostic Checklist
- Consider lymphocele when no obvious change in biopsy accounts for renal transplant dysfunction
  - Particularly when obstructive features are seen
  - Microscopic features include chronic inflammation, edema, and dilated lymphatics

- Renal biopsy may show changes of obstruction
  - Collecting duct dilation
  - Interstitial edema
  - Dilation of lymphatics, present normally along larger vessels
  - Mild interstitial mononuclear inflammation (borderline)
- Microscopic pathologic descriptions are limited

Predominant Pattern/Injury Type
- Inflammatory

DIFFERENTIAL DIAGNOSIS

Abscess
- High numbers of neutrophils are appreciated on aspirate samples
- Cultures of aspirates useful

Hematoma
- Occur earlier, often in immediate postsurgical period

Urine Leak
- Has higher creatinine and potassium concentration and lower sodium concentration

DIAGNOSTIC CHECKLIST

Pathologic Interpretation Pearls
- Lymphocele should be considered when no obvious change in biopsy accounts for renal transplant dysfunction
  - Particularly when obstructive features are seen

SELECTED REFERENCES

1. Colvin RB et al: Renal Transplant Pathology. In Jennette JC et al: Heptinstall's Pathology of the Kidney. 6th ed. Philadelphia: Lippincott Williams & Wilkins. 1347-1490, 2007
2. Król R et al: Did volume of lymphocele after kidney transplantation determine the choice of treatment modality? Transplant Proc. 39(9):2740-3, 2007
3. Friedewald SM et al: Vascular and nonvascular complications of renal transplants: sonographic evaluation and correlation with other imaging modalities, surgery, and pathology. J Clin Ultrasound. 33(3):127-39, 2005
4. Goel M et al: The influence of various maintenance immunosuppressive drugs on lymphocele formation and treatment after kidney transplantation. J Urol. 171(5):1788-92, 2004
5. Bailey SH et al: Laparoscopic treatment of post renal transplant lymphoceles. Surg Endosc. 17(12):1896-9, 2003

IMAGE GALLERY

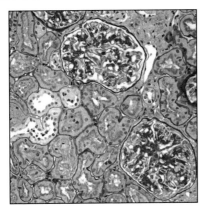 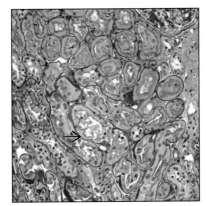 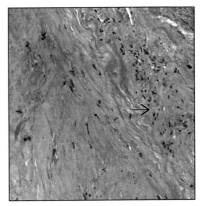

(Left) A medium-power image shows largely unremarkable glomeruli in a case with a lymphocele. *(Center)* The tubules show focal epithelial flattening and nuclear loss ➡, consistent with a mild tubular injury in a lymphocele case. *(Right)* Higher power examination of the lymphocele wall shows that the fibrous tissue lining has focal chronic inflammation ➡.

RENAL ARTERY OR VEIN THROMBOSIS

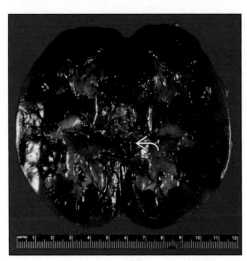

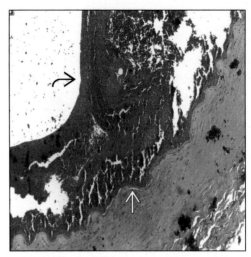

Thrombosis of the renal vein ➔ 2 days post living donor transplant. The cortex is congested. Arterial thrombosis developed hours post transplant. Despite an arterial thrombectomy, RVT ensued.

An acute thrombus ➔ is attached to the internal elastic lamina ➔ of the renal artery with loss of endothelium. No inflammation is evident, in contrast to acute humoral or cellular rejection.

TERMINOLOGY

Abbreviations
- Renal vein thrombosis (RVT)
- Renal artery thrombosis (RAT)

Definitions
- Thrombosis of renal artery or vein

ETIOLOGY/PATHOGENESIS

Surgical Technical Problems
- Intimal injury during procurement
- Difficult anastomosis
- Stenosis of anastomosis
- Trauma to vessels with dissection
- Narrow, twisted, or compressed renal vein

Hypercoagulable State
- Antiphospholipid antibody syndrome
- Nephrotic syndrome
- Factor V Leiden mutation

Risk Factors
- Multiple arteries
  - Especially if accessory artery supplies lower pole or ureter
- Placement of graft on left side

CLINICAL ISSUES

Epidemiology
- Incidence
  - Prevalence highly variable by center
    - Primary arterial thrombosis: 0.4-1.9%
    - Primary venous thrombosis: 0.7-3.4%
  - Arterial thrombosis usually occurs within 30 days of transplant
  - RVT early or late

Site
- Hilar vessels
  - Intraparenchymal arteries and glomeruli are spared
- May extend into inferior vena cava

Presentation
- Macrohematuria
- Proteinuria
- Acute renal failure
- Anuria
  - Sudden decrease in urine output may result from both RVT and RAT
- Pain in transplant
- Graft swelling

Treatment
- Surgical approaches
  - Thrombectomy
  - Revision of anastomosis
- Drugs
  - Thrombolytics
  - Anticoagulation

Prognosis
- Usually causes graft loss
- Early treatment essential

IMAGE FINDINGS

Radiographic Findings
- Angiography demonstrates thrombosis and loss of cortical perfusion, usually wedge-shaped

Ultrasonographic Findings
- Doppler ultrasound may demonstrate thrombus and absent flow
- Renal vein thrombosis
  - Diastolic reversal of flow in renal artery
  - Kidney may be enlarged with surrounding blood

RENAL ARTERY OR VEIN THROMBOSIS

Key Facts

Etiology/Pathogenesis
- Anastomotic problems
- Multiple arteries
- Hypercoagulability

Clinical Issues
- Macrohematuria
- Acute renal failure
- Prevalence highly variable by center
- Early treatment essential

Microscopic Pathology
- Thrombosis in vessel lumina
- Loss of endothelium
- Infarction of cortex
- Sparse neutrophils in capillaries
- Recanalization if chronic

Diagnostic Checklist
- C4d(-) in peritubular capillaries

MACROSCOPIC FEATURES

General Features
- RVT: Engorged and purple
- RAT: Pale, infarcted

MICROSCOPIC PATHOLOGY

Histologic Features
- Arterial thrombosis
  - Loss of endothelium
  - Adherence of platelets
  - Dissection of media
  - Infarction of cortex
  - Recanalization if chronic
- Venous thrombosis
  - Loss of endothelium
  - Adherence of platelets
  - Recanalization if chronic
- Cortex
  - Neutrophils peritubular and glomerular capillaries
  - Edema
  - Congestion

DIFFERENTIAL DIAGNOSIS

Hyperacute and Acute Humoral Rejection
- Usually more neutrophils
- C4d(+) in peritubular capillaries

- Usually no large vessel thrombosis

Acute Cellular Rejection
- Endothelial mononuclear inflammation

DIAGNOSTIC CHECKLIST

Pathologic Interpretation Pearls
- C4d(-) in peritubular capillaries

SELECTED REFERENCES

1. Colvin RB et al: Renal Transplant Pathology. In Jennette JC et al: Heptinstall's Pathology of the Kidney. 6th ed. Philadelphia: Lippincott Williams & Wilkins. 1347-1490, 2007
2. Aschwanden M et al: Renal vein thrombosis after renal transplantation--early diagnosis by duplex sonography prevented fatal outcome. Nephrol Dial Transplant. 21(3):825-6, 2006
3. Osman Y et al: Vascular complications after live donor renal transplantation: study of risk factors and effects on graft and patient survival. J Urol. 169(3):859-62, 2003
4. Bakir N et al: Primary renal graft thrombosis. Nephrol Dial Transplant. 11(1):140-7, 1996

IMAGE GALLERY

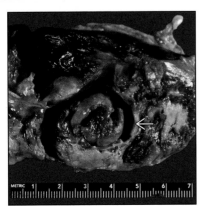 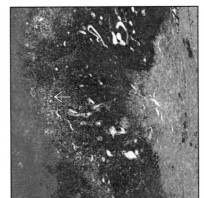 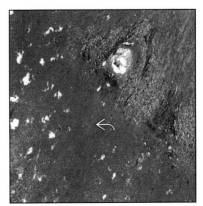

(Left) This nephrectomy of a long-term renal allograft has a chronic renal vein thrombosis ➡. *(Center)* Granulation tissue ➡ is growing into a renal vein thrombosis, indicating that the thrombus is longstanding. *(Right)* The renal parenchyma is hemorrhagic and infarcted ➡.

8

TRANSPLANT RENAL ARTERY STENOSIS

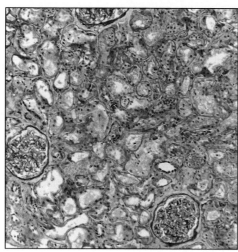

A renal biopsy from a patient with intermittent renal artery stenosis 5 months after renal transplantation shows thinning of the tubules with PAS(+) brush border loss, typical of an acute tubular injury.

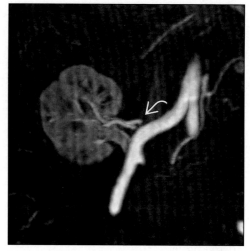

Magnetic resonance angiography shows stenosis ➔ of a donor renal artery at the site of anastomosis in an allograft due to atherosclerosis. A biopsy showed cholesterol emboli and mild tubular atrophy.

TERMINOLOGY

Abbreviations
- Transplant renal artery stenosis (TRAS)

Definitions
- Post-transplant stenosis of major renal arteries, typically causing refractory hypertension due to increased renin production

ETIOLOGY/PATHOGENESIS

Surgical Complication
- Subintimal dissection or flap created at harvest or reanastomosis
- Kinking or twisting of renal artery at transplantation
- End-to-side anastomoses are higher risk than end-to-end anastomoses

Donor Artery Atherosclerosis
- Can be complicated by atherosclerosis in recipient
- Must be distinguished from de novo atherosclerosis and chronic transplant arteriopathy

Chronic Transplant Arteriopathy
- Typically diffuse stenosis
- Episodes of acute rejection more common in recipients with TRAS

CLINICAL ISSUES

Epidemiology
- Incidence
  - Clinically significant in 1-5% of recipients
    - As high as 23% if milder cases are included
  - Most common vascular complication after kidney transplantation

Presentation
- Delayed graft function
- Hypertension
  - Typically refractory to drugs
- Bruit over transplanted kidney
- Renal dysfunction
  - Progressive deterioration
  - May be intermittent

Natural History
- Usually presents 3-24 months after transplantation

Treatment
- Surgical approaches
  - Percutaneous transluminal angioplasty
    - ± stent
  - Saphenous vein or recipient iliac artery grafts
  - Revision of anastomosis

Prognosis
- Percutaneous transluminal angioplasty restenosis rate is 10-60%
- Surgical correction is difficult; graft loss ~ 20%

IMAGE FINDINGS

Ultrasonographic Findings
- Color flow duplex ultrasound reveals flow abnormalities
  - Stenosis may be incidental finding without hypertension or graft dysfunction

MACROSCOPIC FEATURES

General Features
- Stenosis usually occurs near renal-iliac artery anastomosis
- Uniform atrophy

TRANSPLANT RENAL ARTERY STENOSIS

Key Facts

Terminology
- Post-transplant stenosis of major renal arteries, typically causing refractory hypertension due to increased renin production
- Caused by atherosclerosis, intimal flap, kinking, and chronic rejection

Microscopic Pathology
- Cholesterol emboli may be present if stenosis is due to atheroma

- Tubular atrophy with little fibrosis is typical pattern
- Acute tubular injury if acute or intermittent stenosis

Top Differential Diagnoses
- Calcineurin inhibitor toxicity
- Obstruction

Diagnostic Checklist
- Histologic findings bland, subtle, and nonspecific
- Diagnosis easily missed
- Cholesterol emboli provides clue

MICROSCOPIC PATHOLOGY

Histologic Features
- Renal-iliac artery anastomosis
  - Rarely sampled for histology
  - Atherosclerosis
  - Medial dissection
  - Intimal flap
  - Intimal hyperplasia with inflammation (allograft arteriopathy)
- Transplant kidney
  - Tubular atrophy with little fibrosis if stenosis is chronic
  - Acute tubular injury may occur if stenosis is intermittent
  - May have prominent juxtaglomerular apparati
  - Cholesterol emboli may be present if stenosis is due to atheroma
  - Normal glomeruli, arteries and arterioles

Predominant Cell/Compartment Type
- Renal artery, extrarenal
  - Stenosis of renal artery with secondary effects on tubules and glomeruli

DIFFERENTIAL DIAGNOSIS

Calcineurin Inhibitor Toxicity
- Arteriolar hyalinosis
- Isometric tubular vacuolization

Obstruction
- Collecting duct dilation
- Dilated lymphatics
- Leakage of Tamm-Horsfall protein into interstitium

DIAGNOSTIC CHECKLIST

Pathologic Interpretation Pearls
- Histologic findings bland, subtle, and nonspecific
- Diagnosis easily missed
- Acute tubular injury
- Cholesterol emboli provides clue

SELECTED REFERENCES

1. Allen R.D.M. et al: Vascular Complications after Kidney Transplantation. In Morris P.J. et al: Principles and Practice. 6th ed. Philadelphia: Saunders Elsevier. 439-61, 2008
2. Audard V et al: Risk factors and long-term outcome of transplant renal artery stenosis in adult recipients after treatment by percutaneous transluminal angioplasty. Am J Transplant. 6(1):95-9, 2006
3. Beecroft JR et al: renal artery stenosis: outcome after percutaneous intervention. J Vasc Interv Radiol. 15(12):1407-13, 2004
4. Bruno S et al: Transplant renal artery stenosis. J Am Soc Nephrol. 15(1):134-41, 2004
5. Buturović-Ponikvar J: Renal transplant artery stenosis. Nephrol Dial Transplant. 18 Suppl 5:v74-7, 2003

IMAGE GALLERY

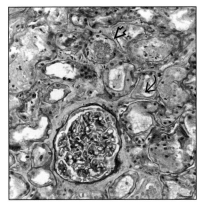 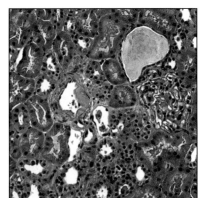 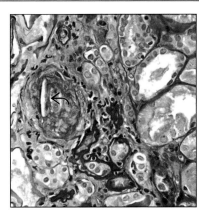

(Left) Periodic acid-Schiff stain of a transplant biopsy from a patient with intermittent renal artery stenosis shows a loss of brush borders, sparse tubular nuclei ⤔, and granular pigmented casts ⧫, indicative of an acute tubular injury. *(Center)* Hematoxylin & eosin shows minimal tubular atrophy in a case of renal artery stenosis of an allograft kidney due to atherosclerosis. *(Right)* Periodic acid-Schiff stain shows a cholesterol cleft ⤔ in an allograft with stenosis due to atherosclerotic disease. Cholesterol emboli provided a clue to the diagnosis.

POST-TRANSPLANT LYMPHOPROLIFERATIVE DISEASE

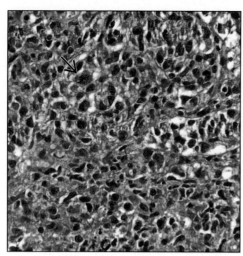

High power of a monomorphic EBV-driven B-cell PTLD shows pleomorphic cells, many of which are enlarged and have irregular nuclear contours, prominent nucleoli, and mitoses ➡.

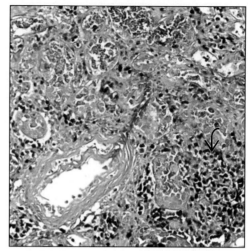

In situ hybridization of Epstein-Barr virus-encoded RNA (EBER) shows that many cells in the lymphoid infiltrate are positive ➡*, indicating that this is a monomorphic EBV-driven B-cell PTLD, diffuse large B-cell lymphoma type.*

TERMINOLOGY

Abbreviations
- Post-transplant lymphoproliferative disease (PTLD)

Synonyms
- Post-transplant lymphoproliferative disorder

Definitions
- Lymphoproliferative proliferation that in many cases manifests as a frank lymphoma arising in immunocompromised hosts who are recipients of solid organ or bone marrow allografts

ETIOLOGY/PATHOGENESIS

Infectious Agents
- Epstein-Barr virus (EBV)
  - Most important risk factor is EBV seronegativity at time of transplantation
    - Primary EBV infection increases the risk for PTLD by 10-76x
  - Risk for PTLD increases with increasing immunosuppression
    - Renal allograft recipients have lowest incidence of PTLD (< 1%)
    - Cardiac allograft recipients have intermediate risk (1-2%)
    - Heart-lung or intestinal allograft recipients have highest frequency (5% or greater)
    - Peripheral blood, stem cell, and bone marrow allograft recipients have low risk of PTLD (< 1%)
  - 70% of PTLD are EBV(+)

B-cell PTLD
- Most PTLD are B-cell type
- Usually driven by EBV
- Monomorphic B-cell PTLD are monoclonal transformed B lymphocytic or plasmacytic proliferations fulfilling diffuse large B-cell lymphoma

criteria (& less commonly Burkitt lymphoma or plasma cell neoplasms)
- Can also be polyclonal

T-cell and NK-cell PTLD
- T/NK-cell PTLD account for 7-15% of PTLDs (larger reported range in 1 Japanese series of 2-45%)
- Occur longer after transplant (median of 66 months) and are usually extranodal
- ~ 1/3 are EBV(+)
- Median survival is 6 months
- EBV(+) cases survive longer
- Types
  - Peripheral T-cell lymphoma, unspecified
  - Hepatosplenic T-cell lymphoma
  - T-cell large granular lymphocytic leukemia (EBV[-])

CLINICAL ISSUES

Epidemiology
- Incidence
  - Estimated to occur in around 1% of renal allograft recipients (1.4% of 25,127 recipients from 1996-2000)
  - In renal allograft patients with PTLD, allograft kidney is affected in > 30% of patients
  - Kidney more often involved in kidney transplant patients (14%) than in heart transplant patients (0.7%)
    - Conversely, heart is involved more in heart (18%) than kidney (7%) transplant patients
    - Suggests immunologic reaction in allograft is pathogenic factor
  - PTLD most often (> 90%) of donor origin
    - Donor origin PTLD appears more commonly in liver and lung allograft recipients and frequently involves allograft
  - Lymphomas account for 15% of tumors among adult transplant recipients (~ 51% in children)

POST-TRANSPLANT LYMPHOPROLIFERATIVE DISEASE

Key Facts

Terminology
- Post-transplant lymphoproliferative disorder (PTLD)
- Frank lymphoma sometimes manifests in immunocompromised hosts in solid organ or bone marrow allograft recipients

Clinical Issues
- Occurs in around 1% of renal allograft recipients
- Treatment
  - Reduction in immunosuppression, antiviral drugs (acyclovir, ganciclovir, α-interferon), chemotherapy, anti-CD20 (rituximab)
- Reported mortality of 40-60%

Macroscopic Features
- Swollen kidneys

- Blurring of corticomedullary junction and diffuse petechiae with vaguely nodular involvement

Microscopic Pathology
- Mononuclear cells ("activated" lymphocytes) with enlarged nuclei, prominent nucleoli, and mitoses
- Cells of PTLD may be monomorphic or polymorphic
- Necrosis, often described as being in serpiginous pattern, is often present

Ancillary Tests
- Most express CD20 (approximately 85-90%)
- Immunohistochemical stains for EBV-associated antigens (such as LMP-1 and EBNA-2)
- In situ hybridization for EBV-encoded RNA (EBER) usually shows prominent staining in atypical lymphoid cells

Presentation
- Malaise
- Weight loss
- Lethargy
- Fever
  - Fever of unknown origin/unexplained fever
- Mononucleosis-type syndrome
  - Fever & malaise
  - Pharyngitis or tonsillitis
    - Sometimes recognized incidentally on tonsillectomy specimens ± lymphadenopathy
- Abdominal mass
- Hepatocellular or pancreatic dysfunction
- Central nervous system disease

Laboratory Tests
- Quantitative EBV viral-load testing with polymerase chain reaction (PCR)
  - Serial assays are more useful in individual patient than specific viral load measurements
  - Assays are not standardized and cannot typically be compared between centers
- Serological testing is not typically thought to be useful

Natural History
- PTLD restricted to kidney transplant (around 12% of cases) tend to occur early (around 5 months) after surgery
- EBV(-) PTLD and T/NK-cell PTLD tend to present later (median time to occurrence 4-5 years and 6.5 years, respectively)

Treatment
- Surgical approaches
  - Surgical excision of affected allograft or ureter may be useful
- Drugs
  - Reduction in immunosuppression.
  - Antiviral drugs (acyclovir, ganciclovir, α-interferon)
  - Chemotherapy

    - Often: CHOP (cyclophosphamide, hydroxydaunomycin, vincristine [Oncovin], prednisone)
  - Anti-CD20 (rituximab)
    - Has helped contribute to complete remission
- Radiation
  - Localized radiation may be combined with chemotherapy
- Cellular immunotherapy to restore EBV-specific cytotoxic T-cell immunity in EBV-driven refractory disease
  - Employs the principle of adoptive immunotherapy with stimulated T cells

Prognosis
- Overall reported mortality of 40-60%
- "Early" lesions tend to regress when immunosuppression is reduced
- Polymorphic and less often monomorphic PTLD may also regress with reduction in immune suppression
- Acute and chronic rejection may occur when immunosuppression is reduced, leading to graft loss and mortality
- Associated with adverse outcome
  - Multiple disease sites (may not be a factor in pediatric patients)
  - Advanced stage
  - Older age at diagnosis
    - Mortality typically thought to be lower in children than adults
  - Late onset disease
  - Higher international prognostic index
  - Elevated lactate dehydrogenase
  - Mortality even higher in bone marrow allograft recipients than solid organ allograft recipients

IMAGE FINDINGS

General Features
- May show up as a mass on radiology studies

POST-TRANSPLANT LYMPHOPROLIFERATIVE DISEASE

MACROSCOPIC FEATURES

General Features
- Swollen kidneys
- Blurring of corticomedullary junction and diffuse petechiae
- Vaguely nodular involvement

MICROSCOPIC PATHOLOGY

Histologic Features
- WHO classification (2008)
  - 4 major categories
    - Early lesions
    - Polymorphic PTLD
    - Monomorphic PTLD (T, B, NK)
    - Classical Hodgkin lymphoma
  - 1st 2 are specific for transplant recipients
- Early lesions
  - Plasmacytic hyperplasia and infectious mononucleosis-like PTLD
  - Involved tissue has architectural preservation
  - Nodal sinuses or tonsillar crypts are still present
  - Follicles are often floridly reactive or hyperplastic
  - In plasmacytic hyperplasia, plasma cells are prominently admixed with small lymphocytes
  - In infectious mononucleosis-like lesion, there is paracortical expansion with numerous immunoblasts admixed with T cells and plasma cells
  - Lesions may form masses
  - Occur at a younger age than other PTLD types (children or adult solid organ recipients who have not had prior EBV infections)
  - Lymph nodes or tonsils are common sites
  - Often EBV(+)
- Polymorphic PTLD
  - Immunoblasts, plasma cells, and small and intermediate-sized lymphoid cells effacing architecture of lymph nodes
  - Full range of B-cell maturation is present
  - Large, bizarre cells may resemble Reed-Sternberg cells (atypical immunoblasts [may be Hodgkin-like])
  - Areas of geographic necrosis may be present
  - Distinction of polymorphic from monomorphic PTLD is not always clear-cut
  - Frequency 20-80% depending on institution
  - Polymorphic variant is most common type in children and frequently follows a primary EBV infection
  - Polymorphic variant is more common in PTLD involving the kidney
  - Often EBV(+)
- Monomorphic PTLD
  - Fulfills criteria for 1 of the B-cell or T/NK-cell neoplasms recognized in immunocompetent hosts
  - Small B-cell lymphoid neoplasms, such as follicular lymphomas or MALT lymphomas, are not designated as PTLD
    - Despite the fact that some have recognized that these occur in post-transplant setting (e.g., MALT lymphoma)

- Monomorphic B-cell PTLD
  - Necrosis, often described as being in serpiginous pattern, is often present
  - Monomorphic B-cell PTLD often fulfill criteria for diffuse large B-cell lymphoma
  - Burkitt lymphoma or plasma cell neoplasms occur less commonly
  - Cells are often collected in vaguely nodular pattern in sheets
  - Mononuclear cells ("activated" lymphocytes) with enlarged nuclei, prominent nucleoli, and mitoses
  - Cells may have blast-like features
  - Term "monomorphic" does not imply cellular monotony since cells may be bizarre, multinucleated, and Reed-Sternberg-like
  - May also be plasmacytic or plasmacytoid features
  - Burkitt lymphomas have monomorphic medium-sized transformed cells, often with multiple small nucleoli and dispersed chromatin, and may posses MYC gene translocations
    - e.g., characteristically t(8;14) but also t(8;22) or t(2;8)
- Monomorphic T/NK-cell PTLD
  - Fulfill criteria for T/NK-cell lymphomas
  - Most present at extranodal sites
  - Largest group consists of peripheral T-cell lymphoma, not otherwise specified (NOS) category
  - Peripheral T-cell lymphoma, NOS has wide range in morphology
  - Peripheral T-cell lymphoma, NOS is often accompanied by eosinophilia, pruritus, or hemophagocytic syndrome
  - Up to 20% of hepatosplenic T-cell lymphomas arise in setting of chronic immunosuppression
    - Mostly long-term immunosuppression for solid organ transplantation in which it is regarded as late-onset PTLD of host orgin
  - Hepatosplenic T-cell lymphoma is thought to arise from cytotoxic T-cells (usually of γ/δ variety)
  - Hepatosplenic T-cell lymphoma demonstrates medium-sized lymphoid cells infiltrating bone marrow, spleen, and liver
- Classical Hodgkin lymphoma (CHL) type PTLD
  - Least common form of PTLD
  - Occurs more commonly in renal transplant patients than in other transplant recipients
  - Reed-Sternberg-like cells may be seen in early, polymorphic, and some monomorphic PTLDs and cause diagnostic confusion
  - Cases should fulfill criteria for CHL
  - Usually both CD15 and CD30 are positive
  - CD15(-) cases can occur but must be distinguished from Hodgkin-like lesions

ANCILLARY TESTS

Immunohistochemistry
- Most are B-cell derived and express B-cell markers
  - CD20 (approximately 85-90%)
  - Others: CD20, CD79a
  - CD30 is positive in many B-cell PTLD cases (± anaplastic morphology)

POST-TRANSPLANT LYMPHOPROLIFERATIVE DISEASE

- ○ CD138(+) in a minority
- ○ EBV(+) cases usually have late germinal center/post germinal center phenotype (CD10[-], Bcl-6[+/-], IRF/MUM1[+])
- ○ EBV(-) cases often have germinal center phenotype (CD10[+/-], Bcl-6[+], IRF/MUM1[-], CD138[-])
- ○ EBV(-) monomorphic PTLD frequently lacks expression of cyclin-dependent kinase inhibitor (CDKN2A [p16INK4A])
- ○ Monotypic immunoglobulin often with expression of γ or α heavy chain in ~ 50% of monomorphic B-cell PTLD
- Classical Hodgkin lymphoma type PTLD
  - ○ Typically CD15(+) and CD30(+) and EBV(+)
  - ○ CD15(-) classical Hodgkin lymphoma case occur and should be distinguished from other Hodgkin-like lesions
  - ○ CD15, when present, often gives Golgi-type pattern of expression
- T/NK-cell PTLD have pan-T-cell and NK-cell antigens
  - ○ CD4 or 8, CD30, ALK, and α/β or γ/δ T cell
    - ■ Hepatosplenic T-cell lymphoma is usually of γ/δ variety
  - ○ Around 1/3 are EBV(+)
- Immunohistochemical stains for EBV-associated antigens (such as LMP-1 and EBNA-2)

Cytogenetics
- Clonal cytogenetic abnormalities are common, particularly in monomorphic PTLD

In Situ Hybridization
- Most EBV(+) (around 85%)
  - ○ In situ hybridization for EBV-encoded RNA (EBER) usually shows prominent staining in atypical lymphoid cells
- In situ hybridization for kappa and lambda light chains may demonstrate light chain restriction
  - ○ Occurs in ~ 50% of monomorphic PTLD and usually only focal in polymorphic PTLD

PCR
- Gene rearrangement studies can demonstrate clonally rearranged immunoglobulin genes
  - ○ Usually a more prominent feature of monomorphic B-cell PTLD
  - ○ Can occur in polymorphic B-cell PTLD
    - ■ Some have reported immunoglobulin gene variable regions without ongoing mutations in 75% of polymorphic PTLDs
- Monomorphic B-cell PTLD has oncogene abnormalities (*PAS*, *TP53*, and *MYC* rearrangements, *BCL6* somatic hypermutation, and aberrant promoter methylation)
- Cases of T-cell origin have clonal T-cell receptor gene rearrangements

Array CGH
- Demonstrate additions, gains, and losses

DIFFERENTIAL DIAGNOSIS

Allograft Rejection
- PTLD may be confused with allograft rejection because features mimicking rejection, such as tubulitis and endarteritis, may be present
- Granulocytes and macrophages are more commonly seen in rejection
- Rejection usually shows predominance of CD3(+) T-lymphocytes and CD68 macrophages
- It has been proposed that concurrent rejection and PTLD may occur

Smooth Muscle Tumors
- Spindle cell neoplasms may be seen in post-transplant setting and may be EBV(+)
- Histologic examination usually confirms prominent spindling, which is not typical of PTLD
- Immunohistochemical studies usually demonstrate smooth muscle differentiation (actin and desmin)

DIAGNOSTIC CHECKLIST

Pathologic Interpretation Pearls
- Detection of rare EBV(+) cells without lymphoid/plasmacytic proliferation is not diagnostic of PTLD

REPORTING CONSIDERATIONS

Key Elements to Report
- Categories of PTLD according to 2008 WHO classification
  - ○ Early lesions
    - ■ Plasmacytic hyperplasia
    - ■ Infectious mononucleosis-like lesion
  - ○ Polymorphic PTLD
  - ○ Monomorphic PTLD
    - ■ B-cell neoplasms: Diffuse large B-cell lymphoma (DLBCL), Burkitt lymphoma, plasma cell myeloma, plasmacytoma-like lesion, other (e.g., indolent small B-cell lymphomas arising in transplant recipients)
    - ■ T-cell neoplasms: Peripheral T-cell lymphoma, NOS; hepatosplenic T-cell lymphoma; other
  - ○ Classical Hodgkin lymphoma-type PTLD

SELECTED REFERENCES

1. Siemer D et al: EBV transformation overrides gene expression patterns of B cell differentiation stages. Mol Immunol. 45(11):3133-41, 2008
2. Swerdlow SH et al: Post-transplant lymphoproliferative disorders. In Swerdlow SH et al: WHO Classification of Tumours of Haematopoietic and Lymphoid Tissues. Lyon: IARC. 343-48, 2008
3. Bakker NA et al: Presentation and early detection of post-transplant lymphoproliferative disorder after solid organ transplantation. Transpl Int. 20(3):207-18, 2007
4. Colvin RB et al: Renal transplant pathology. In Jennette JC et al: Heptinstall's Pathology of the Kidney. 6th ed. Philadelphia: Lippincott Williams & Wilkins. 1347-1490, 2007

POST-TRANSPLANT LYMPHOPROLIFERATIVE DISEASE

Categories and Selected Features of Post-Transplant Lymphoproliferative Disease (PTLD)

Category	Morphology	EBV	Immunophenotype and Genetics
Early lesions			
Plasmacytic hyperplasia	Plasma cells and lymphocytes	Often +	Usually polyclonal
Infectious mononucleosis-like lesion	Mixture: Lymphocytes ± plasma cells, ± immunoblasts	Often +	Usually polyclonal
Polymorphic PTLD	Mixture: Lymphocytes ± plasma cells ± immunoblasts (full spectrum of maturation)	Often +	May have monoclonal B cells
Monomorphic PTLD			
B-cell neoplasms			Express B-cell markers
Diffuse large B-cell lymphoma	Large B cells	Variable	Clonal
Burkitt lymphoma	Medium-sized B cells with multiple nucleoli and finely dispersed chromatin	Variable	Clonal, may have translocations, e.g., t(8;14) but also t(8;22) or t(2;8)
Plasma cell myeloma	Diffuse plasma cell infiltrate with criteria sufficient to diagnose myeloma	Variable	Clonal
Plasmacytoma-like lesion	Localized site with a diffuse plasma cell infiltrate	Usually -	Monotypic immunoglobulin
T-cell neoplasms			Express T-cell (and less commonly NK-cell) markers
Peripheral T-cell lymphoma, NOS	May be polymorphous or polymorphous with medium to large-sized cells and Reed-Sternberg (RS)-type cells	Minority +	Typically clonal with rearranged T-cell receptor genes
Hepatosplenic T-cell lymphoma	Liver, spleen, and bone marrow are diffusely involved with monotonous medium-sized cells with inconspicuous nucleoli	Minority +	Typically clonal with rearranged T-cell receptor genes (usually of the γ/δ type), may have +8 chromosomal modification
Classical Hodgkin lymphoma (CHL)-type PTLD	Fulfills criteria for a diagnosis of CHL and classically may have RS cells	Often +	Clonality usually cannot be shown, e.g., with IgH rearrangement studies

5. Everly MJ et al: Posttransplant lymphoproliferative disorder. Ann Pharmacother. 41(11):1850-8, 2007

6. Fishman JA: Infection in solid-organ transplant recipients. N Engl J Med. 357(25):2601-14, 2007

7. Lee JJ et al: Role of chemotherapy and rituximab for treatment of posttransplant lymphoproliferative disorder in solid organ transplantation. Ann Pharmacother. 41(10):1648-59, 2007

8. Swerdlow SH: T-cell and NK-cell posttransplantation lymphoproliferative disorders. Am J Clin Pathol. 127(6):887-95, 2007

9. Becker YT et al: The emerging role of rituximab in organ transplantation. Transpl Int. 19(8):621-8, 2006

10. Deyrup AT et al: Epstein-Barr virus-associated smooth muscle tumors are distinctive mesenchymal tumors reflecting multiple infection events: a clinicopathologic and molecular analysis of 29 tumors from 19 patients. Am J Surg Pathol. 30(1):75-82, 2006

11. Johnson LR et al: Impact of Epstein-Barr virus in monomorphic B-cell posttransplant lymphoproliferative disorders: a histogenetic study. Am J Surg Pathol. 30(12):1604-12, 2006

12. Blaes AH et al: Rituximab therapy is effective for posttransplant lymphoproliferative disorders after solid organ transplantation: results of a phase II trial. Cancer. 104(8):1661-7, 2005

13. Capello D et al: Post-transplant lymphoproliferative disorders: molecular basis of disease histogenesis and pathogenesis. Hematol Oncol. 23(2):61-7, 2005

14. Novoa-Takara L et al: Histogenetic phenotypes of B cells in posttransplant lymphoproliferative disorders by immunohistochemical analysis correlate with transplant type: solid organ vs hematopoietic stem cell transplantation. Am J Clin Pathol. 123(1):104-12, 2005

15. Oertel SH et al: Effect of anti-CD 20 antibody rituximab in patients with post-transplant lymphoproliferative disorder (PTLD). Am J Transplant. 5(12):2901-6, 2005

16. Abed N et al: Evaluation of histogenesis of B-lymphocytes in pediatric EBV-related post-transplant lymphoproliferative disorders. Bone Marrow Transplant. 33(3):321-7, 2004

17. Gill D et al: Durable and high rates of remission following chemotherapy in posttransplantation lymphoproliferative disorders after renal transplantation. Transplant Proc. 35(1):256-7, 2003

18. Dotti G et al: Epstein-Barr virus-negative lymphoproliferate disorders in long-term survivors after heart, kidney, and liver transplant. Transplantation. 69(5):827-33, 2000

19. Ifthikharuddin JJ et al: CD-20 expression in post-transplant lymphoproliferative disorders: treatment with rituximab. Am J Hematol. 65(2):171-3, 2000

20. Shapiro R et al: Posttransplant lymphoproliferative disorders in adult and pediatric renal transplant patients receiving tacrolimus-based immunosuppression. Transplantation. 68(12):1851-4, 1999

21. Harris NL et al: Posttransplant lymphoproliferative disorders: summary of Society for Hematopathology Workshop. Semin Diagn Pathol. 14(1):8-14, 1997

Early Lesions and Polymorphic PTLD

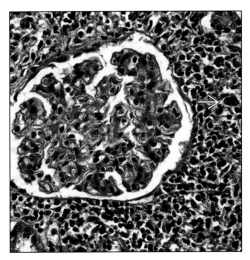

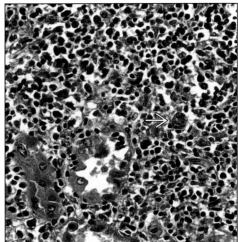

(Left) High power of a renal allograft from the recipient's autopsy shows involvement by immunoblastic plasmacytoid PTLD with large atypical cells ➡. (Courtesy J.A. Ferry, MD.) (Right) High power of the allograft from the autopsy of the recipient of a renal allograft shows involvement by PTLD with large atypical cells ➡ among renal tubules. This PTLD was classified as an immunoblastic plasmacytoid PTLD. (Courtesy J.A. Ferry, MD.)

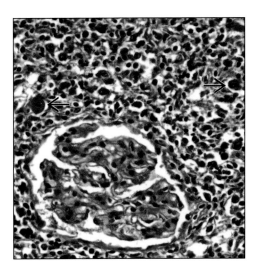

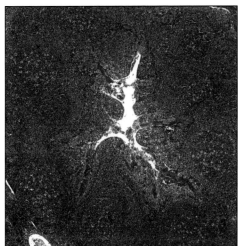

(Left) High power of an allograft shows involvement by PTLD with large atypical cells ➡. This PTLD was classified as an immunoblastic plasmacytoid PTLD. (Courtesy J.A. Ferry, MD.) (Right) Low-power view of a tonsil in a pediatric renal allograft recipient shows involvement by an infectious mononucleosis-like PTLD. The architecture is overall preserved, but it can be appreciated that lymphoid follicles show attenuated mantles. (Courtesy J.A. Ferry, MD.)

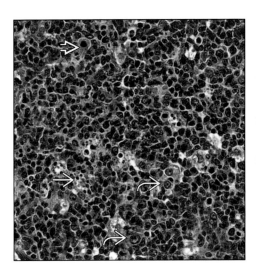

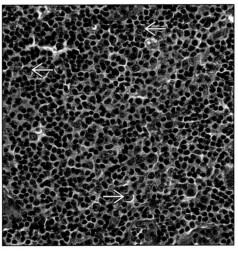

(Left) High-power view of the tonsil involved by mononucleosis-like PTLD shows that lymphoid follicles are floridly reactive with mostly small lymphocytes and scattered tingible body macrophages ➡, immunoblasts ➡, and apoptotic cells ➡. (Courtesy J.A. Ferry, MD.) (Right) Higher power view of the interfollicular area of the tonsil with mononucleosis-like PTLD shows mostly small lymphocytes and scattered immunoblasts ➡. (Courtesy J.A. Ferry, MD.)

Monomorphic PTLD, B-cell

(Left) A gross photograph shows nodular involvement of an allograft kidney by PTLD. *(Courtesy P. Randhawa, MD.)* *(Right)* A low power of the allograft from the autopsy of the recipient of a renal allograft shows involvement by PTLD with an area of necrosis ➡. *(Courtesy J.A. Ferry, MD.)*

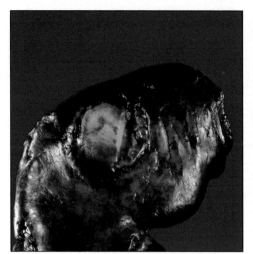 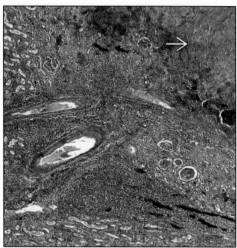

(Left) PAS stain of a monomorphic EBV-driven B-cell PTLD, diffuse large B-cell lymphoma type, shows a relatively normal glomerulus ➡ amidst a necrotic parenchyma ➡ with a dense lymphoid infiltrate ➡. *(Right)* This PTLD shows fatty infiltration in the surrounding soft tissues. *(Courtesy P. Randhawa, MD.)*

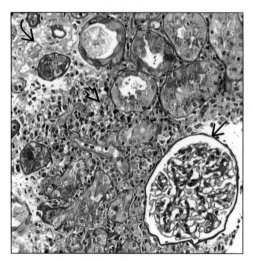 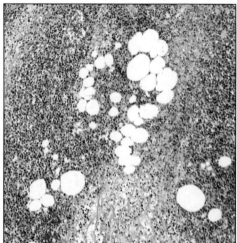

(Left) This B-cell PTLD has foci of tubulitis, illustrating that this pattern can be seen in PTLD as well as cellular rejection. *(Courtesy P. Randhawa, MD.)* *(Right)* EBER RNA stain shows tubulitis with EBV-infected cells, demonstrating that this PTLD is an EBV-driven process. *(Courtesy P. Randhawa, MD.)*

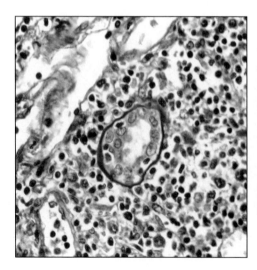 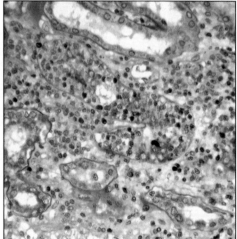

Monomorphic PTLD, B-cell

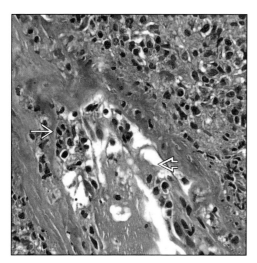 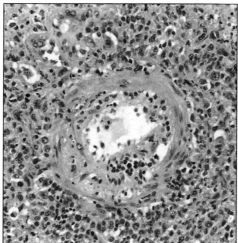

(Left) High-power examination shows an arterial wall involved by monomorphic EBV-driven B-cell PTLD, diffuse large B-cell lymphoma type, with malignant lymphoid cells ➡ and admixed fibrin ➡. *(Right)* Hematoxylin & eosin stain shows vascular involvement by a B-cell PTLD, illustrating the fact that this can occur in PTLD, simulating endarteritis that can be seen in cellular rejection. *(Courtesy P. Randhawa, MD.)*

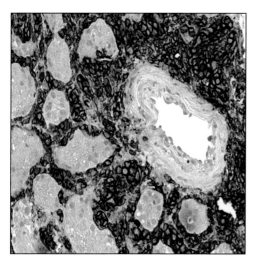 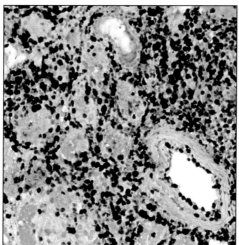

(Left) CD20 immunohistochemistry of a monomorphic EBV-driven B-cell PTLD, diffuse large B-cell lymphoma type, shows that almost all of the atypical lymphoid infiltrate consists of CD20(+) B cells. *(Right)* A Ki-67 immunohistochemical stain is positive in most of the atypical lymphoid infiltrate in this monomorphic EBV-driven B-cell PTLD, diffuse large B-cell lymphoma type, indicating that it is highly proliferative.

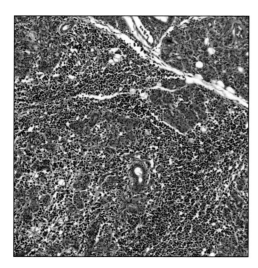 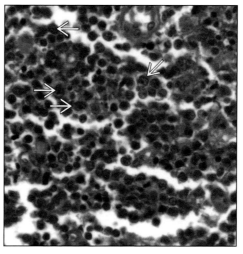

(Left) Low power of a submandibular gland in a patient with history of a renal allograft shows diffuse involvement by a lymphoid infiltrate in a Burkitt lymphoma-type monomorphic PTLD. *(Courtesy J.A. Ferry, MD.)* *(Right)* A Giemsa stain of a Burkitt lymphoma-type PTLD shows that many of the cells have prominent nucleoli ➡. *(Courtesy J.A. Ferry, MD.)*

Monomorphic PTLD, T-cell

(Left) High power shows an atypical lymphoid infiltrate in a case of T-cell PTLD with a mixed pleomorphic cell population, containing a mixture of small and large cells with a variety of shapes. *(Right)* High power of a T-cell PTLD shows large atypical cells ⇥, mitotic figures ⇥, and admixed eosinophils ⇥.

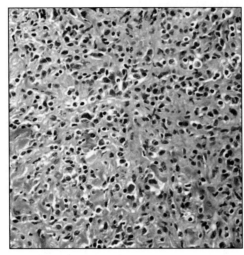
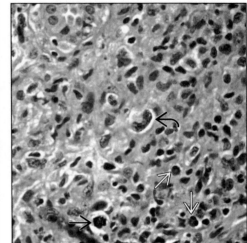

(Left) Immunohistochemical stain of T-cell PTLD shows that most of the atypical infiltrate is composed of CD3(+) T cells with a variety of shapes and sizes. *(Right)* A liver biopsy in a renal allograft recipient with hepatosplenic T-cell lymphoma has diffuse portal and lobular involvement by a lymphoid infiltrate of small to medium lymphoid cells mimicking hepatitis. *(Courtesy J.A. Ferry, MD.)*

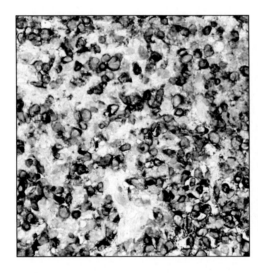
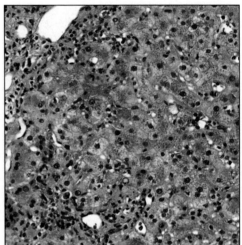

(Left) Lymphoid cells (that were CD3[+], CD8[+] and CD4[-], CD5[-] by immunohistochemistry) are primarily present along liver sinusoids, consistent with a hepatosplenic T-cell lymphoma in a renal allograft recipient. *(Courtesy J.A. Ferry, MD.)* *(Right)* It can be appreciated in this image that the lymphoid cells primarily travel along the hepatic sinusoids ⇥ in the hepatic lobules in a hepatosplenic T-cell lymphoma in a renal allograft recipient. *(Courtesy J.A. Ferry, MD.)*

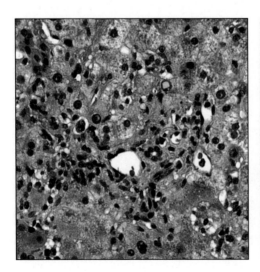
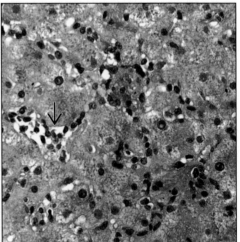

CHL PTLD, Nerve Involvement and Spindle Cell Tumor

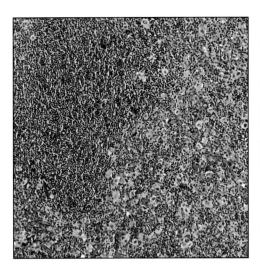

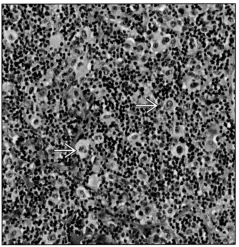

(Left) At low power, a Hodgkin lymphoma-type PTLD involving the tongue base can be appreciated with a heterogeneous cell population. (Courtesy N.L. Harris, MD.) *(Right)* This Hodgkin lymphoma-type PTLD contains many Reed-Sternberg variant cells ➡. (Courtesy N.L. Harris, MD.)

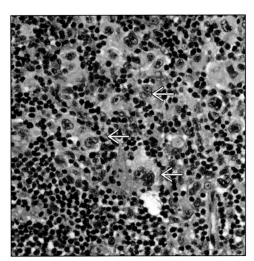

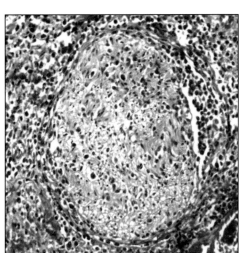

(Left) This Hodgkin lymphoma-type PTLD contains many Reed-Sternberg variant cells ➡. (Courtesy N.L. Harris, MD.) *(Right)* At medium-power examination, one can observe a nerve with involvement by B-cell PTLD. (Courtesy P. Randhawa, MD.)

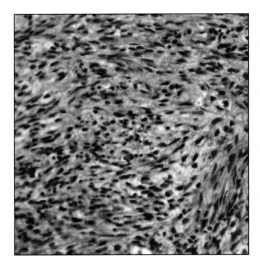

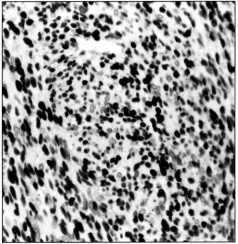

(Left) Light microscopy shows post-transplant spindle cell tumor. In this case, immunohistochemistry showed smooth muscle differentiation. (Courtesy P. Randhawa, MD.) *(Right)* In situ hybridization for EBER shows EBV-infected cells in a spindle cell tumor. Lymphoid markers would demonstrate that this is not a PTLD but rather a post-transplant spindle cell tumor caused by EBV. (Courtesy P. Randhawa, MD.)

PROTOCOL BIOPSIES

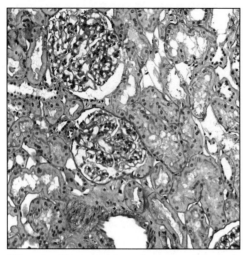

This protocol biopsy specimen shows normal glomeruli, normal tubules and interstitium, and a normal artery, confirming a lack of rejection, de novo or recurrent disease.

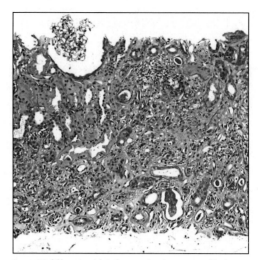

Interstitial fibrosis with inflammation is seen on this 1-year protocol biopsy in a patient with normal renal function. Inflammation in fibrotic areas is associated with increased risk of graft loss.

TERMINOLOGY

Synonyms
- Surveillance biopsies

Definitions
- Renal allograft biopsies performed at predetermined intervals, unrelated to graft dysfunction

CLINICAL IMPLICATIONS

Value of Protocol Biopsies
- Useful in monitoring highly sensitized patients
- Ability to detect and potentially treat subclinical disease when it may be reversible
  - Includes subclinical rejection, infection, and recurrent disease
- Findings on earlier protocol biopsies may identify cause of later graft loss
  - Specific cause of graft loss can be identified in ~ 95% of cases, largely based on earlier biopsies
- Frequency of subclinical rejection low in modern era
  - Other diseases may be detected: Drug toxicity, polyoma infection, recurrent disease
- Clinical trials
  - Document outcome
  - Detect toxicity
- Used more commonly in high-risk (presensitized) patients

Risk of Biopsy Procedure
- 0.4% risk of major complications
  - Hemorrhage
  - Peritonitis from bowel perforation
  - Graft loss (< 0.05%)

Timing
- Donor biopsies (implantation, time zero)
- Early biopsies in highly sensitized patients
- 3-4, 6, 12 months

MICROSCOPIC FINDINGS

General Features
- Variable findings depending on diagnosis

Glomeruli
- Normal
- Duplication of glomerular basement membrane
- Mesangial hypercellularity
- Focal segmental glomerulosclerosis
- Immune complex deposition if recurrent or de novo disease

Tubules
- Normal
- Tubular atrophy
- Tubulitis
- Viral inclusions

Interstitium
- Normal
- Fibrosis
- Inflammation
  - Inflammation in areas of fibrosis associated with increased risk of graft loss
  - Inflammation outside areas of fibrosis may indicate subclinical cellular rejection

Arteries and Arterioles
- Normal
- Arteriosclerosis
- Endarteritis rarely found (~ 0.2% of biopsies)
- Hyalinosis in arterioles

Peritubular Capillaries (PTC)
- Normal
- C4d(+) PTC
- Mononuclear cells in PTC

DIAGNOSES

Normal Histology
- Comprises majority of protocol biopsies

Subclinical Acute Cellular Rejection (ACR)
- 12-17% of protocol biopsies within 1st 6 months post transplant; incidence lower after 1st year and on tacrolimus (5%)
- 5% prevalence on 1-year protocol biopsies
  - Includes borderline/suspicious ACR, type I ACR (tubulointerstitial), and type II ACR (with endothelialitis)

Subclinical BK Polyomavirus Nephropathy
- 5% prevalence on 1-year protocol biopsies

Chronic Calcineurin Inhibitor Toxicity
- Arteriolar hyalinosis in 61.3%, 90.5%, and 100% of biopsies at 1, 5, and 10 years, respectively, in patients on cyclosporine in 1 study
  - Not necessarily specific for CNI toxicity
- Arteriolar hyalinosis may be less prevalent and less severe in patients on tacrolimus or sirolimus vs. cyclosporine
  - In another study, 19% prevalence of moderate to severe hyalinosis on 5-year protocol biopsies in a series of patients on tacrolimus-based immunosuppression
    - 5% of sirolimus-based, CNI-free immunosuppression showed moderate to severe hyalinosis

Arteriosclerosis
- May be donor disease or de novo
  - Comparison to time zero (implantation) biopsy is helpful

Interstitial Fibrosis and Tubular Atrophy (IFTA), NOS
- 81% of cases of graft loss with IFTA have identifiable cause, in part detected on earlier biopsies
- ~ 60% of functioning grafts at 5 years have some IFTA (ct or $ci > 0$)
  - Moderate to severe IFTA (Banff $ci > 1$, $ct > 1$) in 17% of biopsies at 5 years
    - Associated with previous acute cellular rejection and BK polyomavirus infection episodes
- IFTA does not necessarily progress with time
  - In a study of conventional transplants, allografts with mild fibrosis ($ci1$) on 1-year protocol biopsy often had different findings on 5-year biopsy
    - 39% showed no fibrosis ($ci0$) on 5-year biopsy
    - Only 23% showed more severe fibrosis on 5-year biopsy
  - Of patients with moderate fibrosis ($ci2$) on 1-year protocol biopsy, > 50% show mild or no fibrosis at 5 years
  - Findings may in part represent sampling error
- Combination of interstitial fibrosis and mononuclear inflammation increases risk of later graft loss
  - Shown in several independent studies
  - All types of inflammation are considered in Banff ti score

Chronic Humoral Rejection
- ~ 2-5% incidence of transplant glomerulopathy in 1-year protocol biopsies of conventional transplant patients
  - Increased risk in patients with anti-donor HLA antibodies
- Reduced graft survival with TG finding on protocol biopsy

Accommodation
- No active rejection
- C4d(+) PTC
- Common in ABO-blood-group-incompatible transplants

Recurrent Glomerular Disease
- Early recurrent membranous glomerulonephritis and IgA nephropathy are commonly subclinical

De Novo Glomerular Disease
- Focal glomerulosclerosis and membranous glomerulonephritis are most common

SELECTED REFERENCES

1. Park WD et al: Fibrosis with inflammation at one year predicts transplant functional decline. J Am Soc Nephrol. 21(11):1987-97, 2010
2. Stegall MD et al: The histology of solitary renal allografts at 1 and 5 years after transplantation. Am J Transplant. Epub ahead of print, 2010
3. El-Zoghby ZM et al: Identifying specific causes of kidney allograft loss. Am J Transplant. 9(3):527-35, 2009
4. Gloor JM et al: Transplant glomerulopathy: subclinical incidence and association with alloantibody. Am J Transplant. 7(9):2124-32, 2007
5. Mengel M et al: Infiltrates in protocol biopsies from renal allografts. Am J Transplant. 7(2):356-65, 2007
6. Moreso F et al: Subclinical rejection associated with chronic allograft nephropathy in protocol biopsies as a risk factor for late graft loss. Am J Transplant. 6(4):747-52, 2006
7. Cosio FG et al: Predicting subsequent decline in kidney allograft function from early surveillance biopsies. Am J Transplant. 5(10):2464-72, 2005
8. Nankivell BJ et al: Calcineurin inhibitor nephrotoxicity: longitudinal assessment by protocol histology. Transplantation. 78(4):557-65, 2004
9. Furness PN et al: Protocol biopsy of the stable renal transplant: a multicenter study of methods and complication rates. Transplantation. 76(6):969-73, 2003
10. Nankivell BJ et al: The natural history of chronic allograft nephropathy. N Engl J Med. 349(24):2326-33, 2003
11. Shishido S et al: The impact of repeated subclinical acute rejection on the progression of chronic allograft nephropathy. J Am Soc Nephrol. 14(4):1046-52, 2003

Protocol Biopsy Features

(Left) A 1-year protocol biopsy specimen in a patient with normal renal function is shown. The biopsy appears normal. *(Right)* Normal glomerulus by electron microscopy in a protocol biopsy is shown. Podocyte foot processes are preserved ➡. No glomerular basement membrane (GBM) duplication or subendothelial lucency is present. No immune deposits are noted. Endothelial cells appear normal, with preserved fenestrations ➡.

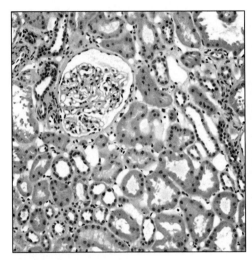
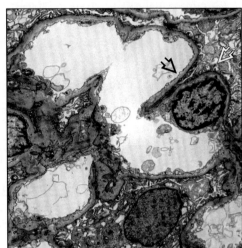

(Left) Normal peritubular capillary by electron microscopy in a protocol biopsy specimen is shown. The capillary shows a single basement membrane layer ➡ and normal-appearing endothelial cells. *(Right)* Rare arterioles show intimal ➡ and peripheral nodular ➡ hyalinosis, likely due to subclinical calcineurin inhibitor toxicity. Arteriolar hyalinosis becomes more common with time in allografts.

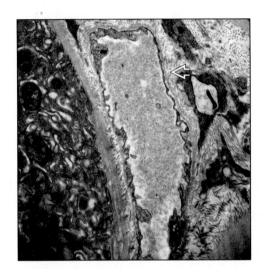
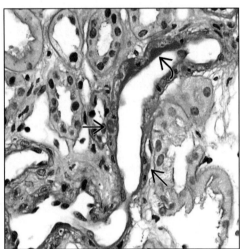

(Left) Peritubular capillaritis ➡ is seen in this protocol biopsy, 4 months post transplant, from a patient with preformed donor-specific antibody and normal renal function. This finding should not be confused with acute cellular rejection. *(Right)* Early, subclinical transplant glomerulopathy is seen in a 1-year protocol biopsy. Glomerulitis ➡ and segmental GBM duplication ➡ are seen. This patient also had preformed donor-specific HLA antibody but normal renal function.

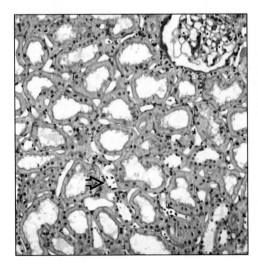
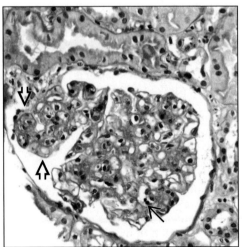

Subclinical Glomerular Disease

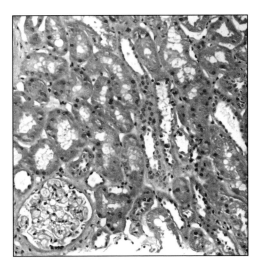

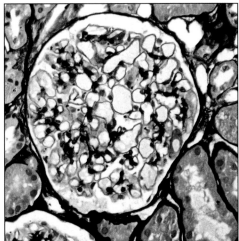

(Left) Early recurrent membranous glomerulonephritis (MGN) is seen on a 4-month protocol biopsy. The biopsy appears normal by light microscopy, but the GBM deposits were readily shown by IF. MGN typically recurs in the 1st year post transplant. (Right) This glomerulus from early recurrent MGN does not show evidence of GBM abnormalities ("spikes" or "pinholes") on high magnification. No deposits were noted on a trichrome stain.

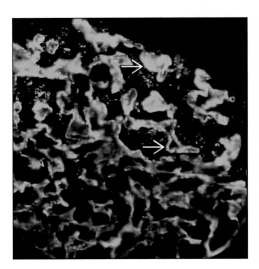

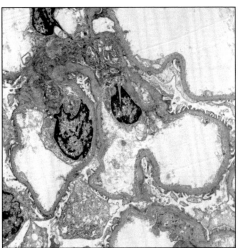

(Left) In early recurrent MGN, IF staining for C4d reveals granular GBM staining in a membranous pattern ➡, in contrast to usual and normal glomerular C4d staining restricted to the mesangium. Similar staining was seen for IgG. (Right) A 4-month protocol biopsy specimen in a patient with early recurrent MGN and minimal proteinuria shows no electron-dense deposits by EM, despite IgG and complement deposits by IF. Podocyte foot processes are intact.

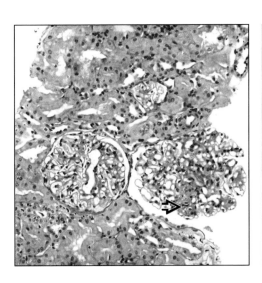

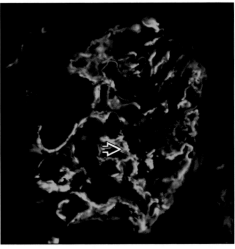

(Left) Subclinical IgA nephropathy 5 years post transplant shows segmental mild to moderate mesangial hypercellularity and mesangial matrix expansion ➡. The patient had stable renal function (Cr 1.5 mg/dL) without hematuria or proteinuria. The original disease was attributed to diabetes and hypertension. The findings here may represent recurrent or de novo IgA nephropathy. (Right) Subclinical IgA nephropathy: Granular mesangial IgA deposits are shown by IF ➡.

ACCOMMODATION

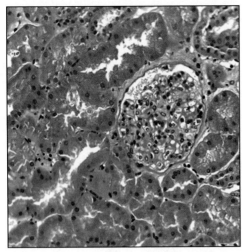

Protocol biopsy is shown from a patient with stable renal function with an HLA-incompatible, ABO-compatible graft. The appearance by light microscopy is entirely normal, although C4d was present in PTC.

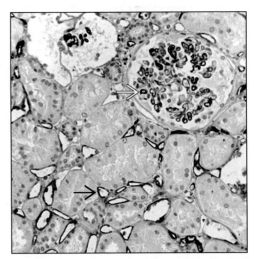

Protocol biopsy is shown from a patient with stable renal function with an HLA-incompatible, ABO-compatible graft. C4d is in the PTC ⇒ and glomerular ➡ basement membranes in the absence of inflammation.

TERMINOLOGY

Definitions
- Accommodation refers to lack of graft injury in presence of donor-reactive immune response, usually detected by circulating anti-donor antibodies
  - Commonly but not always occurring in ABO incompatible grafts
- Corresponding Banff definition: "Presence of peritubular capillary C4d in graft biopsy without evidence of active rejection"

ETIOLOGY/PATHOGENESIS

Response of Endothelium to Antibodies Reactive to Surface Components
- Increased antiapoptotic molecules (Bcl-xL)
- Increased complement regulatory proteins (CD55, decay accelerating factor)
- Increased MUC1

Animal Models
- In nonhuman primates, 4 stages of humoral rejection have been defined
  - Stage I: Circulating donor-specific antibody (DSA) (accommodation 1)
  - Stage II: DSA + C4d in peritubular capillaries (PTC) (accommodation 2)
  - Stage III: DSA + C4d + pathologic changes (subclinical chronic humoral rejection [CHR])
  - Stage IV: DSA + C4d + pathology + functional impairment
- Time course between stages is variable and not predictable

CLINICAL ISSUES

Epidemiology
- Incidence
  - Commonly occurs in ABO blood group-incompatible (ABOi) grafts (> 80%)
  - Incidence in HLA incompatible grafts uncertain (2-4% in early protocol biopsies)

Presentation
- Normal graft function
- Positive circulating DSA either HLA or ABO blood group antibodies

Treatment
- No treatment indicated
- Watchful waiting to monitor possible progression to CHR
  - Circulating HLA antibody
  - Function (Cr, proteinuria)
  - Repeat biopsy if deterioration of function

Prognosis
- In ABOi grafts, no immediate effects on graft survival
  - Long-term effect (years) under evaluation
- In HLA, incompatible grafts with HLA DSA
  - Outcome not well defined
  - May develop chronic graft injury (chronic humoral rejection)

MICROSCOPIC PATHOLOGY

Histologic Features
- Normal graft biopsy
- Glomeruli
  - No glomerulitis
  - No GBM duplication (< 10%)
- Interstitium
  - No interstitial infiltrate (< 10%)
- Tubules

ACCOMMODATION

Key Facts

Terminology
- Lack of graft injury in presence of donor-reactive immune response

Clinical Issues
- Normal graft function
- No treatment indicated
- No immediate effect on graft survival in ABOi grafts
- Outcome not well defined in other settings

Microscopic Pathology
- Normal graft biopsy
- Positive stain for C4d in PTC
- Normal GBM and PTC by electron microscopy

Top Differential Diagnoses
- Chronic humoral rejection
  - EM shows multilamination of PTC basement membrane and GBM
  - Mononuclear cells in PTC (capillaritis)

  - No tubulitis (< 5 cells/tubule)
- Arteries
  - No arteritis
- Peritubular capillaries
  - No capillaritis

ANCILLARY TESTS

Immunohistochemistry
- Positive stain for C4d in peritubular capillaries and glomeruli

Immunofluorescence
- Positive stain for C4d in PTC
- C3d in ABOi correlates with acute inflammation
  - C3d not helpful in ABO-compatible grafts
  - C4d present in TBM confounds interpretation

Electron Microscopy
- Lack of reactive endothelial cells in glomeruli and peritubular capillaries
- Lack of multilamination of peritubular capillary basement membranes
- Lack of glomerular basement membrane duplication

DIFFERENTIAL DIAGNOSIS

Chronic Humoral Rejection
- PTC "capillaritis" and glomerulitis

- Multilamination of PTC basement membrane and GBM

DIAGNOSTIC CHECKLIST

Pathologic Interpretation Pearls
- Stability of accommodation is not known
- Clinicians should not overtreat but should not dismiss findings as totally benign

SELECTED REFERENCES

1. Haas M: The significance of C4d staining with minimal histologic abnormalities. Curr Opin Organ Transplant. 15(1):21-7, 2010
2. Smith RN et al: Four stages and lack of stable accommodation in chronic alloantibody-mediated renal allograft rejection in Cynomolgus monkeys. Am J Transplant. 8(8):1662-72, 2008
3. Colvin RB: Antibody-mediated renal allograft rejection: diagnosis and pathogenesis. J Am Soc Nephrol. 18(4):1046-56, 2007
4. Takahashi K: Recent findings in ABO-incompatible kidney transplantation: classification and therapeutic strategy for acute antibody-mediated rejection due to ABO-blood-group-related antigens during the critical period preceding the establishment of accommodation. Clin Exp Nephrol. 11(2):128-41, 2007
5. Haas M et al: C4d and C3d staining in biopsies of ABO- and HLA-incompatible renal allografts: correlation with histologic findings. Am J Transplant. 6(8):1829-40, 2006

IMAGE GALLERY

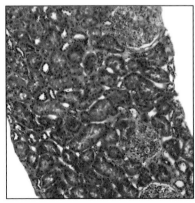 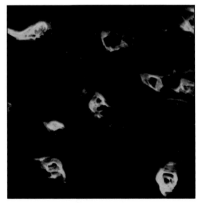 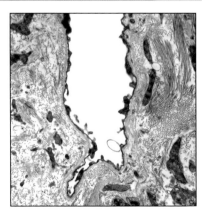

(Left) Protocol biopsy of an ABO-incompatible graft 3 months after transplantation appears entirely normal by light microscopy. *(Center)* Protocol biopsy of an ABO-incompatible graft 3 months after transplantation shows bright and widespread staining of PTC for C4d in the absence of inflammation. *(Right)* Protocol biopsy of a C4d(+), normal-appearing ABO-incompatible graft 3 months after transplantation shows entirely normal PTC endothelium, indicative of accommodation.

Antibody Index

ANTIBODY INDEX

Antibodies Discussed

Antibody Name/ Symbol	Antibody Description	Clones/Alternative Names	Chapters
α-fetoprotein	alpha 1 fetoprotein	AFP, Z5A06, clone C3	Congenital Nephrotic Syndrome of the Finnish Type; Pierson Syndrome
β-2-microglobulin		B2-microglob	Amyloidosis; Lead and Other Heavy Metal Toxins
κ light chain	kappa light chain	KAPPA	Anti-GBM Glomerulonephritis; De Novo Membranous Glomerulonephritis; Differential Diagnosis of Acute Interstitial Nephritis; Fibrillary Glomerulopathy; Henoch-Schönlein Purpura; Hepatitis C Virus; IgA Nephropathy; Immunotactoid Glomerulopathy; Light Chain Fanconi Syndrome; Membranous Glomerulonephritis, Primary; Mixed Cryoglobulinemic Glomerulonephritis; Monoclonal Immunoglobulin Deposition Disease; Myeloma Cast Nephropathy; IgG4-related Systemic Disease; Introduction to Renal Pathology; Secondary Oxalosis
λ light chain	lambda light chain	LAMBDA	Amyloidosis; Anti-GBM Glomerulonephritis; Diseases That Recur in Allografts; Drug-Induced Acute Interstitial Nephritis; Fibrillary Glomerulopathy; Henoch-Schönlein Purpura; Hepatitis C Virus; Hyperoxaluria; IgA Nephropathy; Immunotactoid Glomerulopathy; Membranous Glomerulonephritis, Secondary; De Novo Membranous Glomerulonephritis; Minimal Change Disease; Myeloma Cast Nephropathy
A1AT	alpha-1-antitrypsin	α-1-antitrypsin	Membranoproliferative Glomerulonephritis, Type I/III
AA-protein	acute-phase protein associated with many chronic inflammatory conditions	amyloid fibril protein AA, SAA1	Amyloidosis
Actin-sm	actin, smooth muscle	SMA	Obstructive Nephropathy
AE1/AE3	mixture of 2 anticytokeratin clones that detect a variety of both high- and low-molecular weight cytokeratins		Malakoplakia; Xanthogranulomatous Pyelonephritis
Bartonella henselae	B. henselae	B-henselae, cat scratch fever agent	Acute Postinfectious Glomerulonephritis, Nonstreptococcal; Endocarditis
Beta-catenin	involved in regulation of cell adhesion and in signal transduction through Wnt pathway	β-catenin, clone 14, E-5, RB-9035Po, 17C2, 5H10	Normal Kidney Development
C3b	erythrocyte complement receptor 1, immune adherence receptor, C3b/C4b	CD35, CR1, BER-MAC-DRC, TO5, E11	Collapsing Glomerulopathy
C-reactive protein	Acute phase protein involved in complement activation	CRP	Glomerulonephritis of Chronic Infection Including Shunt Nephritis
C4d	Degradation product of the activated complement factor 4, regarded as an indirect sign of antibody-mediated alloreactivity		Accommodation; Acute Allograft Ischemia; Acute Pyelonephritis; Acute Cellular Rejection; Acute Humoral Rejection; Anti-GBM Disease in Alport Syndrome; Calcineurin Inhibitor Toxicity; Cytomegalovirus Infection; De Novo Membranous Glomerulonephritis; Diseases That Recur in Allografts; Evaluation of the Allograft Kidney; Evaluation of the Donor Kidney; De Novo Focal Segmental Glomerulosclerosis; Hereditary Endotheliopathy, Retinopathy, Nephropathy, and Stroke; Hyperacute Rejection; Introduction to Renal Pathology; Membranoproliferative Glomerulonephritis, Type I/III; Mixed Cryoglobulinemic Glomerulonephritis; mTOR Inhibitor Toxicity; Pathological Classification of Renal Allograft Diseases; Polyomavirus Nephritis; Protocol Biopsies; Systemic Lupus Erythematosus; Thrombotic Microangiopathy, Drugs

CA9	carbonic anhydrase IX	CAIX, M75, NB100-417, ab1508	Acquired Cystic Disease
Carcinoembryonic antigen	glycoprotein involved in cell adhesion and widely used as a tumor marker	CEA-M, mCEA, CEA-B18, CEA-D14, CEA-GOLD 1, T84.6, CEA-GOLD 2, CEA 11, CEA-GOLD 3, CEA 27, CEA-GOLD 4, CEA 41, CEA-GOLD 5, T84.1, CEA-M, A5B7, CEJ065, IL-7, T84.66, TF3H8-1, 0062, D14, alpha-7, PARLAM 1, ZC23, CEM010, A115, COL-1, AF4, 12.140.10, 11-7, M773, CEA-M431_31, CEJO65	Membranous Glomerulonephritis, Secondary
CD2AP	CD2 associated protein		Normal Kidney Structure; Podocin Deficiency
CD3	T-cell receptor	F7238, A0452, CD3-P, CD3-M, SP7, PS1	Chronic Cellular Rejection; Chronic Humoral Rejection; Differential Diagnosis of Acute Interstitial Nephritis; Idiopathic Hypocomplementemic Tubulointerstitial Nephritis; Post-Transplant Lymphoproliferative Disease; Systemic Lupus Erythematosus; Tubulointerstitial Nephritis with Uveitis
CD4	T-cell surface glycoprotein L3T4	IF6, 1290, 4B12	HIV-associated Collapsing Glomerulonephropathy; Miscellaneous HIV-associated Renal Diseases; Post-Transplant Lymphoproliferative Disease; Tubulointerstitial Nephritis with Uveitis
CD8	T-cell coreceptor antigen, Leu2, T-cytotoxic cells	M7103, C8/144, C8/144B	Cytomegalovirus Infection; Hantavirus Nephropathy; HIV-associated Collapsing Glomerulonephropathy; Tubulointerstitial Nephritis with Uveitis
CD10	neutral endopeptidase	CALLA, neprilysin, NEP	Anti-GBM Glomerulonephritis; Drug-induced Acute Interstitial Nephritis; Membranous Glomerulonephritis, Primary; Multilocular Cystic Nephroma; Renal Tubular Dysgenesis
CD15	reacts with Reed-Sternberg cells of Hodgkin disease and with granulocytes	VIM-2,3C4, LEU-M1, TU9, MIV-D5, MY1, CBD1, MMA, 3CD1, Lewis X, SSEA-1	Post-Transplant Lymphoproliferative Disease
CD16	CD 16 (Fc receptor of IgG)		Chronic Humoral Rejection
CD20	membrane spanning 4 domains of B lymphocytes	FB1, B1, L26, MS4A1	Idiopathic Hypocomplementemic Interstitial Nephritis with Extensive Tubulointerstitial Deposits; Post-Transplant Lymphoproliferative Disease; Systemic Lupus Erythematosus
CD21	CR2, complement component receptor 2, Epstein-Barr virus receptor	IF8	Systemic Lupus Erythematosus
CD30	tumor necrosis factor SF8	BER-H2, KI-1, TNFRSF8	Post-Transplant Lymphoproliferative Disease
CD31	platelet endothelial cell adhesion molecule	JC/70, JC/70A, PECAM-1	Idiopathic Nodular Glomerulopathy
CD33	SIGLEC lectin 3	PWS44	Differential Diagnosis of Acute Interstitial Nephritis
CD34	hematopoietic progenitor cell antigen	MY10, IOM34, QBEND10, 8G12, 1309, HPCA-1, NU-4A1, TUK4, clone 581, BI-3c5	Chronic Humoral Rejection; Differential Diagnosis of Acute Interstitial Nephritis; Idiopathic Nodular Glomerulopathy
CD61	cluster of differentiation found on thrombocytes corresponding to glycoprotein IIb/IIIa	Integrin, beta 3 (platelet glycoprotein IIIa), ITGB3, GP3A, GPIIIa, Y2/5, HPA	Calcineurin Inhibitor Toxicity; Hyperacute Rejection; mTOR Inhibitor Toxicity; Radiation Nephropathy; Renal Cortical Necrosis; Renal Vein Thrombosis
CD62	cell adhesion molecule found on leukocytes that acts as a homing receptor	L-selectin,lymphocyte adhesion molecule 1, LAM-1, LAM1, LECAM1, LEU 8	Calcineurin Inhibitor Toxicity
CD68	cytoplasmic granule protein of monocytes, macrophages	pG-M1, KP-1, LN5	Acute Poststreptococcal Glomerulonephritis; Anti-GBM Disease in Alport Syndrome; Anti-GBM Glomerulonephritis; Chronic Humoral Rejection; Giant Cell Arteritis; Malakoplakia; Mixed Cryoglobulinemic Glomerulonephritis; Post-Transplant Lymphoproliferative Disease; Xanthogranulomatous Pyelonephritis
CD138	syndecan; a useful marker for plasma cells	B-B4, AM411-10M, MI15	Differential Diagnosis of Acute Interstitial Nephritis

9

ANTIBODY INDEX

CD163	macrophage hemoglobin scavenging system	10D6	Malakoplakia; Xanthogranulomatous Pyelonephritis
CK7	cytokeratin 7; low molecular weight cytokeratin	K72.7, KS7.18, OVTL 12/30, LDS-68, CK 07	Normal Kidney Structure; Renal Tubular Dysgenesis
CK8/18/CAM5.2	cytokeratin 8/18; simple epithelial-type cytokeratins	5D3, Zym5.2, CAM 5.2, KER 10.11, NCL-5D3, cytokeratin LMW	Xanthogranulomatous Pyelonephritis
CK-PAN	cytokeratin pan (AE1/AE3/LP34); cocktail of high and low molecular weight cytokeratins	keratin pan, MAK-6, K576, LU-5, KL-1, KC-8, MNF 116, pankeratin, pancytokeratin	mTOR Inhibitor Toxicity
CMV	Cytomegalovirus		Acute Cellular Rejection; Antiviral Drug Nephrotoxicity; C1q Nephropathy; Cytomegalovirus Infection; Herpes Simplex Acute Nephritis; Miscellaneous HIV-associated Renal Diseases; Urine Leak
Collagen II	major component of articular and hyaline cartilage	2B1.5	Introduction to Renal Pathology; Type III Collagen Glomerulopathy
Collagen III	fibril-forming interstitial collagen	COL3A1, Collagen alpha 1(III) chain, Collagen III alpha 1 chain precursor, Collagen III alpha 1 polypeptide, Collagen type III alpha 1 (Ehlers Danlos syndrome type IV autosomal dominant), Collagen type III alpha 1, Collagen type III alpha, EDS4A, Ehlers Danlos syndrome type IV, autosomal dominant, Fetal collagen, Type III collagen	Type III Collagen Glomerulopathy
Collagen IV	major constituent of the basement membranes along with laminins, proteoglycans, and enactins	CIV22, COL4A [1-5], collagen α-1(IV) chain	Alport Syndrome; Anti-GBM Disease in Alport Syndrome; Anti-GBM Glomerulonephritis; Hyperperfusion Injury; Loin Pain Hematuria Syndrome; Normal Kidney Structure
COX-2	cyclooxygenase-2	CX229, CLONE 33, COX-2-P	Drug-induced Acute Interstitial Nephritis
cyclin D3	activates cyclin-dependent kinases and thereby promotes G1/S phase transition	DCS-22	Normal Kidney Structure
Cyclooxygenase-2	inducible enzyme/isoenzyme of cyclooxygenase that is abundant in activated macrophages and at sites of inflammation		Drug-induced Minimal Change Disease
Cysteine protease	enzyme that degrades polypeptides	Separase, ESPL1	Anti-tubular Basement Membrane Disease
D2-40	marker for reactive follicular dendritic cells and follicular dendritic cell sarcomas	podoplanin, M2A	Renal Lymphangiectasis
Desmin	class III intermediate filaments found in muscle cells	M760, DE-R-11, D33, DE5, DE-U-10, ZC18	Fibronectin Glomerulopathy
EBER	Epstein-Barr virus-encoded RNA		Acute Cellular Rejection; Post-Transplant Lymphoproliferative Disease
EBV-LMP	Epstein-Barr virus latent membrane protein	LMP1, CS 1-4	Cytomegalovirus Infection; Epstein-Barr Virus Nephritis
Elastase	enzyme that breaks down elastin		ANCA-related Glomerulonephritis; Granulomatosis with Polyangiitis (Wegener)
EMA	epithelial membrane antigen	GP1.4, 214D4, MC5, E29	Renal Tubular Dysgenesis; Xanthogranulomatous Pyelonephritis
ER	estrogen receptor protein	1D5, 6F11, SP1, 15D, H222, TE111, ERP, ER1D5, NCLER611, NCL-ER-LH2, PGP-1A6	Fabry Disease; Familial Juvenile Hyperuricemic Nephropathy
Fibrinogen	soluble plasma glycoprotein made by the liver and involved in blood coagulation		Amyloidosis
Fibronectin	extracellular matrix glycoprotein	FN1, A0245, CIG	Amyloidosis; Diabetic Nephropathy; Fibronectin Glomerulopathy; Idiopathic Nodular Glomerulopathy; Immunotactoid Glomerulopathy; Normal Kidney Structure
FN1	fibronectin	A0245, CIG	Fibronectin Glomerulopathy
FVIIIRAg	factor VIII-related antigen	F8/86, von Willenbrand factor	Thrombotic Microangiopathy, Genetic
HBcAg	hepatitis B core antigen	HBCAG, GBcAg	Hepatitis B Virus
HBsAg	hepatitis B surface antigen	HBSAG, HBsAg, 3E7	Hepatitis B Virus
Helicobacter pylori	H. pylori	H-pylori	Hemolytic Uremic Syndrome, Infection Related; IgG4-related Systemic Disease
HLA-DR	human leukocyte antigen DR	DK22, LN3, TAL.1B5, LK8D3	Anti-GBM Glomerulonephritis; HIV-associated Collapsing

ANTIBODY INDEX

			Glomerulonephropathy; Hyperacute Rejection
HSV1/2	herpes simplex virus 1/2	HSV1/HSV2	Cytomegalovirus Infection; Herpes Simplex Acute Nephritis
Hypoxia inducible factor 1 alpha	oxygen-dependent transcriptonal activator with roles in angiogenesis	HIF-1-α, HIF-1-alpha	von Hippel-Lindau Disease
J chain	immunoglobulin joining segment	J-CHAIN, NFGD11	IgA Nephropathy
Ki-67	marker of cell proliferation	MM1, KI88, IVAK-2, MIB 1	Acquired Cystic Disease; Acute Allograft Ischemia; Collapsing Glomerulopathy; HIV-associated Collapsing Glomerulonephropathy; Pamidronate-induced Collapsing FSGS; Post-Transplant Lymphoproliferative Disease
Laminin	major protein in basal lamina	LAMININ-4C7, 4C12.8, LAM-89	Diabetic Nephropathy; Diffuse Mesangial Sclerosis; Diffuse Mesangial Sclerosis; Frasier Syndrome; Galloway-Mowat Syndrome; Pierson Syndrome
LECT2	leukocyte chemotactic factor 2		Amyloidosis
LH	Luteinizing hormone	beta-LH	Membranous Glomerulonephritis, Primary
Lysozyme	1,4-beta N-acetylmuramidase	Lyz, Lzm, Ec3.2.1.17	Amyloidosis
MPO	myeloperoxidase		ANCA-related Glomerulonephritis; Microscopic Polyangiitis; Granulomatosis with Polyangiitis (Wegener)
MUC1	epithelial membrane antigen	LICR-LON-M8, BC3, DF3, VU3D1, MUSEII, RD-1, MA695, MA552, PS2P446, 115D8	Accommodation
Myoglobin	iron and oxygen-building protein found in muscle tissue	MG-1	Acute Allograft Ischemia; Acute Tubular Necrosis; Classification of Tubulointerstitial Diseases; Evaluation of the Donor Kidney; Hepatorenal Syndrome/Bile Nephrosis; Introduction to Renal Pathology; Leptospirosis; mTOR Inhibitor Toxicity; Myeloma Cast Nephropathy; Myoglobinuria/ Rhabdomyolysis/Hemoglobinuria; Osmotic Tubulopathy
Myosin	motor protein responsible for actin-based motility in striated and smooth muscle cells		Collapsing Glomerulopathy
NCCT	Thiazide-sensitive Na-Cl cotransporter that is primarily expressed in the distal convoluted tubule of the kidney where it accounts for a significant fraction of net renal sodium reabsorption	FLJ96318, NaCL symporter, Na-Cl symporter, NaCl electroneutral thiazide sensitive cotransporter antibody, S12A3, slc12a3, TSC, Thiazide-sensitive sodium chloride cotransporter	Sjögren Syndrome
Neutrophil elastase	serine protease secreted by granulocytes during inflammation	NP57	Granulomatosis with Polyangiitis (Wegener)
P-cadherin	placental dependent adhesion protein	56, clone 56	Normal Kidney Structure
p53	P53 tumor suppressor gene protein	DO7, 21N, BP-53-12-1, AB6, CM1, PAB1801, DO1, BP53-11, PAB240, RSP53, MU195, P53	Aristolochic Acid Nephropathy; Balkan Endemic Nephropathy
pax-2	paired box gene 2	Z-RX2, PAX-2	Denys-Drash Syndrome
PCNA	proliferating cell nuclear antigen	19 A2, PC10	Karyomegalic Interstitial Nephritis
Peanut agglutinin		PNA	Renal Tubular Dysgenesis
Phospholipase A2	Enzyme that releases fatty acids from glycerol to liberate arachidonic acid	PLA2, phosolip A2	Membranous Glomerulonephritis, Primary; Systemic Lupus Erythematosus
Podoplanin	marker for reactive follicular dendritic cells and follicular dendritic cell sarcomas	D2-40, M2A	Renal Lymphangiectasis
Polyomavirus large T antigen	nuclear phosphoprotein that helps to regulate viral replication and gene expression; used for the detection of polyomavirus infected cells		Polyomavirus Nephritis
PR	progesterone receptor protein	10A9, PGR-1A6, KD68, PGR-ICA, PRP-P, PRP, PRI, 1A6, 1AR, HPRA3, PGR-636, 636, PR88, NCL-PGR, PgR	Multilocular Cystic Nephroma; Polyarteritis Nodosa
Prealbumin	carrier protein of thyroxin and retinol; rich in a beta sheet structure	Transthyretin	Amyloidosis
Renin	participates in renin-angiotensinsystem	Angiotensinase	Renal Tubular Dysgenesis

ANTIBODY INDEX

S100	low molecular weight protein normally present in cells derived from neural crest (Schwann cells, melanocytes, and glial cells), chondrocytes, adipocytes, myoepithelial cells, macrophages, Langerhans cells, dendritic cells, and keratinocytes	S-100, A6, 15E2E2, Z311, 4C4.9	Neurofibromatosis
SAP	serum amyloid P component protein		Amyloidosis
SV40	simian virus 40		Adenovirus Infection; Anti-GBM Disease in Alport Syndrome; Cytomegalovirus Infection; Epstein-Barr Virus Nephritis; Herpes Simplex Acute Nephritis; Polyomavirus Nephritis
Synaptopodin	actin-associated protein that may play a role in modulating actin-based shape and motility of dendritic spines and renal podocyte foot processes	SYNPO, KIAA1029	Collapsing Glomerulopathy
THP	Tamm-Horsfall protein	10.32	Obstructive Nephropathy
Thrombomodulin	cofactor in thrombin-induced activation of protein C	1009, 15C8, CD141	Thrombotic Microangiopathy, Genetic
TNF-α	gamma catenin	G-catenin, TNF alpha, alpha alpha	ANCA-Related Glomerulonephritis; Rheumatoid Arthritis
Toxoplasma gondii	*T. Gondii*		Microsporidiosis
VEGF	vascular endothelial growth factor	JH121, 26503.11, VPF, VPF/VEGF, VEGF-A, VEGF-C, RP 077, VEGFR-1, RP 076, VEGFR-2, 9D9, VEGFR-3, FLT-4	Normal Kidney Structure; Pre-eclampsia, Eclampsia, HELLP Syndrome; Thrombotic Microangiopathy, Drugs; von Hippel-Lindau Disease; Epstein-Barr Virus Nephritis; Fibronectin Glomerulopathy; Introduction to Thrombotic Microangiopathies
Villin	protein binding the actin filaments of mesenchymal cells	1D2C3	Fibronectin Glomerulopathy
Vimentin	major subunit protein of intermediate filaments of mesenchymal cells	43BE8, 3B4, V10, V9, VIM-B34, VIM	Normal Kidney Structure
von Willenbrand Factor	factor VIII-related antigen	F8/86, FVIIIRAg	Introduction to Thrombotic Microangiopathies; Postpartum Hemolytic Uremic Syndrome; Thrombotic Microangiopathy, Autoimmune
WT1	Wilms tumor gene 1	6F-H2, C-19	Alpha-Actinin-4 Deficiency; Collapsing Glomerulopathy; Denys-Drash Syndrome; Diffuse Mesangial Sclerosis; Focal Segmental Glomerulosclerosis Classification; Frasier Syndrome; HIV-associated Collapsing Glomerulonephropathy; Normal Kidney Structure

INDEX

A

INDEX

INDEX

INDEX

INDEX

INDEX

INDEX

INDEX

INDEX

INDEX

INDEX

INDEX

INDEX

INDEX

INDEX

INDEX

INDEX

INDEX

INDEX

INDEX

INDEX

INDEX

INDEX

INDEX

INDEX

INDEX